ATLAS OF HUMAN ANATOMY

ATLAS

HUMAN

OF ANATOMY

by FRANK H. NETTER, M.D.

Sharon Colacino, Ph.D., *Consulting Editor*

CIBA–GEIGY CORPORATION

SUMMIT, NEW JERSEY

Copies of *Atlas of Human Anatomy, The CIBA Collection of Medical
Illustrations, Clinical Symposia* reprints and color slides of all
illustrations are available from CIBA–GEIGY Medical Education,
14 Henderson Drive, West Caldwell, NJ 07006

Library of Congress Cataloging-in-Publication Data

Netter, Frank H. (Frank Henry), 1906–
    Atlas of human anatomy / by Frank H. Netter: Sharon Colacino,
  consulting editor.
      p.   cm,
    Includes bibliographies and index.
    ISBN 0-914168-18-5—ISBN 0-914168-19-3 (pbk.)
    1. Anatomy, Human–Atlases.   I. Colacino, Sharon.   II. Title.
    [DNLM: 1. Anatomy–atlases. QS 17 N474a]
  QM25. N46 1989
  611: 0022–dc20
  DNLM/DLC
  for Library of Congress   89-60477
                                                      CIP

First Printing, 1989
Second Printing, 1990
Third Printing, 1990
Fourth Printing, 1991

ISBN 0-914168-19-3
Library of Congress Catalog No: 89-060477

Design and production by Philip Grushkin
Color separations by Daiichi Seihan
Printing by Acme Printing Company, Inc.
Binding by The Riverside Group
Composition by U.S. Lithograph, typographers

To my dear wife, Vera

INTRODUCTION

Other books by FRANK H. NETTER, M.D.

THE CIBA COLLECTION OF MEDICAL ILLUSTRATIONS

Nervous System, Part I: Anatomy and Physiology

Nervous System, Part II: Neurologic and Neuromuscular Disorders

Reproductive System

Digestive System, Part I: Upper Digestive Tract

Digestive System, Part II: Lower Digestive Tract

Digestive System, Part III: Liver, Biliary Tract and Pancreas

Endocrine System and Selected Metabolic Diseases

Heart

Kidney, Ureters, and Urinary Bladder

Respiratory System

Musculoskeletal System, Part I: Anatomy, Physiology, and Metabolic Disorders

Musculoskeletal System, Part II: Developmental Disorders, Tumors,
   Rheumatic Diseases, and Joint Replacement

Musculoskeletal System, Part III: Trauma, Evaluation, and Management
   (*in preparation*)

I have often said that my career as a medical artist for almost 50 years has been a sort of "command performance" in the sense that it has grown in response to the desires and requests of the medical profession. Over these many years, I have produced almost 4,000 illustrations, mostly for *The CIBA Collection of Medical Illustrations* but also for *Clinical Symposia*. These pictures have been concerned with the varied subdivisions of medical knowledge such as gross anatomy, histology, embryology, physiology, pathology, diagnostic modalities, surgical and therapeutic techniques and clinical manifestations of a multitude of diseases. As the years went by, however, there were more and more requests from physicians and students for me to produce an atlas purely of gross anatomy. Thus, this atlas has come about, not through any inspiration on my part but rather, like most of my previous works, as a fulfillment of the desires of the medical profession. I was, however, so occupied with other commitments that it took me a long time to get around to undertaking it. And then when I finally did, I found it to require much more work and time than I had anticipated. It involved going back over all the illustrations I had made over so many years, selecting those pertinent to gross anatomy, classifying them and organizing them by system and region, adapting them to page size and space and arranging them in logical sequence. Anatomy of course does not change, but our understanding of anatomy and its clinical significance does change as do anatomical terminology and nomenclature. This therefore required much updating of many of the older pictures and even revision of a number of them in order to make them more pertinent to today's ever-expanding scope of medical and surgical practice. In addition I found that there were gaps in the portrayal of medical knowledge as pictorialized in the illustrations I had previously done, and this necessitated my making a number of new pictures that are included in this volume.

In creating an atlas such as this, it is important to achieve a happy medium between complexity and simplification. If the pictures are too complex, they may be difficult and confusing to read; if oversimplified, they may not be adequately definitive or may even be misleading. I have therefore striven for a middle course of realism without the clutter of confusing minutiae. I hope that the students and members of the medical and allied professions will find the illustrations readily understandable, yet instructive and useful.

At one point Mr. Flagler, the publisher, and I thought it might be nice to include a foreword by a truly outstanding and renowned anatomist, but there are so many in that category, a considerable number of whom have collaborated with me in the past and who are listed elsewhere in this volume, that we could not make a choice. We did think of men like Vesalius, Leonardo da Vinci, William Hunter and Henry Gray, who of course are unfortunately unavailable, but I do wonder what their comments might have been about this atlas.

Frank H. Netter, M.D.

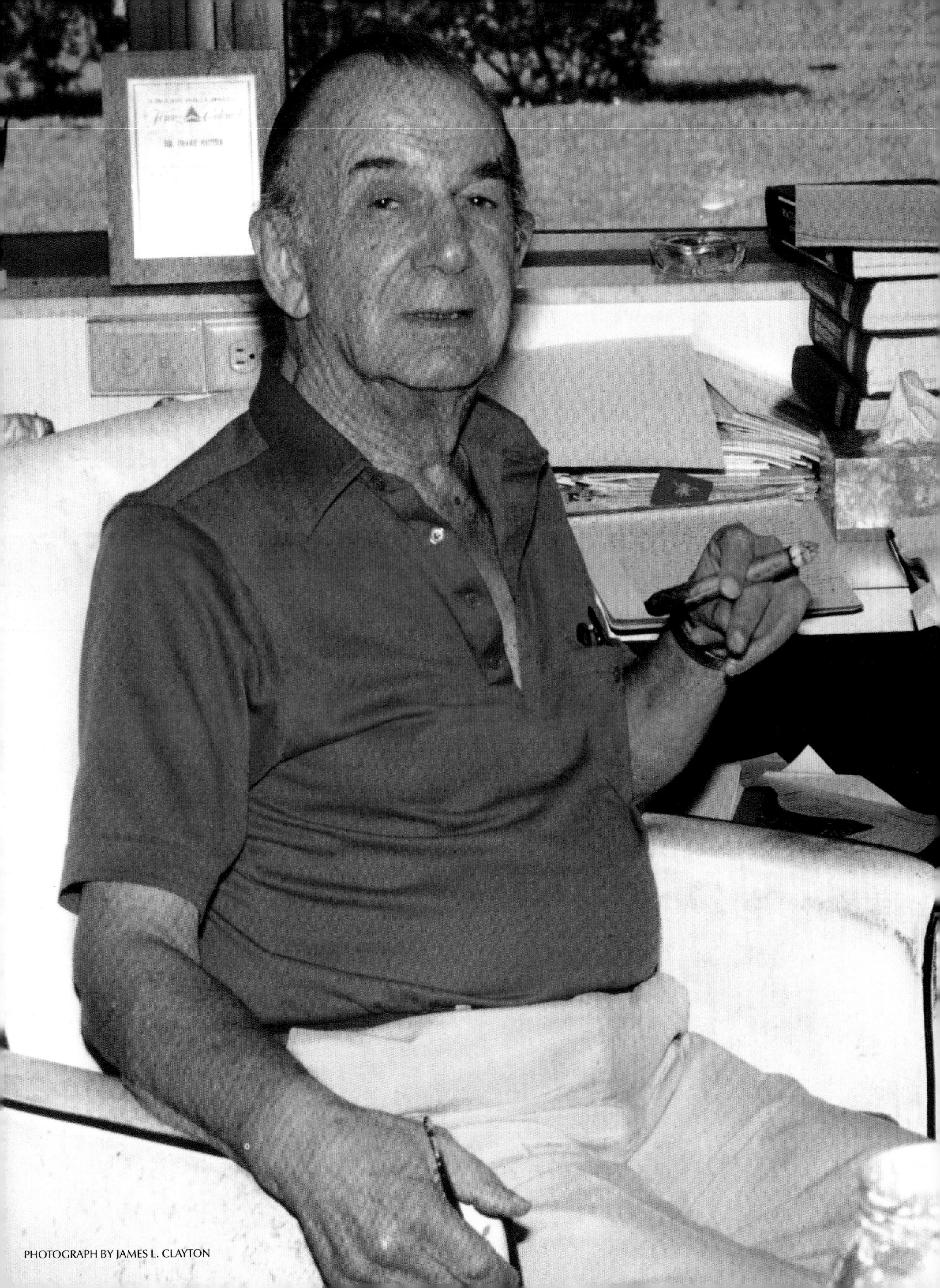

PHOTOGRAPH BY JAMES L. CLAYTON

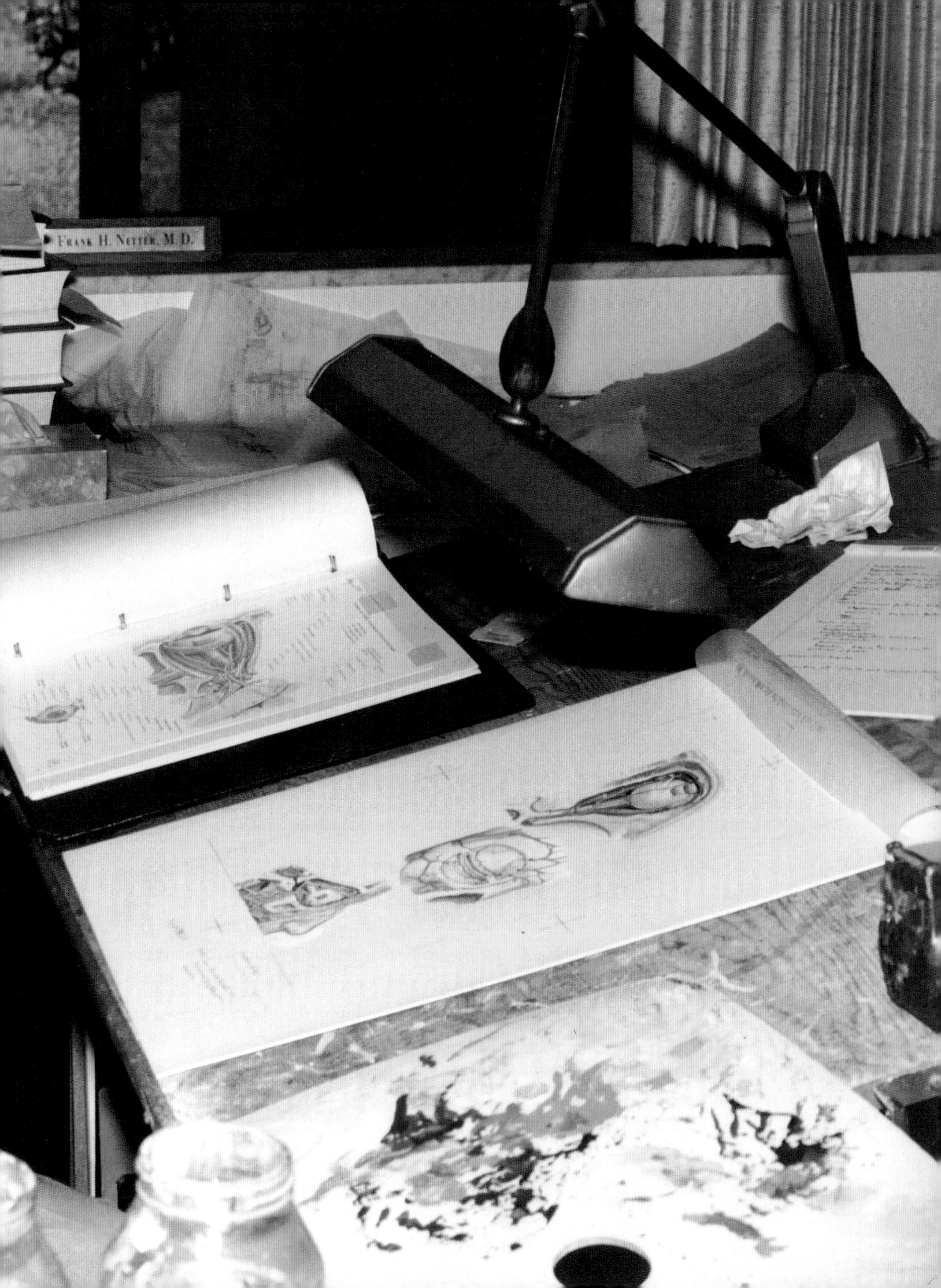

ACKNOWLEDGMENTS

I have not been alone in this entire venture of medical pictorialization. There has been first and foremost the CIBA Pharmaceutical Company (now the CIBA–GEIGY Corporation) that has sponsored the creation of *The CIBA Collection of Medical Illustrations* as well as of this *Atlas of Human Anatomy*, which has grown out of it. Ours has been a long, happy and productive association. Very significant in this connection was a very special person and good friend, Mr. Paul Roder, then a CIBA executive, who early recognized the artistic and educational value of my pictures, and who was a major influence in CIBA's undertaking their sponsorship, as well as in encouraging me to do more. Another person who was most important in these respects was the late Dr. Ernst Oppenheimer, then chief pharmacologist at CIBA, who edited the first three volumes of *The CIBA Collection*.

In the creation of this specific *Atlas of Human Anatomy*, Dr. Sharon Colacino, assistant professor of anatomy at the College of Physicians and Surgeons, Columbia University, and consulting editor of this volume, played so vital and diversified a role that I cannot find words to adequately describe it. I can only express my heartfelt thanks for her help in many, many ways such as in organization of the atlas, in proposing modification of many of the old plates, in suggesting additional new ones, in checking on anatomical details and nomenclature, in planning sectional and subsectional divisions of the book and, in general, for her tireless and dedicated devotion to the project.

I furthermore express herewith my admiration for the artistry and skill of Mr. Philip Grushkin, who did the overall and typographic design, made the mechanicals and oversaw the entire production and printing of this atlas. Its visual appeal, readability and fine quality of pictorial reproduction are largely attributable to him, and his efficiency of operation greatly expedited its production.

I thank also dear Ms. Jeffie Lemons, who kept track of the over 500 illustrations with numerous type overlays for each, and the multitude of typographic and organizational changes as we went along, and who made up the preliminary and revised dummies that were necessary. Her pleasantness and efficiency in handling these almost overwhelming detailed responsibilities were a delight to me.

Thanks as well to Ms. Sally Chichester without whose editorial expertise this book would not have been possible.

Finally I must give great credit to Mr. Philip Flagler, who kept the whole project moving along and the entire team working together, and on whom it befell to make many production and financial decisions; to Dr. Milton Donin and Dr. Roy A. Ellis, who both did much in initiating this undertaking; and to a great many others of the CIBA organization for their supporting roles.

Many of the illustrations in this atlas have been published previously in various volumes of *The CIBA Collection of Medical Illustrations* or *Clinical Symposia*. In creating those illustrations, I had the pleasure and benefit of collaborating with a number of outstanding anatomists from various parts of the world, some of whom are now deceased. Many of these knowledgeable people are listed below, but there were also many others who gave to me of their advice and criticism and I thank them all very much.

Frank H. Netter, M.D.

Jay B. Angevine, Jr., Ph.D.

Louis L. Bergmann, M.D.

Hyun Taik Cho, M.D.

Eugene Cliffton, M.D.

Edmund S. Crelin, Ph.D., D.Sc.

Calvin Ezrin, M.D.

Joseph A. Gaines, M.D.

Charles F. Geschickter, M.D.

Rudolph V. Gorsch, M.D.

Brian F. Hoffman, M.D.

John Franklin Huber, M.D., Ph.D.

W.R. Ingram, Ph.D.

Abraham Kaplan, M.D.

Albert Kuntz, Ph.D, M.D.

Nicholas A. Michels, M.A., D.Sc.

G.A.G. Mitchell, Ch.M., D.Sc., F.R.C.S.

Barry W. Peterson, Ph.D.

Hans Popper, M.D.

Lynne M. Reid, M.D.

Johannes A.G. Rhodin, M.D., Ph.D.

I.C. Rubin, M.D.

Jerome J. Sheldon, M.D.

Max L. Som, M.D.

F. Mason Sones, Jr., M.D.

Somers H. Sturgis, M.D.

Lodewyk H.S. Van Mierop, M.D.

Samuel A. Vest, M.D.

Gerhardt von Bonin, M.D.

Bernard S. Wolf, M.D.

Gerhard Wolf-Heidegger, M.D., Ph.D.

Russell T. Woodburne, M.A., Ph.D.

PUBLISHER'S NOTE

Completion of a project as large and complex as this atlas requires the work of many people with diverse skills, a wealth of talent and single-minded dedication to see their tasks through to the end. We have been most fortunate to have just such a group working together with Dr. Netter to publish this book, and they have done it with enthusiasm, tenacity and great care. I extend to them my personal thanks as well as those of CIBA–GEIGY.

Dr. Netter has worked primarily with his collaborators, our consultants and the editorial staff, all of whom he has thanked in his own acknowledgments. I am delighted to second that thanks. Many others were involved in important ways, however, and their contributions must also be acknowledged.

Between the editorial and production functions lies a land of unsung heroes, several of whom should be recognized by name. Proofreaders Jo Sacher and Robin Snowden provided invaluable assistance, as anyone who looks at the legends on the pictures will agree. Designer Clark Carroll assisted Philip Grushkin in the preparation of mechanicals, brackets, special figures and many of the leader lines. Editorial Assistant Nicole Friedman, though not officially assigned to the project, became involved frequently—and willingly.

I would be remiss not to mention an important attribute of this atlas, which along with so many other jobs, was taken on as a special project by Dr. Colacino, Sally Chichester and Jeffie Lemons. I think you will find that every legend on every painting in the book has been called out in the index—and in a very usable way too. An index of 36 pages is a book in itself, and it took many late nights with the exercise of infinite patience to prepare.

The paintings are reproduced with a clarity and accuracy never before possible, and this is due to the work of two companies whose people became full partners with us in this project. Don Sigovich and his staff at Gamma One Conversions in New York City photographed all of the paintings, both old and new, using a process that captures on film the colors, densities, shapes and textures of Dr. Netter's originals. These transparencies, color corrected by hand to precisely match the art, became the starting point in the reproduction process.

The transparencies, in turn, were handed over to Daiichi Seihan, who produced the color separations from which the printing plates were made and who also printed and bound the finished work. Tomeji Maruyama personally oversaw each step in the difficult process of color separation both here in the United States and in Japan where the films were physically prepared. His application of time, talent, patience, organization and hard work was extraordinary. Tomeji was assisted in these steps by Bill Bianco, also of Daiichi Seihan, and the company's staff in Japan (who at this writing I have not met, but who certainly will become colleagues and friends before the ink is dry and the covers are attached).

Finally, of course, we at CIBA–GEIGY thank Frank H. Netter, M.D., our friend, our colleague and our inspiration. We hope he has found as much satisfaction and pleasure in preparing this atlas as each of us has found in working with him. At 83, he is still the master artist, the master teacher and the master physician, and he can still outwork all of us. As we go to press with this atlas, he is ready with all the paintings for the next addition to *The CIBA Collection of Medical Illustrations, Musculoskeletal System*, Part II (tentative publishing date, September 1990), as well as many of the paintings for *Musculoskeletal System*, Part III. Perhaps we should say he is the master of productivity as well!

Again, many thanks to all who have had a hand in bringing this very special book to life. It is our hope it will help countless generations of students learn the complexities of human anatomy and find a place as a reference wherever the intricacies of the human body are studied and discussed.

Philip Flagler
Director
Medical Education

CONTENTS

NOMENCLATURE

The *Atlas of Human Anatomy* follows the nomenclature
adopted by the Eleventh International Congress of Anatomists
in 1980. In accordance with the recommendation of the
International Anatomical Nomenclature Committee, the
terminology in this book departs from the strict Latin in many
cases by either anglicizing names or by using direct English
translations. If the adopted *Nomina Anatomica* terms differ
substantially from the older terms or if eponyms and older
terms are still in common use by the medical community,
these alternate terms are given in parentheses.

Section I

HEAD AND NECK

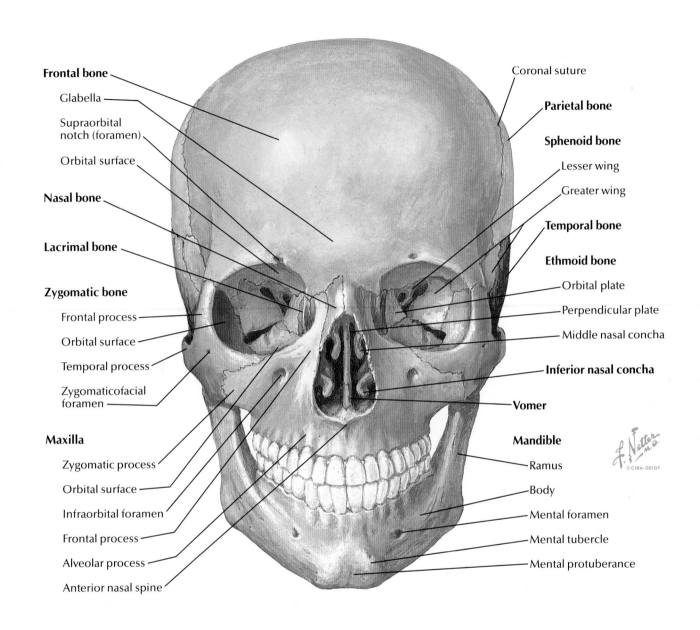

Frontal bone

Glabella

Supraorbital notch (foramen)

Orbital surface

Nasal bone

Lacrimal bone

Zygomatic bone

Frontal process

Orbital surface

Temporal process

Zygomaticofacial foramen

Maxilla

Zygomatic process

Orbital surface

Infraorbital foramen

Frontal process

Alveolar process

Anterior nasal spine

Coronal suture

Parietal bone

Sphenoid bone

Lesser wing

Greater wing

Temporal bone

Ethmoid bone

Orbital plate

Perpendicular plate

Middle nasal concha

Inferior nasal concha

Vomer

Mandible

Ramus

Body

Mental foramen

Mental tubercle

Mental protuberance

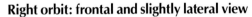

Right orbit: frontal and slightly lateral view

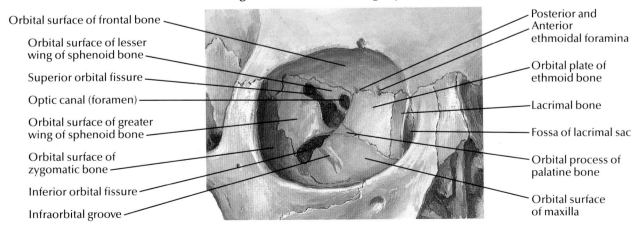

Orbital surface of frontal bone

Orbital surface of lesser wing of sphenoid bone

Superior orbital fissure

Optic canal (foramen)

Orbital surface of greater wing of sphenoid bone

Orbital surface of zygomatic bone

Inferior orbital fissure

Infraorbital groove

Posterior and Anterior ethmoidal foramina

Orbital plate of ethmoid bone

Lacrimal bone

Fossa of lacrimal sac

Orbital process of palatine bone

Orbital surface of maxilla

BONES AND LIGAMENTS

PLATE 1

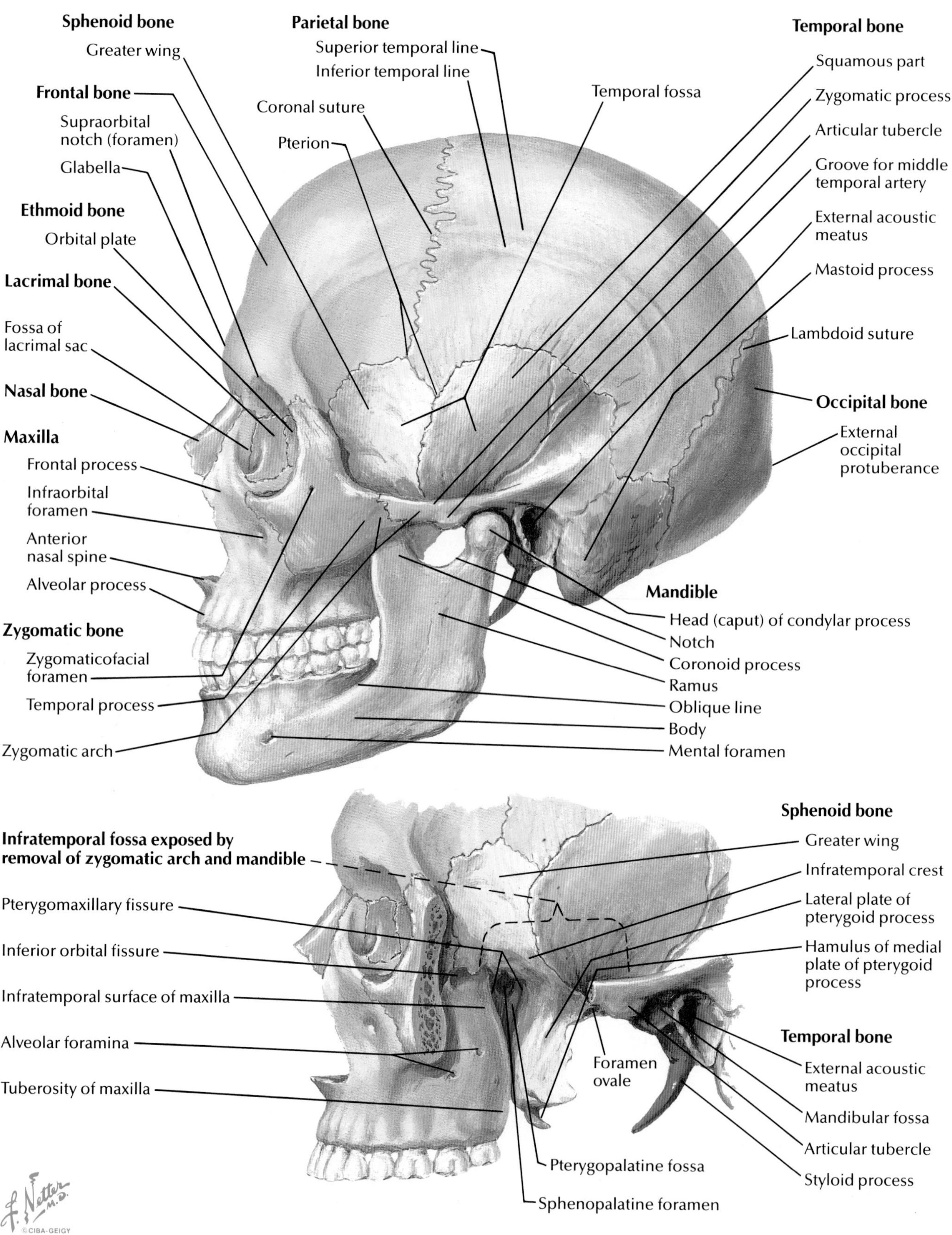

Sphenoid bone
Greater wing

Frontal bone
Supraorbital notch (foramen)
Glabella

Ethmoid bone
Orbital plate

Lacrimal bone
Fossa of lacrimal sac

Nasal bone

Maxilla
Frontal process
Infraorbital foramen
Anterior nasal spine
Alveolar process

Zygomatic bone
Zygomaticofacial foramen
Temporal process
Zygomatic arch

Parietal bone
Superior temporal line
Inferior temporal line
Coronal suture
Pterion

Temporal fossa

Temporal bone
Squamous part
Zygomatic process
Articular tubercle
Groove for middle temporal artery
External acoustic meatus
Mastoid process
Lambdoid suture

Occipital bone
External occipital protuberance

Mandible
Head (caput) of condylar process
Notch
Coronoid process
Ramus
Oblique line
Body
Mental foramen

Infratemporal fossa exposed by removal of zygomatic arch and mandible
Pterygomaxillary fissure
Inferior orbital fissure
Infratemporal surface of maxilla
Alveolar foramina
Tuberosity of maxilla

Foramen ovale

Pterygopalatine fossa
Sphenopalatine foramen

Sphenoid bone
Greater wing
Infratemporal crest
Lateral plate of pterygoid process
Hamulus of medial plate of pterygoid process

Temporal bone
External acoustic meatus
Mandibular fossa
Articular tubercle
Styloid process

PLATE 2

HEAD AND NECK

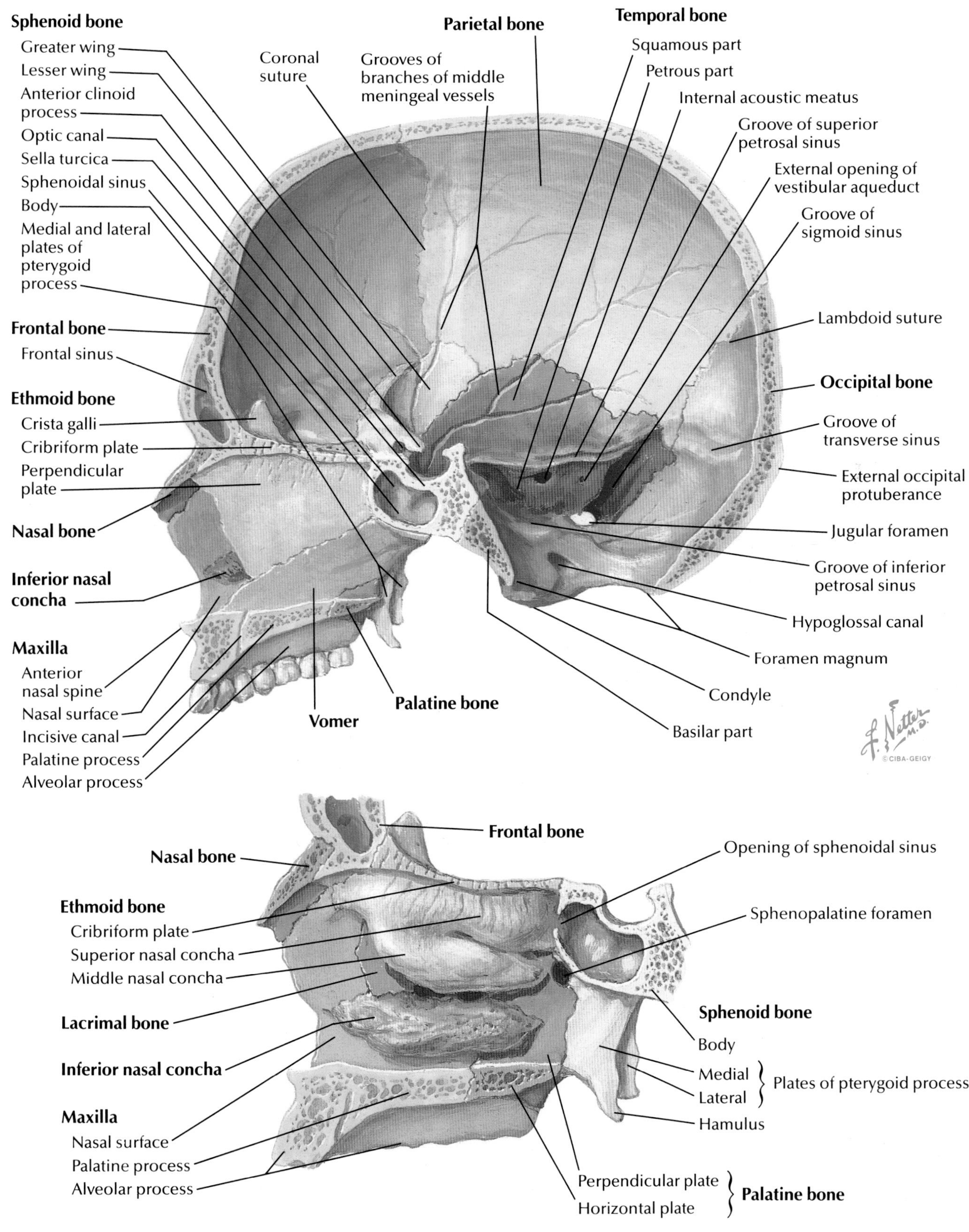

Sphenoid bone
- Greater wing
- Lesser wing
- Anterior clinoid process
- Optic canal
- Sella turcica
- Sphenoidal sinus
- Body
- Medial and lateral plates of pterygoid process

Frontal bone
- Frontal sinus

Ethmoid bone
- Crista galli
- Cribriform plate
- Perpendicular plate

Nasal bone

Inferior nasal concha

Maxilla
- Anterior nasal spine
- Nasal surface
- Incisive canal
- Palatine process
- Alveolar process

Coronal suture

Grooves of branches of middle meningeal vessels

Parietal bone

Temporal bone
- Squamous part
- Petrous part
- Internal acoustic meatus
- Groove of superior petrosal sinus
- External opening of vestibular aqueduct
- Groove of sigmoid sinus

Lambdoid suture

Occipital bone
- Groove of transverse sinus
- External occipital protuberance
- Jugular foramen
- Groove of inferior petrosal sinus
- Hypoglossal canal
- Foramen magnum
- Condyle
- Basilar part

Vomer

Palatine bone

Frontal bone

Nasal bone

Ethmoid bone
- Cribriform plate
- Superior nasal concha
- Middle nasal concha

Lacrimal bone

Inferior nasal concha

Maxilla
- Nasal surface
- Palatine process
- Alveolar process

Opening of sphenoidal sinus

Sphenopalatine foramen

Sphenoid bone
- Body
- Medial } Plates of pterygoid process
- Lateral }
- Hamulus

Perpendicular plate } **Palatine bone**
Horizontal plate }

Calvaria

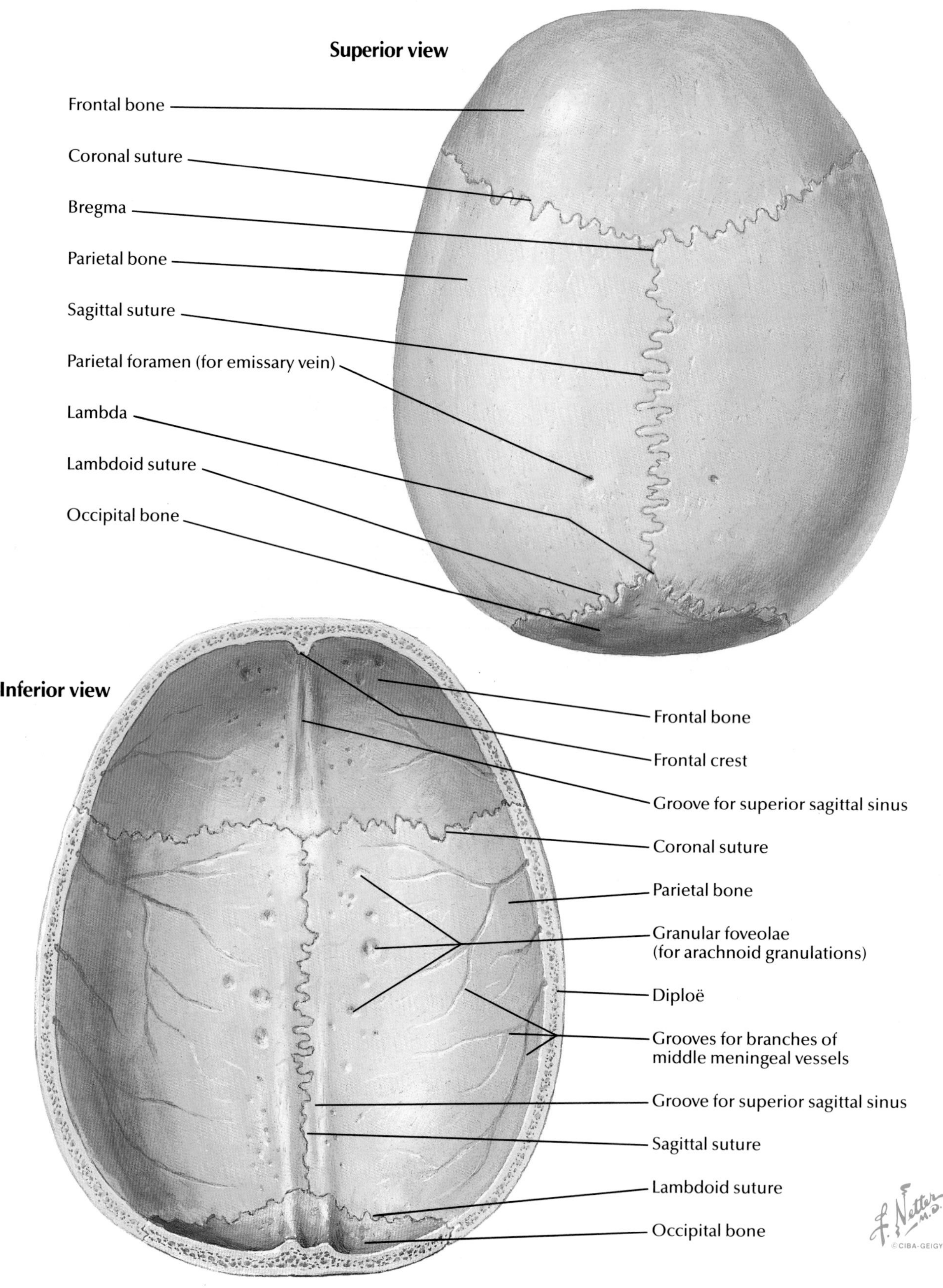

Superior view

Frontal bone

Coronal suture

Bregma

Parietal bone

Sagittal suture

Parietal foramen (for emissary vein)

Lambda

Lambdoid suture

Occipital bone

Inferior view

Frontal bone

Frontal crest

Groove for superior sagittal sinus

Coronal suture

Parietal bone

Granular foveolae (for arachnoid granulations)

Diploë

Grooves for branches of middle meningeal vessels

Groove for superior sagittal sinus

Sagittal suture

Lambdoid suture

Occipital bone

PLATE 4

HEAD AND NECK

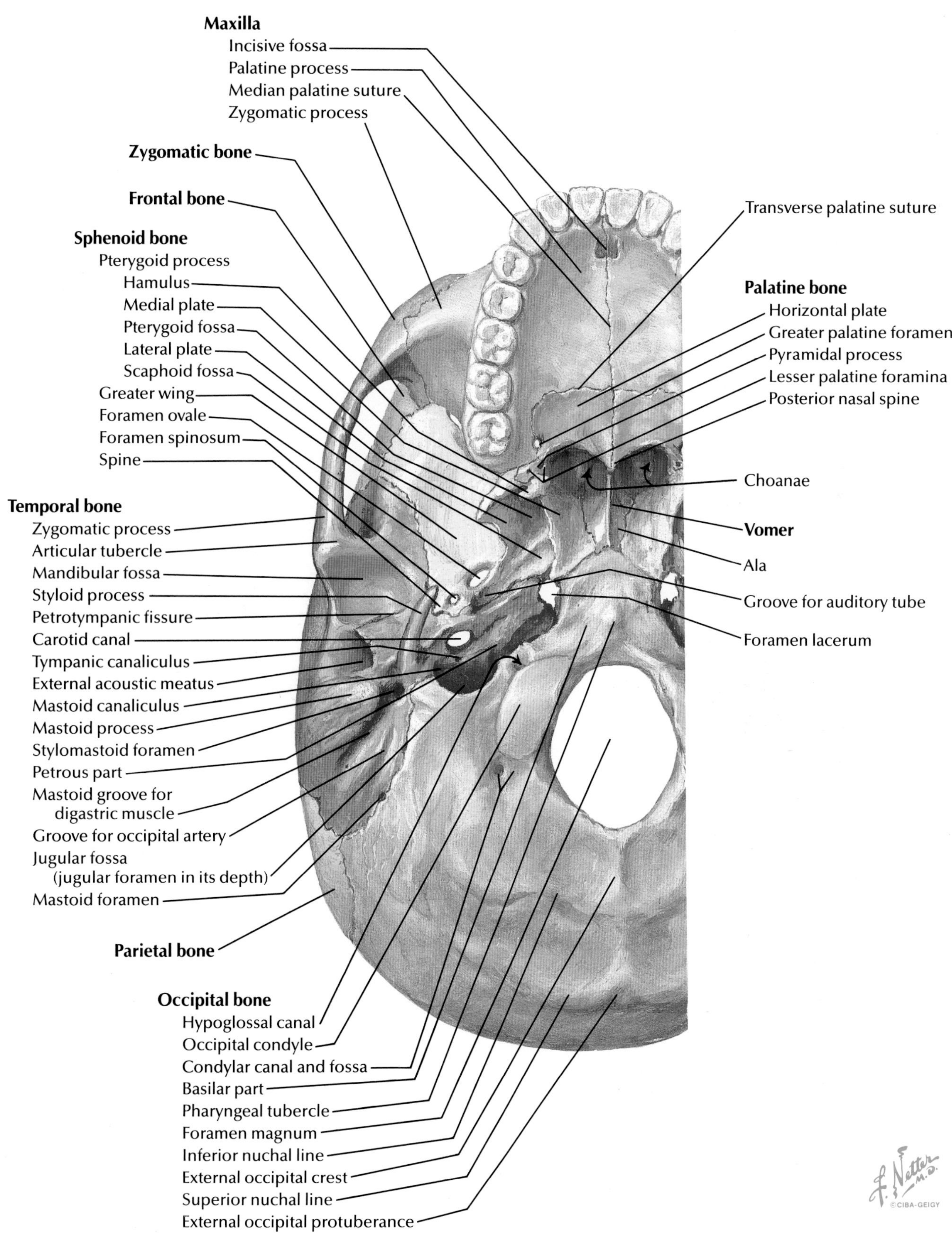

Maxilla
Incisive fossa
Palatine process
Median palatine suture
Zygomatic process

Zygomatic bone

Frontal bone

Sphenoid bone
Pterygoid process
Hamulus
Medial plate
Pterygoid fossa
Lateral plate
Scaphoid fossa
Greater wing
Foramen ovale
Foramen spinosum
Spine

Temporal bone
Zygomatic process
Articular tubercle
Mandibular fossa
Styloid process
Petrotympanic fissure
Carotid canal
Tympanic canaliculus
External acoustic meatus
Mastoid canaliculus
Mastoid process
Stylomastoid foramen
Petrous part
Mastoid groove for
 digastric muscle
Groove for occipital artery
Jugular fossa
 (jugular foramen in its depth)
Mastoid foramen

Parietal bone

Occipital bone
Hypoglossal canal
Occipital condyle
Condylar canal and fossa
Basilar part
Pharyngeal tubercle
Foramen magnum
Inferior nuchal line
External occipital crest
Superior nuchal line
External occipital protuberance

Transverse palatine suture

Palatine bone
Horizontal plate
Greater palatine foramen
Pyramidal process
Lesser palatine foramina
Posterior nasal spine

Choanae

Vomer

Ala

Groove for auditory tube

Foramen lacerum

Frontal bone
- Groove for superior sagittal sinus
- Frontal crest
- Groove for anterior meningeal vessels
- Foramen cecum
- Superior surface of orbital part

Ethmoid bone
- Crista galli
- Cribriform plate

Sphenoid bone
- Lesser wing
  - Anterior clinoid process
- Greater wing
  - Groove for middle meningeal vessels (frontal branches)
- Body
  - Jugum
  - Chiasmatic groove
  - Sella turcica
    - Tuberculum sellae
    - Hypophyseal fossa
    - Dorsum sellae
    - Posterior clinoid process
  - Groove for internal carotid artery
  - Clivus

Temporal bone
- Squamous part
- Petrous part
  - Groove for lesser petrosal nerve
  - Groove for greater petrosal nerve
  - Arcuate eminence
  - Depression for trigeminal ganglion
  - Groove for superior petrosal sinus
  - Groove for sigmoid sinus

Parietal bone
- Groove for middle meningeal vessels (parietal branches)
- Mastoid angle

Occipital bone
- Clivus
- Groove for inferior petrosal sinus
- Basilar part
- Groove for posterior meningeal vessels
- Condyle
- Groove for transverse sinus
- Groove for occipital sinus
- Internal occipital crest
- Internal occipital protuberance
- Groove for superior sagittal sinus

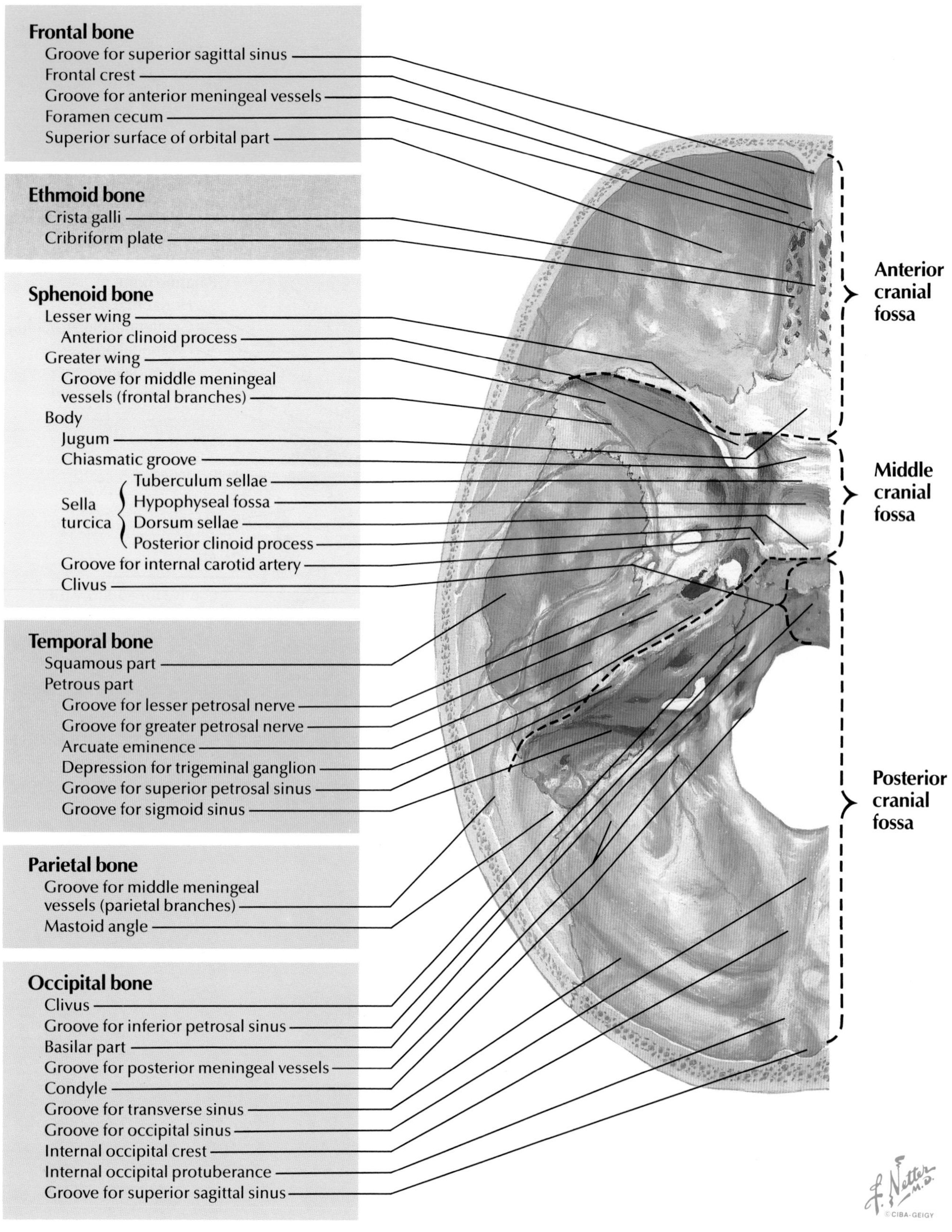

Anterior cranial fossa

Middle cranial fossa

Posterior cranial fossa

PLATE 6   **HEAD AND NECK**

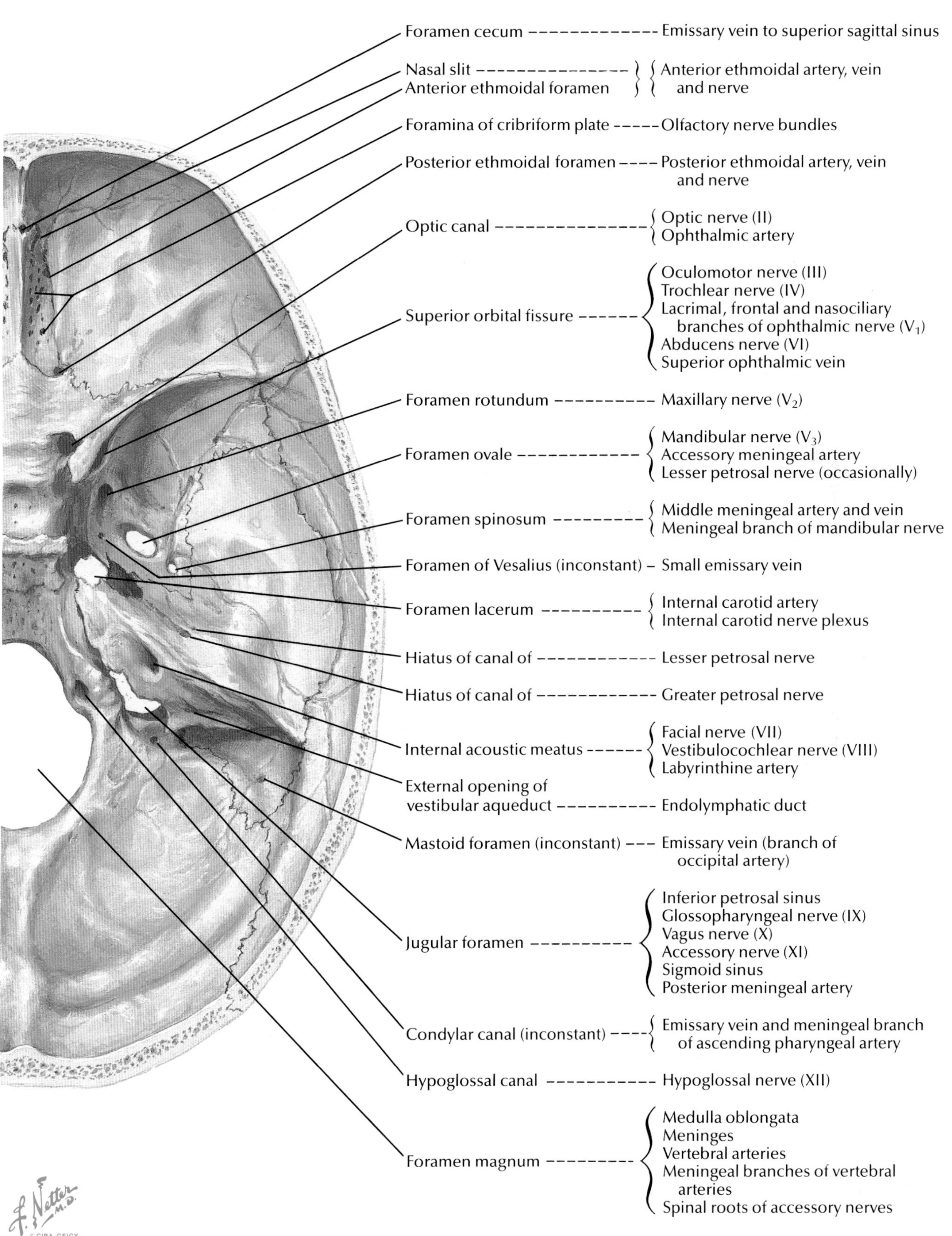

Foramen cecum ------------ Emissary vein to superior sagittal sinus

Nasal slit -------------- } { Anterior ethmoidal artery, vein
Anterior ethmoidal foramen } {   and nerve

Foramina of cribriform plate -----Olfactory nerve bundles

Posterior ethmoidal foramen ---- Posterior ethmoidal artery, vein
    and nerve

Optic canal --------------- { Optic nerve (II)
{ Ophthalmic artery

Superior orbital fissure ------ { Oculomotor nerve (III)
Trochlear nerve (IV)
Lacrimal, frontal and nasociliary
    branches of ophthalmic nerve (V_1)
Abducens nerve (VI)
Superior ophthalmic vein

Foramen rotundum --------- Maxillary nerve (V_2)

Foramen ovale ----------- { Mandibular nerve (V_3)
Accessory meningeal artery
Lesser petrosal nerve (occasionally)

Foramen spinosum -------- { Middle meningeal artery and vein
{ Meningeal branch of mandibular nerve

Foramen of Vesalius (inconstant) - Small emissary vein

Foramen lacerum ---------- { Internal carotid artery
{ Internal carotid nerve plexus

Hiatus of canal of ----------- Lesser petrosal nerve

Hiatus of canal of ----------- Greater petrosal nerve

Internal acoustic meatus ------ { Facial nerve (VII)
Vestibulocochlear nerve (VIII)
Labyrinthine artery

External opening of
vestibular aqueduct --------- Endolymphatic duct

Mastoid foramen (inconstant) --- Emissary vein (branch of
    occipital artery)

Jugular foramen ---------- { Inferior petrosal sinus
Glossopharyngeal nerve (IX)
Vagus nerve (X)
Accessory nerve (XI)
Sigmoid sinus
Posterior meningeal artery

Condylar canal (inconstant) ----{ Emissary vein and meningeal branch
    of ascending pharyngeal artery

Hypoglossal canal ---------- Hypoglossal nerve (XII)

Foramen magnum -------- { Medulla oblongata
Meninges
Vertebral arteries
Meningeal branches of vertebral
    arteries
Spinal roots of accessory nerves

Skull of Newborn

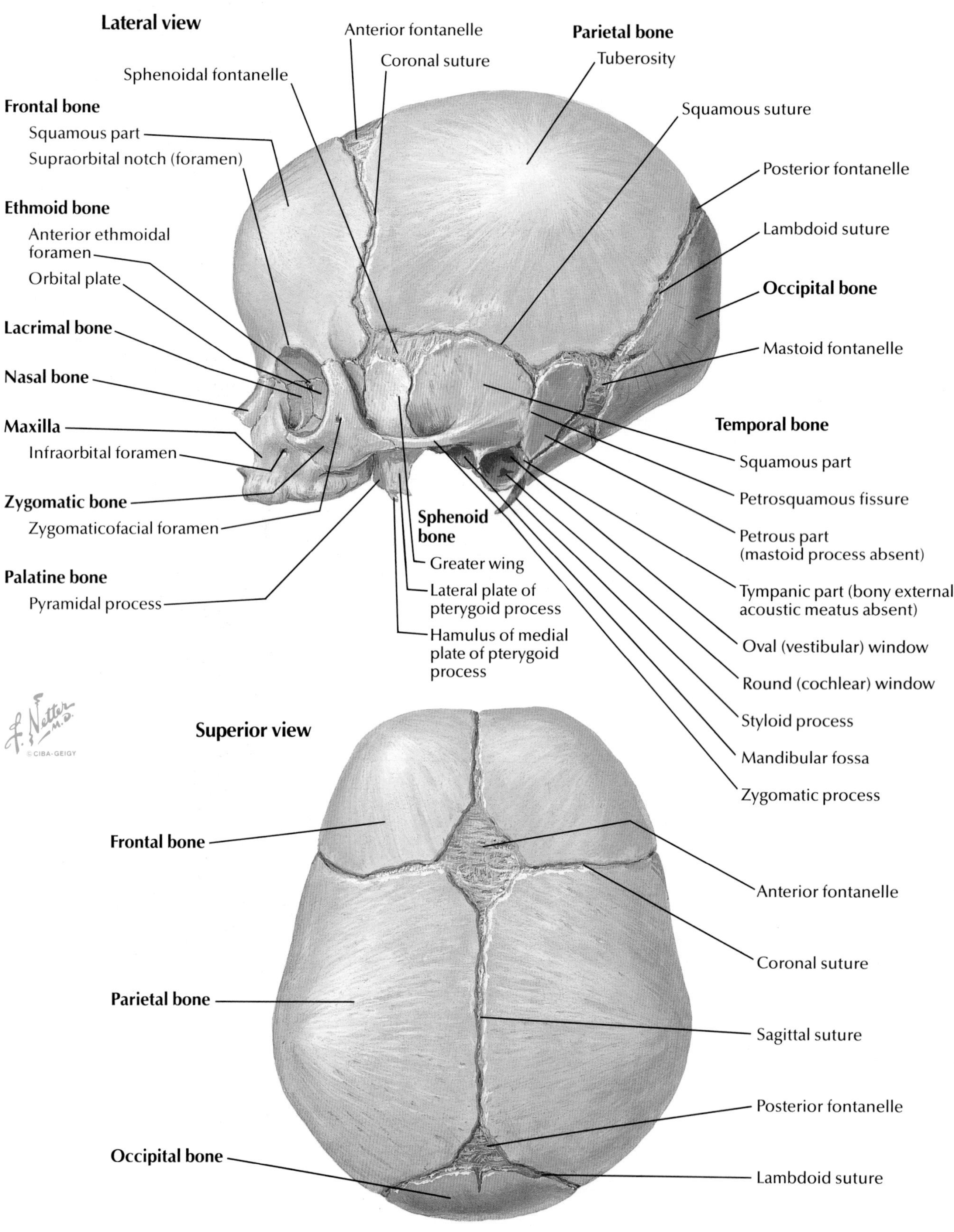

Lateral view

Anterior fontanelle

Coronal suture

Sphenoidal fontanelle

Parietal bone

Tuberosity

Frontal bone

Squamous part

Supraorbital notch (foramen)

Squamous suture

Posterior fontanelle

Ethmoid bone

Anterior ethmoidal foramen

Orbital plate

Lambdoid suture

Occipital bone

Lacrimal bone

Mastoid fontanelle

Nasal bone

Maxilla

Infraorbital foramen

Temporal bone

Squamous part

Petrosquamous fissure

Zygomatic bone

Zygomaticofacial foramen

Petrous part (mastoid process absent)

Sphenoid bone

Greater wing

Tympanic part (bony external acoustic meatus absent)

Palatine bone

Pyramidal process

Lateral plate of pterygoid process

Oval (vestibular) window

Hamulus of medial plate of pterygoid process

Round (cochlear) window

Styloid process

Mandibular fossa

Zygomatic process

Superior view

Frontal bone

Anterior fontanelle

Coronal suture

Parietal bone

Sagittal suture

Posterior fontanelle

Occipital bone

Lambdoid suture

PLATE 8

HEAD AND NECK

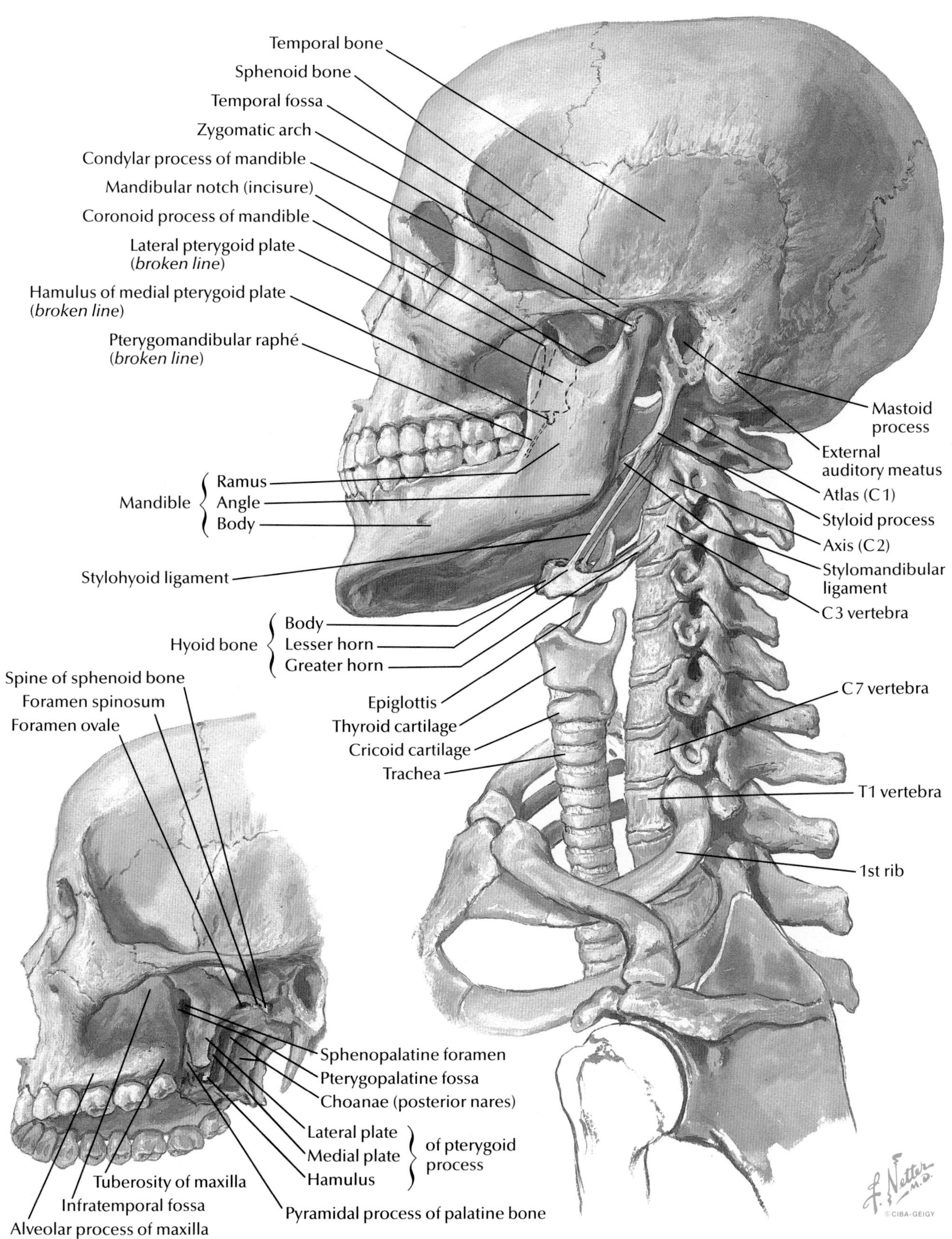

Temporal bone
Sphenoid bone
Temporal fossa
Zygomatic arch
Condylar process of mandible
Mandibular notch (incisure)
Coronoid process of mandible
Lateral pterygoid plate (*broken line*)
Hamulus of medial pterygoid plate (*broken line*)
Pterygomandibular raphé (*broken line*)

Mandible { Ramus / Angle / Body }

Stylohyoid ligament

Hyoid bone { Body / Lesser horn / Greater horn }

Spine of sphenoid bone
Foramen spinosum
Foramen ovale

Epiglottis
Thyroid cartilage
Cricoid cartilage
Trachea

Mastoid process
External auditory meatus
Atlas (C 1)
Styloid process
Axis (C 2)
Stylomandibular ligament
C 3 vertebra

C 7 vertebra

T 1 vertebra

1st rib

Sphenopalatine foramen
Pterygopalatine fossa
Choanae (posterior nares)
Lateral plate } of pterygoid process
Medial plate
Hamulus
Pyramidal process of palatine bone

Tuberosity of maxilla
Infratemporal fossa
Alveolar process of maxilla

Mandible

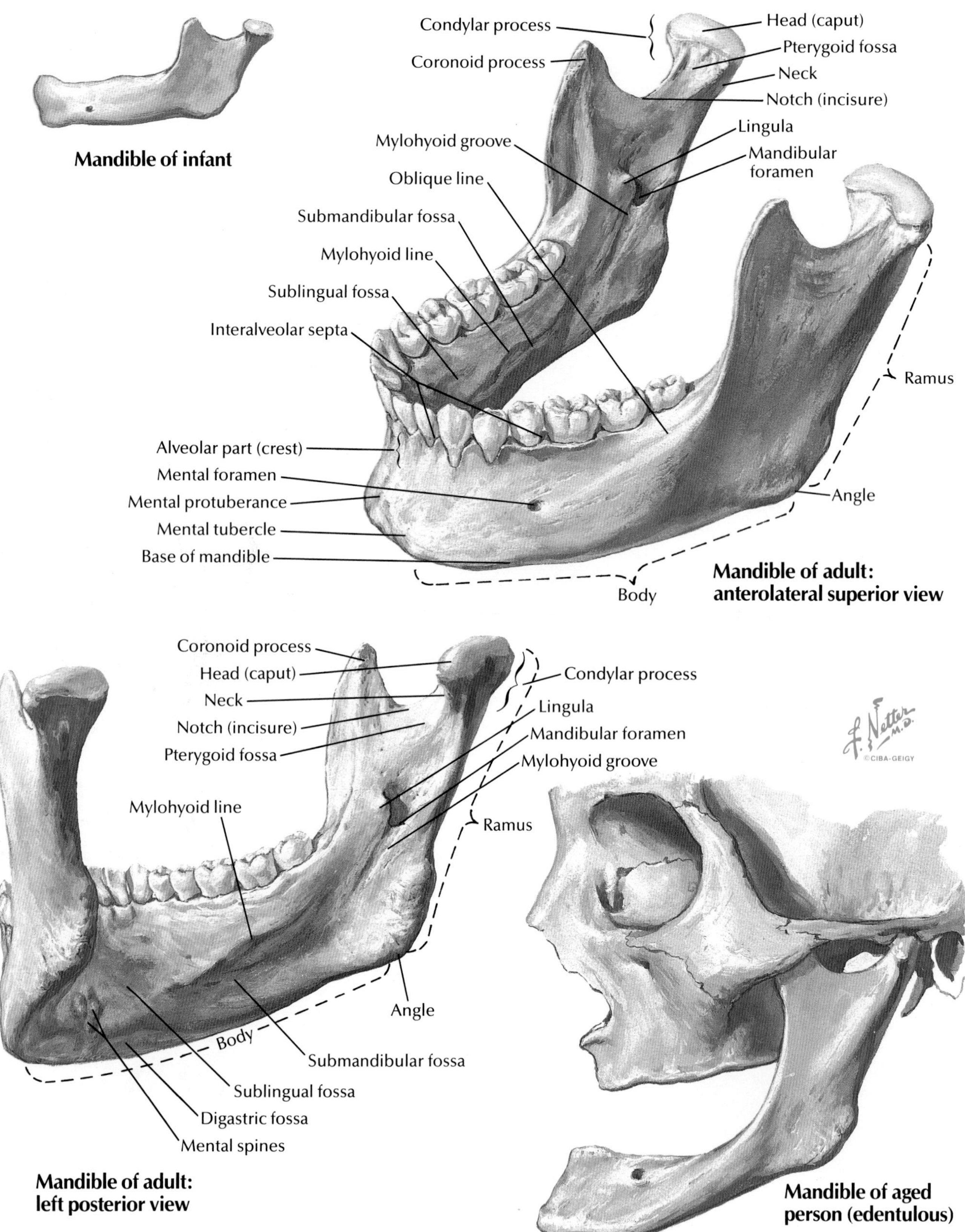

Mandible of infant

Condylar process

Coronoid process

Head (caput)

Pterygoid fossa

Neck

Notch (incisure)

Lingula

Mandibular foramen

Mylohyoid groove

Oblique line

Submandibular fossa

Mylohyoid line

Sublingual fossa

Interalveolar septa

Alveolar part (crest)

Mental foramen

Mental protuberance

Mental tubercle

Base of mandible

Ramus

Angle

Body

**Mandible of adult:
anterolateral superior view**

Coronoid process

Head (caput)

Neck

Notch (incisure)

Pterygoid fossa

Condylar process

Lingula

Mandibular foramen

Mylohyoid groove

Mylohyoid line

Ramus

Angle

Body

Submandibular fossa

Sublingual fossa

Digastric fossa

Mental spines

**Mandible of adult:
left posterior view**

**Mandible of aged
person (edentulous)**

PLATE 10

HEAD AND NECK

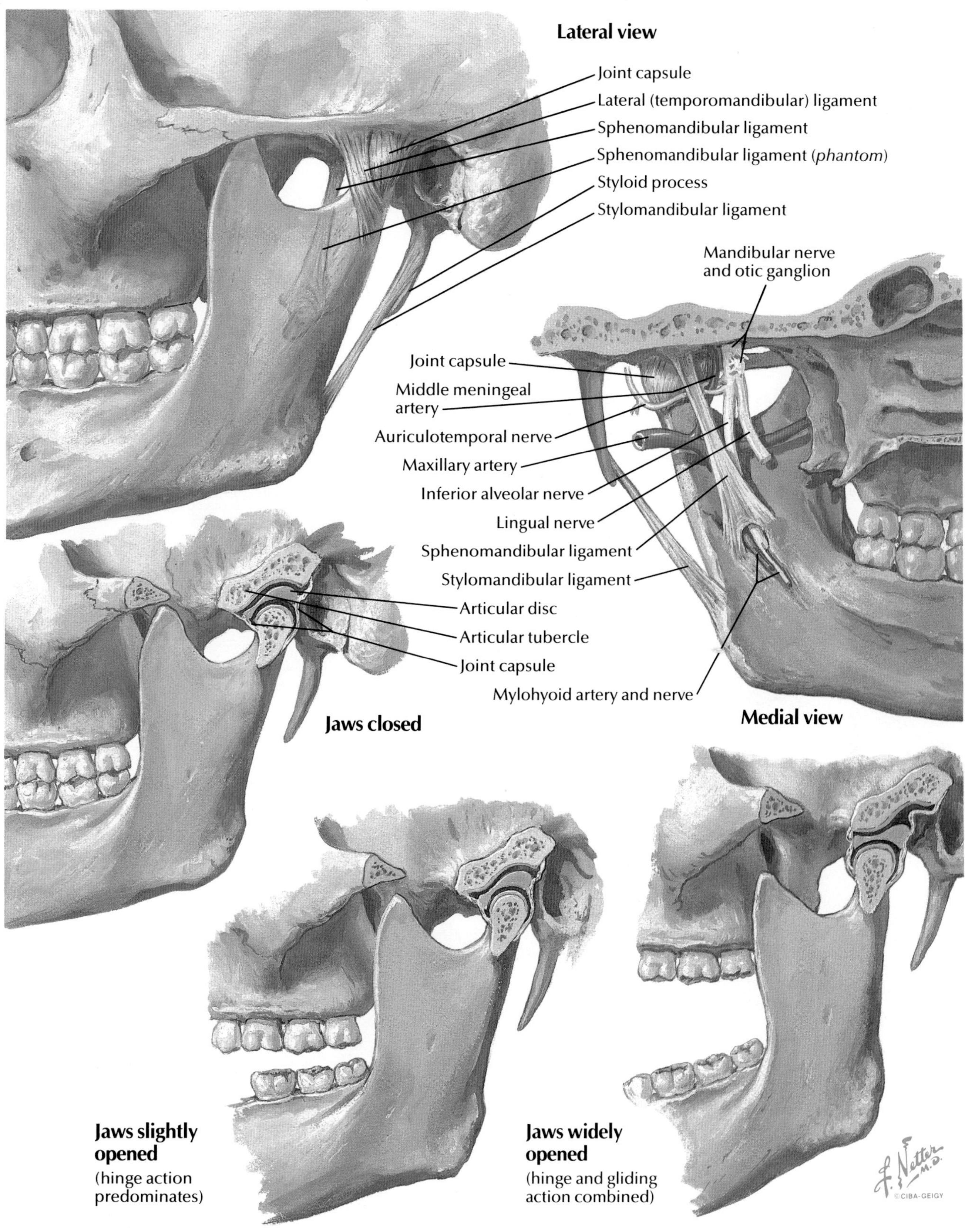

Lateral view

- Joint capsule
- Lateral (temporomandibular) ligament
- Sphenomandibular ligament
- Sphenomandibular ligament (*phantom*)
- Styloid process
- Stylomandibular ligament

Mandibular nerve and otic ganglion

- Joint capsule
- Middle meningeal artery
- Auriculotemporal nerve
- Maxillary artery
- Inferior alveolar nerve
- Lingual nerve
- Sphenomandibular ligament
- Stylomandibular ligament
- Articular disc
- Articular tubercle
- Joint capsule
- Mylohyoid artery and nerve

Medial view

Jaws closed

Jaws slightly opened
(hinge action predominates)

Jaws widely opened
(hinge and gliding action combined)

Cervical Vertebrae: Atlas and Axis

SEE ALSO PLATES 9, 142

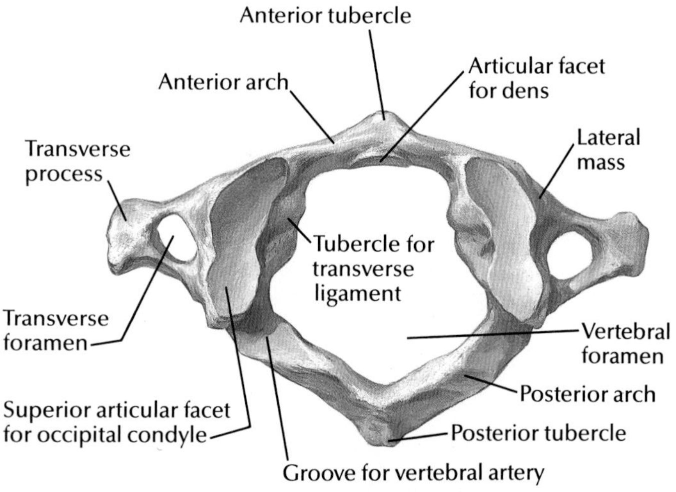

Atlas (C 1): superior view

Anterior tubercle
Anterior arch
Articular facet for dens
Transverse process
Lateral mass
Tubercle for transverse ligament
Transverse foramen
Vertebral foramen
Superior articular facet for occipital condyle
Posterior arch
Posterior tubercle
Groove for vertebral artery

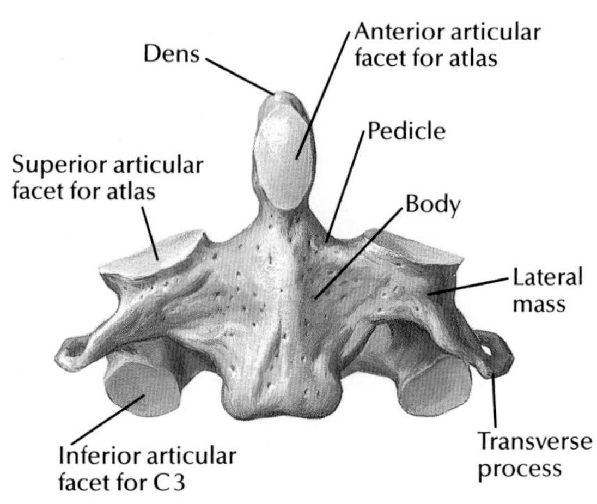

Axis (C 2): anterior view

Dens
Anterior articular facet for atlas
Pedicle
Superior articular facet for atlas
Body
Lateral mass
Transverse process
Inferior articular facet for C 3

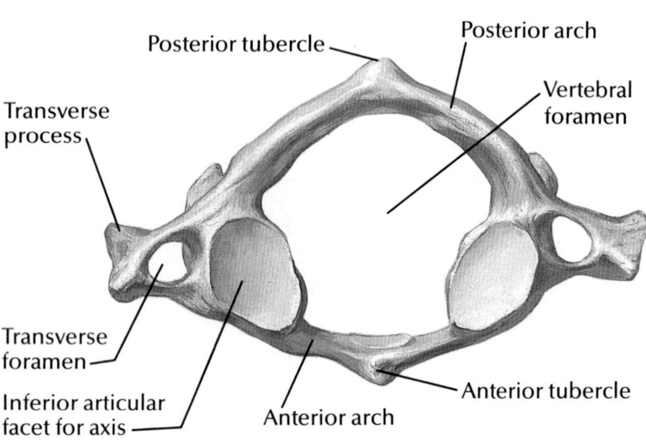

Atlas (C 1): inferior view

Posterior tubercle
Posterior arch
Vertebral foramen
Transverse process
Transverse foramen
Inferior articular facet for axis
Anterior arch
Anterior tubercle

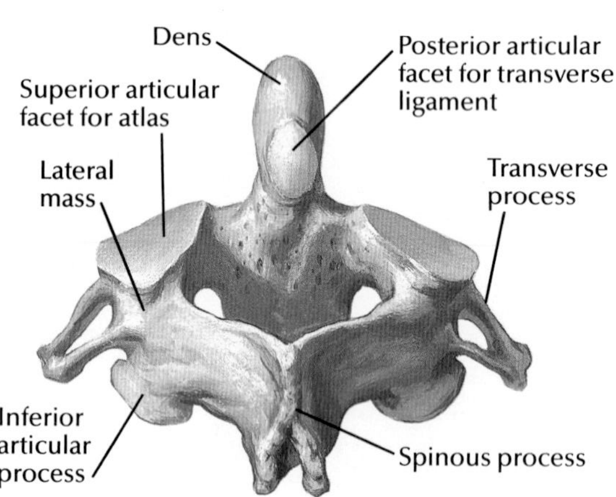

Axis (C 2): posterosuperior view

Dens
Posterior articular facet for transverse ligament
Superior articular facet for atlas
Lateral mass
Transverse process
Inferior articular process
Spinous process

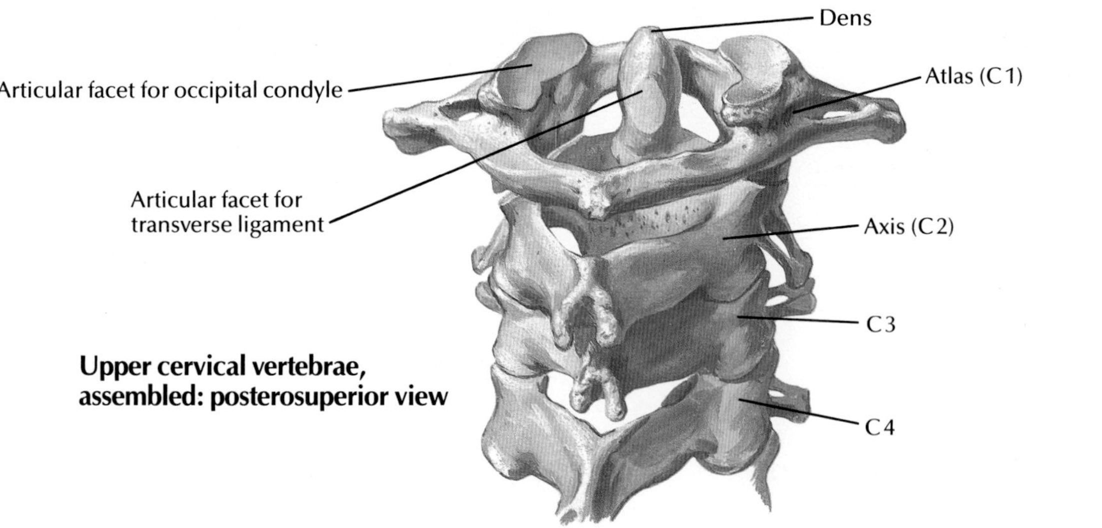

Upper cervical vertebrae, assembled: posterosuperior view

Dens
Articular facet for occipital condyle
Atlas (C 1)
Articular facet for transverse ligament
Axis (C 2)
C 3
C 4

PLATE 12

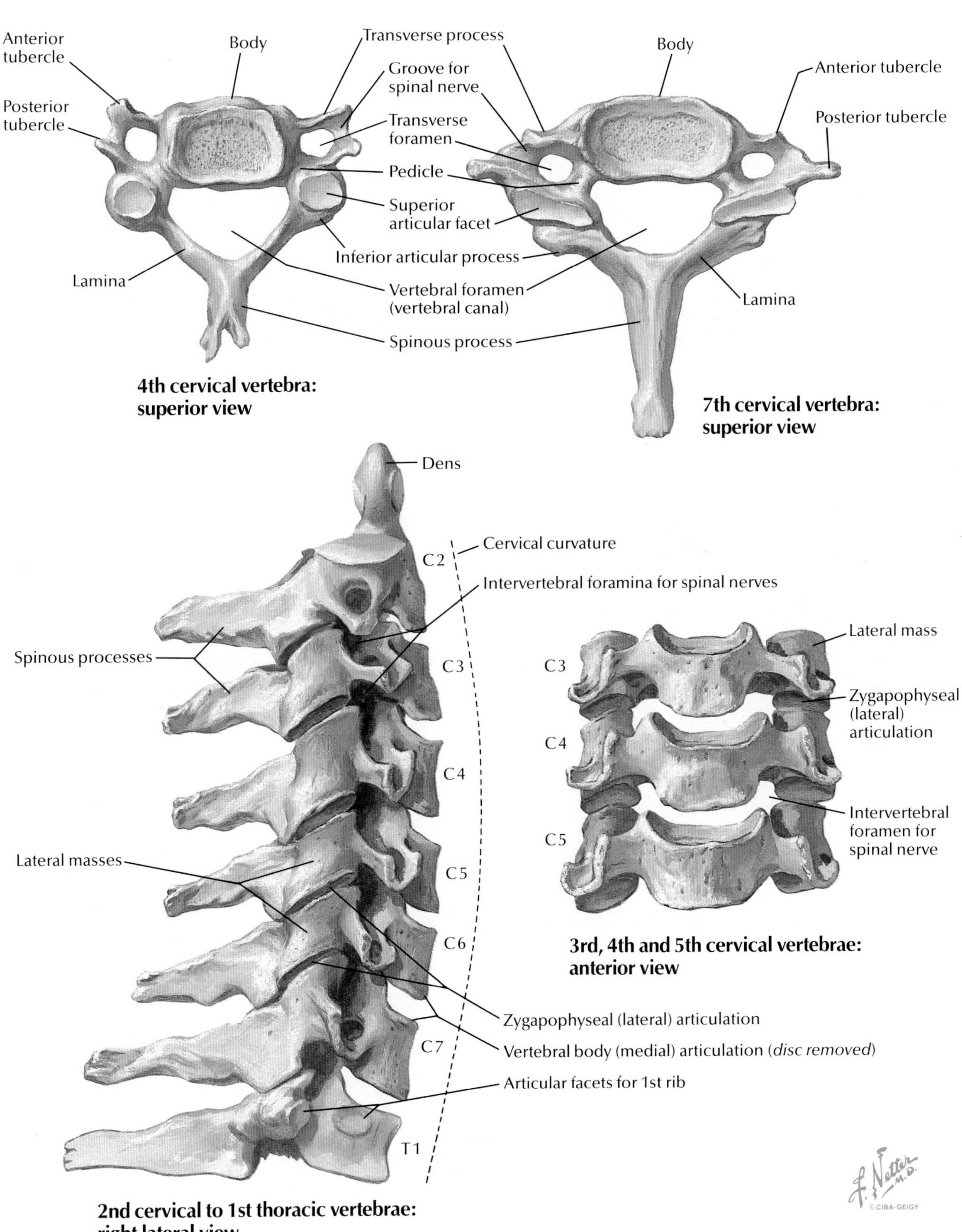

Anterior tubercle

Body

Transverse process

Groove for spinal nerve

Transverse foramen

Pedicle

Posterior tubercle

Superior articular facet

Inferior articular process

Lamina

Vertebral foramen (vertebral canal)

Spinous process

4th cervical vertebra: superior view

Body

Anterior tubercle

Posterior tubercle

Lamina

7th cervical vertebra: superior view

Dens

Cervical curvature

Intervertebral foramina for spinal nerves

C2

C3

C4

C5

C6

C7

T1

Spinous processes

Lateral masses

Zygapophyseal (lateral) articulation

Vertebral body (medial) articulation (*disc removed*)

Articular facets for 1st rib

2nd cervical to 1st thoracic vertebrae: right lateral view

C3

C4

C5

Lateral mass

Zygapophyseal (lateral) articulation

Intervertebral foramen for spinal nerve

3rd, 4th and 5th cervical vertebrae: anterior view

External Craniocervical Ligaments

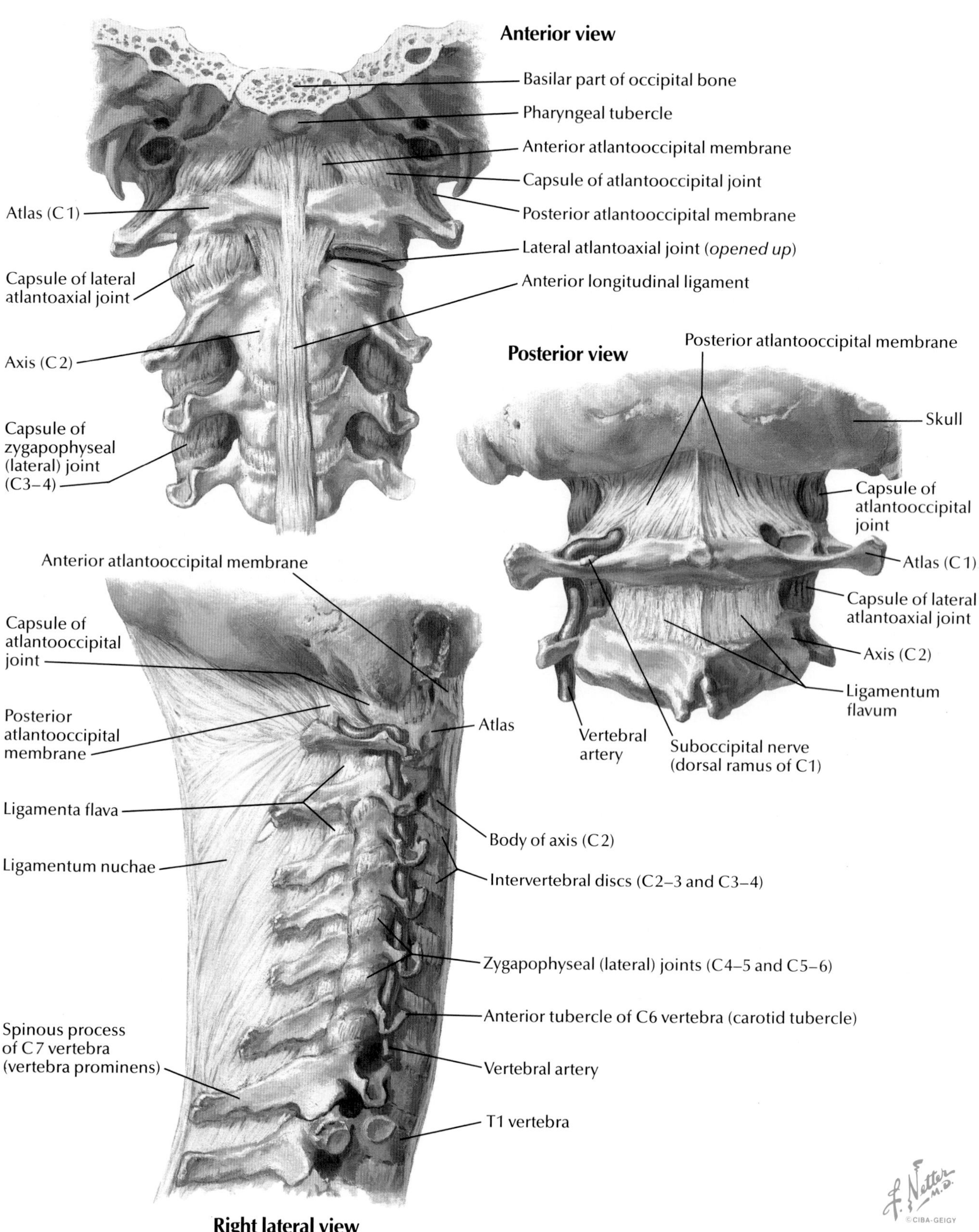

Anterior view

Basilar part of occipital bone

Pharyngeal tubercle

Anterior atlantooccipital membrane

Capsule of atlantooccipital joint

Posterior atlantooccipital membrane

Lateral atlantoaxial joint (*opened up*)

Anterior longitudinal ligament

Atlas (C 1)

Capsule of lateral atlantoaxial joint

Axis (C 2)

Capsule of zygapophyseal (lateral) joint (C3–4)

Posterior view

Posterior atlantooccipital membrane

Skull

Capsule of atlantooccipital joint

Atlas (C 1)

Capsule of lateral atlantoaxial joint

Axis (C 2)

Ligamentum flavum

Vertebral artery

Suboccipital nerve (dorsal ramus of C1)

Anterior atlantooccipital membrane

Capsule of atlantooccipital joint

Posterior atlantooccipital membrane

Ligamenta flava

Ligamentum nuchae

Atlas

Body of axis (C 2)

Intervertebral discs (C2–3 and C3–4)

Zygapophyseal (lateral) joints (C4–5 and C5–6)

Anterior tubercle of C6 vertebra (carotid tubercle)

Vertebral artery

Spinous process of C7 vertebra (vertebra prominens)

T1 vertebra

Right lateral view

PLATE 14

HEAD AND NECK

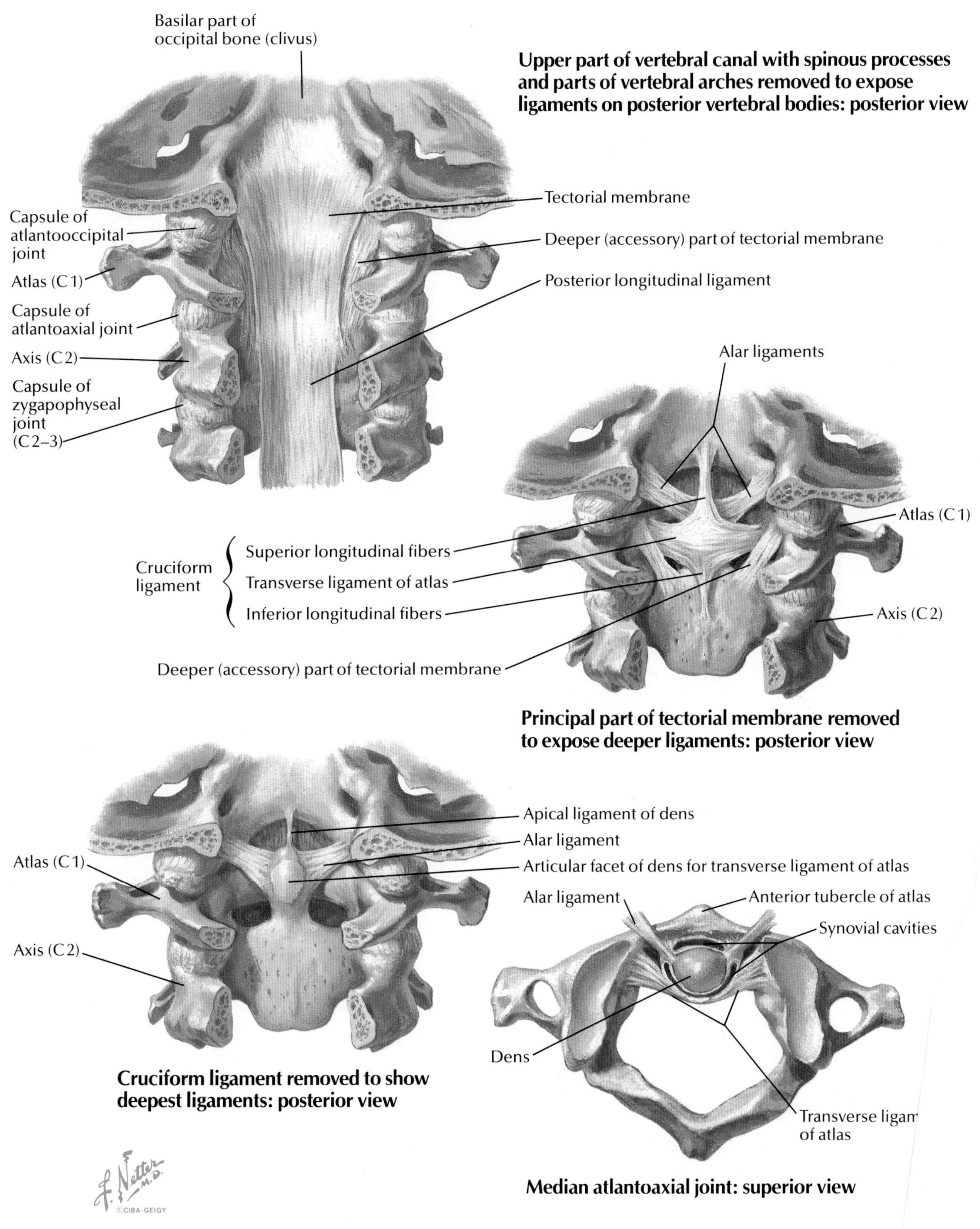

Basilar part of
occipital bone (clivus)

**Upper part of vertebral canal with spinous processes
and parts of vertebral arches removed to expose
ligaments on posterior vertebral bodies: posterior view**

Capsule of
atlantooccipital
joint

Atlas (C1)

Capsule of
atlantoaxial joint

Axis (C2)

Capsule of
zygapophyseal
joint
(C2–3)

Tectorial membrane

Deeper (accessory) part of tectorial membrane

Posterior longitudinal ligament

Alar ligaments

Atlas (C1)

Axis (C2)

Cruciform
ligament
{
Superior longitudinal fibers

Transverse ligament of atlas

Inferior longitudinal fibers
}

Deeper (accessory) part of tectorial membrane

**Principal part of tectorial membrane removed
to expose deeper ligaments: posterior view**

Atlas (C1)

Axis (C2)

Apical ligament of dens

Alar ligament

Articular facet of dens for transverse ligament of atlas

Alar ligament

Anterior tubercle of atlas

Synovial cavities

Dens

Transverse ligament
of atlas

**Cruciform ligament removed to show
deepest ligaments: posterior view**

Median atlantoaxial joint: superior view

Atlantooccipital Junction

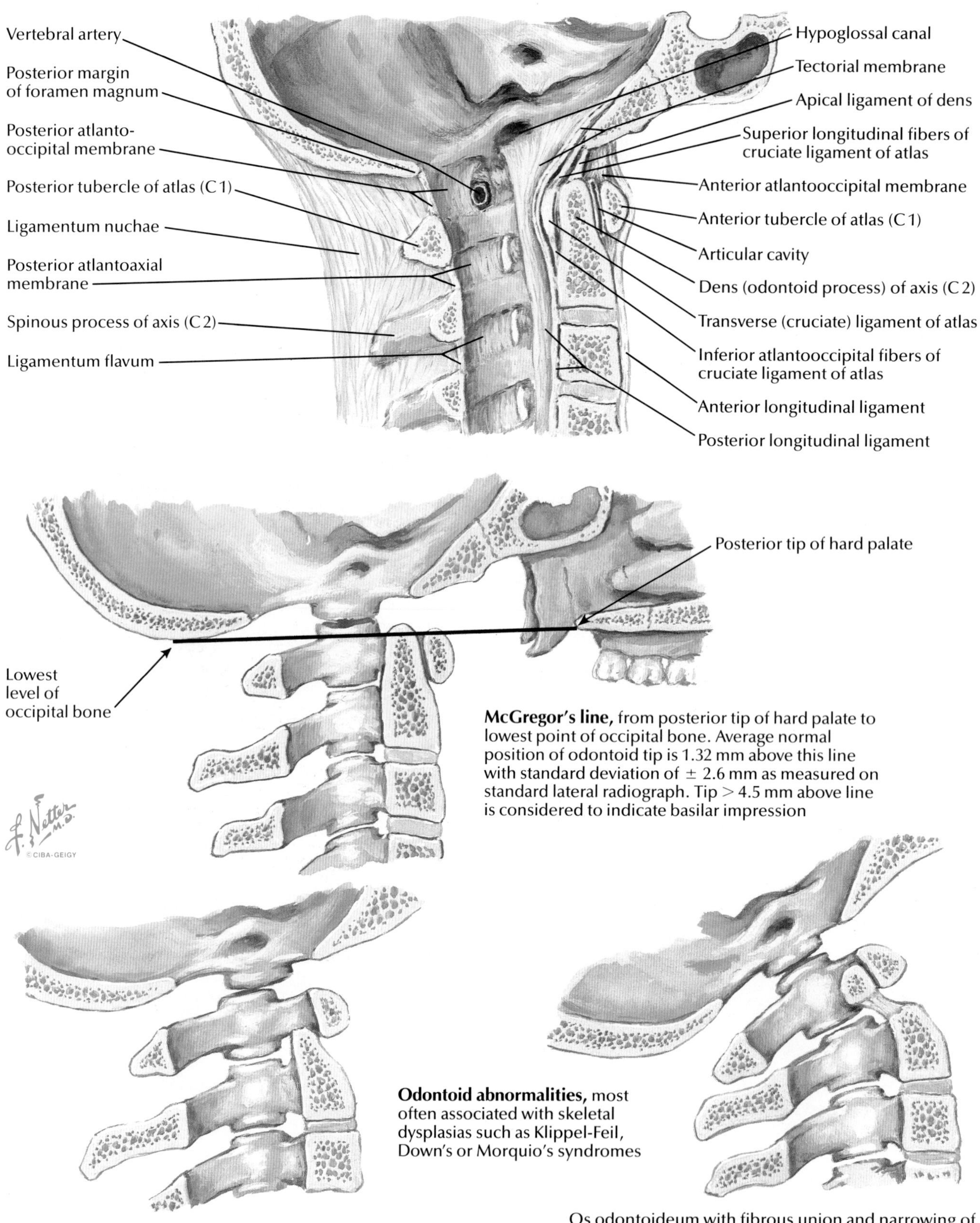

Vertebral artery

Posterior margin of foramen magnum

Posterior atlanto-occipital membrane

Posterior tubercle of atlas (C 1)

Ligamentum nuchae

Posterior atlantoaxial membrane

Spinous process of axis (C 2)

Ligamentum flavum

Hypoglossal canal

Tectorial membrane

Apical ligament of dens

Superior longitudinal fibers of cruciate ligament of atlas

Anterior atlantooccipital membrane

Anterior tubercle of atlas (C 1)

Articular cavity

Dens (odontoid process) of axis (C 2)

Transverse (cruciate) ligament of atlas

Inferior atlantooccipital fibers of cruciate ligament of atlas

Anterior longitudinal ligament

Posterior longitudinal ligament

Posterior tip of hard palate

Lowest level of occipital bone

McGregor's line, from posterior tip of hard palate to lowest point of occipital bone. Average normal position of odontoid tip is 1.32 mm above this line with standard deviation of ± 2.6 mm as measured on standard lateral radiograph. Tip > 4.5 mm above line is considered to indicate basilar impression

Odontoid abnormalities, most often associated with skeletal dysplasias such as Klippel-Feil, Down's or Morquio's syndromes

Hypoplastic dens (odontoid process)

Os odontoideum with fibrous union and narrowing of vertebral canal with head in extension

PLATE 16

HEAD AND NECK

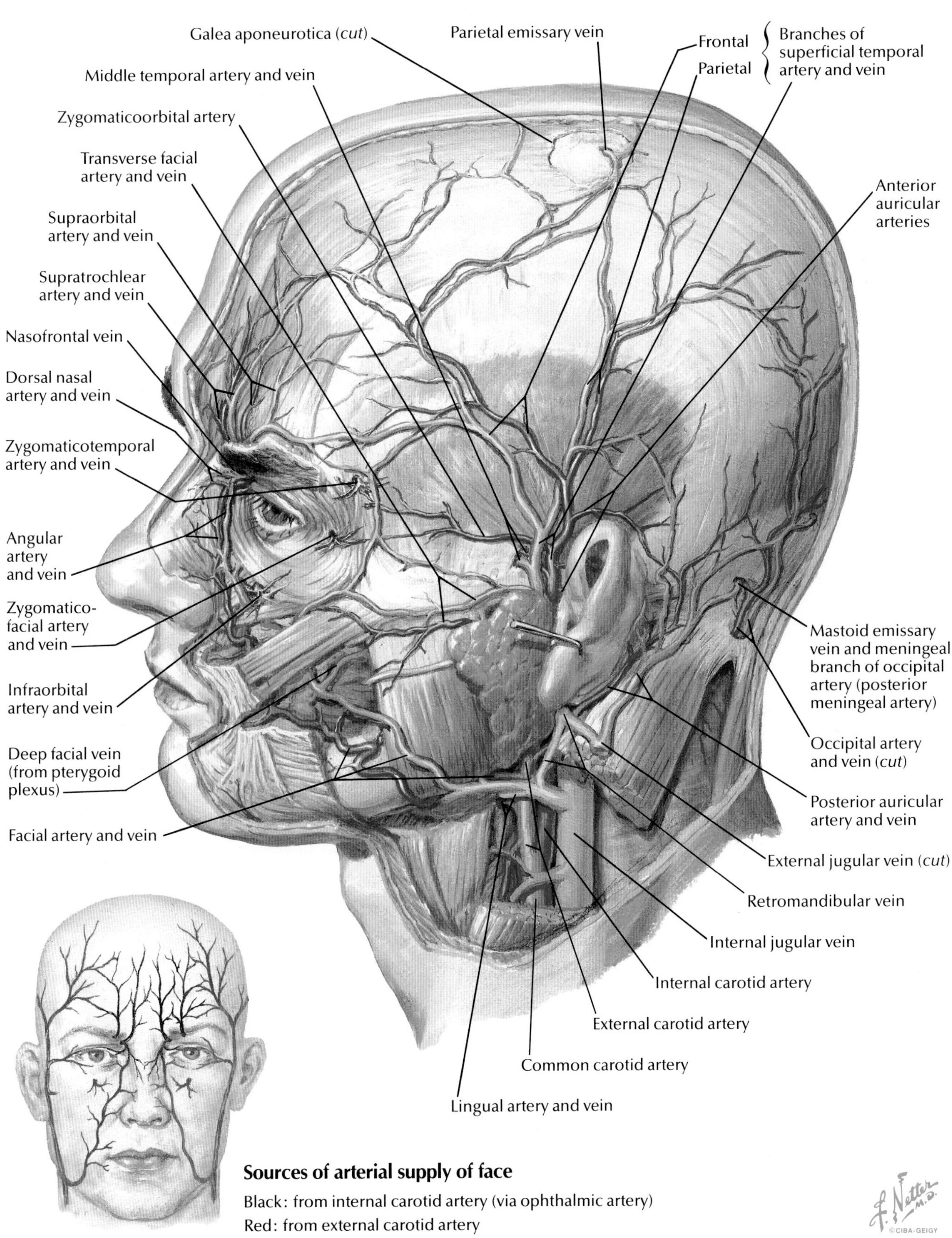

Galea aponeurotica (*cut*)

Parietal emissary vein

Frontal

Parietal

Branches of superficial temporal artery and vein

Middle temporal artery and vein

Zygomaticoorbital artery

Transverse facial artery and vein

Supraorbital artery and vein

Supratrochlear artery and vein

Nasofrontal vein

Dorsal nasal artery and vein

Zygomaticotemporal artery and vein

Angular artery and vein

Zygomatico-facial artery and vein

Infraorbital artery and vein

Deep facial vein (from pterygoid plexus)

Facial artery and vein

Anterior auricular arteries

Mastoid emissary vein and meningeal branch of occipital artery (posterior meningeal artery)

Occipital artery and vein (*cut*)

Posterior auricular artery and vein

External jugular vein (*cut*)

Retromandibular vein

Internal jugular vein

Internal carotid artery

External carotid artery

Common carotid artery

Lingual artery and vein

Sources of arterial supply of face

Black: from internal carotid artery (via ophthalmic artery)
Red: from external carotid artery

Cutaneous Nerves of Head and Neck

SEE ALSO PLATES 27, 31, 40, 41, 116

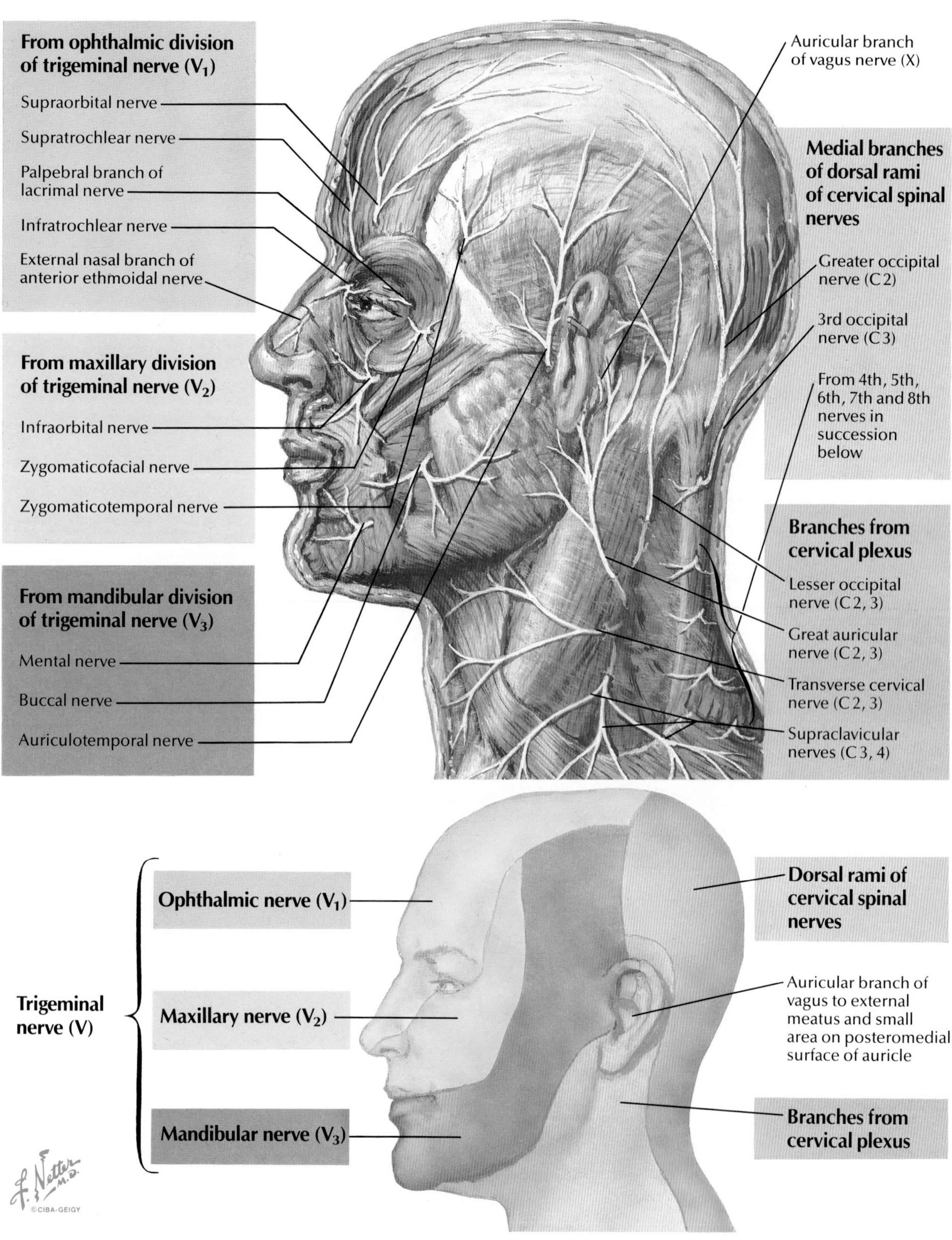

From ophthalmic division of trigeminal nerve (V₁)

Supraorbital nerve

Supratrochlear nerve

Palpebral branch of lacrimal nerve

Infratrochlear nerve

External nasal branch of anterior ethmoidal nerve

From maxillary division of trigeminal nerve (V₂)

Infraorbital nerve

Zygomaticofacial nerve

Zygomaticotemporal nerve

From mandibular division of trigeminal nerve (V₃)

Mental nerve

Buccal nerve

Auriculotemporal nerve

Auricular branch of vagus nerve (X)

Medial branches of dorsal rami of cervical spinal nerves

Greater occipital nerve (C 2)

3rd occipital nerve (C 3)

From 4th, 5th, 6th, 7th and 8th nerves in succession below

Branches from cervical plexus

Lesser occipital nerve (C 2, 3)

Great auricular nerve (C 2, 3)

Transverse cervical nerve (C 2, 3)

Supraclavicular nerves (C 3, 4)

Trigeminal nerve (V)

Ophthalmic nerve (V₁)

Maxillary nerve (V₂)

Mandibular nerve (V₃)

Dorsal rami of cervical spinal nerves

Auricular branch of vagus to external meatus and small area on posteromedial surface of auricle

Branches from cervical plexus

PLATE 18   **HEAD AND NECK**

Facial Nerve Branches and Parotid Gland

SEE ALSO PLATE 117

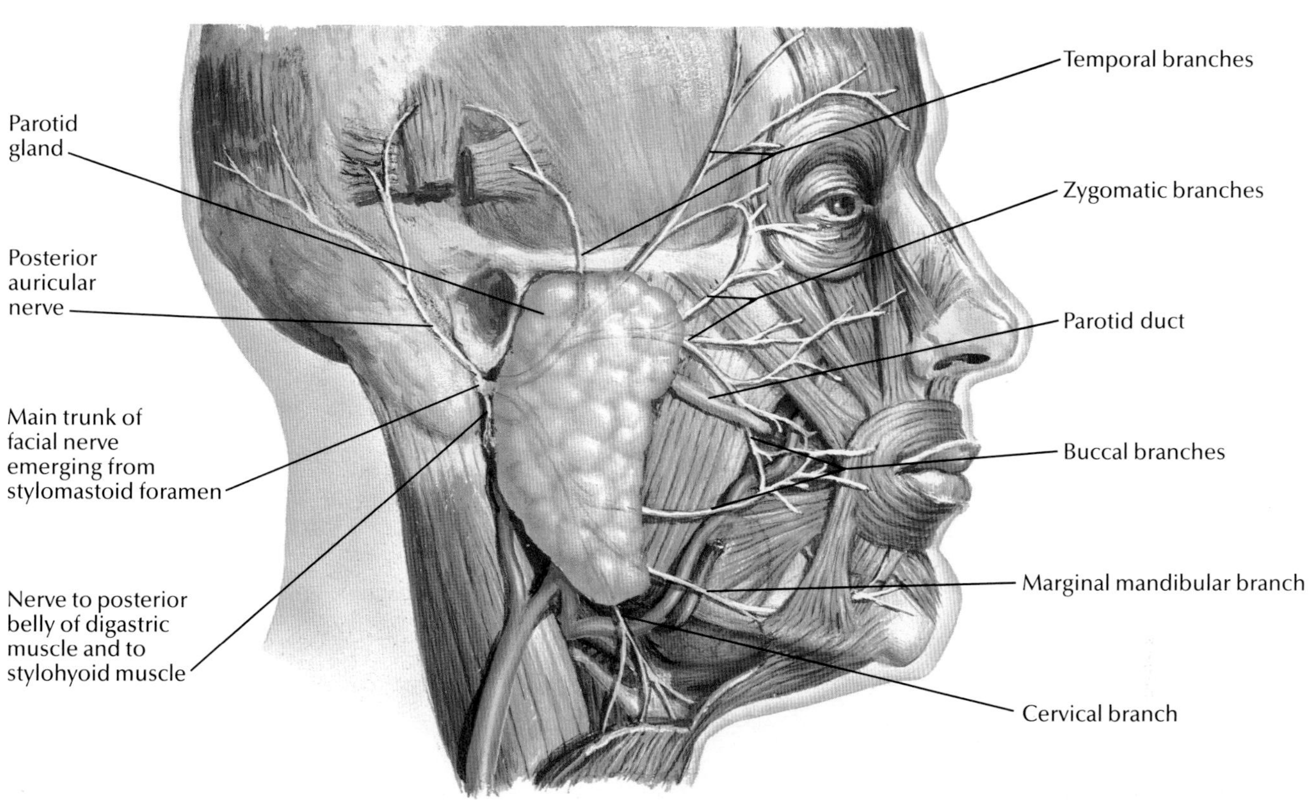

Temporal branches

Zygomatic branches

Parotid gland

Posterior auricular nerve

Parotid duct

Main trunk of facial nerve emerging from stylomastoid foramen

Buccal branches

Marginal mandibular branch

Nerve to posterior belly of digastric muscle and to stylohyoid muscle

Cervical branch

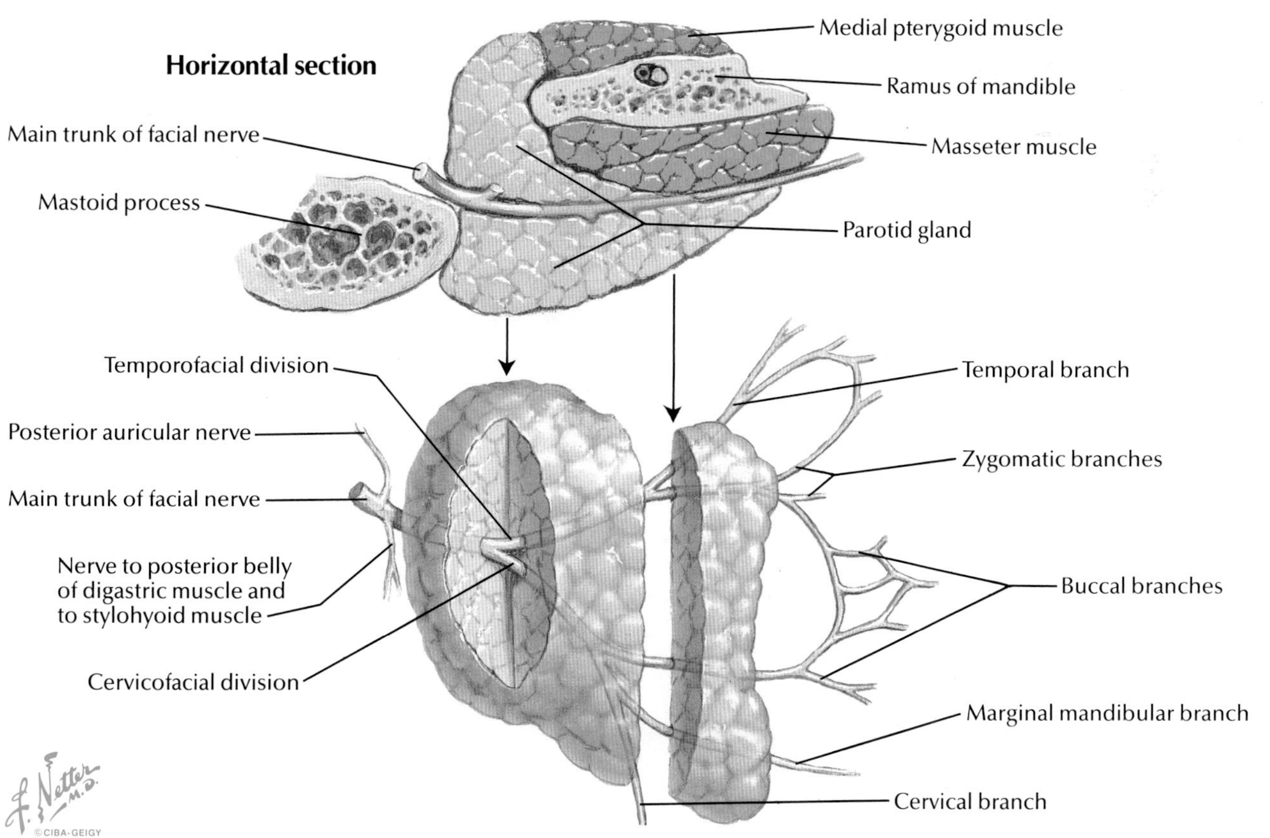

Horizontal section

Medial pterygoid muscle

Ramus of mandible

Main trunk of facial nerve

Masseter muscle

Mastoid process

Parotid gland

Temporofacial division

Temporal branch

Posterior auricular nerve

Zygomatic branches

Main trunk of facial nerve

Nerve to posterior belly of digastric muscle and to stylohyoid muscle

Buccal branches

Cervicofacial division

Marginal mandibular branch

Cervical branch

SUPERFICIAL FACE

PLATE 19

Muscles of Facial Expression: Anterior View

SEE ALSO PLATE 48

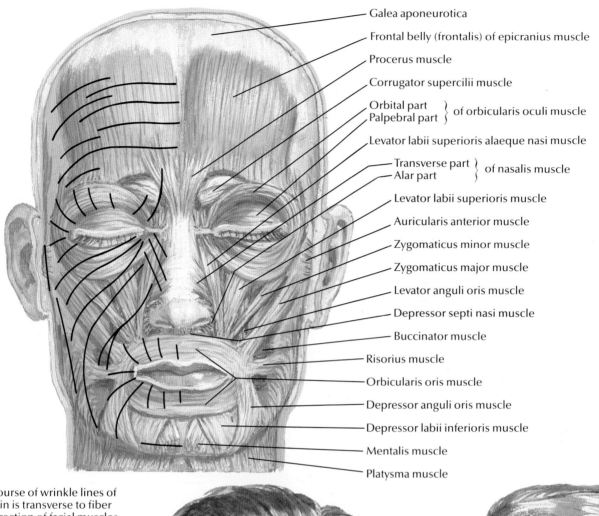

Galea aponeurotica

Frontal belly (frontalis) of epicranius muscle

Procerus muscle

Corrugator supercilii muscle

Orbital part
Palpebral part } of orbicularis oculi muscle

Levator labii superioris alaeque nasi muscle

Transverse part } of nasalis muscle
Alar part

Levator labii superioris muscle

Auricularis anterior muscle

Zygomaticus minor muscle

Zygomaticus major muscle

Levator anguli oris muscle

Depressor septi nasi muscle

Buccinator muscle

Risorius muscle

Orbicularis oris muscle

Depressor anguli oris muscle

Depressor labii inferioris muscle

Mentalis muscle

Platysma muscle

Course of wrinkle lines of skin is transverse to fiber direction of facial muscles. Elliptical incisions for removal of skin tumors conform to direction of wrinkle lines

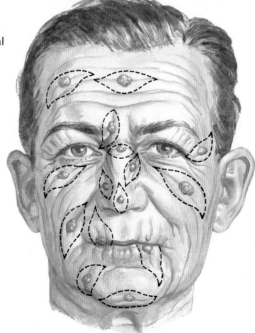

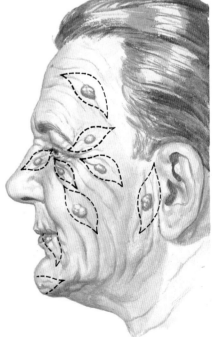

PLATE 20

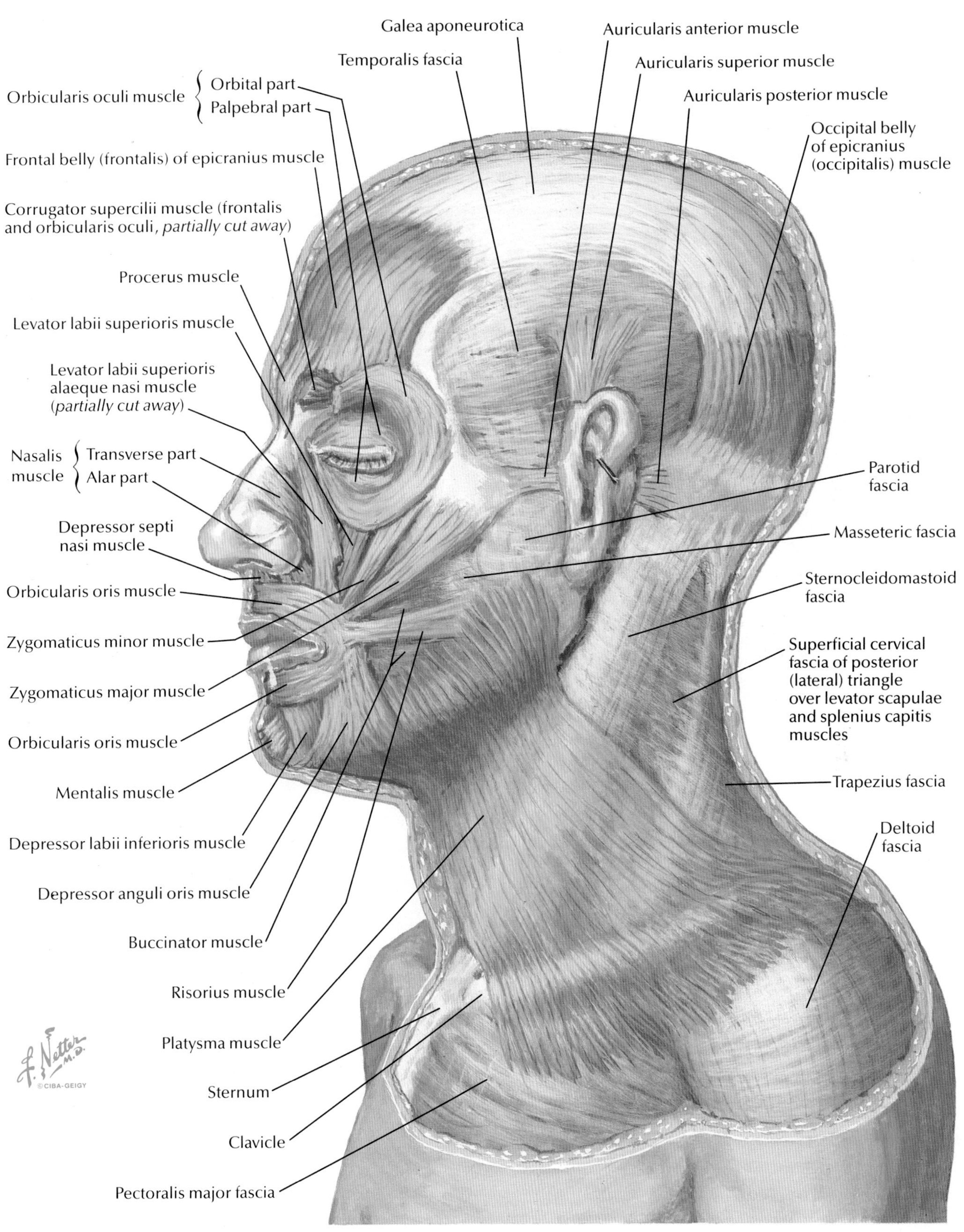

Galea aponeurotica

Temporalis fascia

Auricularis anterior muscle

Auricularis superior muscle

Auricularis posterior muscle

Occipital belly
of epicranius
(occipitalis) muscle

Orbicularis oculi muscle { Orbital part
Palpebral part

Frontal belly (frontalis) of epicranius muscle

Corrugator supercilii muscle (frontalis
and orbicularis oculi, *partially cut away*)

Procerus muscle

Levator labii superioris muscle

Levator labii superioris
alaeque nasi muscle
(*partially cut away*)

Nasalis { Transverse part
muscle { Alar part

Depressor septi
nasi muscle

Orbicularis oris muscle

Zygomaticus minor muscle

Zygomaticus major muscle

Orbicularis oris muscle

Mentalis muscle

Depressor labii inferioris muscle

Depressor anguli oris muscle

Buccinator muscle

Risorius muscle

Platysma muscle

Sternum

Clavicle

Pectoralis major fascia

Parotid
fascia

Masseteric fascia

Sternocleidomastoid
fascia

Superficial cervical
fascia of posterior
(lateral) triangle
over levator scapulae
and splenius capitis
muscles

Trapezius fascia

Deltoid
fascia

f. Netter
©CIBA-GEIGY

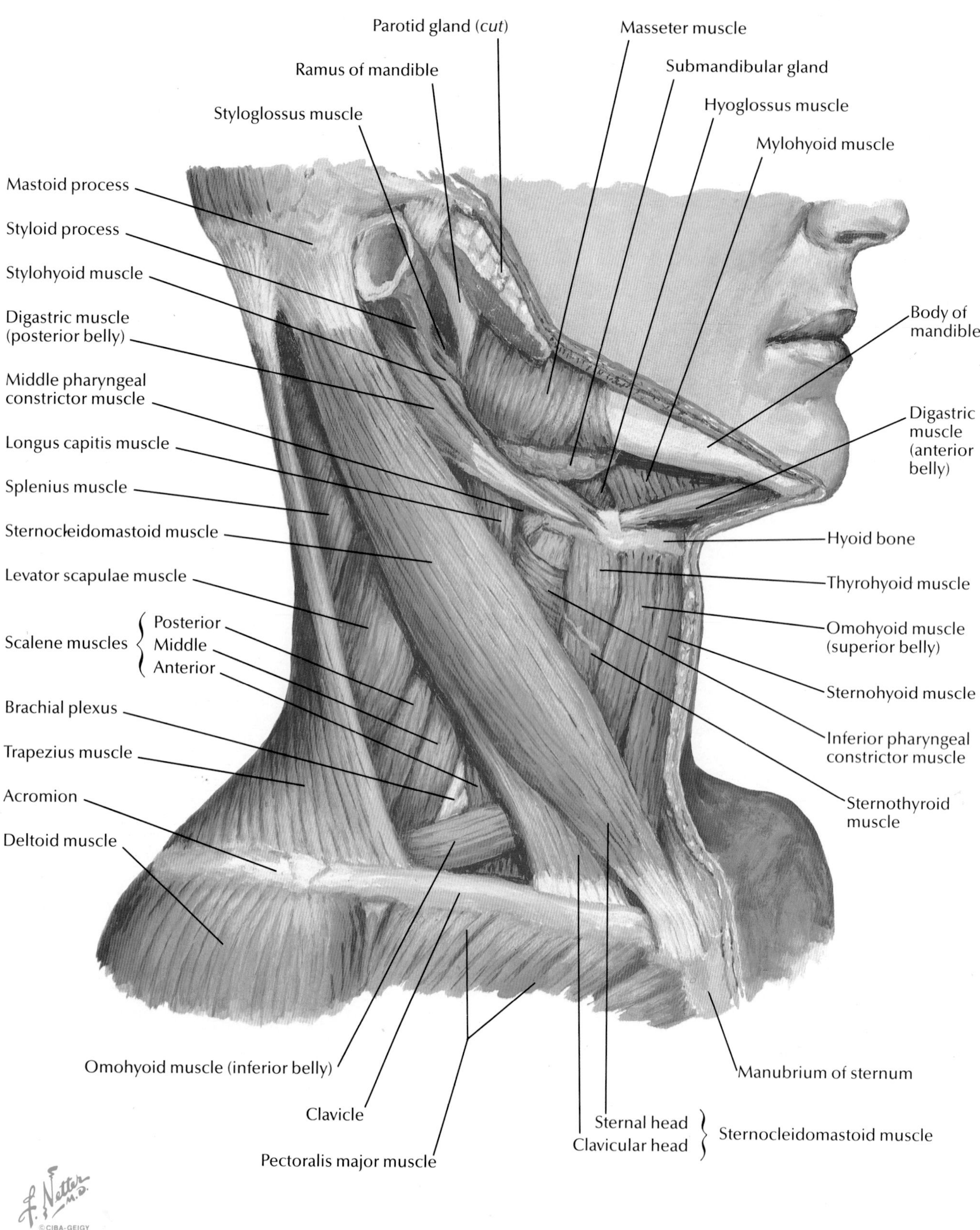

Parotid gland (*cut*)

Masseter muscle

Ramus of mandible

Submandibular gland

Styloglossus muscle

Hyoglossus muscle

Mylohyoid muscle

Mastoid process

Styloid process

Stylohyoid muscle

Digastric muscle (posterior belly)

Middle pharyngeal constrictor muscle

Longus capitis muscle

Splenius muscle

Sternocleidomastoid muscle

Levator scapulae muscle

Scalene muscles {
Posterior
Middle
Anterior

Brachial plexus

Trapezius muscle

Acromion

Deltoid muscle

Body of mandible

Digastric muscle (anterior belly)

Hyoid bone

Thyrohyoid muscle

Omohyoid muscle (superior belly)

Sternohyoid muscle

Inferior pharyngeal constrictor muscle

Sternothyroid muscle

Omohyoid muscle (inferior belly)

Clavicle

Pectoralis major muscle

Sternal head }
Clavicular head }
Sternocleidomastoid muscle

Manubrium of sternum

PLATE 22

HEAD AND NECK

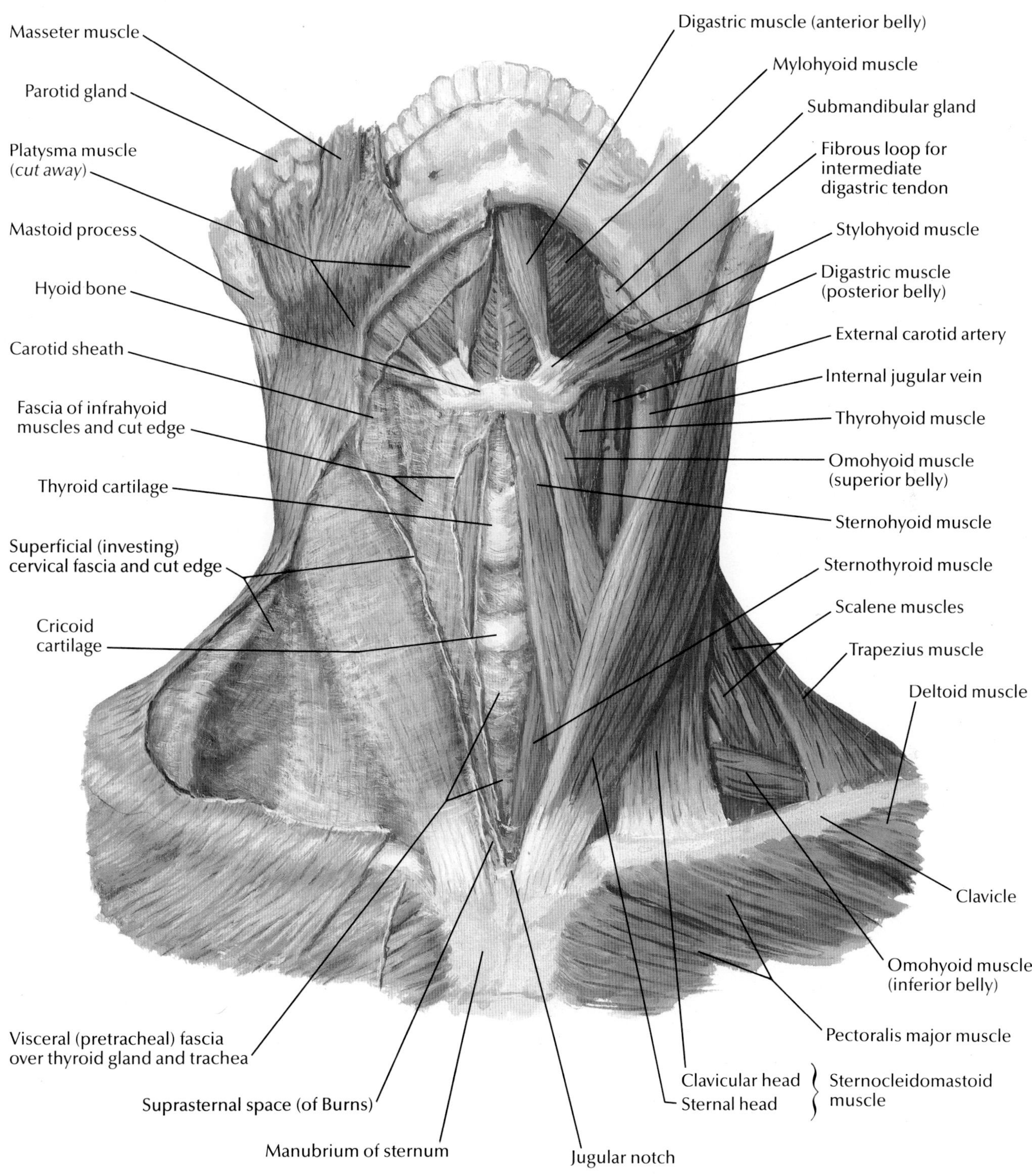

Masseter muscle

Parotid gland

Platysma muscle
(*cut away*)

Mastoid process

Hyoid bone

Carotid sheath

Fascia of infrahyoid
muscles and cut edge

Thyroid cartilage

Superficial (investing)
cervical fascia and cut edge

Cricoid
cartilage

Digastric muscle (anterior belly)

Mylohyoid muscle

Submandibular gland

Fibrous loop for
intermediate
digastric tendon

Stylohyoid muscle

Digastric muscle
(posterior belly)

External carotid artery

Internal jugular vein

Thyrohyoid muscle

Omohyoid muscle
(superior belly)

Sternohyoid muscle

Sternothyroid muscle

Scalene muscles

Trapezius muscle

Deltoid muscle

Clavicle

Omohyoid muscle
(inferior belly)

Pectoralis major muscle

Clavicular head } Sternocleidomastoid
Sternal head } muscle

Visceral (pretracheal) fascia
over thyroid gland and trachea

Suprasternal space (of Burns)

Manubrium of sternum

Jugular notch

Infrahyoid and Suprahyoid Muscles

SEE ALSO PLATE 47

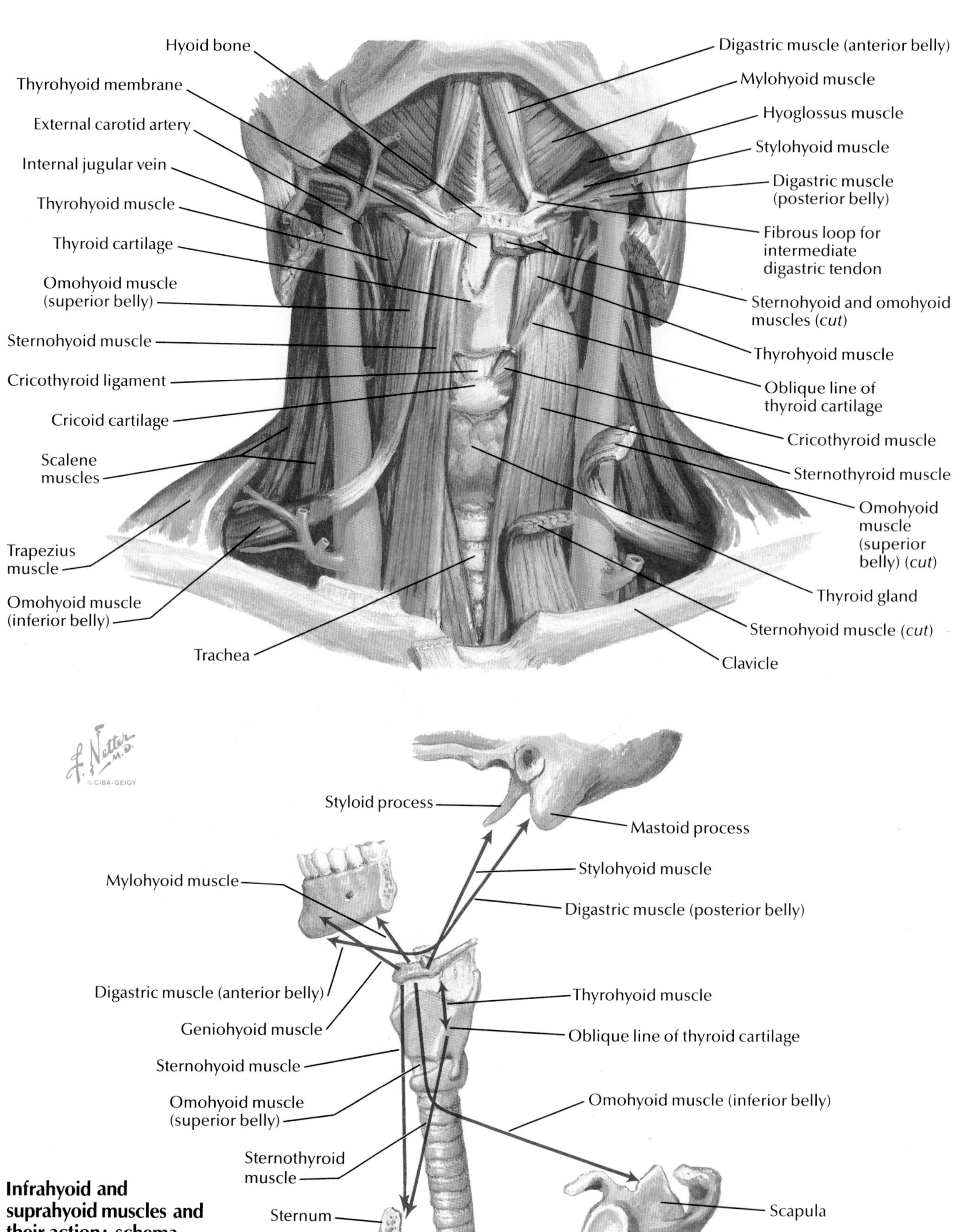

Hyoid bone

Thyrohyoid membrane

External carotid artery

Internal jugular vein

Thyrohyoid muscle

Thyroid cartilage

Omohyoid muscle (superior belly)

Sternohyoid muscle

Cricothyroid ligament

Cricoid cartilage

Scalene muscles

Trapezius muscle

Omohyoid muscle (inferior belly)

Trachea

Digastric muscle (anterior belly)

Mylohyoid muscle

Hyoglossus muscle

Stylohyoid muscle

Digastric muscle (posterior belly)

Fibrous loop for intermediate digastric tendon

Sternohyoid and omohyoid muscles (*cut*)

Thyrohyoid muscle

Oblique line of thyroid cartilage

Cricothyroid muscle

Sternothyroid muscle

Omohyoid muscle (superior belly) (*cut*)

Thyroid gland

Sternohyoid muscle (*cut*)

Clavicle

Styloid process

Mastoid process

Stylohyoid muscle

Digastric muscle (posterior belly)

Mylohyoid muscle

Digastric muscle (anterior belly)

Geniohyoid muscle

Sternohyoid muscle

Omohyoid muscle (superior belly)

Sternothyroid muscle

Sternum

Thyrohyoid muscle

Oblique line of thyroid cartilage

Omohyoid muscle (inferior belly)

Scapula

Infrahyoid and suprahyoid muscles and their action: schema

PLATE 24

HEAD AND NECK

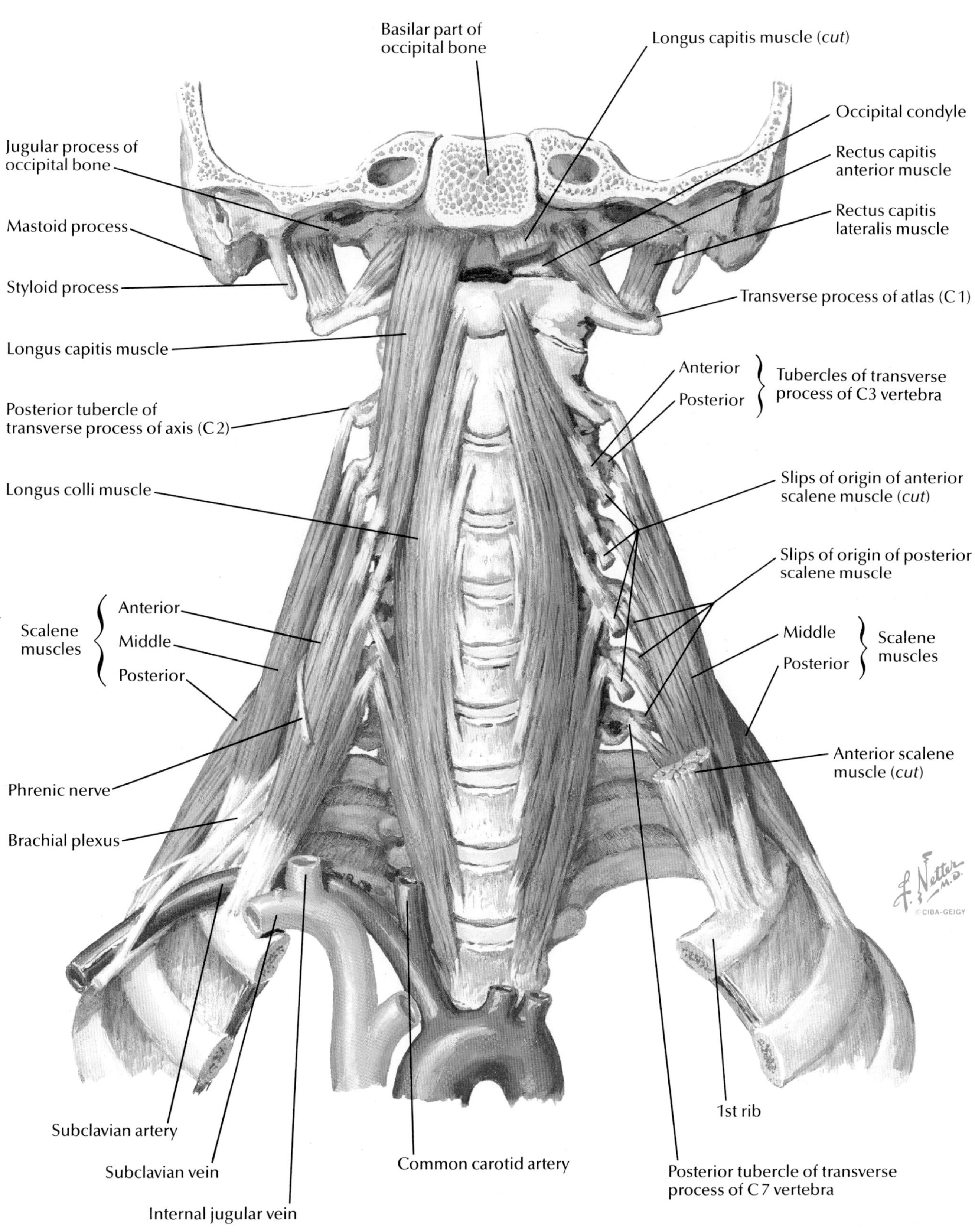

Basilar part of
occipital bone

Longus capitis muscle (*cut*)

Occipital condyle

Jugular process of
occipital bone

Rectus capitis
anterior muscle

Mastoid process

Rectus capitis
lateralis muscle

Styloid process

Transverse process of atlas (C 1)

Longus capitis muscle

Anterior
Posterior } Tubercles of transverse
process of C3 vertebra

Posterior tubercle of
transverse process of axis (C 2)

Slips of origin of anterior
scalene muscle (*cut*)

Longus colli muscle

Slips of origin of posterior
scalene muscle

Scalene
muscles { Anterior
Middle
Posterior

Middle
Posterior } Scalene
muscles

Phrenic nerve

Anterior scalene
muscle (*cut*)

Brachial plexus

Subclavian artery

1st rib

Subclavian vein

Posterior tubercle of transverse
process of C 7 vertebra

Common carotid artery

Internal jugular vein

Superficial Veins and Cutaneous Nerves of Neck

FOR DEEP VEINS OF NECK SEE PLATE 64

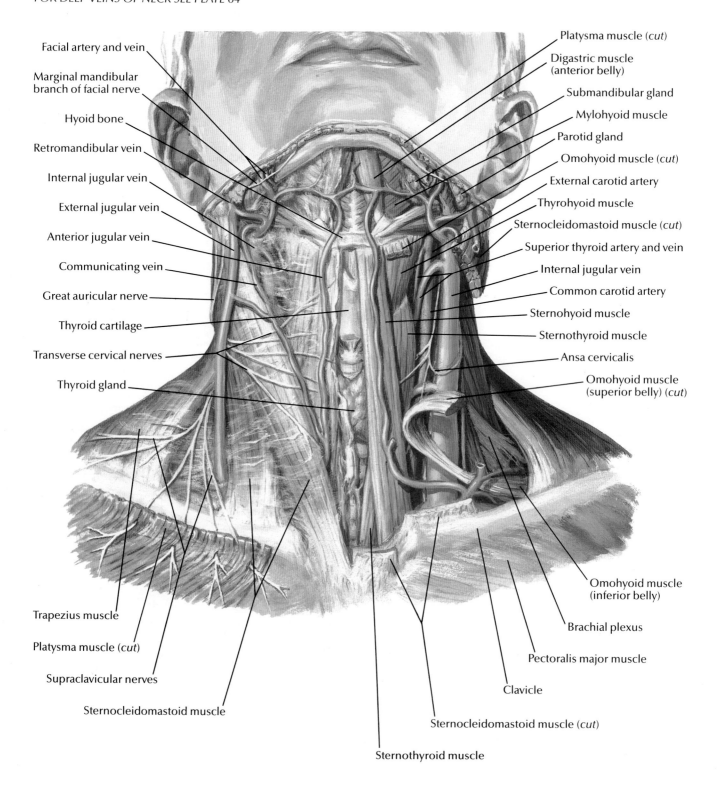

Facial artery and vein

Marginal mandibular branch of facial nerve

Hyoid bone

Retromandibular vein

Internal jugular vein

External jugular vein

Anterior jugular vein

Communicating vein

Great auricular nerve

Thyroid cartilage

Transverse cervical nerves

Thyroid gland

Trapezius muscle

Platysma muscle (*cut*)

Supraclavicular nerves

Sternocleidomastoid muscle

Sternothyroid muscle

Platysma muscle (*cut*)

Digastric muscle (anterior belly)

Submandibular gland

Mylohyoid muscle

Parotid gland

Omohyoid muscle (*cut*)

External carotid artery

Thyrohyoid muscle

Sternocleidomastoid muscle (*cut*)

Superior thyroid artery and vein

Internal jugular vein

Common carotid artery

Sternohyoid muscle

Sternothyroid muscle

Ansa cervicalis

Omohyoid muscle (superior belly) (*cut*)

Omohyoid muscle (inferior belly)

Brachial plexus

Pectoralis major muscle

Clavicle

Sternocleidomastoid muscle (*cut*)

PLATE 26

HEAD AND NECK

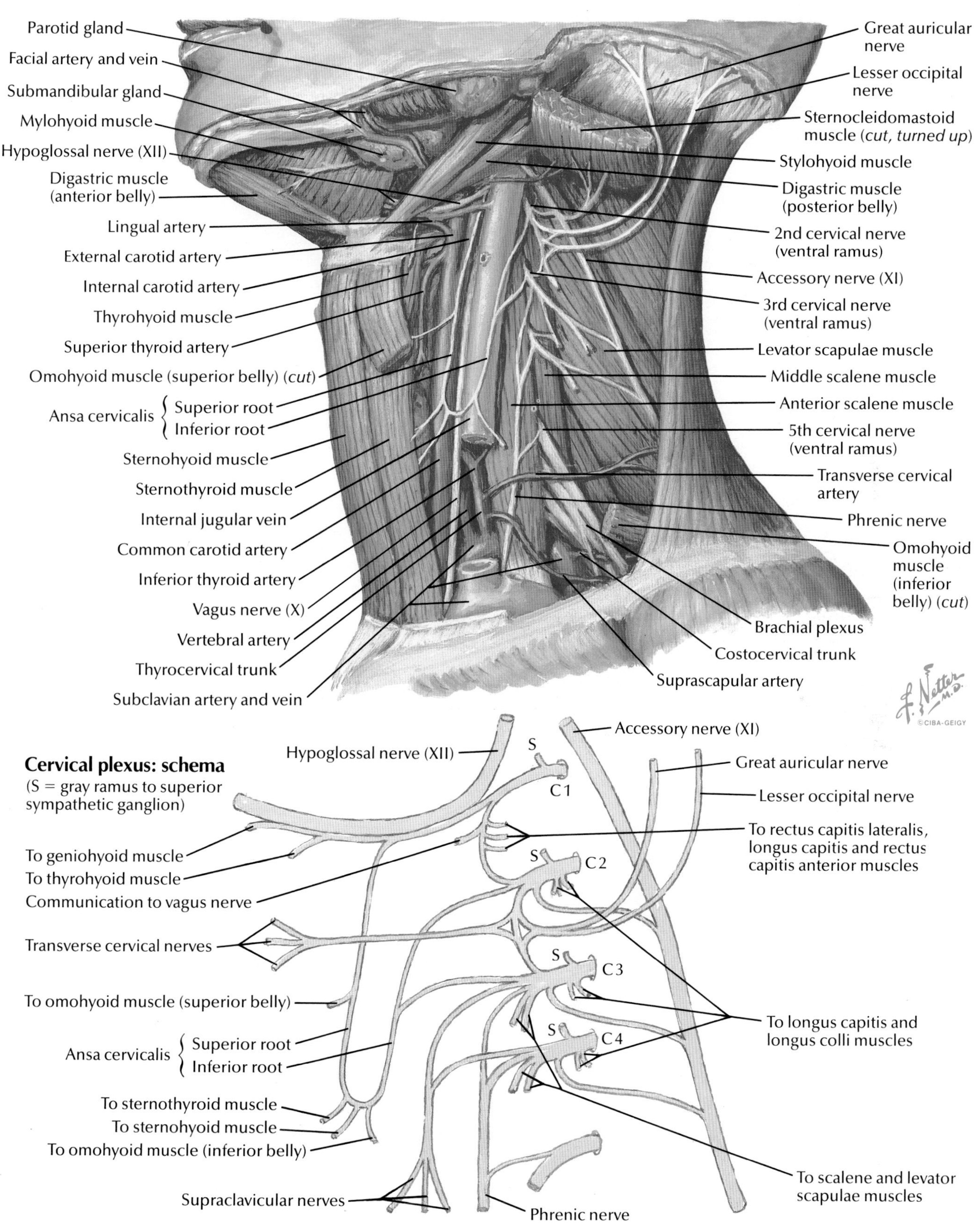

Parotid gland

Facial artery and vein

Submandibular gland

Mylohyoid muscle

Hypoglossal nerve (XII)

Digastric muscle (anterior belly)

Lingual artery

External carotid artery

Internal carotid artery

Thyrohyoid muscle

Superior thyroid artery

Omohyoid muscle (superior belly) (*cut*)

Ansa cervicalis { Superior root / Inferior root

Sternohyoid muscle

Sternothyroid muscle

Internal jugular vein

Common carotid artery

Inferior thyroid artery

Vagus nerve (X)

Vertebral artery

Thyrocervical trunk

Subclavian artery and vein

Great auricular nerve

Lesser occipital nerve

Sternocleidomastoid muscle (*cut, turned up*)

Stylohyoid muscle

Digastric muscle (posterior belly)

2nd cervical nerve (ventral ramus)

Accessory nerve (XI)

3rd cervical nerve (ventral ramus)

Levator scapulae muscle

Middle scalene muscle

Anterior scalene muscle

5th cervical nerve (ventral ramus)

Transverse cervical artery

Phrenic nerve

Omohyoid muscle (inferior belly) (*cut*)

Brachial plexus

Costocervical trunk

Suprascapular artery

Cervical plexus: schema
(S = gray ramus to superior sympathetic ganglion)

To geniohyoid muscle

To thyrohyoid muscle

Communication to vagus nerve

Transverse cervical nerves

To omohyoid muscle (superior belly)

Ansa cervicalis { Superior root / Inferior root

To sternothyroid muscle

To sternohyoid muscle

To omohyoid muscle (inferior belly)

Supraclavicular nerves

Hypoglossal nerve (XII)

Accessory nerve (XI)

Great auricular nerve

Lesser occipital nerve

To rectus capitis lateralis, longus capitis and rectus capitis anterior muscles

To longus capitis and longus colli muscles

To scalene and levator scapulae muscles

Phrenic nerve

S

C1

S

C2

S

C3

S

C4

Subclavian Artery

SEE ALSO PLATE 402

Right anterior dissection

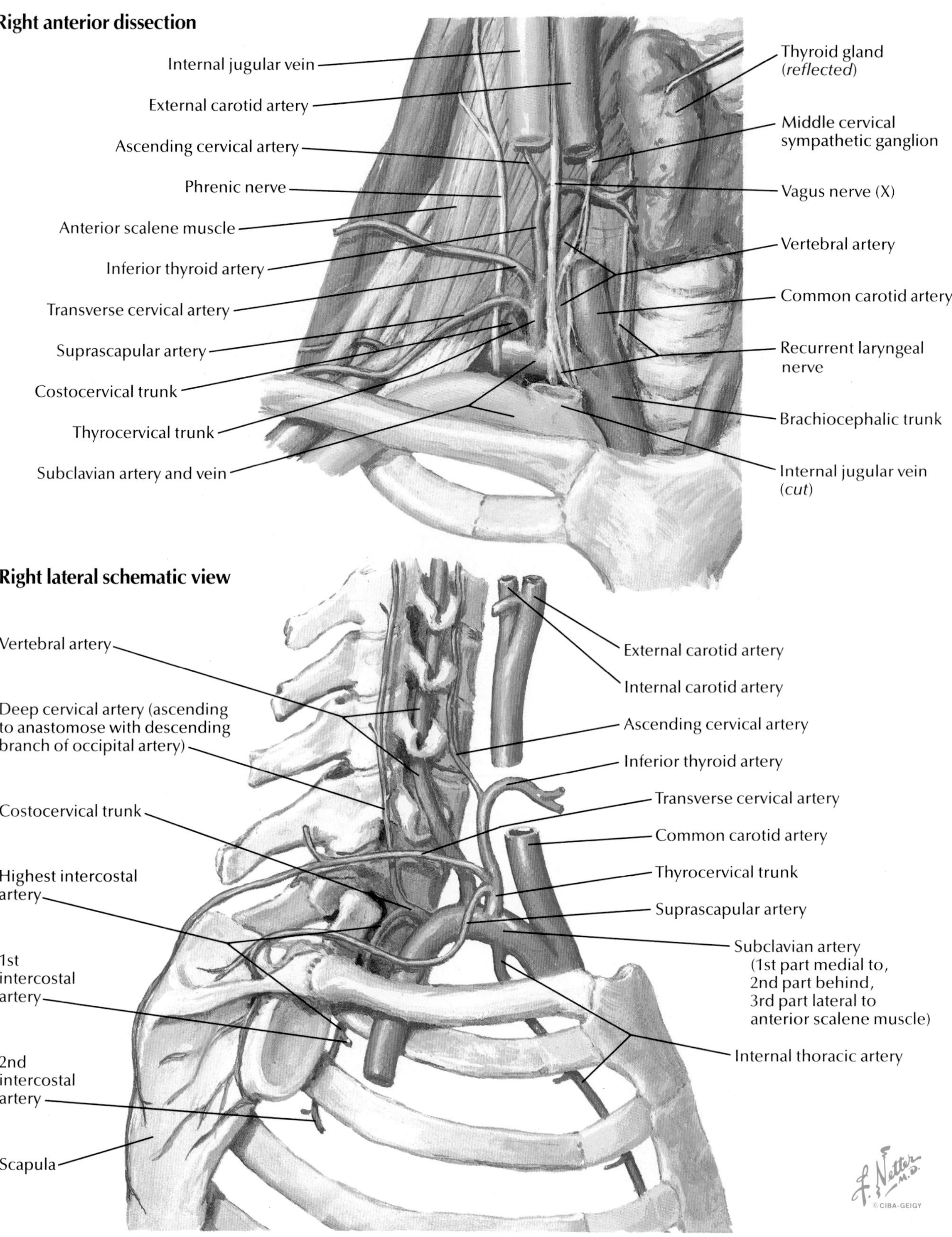

Internal jugular vein

External carotid artery

Ascending cervical artery

Phrenic nerve

Anterior scalene muscle

Inferior thyroid artery

Transverse cervical artery

Suprascapular artery

Costocervical trunk

Thyrocervical trunk

Subclavian artery and vein

Thyroid gland (*reflected*)

Middle cervical sympathetic ganglion

Vagus nerve (X)

Vertebral artery

Common carotid artery

Recurrent laryngeal nerve

Brachiocephalic trunk

Internal jugular vein (*cut*)

Right lateral schematic view

Vertebral artery

Deep cervical artery (ascending to anastomose with descending branch of occipital artery)

Costocervical trunk

Highest intercostal artery

1st intercostal artery

2nd intercostal artery

Scapula

External carotid artery

Internal carotid artery

Ascending cervical artery

Inferior thyroid artery

Transverse cervical artery

Common carotid artery

Thyrocervical trunk

Suprascapular artery

Subclavian artery (1st part medial to, 2nd part behind, 3rd part lateral to anterior scalene muscle)

Internal thoracic artery

PLATE 28

HEAD AND NECK

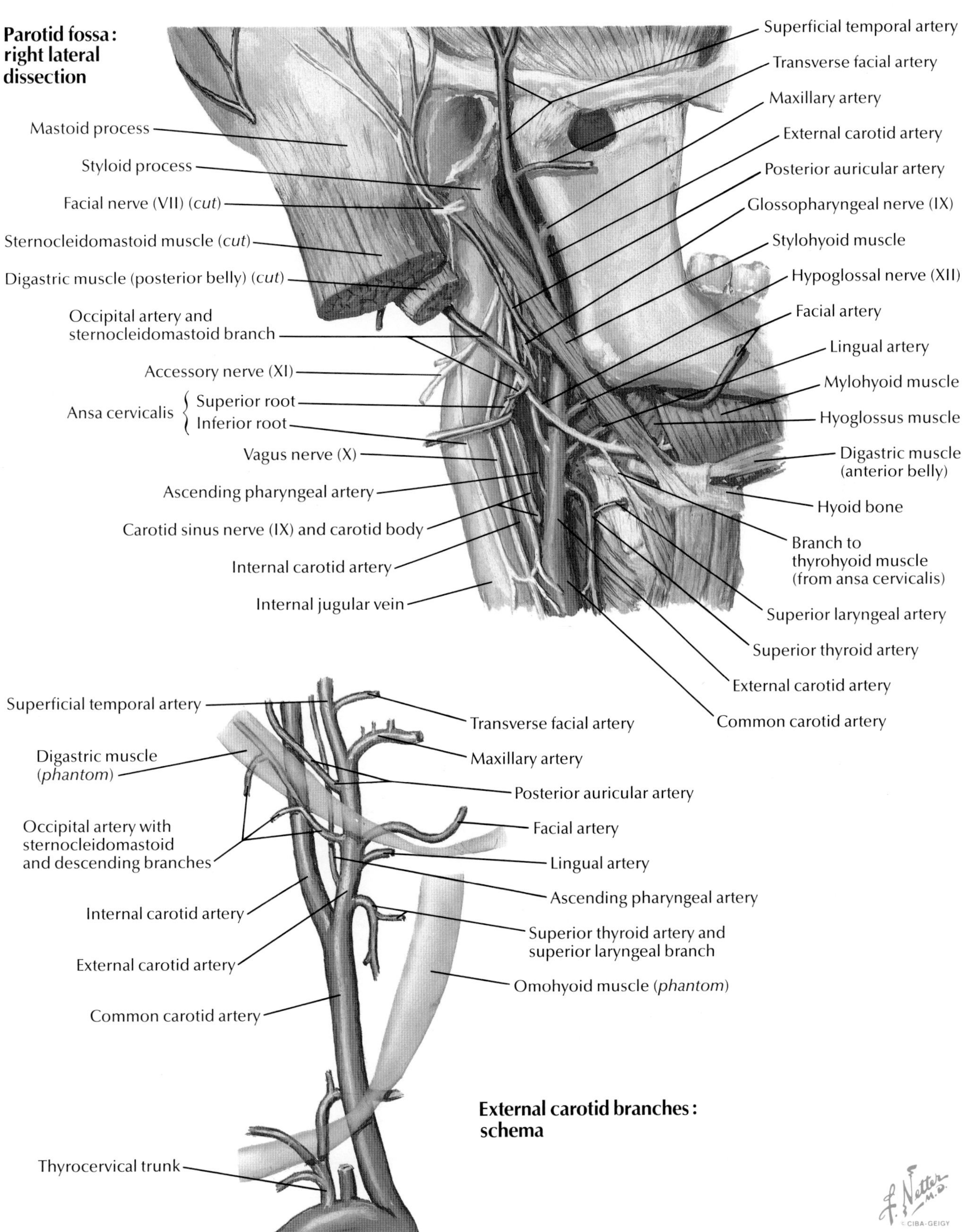

**Parotid fossa:
right lateral
dissection**

Mastoid process

Styloid process

Facial nerve (VII) (*cut*)

Sternocleidomastoid muscle (*cut*)

Digastric muscle (posterior belly) (*cut*)

Occipital artery and
sternocleidomastoid branch

Accessory nerve (XI)

Ansa cervicalis { Superior root
Inferior root

Vagus nerve (X)

Ascending pharyngeal artery

Carotid sinus nerve (IX) and carotid body

Internal carotid artery

Internal jugular vein

Superficial temporal artery

Transverse facial artery

Maxillary artery

External carotid artery

Posterior auricular artery

Glossopharyngeal nerve (IX)

Stylohyoid muscle

Hypoglossal nerve (XII)

Facial artery

Lingual artery

Mylohyoid muscle

Hyoglossus muscle

Digastric muscle
(anterior belly)

Hyoid bone

Branch to
thyrohyoid muscle
(from ansa cervicalis)

Superior laryngeal artery

Superior thyroid artery

External carotid artery

Common carotid artery

Superficial temporal artery

Digastric muscle
(*phantom*)

Occipital artery with
sternocleidomastoid
and descending branches

Internal carotid artery

External carotid artery

Common carotid artery

Thyrocervical trunk

Transverse facial artery

Maxillary artery

Posterior auricular artery

Facial artery

Lingual artery

Ascending pharyngeal artery

Superior thyroid artery and
superior laryngeal branch

Omohyoid muscle (*phantom*)

**External carotid branches:
schema**

Fascial Layers of Neck

FOR CONTENTS OF CAROTID SHEATH SEE PLATES 63, 64, 65

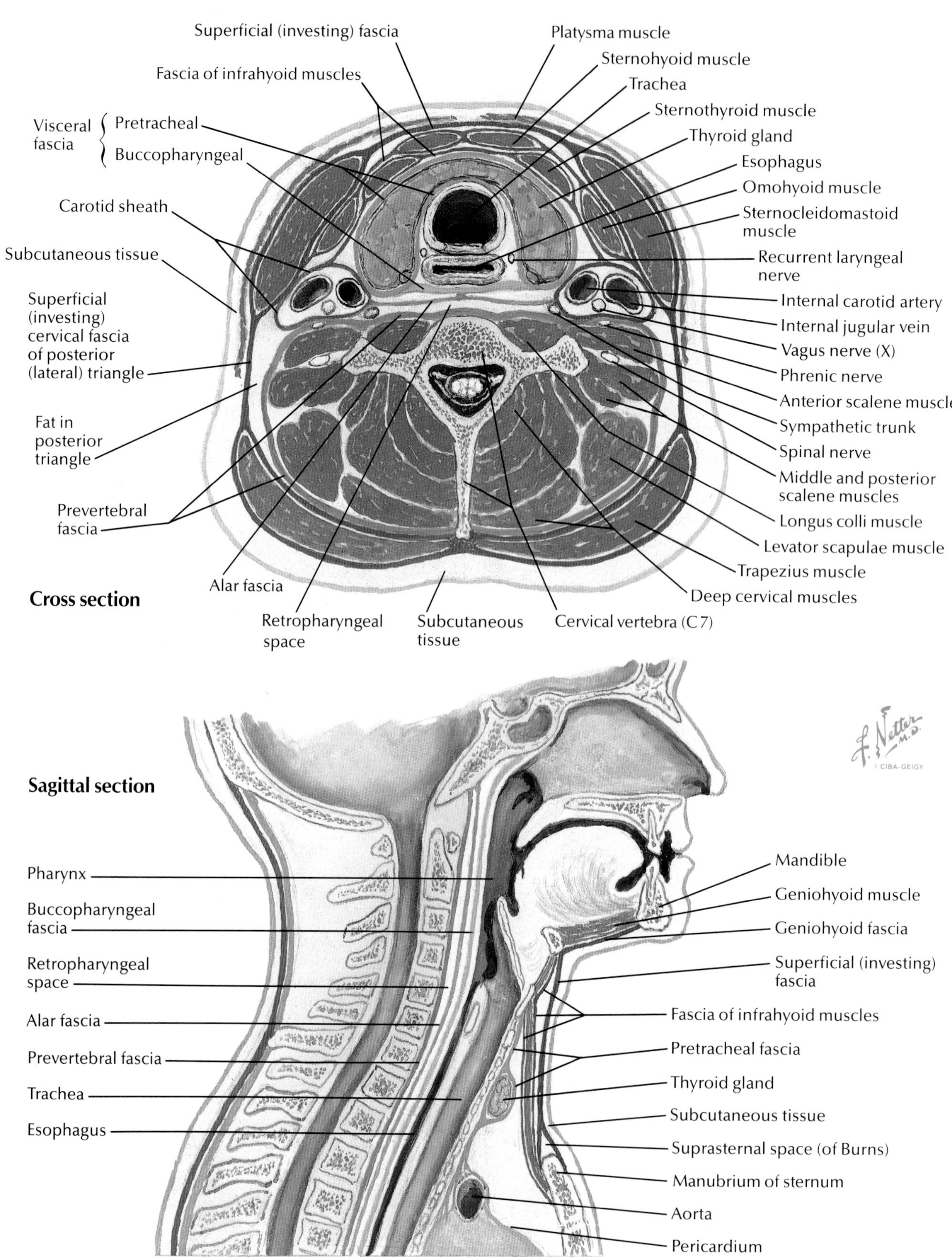

Cross section

Superficial (investing) fascia

Fascia of infrahyoid muscles

Visceral fascia
— Pretracheal
— Buccopharyngeal

Carotid sheath

Subcutaneous tissue

Superficial (investing) cervical fascia of posterior (lateral) triangle

Fat in posterior triangle

Prevertebral fascia

Alar fascia

Retropharyngeal space

Subcutaneous tissue

Cervical vertebra (C 7)

Platysma muscle

Sternohyoid muscle

Trachea

Sternothyroid muscle

Thyroid gland

Esophagus

Omohyoid muscle

Sternocleidomastoid muscle

Recurrent laryngeal nerve

Internal carotid artery

Internal jugular vein

Vagus nerve (X)

Phrenic nerve

Anterior scalene muscle

Sympathetic trunk

Spinal nerve

Middle and posterior scalene muscles

Longus colli muscle

Levator scapulae muscle

Trapezius muscle

Deep cervical muscles

Sagittal section

Pharynx

Buccopharyngeal fascia

Retropharyngeal space

Alar fascia

Prevertebral fascia

Trachea

Esophagus

Mandible

Geniohyoid muscle

Geniohyoid fascia

Superficial (investing) fascia

Fascia of infrahyoid muscles

Pretracheal fascia

Thyroid gland

Subcutaneous tissue

Suprasternal space (of Burns)

Manubrium of sternum

Aorta

Pericardium

PLATE 30

HEAD AND NECK

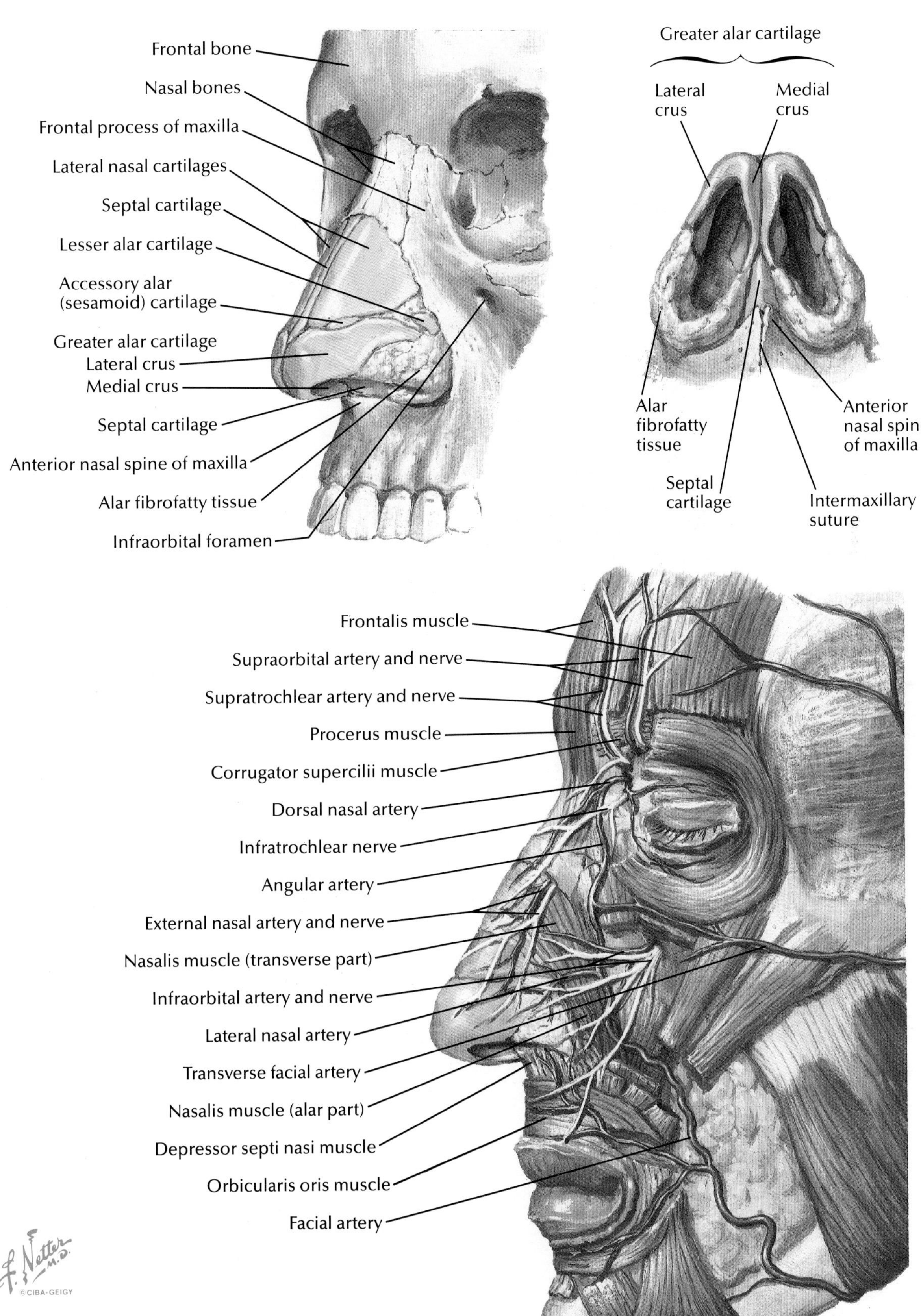

Frontal bone

Nasal bones

Frontal process of maxilla

Lateral nasal cartilages

Septal cartilage

Lesser alar cartilage

Accessory alar (sesamoid) cartilage

Greater alar cartilage

Lateral crus

Medial crus

Septal cartilage

Anterior nasal spine of maxilla

Alar fibrofatty tissue

Infraorbital foramen

Greater alar cartilage

Lateral crus

Medial crus

Alar fibrofatty tissue

Septal cartilage

Anterior nasal spine of maxilla

Intermaxillary suture

Frontalis muscle

Supraorbital artery and nerve

Supratrochlear artery and nerve

Procerus muscle

Corrugator supercilii muscle

Dorsal nasal artery

Infratrochlear nerve

Angular artery

External nasal artery and nerve

Nasalis muscle (transverse part)

Infraorbital artery and nerve

Lateral nasal artery

Transverse facial artery

Nasalis muscle (alar part)

Depressor septi nasi muscle

Orbicularis oris muscle

Facial artery

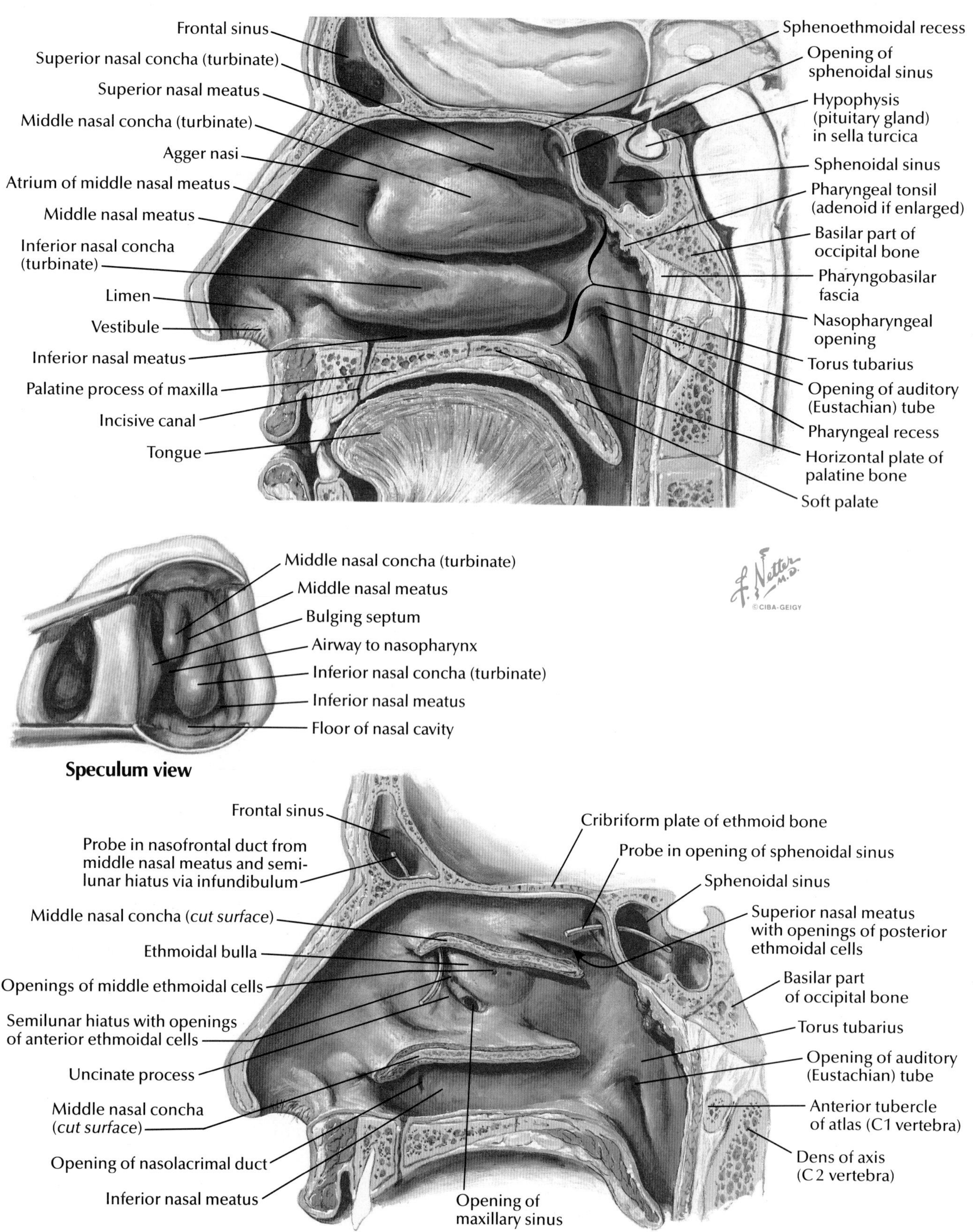

Frontal sinus

Superior nasal concha (turbinate)

Superior nasal meatus

Middle nasal concha (turbinate)

Agger nasi

Atrium of middle nasal meatus

Middle nasal meatus

Inferior nasal concha (turbinate)

Limen

Vestibule

Inferior nasal meatus

Palatine process of maxilla

Incisive canal

Tongue

Sphenoethmoidal recess

Opening of sphenoidal sinus

Hypophysis (pituitary gland) in sella turcica

Sphenoidal sinus

Pharyngeal tonsil (adenoid if enlarged)

Basilar part of occipital bone

Pharyngobasilar fascia

Nasopharyngeal opening

Torus tubarius

Opening of auditory (Eustachian) tube

Pharyngeal recess

Horizontal plate of palatine bone

Soft palate

Middle nasal concha (turbinate)

Middle nasal meatus

Bulging septum

Airway to nasopharynx

Inferior nasal concha (turbinate)

Inferior nasal meatus

Floor of nasal cavity

Speculum view

Frontal sinus

Probe in nasofrontal duct from middle nasal meatus and semilunar hiatus via infundibulum

Middle nasal concha (*cut surface*)

Ethmoidal bulla

Openings of middle ethmoidal cells

Semilunar hiatus with openings of anterior ethmoidal cells

Uncinate process

Middle nasal concha (*cut surface*)

Opening of nasolacrimal duct

Inferior nasal meatus

Cribriform plate of ethmoid bone

Probe in opening of sphenoidal sinus

Sphenoidal sinus

Superior nasal meatus with openings of posterior ethmoidal cells

Basilar part of occipital bone

Torus tubarius

Opening of auditory (Eustachian) tube

Anterior tubercle of atlas (C 1 vertebra)

Dens of axis (C 2 vertebra)

Opening of maxillary sinus

PLATE 32

HEAD AND NECK

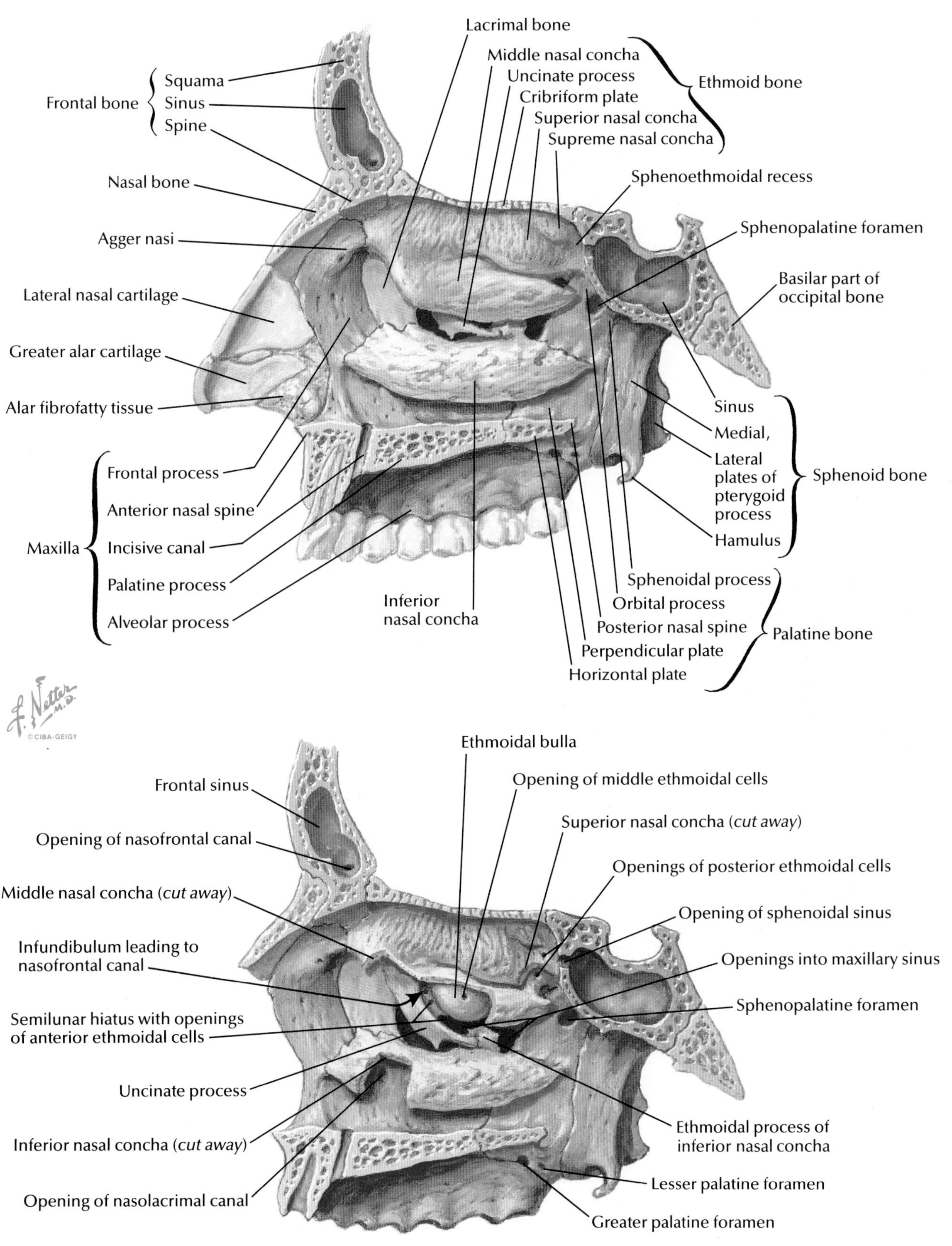

Lacrimal bone

Frontal bone { Squama / Sinus / Spine

Middle nasal concha

Uncinate process

Cribriform plate

Superior nasal concha

Supreme nasal concha

Ethmoid bone

Nasal bone

Agger nasi

Lateral nasal cartilage

Greater alar cartilage

Alar fibrofatty tissue

Sphenoethmoidal recess

Sphenopalatine foramen

Basilar part of occipital bone

Sinus

Medial,

Lateral plates of pterygoid process

Sphenoid bone

Hamulus

Maxilla { Frontal process / Anterior nasal spine / Incisive canal / Palatine process / Alveolar process

Inferior nasal concha

Sphenoidal process

Orbital process

Posterior nasal spine

Perpendicular plate

Horizontal plate

Palatine bone

Ethmoidal bulla

Opening of middle ethmoidal cells

Frontal sinus

Opening of nasofrontal canal

Middle nasal concha (*cut away*)

Infundibulum leading to nasofrontal canal

Semilunar hiatus with openings of anterior ethmoidal cells

Uncinate process

Inferior nasal concha (*cut away*)

Opening of nasolacrimal canal

Superior nasal concha (*cut away*)

Openings of posterior ethmoidal cells

Opening of sphenoidal sinus

Openings into maxillary sinus

Sphenopalatine foramen

Ethmoidal process of inferior nasal concha

Lesser palatine foramen

Greater palatine foramen

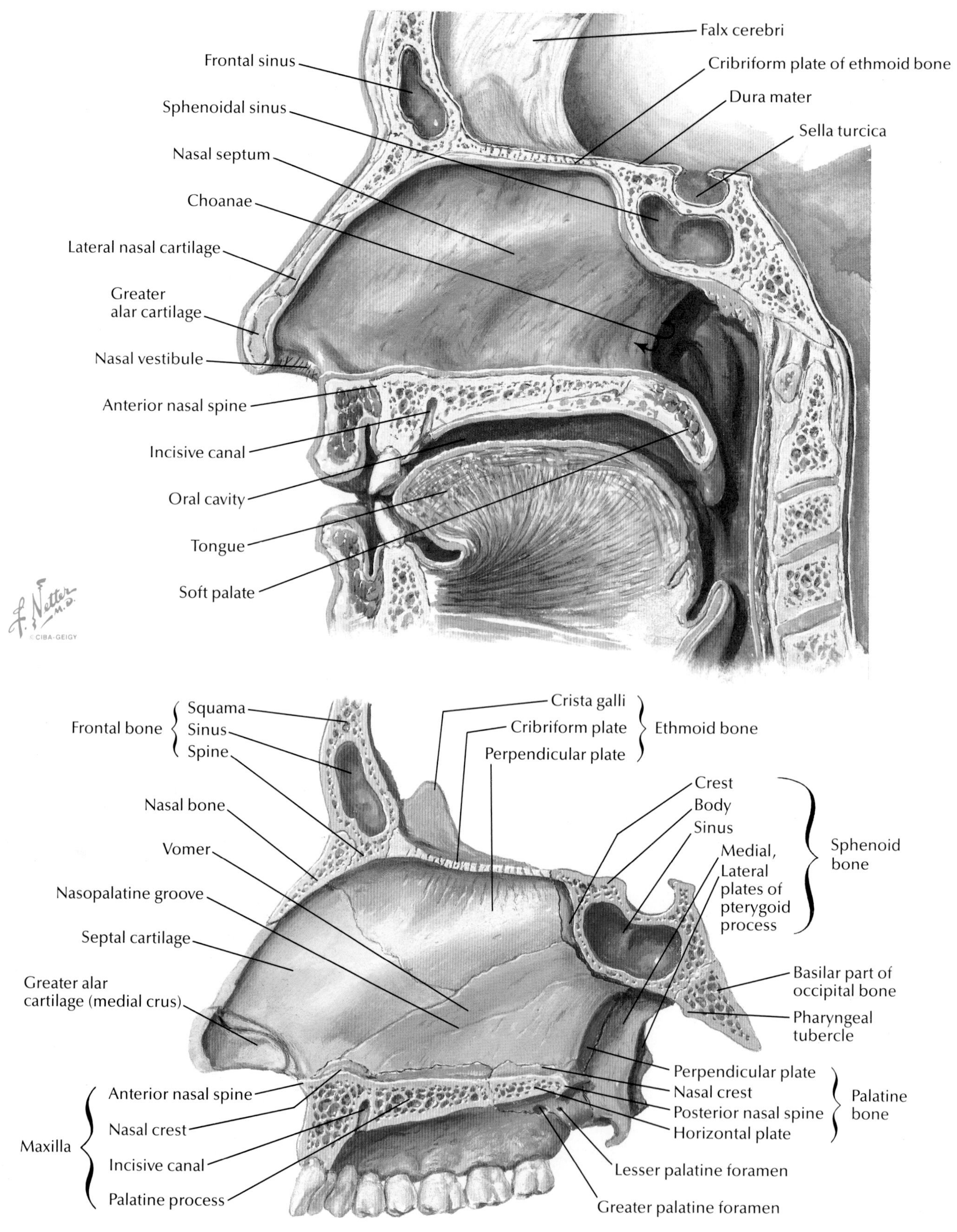

Falx cerebri

Frontal sinus

Cribriform plate of ethmoid bone

Sphenoidal sinus

Dura mater

Nasal septum

Sella turcica

Choanae

Lateral nasal cartilage

Greater alar cartilage

Nasal vestibule

Anterior nasal spine

Incisive canal

Oral cavity

Tongue

Soft palate

Crista galli

Squama

Frontal bone { Sinus

Cribriform plate } Ethmoid bone

Spine

Perpendicular plate

Nasal bone

Crest

Body

Vomer

Sinus

Nasopalatine groove

Medial, Lateral plates of pterygoid process } Sphenoid bone

Septal cartilage

Greater alar cartilage (medial crus)

Basilar part of occipital bone

Pharyngeal tubercle

Perpendicular plate

Anterior nasal spine

Nasal crest } Palatine bone

Nasal crest

Posterior nasal spine

Maxilla {

Incisive canal

Horizontal plate

Palatine process

Lesser palatine foramen

Greater palatine foramen

PLATE 34

HEAD AND NECK

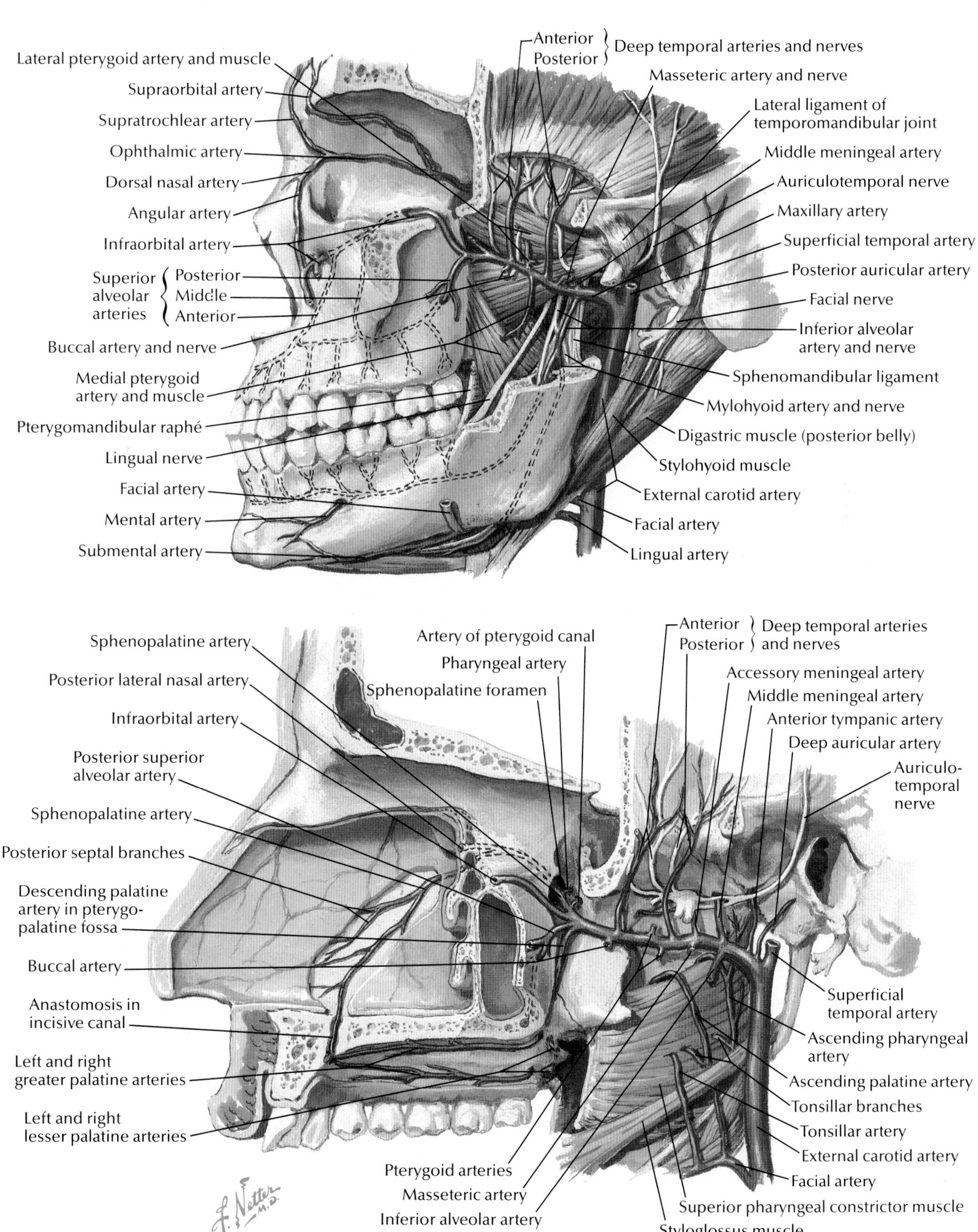

Lateral pterygoid artery and muscle
Supraorbital artery
Supratrochlear artery
Ophthalmic artery
Dorsal nasal artery
Angular artery
Infraorbital artery
Superior { Posterior
alveolar { Middle
arteries { Anterior
Buccal artery and nerve
Medial pterygoid artery and muscle
Pterygomandibular raphé
Lingual nerve
Facial artery
Mental artery
Submental artery

Anterior } Deep temporal arteries and nerves
Posterior }
Masseteric artery and nerve
Lateral ligament of temporomandibular joint
Middle meningeal artery
Auriculotemporal nerve
Maxillary artery
Superficial temporal artery
Posterior auricular artery
Facial nerve
Inferior alveolar artery and nerve
Sphenomandibular ligament
Mylohyoid artery and nerve
Digastric muscle (posterior belly)
Stylohyoid muscle
External carotid artery
Facial artery
Lingual artery

Sphenopalatine artery
Posterior lateral nasal artery
Infraorbital artery
Posterior superior alveolar artery
Sphenopalatine artery
Posterior septal branches
Descending palatine artery in pterygo-palatine fossa
Buccal artery
Anastomosis in incisive canal
Left and right greater palatine arteries
Left and right lesser palatine arteries

Artery of pterygoid canal
Pharyngeal artery
Sphenopalatine foramen

Anterior } Deep temporal arteries
Posterior } and nerves
Accessory meningeal artery
Middle meningeal artery
Anterior tympanic artery
Deep auricular artery
Auriculo-temporal nerve
Superficial temporal artery
Ascending pharyngeal artery
Ascending palatine artery
Tonsillar branches
Tonsillar artery
External carotid artery
Facial artery

Pterygoid arteries
Masseteric artery
Inferior alveolar artery
Superior pharyngeal constrictor muscle
Styloglossus muscle

Arteries of Nasal Cavity

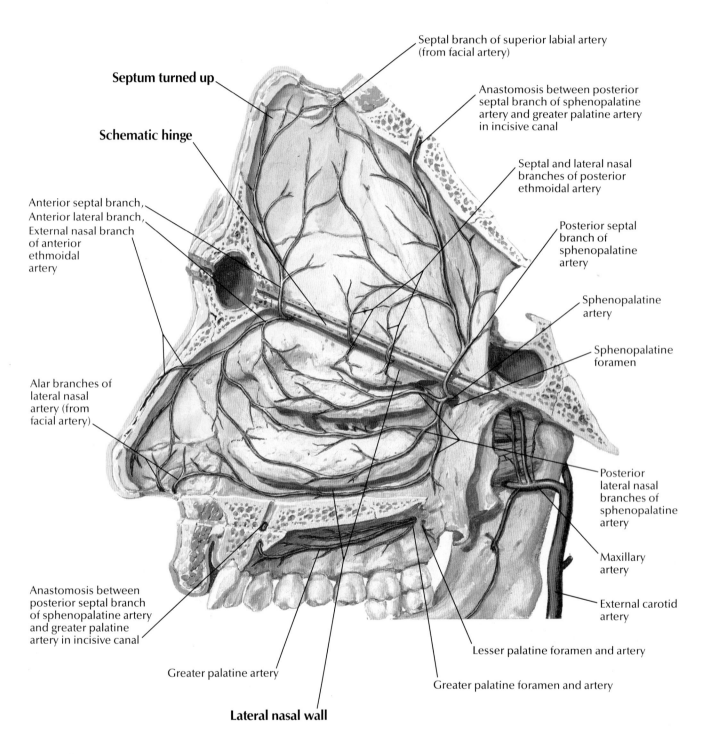

Septal branch of superior labial artery (from facial artery)

Septum turned up

Anastomosis between posterior septal branch of sphenopalatine artery and greater palatine artery in incisive canal

Schematic hinge

Septal and lateral nasal branches of posterior ethmoidal artery

Anterior septal branch, Anterior lateral branch, External nasal branch of anterior ethmoidal artery

Posterior septal branch of sphenopalatine artery

Sphenopalatine artery

Sphenopalatine foramen

Alar branches of lateral nasal artery (from facial artery)

Posterior lateral nasal branches of sphenopalatine artery

Maxillary artery

Anastomosis between posterior septal branch of sphenopalatine artery and greater palatine artery in incisive canal

External carotid artery

Greater palatine artery

Lesser palatine foramen and artery

Greater palatine foramen and artery

Lateral nasal wall

PLATE 36

HEAD AND NECK

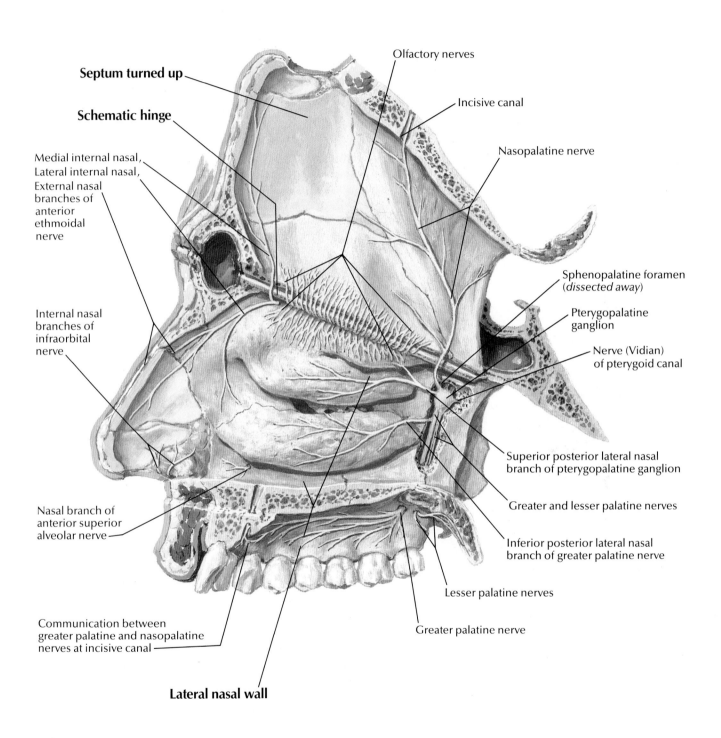

Olfactory nerves

Incisive canal

Nasopalatine nerve

Septum turned up

Schematic hinge

Medial internal nasal,
Lateral internal nasal,
External nasal
branches of
anterior
ethmoidal
nerve

Internal nasal
branches of
infraorbital
nerve

Sphenopalatine foramen
(*dissected away*)

Pterygopalatine
ganglion

Nerve (Vidian)
of pterygoid canal

Superior posterior lateral nasal
branch of pterygopalatine ganglion

Greater and lesser palatine nerves

Inferior posterior lateral nasal
branch of greater palatine nerve

Nasal branch of
anterior superior
alveolar nerve

Lesser palatine nerves

Greater palatine nerve

Communication between
greater palatine and nasopalatine
nerves at incisive canal

Lateral nasal wall

Nerves of Nasal Cavity (continued)

SEE ALSO PLATE 113

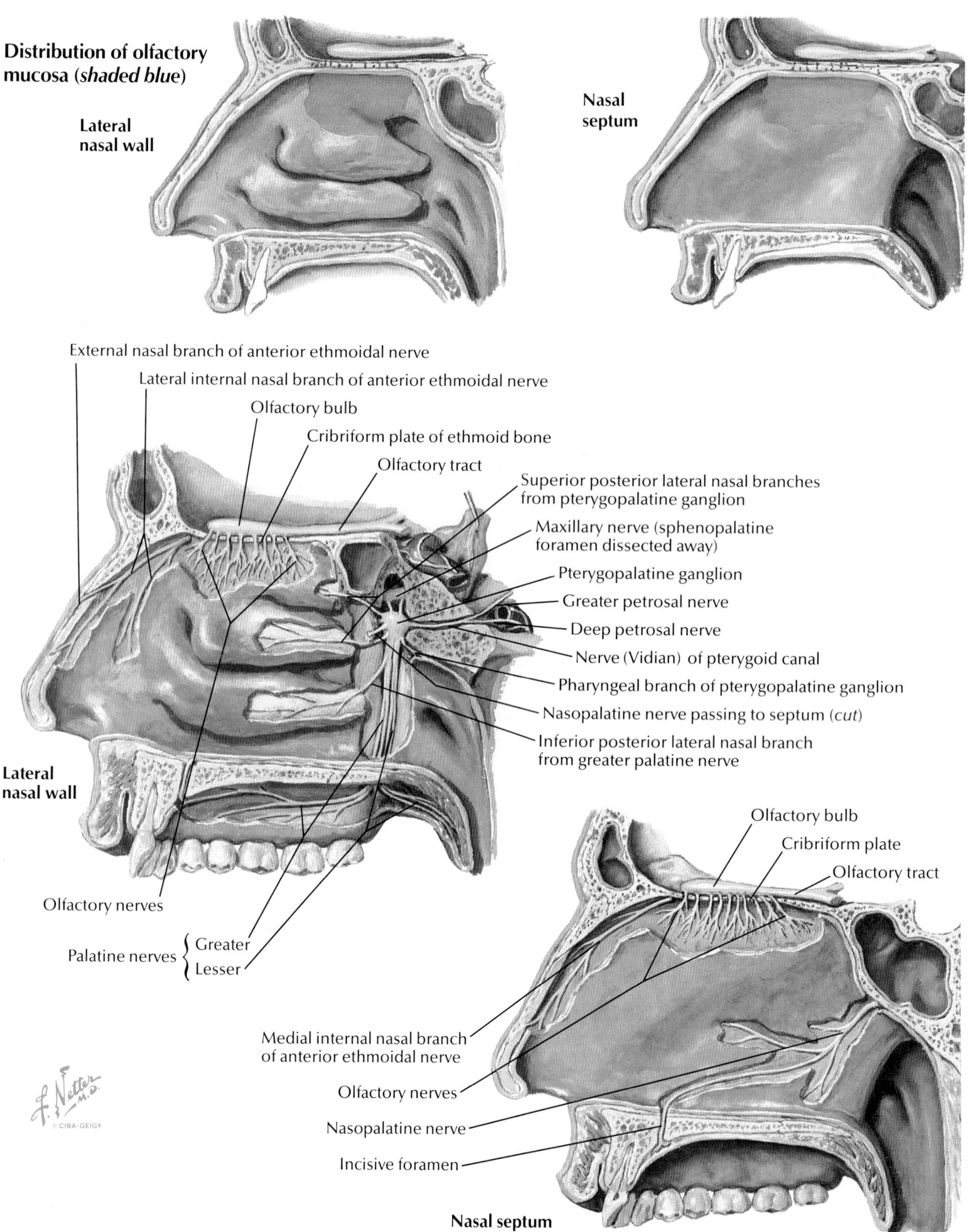

Distribution of olfactory mucosa (*shaded blue*)

Lateral nasal wall

Nasal septum

External nasal branch of anterior ethmoidal nerve

Lateral internal nasal branch of anterior ethmoidal nerve

Olfactory bulb

Cribriform plate of ethmoid bone

Olfactory tract

Superior posterior lateral nasal branches from pterygopalatine ganglion

Maxillary nerve (sphenopalatine foramen dissected away)

Pterygopalatine ganglion

Greater petrosal nerve

Deep petrosal nerve

Nerve (Vidian) of pterygoid canal

Pharyngeal branch of pterygopalatine ganglion

Nasopalatine nerve passing to septum (*cut*)

Inferior posterior lateral nasal branch from greater palatine nerve

Lateral nasal wall

Olfactory nerves

Palatine nerves { Greater / Lesser

Olfactory bulb

Cribriform plate

Olfactory tract

Medial internal nasal branch of anterior ethmoidal nerve

Olfactory nerves

Nasopalatine nerve

Incisive foramen

Nasal septum

PLATE 38

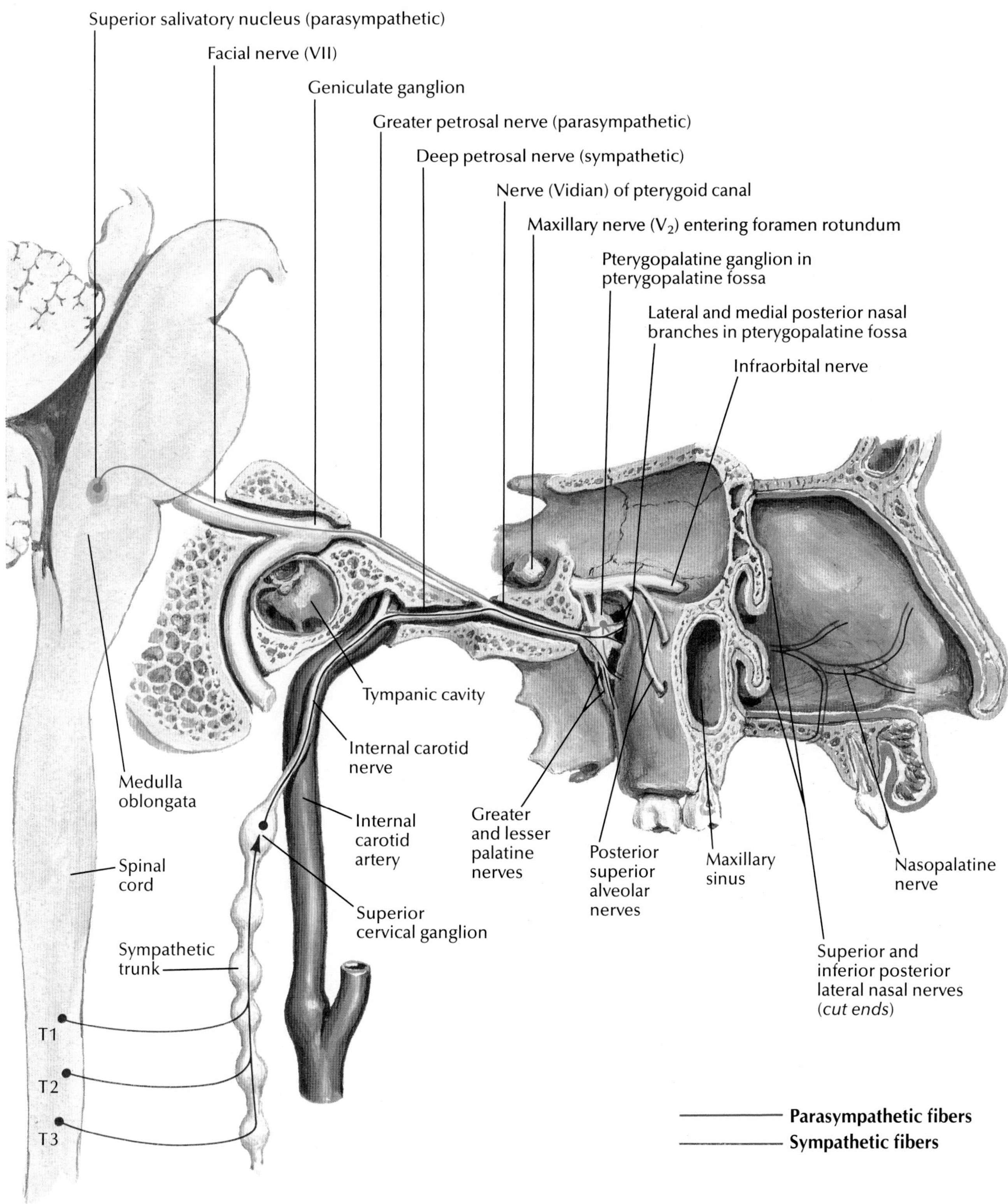

Superior salivatory nucleus (parasympathetic)

Facial nerve (VII)

Geniculate ganglion

Greater petrosal nerve (parasympathetic)

Deep petrosal nerve (sympathetic)

Nerve (Vidian) of pterygoid canal

Maxillary nerve (V_2) entering foramen rotundum

Pterygopalatine ganglion in pterygopalatine fossa

Lateral and medial posterior nasal branches in pterygopalatine fossa

Infraorbital nerve

Tympanic cavity

Internal carotid nerve

Medulla oblongata

Internal carotid artery

Spinal cord

Greater and lesser palatine nerves

Posterior superior alveolar nerves

Maxillary sinus

Nasopalatine nerve

Superior cervical ganglion

Sympathetic trunk

T1

T2

T3

Superior and inferior posterior lateral nasal nerves (*cut ends*)

—————— **Parasympathetic fibers**

—————— **Sympathetic fibers**

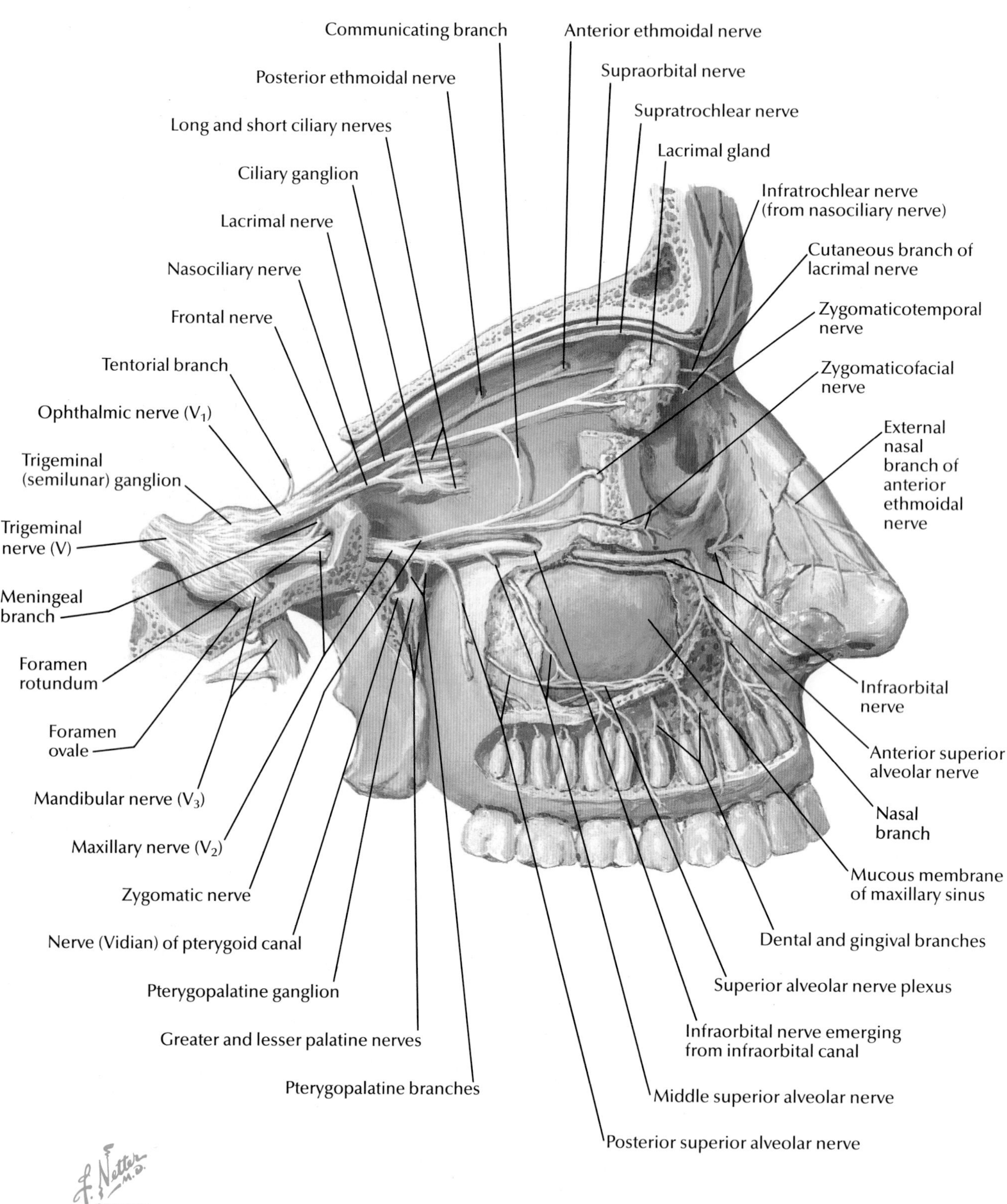

Communicating branch

Posterior ethmoidal nerve

Long and short ciliary nerves

Ciliary ganglion

Lacrimal nerve

Nasociliary nerve

Frontal nerve

Tentorial branch

Ophthalmic nerve (V₁)

Trigeminal (semilunar) ganglion

Trigeminal nerve (V)

Meningeal branch

Foramen rotundum

Foramen ovale

Mandibular nerve (V₃)

Maxillary nerve (V₂)

Zygomatic nerve

Nerve (Vidian) of pterygoid canal

Pterygopalatine ganglion

Greater and lesser palatine nerves

Pterygopalatine branches

Anterior ethmoidal nerve

Supraorbital nerve

Supratrochlear nerve

Lacrimal gland

Infratrochlear nerve (from nasociliary nerve)

Cutaneous branch of lacrimal nerve

Zygomaticotemporal nerve

Zygomaticofacial nerve

External nasal branch of anterior ethmoidal nerve

Infraorbital nerve

Anterior superior alveolar nerve

Nasal branch

Mucous membrane of maxillary sinus

Dental and gingival branches

Superior alveolar nerve plexus

Infraorbital nerve emerging from infraorbital canal

Middle superior alveolar nerve

Posterior superior alveolar nerve

PLATE 40

HEAD AND NECK

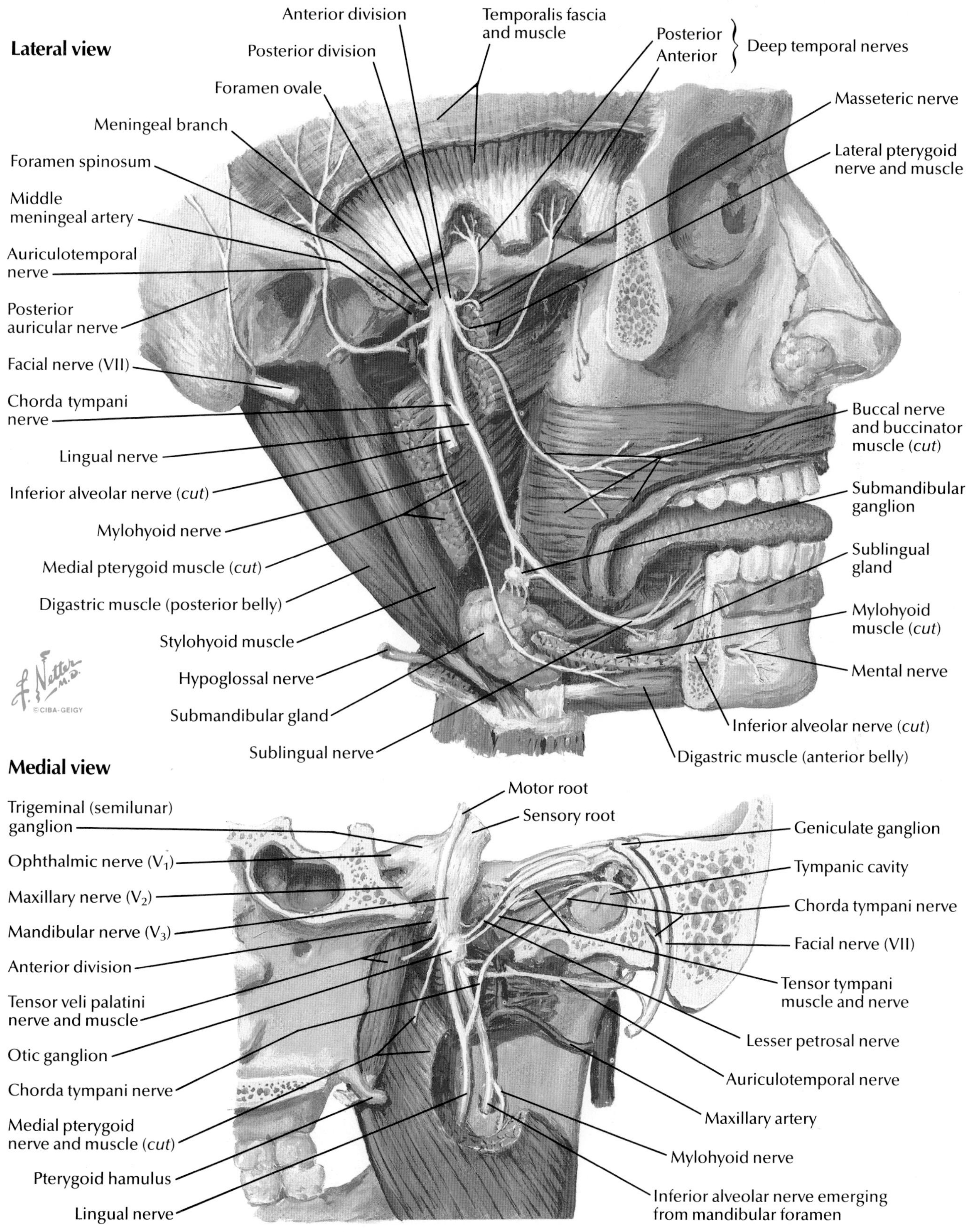

Lateral view

Anterior division
Posterior division
Foramen ovale
Meningeal branch
Foramen spinosum
Middle meningeal artery
Auriculotemporal nerve
Posterior auricular nerve
Facial nerve (VII)
Chorda tympani nerve
Lingual nerve
Inferior alveolar nerve (cut)
Mylohyoid nerve
Medial pterygoid muscle (cut)
Digastric muscle (posterior belly)
Stylohyoid muscle
Hypoglossal nerve
Submandibular gland
Sublingual nerve

Temporalis fascia and muscle
Posterior
Anterior } Deep temporal nerves
Masseteric nerve
Lateral pterygoid nerve and muscle
Buccal nerve and buccinator muscle (cut)
Submandibular ganglion
Sublingual gland
Mylohyoid muscle (cut)
Mental nerve
Inferior alveolar nerve (cut)
Digastric muscle (anterior belly)

Medial view

Trigeminal (semilunar) ganglion
Ophthalmic nerve (V₁)
Maxillary nerve (V₂)
Mandibular nerve (V₃)
Anterior division
Tensor veli palatini nerve and muscle
Otic ganglion
Chorda tympani nerve
Medial pterygoid nerve and muscle (cut)
Pterygoid hamulus
Lingual nerve

Motor root
Sensory root
Geniculate ganglion
Tympanic cavity
Chorda tympani nerve
Facial nerve (VII)
Tensor tympani muscle and nerve
Lesser petrosal nerve
Auriculotemporal nerve
Maxillary artery
Mylohyoid nerve
Inferior alveolar nerve emerging from mandibular foramen

Paranasal Sinuses

Coronal section

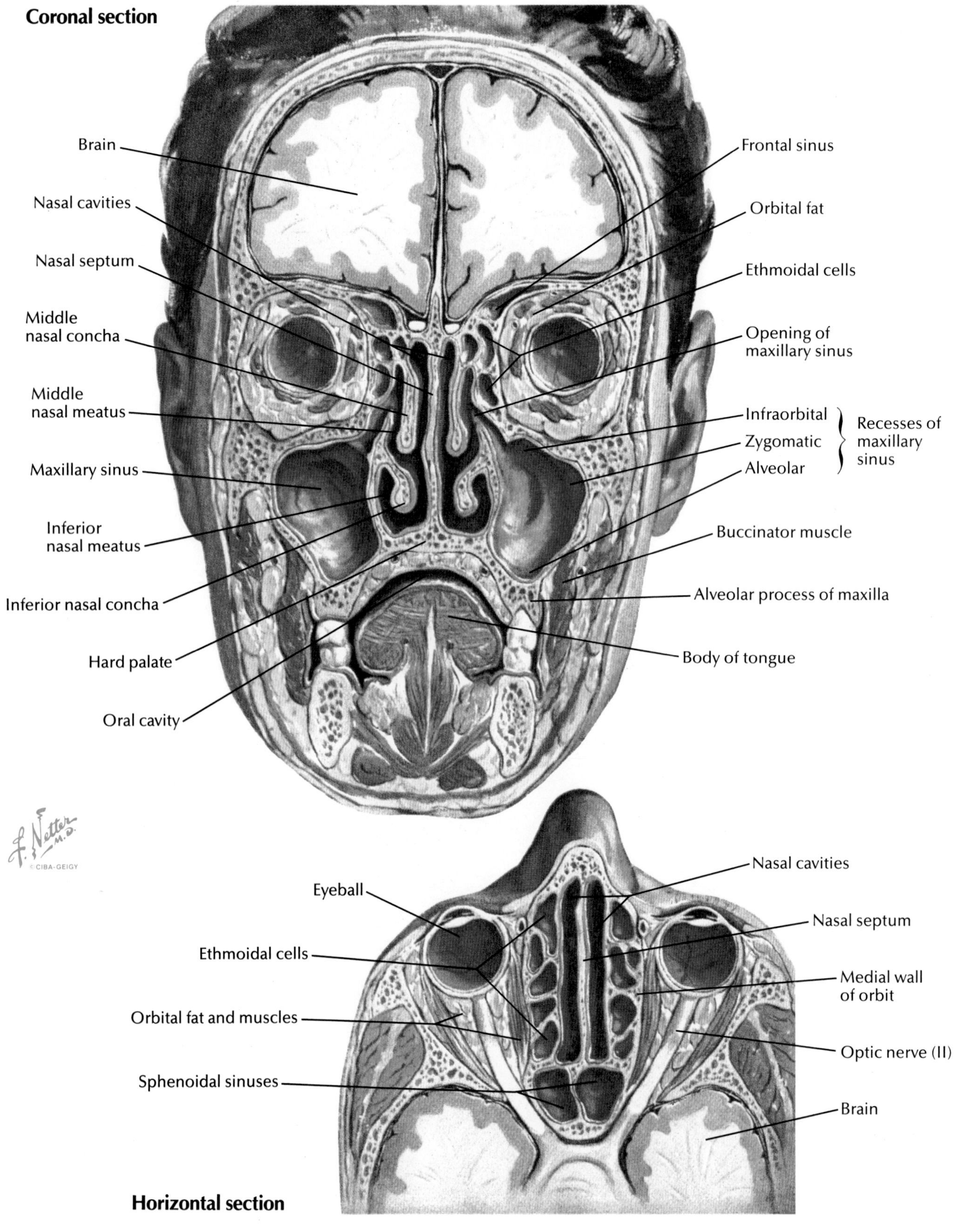

Brain

Nasal cavities

Nasal septum

Middle nasal concha

Middle nasal meatus

Maxillary sinus

Inferior nasal meatus

Inferior nasal concha

Hard palate

Oral cavity

Frontal sinus

Orbital fat

Ethmoidal cells

Opening of maxillary sinus

Infraorbital ⎫
Zygomatic ⎬ Recesses of maxillary sinus
Alveolar   ⎭

Buccinator muscle

Alveolar process of maxilla

Body of tongue

Eyeball

Ethmoidal cells

Orbital fat and muscles

Sphenoidal sinuses

Nasal cavities

Nasal septum

Medial wall of orbit

Optic nerve (II)

Brain

Horizontal section

PLATE 42

HEAD AND NECK

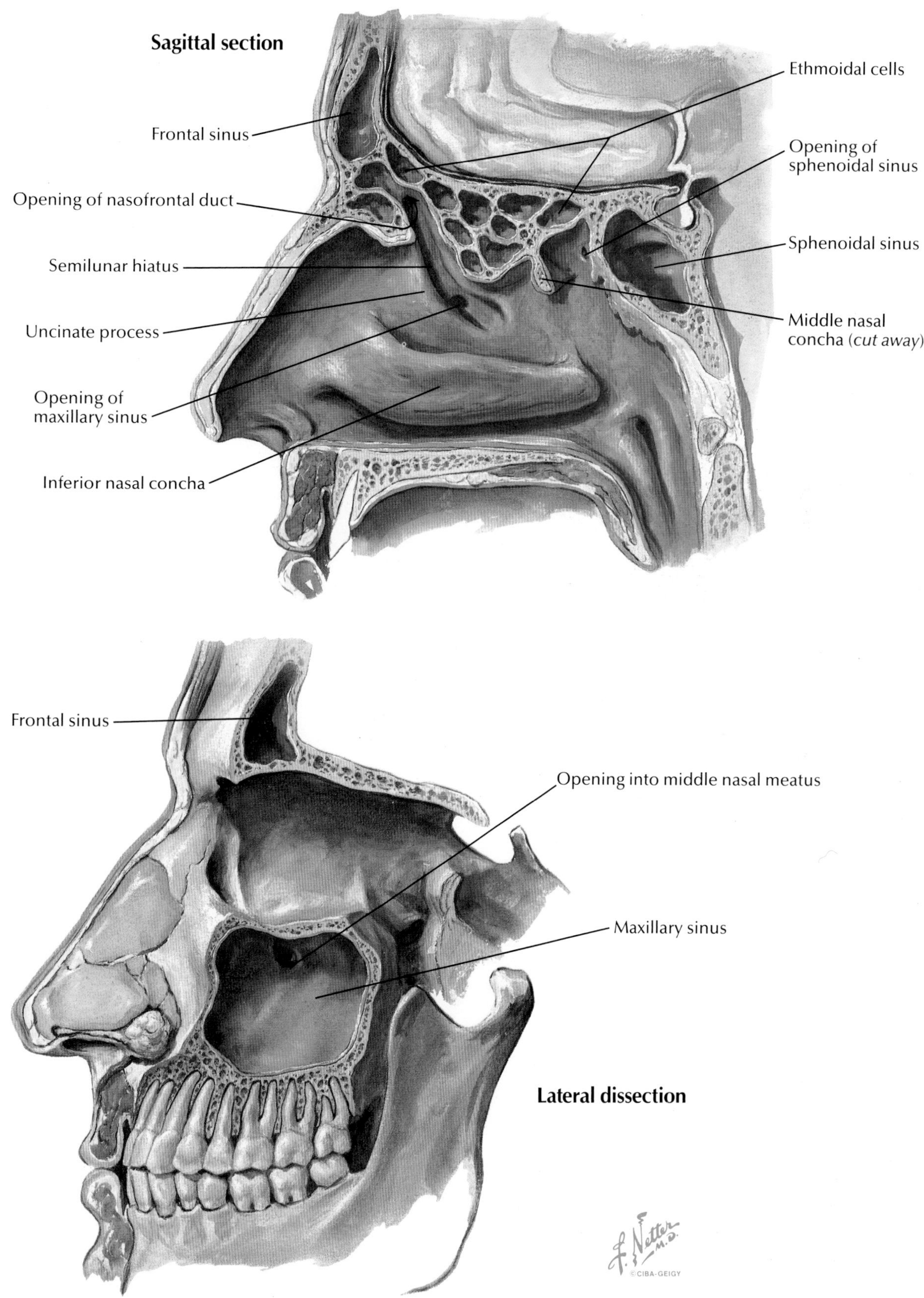

Sagittal section

Frontal sinus

Opening of nasofrontal duct

Semilunar hiatus

Uncinate process

Opening of maxillary sinus

Inferior nasal concha

Ethmoidal cells

Opening of sphenoidal sinus

Sphenoidal sinus

Middle nasal concha (*cut away*)

Frontal sinus

Opening into middle nasal meatus

Maxillary sinus

Lateral dissection

Paranasal Sinuses: Changes With Age

Bones of nasal cavity and paranasal sinuses at birth

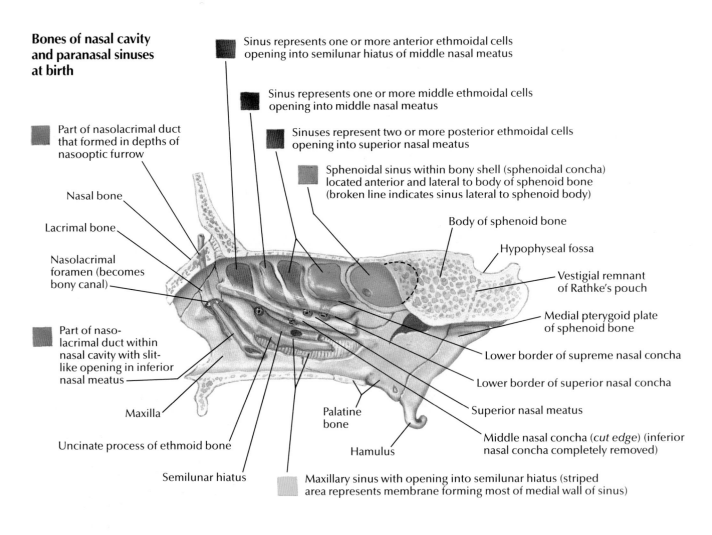

Sinus represents one or more anterior ethmoidal cells opening into semilunar hiatus of middle nasal meatus

Sinus represents one or more middle ethmoidal cells opening into middle nasal meatus

Sinuses represent two or more posterior ethmoidal cells opening into superior nasal meatus

Sphenoidal sinus within bony shell (sphenoidal concha) located anterior and lateral to body of sphenoid bone (broken line indicates sinus lateral to sphenoid body)

Part of nasolacrimal duct that formed in depths of nasooptic furrow

Nasal bone

Lacrimal bone

Nasolacrimal foramen (becomes bony canal)

Body of sphenoid bone

Hypophyseal fossa

Vestigial remnant of Rathke's pouch

Medial pterygoid plate of sphenoid bone

Part of naso-lacrimal duct within nasal cavity with slit-like opening in inferior nasal meatus

Lower border of supreme nasal concha

Lower border of superior nasal concha

Maxilla

Palatine bone

Superior nasal meatus

Uncinate process of ethmoid bone

Hamulus

Middle nasal concha (*cut edge*) (inferior nasal concha completely removed)

Semilunar hiatus

Maxillary sinus with opening into semilunar hiatus (striped area represents membrane forming most of medial wall of sinus)

Growth of frontal and maxillary sinuses throughout life

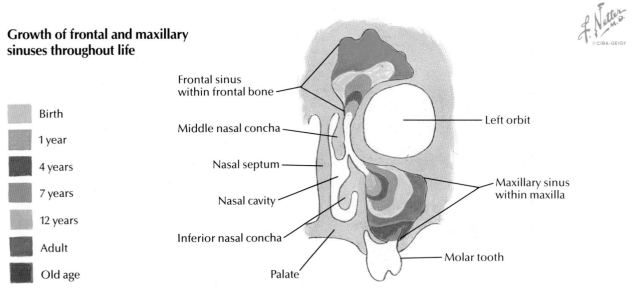

Birth

1 year

4 years

7 years

12 years

Adult

Old age

Frontal sinus within frontal bone

Middle nasal concha

Nasal septum

Nasal cavity

Inferior nasal concha

Palate

Left orbit

Maxillary sinus within maxilla

Molar tooth

PLATE 44

HEAD AND NECK

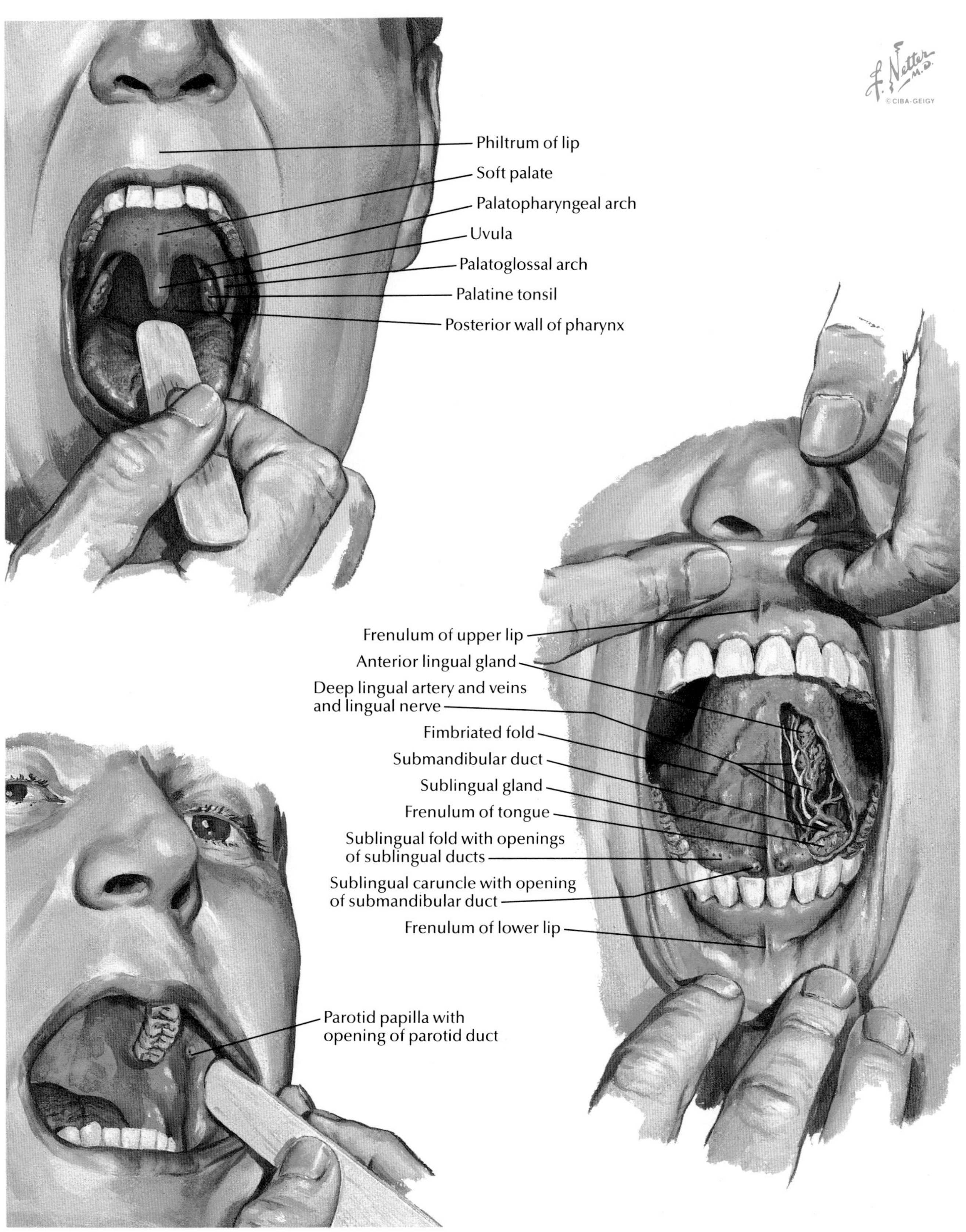

Philtrum of lip

Soft palate

Palatopharyngeal arch

Uvula

Palatoglossal arch

Palatine tonsil

Posterior wall of pharynx

Frenulum of upper lip

Anterior lingual gland

Deep lingual artery and veins
and lingual nerve

Fimbriated fold

Submandibular duct

Sublingual gland

Frenulum of tongue

Sublingual fold with openings
of sublingual ducts

Sublingual caruncle with opening
of submandibular duct

Frenulum of lower lip

Parotid papilla with
opening of parotid duct

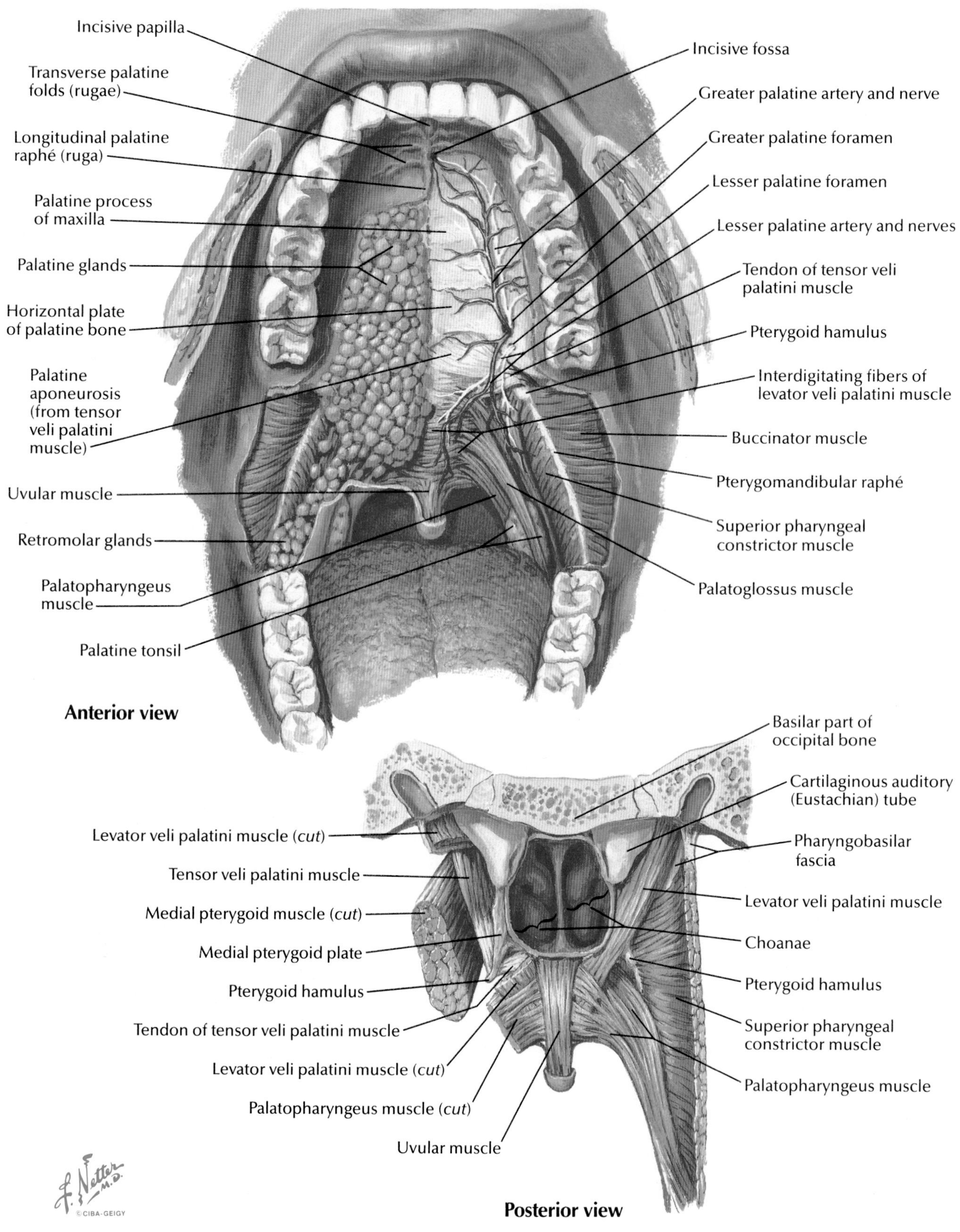

Incisive papilla

Transverse palatine folds (rugae)

Longitudinal palatine raphé (ruga)

Palatine process of maxilla

Palatine glands

Horizontal plate of palatine bone

Palatine aponeurosis (from tensor veli palatini muscle)

Uvular muscle

Retromolar glands

Palatopharyngeus muscle

Palatine tonsil

Incisive fossa

Greater palatine artery and nerve

Greater palatine foramen

Lesser palatine foramen

Lesser palatine artery and nerves

Tendon of tensor veli palatini muscle

Pterygoid hamulus

Interdigitating fibers of levator veli palatini muscle

Buccinator muscle

Pterygomandibular raphé

Superior pharyngeal constrictor muscle

Palatoglossus muscle

Anterior view

Levator veli palatini muscle (*cut*)

Tensor veli palatini muscle

Medial pterygoid muscle (*cut*)

Medial pterygoid plate

Pterygoid hamulus

Tendon of tensor veli palatini muscle

Levator veli palatini muscle (*cut*)

Palatopharyngeus muscle (*cut*)

Uvular muscle

Basilar part of occipital bone

Cartilaginous auditory (Eustachian) tube

Pharyngobasilar fascia

Levator veli palatini muscle

Choanae

Pterygoid hamulus

Superior pharyngeal constrictor muscle

Palatopharyngeus muscle

Posterior view

PLATE 46

HEAD AND NECK

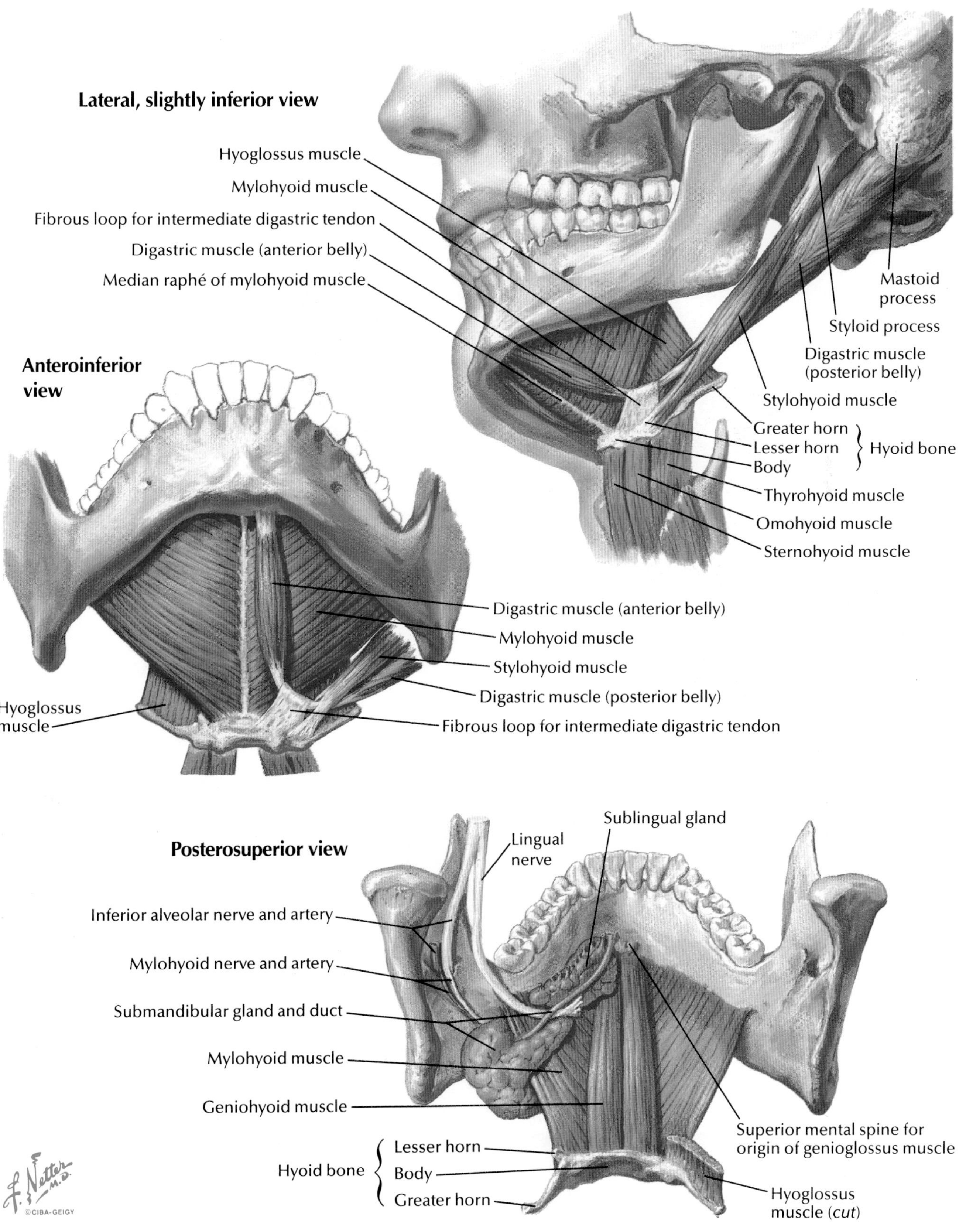

Lateral, slightly inferior view

Hyoglossus muscle

Mylohyoid muscle

Fibrous loop for intermediate digastric tendon

Digastric muscle (anterior belly)

Median raphé of mylohyoid muscle

Mastoid process

Styloid process

Digastric muscle (posterior belly)

Stylohyoid muscle

Greater horn ⎫
Lesser horn ⎬ Hyoid bone
Body ⎭

Thyrohyoid muscle

Omohyoid muscle

Sternohyoid muscle

Anteroinferior view

Digastric muscle (anterior belly)

Mylohyoid muscle

Stylohyoid muscle

Digastric muscle (posterior belly)

Fibrous loop for intermediate digastric tendon

Hyoglossus muscle

Posterosuperior view

Lingual nerve

Sublingual gland

Inferior alveolar nerve and artery

Mylohyoid nerve and artery

Submandibular gland and duct

Mylohyoid muscle

Geniohyoid muscle

Hyoid bone ⎧ Lesser horn
⎨ Body
⎩ Greater horn

Superior mental spine for origin of genioglossus muscle

Hyoglossus muscle (*cut*)

Muscles Involved in Mastication

FOR FACIAL MUSCLES SEE PLATES 20, 21

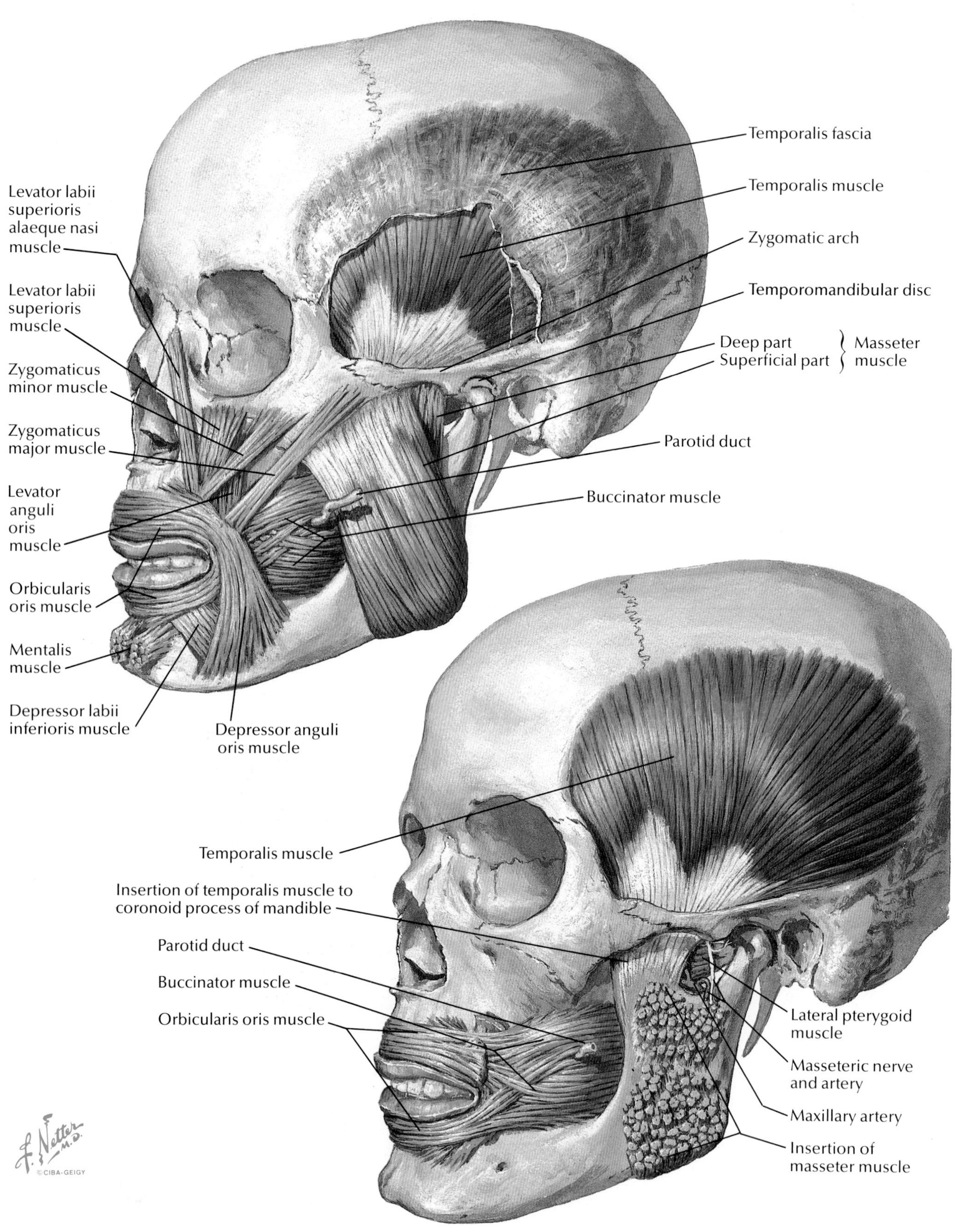

Temporalis fascia

Temporalis muscle

Zygomatic arch

Temporomandibular disc

Deep part ⎫ Masseter
Superficial part ⎭ muscle

Parotid duct

Buccinator muscle

Levator labii
superioris
alaeque nasi
muscle

Levator labii
superioris
muscle

Zygomaticus
minor muscle

Zygomaticus
major muscle

Levator
anguli
oris
muscle

Orbicularis
oris muscle

Mentalis
muscle

Depressor labii
inferioris muscle

Depressor anguli
oris muscle

Temporalis muscle

Insertion of temporalis muscle to
coronoid process of mandible

Parotid duct

Buccinator muscle

Orbicularis oris muscle

Lateral pterygoid
muscle

Masseteric nerve
and artery

Maxillary artery

Insertion of
masseter muscle

PLATE 48   **HEAD AND NECK**

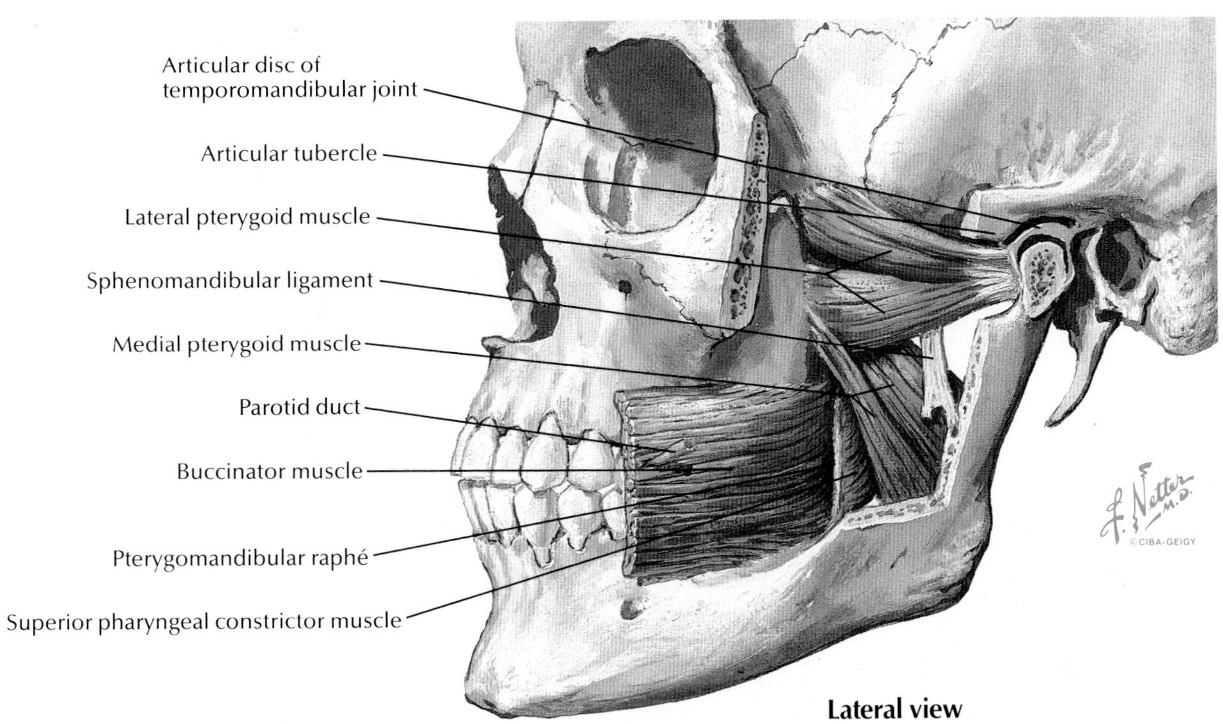

Articular disc of temporomandibular joint

Articular tubercle

Lateral pterygoid muscle

Sphenomandibular ligament

Medial pterygoid muscle

Parotid duct

Buccinator muscle

Pterygomandibular raphé

Superior pharyngeal constrictor muscle

Lateral view

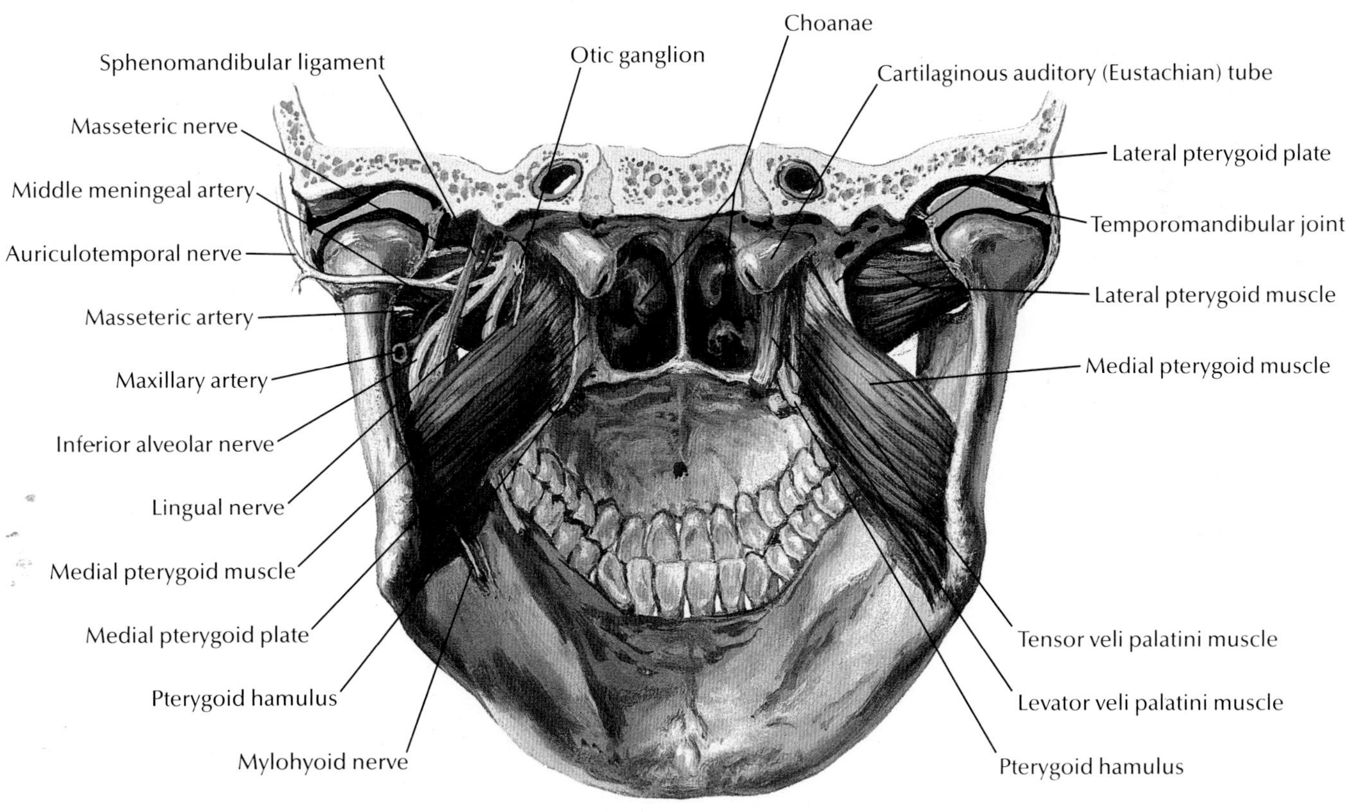

Sphenomandibular ligament

Masseteric nerve

Middle meningeal artery

Auriculotemporal nerve

Masseteric artery

Maxillary artery

Inferior alveolar nerve

Lingual nerve

Medial pterygoid muscle

Medial pterygoid plate

Pterygoid hamulus

Mylohyoid nerve

Otic ganglion

Choanae

Cartilaginous auditory (Eustachian) tube

Lateral pterygoid plate

Temporomandibular joint

Lateral pterygoid muscle

Medial pterygoid muscle

Tensor veli palatini muscle

Levator veli palatini muscle

Pterygoid hamulus

Posterior view

Teeth

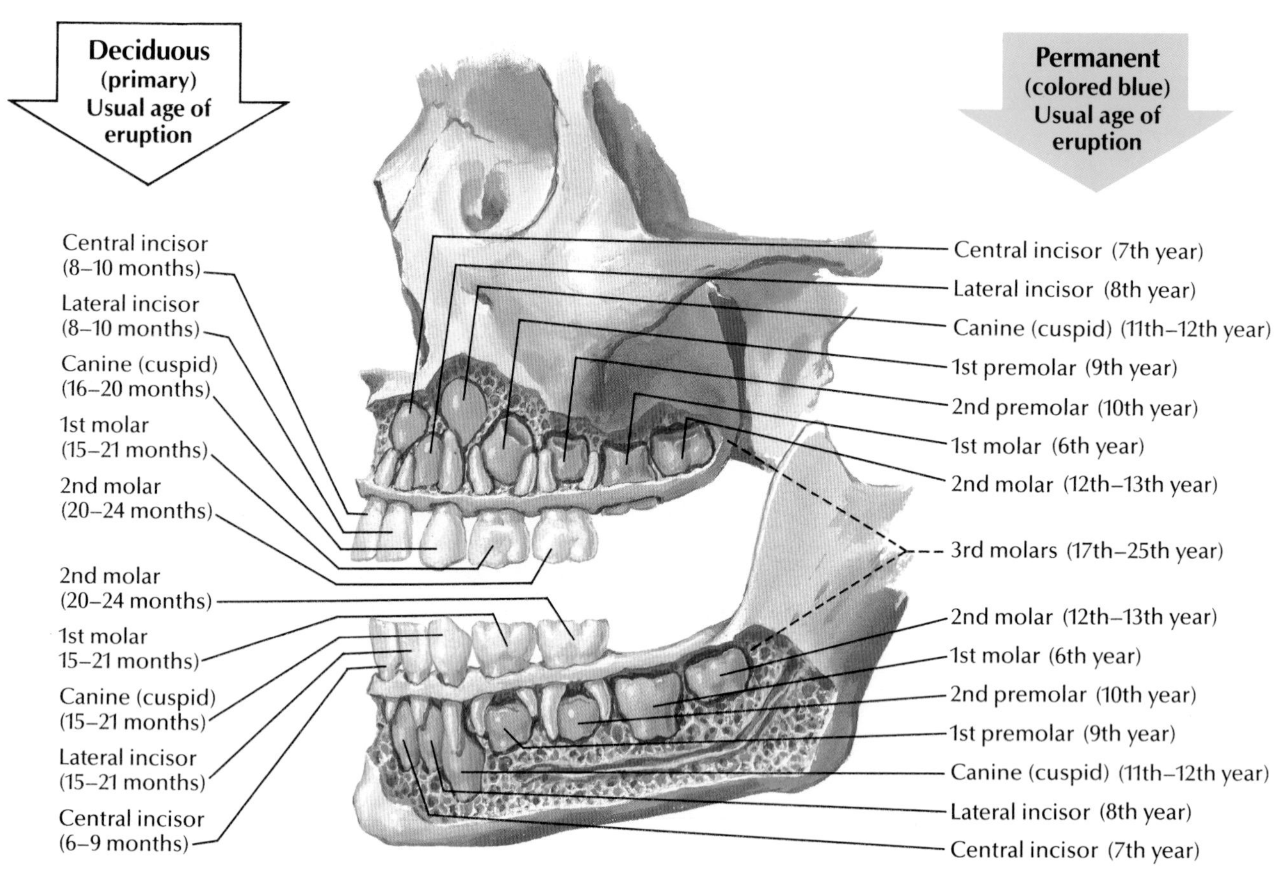

Deciduous (primary) Usual age of eruption

Central incisor (8–10 months)
Lateral incisor (8–10 months)
Canine (cuspid) (16–20 months)
1st molar (15–21 months)
2nd molar (20–24 months)

2nd molar (20–24 months)
1st molar 15–21 months)
Canine (cuspid) (15–21 months)
Lateral incisor (15–21 months)
Central incisor (6–9 months)

Permanent (colored blue) Usual age of eruption

Central incisor (7th year)
Lateral incisor (8th year)
Canine (cuspid) (11th–12th year)
1st premolar (9th year)
2nd premolar (10th year)
1st molar (6th year)
2nd molar (12th–13th year)
3rd molars (17th–25th year)
2nd molar (12th–13th year)
1st molar (6th year)
2nd premolar (10th year)
1st premolar (9th year)
Canine (cuspid) (11th–12th year)
Lateral incisor (8th year)
Central incisor (7th year)

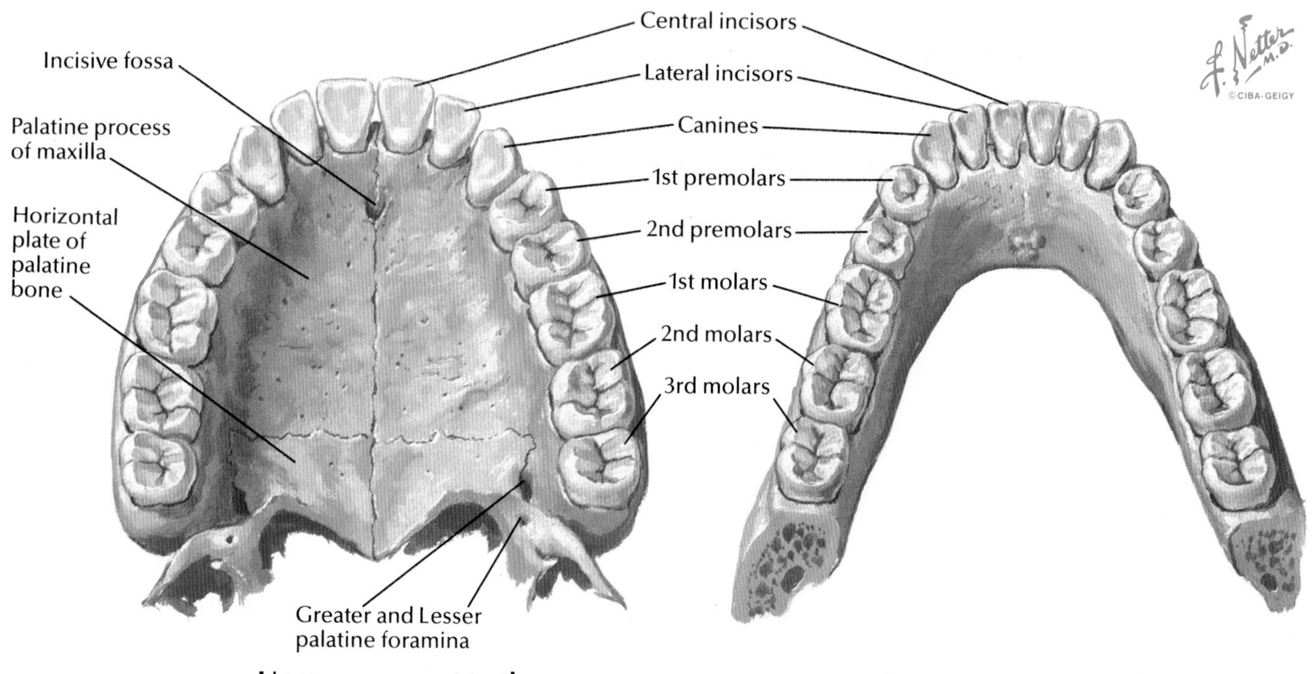

Incisive fossa
Palatine process of maxilla
Horizontal plate of palatine bone

Central incisors
Lateral incisors
Canines
1st premolars
2nd premolars
1st molars
2nd molars
3rd molars

Greater and Lesser palatine foramina

Upper permanent teeth

Lower permanent teeth

PLATE 50

HEAD AND NECK

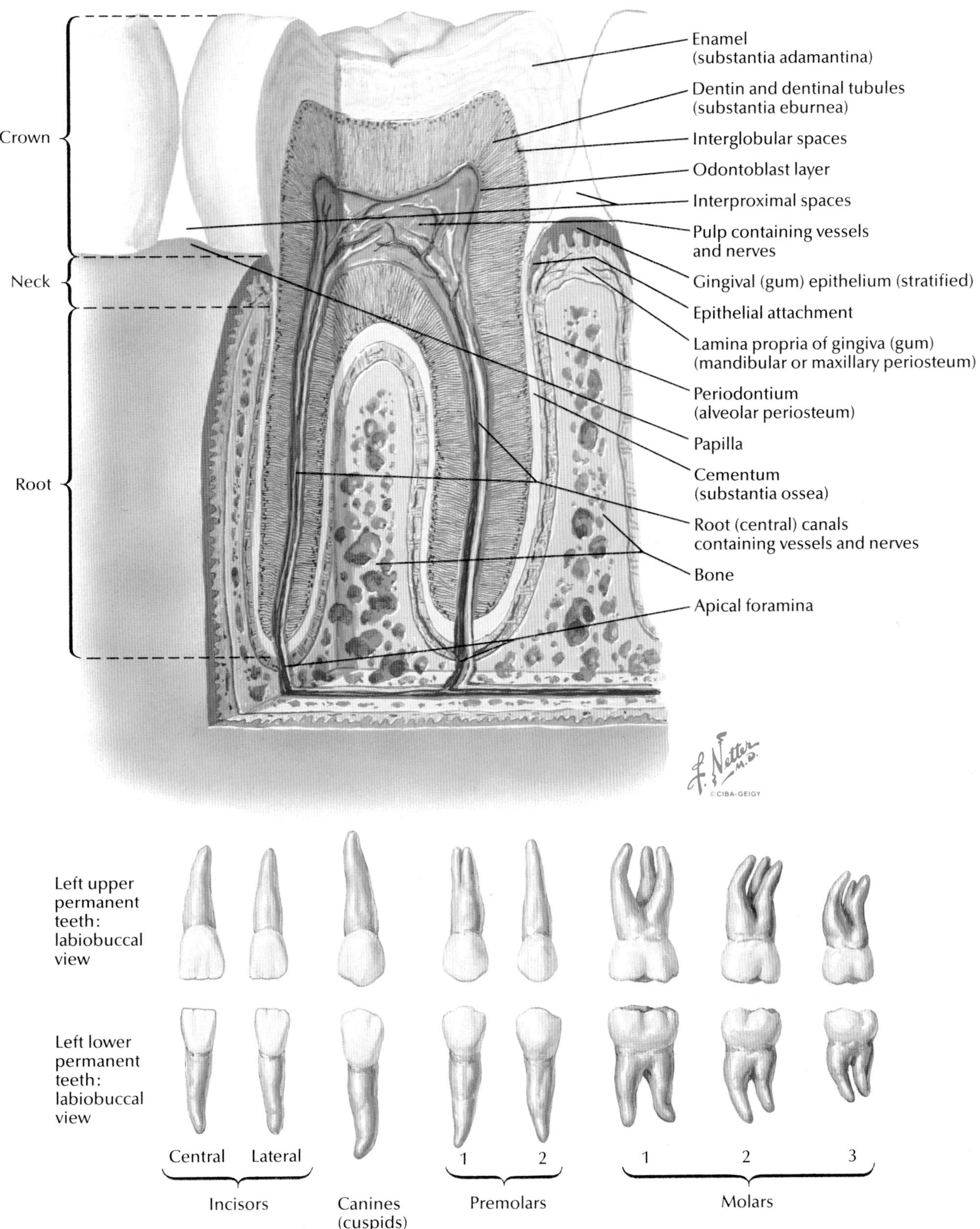

Crown

Neck

Root

Enamel
(substantia adamantina)

Dentin and dentinal tubules
(substantia eburnea)

Interglobular spaces

Odontoblast layer

Interproximal spaces

Pulp containing vessels
and nerves

Gingival (gum) epithelium (stratified)

Epithelial attachment

Lamina propria of gingiva (gum)
(mandibular or maxillary periosteum)

Periodontium
(alveolar periosteum)

Papilla

Cementum
(substantia ossea)

Root (central) canals
containing vessels and nerves

Bone

Apical foramina

Left upper
permanent
teeth:
labiobuccal
view

Left lower
permanent
teeth:
labiobuccal
view

Central   Lateral

Incisors

Canines
(cuspids)

1   2

Premolars

1   2   3

Molars

Tongue

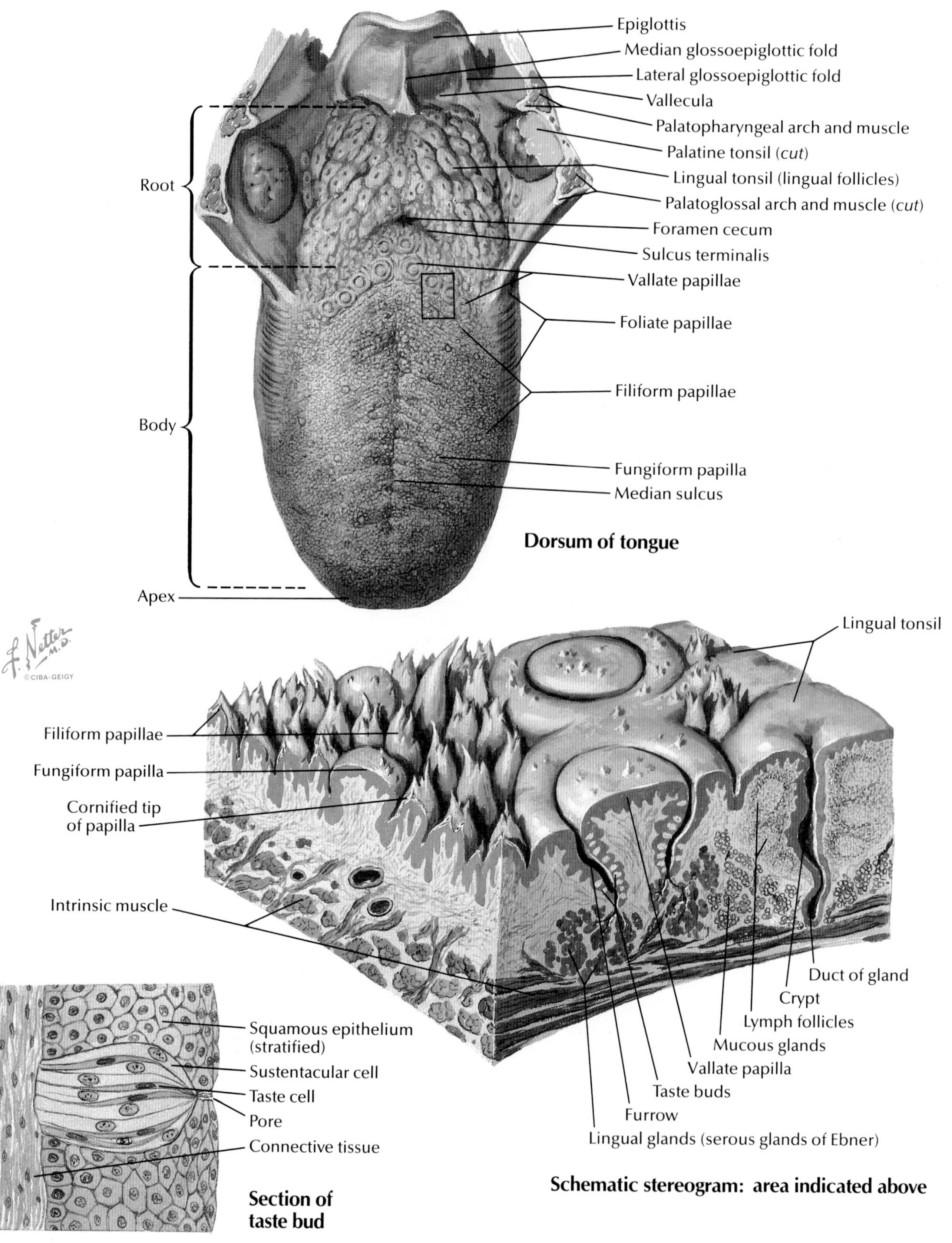

Epiglottis

Median glossoepiglottic fold

Lateral glossoepiglottic fold

Vallecula

Palatopharyngeal arch and muscle

Palatine tonsil (*cut*)

Lingual tonsil (lingual follicles)

Palatoglossal arch and muscle (*cut*)

Foramen cecum

Sulcus terminalis

Vallate papillae

Foliate papillae

Filiform papillae

Fungiform papilla

Median sulcus

Root

Body

Apex

Dorsum of tongue

Lingual tonsil

Filiform papillae

Fungiform papilla

Cornified tip of papilla

Intrinsic muscle

Squamous epithelium (stratified)

Sustentacular cell

Taste cell

Pore

Connective tissue

Section of taste bud

Duct of gland

Crypt

Lymph follicles

Mucous glands

Vallate papilla

Taste buds

Furrow

Lingual glands (serous glands of Ebner)

Schematic stereogram: area indicated above

PLATE 52

HEAD AND NECK

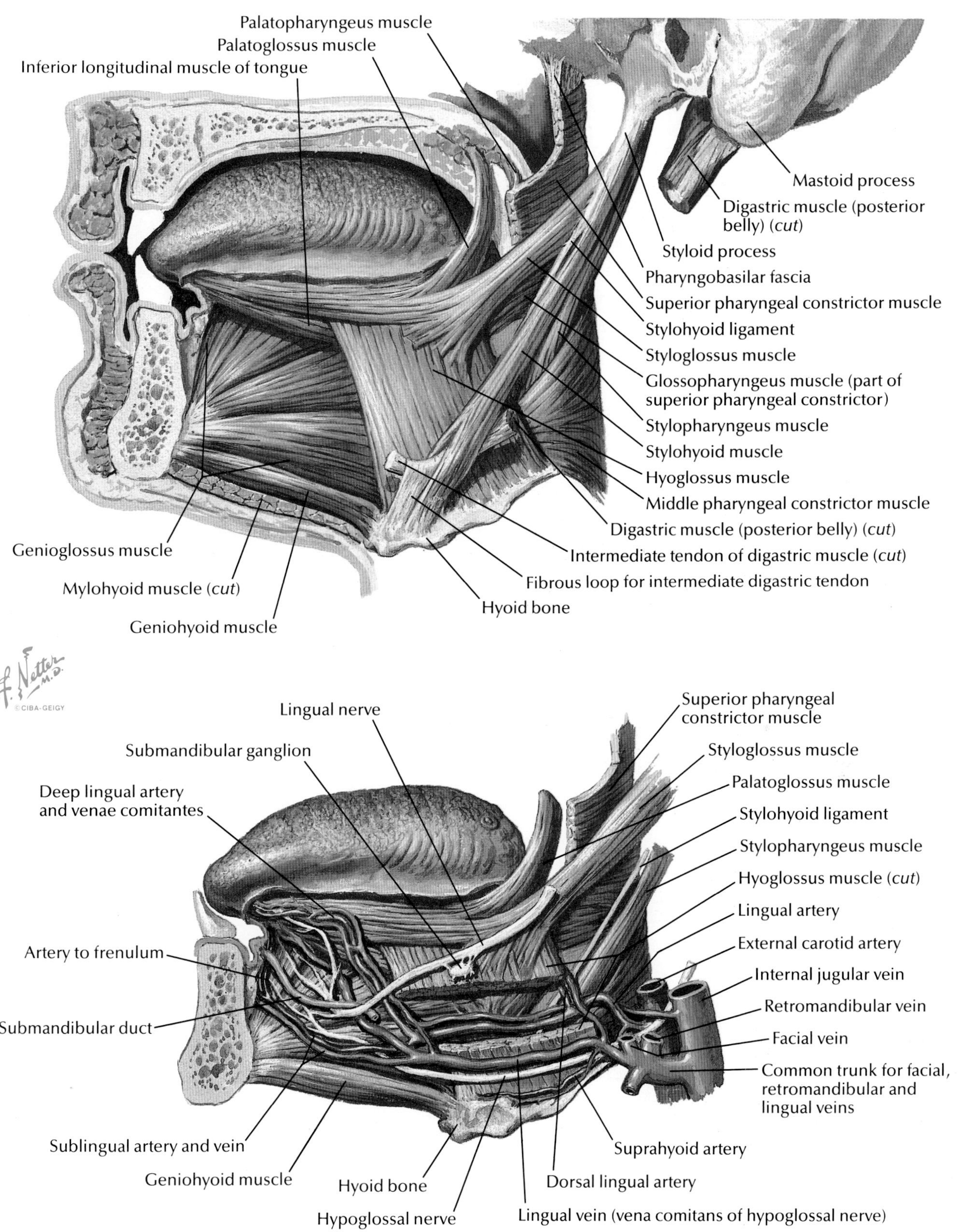

Palatopharyngeus muscle
Palatoglossus muscle
Inferior longitudinal muscle of tongue

Mastoid process
Digastric muscle (posterior belly) (*cut*)
Styloid process
Pharyngobasilar fascia
Superior pharyngeal constrictor muscle
Stylohyoid ligament
Styloglossus muscle
Glossopharyngeus muscle (part of superior pharyngeal constrictor)
Stylopharyngeus muscle
Stylohyoid muscle
Hyoglossus muscle
Middle pharyngeal constrictor muscle
Digastric muscle (posterior belly) (*cut*)
Intermediate tendon of digastric muscle (*cut*)
Fibrous loop for intermediate digastric tendon
Hyoid bone

Genioglossus muscle
Mylohyoid muscle (*cut*)
Geniohyoid muscle

Lingual nerve
Submandibular ganglion
Deep lingual artery and venae comitantes

Superior pharyngeal constrictor muscle
Styloglossus muscle
Palatoglossus muscle
Stylohyoid ligament
Stylopharyngeus muscle
Hyoglossus muscle (*cut*)
Lingual artery
External carotid artery
Internal jugular vein
Retromandibular vein
Facial vein
Common trunk for facial, retromandibular and lingual veins

Artery to frenulum
Submandibular duct

Sublingual artery and vein
Geniohyoid muscle
Hyoid bone
Hypoglossal nerve
Dorsal lingual artery
Suprahyoid artery
Lingual vein (vena comitans of hypoglossal nerve)

Tongue and Mouth: Sections

Horizontal section below lingula of mandible: superior view

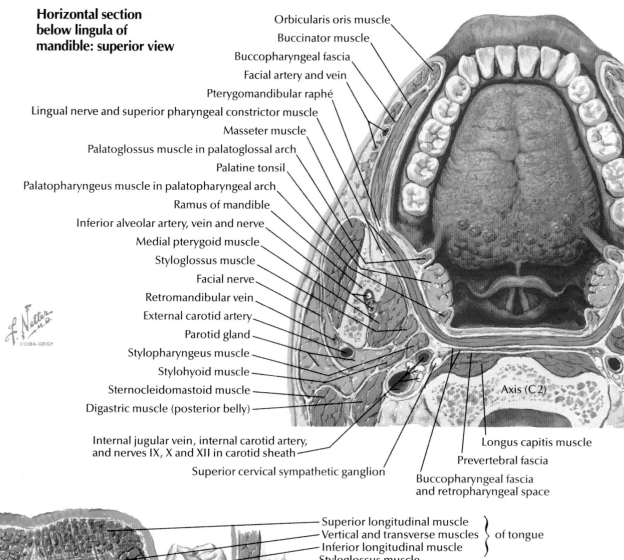

Orbicularis oris muscle

Buccinator muscle

Buccopharyngeal fascia

Facial artery and vein

Pterygomandibular raphé

Lingual nerve and superior pharyngeal constrictor muscle

Masseter muscle

Palatoglossus muscle in palatoglossal arch

Palatine tonsil

Palatopharyngeus muscle in palatopharyngeal arch

Ramus of mandible

Inferior alveolar artery, vein and nerve

Medial pterygoid muscle

Styloglossus muscle

Facial nerve

Retromandibular vein

External carotid artery

Parotid gland

Stylopharyngeus muscle

Stylohyoid muscle

Sternocleidomastoid muscle

Digastric muscle (posterior belly)

Internal jugular vein, internal carotid artery, and nerves IX, X and XII in carotid sheath

Superior cervical sympathetic ganglion

Axis (C2)

Longus capitis muscle

Prevertebral fascia

Buccopharyngeal fascia and retropharyngeal space

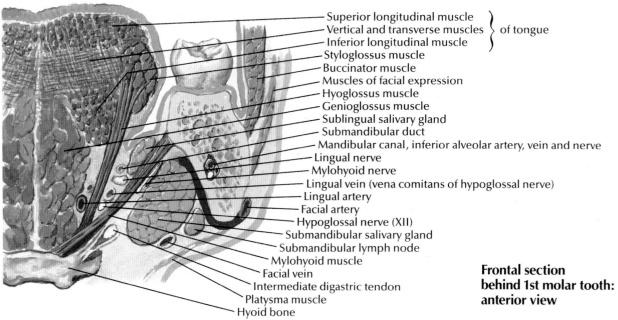

Superior longitudinal muscle
Vertical and transverse muscles } of tongue
Inferior longitudinal muscle
Styloglossus muscle
Buccinator muscle
Muscles of facial expression
Hyoglossus muscle
Genioglossus muscle
Sublingual salivary gland
Submandibular duct
Mandibular canal, inferior alveolar artery, vein and nerve
Lingual nerve
Mylohyoid nerve
Lingual vein (vena comitans of hypoglossal nerve)
Lingual artery
Facial artery
Hypoglossal nerve (XII)
Submandibular salivary gland
Submandibular lymph node
Mylohyoid muscle
Facial vein
Intermediate digastric tendon
Platysma muscle
Hyoid bone

Frontal section behind 1st molar tooth: anterior view

PLATE 54

HEAD AND NECK

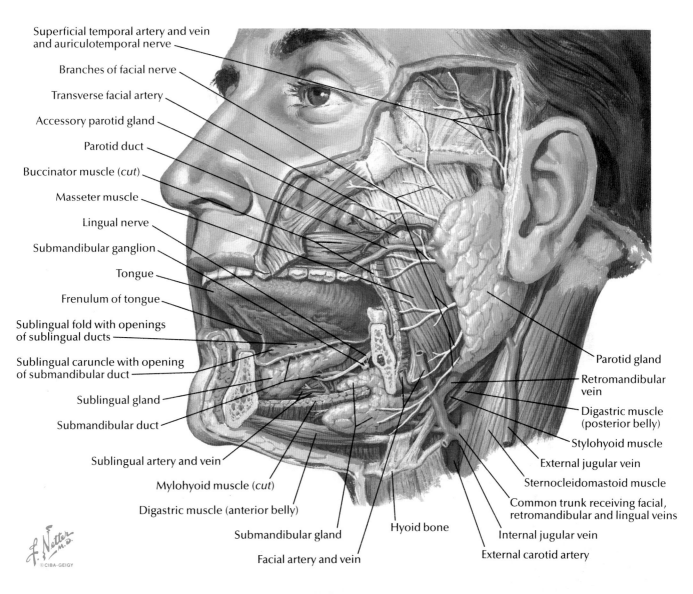

Superficial temporal artery and vein and auriculotemporal nerve

Branches of facial nerve

Transverse facial artery

Accessory parotid gland

Parotid duct

Buccinator muscle (*cut*)

Masseter muscle

Lingual nerve

Submandibular ganglion

Tongue

Frenulum of tongue

Sublingual fold with openings of sublingual ducts

Sublingual caruncle with opening of submandibular duct

Sublingual gland

Submandibular duct

Sublingual artery and vein

Mylohyoid muscle (*cut*)

Digastric muscle (anterior belly)

Submandibular gland

Facial artery and vein

Hyoid bone

Parotid gland

Retromandibular vein

Digastric muscle (posterior belly)

Stylohyoid muscle

External jugular vein

Sternocleidomastoid muscle

Common trunk receiving facial, retromandibular and lingual veins

Internal jugular vein

External carotid artery

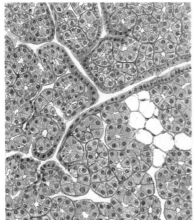

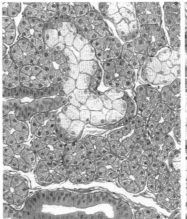

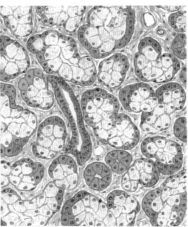

Parotid gland: totally serous

Submandibular gland: mostly serous, partially mucous

Sublingual gland: almost completely mucous

Afferent Innervation of Mouth and Pharynx

SEE ALSO PLATES 41, 46, 53, 58, 116, 117, 119, 127, 129

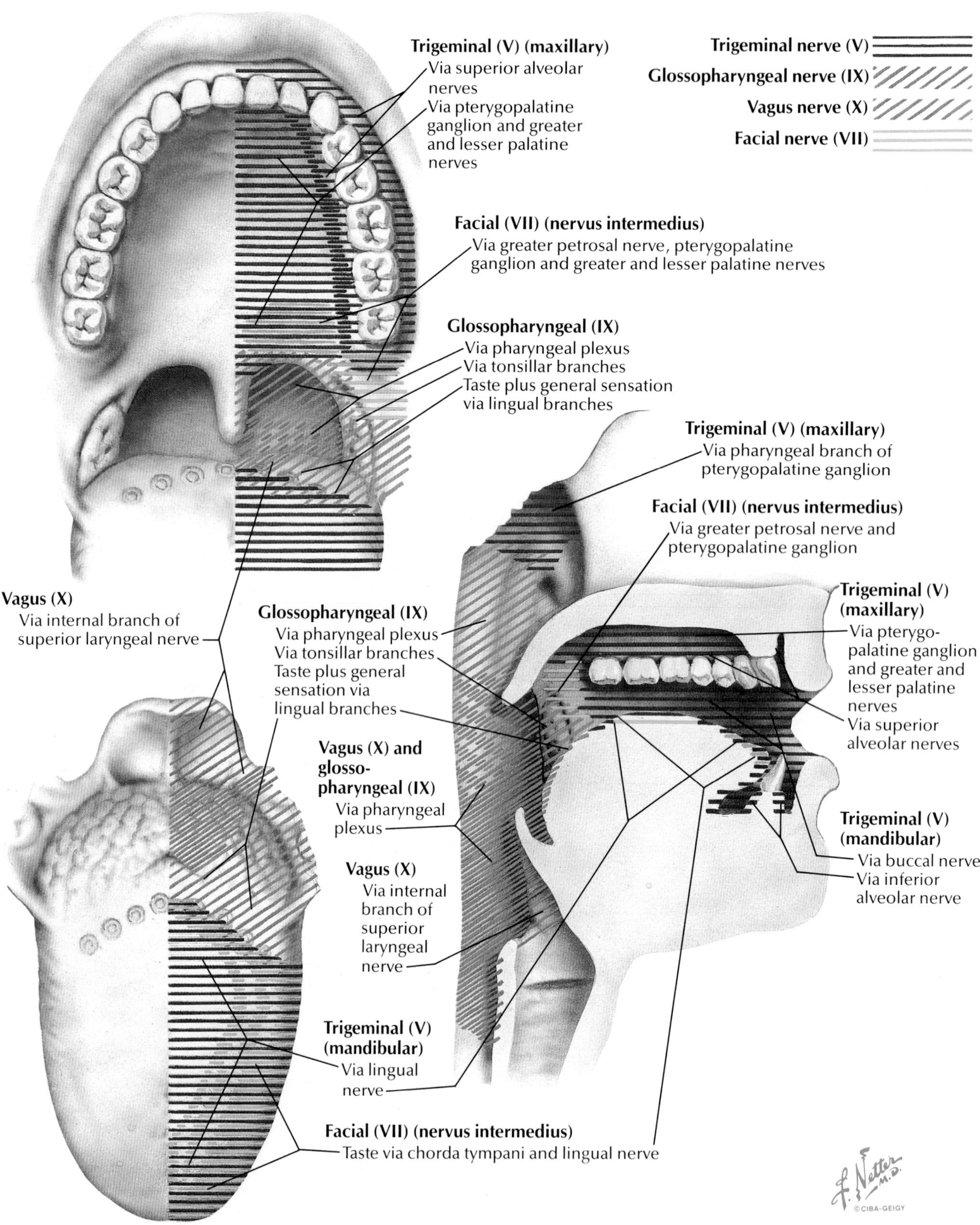

Trigeminal (V) (maxillary)
Via superior alveolar nerves
Via pterygopalatine ganglion and greater and lesser palatine nerves

Trigeminal nerve (V)
Glossopharyngeal nerve (IX)
Vagus nerve (X)
Facial nerve (VII)

Facial (VII) (nervus intermedius)
Via greater petrosal nerve, pterygopalatine ganglion and greater and lesser palatine nerves

Glossopharyngeal (IX)
Via pharyngeal plexus
Via tonsillar branches
Taste plus general sensation via lingual branches

Trigeminal (V) (maxillary)
Via pharyngeal branch of pterygopalatine ganglion

Facial (VII) (nervus intermedius)
Via greater petrosal nerve and pterygopalatine ganglion

Vagus (X)
Via internal branch of superior laryngeal nerve

Glossopharyngeal (IX)
Via pharyngeal plexus
Via tonsillar branches
Taste plus general sensation via lingual branches

Trigeminal (V) (maxillary)
Via pterygo-palatine ganglion and greater and lesser palatine nerves
Via superior alveolar nerves

Vagus (X) and glosso-pharyngeal (IX)
Via pharyngeal plexus

Vagus (X)
Via internal branch of superior laryngeal nerve

Trigeminal (V) (mandibular)
Via buccal nerve
Via inferior alveolar nerve

Trigeminal (V) (mandibular)
Via lingual nerve

Facial (VII) (nervus intermedius)
Taste via chorda tympani and lingual nerve

PLATE 56

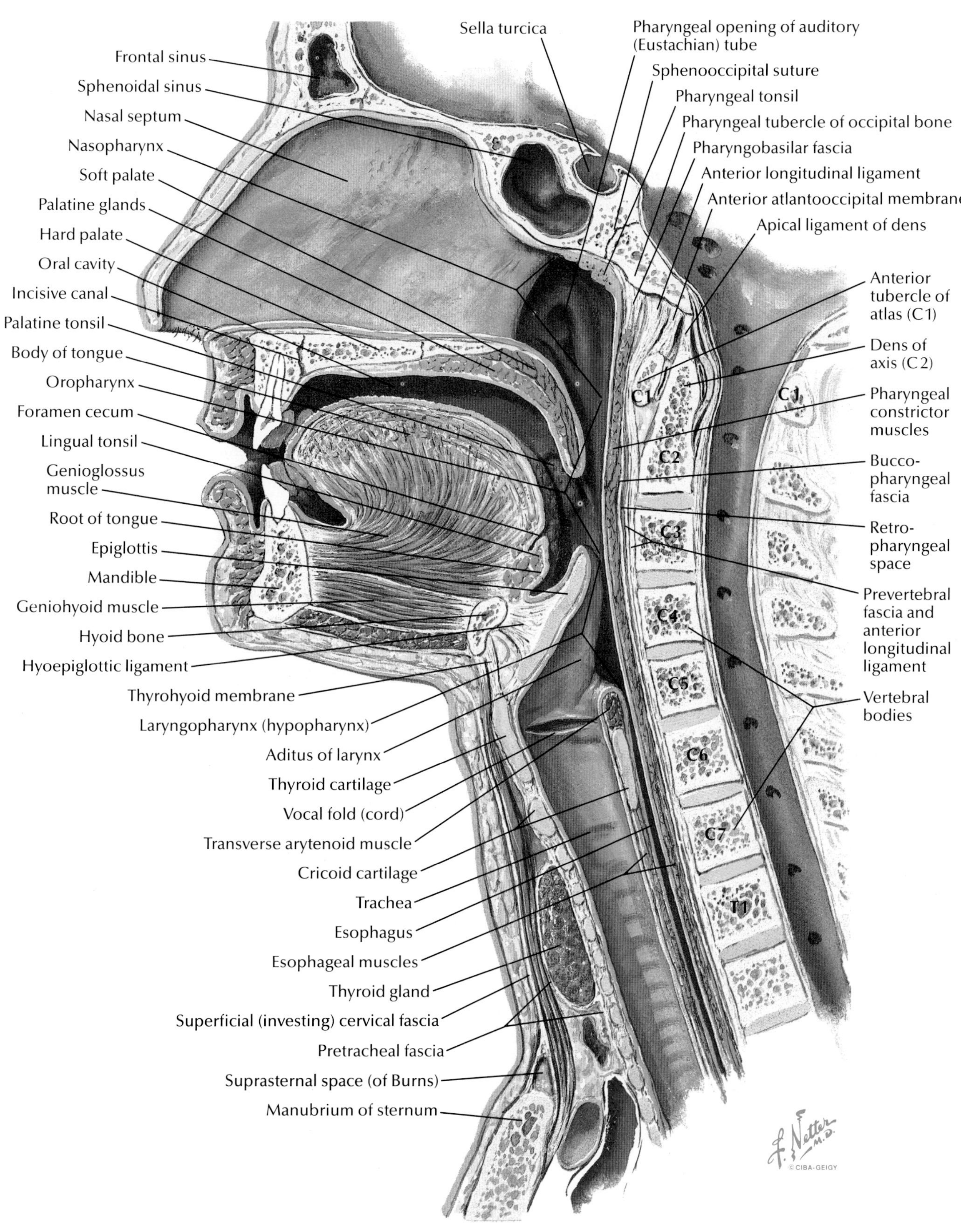

Frontal sinus
Sphenoidal sinus
Nasal septum
Nasopharynx
Soft palate
Palatine glands
Hard palate
Oral cavity
Incisive canal
Palatine tonsil
Body of tongue
Oropharynx
Foramen cecum
Lingual tonsil
Genioglossus muscle
Root of tongue
Epiglottis
Mandible
Geniohyoid muscle
Hyoid bone
Hyoepiglottic ligament
Thyrohyoid membrane
Laryngopharynx (hypopharynx)
Aditus of larynx
Thyroid cartilage
Vocal fold (cord)
Transverse arytenoid muscle
Cricoid cartilage
Trachea
Esophagus
Esophageal muscles
Thyroid gland
Superficial (investing) cervical fascia
Pretracheal fascia
Suprasternal space (of Burns)
Manubrium of sternum

Sella turcica
Pharyngeal opening of auditory (Eustachian) tube
Sphenooccipital suture
Pharyngeal tonsil
Pharyngeal tubercle of occipital bone
Pharyngobasilar fascia
Anterior longitudinal ligament
Anterior atlantooccipital membrane
Apical ligament of dens
Anterior tubercle of atlas (C1)
Dens of axis (C2)
Pharyngeal constrictor muscles
Bucco-pharyngeal fascia
Retro-pharyngeal space
Prevertebral fascia and anterior longitudinal ligament
Vertebral bodies

C1
C1
C2
C3
C4
C5
C6
C7
T1

Fauces

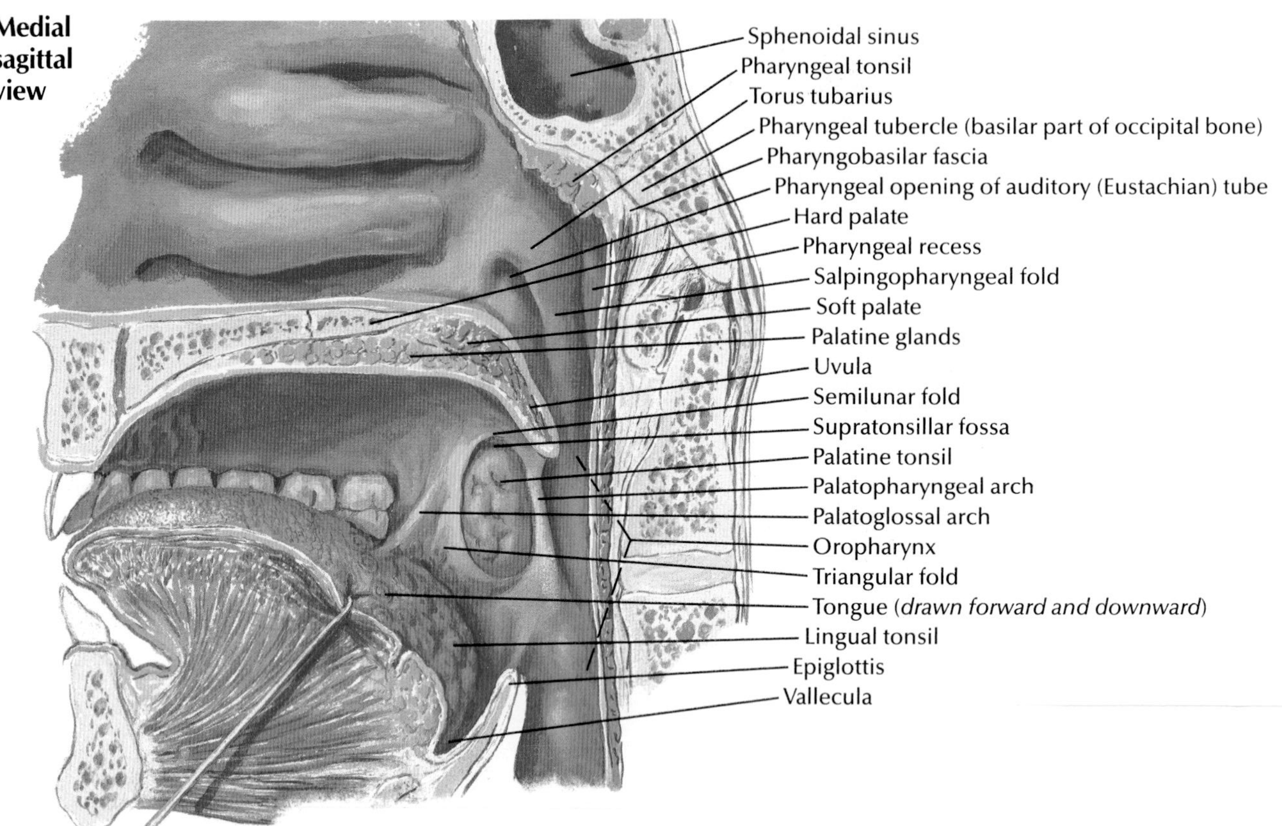

- Sphenoidal sinus
- Pharyngeal tonsil
- Torus tubarius
- Pharyngeal tubercle (basilar part of occipital bone)
- Pharyngobasilar fascia
- Pharyngeal opening of auditory (Eustachian) tube
- Hard palate
- Pharyngeal recess
- Salpingopharyngeal fold
- Soft palate
- Palatine glands
- Uvula
- Semilunar fold
- Supratonsillar fossa
- Palatine tonsil
- Palatopharyngeal arch
- Palatoglossal arch
- Oropharynx
- Triangular fold
- Tongue (*drawn forward and downward*)
- Lingual tonsil
- Epiglottis
- Vallecula

Pharyngeal mucosa removed

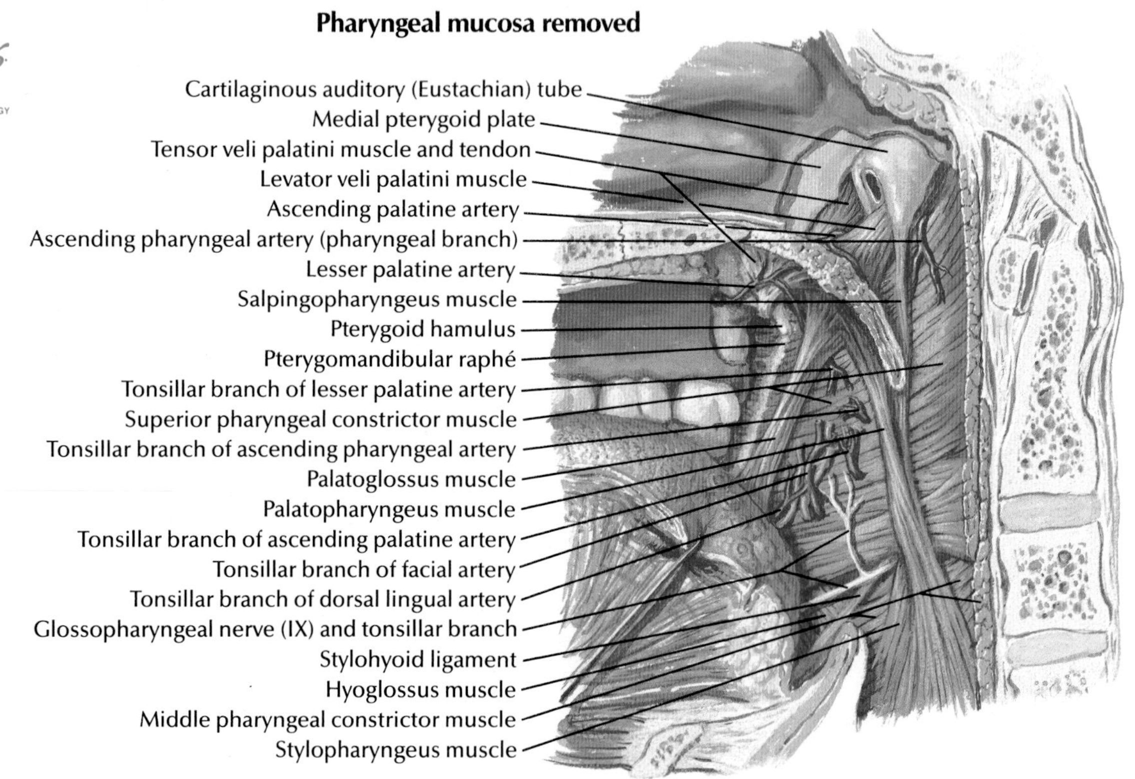

- Cartilaginous auditory (Eustachian) tube
- Medial pterygoid plate
- Tensor veli palatini muscle and tendon
- Levator veli palatini muscle
- Ascending palatine artery
- Ascending pharyngeal artery (pharyngeal branch)
- Lesser palatine artery
- Salpingopharyngeus muscle
- Pterygoid hamulus
- Pterygomandibular raphé
- Tonsillar branch of lesser palatine artery
- Superior pharyngeal constrictor muscle
- Tonsillar branch of ascending pharyngeal artery
- Palatoglossus muscle
- Palatopharyngeus muscle
- Tonsillar branch of ascending palatine artery
- Tonsillar branch of facial artery
- Tonsillar branch of dorsal lingual artery
- Glossopharyngeal nerve (IX) and tonsillar branch
- Stylohyoid ligament
- Hyoglossus muscle
- Middle pharyngeal constrictor muscle
- Stylopharyngeus muscle

PLATE 58

HEAD AND NECK

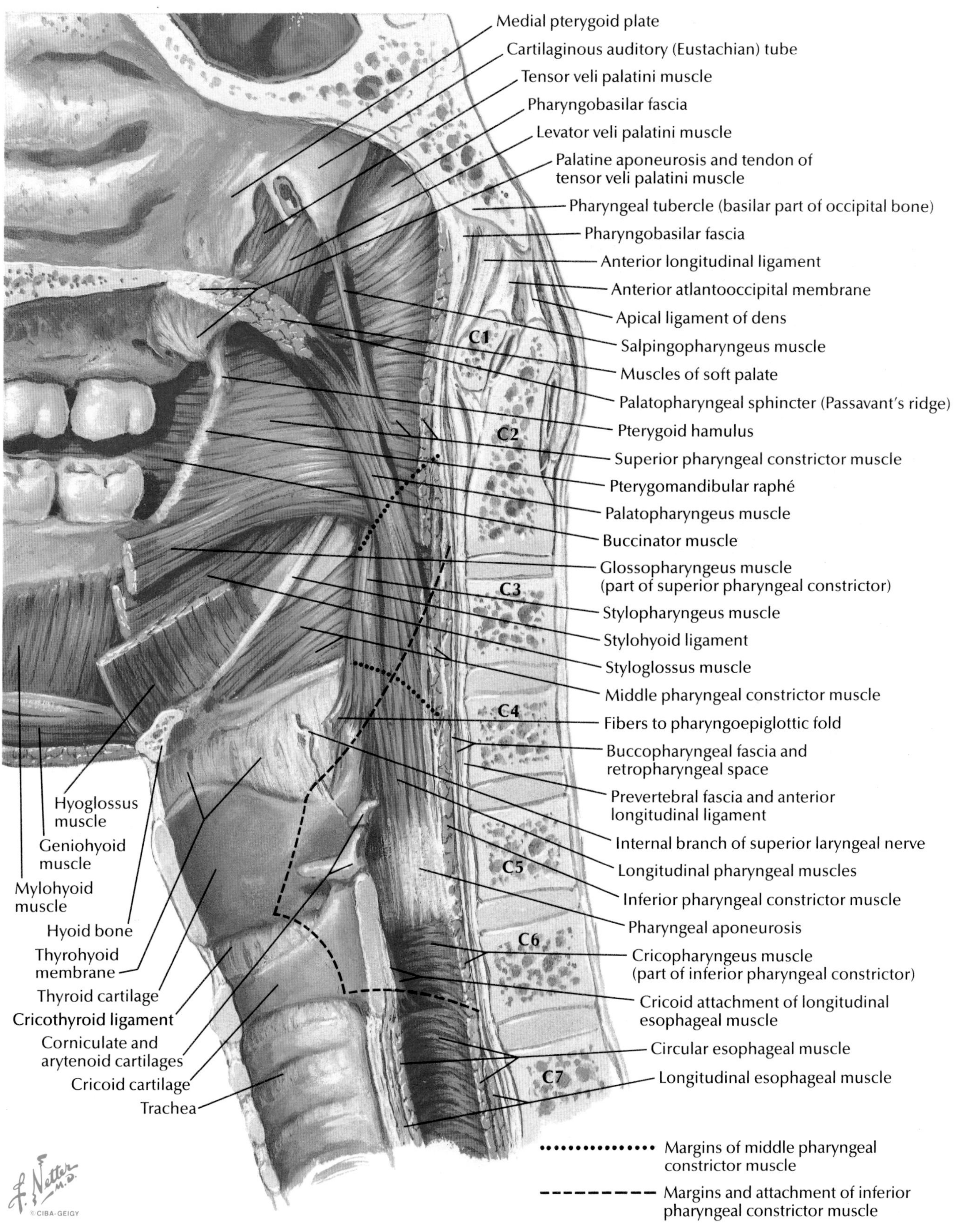

Medial pterygoid plate

Cartilaginous auditory (Eustachian) tube

Tensor veli palatini muscle

Pharyngobasilar fascia

Levator veli palatini muscle

Palatine aponeurosis and tendon of tensor veli palatini muscle

Pharyngeal tubercle (basilar part of occipital bone)

Pharyngobasilar fascia

Anterior longitudinal ligament

Anterior atlantooccipital membrane

Apical ligament of dens

Salpingopharyngeus muscle

Muscles of soft palate

Palatopharyngeal sphincter (Passavant's ridge)

Pterygoid hamulus

Superior pharyngeal constrictor muscle

Pterygomandibular raphé

Palatopharyngeus muscle

Buccinator muscle

Glossopharyngeus muscle (part of superior pharyngeal constrictor)

Stylopharyngeus muscle

Stylohyoid ligament

Styloglossus muscle

Middle pharyngeal constrictor muscle

Fibers to pharyngoepiglottic fold

Buccopharyngeal fascia and retropharyngeal space

Prevertebral fascia and anterior longitudinal ligament

Internal branch of superior laryngeal nerve

Longitudinal pharyngeal muscles

Inferior pharyngeal constrictor muscle

Pharyngeal aponeurosis

Cricopharyngeus muscle (part of inferior pharyngeal constrictor)

Cricoid attachment of longitudinal esophageal muscle

Circular esophageal muscle

Longitudinal esophageal muscle

C1
C2
C3
C4
C5
C6
C7

Hyoglossus muscle

Geniohyoid muscle

Mylohyoid muscle

Hyoid bone

Thyrohyoid membrane

Thyroid cartilage

Cricothyroid ligament

Corniculate and arytenoid cartilages

Cricoid cartilage

Trachea

•••••••••••• Margins of middle pharyngeal constrictor muscle

– – – – – – – Margins and attachment of inferior pharyngeal constrictor muscle

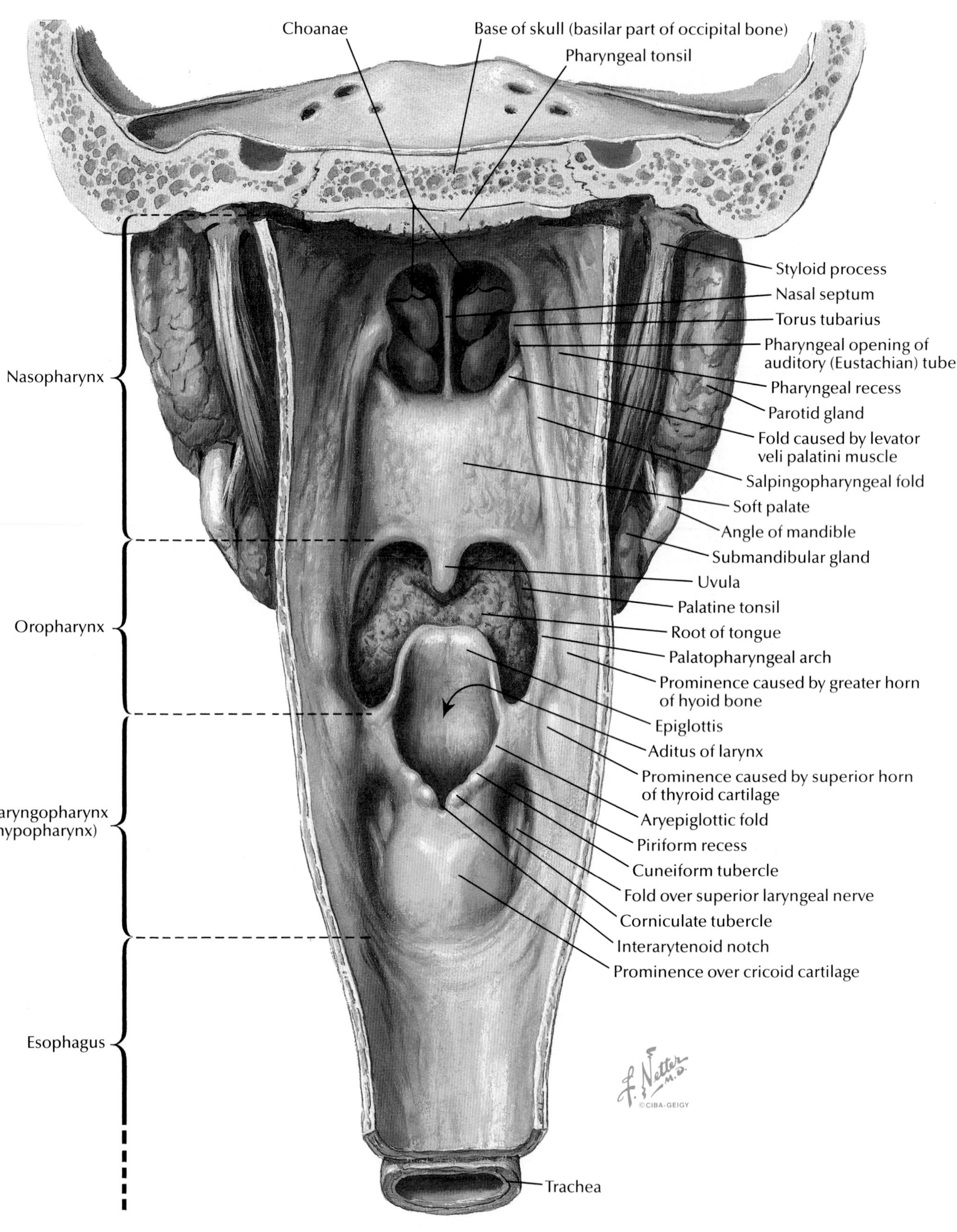

Choanae

Base of skull (basilar part of occipital bone)

Pharyngeal tonsil

Styloid process

Nasal septum

Torus tubarius

Pharyngeal opening of auditory (Eustachian) tube

Pharyngeal recess

Parotid gland

Fold caused by levator veli palatini muscle

Salpingopharyngeal fold

Soft palate

Angle of mandible

Submandibular gland

Uvula

Palatine tonsil

Root of tongue

Palatopharyngeal arch

Prominence caused by greater horn of hyoid bone

Epiglottis

Aditus of larynx

Prominence caused by superior horn of thyroid cartilage

Aryepiglottic fold

Piriform recess

Cuneiform tubercle

Fold over superior laryngeal nerve

Corniculate tubercle

Interarytenoid notch

Prominence over cricoid cartilage

Nasopharynx

Oropharynx

Laryngopharynx (hypopharynx)

Esophagus

Trachea

PLATE 60

HEAD AND NECK

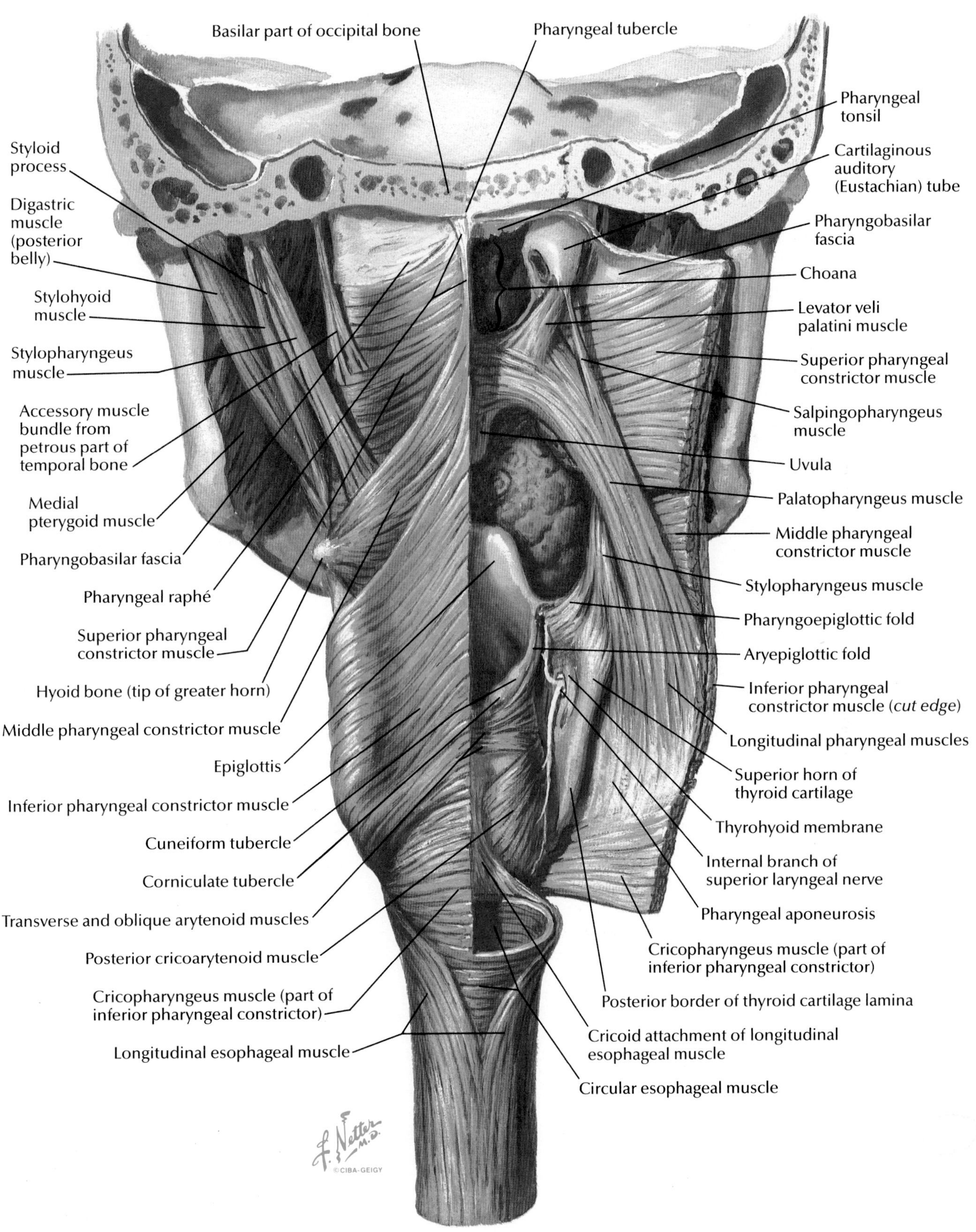

Basilar part of occipital bone

Pharyngeal tubercle

Styloid process

Digastric muscle (posterior belly)

Stylohyoid muscle

Stylopharyngeus muscle

Accessory muscle bundle from petrous part of temporal bone

Medial pterygoid muscle

Pharyngobasilar fascia

Pharyngeal raphé

Superior pharyngeal constrictor muscle

Hyoid bone (tip of greater horn)

Middle pharyngeal constrictor muscle

Epiglottis

Inferior pharyngeal constrictor muscle

Cuneiform tubercle

Corniculate tubercle

Transverse and oblique arytenoid muscles

Posterior cricoarytenoid muscle

Cricopharyngeus muscle (part of inferior pharyngeal constrictor)

Longitudinal esophageal muscle

Pharyngeal tonsil

Cartilaginous auditory (Eustachian) tube

Pharyngobasilar fascia

Choana

Levator veli palatini muscle

Superior pharyngeal constrictor muscle

Salpingopharyngeus muscle

Uvula

Palatopharyngeus muscle

Middle pharyngeal constrictor muscle

Stylopharyngeus muscle

Pharyngoepiglottic fold

Aryepiglottic fold

Inferior pharyngeal constrictor muscle (cut edge)

Longitudinal pharyngeal muscles

Superior horn of thyroid cartilage

Thyrohyoid membrane

Internal branch of superior laryngeal nerve

Pharyngeal aponeurosis

Cricopharyngeus muscle (part of inferior pharyngeal constrictor)

Posterior border of thyroid cartilage lamina

Cricoid attachment of longitudinal esophageal muscle

Circular esophageal muscle

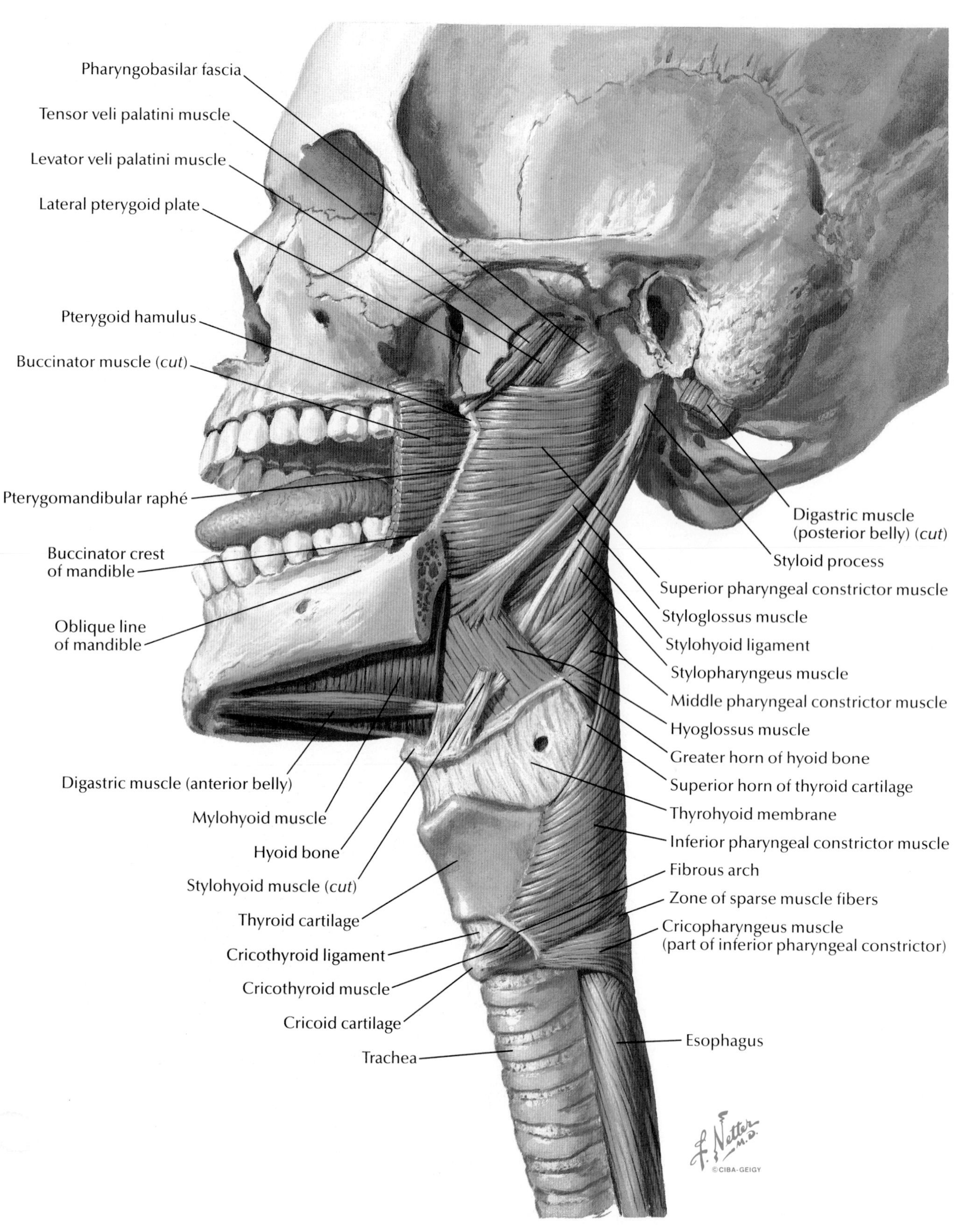

Pharyngobasilar fascia

Tensor veli palatini muscle

Levator veli palatini muscle

Lateral pterygoid plate

Pterygoid hamulus

Buccinator muscle (*cut*)

Pterygomandibular raphé

Buccinator crest of mandible

Oblique line of mandible

Digastric muscle (anterior belly)

Mylohyoid muscle

Hyoid bone

Stylohyoid muscle (*cut*)

Thyroid cartilage

Cricothyroid ligament

Cricothyroid muscle

Cricoid cartilage

Trachea

Digastric muscle (posterior belly) (*cut*)

Styloid process

Superior pharyngeal constrictor muscle

Styloglossus muscle

Stylohyoid ligament

Stylopharyngeus muscle

Middle pharyngeal constrictor muscle

Hyoglossus muscle

Greater horn of hyoid bone

Superior horn of thyroid cartilage

Thyrohyoid membrane

Inferior pharyngeal constrictor muscle

Fibrous arch

Zone of sparse muscle fibers

Cricopharyngeus muscle (part of inferior pharyngeal constrictor)

Esophagus

PLATE 62

HEAD AND NECK

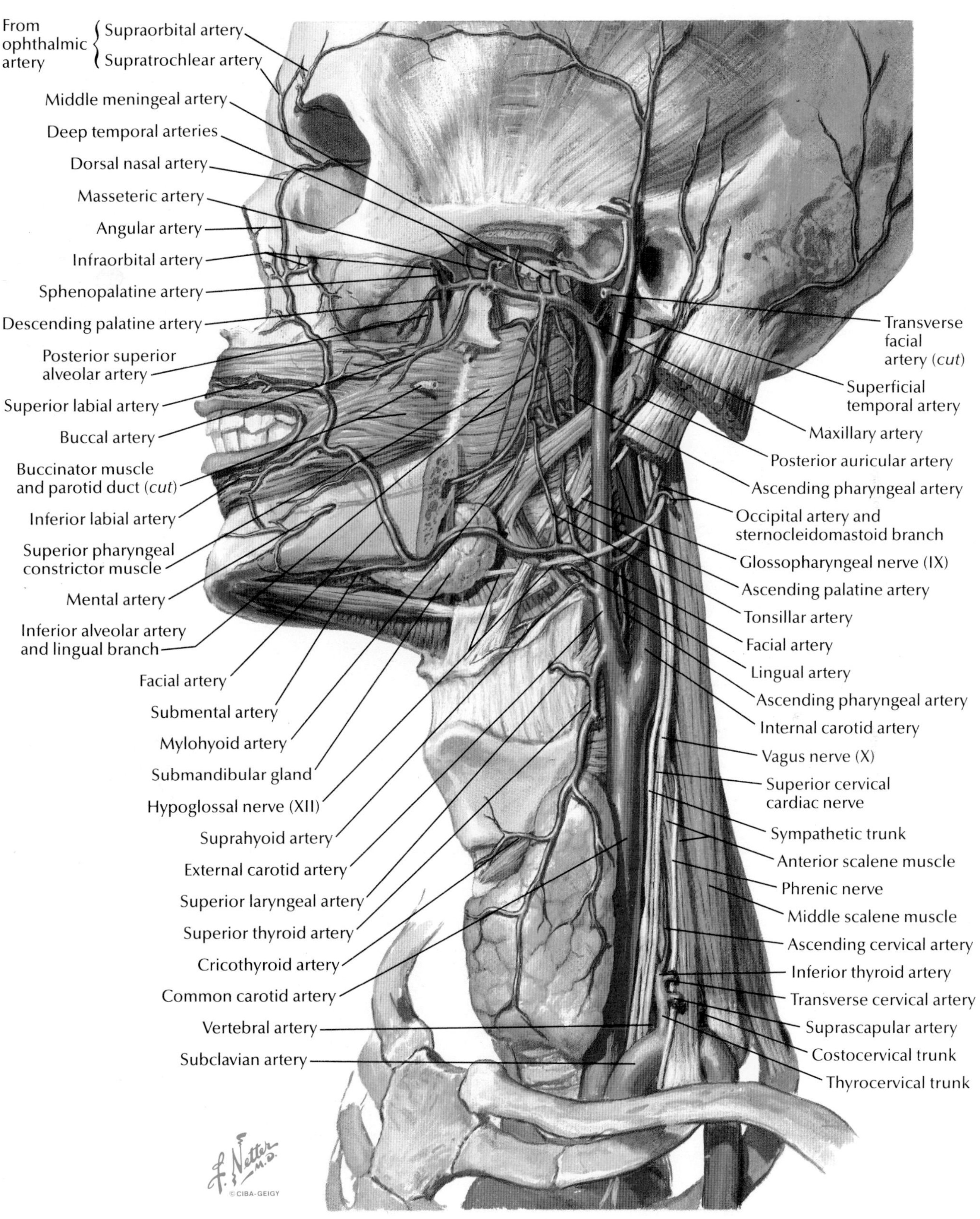

From ophthalmic artery
{ Supraorbital artery
Supratrochlear artery

Middle meningeal artery

Deep temporal arteries

Dorsal nasal artery

Masseteric artery

Angular artery

Infraorbital artery

Sphenopalatine artery

Descending palatine artery

Posterior superior alveolar artery

Superior labial artery

Buccal artery

Buccinator muscle and parotid duct (cut)

Inferior labial artery

Superior pharyngeal constrictor muscle

Mental artery

Inferior alveolar artery and lingual branch

Facial artery

Submental artery

Mylohyoid artery

Submandibular gland

Hypoglossal nerve (XII)

Suprahyoid artery

External carotid artery

Superior laryngeal artery

Superior thyroid artery

Cricothyroid artery

Common carotid artery

Vertebral artery

Subclavian artery

Transverse facial artery (cut)

Superficial temporal artery

Maxillary artery

Posterior auricular artery

Ascending pharyngeal artery

Occipital artery and sternocleidomastoid branch

Glossopharyngeal nerve (IX)

Ascending palatine artery

Tonsillar artery

Facial artery

Lingual artery

Ascending pharyngeal artery

Internal carotid artery

Vagus nerve (X)

Superior cervical cardiac nerve

Sympathetic trunk

Anterior scalene muscle

Phrenic nerve

Middle scalene muscle

Ascending cervical artery

Inferior thyroid artery

Transverse cervical artery

Suprascapular artery

Costocervical trunk

Thyrocervical trunk

Veins of Oral and Pharyngeal Regions

SEE ALSO PLATES 17, 26, 98

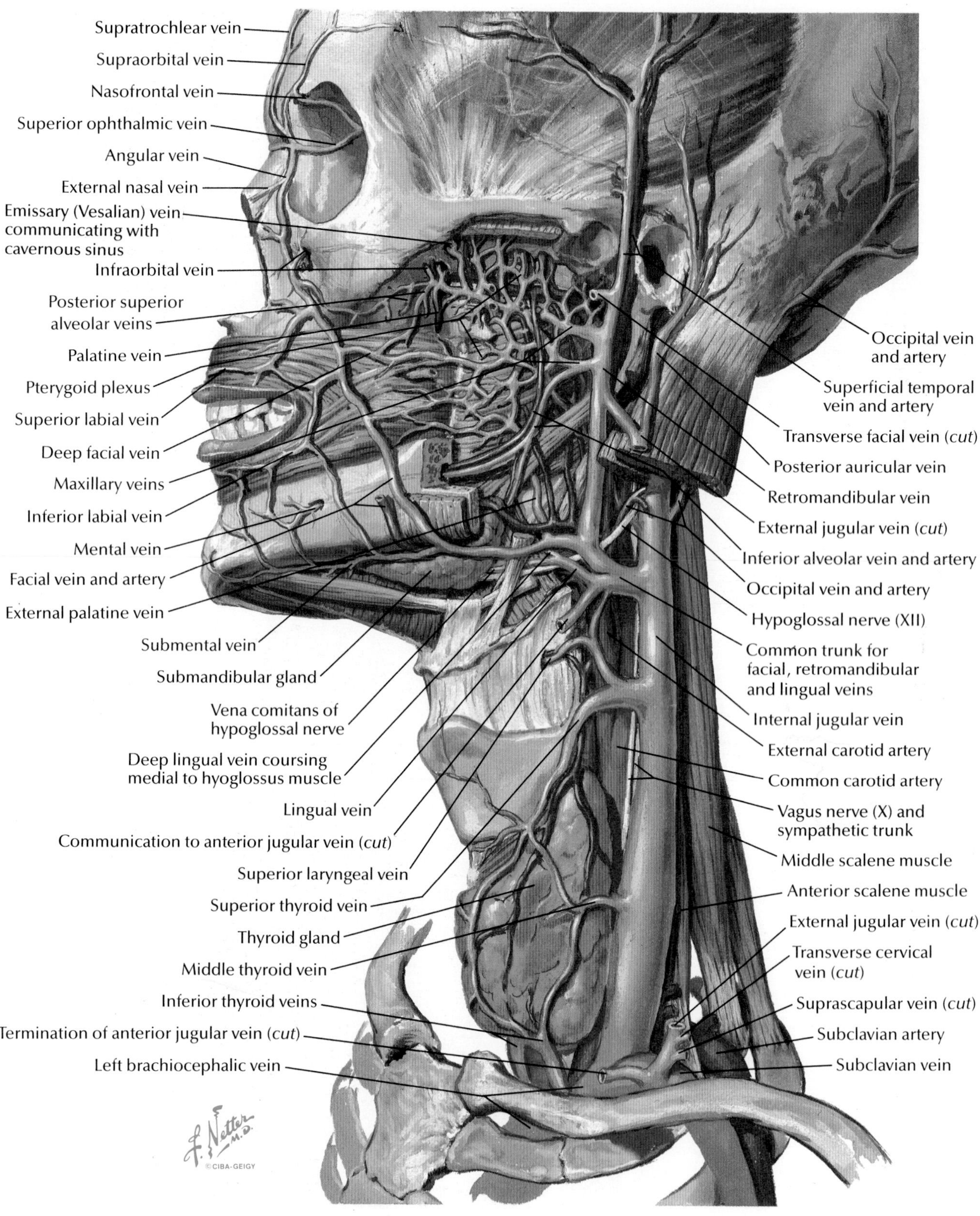

Supratrochlear vein

Supraorbital vein

Nasofrontal vein

Superior ophthalmic vein

Angular vein

External nasal vein

Emissary (Vesalian) vein communicating with cavernous sinus

Infraorbital vein

Posterior superior alveolar veins

Palatine vein

Pterygoid plexus

Superior labial vein

Deep facial vein

Maxillary veins

Inferior labial vein

Mental vein

Facial vein and artery

External palatine vein

Submental vein

Submandibular gland

Vena comitans of hypoglossal nerve

Deep lingual vein coursing medial to hyoglossus muscle

Lingual vein

Communication to anterior jugular vein (cut)

Superior laryngeal vein

Superior thyroid vein

Thyroid gland

Middle thyroid vein

Inferior thyroid veins

Termination of anterior jugular vein (cut)

Left brachiocephalic vein

Occipital vein and artery

Superficial temporal vein and artery

Transverse facial vein (cut)

Posterior auricular vein

Retromandibular vein

External jugular vein (cut)

Inferior alveolar vein and artery

Occipital vein and artery

Hypoglossal nerve (XII)

Common trunk for facial, retromandibular and lingual veins

Internal jugular vein

External carotid artery

Common carotid artery

Vagus nerve (X) and sympathetic trunk

Middle scalene muscle

Anterior scalene muscle

External jugular vein (cut)

Transverse cervical vein (cut)

Suprascapular vein (cut)

Subclavian artery

Subclavian vein

PLATE 64

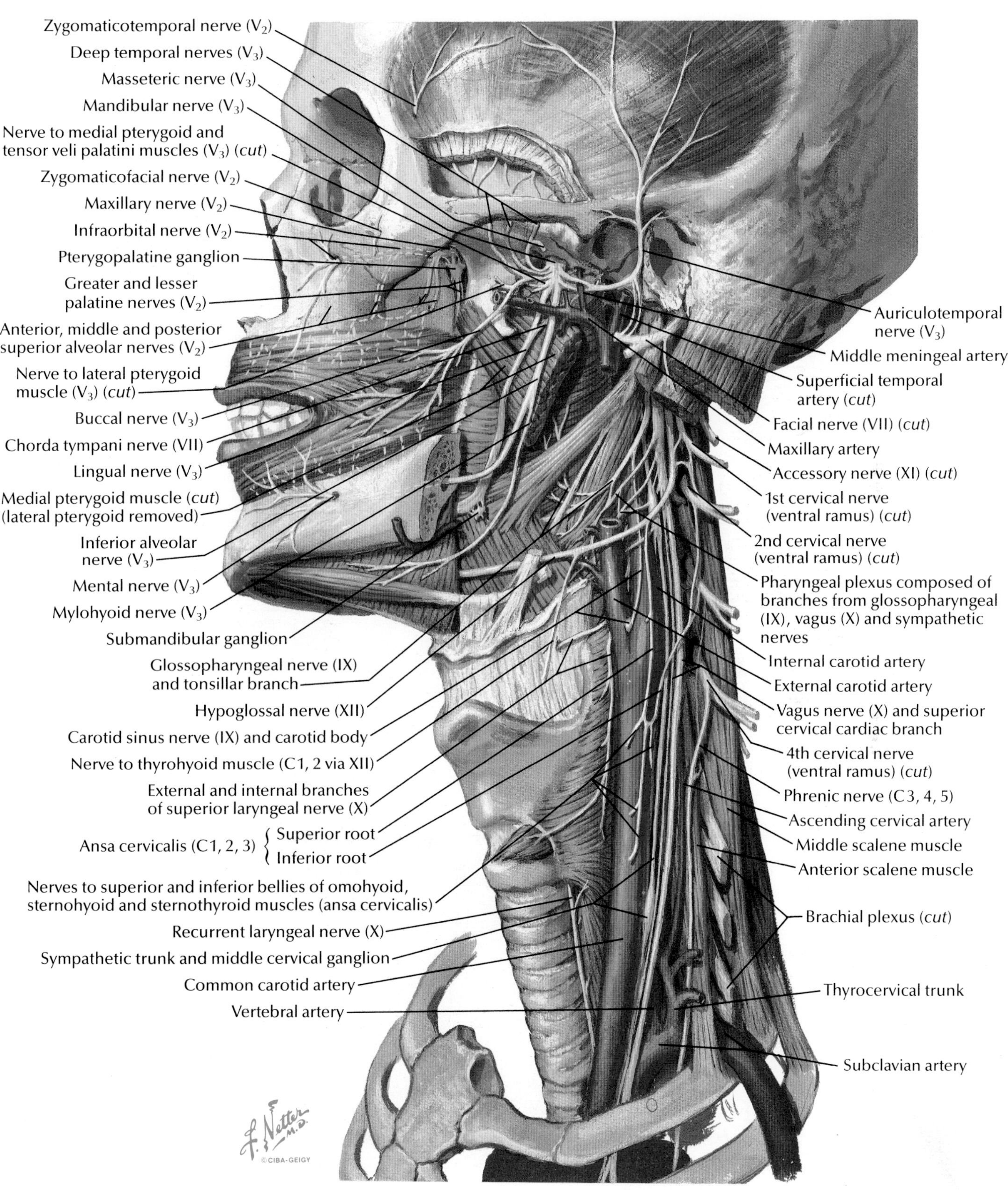

Zygomaticotemporal nerve (V₂)

Deep temporal nerves (V₃)

Masseteric nerve (V₃)

Mandibular nerve (V₃)

Nerve to medial pterygoid and tensor veli palatini muscles (V₃) (*cut*)

Zygomaticofacial nerve (V₂)

Maxillary nerve (V₂)

Infraorbital nerve (V₂)

Pterygopalatine ganglion

Greater and lesser palatine nerves (V₂)

Anterior, middle and posterior superior alveolar nerves (V₂)

Nerve to lateral pterygoid muscle (V₃) (*cut*)

Buccal nerve (V₃)

Chorda tympani nerve (VII)

Lingual nerve (V₃)

Medial pterygoid muscle (*cut*) (lateral pterygoid removed)

Inferior alveolar nerve (V₃)

Mental nerve (V₃)

Mylohyoid nerve (V₃)

Submandibular ganglion

Glossopharyngeal nerve (IX) and tonsillar branch

Hypoglossal nerve (XII)

Carotid sinus nerve (IX) and carotid body

Nerve to thyrohyoid muscle (C1, 2 via XII)

External and internal branches of superior laryngeal nerve (X)

Ansa cervicalis (C1, 2, 3) { Superior root / Inferior root }

Nerves to superior and inferior bellies of omohyoid, sternohyoid and sternothyroid muscles (ansa cervicalis)

Recurrent laryngeal nerve (X)

Sympathetic trunk and middle cervical ganglion

Common carotid artery

Vertebral artery

Auriculotemporal nerve (V₃)

Middle meningeal artery

Superficial temporal artery (*cut*)

Facial nerve (VII) (*cut*)

Maxillary artery

Accessory nerve (XI) (*cut*)

1st cervical nerve (ventral ramus) (*cut*)

2nd cervical nerve (ventral ramus) (*cut*)

Pharyngeal plexus composed of branches from glossopharyngeal (IX), vagus (X) and sympathetic nerves

Internal carotid artery

External carotid artery

Vagus nerve (X) and superior cervical cardiac branch

4th cervical nerve (ventral ramus) (*cut*)

Phrenic nerve (C3, 4, 5)

Ascending cervical artery

Middle scalene muscle

Anterior scalene muscle

Brachial plexus (*cut*)

Thyrocervical trunk

Subclavian artery

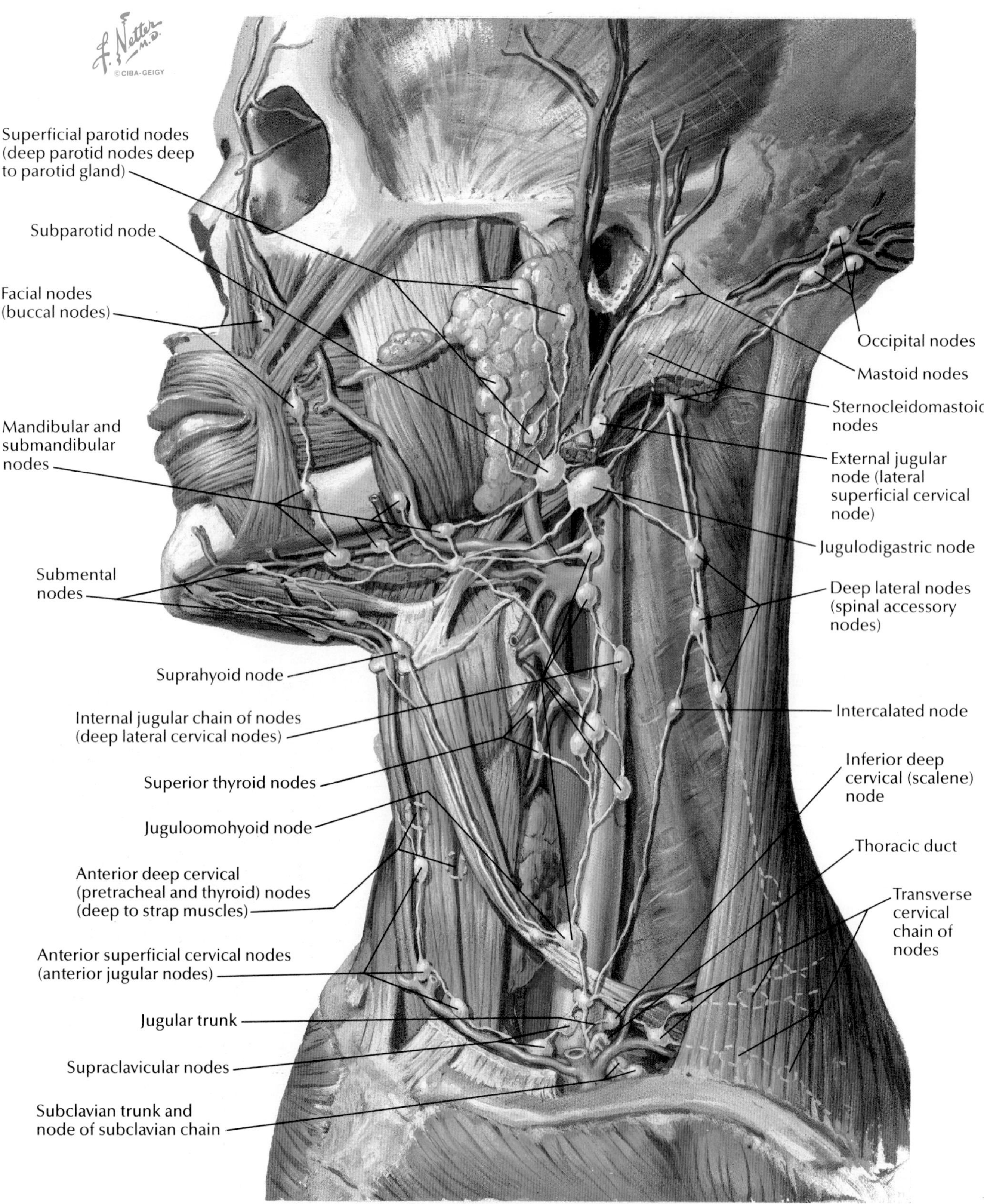

Superficial parotid nodes
(deep parotid nodes deep
to parotid gland)

Subparotid node

Facial nodes
(buccal nodes)

Mandibular and
submandibular
nodes

Submental
nodes

Suprahyoid node

Internal jugular chain of nodes
(deep lateral cervical nodes)

Superior thyroid nodes

Juguloomohyoid node

Anterior deep cervical
(pretracheal and thyroid) nodes
(deep to strap muscles)

Anterior superficial cervical nodes
(anterior jugular nodes)

Jugular trunk

Supraclavicular nodes

Subclavian trunk and
node of subclavian chain

Occipital nodes

Mastoid nodes

Sternocleidomastoid
nodes

External jugular
node (lateral
superficial cervical
node)

Jugulodigastric node

Deep lateral nodes
(spinal accessory
nodes)

Intercalated node

Inferior deep
cervical (scalene)
node

Thoracic duct

Transverse
cervical
chain of
nodes

PLATE 66

HEAD AND NECK

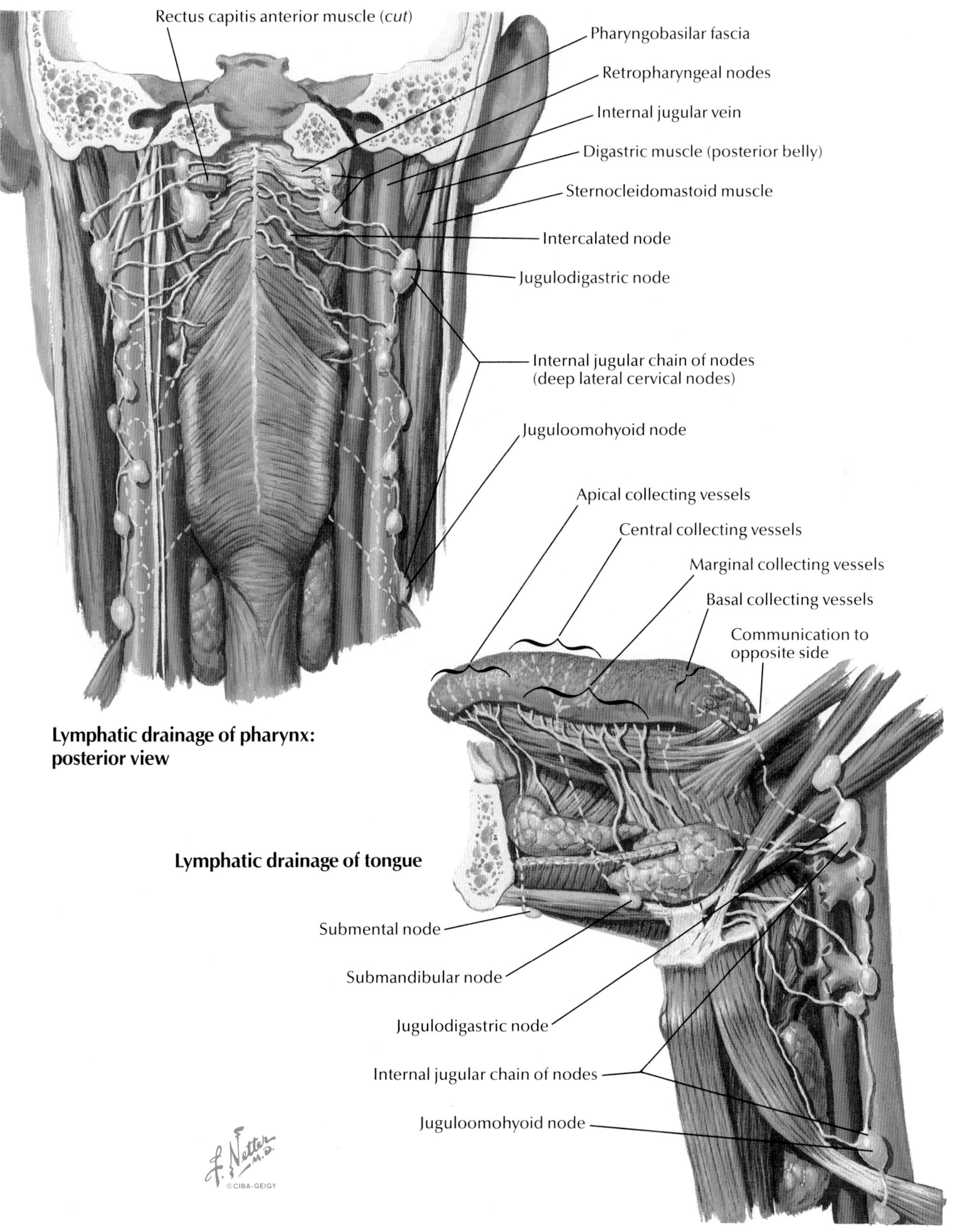

Rectus capitis anterior muscle (*cut*)

Pharyngobasilar fascia

Retropharyngeal nodes

Internal jugular vein

Digastric muscle (posterior belly)

Sternocleidomastoid muscle

Intercalated node

Jugulodigastric node

Internal jugular chain of nodes
(deep lateral cervical nodes)

Juguloomohyoid node

Apical collecting vessels

Central collecting vessels

Marginal collecting vessels

Basal collecting vessels

Communication to
opposite side

**Lymphatic drainage of pharynx:
posterior view**

Lymphatic drainage of tongue

Submental node

Submandibular node

Jugulodigastric node

Internal jugular chain of nodes

Juguloomohyoid node

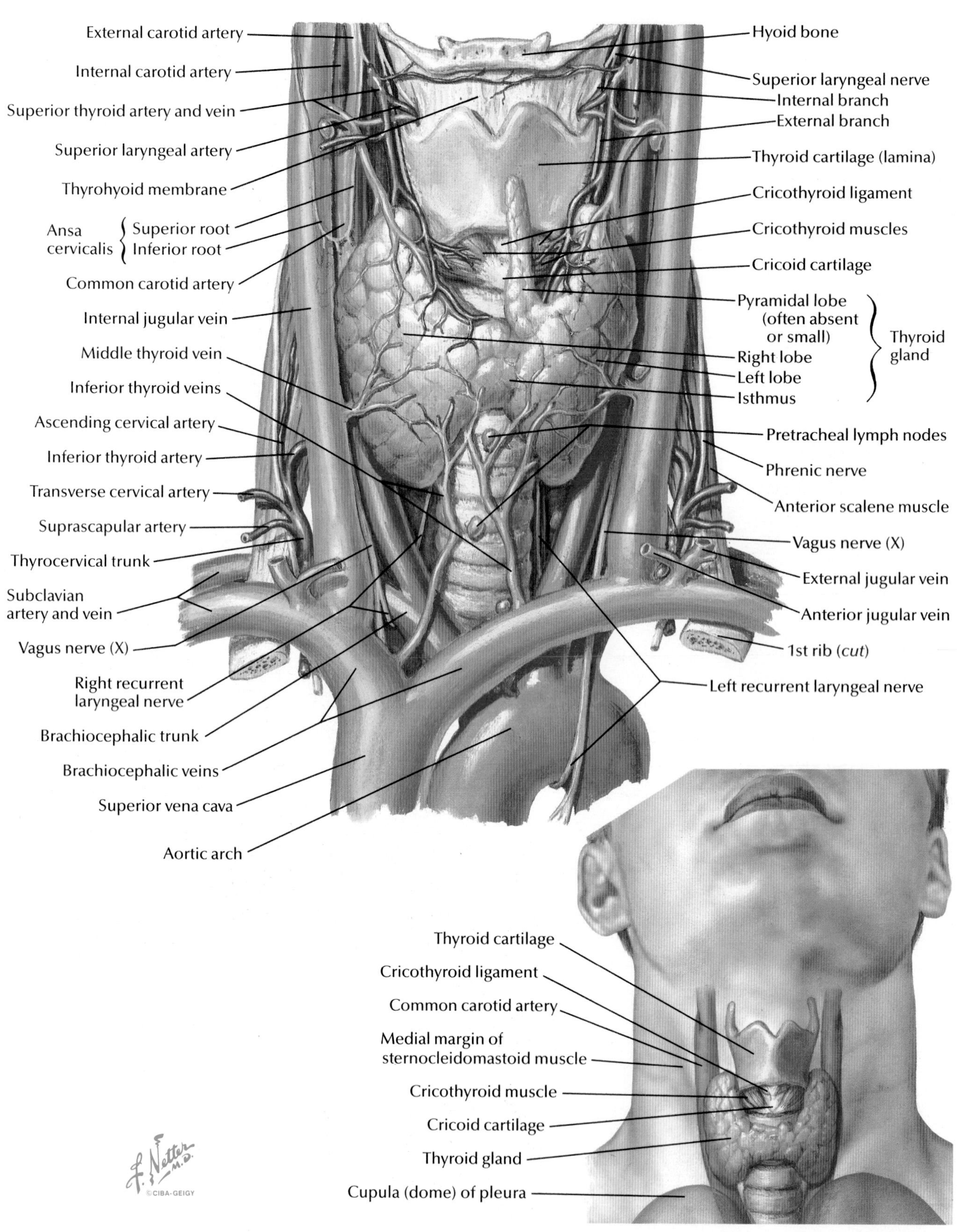

External carotid artery

Internal carotid artery

Superior thyroid artery and vein

Superior laryngeal artery

Thyrohyoid membrane

Ansa cervicalis { Superior root / Inferior root }

Common carotid artery

Internal jugular vein

Middle thyroid vein

Inferior thyroid veins

Ascending cervical artery

Inferior thyroid artery

Transverse cervical artery

Suprascapular artery

Thyrocervical trunk

Subclavian artery and vein

Vagus nerve (X)

Right recurrent laryngeal nerve

Brachiocephalic trunk

Brachiocephalic veins

Superior vena cava

Aortic arch

Hyoid bone

Superior laryngeal nerve
Internal branch
External branch

Thyroid cartilage (lamina)

Cricothyroid ligament

Cricothyroid muscles

Cricoid cartilage

Pyramidal lobe (often absent or small)
Right lobe
Left lobe
Isthmus
} Thyroid gland

Pretracheal lymph nodes

Phrenic nerve

Anterior scalene muscle

Vagus nerve (X)

External jugular vein

Anterior jugular vein

1st rib (*cut*)

Left recurrent laryngeal nerve

Thyroid cartilage

Cricothyroid ligament

Common carotid artery

Medial margin of sternocleidomastoid muscle

Cricothyroid muscle

Cricoid cartilage

Thyroid gland

Cupula (dome) of pleura

PLATE 68

HEAD AND NECK

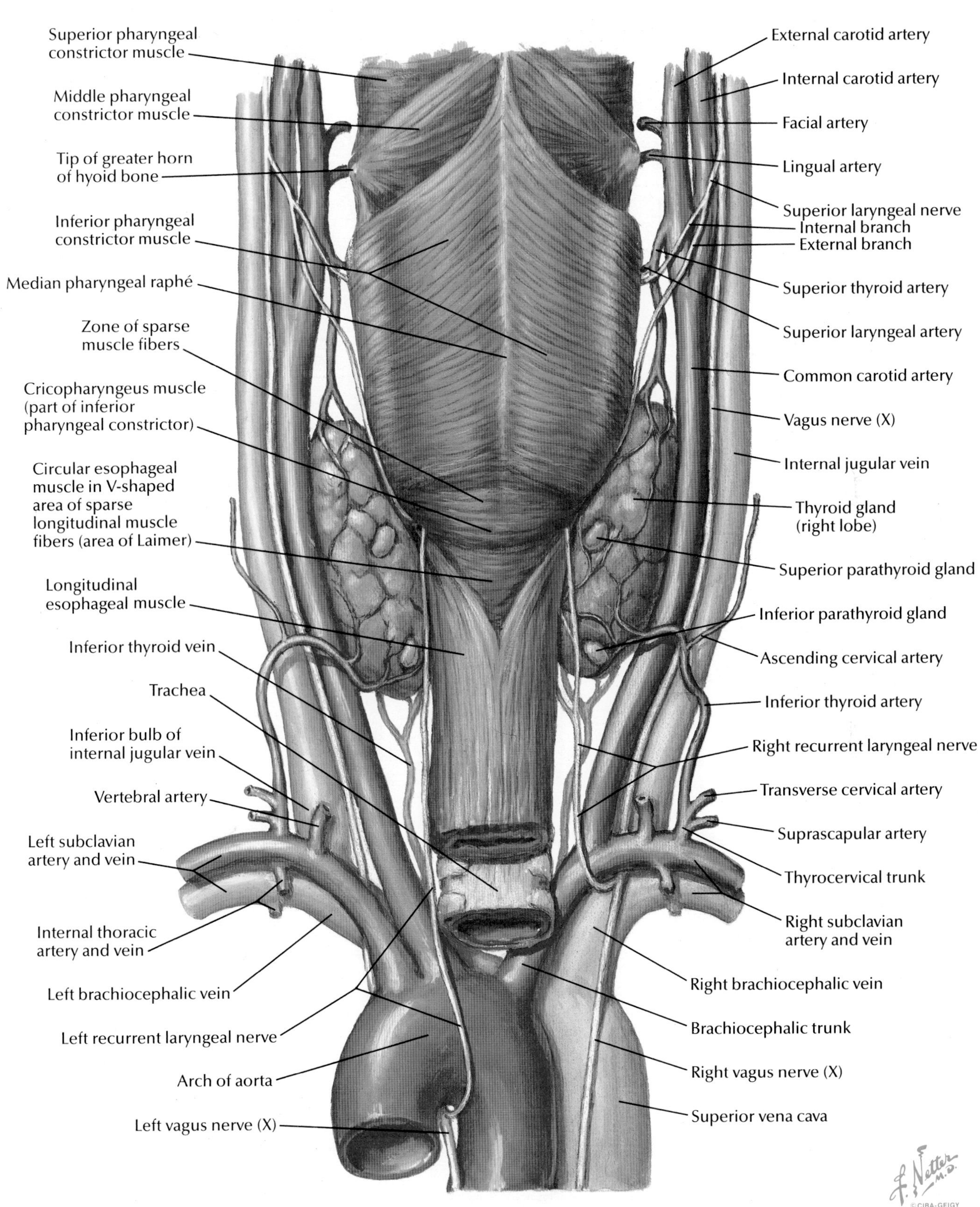

Superior pharyngeal constrictor muscle

Middle pharyngeal constrictor muscle

Tip of greater horn of hyoid bone

Inferior pharyngeal constrictor muscle

Median pharyngeal raphé

Zone of sparse muscle fibers

Cricopharyngeus muscle (part of inferior pharyngeal constrictor)

Circular esophageal muscle in V-shaped area of sparse longitudinal muscle fibers (area of Laimer)

Longitudinal esophageal muscle

Inferior thyroid vein

Trachea

Inferior bulb of internal jugular vein

Vertebral artery

Left subclavian artery and vein

Internal thoracic artery and vein

Left brachiocephalic vein

Left recurrent laryngeal nerve

Arch of aorta

Left vagus nerve (X)

External carotid artery

Internal carotid artery

Facial artery

Lingual artery

Superior laryngeal nerve
Internal branch
External branch

Superior thyroid artery

Superior laryngeal artery

Common carotid artery

Vagus nerve (X)

Internal jugular vein

Thyroid gland (right lobe)

Superior parathyroid gland

Inferior parathyroid gland

Ascending cervical artery

Inferior thyroid artery

Right recurrent laryngeal nerve

Transverse cervical artery

Suprascapular artery

Thyrocervical trunk

Right subclavian artery and vein

Right brachiocephalic vein

Brachiocephalic trunk

Right vagus nerve (X)

Superior vena cava

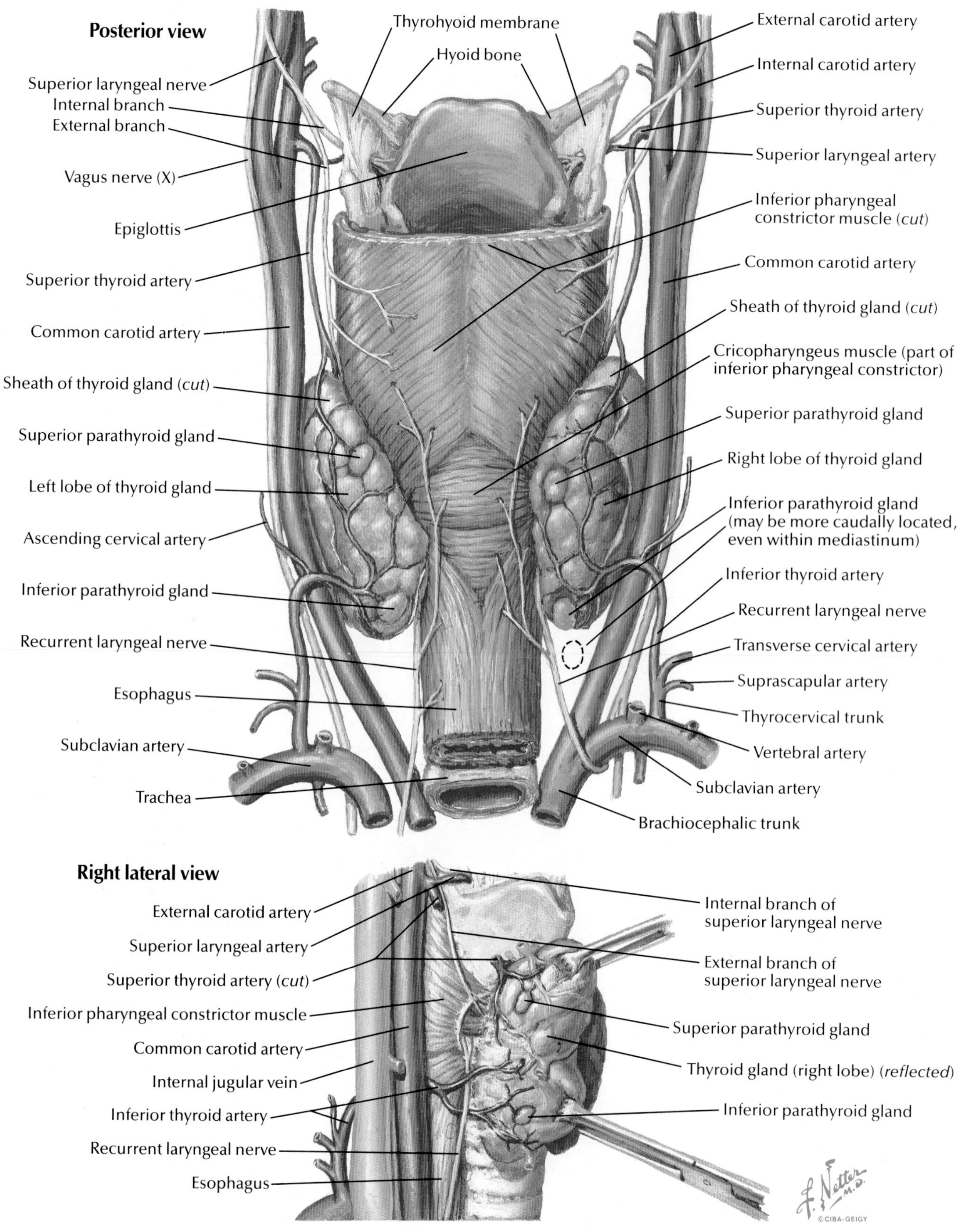

Posterior view

Superior laryngeal nerve
Internal branch
External branch

Vagus nerve (X)

Epiglottis

Superior thyroid artery

Common carotid artery

Sheath of thyroid gland (*cut*)

Superior parathyroid gland

Left lobe of thyroid gland

Ascending cervical artery

Inferior parathyroid gland

Recurrent laryngeal nerve

Esophagus

Subclavian artery

Trachea

Thyrohyoid membrane
Hyoid bone

External carotid artery

Internal carotid artery

Superior thyroid artery

Superior laryngeal artery

Inferior pharyngeal constrictor muscle (*cut*)

Common carotid artery

Sheath of thyroid gland (*cut*)

Cricopharyngeus muscle (part of inferior pharyngeal constrictor)

Superior parathyroid gland

Right lobe of thyroid gland

Inferior parathyroid gland (may be more caudally located, even within mediastinum)

Inferior thyroid artery

Recurrent laryngeal nerve

Transverse cervical artery

Suprascapular artery

Thyrocervical trunk

Vertebral artery

Subclavian artery

Brachiocephalic trunk

Right lateral view

External carotid artery

Superior laryngeal artery

Superior thyroid artery (*cut*)

Inferior pharyngeal constrictor muscle

Common carotid artery

Internal jugular vein

Inferior thyroid artery

Recurrent laryngeal nerve

Esophagus

Internal branch of superior laryngeal nerve

External branch of superior laryngeal nerve

Superior parathyroid gland

Thyroid gland (right lobe) (*reflected*)

Inferior parathyroid gland

PLATE 70

HEAD AND NECK

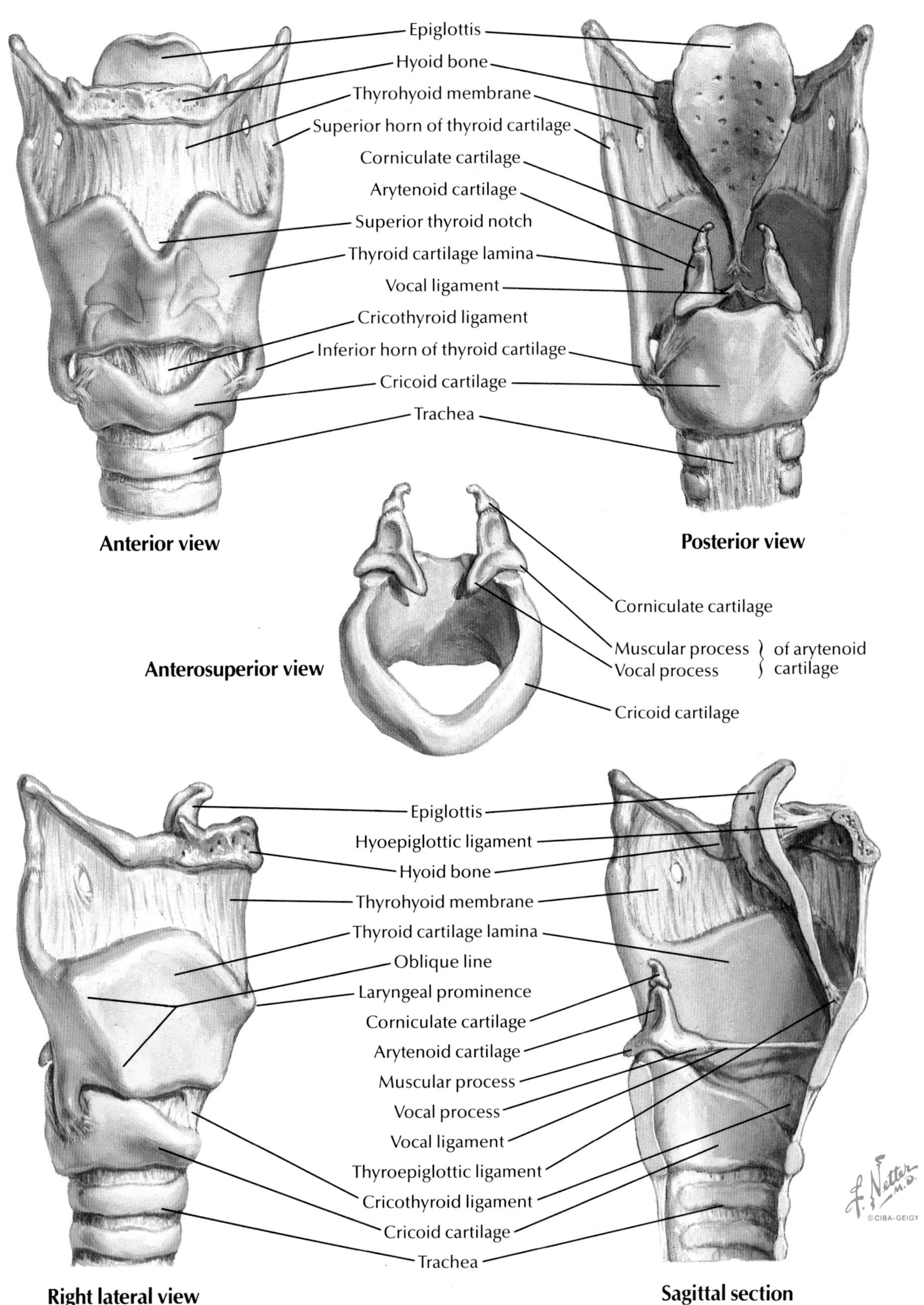

Epiglottis
Hyoid bone
Thyrohyoid membrane
Superior horn of thyroid cartilage
Corniculate cartilage
Arytenoid cartilage
Superior thyroid notch
Thyroid cartilage lamina
Vocal ligament
Cricothyroid ligament
Inferior horn of thyroid cartilage
Cricoid cartilage
Trachea

Anterior view

Posterior view

Anterosuperior view

Corniculate cartilage
Muscular process } of arytenoid
Vocal process } cartilage
Cricoid cartilage

Epiglottis
Hyoepiglottic ligament
Hyoid bone
Thyrohyoid membrane
Thyroid cartilage lamina
Oblique line
Laryngeal prominence
Corniculate cartilage
Arytenoid cartilage
Muscular process
Vocal process
Vocal ligament
Thyroepiglottic ligament
Cricothyroid ligament
Cricoid cartilage
Trachea

Right lateral view

Sagittal section

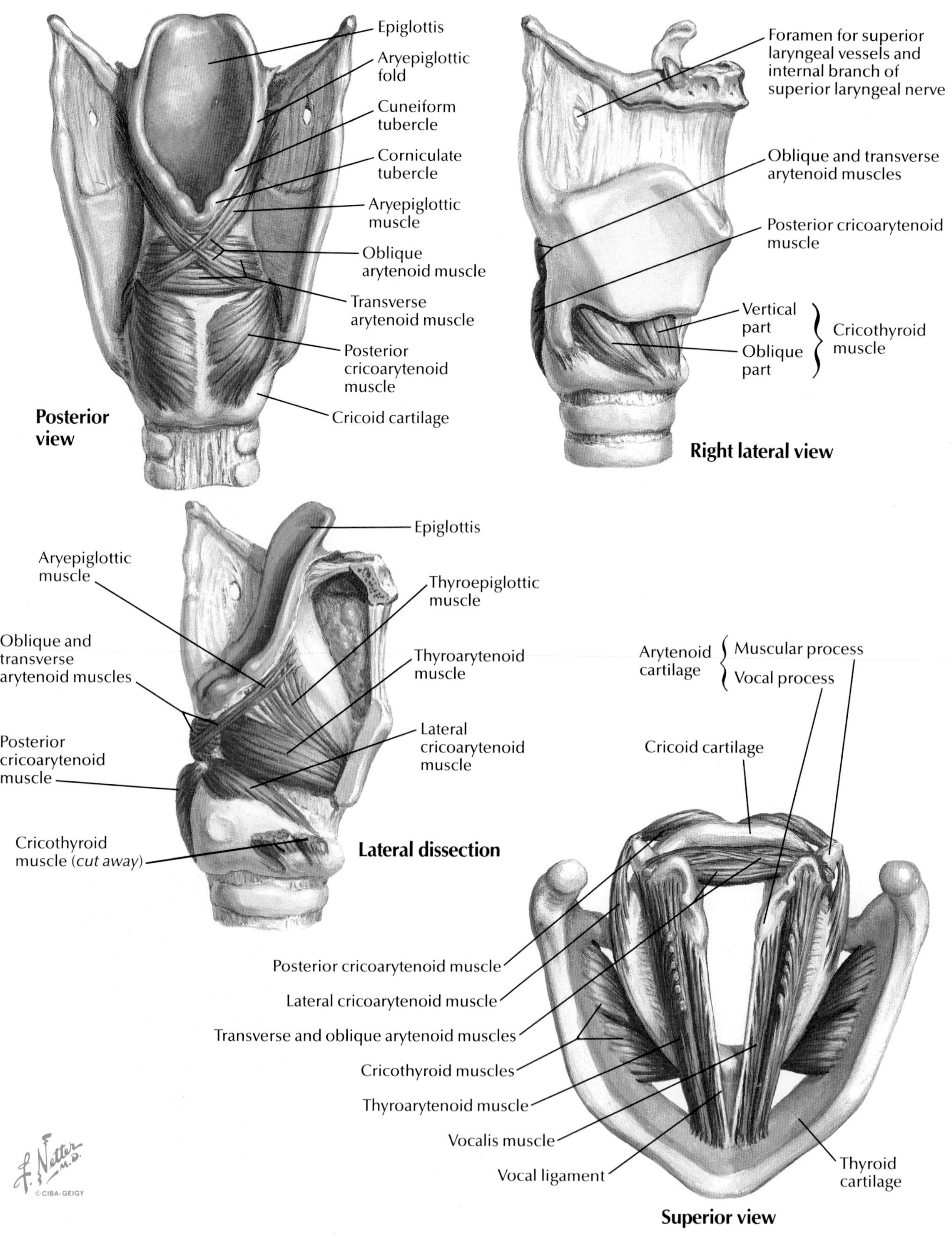

Epiglottis

Aryepiglottic fold

Cuneiform tubercle

Corniculate tubercle

Aryepiglottic muscle

Oblique arytenoid muscle

Transverse arytenoid muscle

Posterior cricoarytenoid muscle

Cricoid cartilage

Posterior view

Foramen for superior laryngeal vessels and internal branch of superior laryngeal nerve

Oblique and transverse arytenoid muscles

Posterior cricoarytenoid muscle

Vertical part

Oblique part

Cricothyroid muscle

Right lateral view

Aryepiglottic muscle

Oblique and transverse arytenoid muscles

Posterior cricoarytenoid muscle

Cricothyroid muscle (*cut away*)

Epiglottis

Thyroepiglottic muscle

Thyroarytenoid muscle

Lateral cricoarytenoid muscle

Lateral dissection

Arytenoid cartilage { Muscular process / Vocal process

Cricoid cartilage

Posterior cricoarytenoid muscle

Lateral cricoarytenoid muscle

Transverse and oblique arytenoid muscles

Cricothyroid muscles

Thyroarytenoid muscle

Vocalis muscle

Vocal ligament

Thyroid cartilage

Superior view

© CIBA-GEIGY

PLATE 72   **HEAD AND NECK**

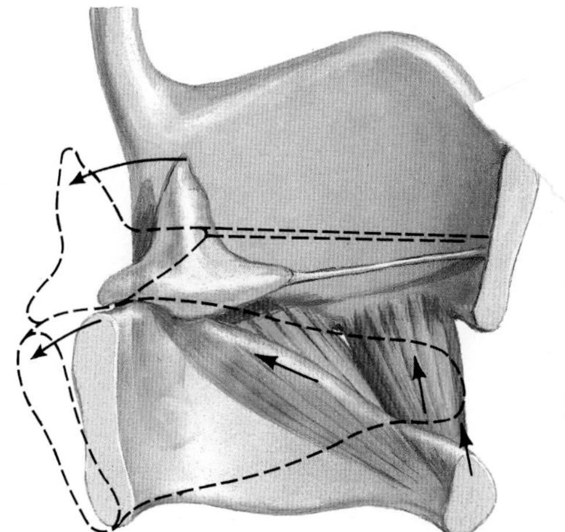

Action of cricothyroid muscles

Lengthening (tension) of vocal folds

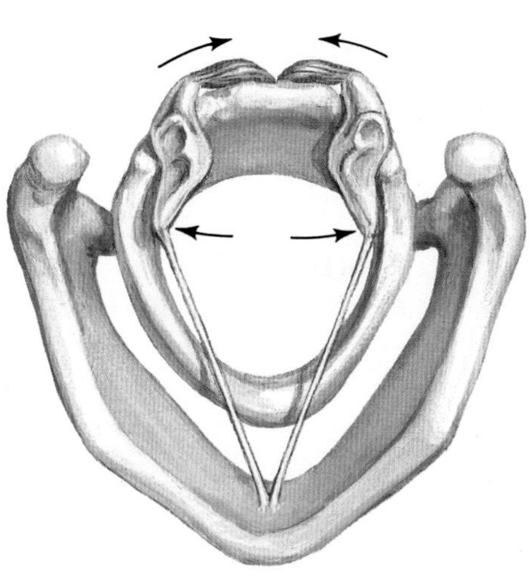

Action of posterior cricoarytenoid muscles

Abduction of vocal folds

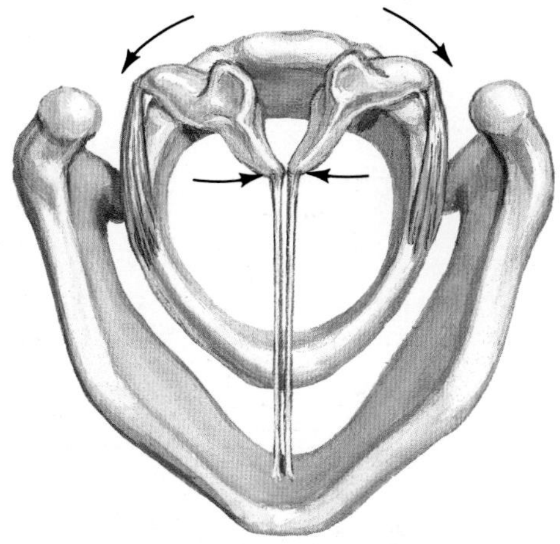

Action of lateral cricoarytenoid muscles

Adduction of vocal folds

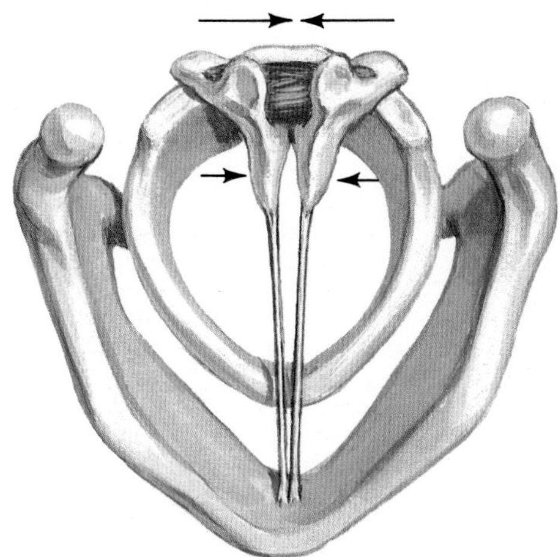

Action of transverse arytenoid muscle

Adduction of vocal folds

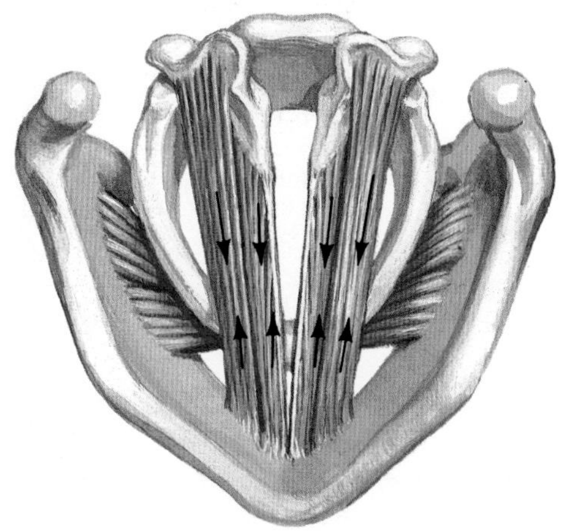

Action of vocalis and thyroarytenoid muscles

Shortening (relaxation) of vocal folds

Nerves of Larynx

SEE ALSO PLATES 68, 69, 70, 223

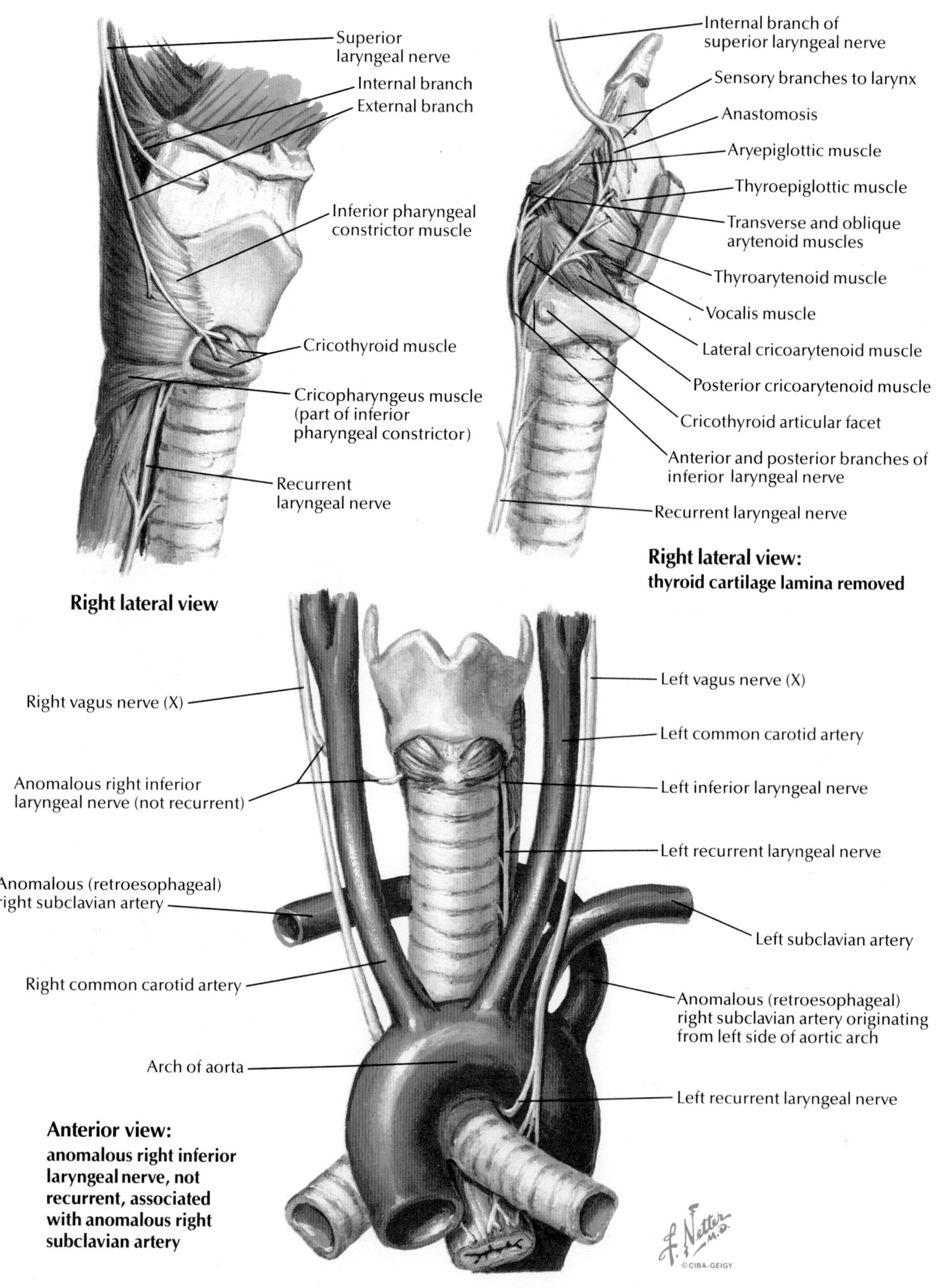

Superior laryngeal nerve

Internal branch

External branch

Inferior pharyngeal constrictor muscle

Cricothyroid muscle

Cricopharyngeus muscle (part of inferior pharyngeal constrictor)

Recurrent laryngeal nerve

Right lateral view

Internal branch of superior laryngeal nerve

Sensory branches to larynx

Anastomosis

Aryepiglottic muscle

Thyroepiglottic muscle

Transverse and oblique arytenoid muscles

Thyroarytenoid muscle

Vocalis muscle

Lateral cricoarytenoid muscle

Posterior cricoarytenoid muscle

Cricothyroid articular facet

Anterior and posterior branches of inferior laryngeal nerve

Recurrent laryngeal nerve

Right lateral view: thyroid cartilage lamina removed

Right vagus nerve (X)

Anomalous right inferior laryngeal nerve (not recurrent)

Anomalous (retroesophageal) right subclavian artery

Right common carotid artery

Arch of aorta

Anterior view: anomalous right inferior laryngeal nerve, not recurrent, associated with anomalous right subclavian artery

Left vagus nerve (X)

Left common carotid artery

Left inferior laryngeal nerve

Left recurrent laryngeal nerve

Left subclavian artery

Anomalous (retroesophageal) right subclavian artery originating from left side of aortic arch

Left recurrent laryngeal nerve

PLATE 74

HEAD AND NECK

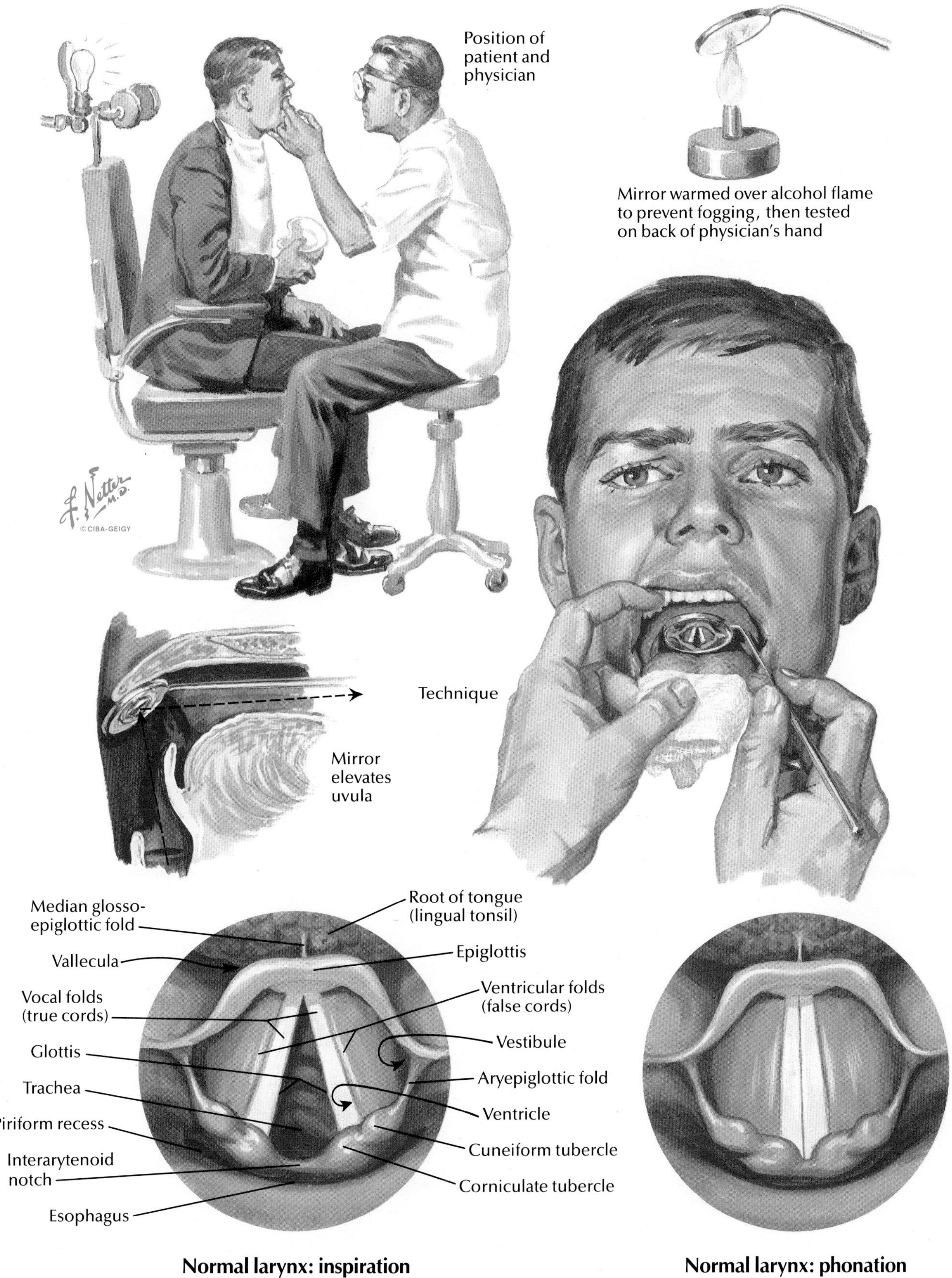

Position of patient and physician

Mirror warmed over alcohol flame to prevent fogging, then tested on back of physician's hand

Technique

Mirror elevates uvula

Normal larynx: inspiration

Median glosso-epiglottic fold

Vallecula

Vocal folds (true cords)

Glottis

Trachea

Piriform recess

Interarytenoid notch

Esophagus

Root of tongue (lingual tonsil)

Epiglottis

Ventricular folds (false cords)

Vestibule

Aryepiglottic fold

Ventricle

Cuneiform tubercle

Corniculate tubercle

Normal larynx: phonation

Eyelids

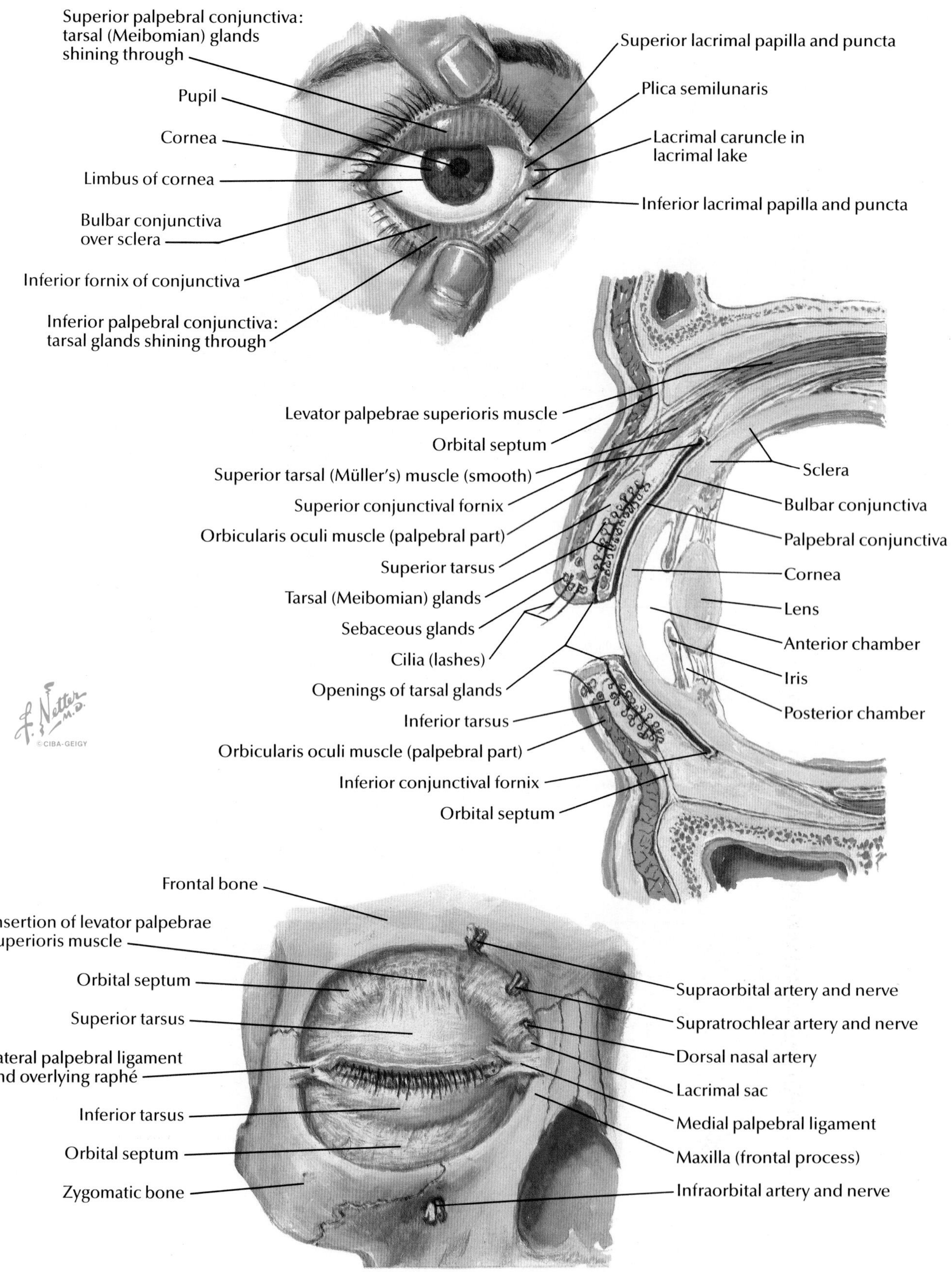

Superior palpebral conjunctiva: tarsal (Meibomian) glands shining through

Pupil

Cornea

Limbus of cornea

Bulbar conjunctiva over sclera

Inferior fornix of conjunctiva

Inferior palpebral conjunctiva: tarsal glands shining through

Superior lacrimal papilla and puncta

Plica semilunaris

Lacrimal caruncle in lacrimal lake

Inferior lacrimal papilla and puncta

Levator palpebrae superioris muscle

Orbital septum

Superior tarsal (Müller's) muscle (smooth)

Superior conjunctival fornix

Orbicularis oculi muscle (palpebral part)

Superior tarsus

Tarsal (Meibomian) glands

Sebaceous glands

Cilia (lashes)

Openings of tarsal glands

Inferior tarsus

Orbicularis oculi muscle (palpebral part)

Inferior conjunctival fornix

Orbital septum

Sclera

Bulbar conjunctiva

Palpebral conjunctiva

Cornea

Lens

Anterior chamber

Iris

Posterior chamber

Frontal bone

Insertion of levator palpebrae superioris muscle

Orbital septum

Superior tarsus

Lateral palpebral ligament and overlying raphé

Inferior tarsus

Orbital septum

Zygomatic bone

Supraorbital artery and nerve

Supratrochlear artery and nerve

Dorsal nasal artery

Lacrimal sac

Medial palpebral ligament

Maxilla (frontal process)

Infraorbital artery and nerve

PLATE 76   **HEAD AND NECK**

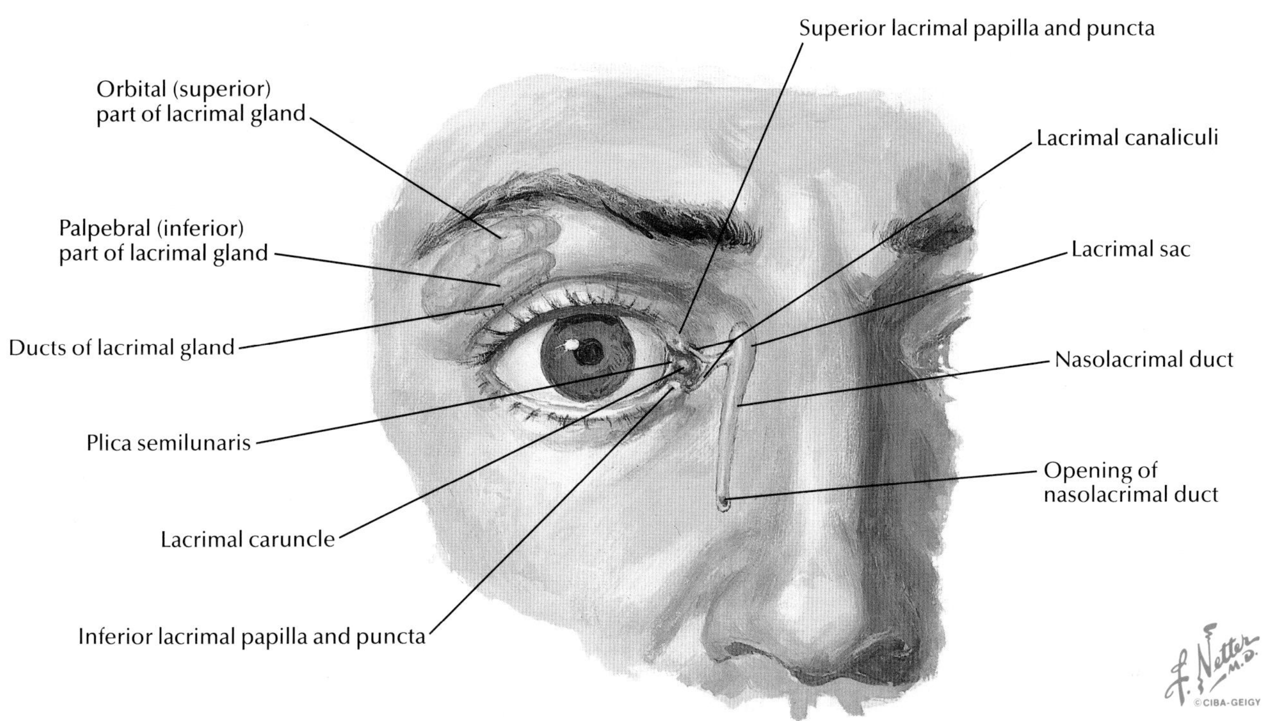

Orbital (superior) part of lacrimal gland

Palpebral (inferior) part of lacrimal gland

Ducts of lacrimal gland

Plica semilunaris

Lacrimal caruncle

Inferior lacrimal papilla and puncta

Superior lacrimal papilla and puncta

Lacrimal canaliculi

Lacrimal sac

Nasolacrimal duct

Opening of nasolacrimal duct

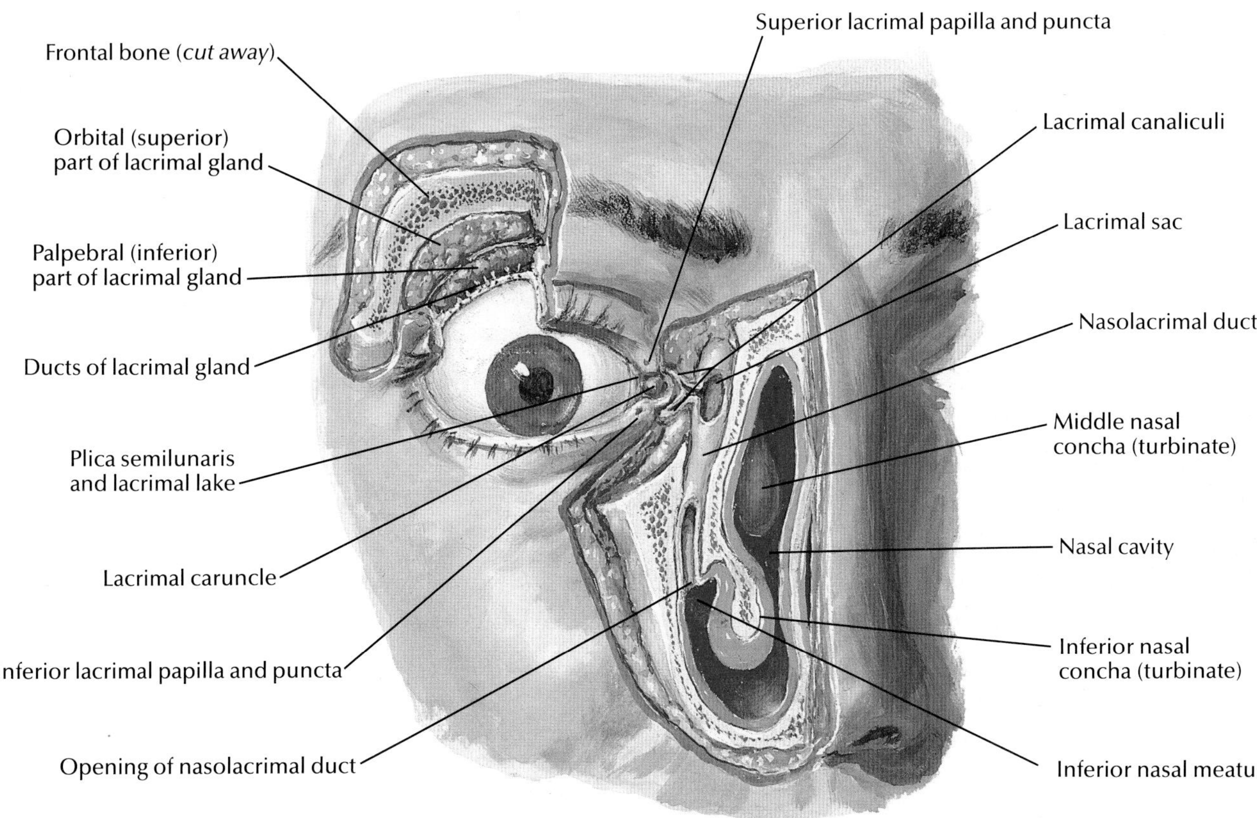

Frontal bone (*cut away*)

Orbital (superior) part of lacrimal gland

Palpebral (inferior) part of lacrimal gland

Ducts of lacrimal gland

Plica semilunaris and lacrimal lake

Lacrimal caruncle

Inferior lacrimal papilla and puncta

Opening of nasolacrimal duct

Superior lacrimal papilla and puncta

Lacrimal canaliculi

Lacrimal sac

Nasolacrimal duct

Middle nasal concha (turbinate)

Nasal cavity

Inferior nasal concha (turbinate)

Inferior nasal meatus

Fascia of Orbit and Eyeball

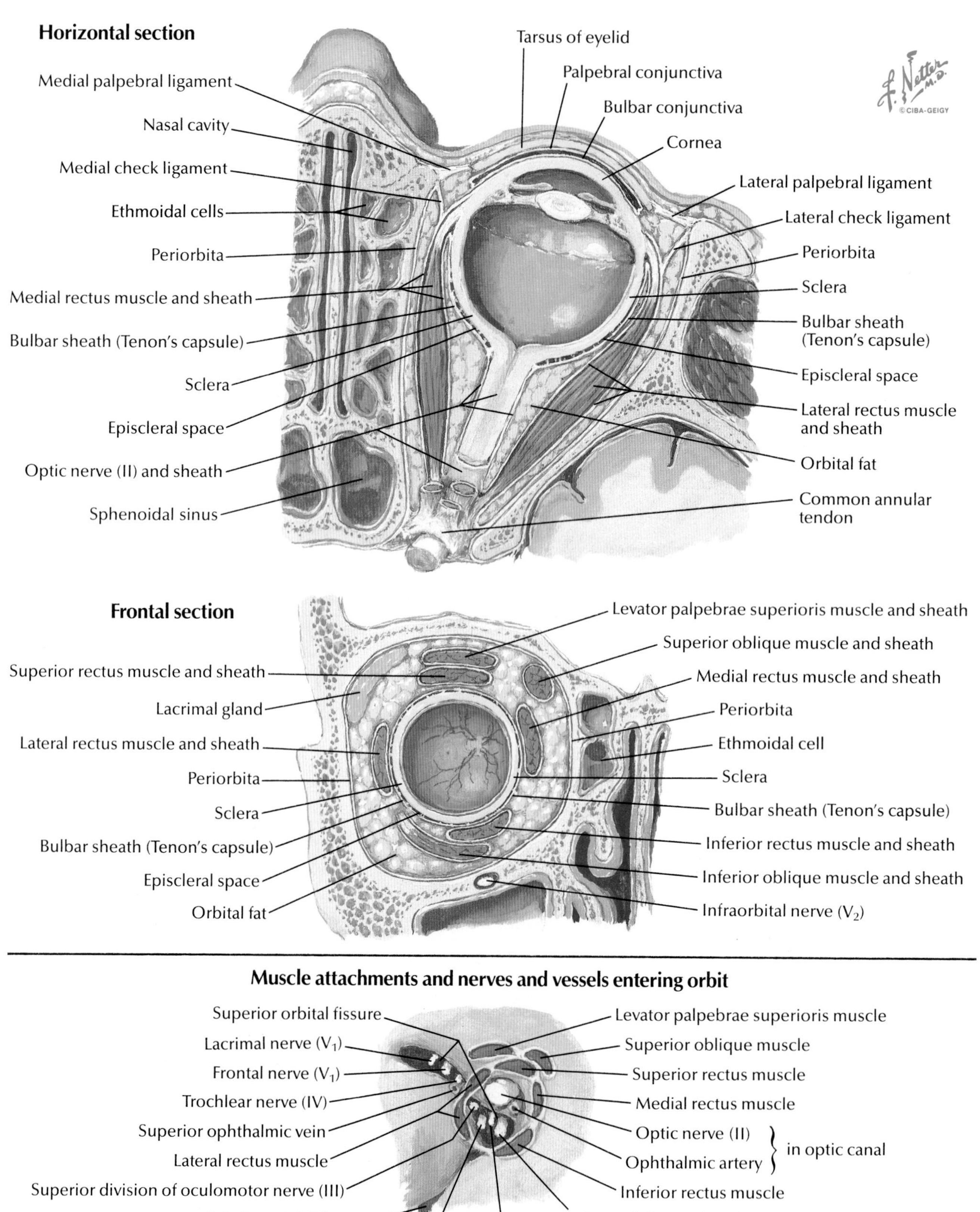

Horizontal section

Medial palpebral ligament
Nasal cavity
Medial check ligament
Ethmoidal cells
Periorbita
Medial rectus muscle and sheath
Bulbar sheath (Tenon's capsule)
Sclera
Episcleral space
Optic nerve (II) and sheath
Sphenoidal sinus

Tarsus of eyelid
Palpebral conjunctiva
Bulbar conjunctiva
Cornea
Lateral palpebral ligament
Lateral check ligament
Periorbita
Sclera
Bulbar sheath (Tenon's capsule)
Episcleral space
Lateral rectus muscle and sheath
Orbital fat
Common annular tendon

Frontal section

Superior rectus muscle and sheath
Lacrimal gland
Lateral rectus muscle and sheath
Periorbita
Sclera
Bulbar sheath (Tenon's capsule)
Episcleral space
Orbital fat

Levator palpebrae superioris muscle and sheath
Superior oblique muscle and sheath
Medial rectus muscle and sheath
Periorbita
Ethmoidal cell
Sclera
Bulbar sheath (Tenon's capsule)
Inferior rectus muscle and sheath
Inferior oblique muscle and sheath
Infraorbital nerve (V$_2$)

Muscle attachments and nerves and vessels entering orbit

Superior orbital fissure
Lacrimal nerve (V$_1$)
Frontal nerve (V$_1$)
Trochlear nerve (IV)
Superior ophthalmic vein
Lateral rectus muscle
Superior division of oculomotor nerve (III)
Inferior orbital fissure
Abducens nerve (VI)

Levator palpebrae superioris muscle
Superior oblique muscle
Superior rectus muscle
Medial rectus muscle
Optic nerve (II)
Ophthalmic artery } in optic canal
Inferior rectus muscle
Inferior division of oculomotor nerve (III)
Nasociliary nerve (V$_1$)

PLATE 78

HEAD AND NECK

Right lateral view

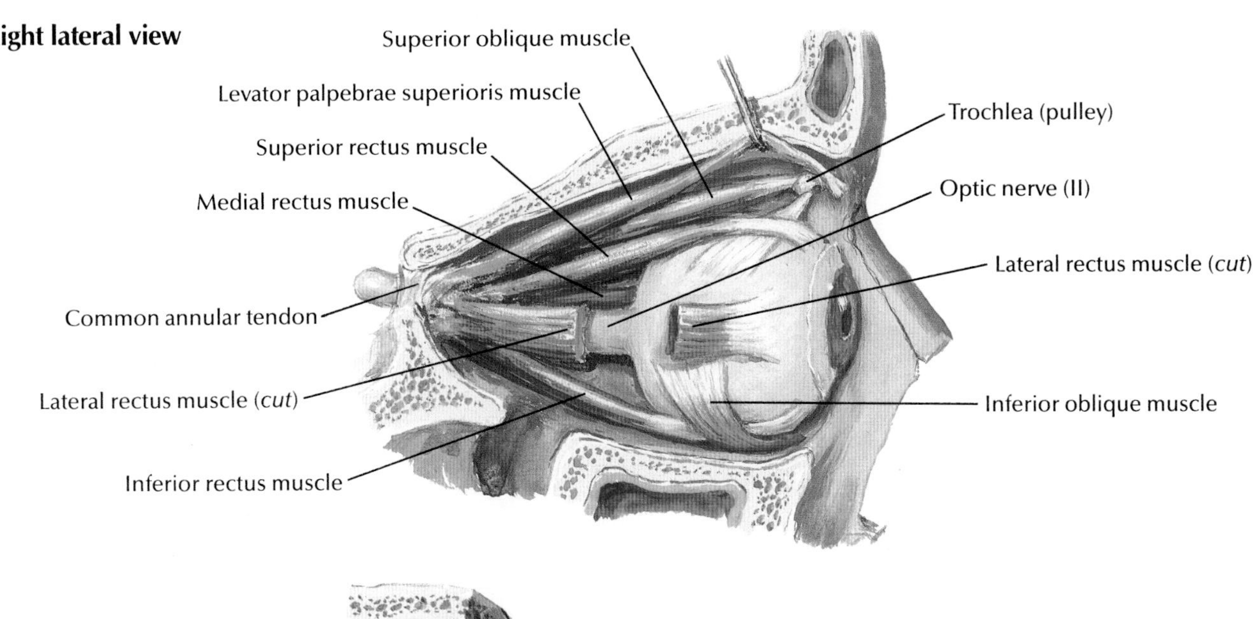

Superior oblique muscle

Levator palpebrae superioris muscle

Superior rectus muscle

Medial rectus muscle

Trochlea (pulley)

Optic nerve (II)

Lateral rectus muscle (*cut*)

Common annular tendon

Lateral rectus muscle (*cut*)

Inferior oblique muscle

Inferior rectus muscle

Superior view

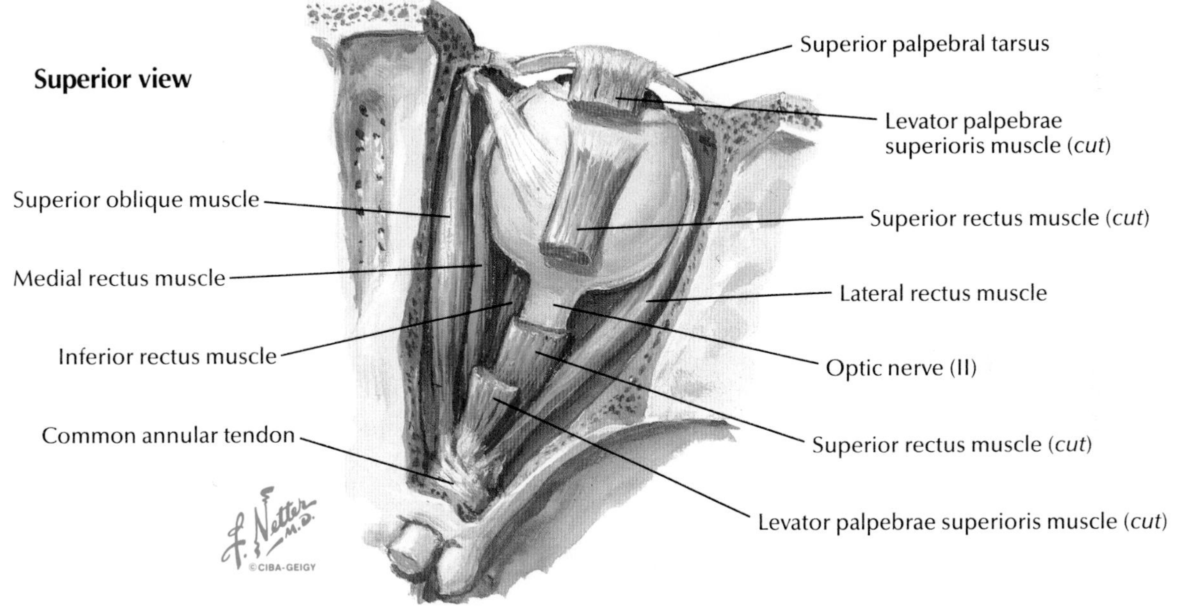

Superior palpebral tarsus

Levator palpebrae superioris muscle (*cut*)

Superior oblique muscle

Medial rectus muscle

Superior rectus muscle (*cut*)

Inferior rectus muscle

Lateral rectus muscle

Common annular tendon

Optic nerve (II)

Superior rectus muscle (*cut*)

Levator palpebrae superioris muscle (*cut*)

Innervation and action of extrinsic eye muscles: anterior view

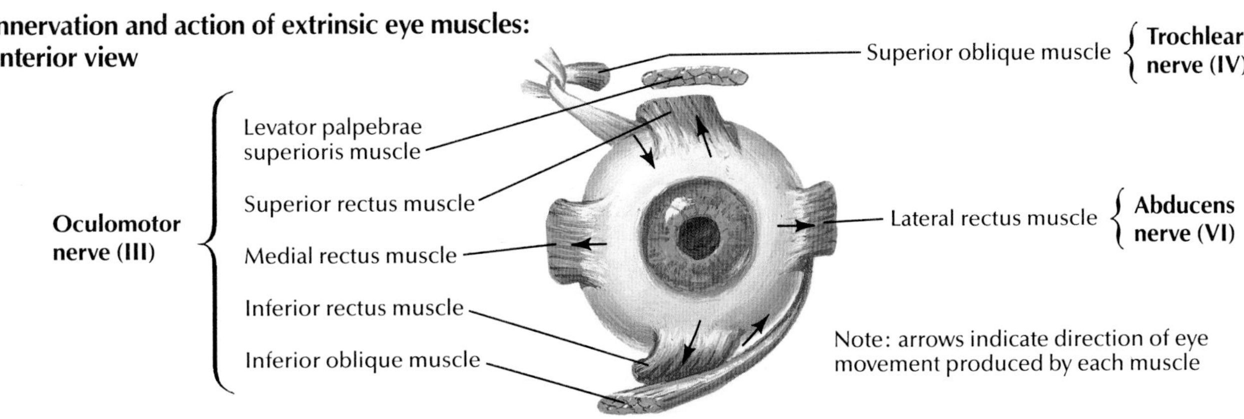

Superior oblique muscle { **Trochlear nerve (IV)**

Levator palpebrae superioris muscle

Superior rectus muscle

Oculomotor nerve (III)

Medial rectus muscle

Lateral rectus muscle { **Abducens nerve (VI)**

Inferior rectus muscle

Inferior oblique muscle

Note: arrows indicate direction of eye movement produced by each muscle

Arteries and Veins of Orbit and Eyelids

SEE ALSO PLATES 17, 98

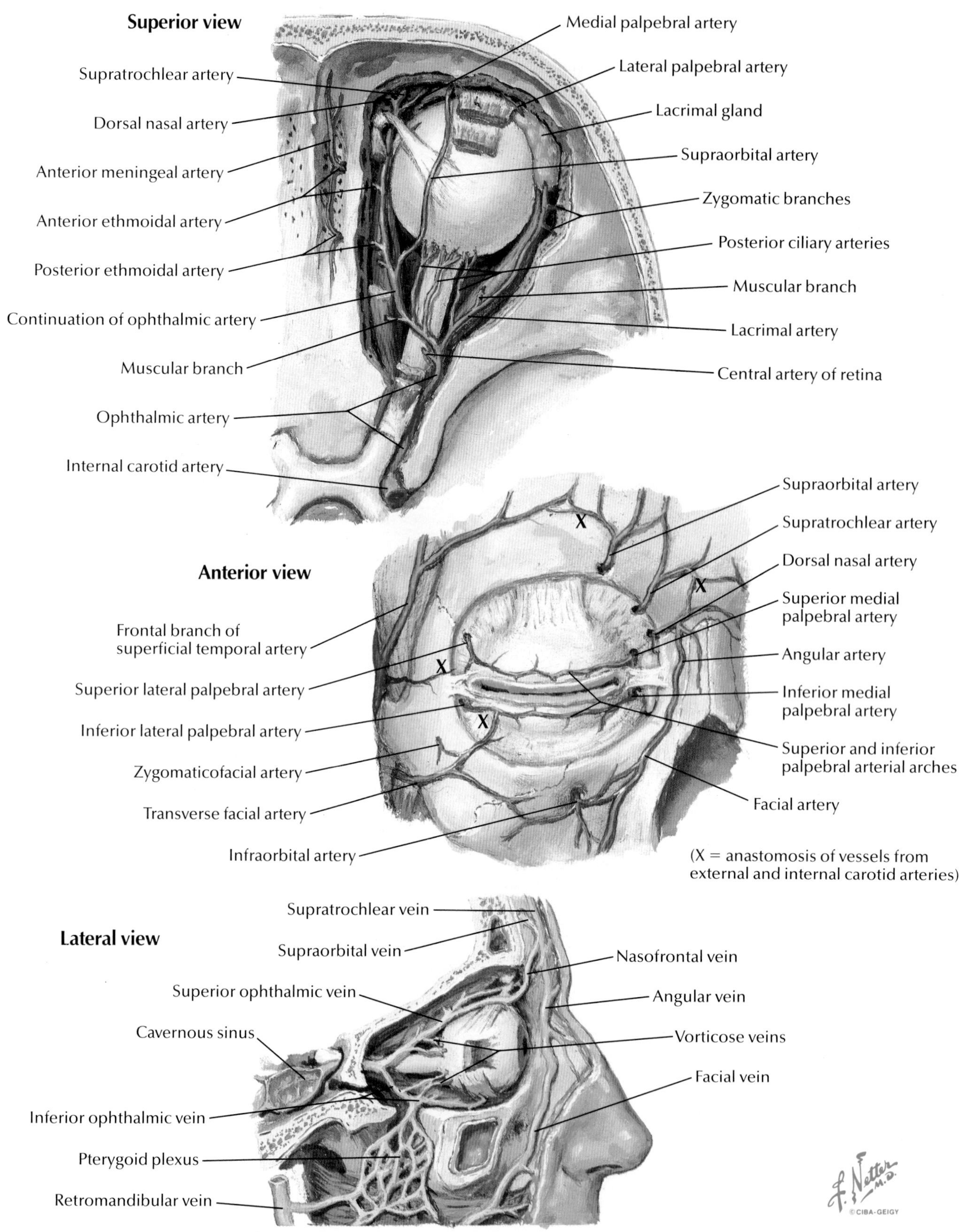

Superior view

Supratrochlear artery

Dorsal nasal artery

Anterior meningeal artery

Anterior ethmoidal artery

Posterior ethmoidal artery

Continuation of ophthalmic artery

Muscular branch

Ophthalmic artery

Internal carotid artery

Medial palpebral artery

Lateral palpebral artery

Lacrimal gland

Supraorbital artery

Zygomatic branches

Posterior ciliary arteries

Muscular branch

Lacrimal artery

Central artery of retina

Anterior view

Frontal branch of superficial temporal artery

Superior lateral palpebral artery

Inferior lateral palpebral artery

Zygomaticofacial artery

Transverse facial artery

Infraorbital artery

Supraorbital artery

Supratrochlear artery

Dorsal nasal artery

Superior medial palpebral artery

Angular artery

Inferior medial palpebral artery

Superior and inferior palpebral arterial arches

Facial artery

(X = anastomosis of vessels from external and internal carotid arteries)

Lateral view

Supratrochlear vein

Supraorbital vein

Superior ophthalmic vein

Cavernous sinus

Inferior ophthalmic vein

Pterygoid plexus

Retromandibular vein

Nasofrontal vein

Angular vein

Vorticose veins

Facial vein

Nerves of Orbit

SEE ALSO PLATES 40, 115, 126

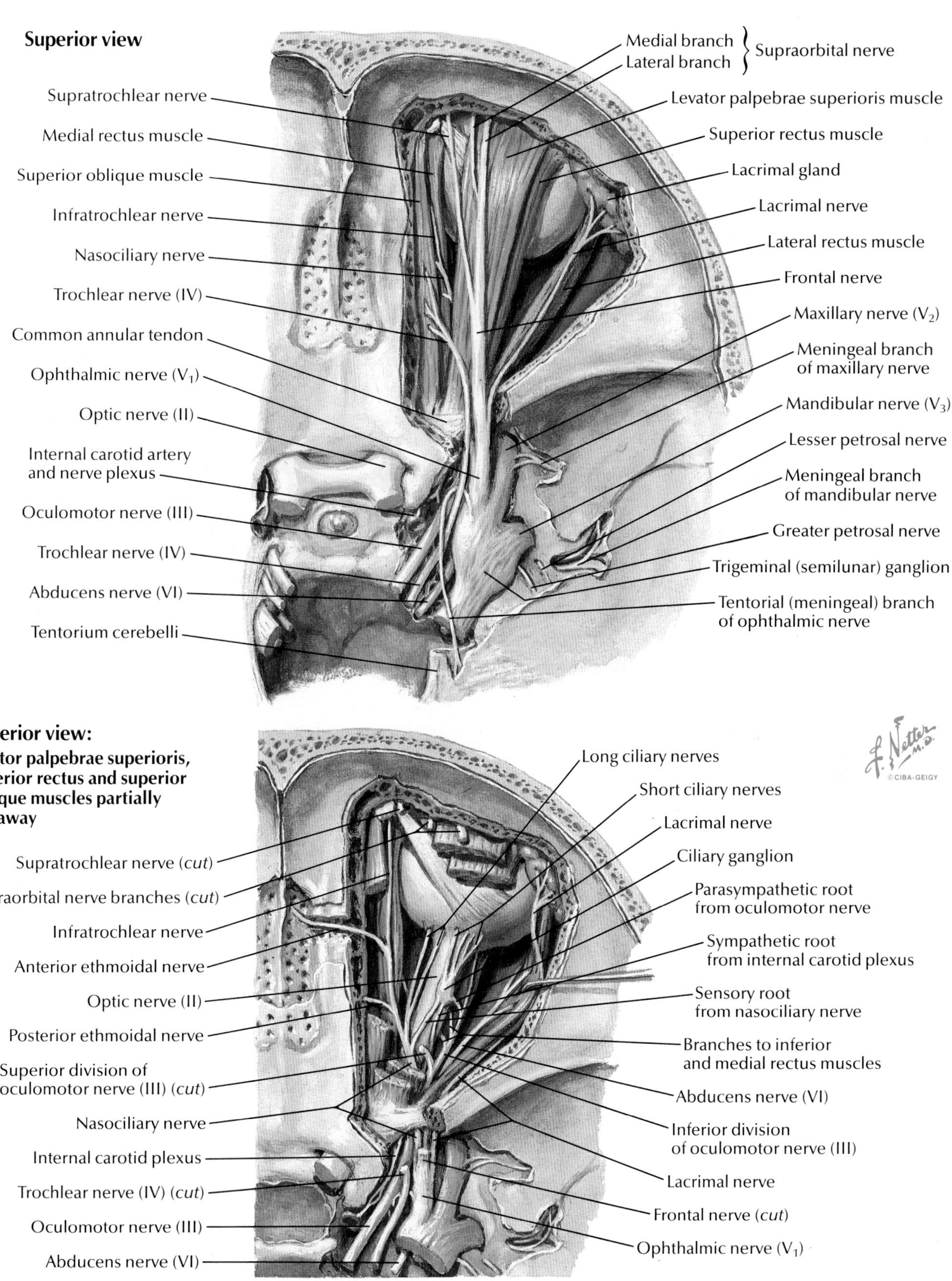

Superior view

Supratrochlear nerve

Medial rectus muscle

Superior oblique muscle

Infratrochlear nerve

Nasociliary nerve

Trochlear nerve (IV)

Common annular tendon

Ophthalmic nerve (V₁)

Optic nerve (II)

Internal carotid artery and nerve plexus

Oculomotor nerve (III)

Trochlear nerve (IV)

Abducens nerve (VI)

Tentorium cerebelli

Medial branch
Lateral branch } Supraorbital nerve

Levator palpebrae superioris muscle

Superior rectus muscle

Lacrimal gland

Lacrimal nerve

Lateral rectus muscle

Frontal nerve

Maxillary nerve (V₂)

Meningeal branch of maxillary nerve

Mandibular nerve (V₃)

Lesser petrosal nerve

Meningeal branch of mandibular nerve

Greater petrosal nerve

Trigeminal (semilunar) ganglion

Tentorial (meningeal) branch of ophthalmic nerve

Superior view:
levator palpebrae superioris, superior rectus and superior oblique muscles partially cut away

Supratrochlear nerve (*cut*)

Supraorbital nerve branches (*cut*)

Infratrochlear nerve

Anterior ethmoidal nerve

Optic nerve (II)

Posterior ethmoidal nerve

Superior division of oculomotor nerve (III) (*cut*)

Nasociliary nerve

Internal carotid plexus

Trochlear nerve (IV) (*cut*)

Oculomotor nerve (III)

Abducens nerve (VI)

Long ciliary nerves

Short ciliary nerves

Lacrimal nerve

Ciliary ganglion

Parasympathetic root from oculomotor nerve

Sympathetic root from internal carotid plexus

Sensory root from nasociliary nerve

Branches to inferior and medial rectus muscles

Abducens nerve (VI)

Inferior division of oculomotor nerve (III)

Lacrimal nerve

Frontal nerve (*cut*)

Ophthalmic nerve (V₁)

ORBIT AND CONTENTS

PLATE 81

Eyeball

Horizontal section

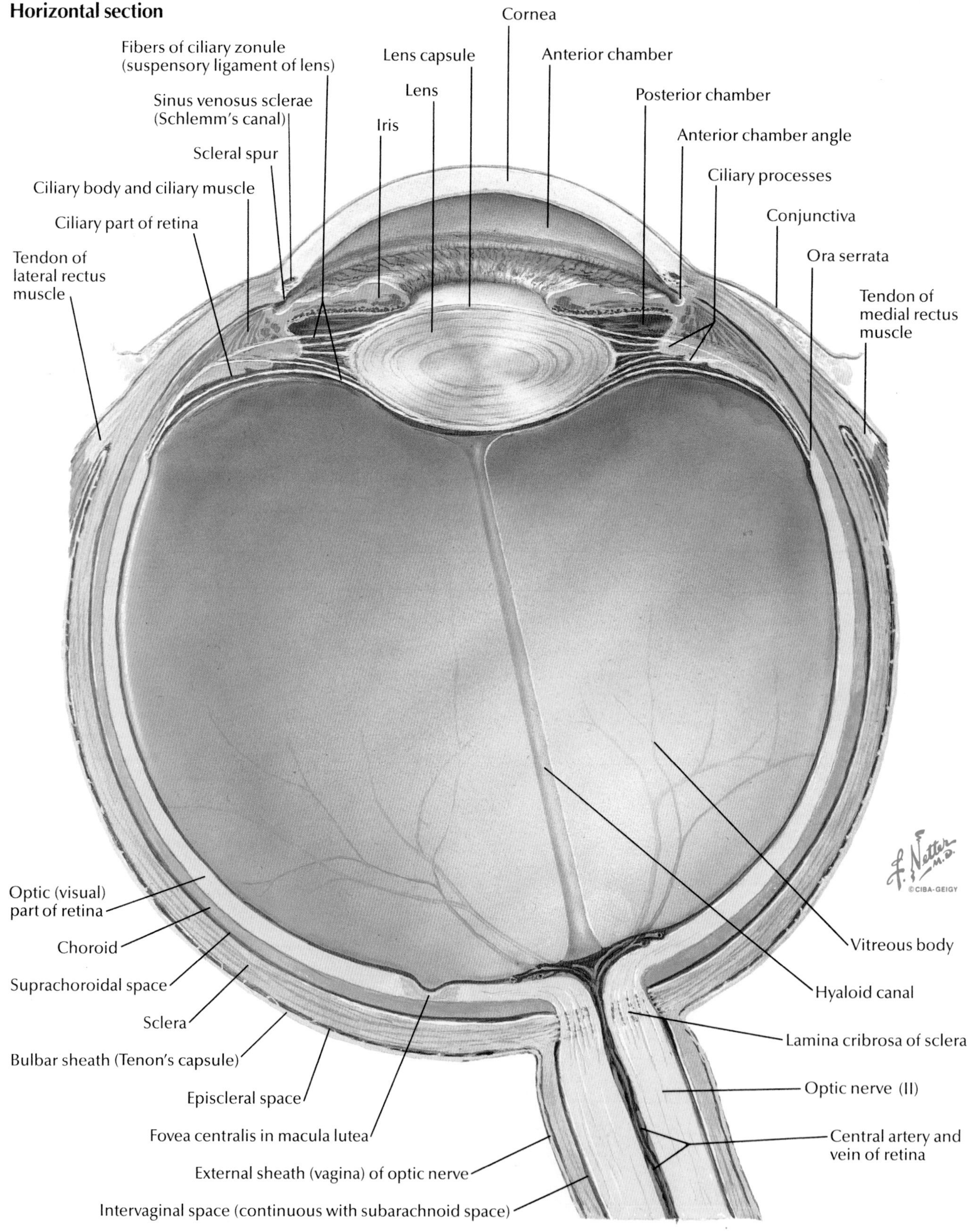

Fibers of ciliary zonule (suspensory ligament of lens)

Sinus venosus sclerae (Schlemm's canal)

Scleral spur

Ciliary body and ciliary muscle

Ciliary part of retina

Tendon of lateral rectus muscle

Iris

Lens

Lens capsule

Cornea

Anterior chamber

Posterior chamber

Anterior chamber angle

Ciliary processes

Conjunctiva

Ora serrata

Tendon of medial rectus muscle

Optic (visual) part of retina

Choroid

Suprachoroidal space

Sclera

Bulbar sheath (Tenon's capsule)

Episcleral space

Fovea centralis in macula lutea

External sheath (vagina) of optic nerve

Intervaginal space (continuous with subarachnoid space)

Vitreous body

Hyaloid canal

Lamina cribrosa of sclera

Optic nerve (II)

Central artery and vein of retina

PLATE 82   **HEAD AND NECK**

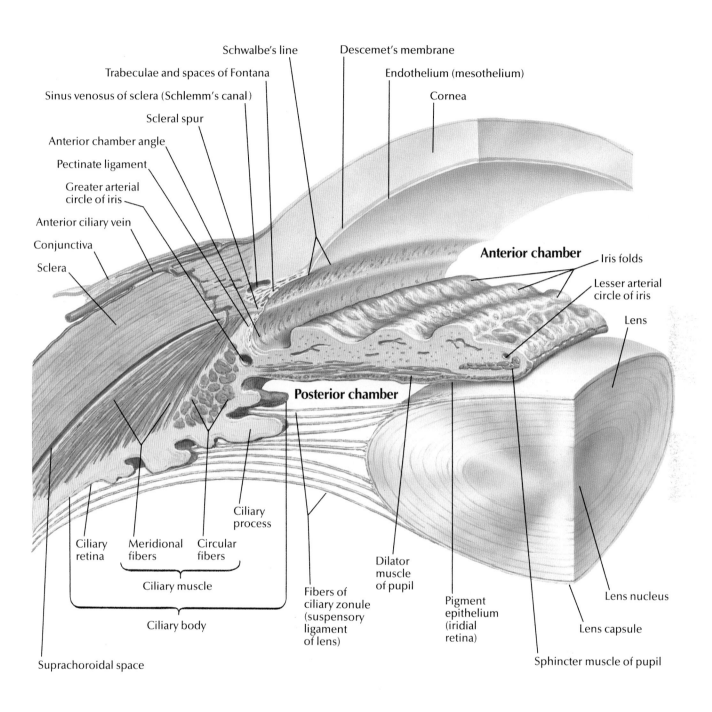

Schwalbe's line

Descemet's membrane

Trabeculae and spaces of Fontana

Endothelium (mesothelium)

Sinus venosus of sclera (Schlemm's canal)

Cornea

Scleral spur

Anterior chamber angle

Pectinate ligament

Greater arterial circle of iris

Anterior chamber

Iris folds

Anterior ciliary vein

Lesser arterial circle of iris

Conjunctiva

Lens

Sclera

Posterior chamber

Ciliary process

Ciliary retina

Meridional fibers

Circular fibers

Dilator muscle of pupil

Lens nucleus

Ciliary muscle

Ciliary body

Fibers of ciliary zonule (suspensory ligament of lens)

Pigment epithelium (iridial retina)

Lens capsule

Sphincter muscle of pupil

Suprachoroidal space

Note: for clarity only single plane of zonular fibers shown; actually fibers surround entire circumference of lens

Anterior Chamber Angle of Eye

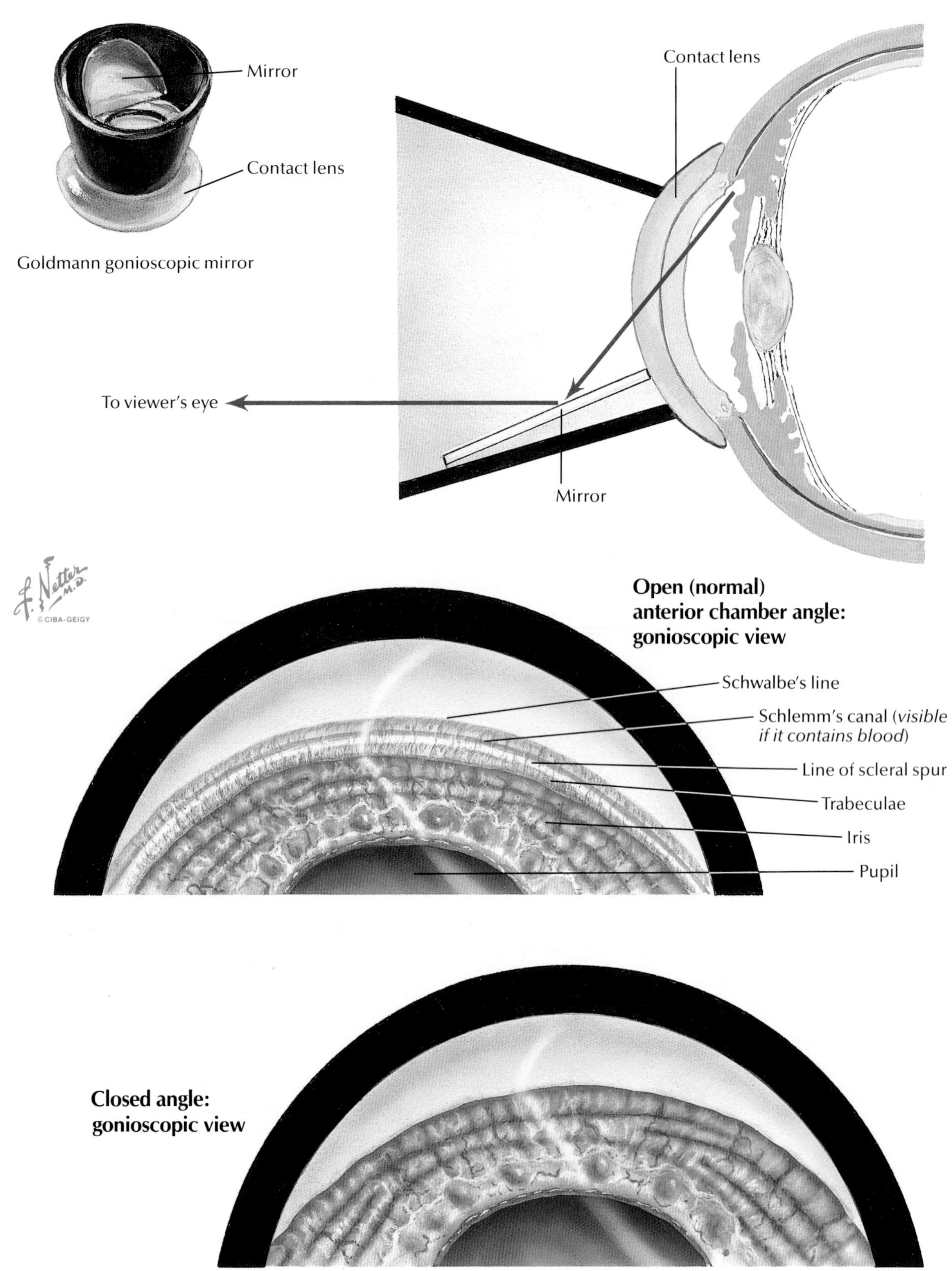

Mirror

Contact lens

Goldmann gonioscopic mirror

Contact lens

To viewer's eye

Mirror

Open (normal) anterior chamber angle: gonioscopic view

Schwalbe's line

Schlemm's canal (*visible if it contains blood*)

Line of scleral spur

Trabeculae

Iris

Pupil

Closed angle: gonioscopic view

PLATE 84

HEAD AND NECK

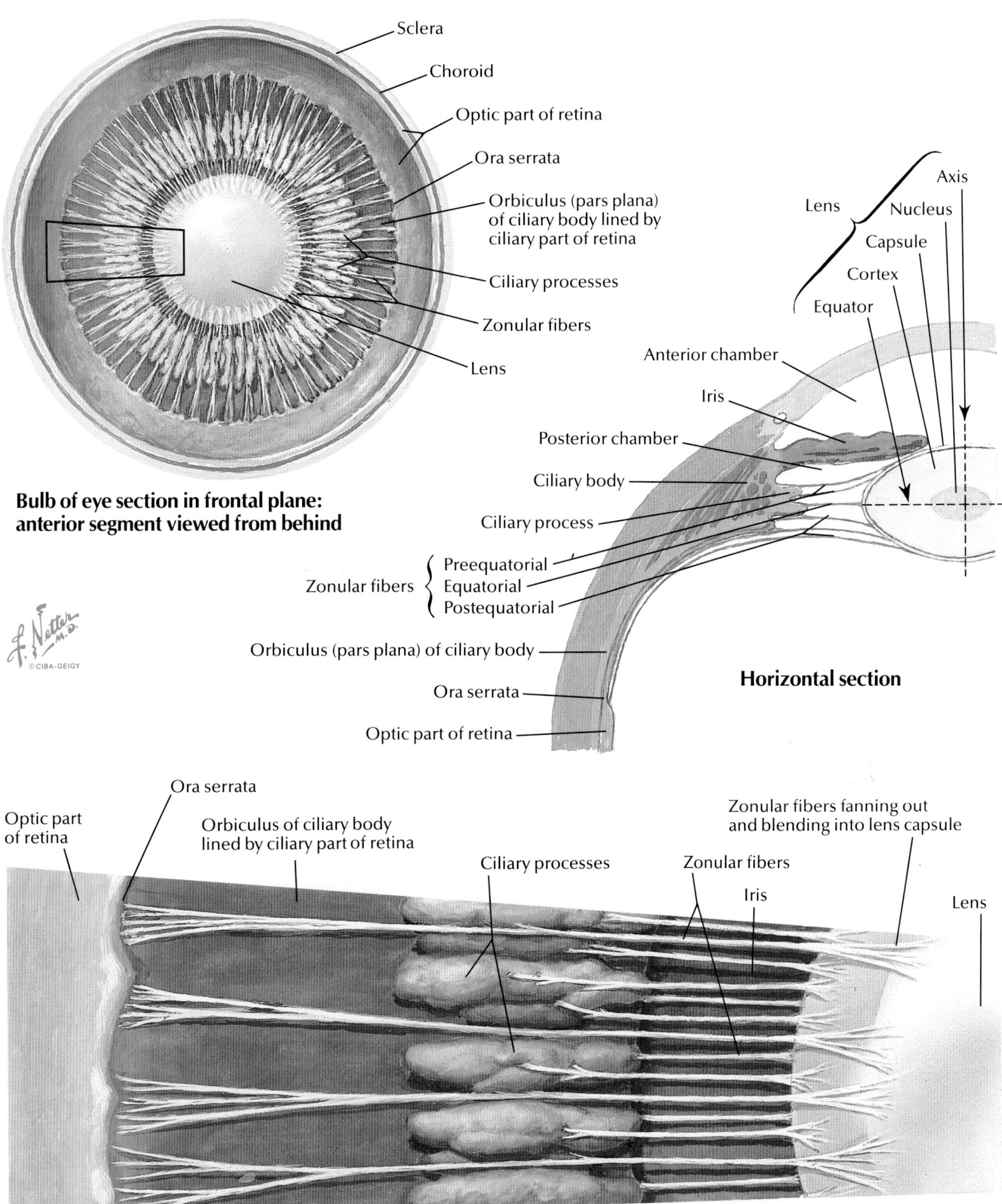

Sclera
Choroid
Optic part of retina
Ora serrata
Orbiculus (pars plana) of ciliary body lined by ciliary part of retina
Ciliary processes
Zonular fibers
Lens

Bulb of eye section in frontal plane: anterior segment viewed from behind

Axis
Lens
Nucleus
Capsule
Cortex
Equator
Anterior chamber
Iris
Posterior chamber
Ciliary body
Ciliary process
Zonular fibers { Preequatorial / Equatorial / Postequatorial
Orbiculus (pars plana) of ciliary body
Ora serrata
Optic part of retina

Horizontal section

Ora serrata
Optic part of retina
Orbiculus of ciliary body lined by ciliary part of retina
Ciliary processes
Zonular fibers fanning out and blending into lens capsule
Zonular fibers
Iris
Lens

Segment outlined in top illustration magnified to ultramicroscopic scale (semischematic)

Intrinsic Arteries and Veins of Eye

SEE ALSO PLATE 80

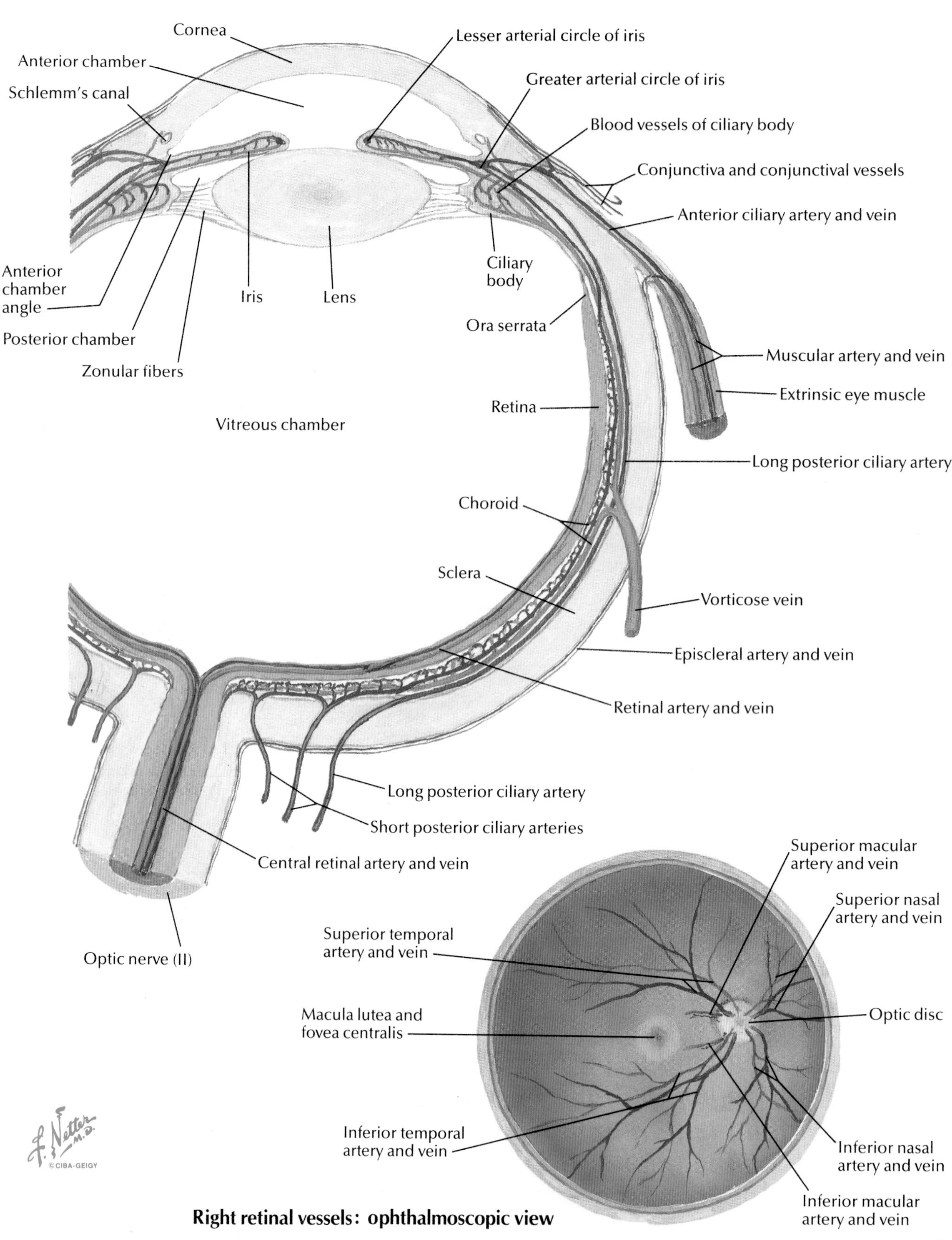

Cornea

Anterior chamber

Schlemm's canal

Anterior chamber angle

Posterior chamber

Zonular fibers

Iris

Lens

Vitreous chamber

Lesser arterial circle of iris

Greater arterial circle of iris

Blood vessels of ciliary body

Conjunctiva and conjunctival vessels

Anterior ciliary artery and vein

Ciliary body

Ora serrata

Retina

Muscular artery and vein

Extrinsic eye muscle

Long posterior ciliary artery

Choroid

Sclera

Vorticose vein

Episcleral artery and vein

Retinal artery and vein

Long posterior ciliary artery

Short posterior ciliary arteries

Central retinal artery and vein

Optic nerve (II)

Superior macular artery and vein

Superior nasal artery and vein

Superior temporal artery and vein

Macula lutea and fovea centralis

Optic disc

Inferior temporal artery and vein

Inferior nasal artery and vein

Inferior macular artery and vein

Right retinal vessels: ophthalmoscopic view

PLATE 86

HEAD AND NECK

Frontal section

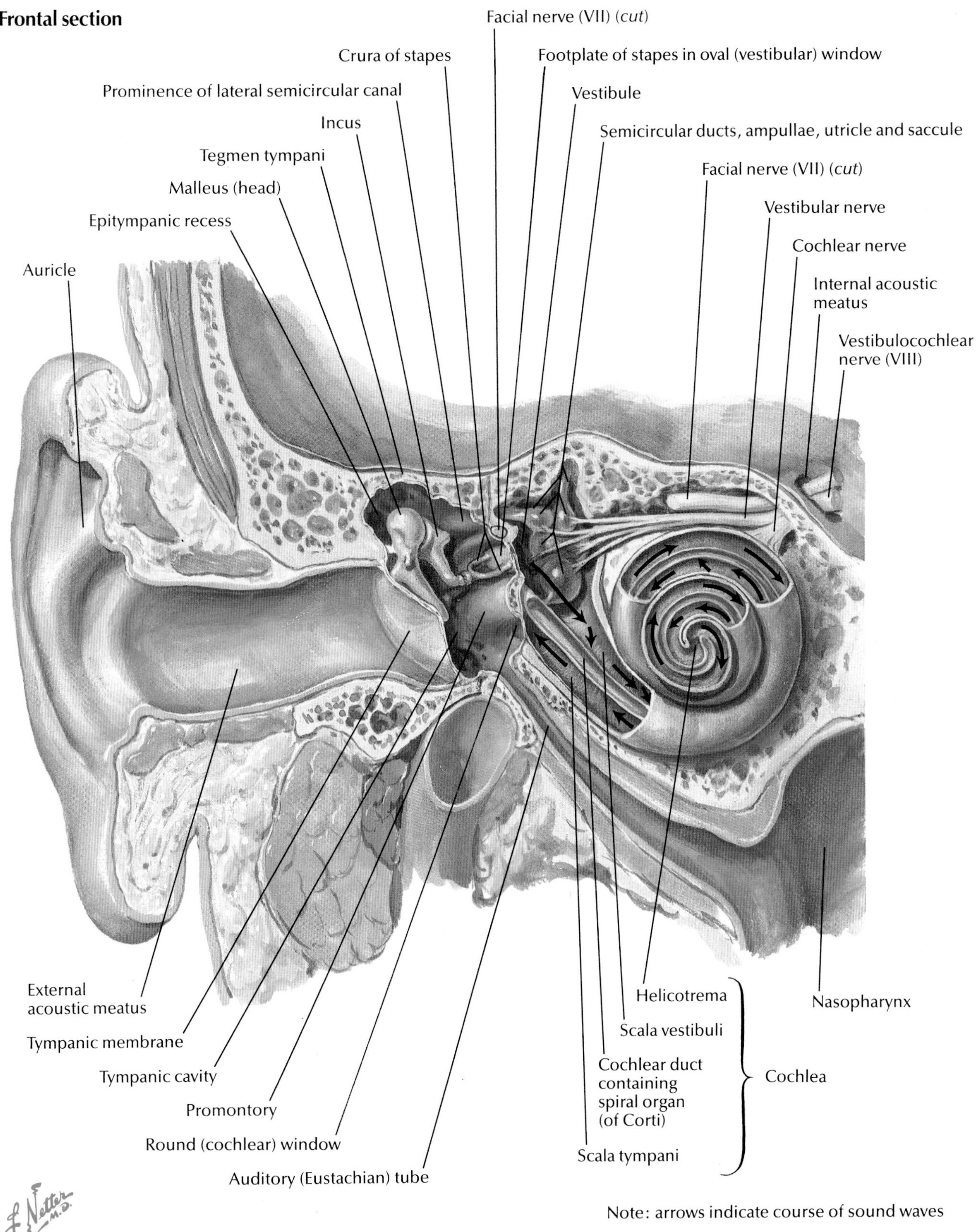

Facial nerve (VII) (*cut*)

Crura of stapes

Footplate of stapes in oval (vestibular) window

Prominence of lateral semicircular canal

Vestibule

Incus

Semicircular ducts, ampullae, utricle and saccule

Tegmen tympani

Facial nerve (VII) (*cut*)

Malleus (head)

Vestibular nerve

Epitympanic recess

Cochlear nerve

Internal acoustic meatus

Auricle

Vestibulocochlear nerve (VIII)

External acoustic meatus

Helicotrema

Nasopharynx

Tympanic membrane

Scala vestibuli

Tympanic cavity

Cochlear duct containing spiral organ (of Corti)

Cochlea

Promontory

Round (cochlear) window

Scala tympani

Auditory (Eustachian) tube

Note: arrows indicate course of sound waves

EAR

PLATE 87

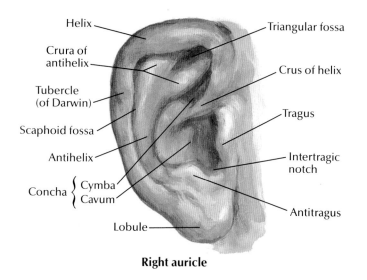

Right auricle

Helix
Crura of antihelix
Tubercle (of Darwin)
Scaphoid fossa
Antihelix
Concha { Cymba / Cavum
Lobule
Triangular fossa
Crus of helix
Tragus
Intertragic notch
Antitragus

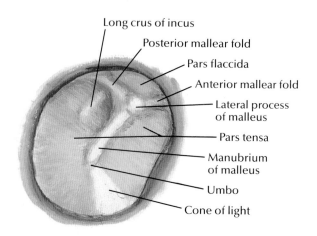

Right tympanic membrane (eardrum) viewed through speculum

Long crus of incus
Posterior mallear fold
Pars flaccida
Anterior mallear fold
Lateral process of malleus
Pars tensa
Manubrium of malleus
Umbo
Cone of light

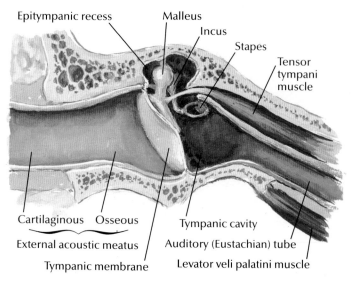

Sagittal section of external acoustic meatus and middle ear

Epitympanic recess
Malleus
Incus
Stapes
Tensor tympani muscle
Cartilaginous
Osseous
External acoustic meatus
Tympanic membrane
Tympanic cavity
Auditory (Eustachian) tube
Levator veli palatini muscle

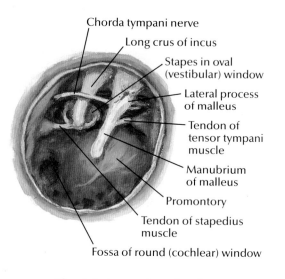

View into tympanic cavity after removal of tympanic membrane

Chorda tympani nerve
Long crus of incus
Stapes in oval (vestibular) window
Lateral process of malleus
Tendon of tensor tympani muscle
Manubrium of malleus
Promontory
Tendon of stapedius muscle
Fossa of round (cochlear) window

Auditory ossicles

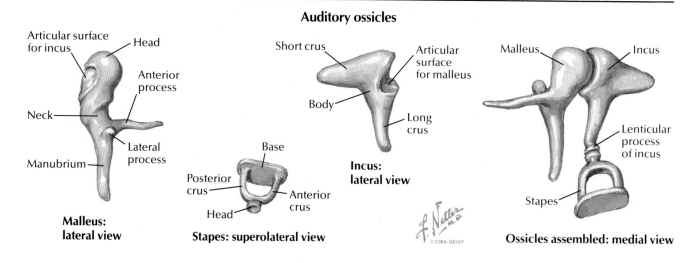

Articular surface for incus
Head
Anterior process
Neck
Manubrium
Lateral process

Malleus: lateral view

Base
Posterior crus
Anterior crus
Head

Stapes: superolateral view

Short crus
Articular surface for malleus
Body
Long crus

Incus: lateral view

Malleus
Incus
Lenticular process of incus
Stapes

Ossicles assembled: medial view

PLATE 88

HEAD AND NECK

Lateral wall of tympanic cavity: medial (internal) view

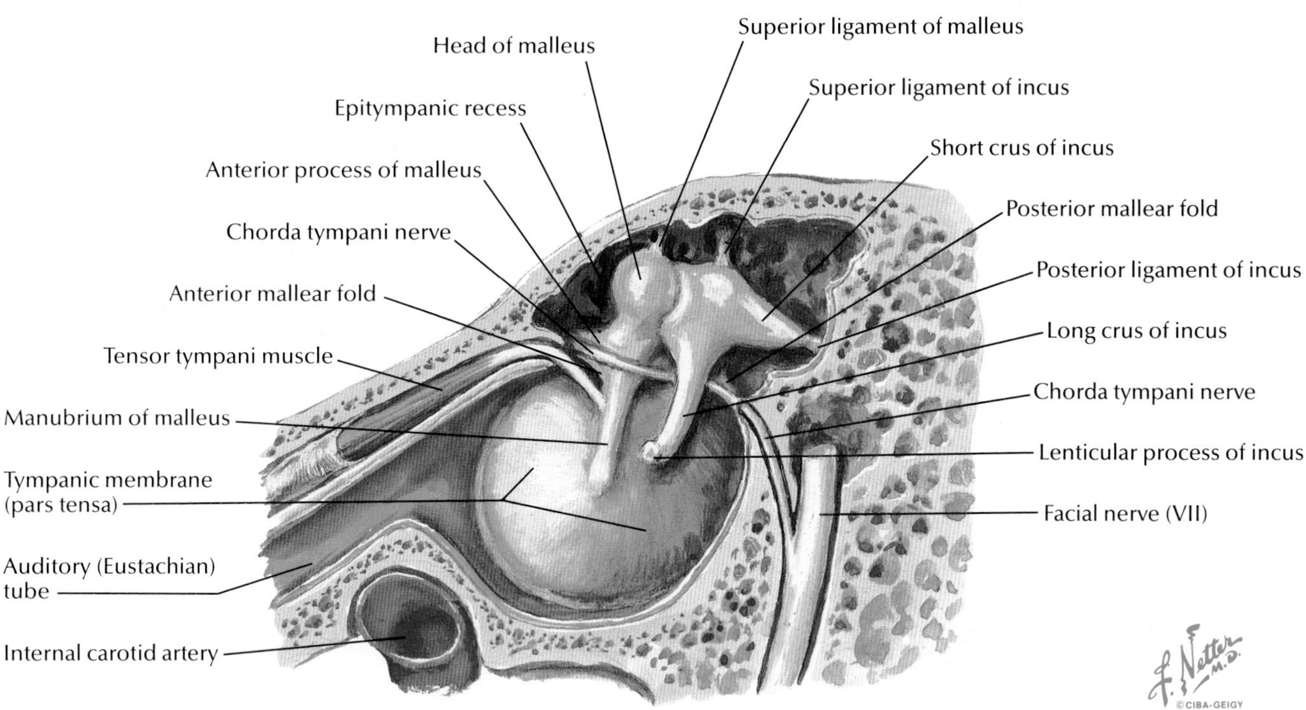

Head of malleus

Epitympanic recess

Anterior process of malleus

Chorda tympani nerve

Anterior mallear fold

Tensor tympani muscle

Manubrium of malleus

Tympanic membrane (pars tensa)

Auditory (Eustachian) tube

Internal carotid artery

Superior ligament of malleus

Superior ligament of incus

Short crus of incus

Posterior mallear fold

Posterior ligament of incus

Long crus of incus

Chorda tympani nerve

Lenticular process of incus

Facial nerve (VII)

Medial wall of tympanic cavity: lateral view

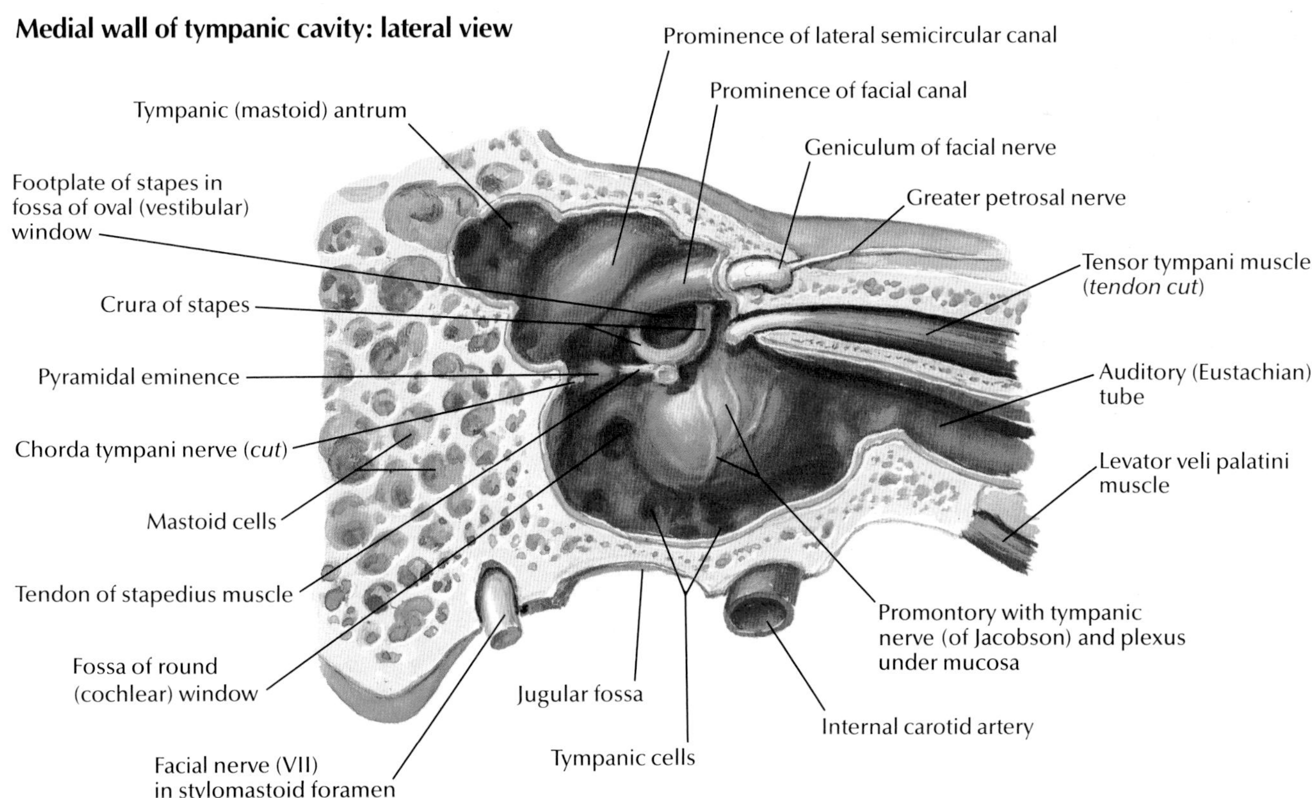

Tympanic (mastoid) antrum

Footplate of stapes in fossa of oval (vestibular) window

Crura of stapes

Pyramidal eminence

Chorda tympani nerve (cut)

Mastoid cells

Tendon of stapedius muscle

Fossa of round (cochlear) window

Facial nerve (VII) in stylomastoid foramen

Jugular fossa

Tympanic cells

Prominence of lateral semicircular canal

Prominence of facial canal

Geniculum of facial nerve

Greater petrosal nerve

Tensor tympani muscle (*tendon cut*)

Auditory (Eustachian) tube

Levator veli palatini muscle

Promontory with tympanic nerve (of Jacobson) and plexus under mucosa

Internal carotid artery

Osseous and Membranous Labyrinths

SEE ALSO PLATE 118

Right osseous labyrinth, anterolateral view: surrounding cancellous bone removed

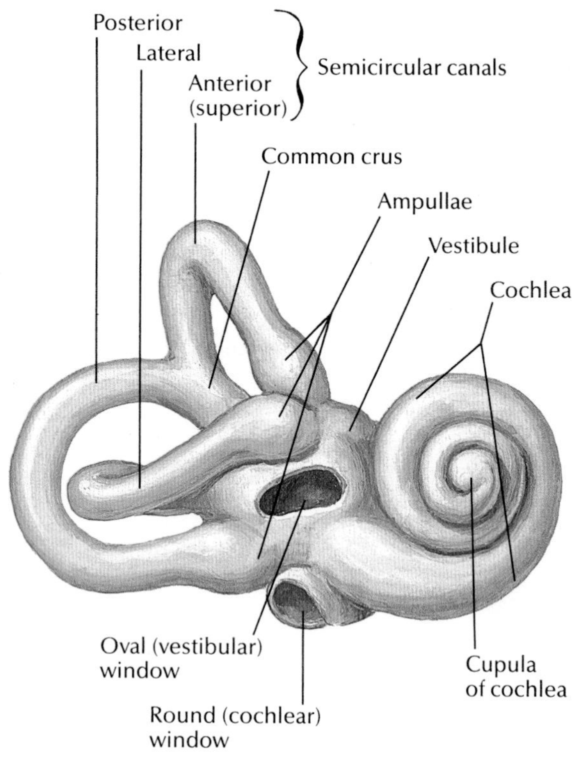

Posterior
Lateral
Anterior (superior)
} Semicircular canals

Common crus

Ampullae

Vestibule

Cochlea

Oval (vestibular) window

Round (cochlear) window

Cupula of cochlea

Dissected right osseous labyrinth: membranous labyrinth removed

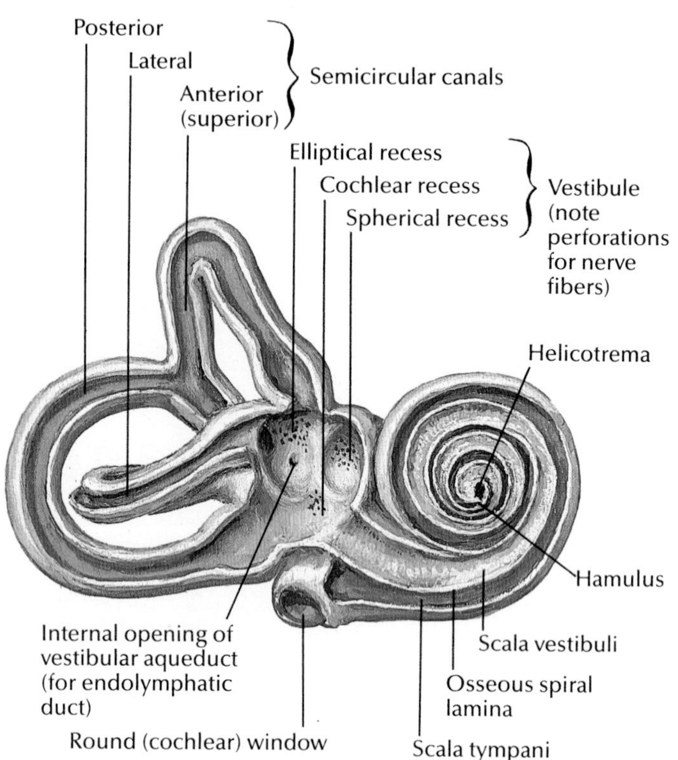

Posterior
Lateral
Anterior (superior)
} Semicircular canals

Elliptical recess
Cochlear recess
Spherical recess
} Vestibule (note perforations for nerve fibers)

Helicotrema

Hamulus

Scala vestibuli

Osseous spiral lamina

Scala tympani

Internal opening of vestibular aqueduct (for endolymphatic duct)

Round (cochlear) window

Right membranous labyrinth with nerves: posteromedial view

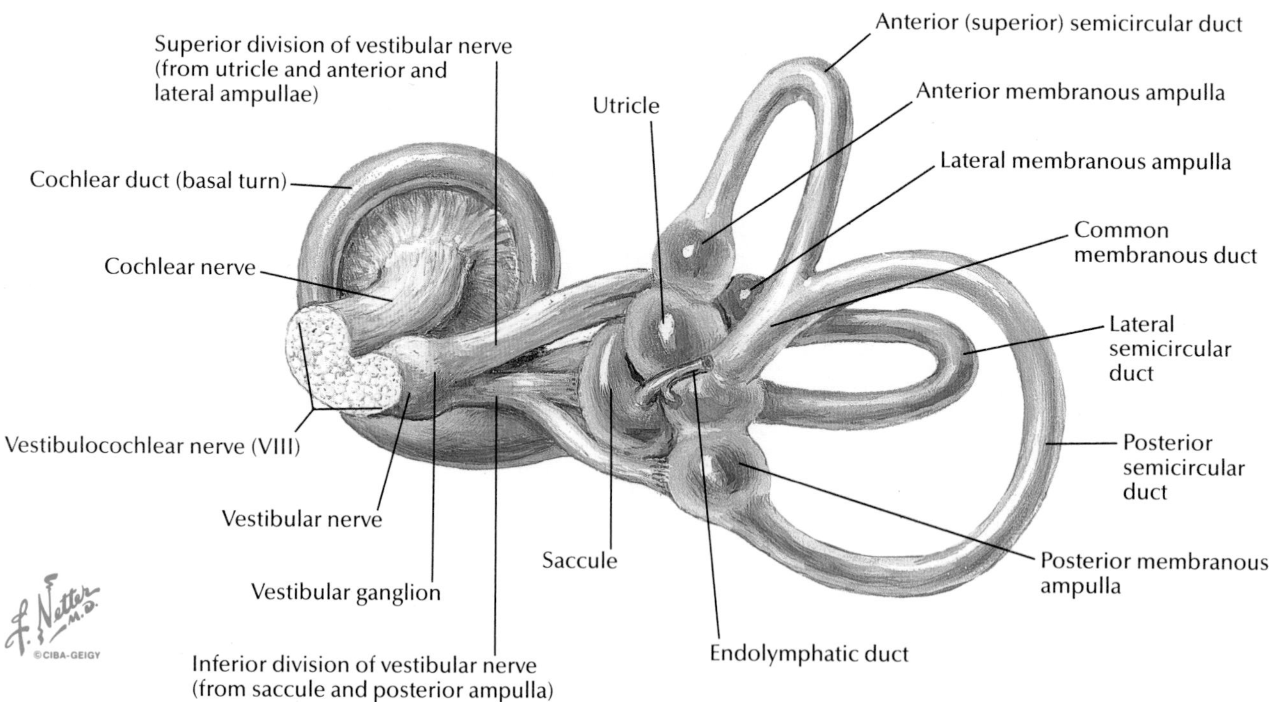

Superior division of vestibular nerve (from utricle and anterior and lateral ampullae)

Cochlear duct (basal turn)

Cochlear nerve

Vestibulocochlear nerve (VIII)

Vestibular nerve

Vestibular ganglion

Inferior division of vestibular nerve (from saccule and posterior ampulla)

Saccule

Endolymphatic duct

Utricle

Anterior (superior) semicircular duct

Anterior membranous ampulla

Lateral membranous ampulla

Common membranous duct

Lateral semicircular duct

Posterior semicircular duct

Posterior membranous ampulla

PLATE 90

HEAD AND NECK

Osseous and membranous labyrinths: schema

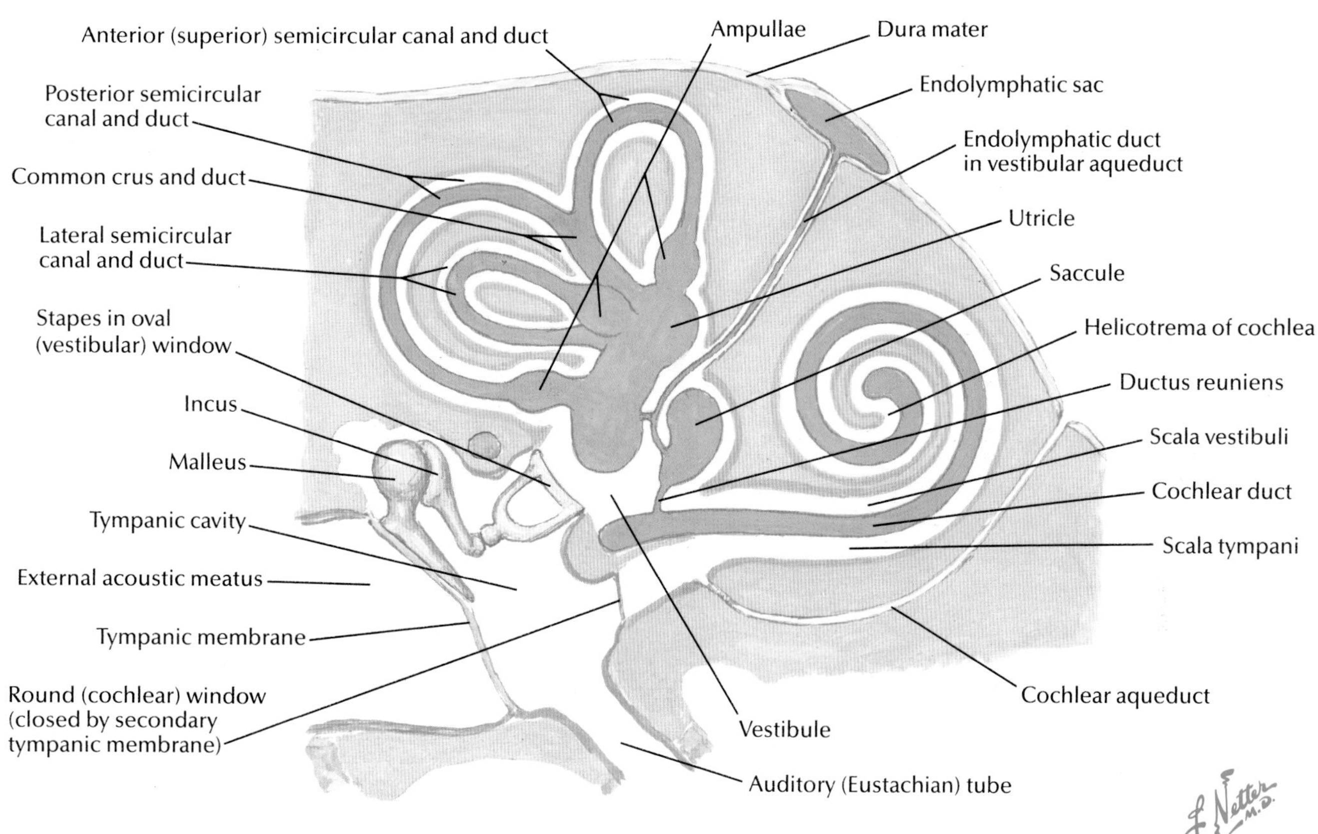

Anterior (superior) semicircular canal and duct

Posterior semicircular canal and duct

Common crus and duct

Lateral semicircular canal and duct

Stapes in oval (vestibular) window

Incus

Malleus

Tympanic cavity

External acoustic meatus

Tympanic membrane

Round (cochlear) window (closed by secondary tympanic membrane)

Ampullae

Dura mater

Endolymphatic sac

Endolymphatic duct in vestibular aqueduct

Utricle

Saccule

Helicotrema of cochlea

Ductus reuniens

Scala vestibuli

Cochlear duct

Scala tympani

Cochlear aqueduct

Vestibule

Auditory (Eustachian) tube

Section through turn of cochlea

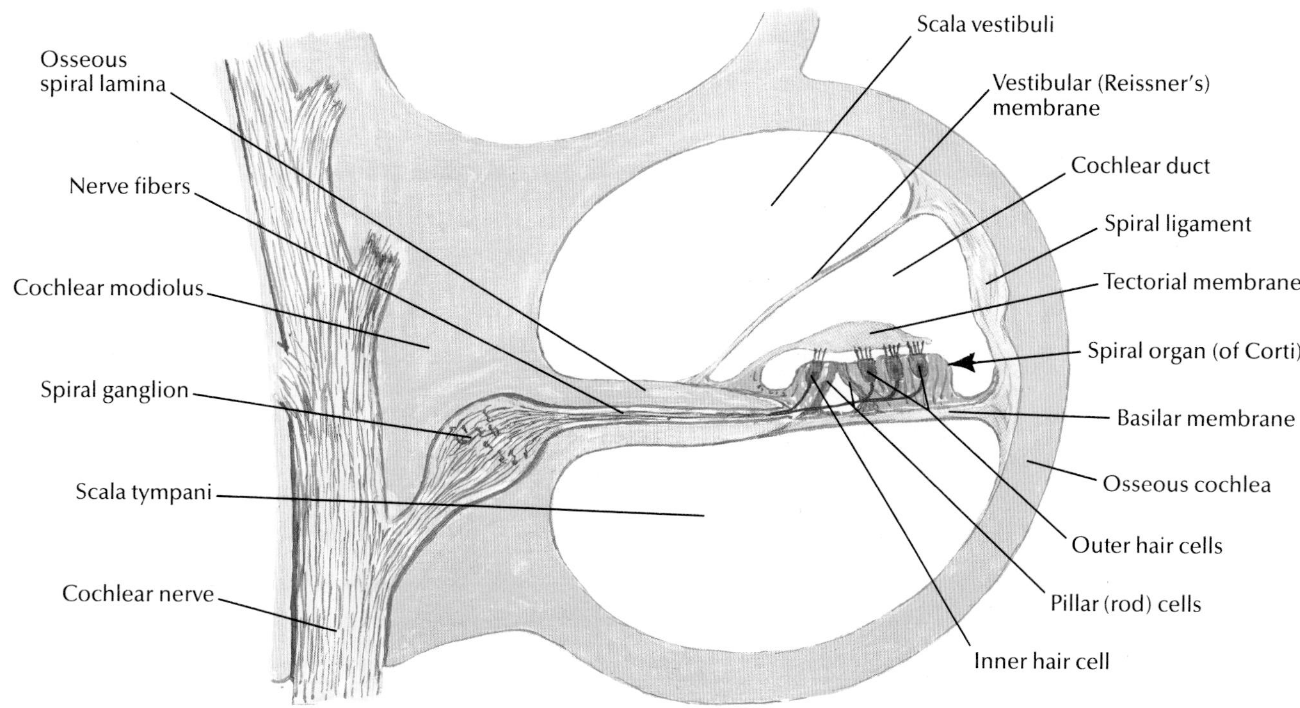

Osseous spiral lamina

Nerve fibers

Cochlear modiolus

Spiral ganglion

Scala tympani

Cochlear nerve

Scala vestibuli

Vestibular (Reissner's) membrane

Cochlear duct

Spiral ligament

Tectorial membrane

Spiral organ (of Corti)

Basilar membrane

Osseous cochlea

Outer hair cells

Pillar (rod) cells

Inner hair cell

Orientation of Labyrinth in Skull

Superior projection of right osseous labyrinth on floor of skull

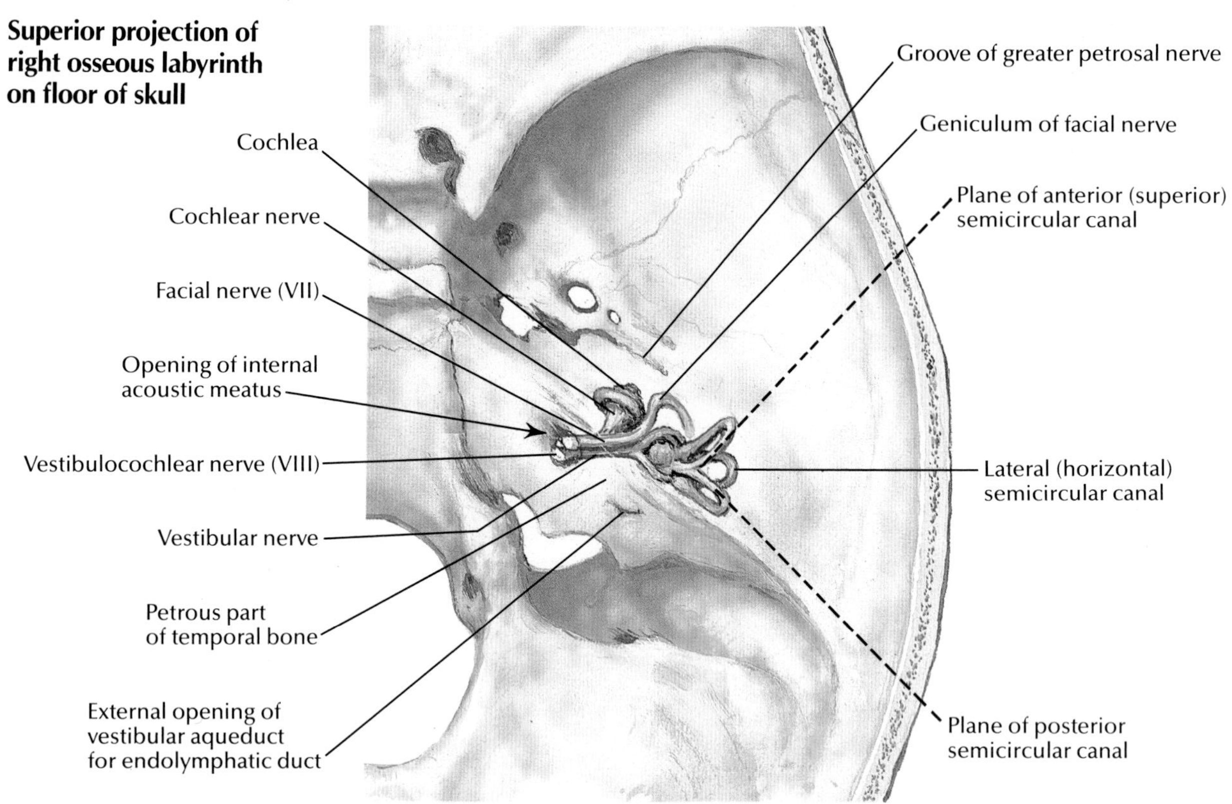

Cochlea

Cochlear nerve

Facial nerve (VII)

Opening of internal acoustic meatus

Vestibulocochlear nerve (VIII)

Vestibular nerve

Petrous part of temporal bone

External opening of vestibular aqueduct for endolymphatic duct

Groove of greater petrosal nerve

Geniculum of facial nerve

Plane of anterior (superior) semicircular canal

Lateral (horizontal) semicircular canal

Plane of posterior semicircular canal

Lateral projection of right membranous labyrinth

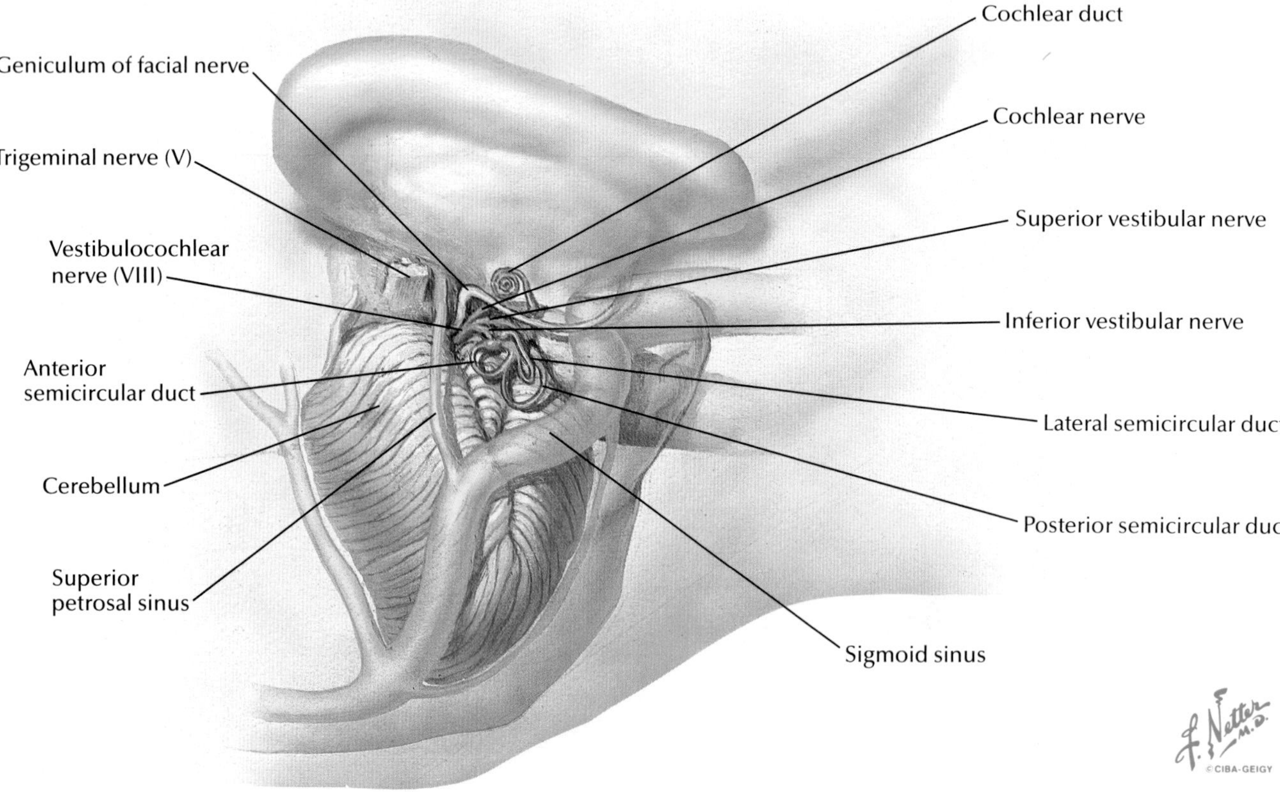

Geniculum of facial nerve

Trigeminal nerve (V)

Vestibulocochlear nerve (VIII)

Anterior semicircular duct

Cerebellum

Superior petrosal sinus

Cochlear duct

Cochlear nerve

Superior vestibular nerve

Inferior vestibular nerve

Lateral semicircular duct

Posterior semicircular duct

Sigmoid sinus

PLATE 92

HEAD AND NECK

**Cartilage of auditory tube
at base of skull: inferior view**

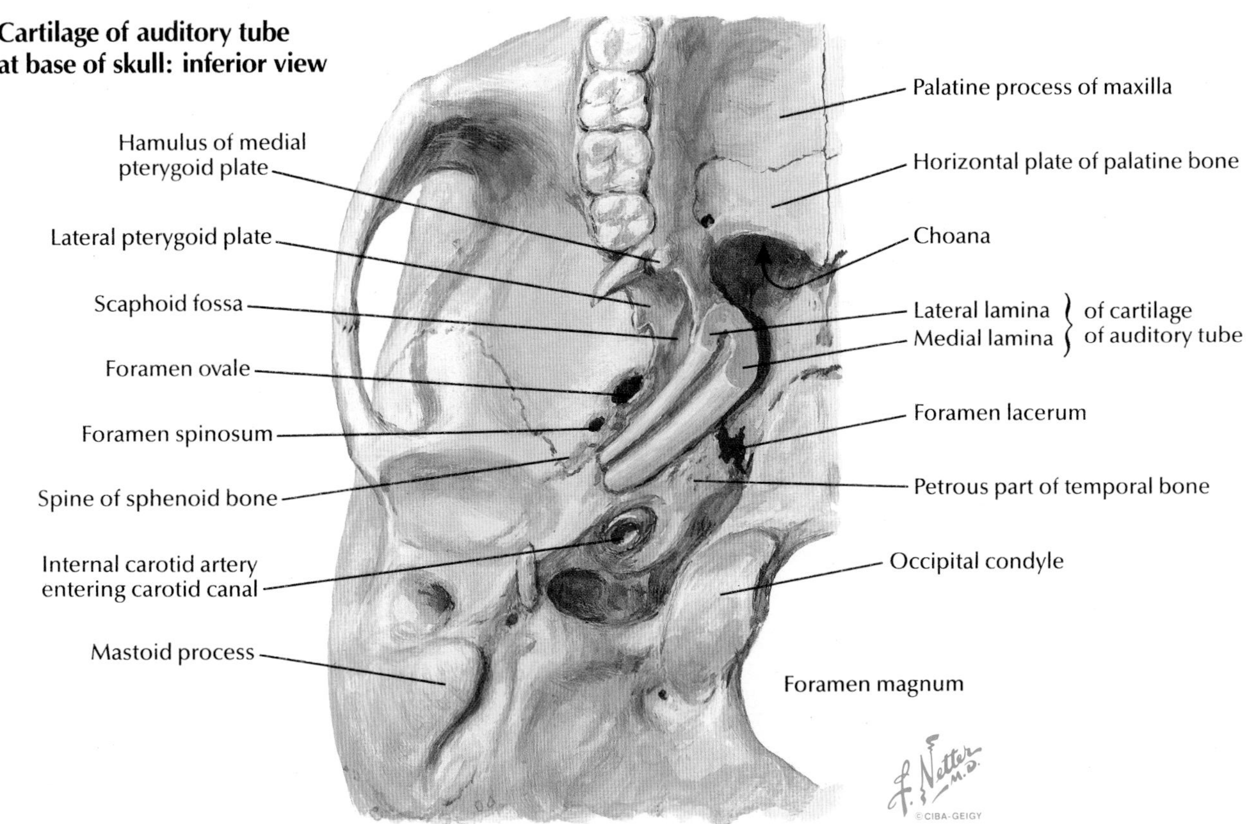

Hamulus of medial
pterygoid plate

Lateral pterygoid plate

Scaphoid fossa

Foramen ovale

Foramen spinosum

Spine of sphenoid bone

Internal carotid artery
entering carotid canal

Mastoid process

Palatine process of maxilla

Horizontal plate of palatine bone

Choana

Lateral lamina ⎫ of cartilage
Medial lamina ⎭ of auditory tube

Foramen lacerum

Petrous part of temporal bone

Occipital condyle

Foramen magnum

**Section through cartilage of auditory tube
with tube closed**

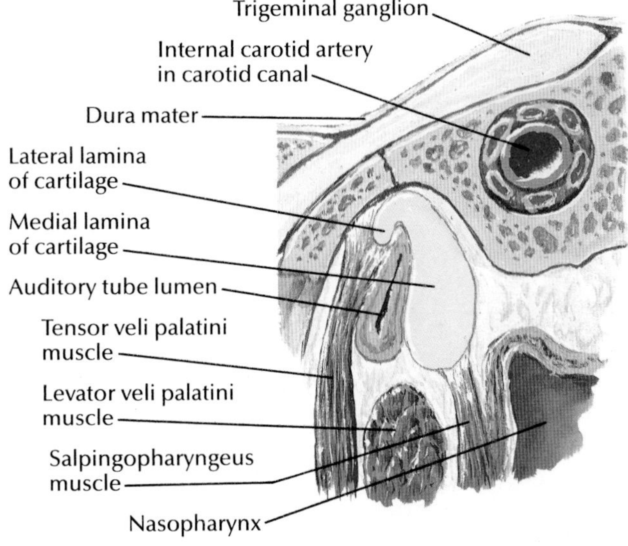

Trigeminal ganglion

Internal carotid artery
in carotid canal

Dura mater

Lateral lamina
of cartilage

Medial lamina
of cartilage

Auditory tube lumen

Tensor veli palatini
muscle

Levator veli palatini
muscle

Salpingopharyngeus
muscle

Nasopharynx

Auditory tube closed by elastic recoil of
cartilage, tissue turgidity and tension of
salpingopharyngeus muscles

**Section through cartilage of auditory tube
with tube open**

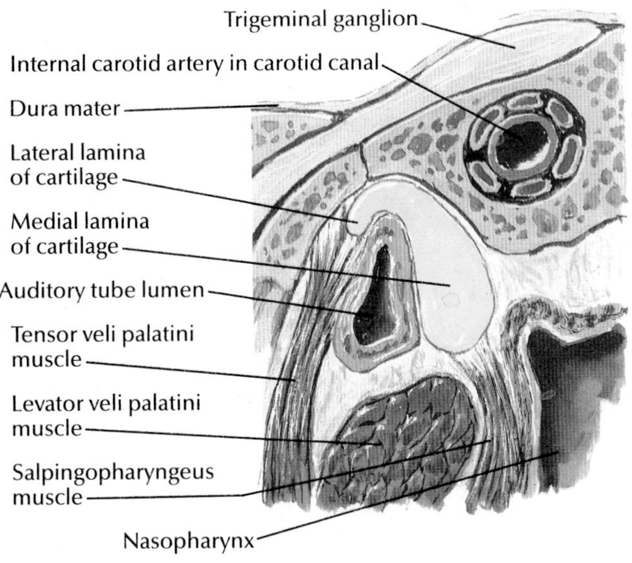

Trigeminal ganglion

Internal carotid artery in carotid canal

Dura mater

Lateral lamina
of cartilage

Medial lamina
of cartilage

Auditory tube lumen

Tensor veli palatini
muscle

Levator veli palatini
muscle

Salpingopharyngeus
muscle

Nasopharynx

Lumen opened chiefly when attachment
of tensor veli palatini muscle pulls wall
of tube laterally during swallowing

Meninges and Diploic Veins

SEE ALSO PLATE 17

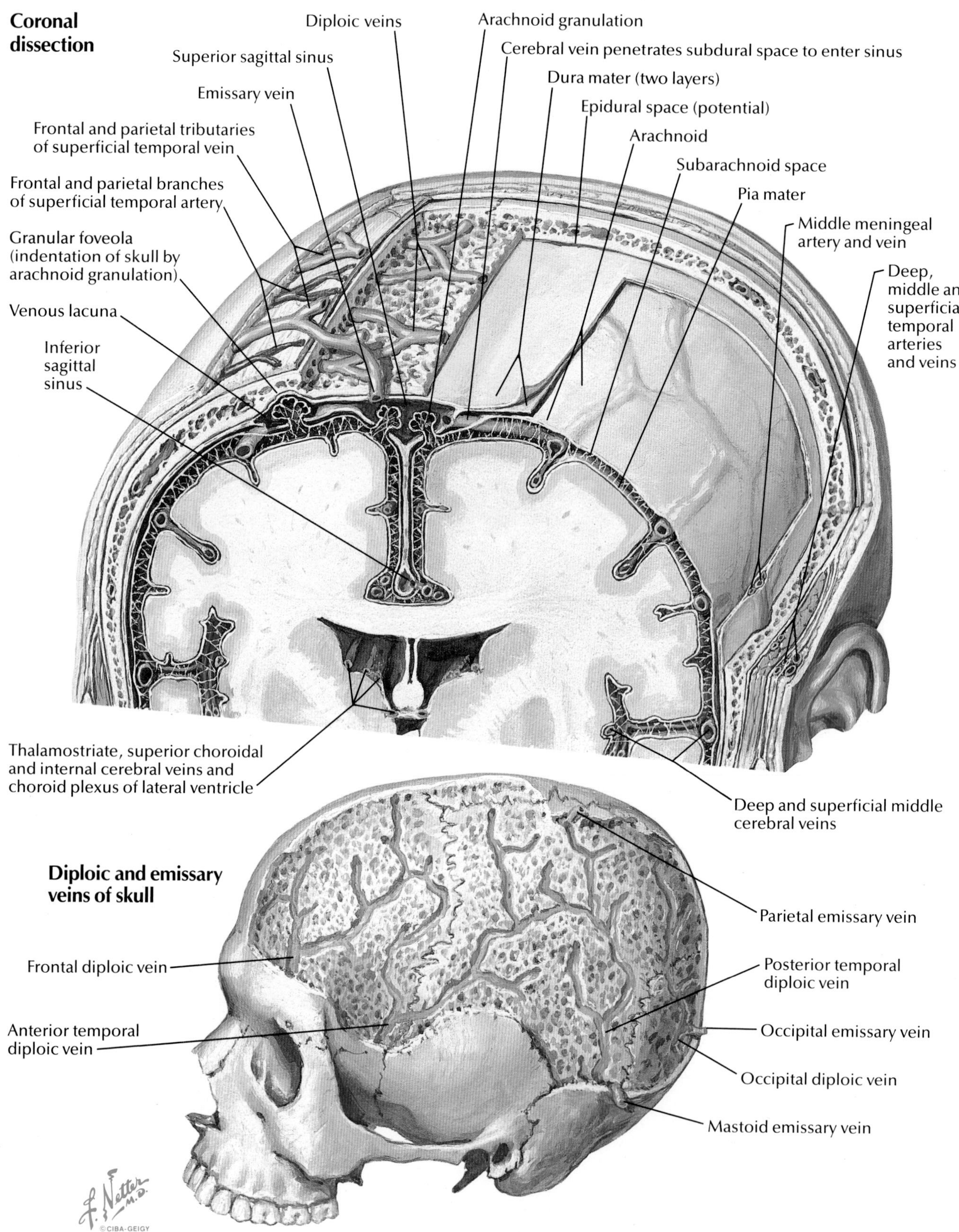

Coronal dissection

Diploic veins

Arachnoid granulation

Cerebral vein penetrates subdural space to enter sinus

Superior sagittal sinus

Dura mater (two layers)

Emissary vein

Epidural space (potential)

Frontal and parietal tributaries of superficial temporal vein

Arachnoid

Frontal and parietal branches of superficial temporal artery

Subarachnoid space

Pia mater

Granular foveola (indentation of skull by arachnoid granulation)

Middle meningeal artery and vein

Venous lacuna

Deep, middle and superficial temporal arteries and veins

Inferior sagittal sinus

Thalamostriate, superior choroidal and internal cerebral veins and choroid plexus of lateral ventricle

Deep and superficial middle cerebral veins

Diploic and emissary veins of skull

Parietal emissary vein

Frontal diploic vein

Posterior temporal diploic vein

Anterior temporal diploic vein

Occipital emissary vein

Occipital diploic vein

Mastoid emissary vein

PLATE 94

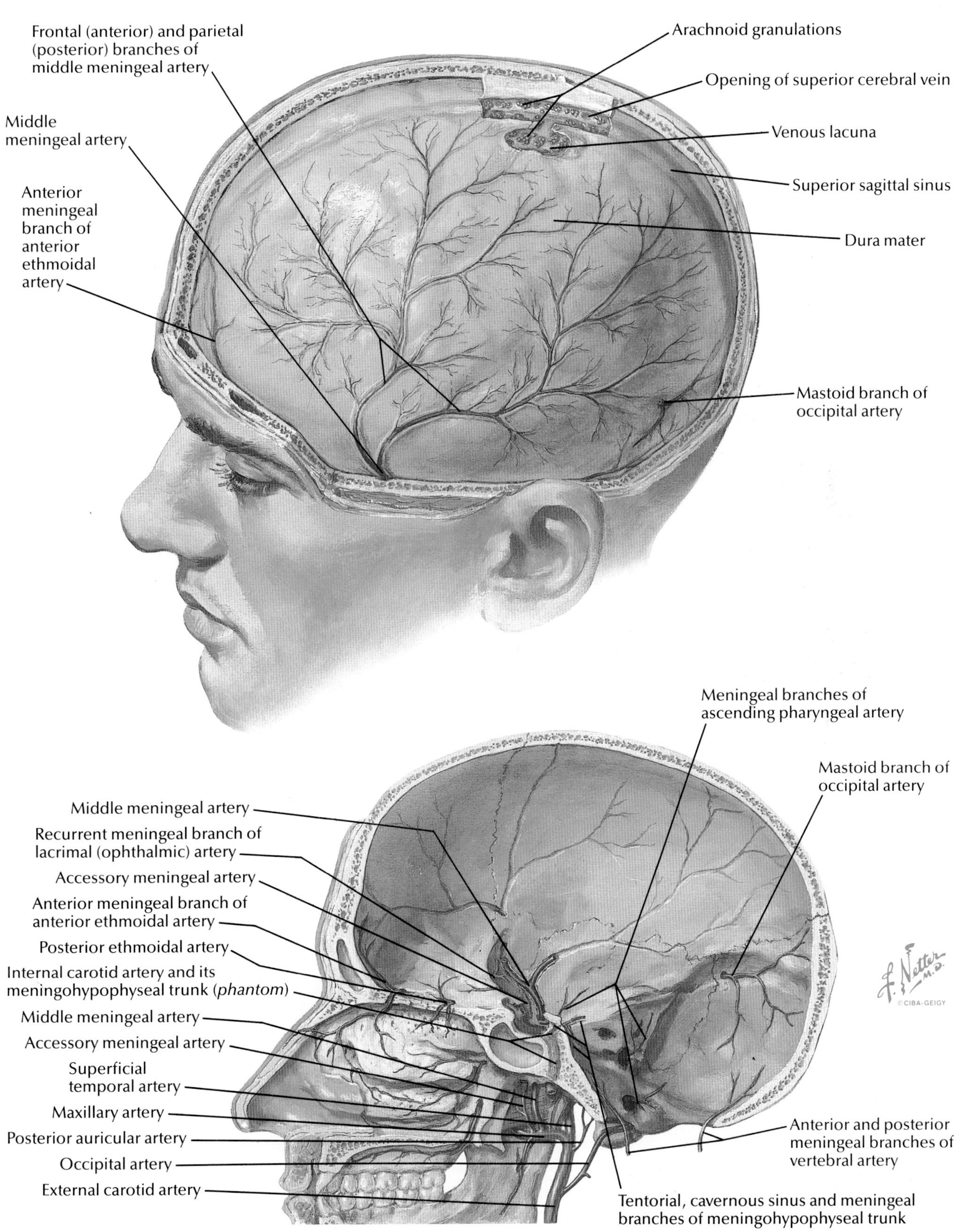

Frontal (anterior) and parietal (posterior) branches of middle meningeal artery

Middle meningeal artery

Anterior meningeal branch of anterior ethmoidal artery

Arachnoid granulations

Opening of superior cerebral vein

Venous lacuna

Superior sagittal sinus

Dura mater

Mastoid branch of occipital artery

Meningeal branches of ascending pharyngeal artery

Mastoid branch of occipital artery

Middle meningeal artery

Recurrent meningeal branch of lacrimal (ophthalmic) artery

Accessory meningeal artery

Anterior meningeal branch of anterior ethmoidal artery

Posterior ethmoidal artery

Internal carotid artery and its meningohypophyseal trunk (*phantom*)

Middle meningeal artery

Accessory meningeal artery

Superficial temporal artery

Maxillary artery

Posterior auricular artery

Occipital artery

External carotid artery

Anterior and posterior meningeal branches of vertebral artery

Tentorial, cavernous sinus and meningeal branches of meningohypophyseal trunk

MENINGES AND BRAIN

PLATE 95

Meninges and Superficial Cerebral Veins

FOR DEEP VEINS OF BRAIN SEE PLATE 138

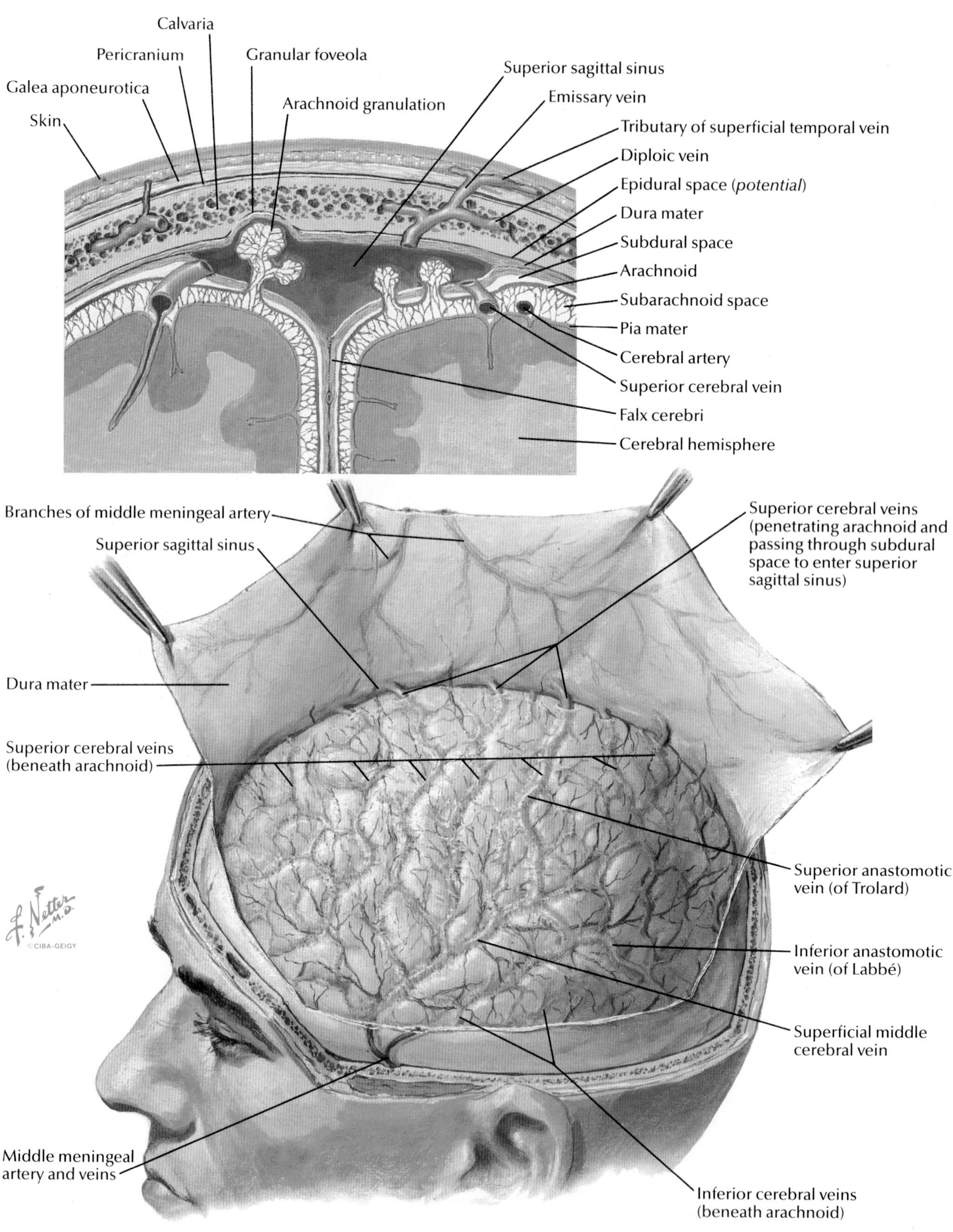

Calvaria

Pericranium

Granular foveola

Galea aponeurotica

Arachnoid granulation

Skin

Superior sagittal sinus

Emissary vein

Tributary of superficial temporal vein

Diploic vein

Epidural space (*potential*)

Dura mater

Subdural space

Arachnoid

Subarachnoid space

Pia mater

Cerebral artery

Superior cerebral vein

Falx cerebri

Cerebral hemisphere

Branches of middle meningeal artery

Superior sagittal sinus

Dura mater

Superior cerebral veins (beneath arachnoid)

Superior cerebral veins (penetrating arachnoid and passing through subdural space to enter superior sagittal sinus)

Superior anastomotic vein (of Trolard)

Inferior anastomotic vein (of Labbé)

Superficial middle cerebral vein

Middle meningeal artery and veins

Inferior cerebral veins (beneath arachnoid)

PLATE 96

HEAD AND NECK

Sagittal section

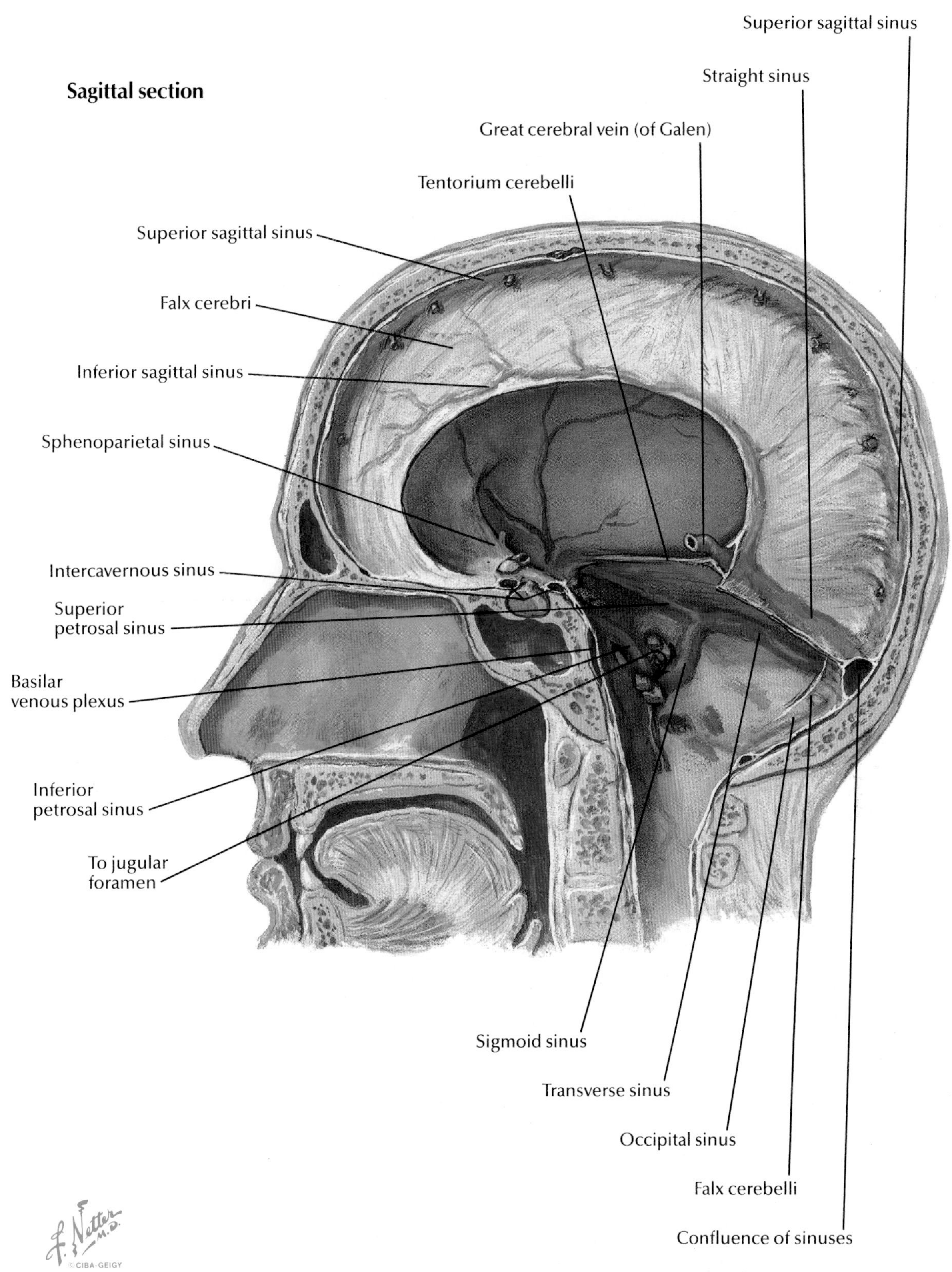

Superior sagittal sinus

Straight sinus

Great cerebral vein (of Galen)

Tentorium cerebelli

Superior sagittal sinus

Falx cerebri

Inferior sagittal sinus

Sphenoparietal sinus

Intercavernous sinus

Superior petrosal sinus

Basilar venous plexus

Inferior petrosal sinus

To jugular foramen

Sigmoid sinus

Transverse sinus

Occipital sinus

Falx cerebelli

Confluence of sinuses

Horizontal section: superior view

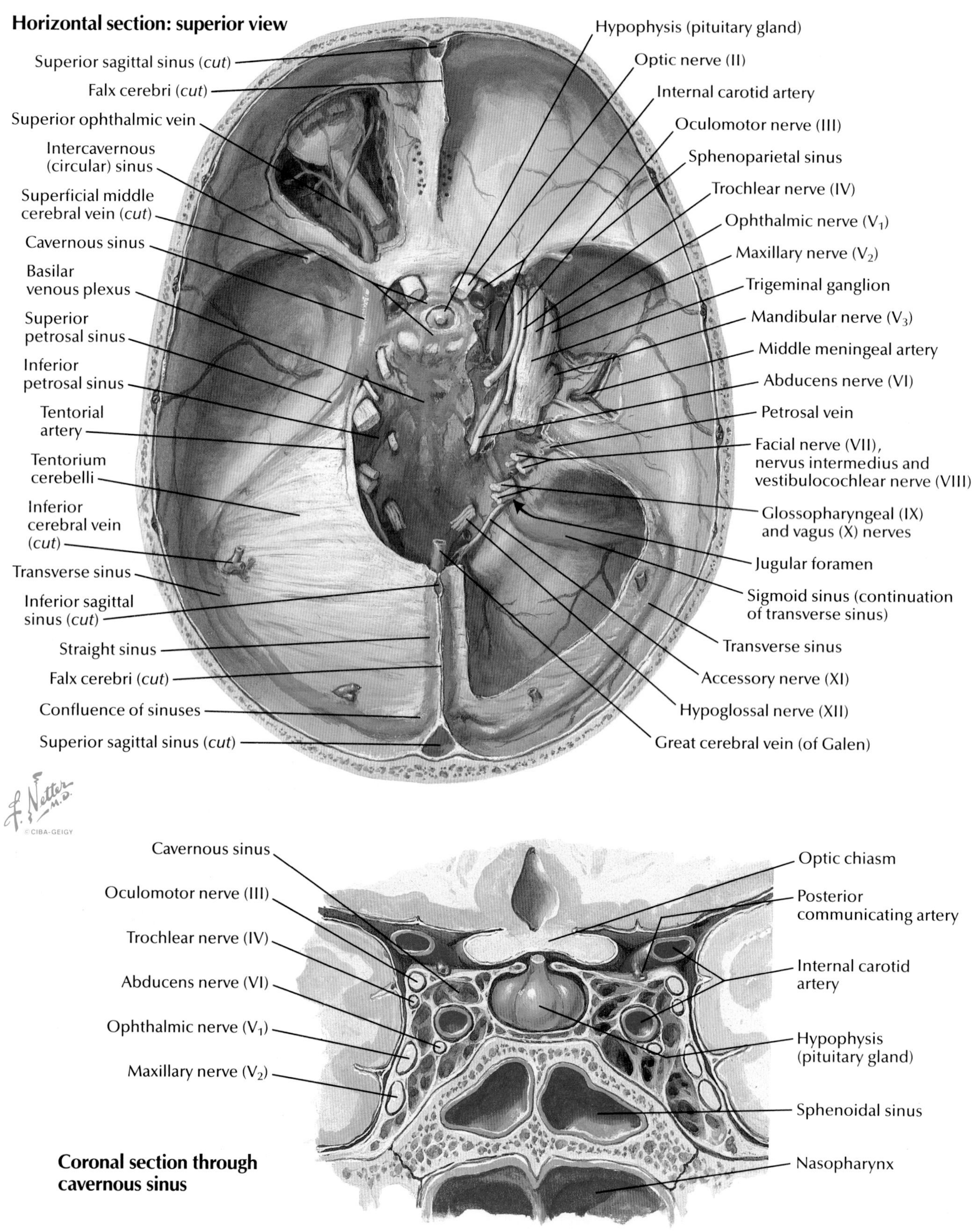

Superior sagittal sinus (*cut*)

Falx cerebri (*cut*)

Superior ophthalmic vein

Intercavernous (circular) sinus

Superficial middle cerebral vein (*cut*)

Cavernous sinus

Basilar venous plexus

Superior petrosal sinus

Inferior petrosal sinus

Tentorial artery

Tentorium cerebelli

Inferior cerebral vein (*cut*)

Transverse sinus

Inferior sagittal sinus (*cut*)

Straight sinus

Falx cerebri (*cut*)

Confluence of sinuses

Superior sagittal sinus (*cut*)

Hypophysis (pituitary gland)

Optic nerve (II)

Internal carotid artery

Oculomotor nerve (III)

Sphenoparietal sinus

Trochlear nerve (IV)

Ophthalmic nerve (V₁)

Maxillary nerve (V₂)

Trigeminal ganglion

Mandibular nerve (V₃)

Middle meningeal artery

Abducens nerve (VI)

Petrosal vein

Facial nerve (VII), nervus intermedius and vestibulocochlear nerve (VIII)

Glossopharyngeal (IX) and vagus (X) nerves

Jugular foramen

Sigmoid sinus (continuation of transverse sinus)

Transverse sinus

Accessory nerve (XI)

Hypoglossal nerve (XII)

Great cerebral vein (of Galen)

Cavernous sinus

Oculomotor nerve (III)

Trochlear nerve (IV)

Abducens nerve (VI)

Ophthalmic nerve (V₁)

Maxillary nerve (V₂)

Coronal section through cavernous sinus

Optic chiasm

Posterior communicating artery

Internal carotid artery

Hypophysis (pituitary gland)

Sphenoidal sinus

Nasopharynx

PLATE 98

HEAD AND NECK

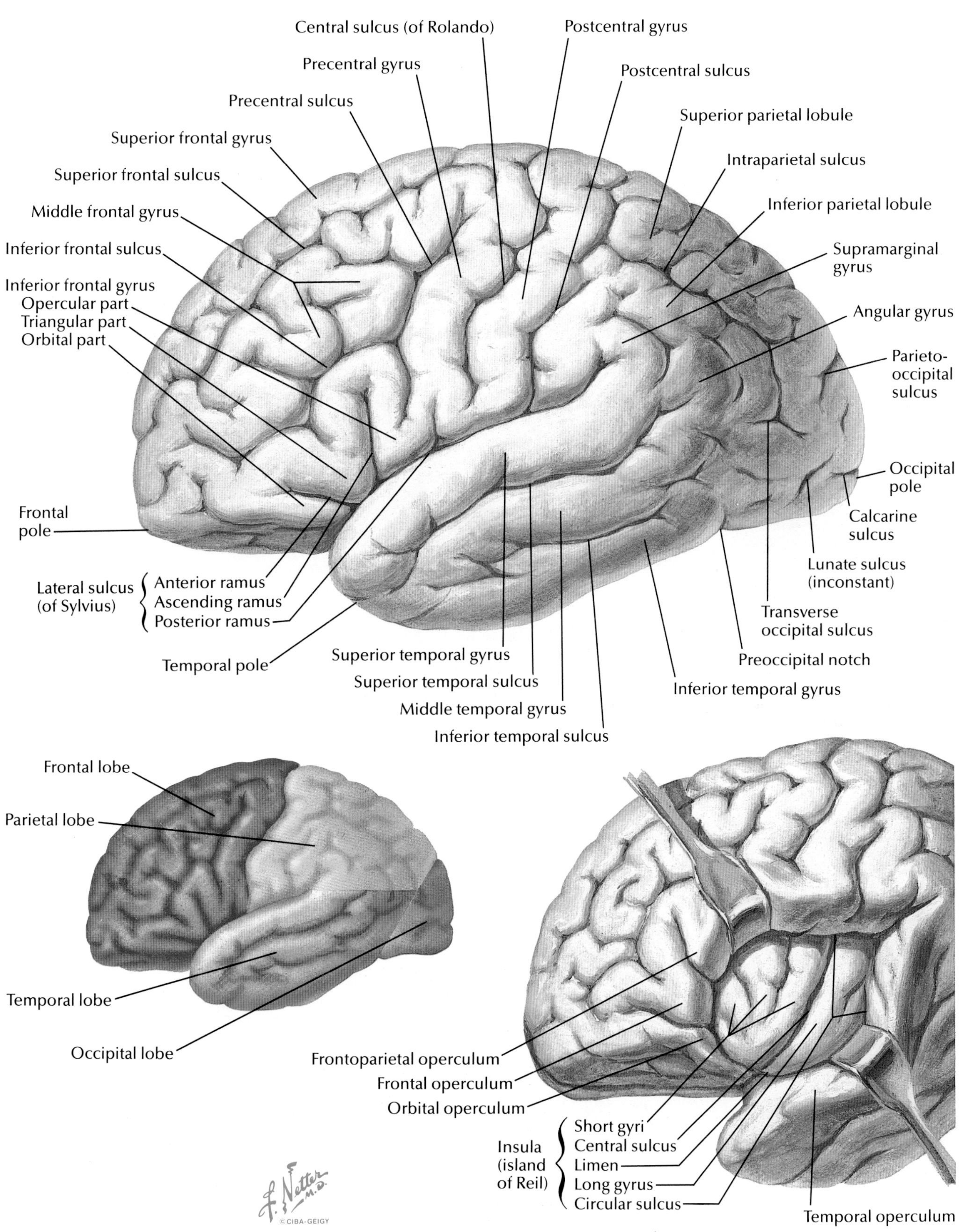

Central sulcus (of Rolando)
Precentral gyrus
Precentral sulcus
Superior frontal gyrus
Superior frontal sulcus
Middle frontal gyrus
Inferior frontal sulcus
Inferior frontal gyrus
Opercular part
Triangular part
Orbital part
Frontal pole
Lateral sulcus (of Sylvius) { Anterior ramus / Ascending ramus / Posterior ramus }
Temporal pole
Superior temporal gyrus
Superior temporal sulcus
Middle temporal gyrus
Inferior temporal sulcus

Postcentral gyrus
Postcentral sulcus
Superior parietal lobule
Intraparietal sulcus
Inferior parietal lobule
Supramarginal gyrus
Angular gyrus
Parieto-occipital sulcus
Occipital pole
Calcarine sulcus
Lunate sulcus (inconstant)
Transverse occipital sulcus
Preoccipital notch
Inferior temporal gyrus

Frontal lobe
Parietal lobe
Temporal lobe
Occipital lobe

Frontoparietal operculum
Frontal operculum
Orbital operculum
Insula (island of Reil) { Short gyri / Central sulcus / Limen / Long gyrus / Circular sulcus }
Temporal operculum

Cerebrum: Medial Views

FOR HYPOPHYSIS SEE PLATE 140

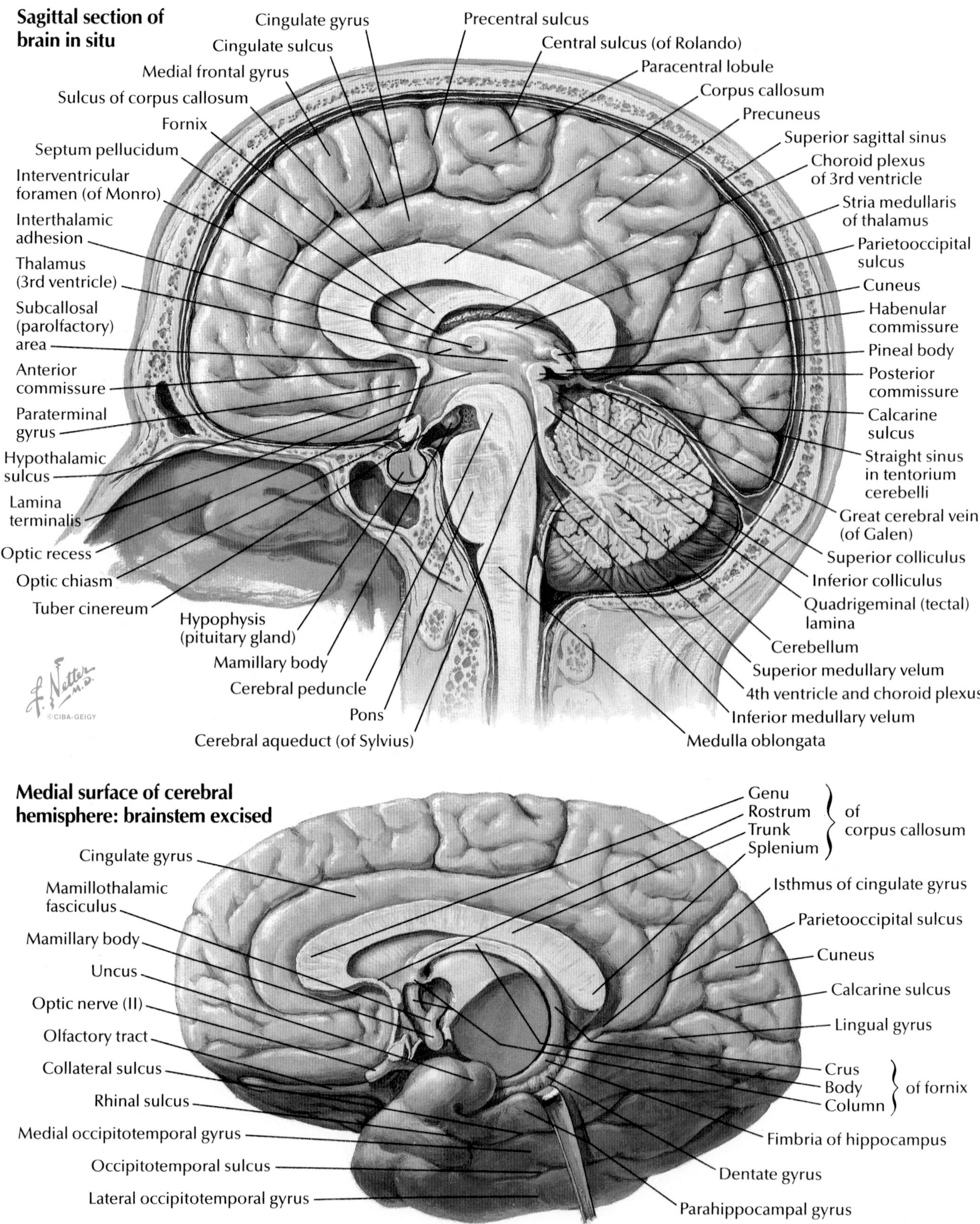

Sagittal section of brain in situ

Cingulate gyrus
Cingulate sulcus
Medial frontal gyrus
Sulcus of corpus callosum
Fornix
Septum pellucidum
Interventricular foramen (of Monro)
Interthalamic adhesion
Thalamus (3rd ventricle)
Subcallosal (parolfactory) area
Anterior commissure
Paraterminal gyrus
Hypothalamic sulcus
Lamina terminalis
Optic recess
Optic chiasm
Tuber cinereum
Hypophysis (pituitary gland)
Mamillary body
Cerebral peduncle
Pons
Cerebral aqueduct (of Sylvius)

Precentral sulcus
Central sulcus (of Rolando)
Paracentral lobule
Corpus callosum
Precuneus
Superior sagittal sinus
Choroid plexus of 3rd ventricle
Stria medullaris of thalamus
Parietooccipital sulcus
Cuneus
Habenular commissure
Pineal body
Posterior commissure
Calcarine sulcus
Straight sinus in tentorium cerebelli
Great cerebral vein (of Galen)
Superior colliculus
Inferior colliculus
Quadrigeminal (tectal) lamina
Cerebellum
Superior medullary velum
4th ventricle and choroid plexus
Inferior medullary velum
Medulla oblongata

Medial surface of cerebral hemisphere: brainstem excised

Cingulate gyrus
Mamillothalamic fasciculus
Mamillary body
Uncus
Optic nerve (II)
Olfactory tract
Collateral sulcus
Rhinal sulcus
Medial occipitotemporal gyrus
Occipitotemporal sulcus
Lateral occipitotemporal gyrus

Genu
Rostrum
Trunk
Splenium
} of corpus callosum

Isthmus of cingulate gyrus
Parietooccipital sulcus
Cuneus
Calcarine sulcus
Lingual gyrus
Crus
Body
Column
} of fornix
Fimbria of hippocampus
Dentate gyrus
Parahippocampal gyrus

PLATE 100

HEAD AND NECK

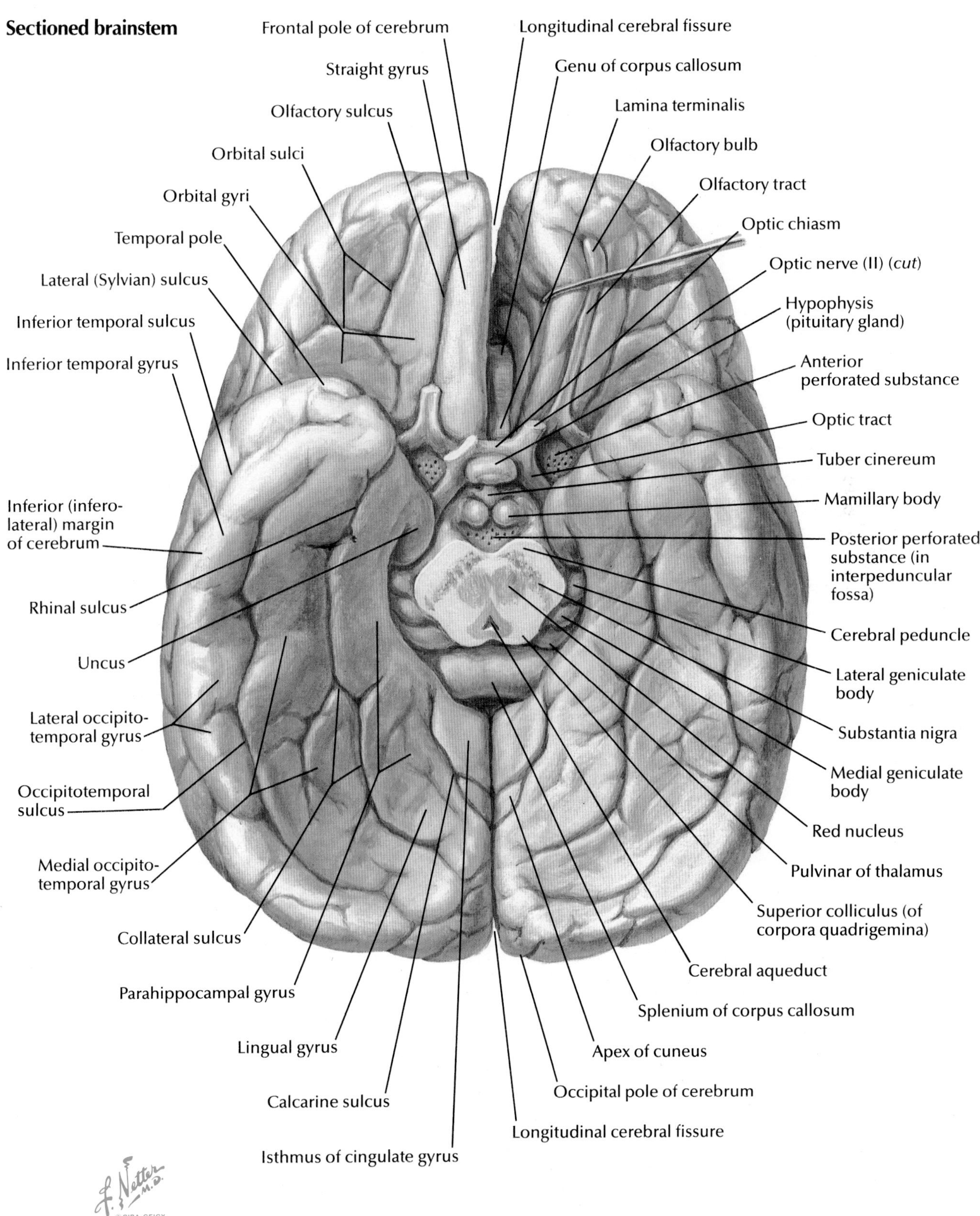

Sectioned brainstem

Frontal pole of cerebrum

Straight gyrus

Olfactory sulcus

Orbital sulci

Orbital gyri

Temporal pole

Lateral (Sylvian) sulcus

Inferior temporal sulcus

Inferior temporal gyrus

Inferior (infero-lateral) margin of cerebrum

Rhinal sulcus

Uncus

Lateral occipito-temporal gyrus

Occipitotemporal sulcus

Medial occipito-temporal gyrus

Collateral sulcus

Parahippocampal gyrus

Lingual gyrus

Calcarine sulcus

Isthmus of cingulate gyrus

Longitudinal cerebral fissure

Genu of corpus callosum

Lamina terminalis

Olfactory bulb

Olfactory tract

Optic chiasm

Optic nerve (II) (*cut*)

Hypophysis (pituitary gland)

Anterior perforated substance

Optic tract

Tuber cinereum

Mamillary body

Posterior perforated substance (in interpeduncular fossa)

Cerebral peduncle

Lateral geniculate body

Substantia nigra

Medial geniculate body

Red nucleus

Pulvinar of thalamus

Superior colliculus (of corpora quadrigemina)

Cerebral aqueduct

Splenium of corpus callosum

Apex of cuneus

Occipital pole of cerebrum

Longitudinal cerebral fissure

Ventricles of Brain

Left lateral phantom view

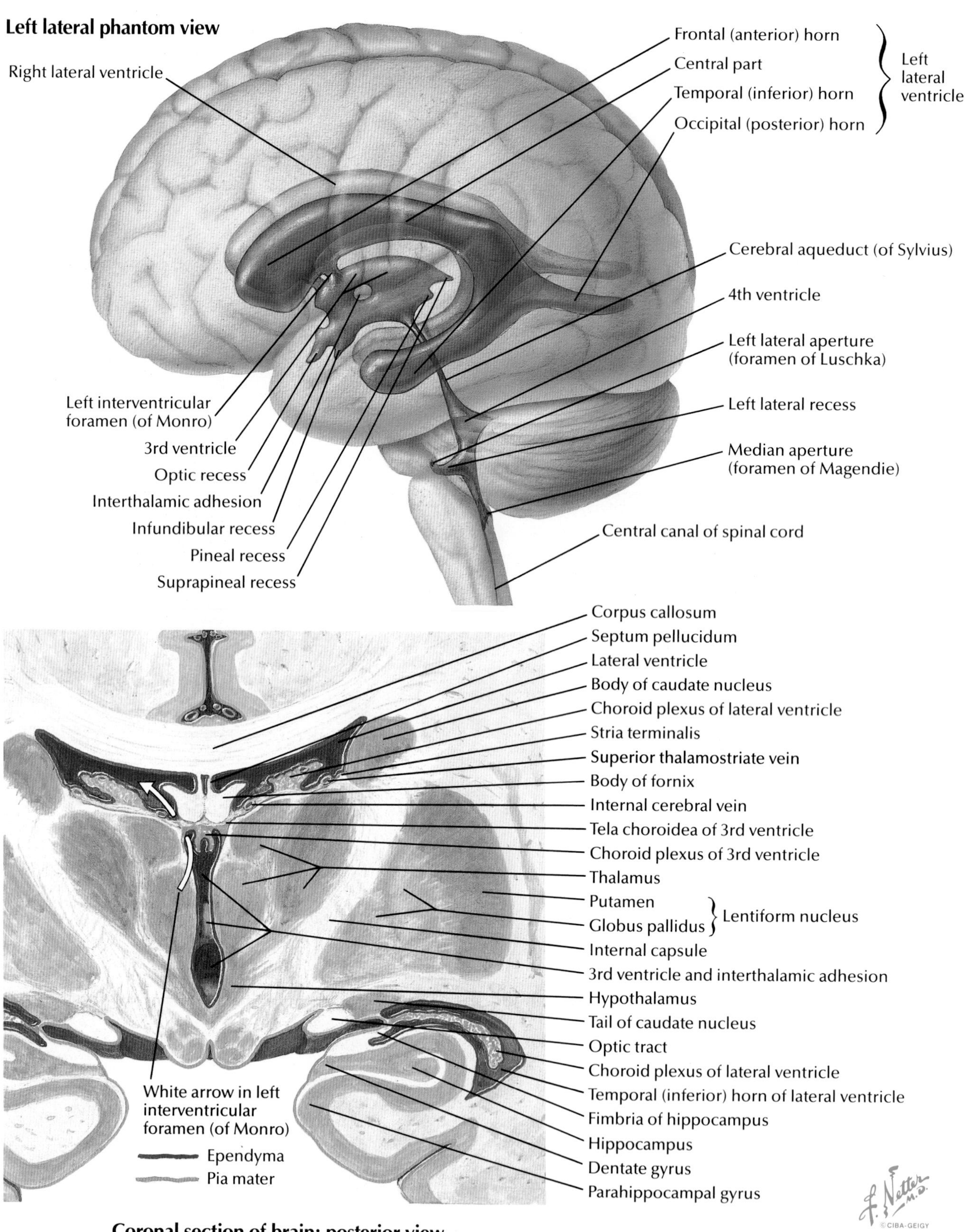

Right lateral ventricle

Frontal (anterior) horn
Central part
Temporal (inferior) horn
Occipital (posterior) horn
} Left lateral ventricle

Cerebral aqueduct (of Sylvius)

4th ventricle

Left lateral aperture (foramen of Luschka)

Left lateral recess

Median aperture (foramen of Magendie)

Left interventricular foramen (of Monro)

3rd ventricle

Optic recess

Interthalamic adhesion

Infundibular recess

Pineal recess

Suprapineal recess

Central canal of spinal cord

Corpus callosum
Septum pellucidum
Lateral ventricle
Body of caudate nucleus
Choroid plexus of lateral ventricle
Stria terminalis
Superior thalamostriate vein
Body of fornix
Internal cerebral vein
Tela choroidea of 3rd ventricle
Choroid plexus of 3rd ventricle
Thalamus
Putamen
Globus pallidus } Lentiform nucleus
Internal capsule
3rd ventricle and interthalamic adhesion
Hypothalamus
Tail of caudate nucleus
Optic tract
Choroid plexus of lateral ventricle
Temporal (inferior) horn of lateral ventricle
Fimbria of hippocampus
Hippocampus
Dentate gyrus
Parahippocampal gyrus

White arrow in left interventricular foramen (of Monro)

Ependyma
Pia mater

Coronal section of brain: posterior view

PLATE 102

HEAD AND NECK

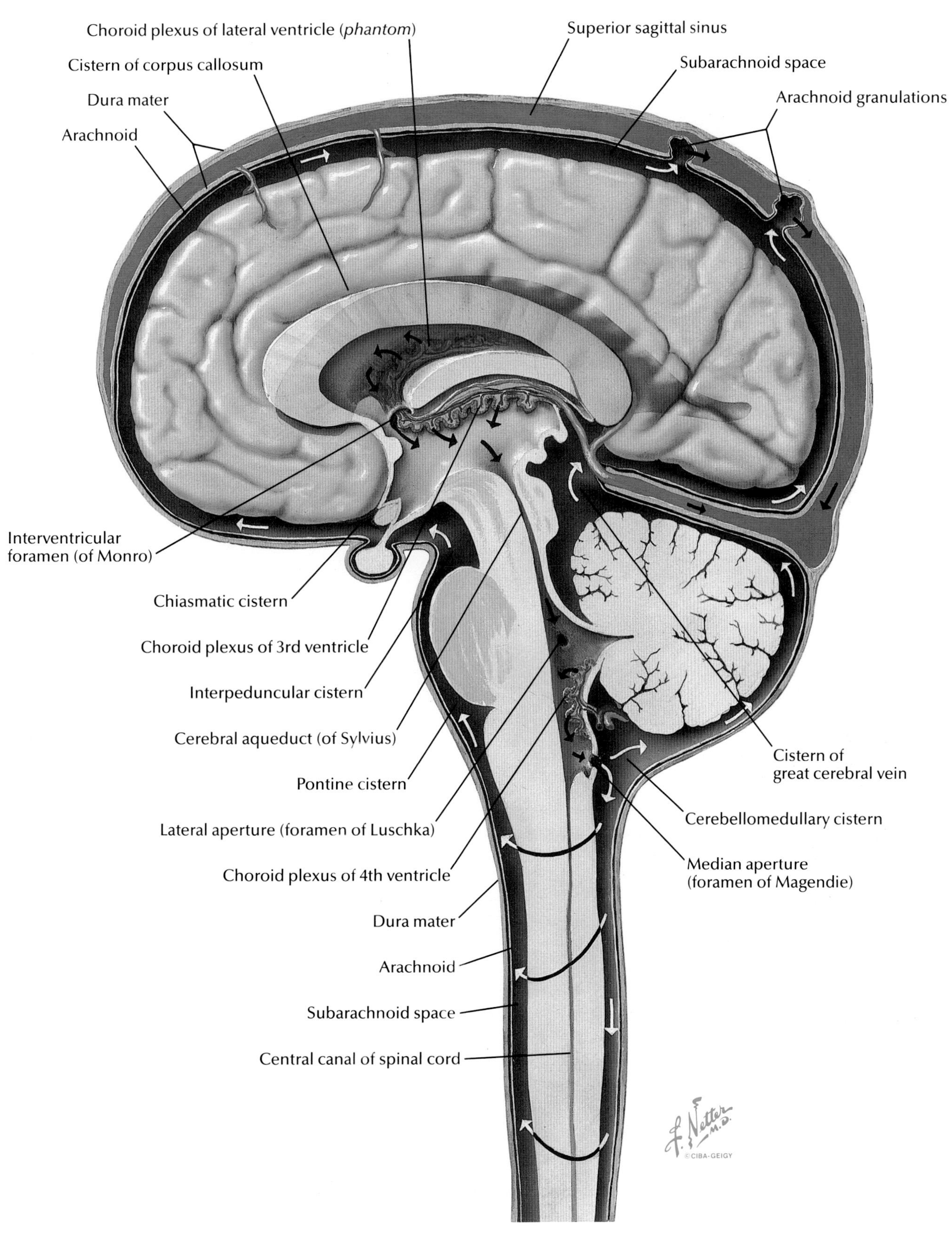

Choroid plexus of lateral ventricle (*phantom*)

Cistern of corpus callosum

Dura mater

Arachnoid

Superior sagittal sinus

Subarachnoid space

Arachnoid granulations

Interventricular foramen (of Monro)

Chiasmatic cistern

Choroid plexus of 3rd ventricle

Interpeduncular cistern

Cerebral aqueduct (of Sylvius)

Pontine cistern

Lateral aperture (foramen of Luschka)

Choroid plexus of 4th ventricle

Dura mater

Arachnoid

Subarachnoid space

Central canal of spinal cord

Cistern of great cerebral vein

Cerebellomedullary cistern

Median aperture (foramen of Magendie)

Basal Ganglia

Horizontal sections through cerebrum

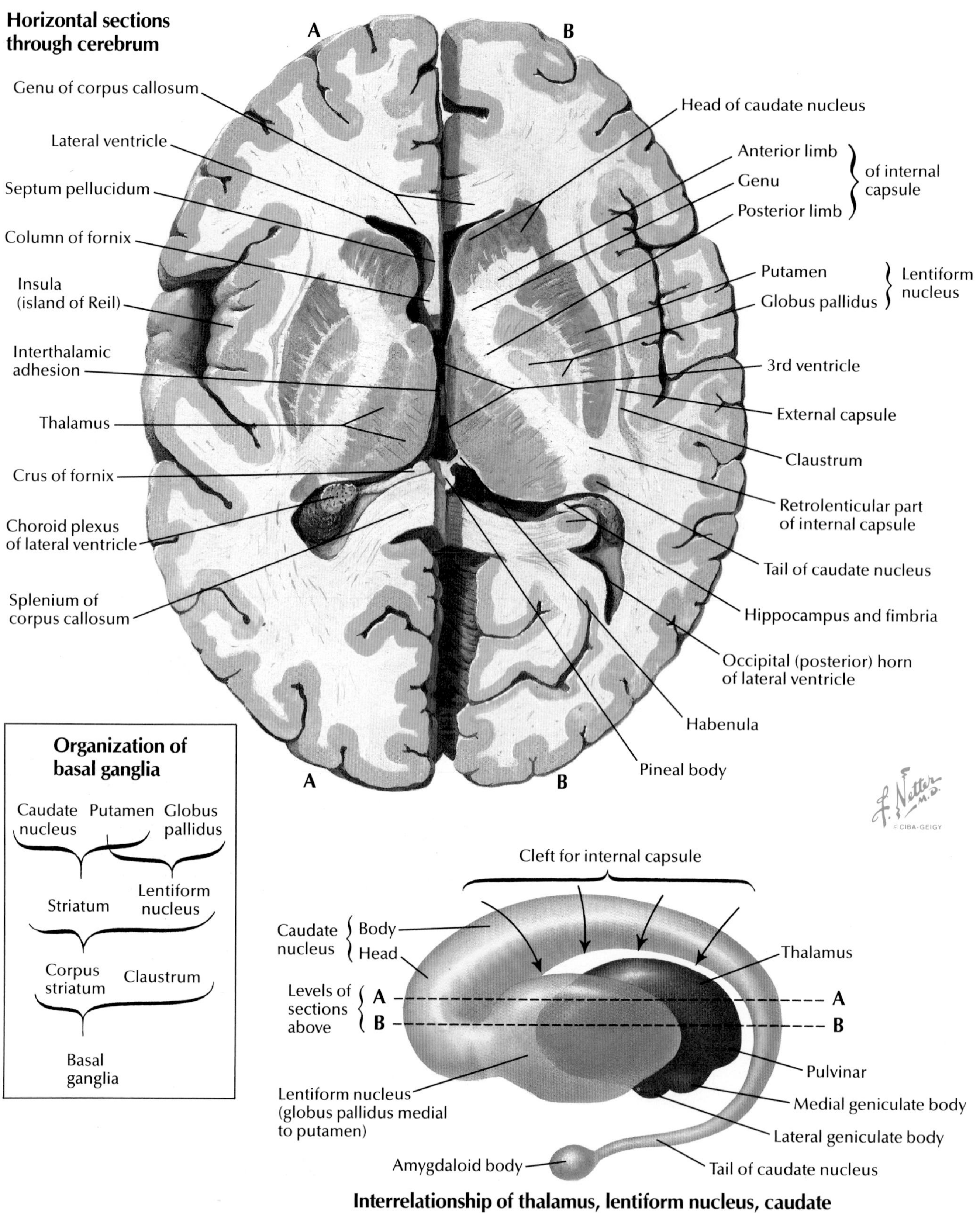

Genu of corpus callosum

Lateral ventricle

Septum pellucidum

Column of fornix

Insula (island of Reil)

Interthalamic adhesion

Thalamus

Crus of fornix

Choroid plexus of lateral ventricle

Splenium of corpus callosum

Head of caudate nucleus

Anterior limb
Genu
Posterior limb
} of internal capsule

Putamen
Globus pallidus
} Lentiform nucleus

3rd ventricle

External capsule

Claustrum

Retrolenticular part of internal capsule

Tail of caudate nucleus

Hippocampus and fimbria

Occipital (posterior) horn of lateral ventricle

Habenula

Pineal body

Organization of basal ganglia

Caudate nucleus   Putamen   Globus pallidus

Striatum   Lentiform nucleus

Corpus striatum   Claustrum

Basal ganglia

Cleft for internal capsule

Caudate nucleus { Body, Head }

Levels of sections above { A, B }

Thalamus

A

B

Lentiform nucleus (globus pallidus medial to putamen)

Pulvinar

Medial geniculate body

Lateral geniculate body

Tail of caudate nucleus

Amygdaloid body

Interrelationship of thalamus, lentiform nucleus, caudate nucleus and amygdaloid body (schema): left lateral view

PLATE 104

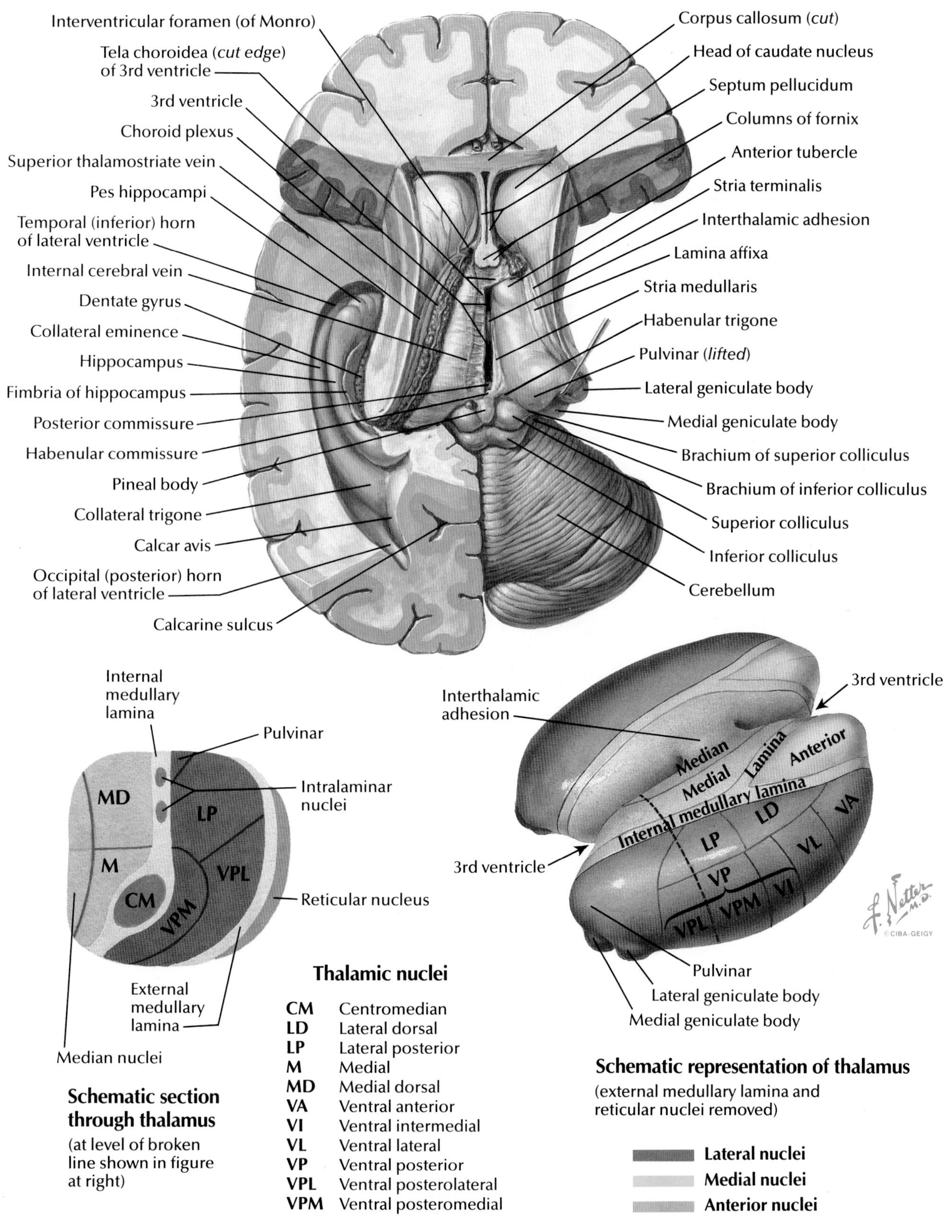

Interventricular foramen (of Monro)
Tela choroidea (*cut edge*) of 3rd ventricle
3rd ventricle
Choroid plexus
Superior thalamostriate vein
Pes hippocampi
Temporal (inferior) horn of lateral ventricle
Internal cerebral vein
Dentate gyrus
Collateral eminence
Hippocampus
Fimbria of hippocampus
Posterior commissure
Habenular commissure
Pineal body
Collateral trigone
Calcar avis
Occipital (posterior) horn of lateral ventricle
Calcarine sulcus

Corpus callosum (*cut*)
Head of caudate nucleus
Septum pellucidum
Columns of fornix
Anterior tubercle
Stria terminalis
Interthalamic adhesion
Lamina affixa
Stria medullaris
Habenular trigone
Pulvinar (*lifted*)
Lateral geniculate body
Medial geniculate body
Brachium of superior colliculus
Brachium of inferior colliculus
Superior colliculus
Inferior colliculus
Cerebellum

Internal medullary lamina
Pulvinar
Intralaminar nuclei
Reticular nucleus
External medullary lamina
Median nuclei

MD
LP
M
VPL
CM
VPM

Interthalamic adhesion
3rd ventricle
3rd ventricle
Median
Medial
Lamina
Anterior
Internal medullary lamina
LP
LD
VA
VP
VL
VPL
VPM
VI
Pulvinar
Lateral geniculate body
Medial geniculate body

Thalamic nuclei

CM	Centromedian
LD	Lateral dorsal
LP	Lateral posterior
M	Medial
MD	Medial dorsal
VA	Ventral anterior
VI	Ventral intermedial
VL	Ventral lateral
VP	Ventral posterior
VPL	Ventral posterolateral
VPM	Ventral posteromedial

Schematic section through thalamus
(at level of broken line shown in figure at right)

Schematic representation of thalamus
(external medullary lamina and reticular nuclei removed)

Lateral nuclei
Medial nuclei
Anterior nuclei

Hippocampus and Fornix

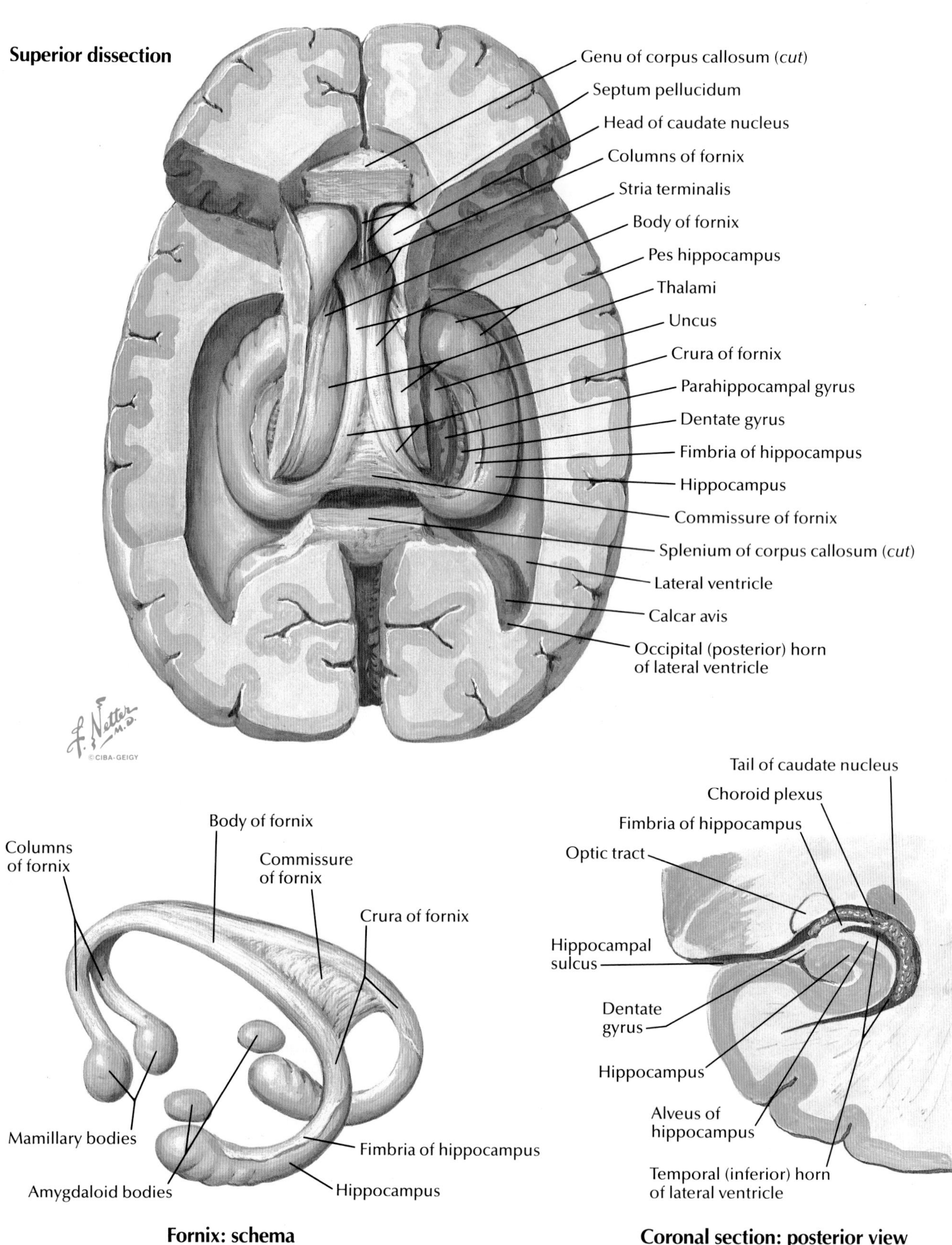

Superior dissection

Genu of corpus callosum (*cut*)
Septum pellucidum
Head of caudate nucleus
Columns of fornix
Stria terminalis
Body of fornix
Pes hippocampus
Thalami
Uncus
Crura of fornix
Parahippocampal gyrus
Dentate gyrus
Fimbria of hippocampus
Hippocampus
Commissure of fornix
Splenium of corpus callosum (*cut*)
Lateral ventricle
Calcar avis
Occipital (posterior) horn of lateral ventricle

Columns of fornix
Body of fornix
Commissure of fornix
Crura of fornix
Mamillary bodies
Amygdaloid bodies
Fimbria of hippocampus
Hippocampus

Fornix: schema

Tail of caudate nucleus
Choroid plexus
Fimbria of hippocampus
Optic tract
Hippocampal sulcus
Dentate gyrus
Hippocampus
Alveus of hippocampus
Temporal (inferior) horn of lateral ventricle

Coronal section: posterior view

PLATE 106

HEAD AND NECK

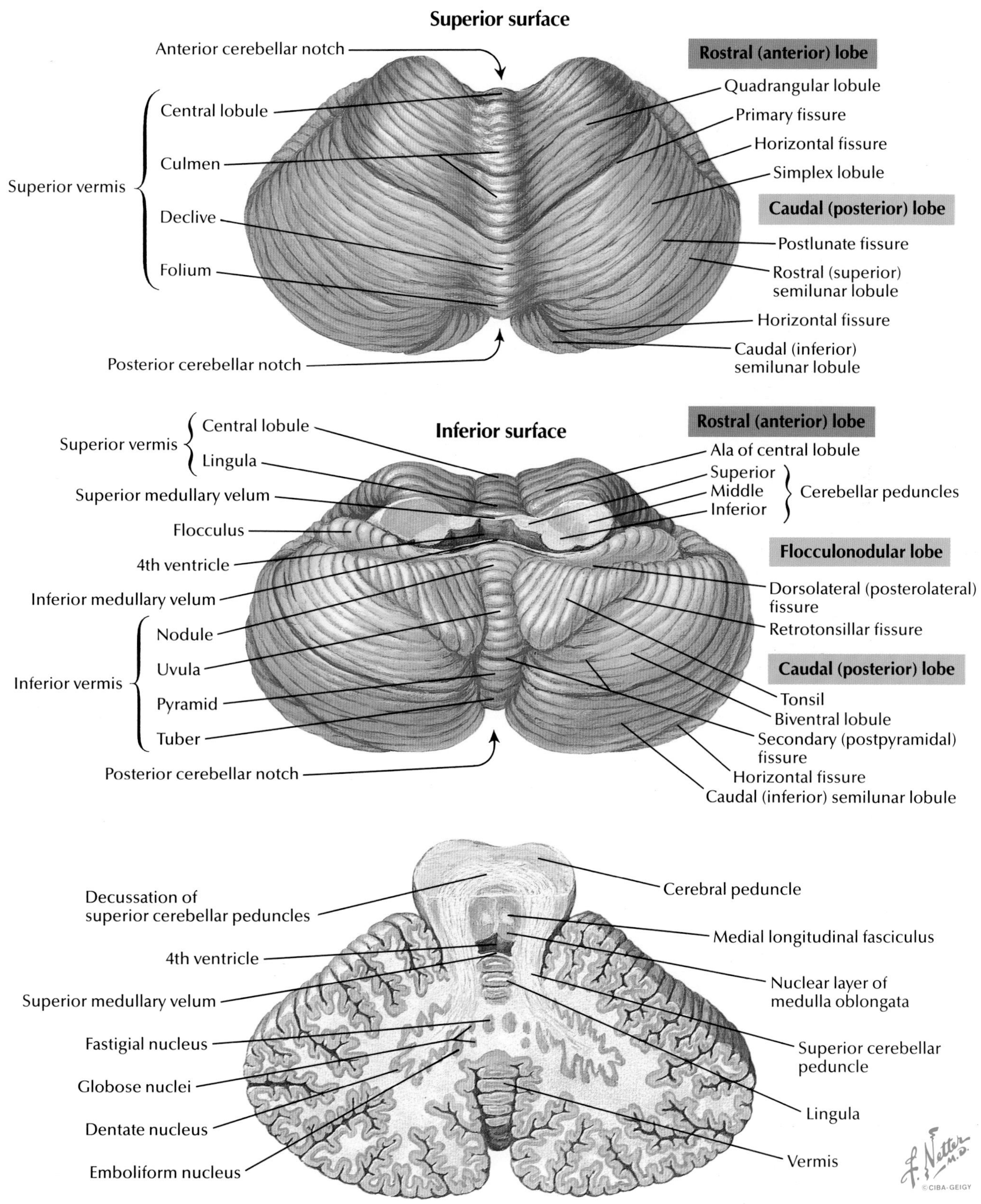

Superior surface

Anterior cerebellar notch

Central lobule

Culmen

Superior vermis {

Declive

Folium

Posterior cerebellar notch

Rostral (anterior) lobe

Quadrangular lobule

Primary fissure

Horizontal fissure

Simplex lobule

Caudal (posterior) lobe

Postlunate fissure

Rostral (superior) semilunar lobule

Horizontal fissure

Caudal (inferior) semilunar lobule

Inferior surface

Superior vermis { Central lobule

Lingula

Superior medullary velum

Flocculus

4th ventricle

Inferior medullary velum

Inferior vermis {

Nodule

Uvula

Pyramid

Tuber

Posterior cerebellar notch

Rostral (anterior) lobe

Ala of central lobule

Superior }

Middle } Cerebellar peduncles

Inferior }

Flocculonodular lobe

Dorsolateral (posterolateral) fissure

Retrotonsillar fissure

Caudal (posterior) lobe

Tonsil

Biventral lobule

Secondary (postpyramidal) fissure

Horizontal fissure

Caudal (inferior) semilunar lobule

Decussation of superior cerebellar peduncles

4th ventricle

Superior medullary velum

Fastigial nucleus

Globose nuclei

Dentate nucleus

Emboliform nucleus

Cerebral peduncle

Medial longitudinal fasciculus

Nuclear layer of medulla oblongata

Superior cerebellar peduncle

Lingula

Vermis

Section in plane of superior cerebellar peduncle

Brainstem

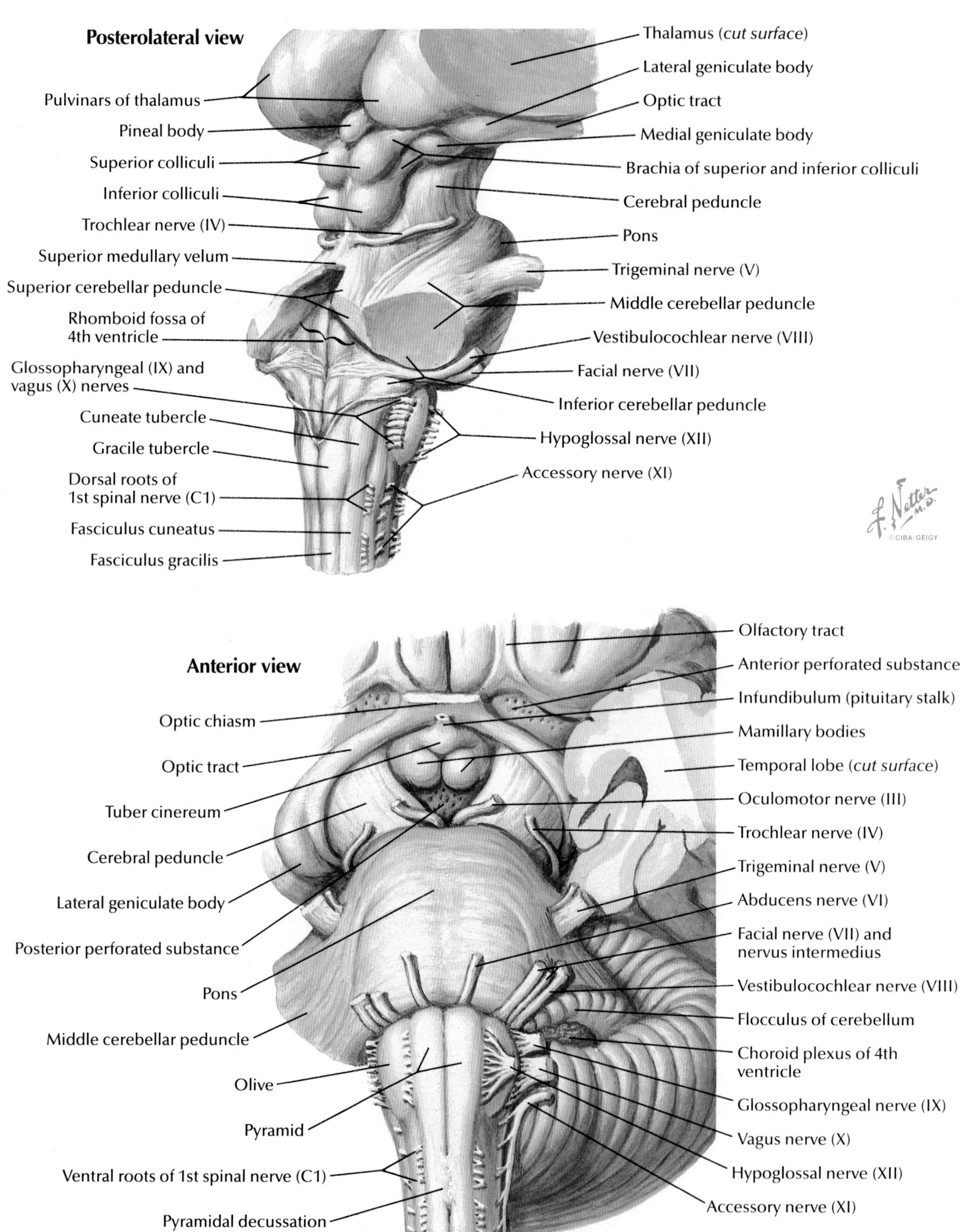

Posterolateral view

Pulvinars of thalamus

Pineal body

Superior colliculi

Inferior colliculi

Trochlear nerve (IV)

Superior medullary velum

Superior cerebellar peduncle

Rhomboid fossa of 4th ventricle

Glossopharyngeal (IX) and vagus (X) nerves

Cuneate tubercle

Gracile tubercle

Dorsal roots of 1st spinal nerve (C1)

Fasciculus cuneatus

Fasciculus gracilis

Thalamus (*cut surface*)

Lateral geniculate body

Optic tract

Medial geniculate body

Brachia of superior and inferior colliculi

Cerebral peduncle

Pons

Trigeminal nerve (V)

Middle cerebellar peduncle

Vestibulocochlear nerve (VIII)

Facial nerve (VII)

Inferior cerebellar peduncle

Hypoglossal nerve (XII)

Accessory nerve (XI)

Anterior view

Optic chiasm

Optic tract

Tuber cinereum

Cerebral peduncle

Lateral geniculate body

Posterior perforated substance

Pons

Middle cerebellar peduncle

Olive

Pyramid

Ventral roots of 1st spinal nerve (C1)

Pyramidal decussation

Olfactory tract

Anterior perforated substance

Infundibulum (pituitary stalk)

Mamillary bodies

Temporal lobe (*cut surface*)

Oculomotor nerve (III)

Trochlear nerve (IV)

Trigeminal nerve (V)

Abducens nerve (VI)

Facial nerve (VII) and nervus intermedius

Vestibulocochlear nerve (VIII)

Flocculus of cerebellum

Choroid plexus of 4th ventricle

Glossopharyngeal nerve (IX)

Vagus nerve (X)

Hypoglossal nerve (XII)

Accessory nerve (XI)

PLATE 108

HEAD AND NECK

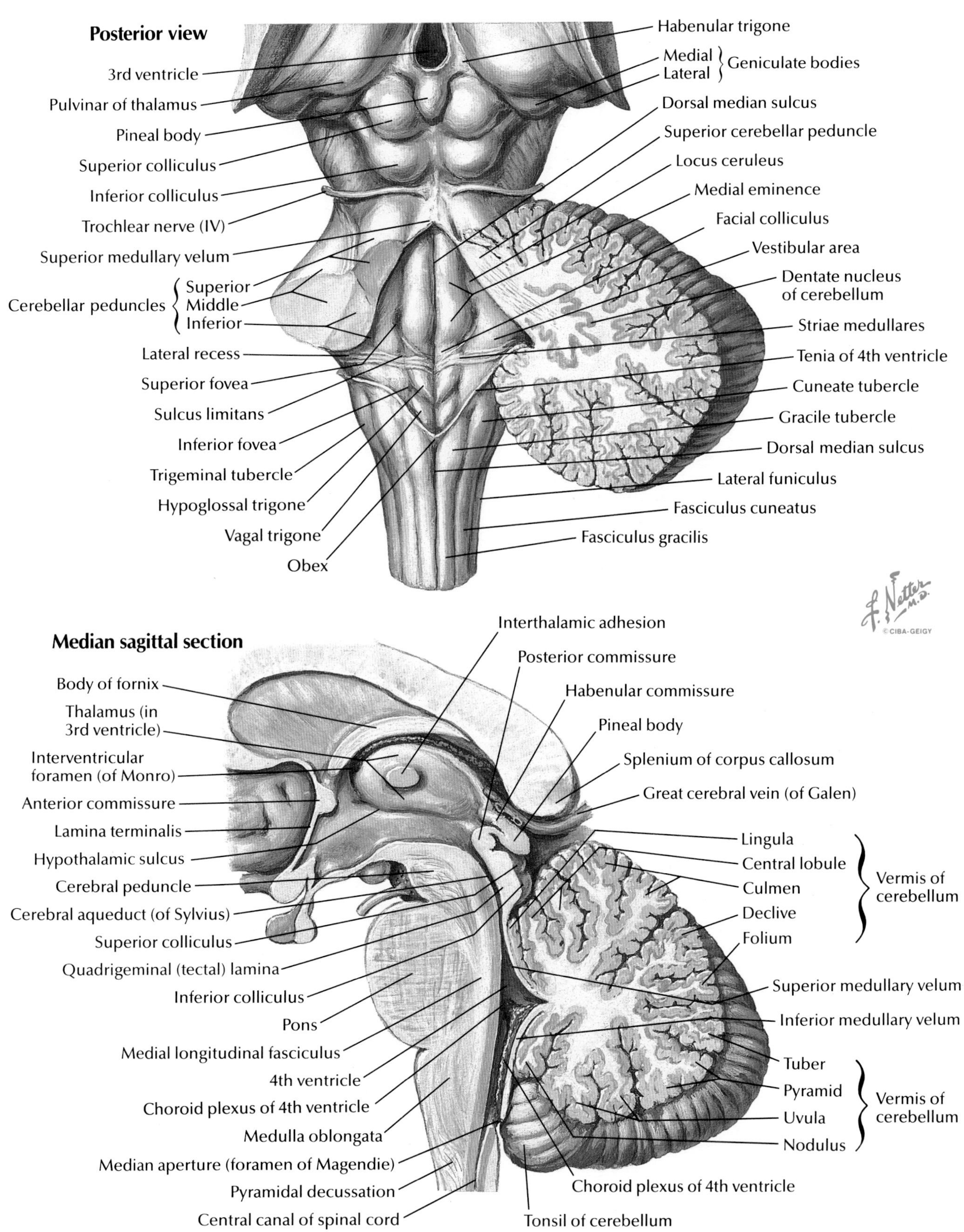

Posterior view

- Habenular trigone
- Medial } Geniculate bodies
- Lateral }
- 3rd ventricle
- Pulvinar of thalamus
- Dorsal median sulcus
- Pineal body
- Superior cerebellar peduncle
- Superior colliculus
- Locus ceruleus
- Inferior colliculus
- Medial eminence
- Trochlear nerve (IV)
- Facial colliculus
- Superior medullary velum
- Vestibular area
- Cerebellar peduncles { Superior / Middle / Inferior }
- Dentate nucleus of cerebellum
- Lateral recess
- Striae medullares
- Superior fovea
- Tenia of 4th ventricle
- Sulcus limitans
- Cuneate tubercle
- Inferior fovea
- Gracile tubercle
- Trigeminal tubercle
- Dorsal median sulcus
- Hypoglossal trigone
- Lateral funiculus
- Vagal trigone
- Fasciculus cuneatus
- Obex
- Fasciculus gracilis

Median sagittal section

- Interthalamic adhesion
- Posterior commissure
- Body of fornix
- Habenular commissure
- Thalamus (in 3rd ventricle)
- Pineal body
- Interventricular foramen (of Monro)
- Splenium of corpus callosum
- Anterior commissure
- Great cerebral vein (of Galen)
- Lamina terminalis
- Lingula
- Hypothalamic sulcus
- Central lobule
- Cerebral peduncle
- Culmen } Vermis of cerebellum
- Cerebral aqueduct (of Sylvius)
- Declive
- Superior colliculus
- Folium
- Quadrigeminal (tectal) lamina
- Inferior colliculus
- Superior medullary velum
- Pons
- Inferior medullary velum
- Medial longitudinal fasciculus
- Tuber
- 4th ventricle
- Pyramid } Vermis of cerebellum
- Choroid plexus of 4th ventricle
- Uvula
- Medulla oblongata
- Nodulus
- Median aperture (foramen of Magendie)
- Pyramidal decussation
- Choroid plexus of 4th ventricle
- Central canal of spinal cord
- Tonsil of cerebellum

Cranial Nerve Nuclei in Brainstem: Schema

Posterior phantom view

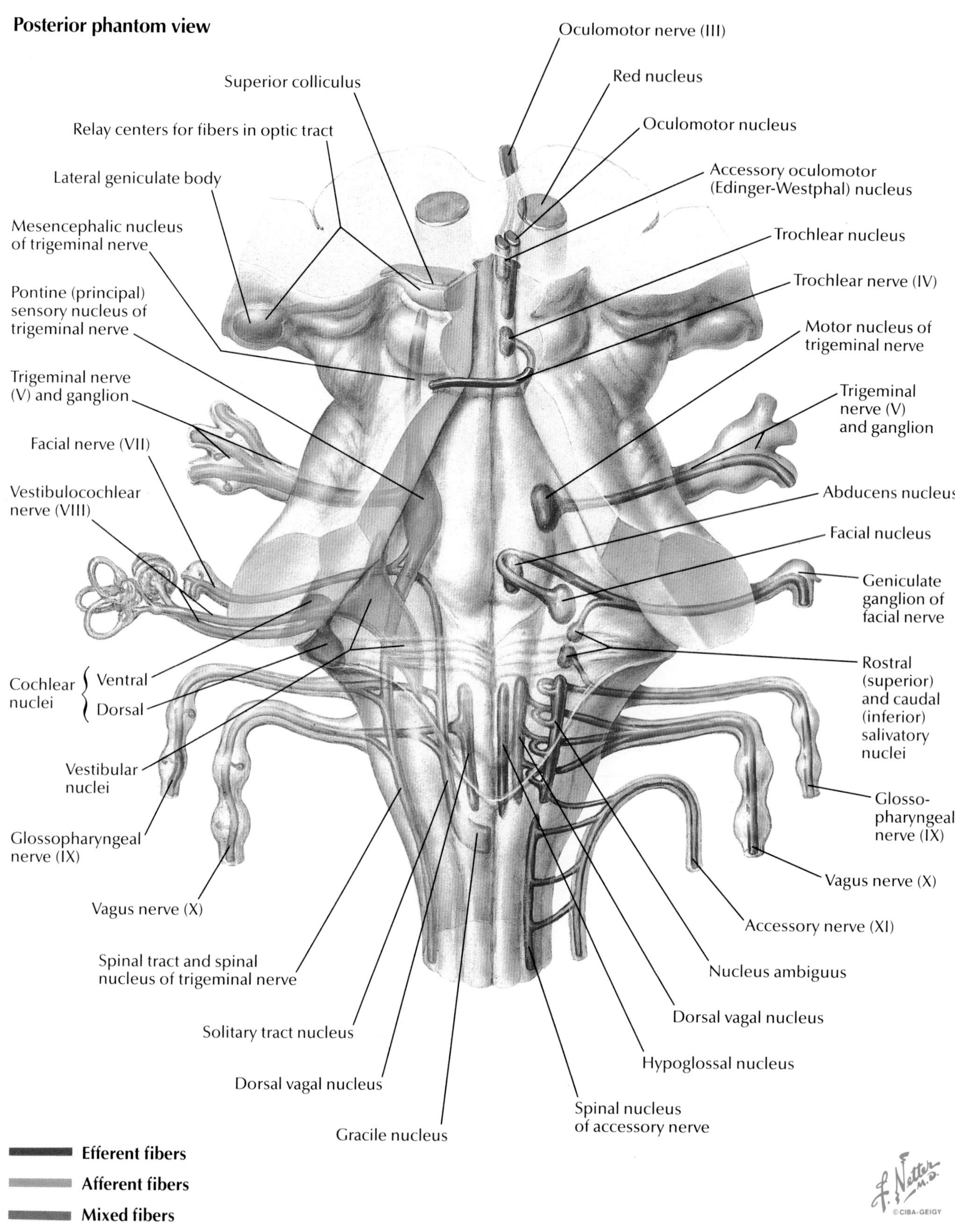

Superior colliculus

Relay centers for fibers in optic tract

Lateral geniculate body

Mesencephalic nucleus of trigeminal nerve

Pontine (principal) sensory nucleus of trigeminal nerve

Trigeminal nerve (V) and ganglion

Facial nerve (VII)

Vestibulocochlear nerve (VIII)

Cochlear { Ventral
nuclei { Dorsal

Vestibular nuclei

Glossopharyngeal nerve (IX)

Vagus nerve (X)

Spinal tract and spinal nucleus of trigeminal nerve

Solitary tract nucleus

Dorsal vagal nucleus

Gracile nucleus

Oculomotor nerve (III)

Red nucleus

Oculomotor nucleus

Accessory oculomotor (Edinger-Westphal) nucleus

Trochlear nucleus

Trochlear nerve (IV)

Motor nucleus of trigeminal nerve

Trigeminal nerve (V) and ganglion

Abducens nucleus

Facial nucleus

Geniculate ganglion of facial nerve

Rostral (superior) and caudal (inferior) salivatory nuclei

Glosso-pharyngeal nerve (IX)

Vagus nerve (X)

Accessory nerve (XI)

Nucleus ambiguus

Dorsal vagal nucleus

Hypoglossal nucleus

Spinal nucleus of accessory nerve

Efferent fibers
Afferent fibers
Mixed fibers

PLATE 110

HEAD AND NECK

Medial dissection

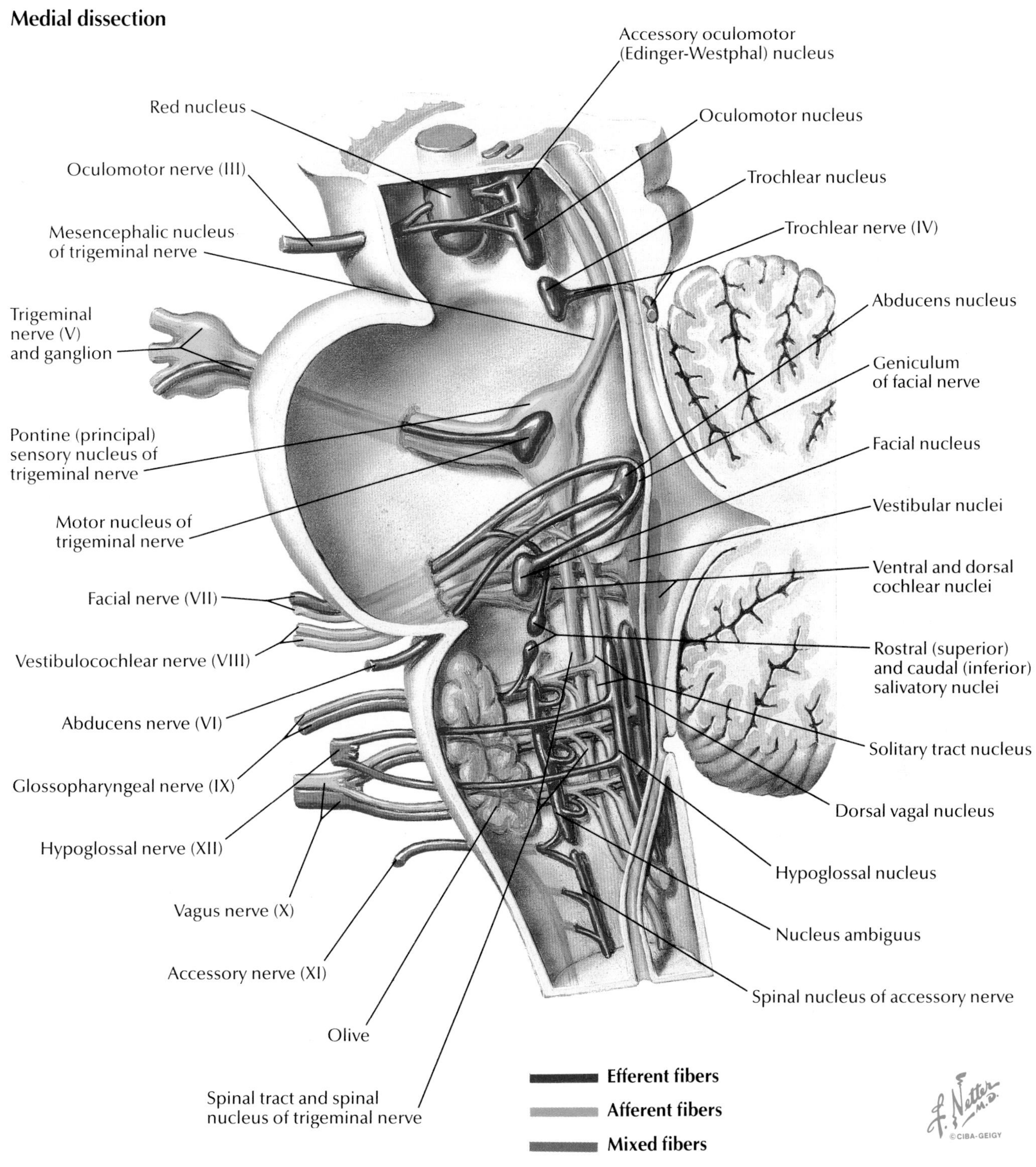

Accessory oculomotor (Edinger-Westphal) nucleus

Red nucleus

Oculomotor nucleus

Oculomotor nerve (III)

Trochlear nucleus

Mesencephalic nucleus of trigeminal nerve

Trochlear nerve (IV)

Trigeminal nerve (V) and ganglion

Abducens nucleus

Geniculum of facial nerve

Pontine (principal) sensory nucleus of trigeminal nerve

Facial nucleus

Vestibular nuclei

Motor nucleus of trigeminal nerve

Ventral and dorsal cochlear nuclei

Facial nerve (VII)

Rostral (superior) and caudal (inferior) salivatory nuclei

Vestibulocochlear nerve (VIII)

Abducens nerve (VI)

Solitary tract nucleus

Glossopharyngeal nerve (IX)

Dorsal vagal nucleus

Hypoglossal nerve (XII)

Hypoglossal nucleus

Vagus nerve (X)

Nucleus ambiguus

Accessory nerve (XI)

Spinal nucleus of accessory nerve

Olive

Spinal tract and spinal nucleus of trigeminal nerve

▬ **Efferent fibers**

▬ **Afferent fibers**

▬ **Mixed fibers**

Cranial Nerves (Motor and Sensory Distribution): Schema

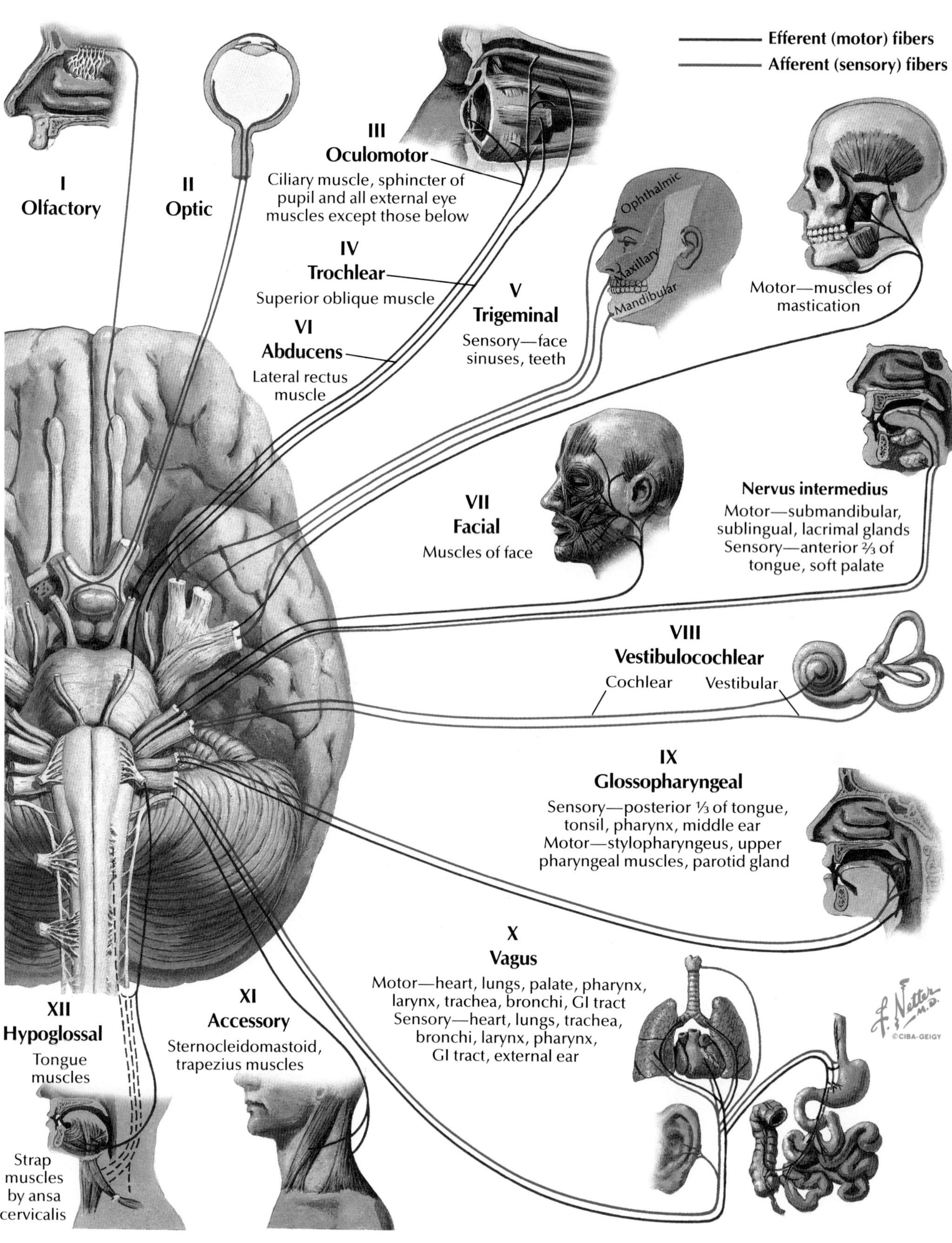

Efferent (motor) fibers
Afferent (sensory) fibers

I Olfactory

II Optic

III Oculomotor
Ciliary muscle, sphincter of pupil and all external eye muscles except those below

IV Trochlear
Superior oblique muscle

VI Abducens
Lateral rectus muscle

V Trigeminal
Sensory—face sinuses, teeth

Ophthalmic
Maxillary
Mandibular

Motor—muscles of mastication

VII Facial
Muscles of face

Nervus intermedius
Motor—submandibular, sublingual, lacrimal glands
Sensory—anterior ⅔ of tongue, soft palate

VIII Vestibulocochlear
Cochlear   Vestibular

IX Glossopharyngeal
Sensory—posterior ⅓ of tongue, tonsil, pharynx, middle ear
Motor—stylopharyngeus, upper pharyngeal muscles, parotid gland

X Vagus
Motor—heart, lungs, palate, pharynx, larynx, trachea, bronchi, GI tract
Sensory—heart, lungs, trachea, bronchi, larynx, pharynx, GI tract, external ear

XII Hypoglossal
Tongue muscles

Strap muscles by ansa cervicalis

XI Accessory
Sternocleidomastoid, trapezius muscles

PLATE 112

HEAD AND NECK

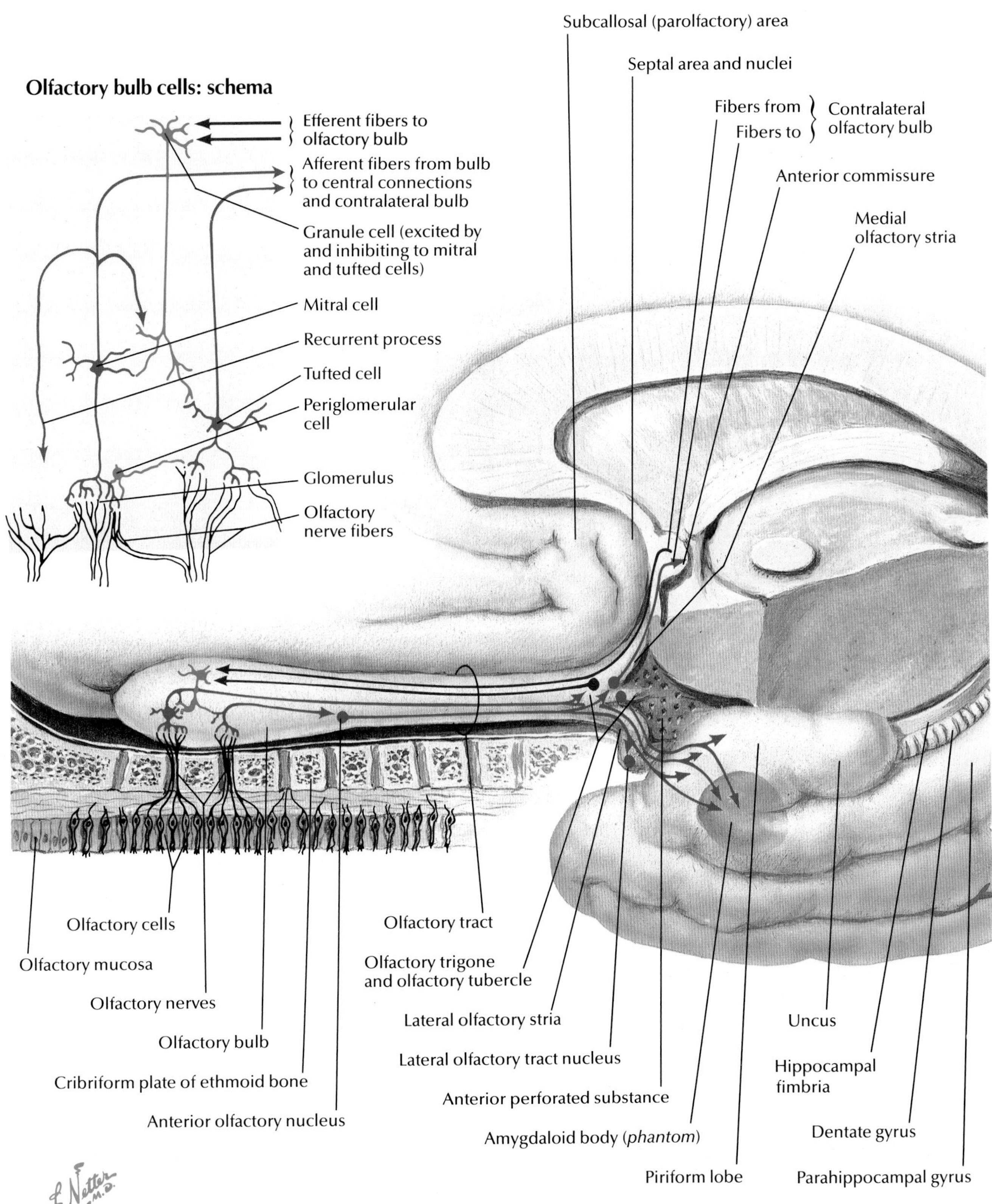

Olfactory bulb cells: schema

Efferent fibers to olfactory bulb

Afferent fibers from bulb to central connections and contralateral bulb

Granule cell (excited by and inhibiting to mitral and tufted cells)

Mitral cell

Recurrent process

Tufted cell

Periglomerular cell

Glomerulus

Olfactory nerve fibers

Subcallosal (parolfactory) area

Septal area and nuclei

Fibers from } Contralateral
Fibers to } olfactory bulb

Anterior commissure

Medial olfactory stria

Olfactory cells

Olfactory mucosa

Olfactory nerves

Olfactory bulb

Cribriform plate of ethmoid bone

Anterior olfactory nucleus

Olfactory tract

Olfactory trigone and olfactory tubercle

Lateral olfactory stria

Lateral olfactory tract nucleus

Anterior perforated substance

Amygdaloid body (*phantom*)

Piriform lobe

Uncus

Hippocampal fimbria

Dentate gyrus

Parahippocampal gyrus

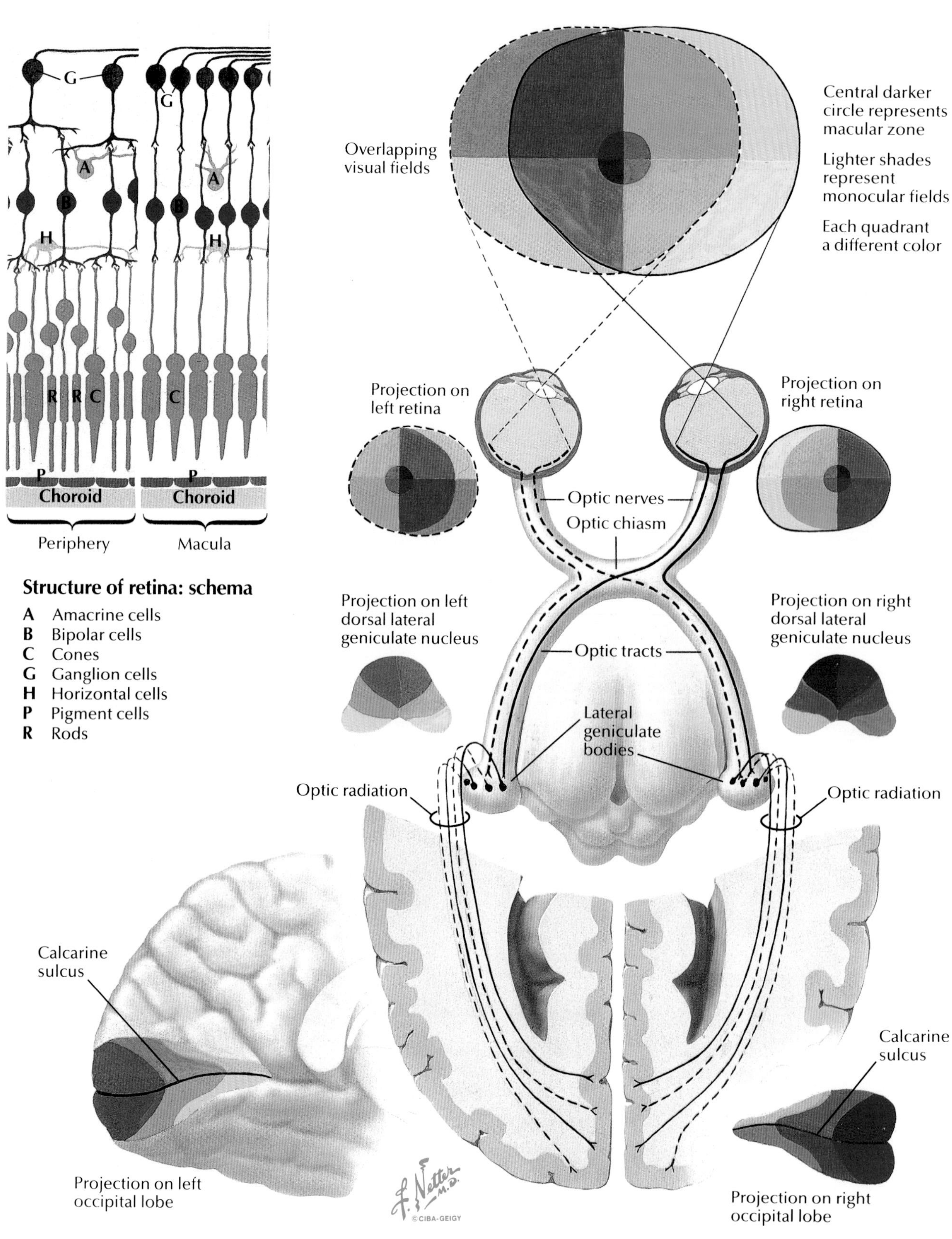

Structure of retina: schema

A Amacrine cells
B Bipolar cells
C Cones
G Ganglion cells
H Horizontal cells
P Pigment cells
R Rods

Periphery   Macula

Overlapping visual fields

Central darker circle represents macular zone

Lighter shades represent monocular fields

Each quadrant a different color

Projection on left retina

Projection on right retina

Optic nerves
Optic chiasm

Projection on left dorsal lateral geniculate nucleus

Projection on right dorsal lateral geniculate nucleus

Optic tracts

Lateral geniculate bodies

Optic radiation

Optic radiation

Calcarine sulcus

Calcarine sulcus

Projection on left occipital lobe

Projection on right occipital lobe

PLATE 114

HEAD AND NECK

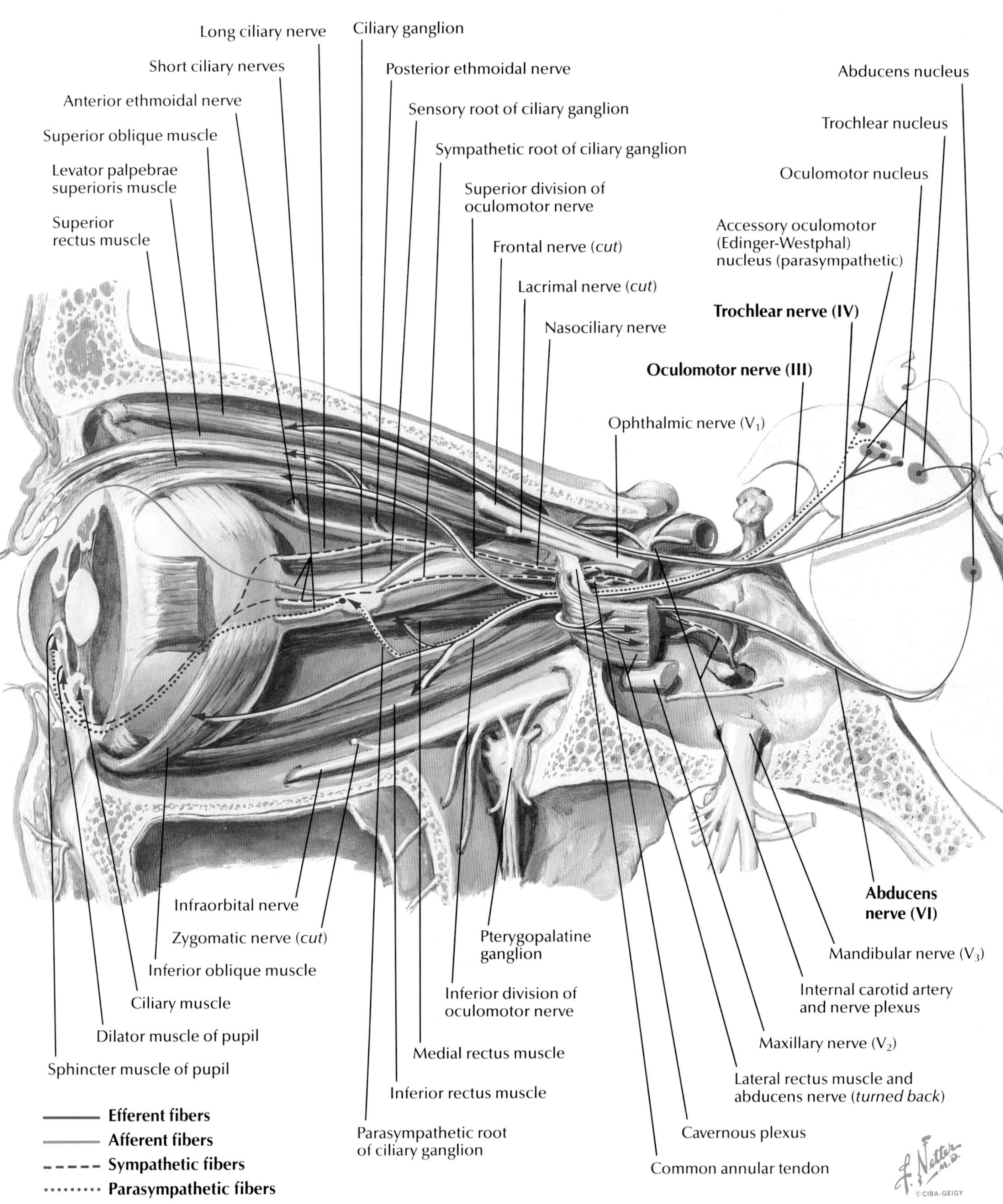

Long ciliary nerve

Short ciliary nerves

Anterior ethmoidal nerve

Superior oblique muscle

Levator palpebrae superioris muscle

Superior rectus muscle

Ciliary ganglion

Posterior ethmoidal nerve

Sensory root of ciliary ganglion

Sympathetic root of ciliary ganglion

Superior division of oculomotor nerve

Frontal nerve (cut)

Lacrimal nerve (cut)

Nasociliary nerve

Abducens nucleus

Trochlear nucleus

Oculomotor nucleus

Accessory oculomotor (Edinger-Westphal) nucleus (parasympathetic)

Trochlear nerve (IV)

Oculomotor nerve (III)

Ophthalmic nerve (V₁)

Infraorbital nerve

Zygomatic nerve (cut)

Inferior oblique muscle

Ciliary muscle

Dilator muscle of pupil

Sphincter muscle of pupil

Pterygopalatine ganglion

Inferior division of oculomotor nerve

Medial rectus muscle

Inferior rectus muscle

Parasympathetic root of ciliary ganglion

Abducens nerve (VI)

Mandibular nerve (V₃)

Internal carotid artery and nerve plexus

Maxillary nerve (V₂)

Lateral rectus muscle and abducens nerve (turned back)

Cavernous plexus

Common annular tendon

—— **Efferent fibers**
—— **Afferent fibers**
- - - **Sympathetic fibers**
······ **Parasympathetic fibers**

Trigeminal Nerve: Schema

SEE ALSO PLATES 18, 37, 38, 40, 41, 153

—— **Efferent fibers**
—— **Afferent fibers**
······ **Proprioceptive fibers**
······ **Parasympathetic fibers**
- - - - **Sympathetic fibers**

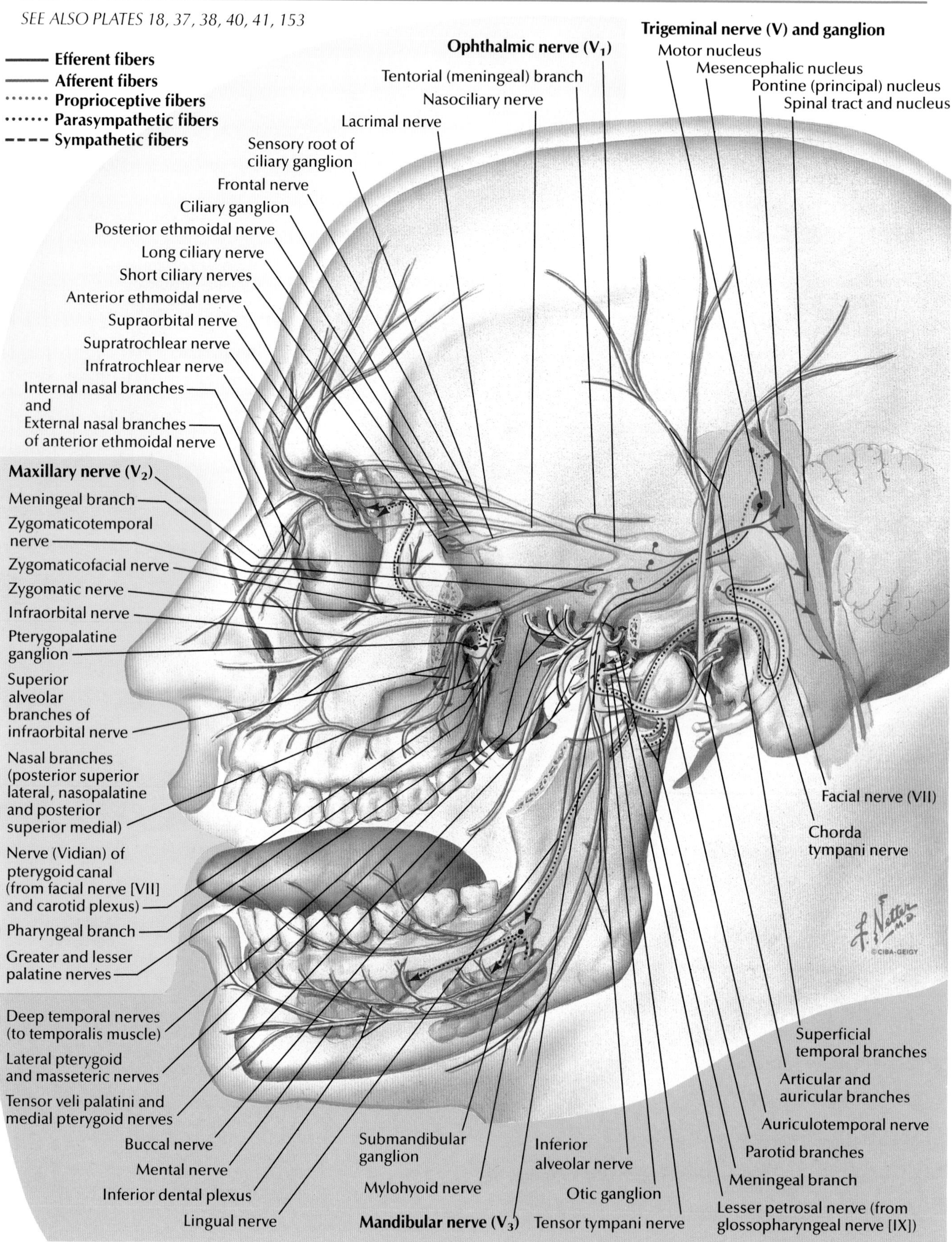

Ophthalmic nerve (V₁)

Tentorial (meningeal) branch
Nasociliary nerve
Lacrimal nerve
Sensory root of ciliary ganglion
Frontal nerve
Ciliary ganglion
Posterior ethmoidal nerve
Long ciliary nerve
Short ciliary nerves
Anterior ethmoidal nerve
Supraorbital nerve
Supratrochlear nerve
Infratrochlear nerve
Internal nasal branches and
External nasal branches of anterior ethmoidal nerve

Maxillary nerve (V₂)

Meningeal branch
Zygomaticotemporal nerve
Zygomaticofacial nerve
Zygomatic nerve
Infraorbital nerve
Pterygopalatine ganglion
Superior alveolar branches of infraorbital nerve
Nasal branches (posterior superior lateral, nasopalatine and posterior superior medial)
Nerve (Vidian) of pterygoid canal (from facial nerve [VII] and carotid plexus)
Pharyngeal branch
Greater and lesser palatine nerves

Deep temporal nerves (to temporalis muscle)
Lateral pterygoid and masseteric nerves
Tensor veli palatini and medial pterygoid nerves
Buccal nerve
Mental nerve
Inferior dental plexus
Lingual nerve

Trigeminal nerve (V) and ganglion
Motor nucleus
Mesencephalic nucleus
Pontine (principal) nucleus
Spinal tract and nucleus

Facial nerve (VII)
Chorda tympani nerve

Superficial temporal branches
Articular and auricular branches
Auriculotemporal nerve
Parotid branches
Meningeal branch
Lesser petrosal nerve (from glossopharyngeal nerve [IX])

Submandibular ganglion
Mylohyoid nerve
Mandibular nerve (V₃)
Inferior alveolar nerve
Otic ganglion
Tensor tympani nerve

PLATE 116

HEAD AND NECK

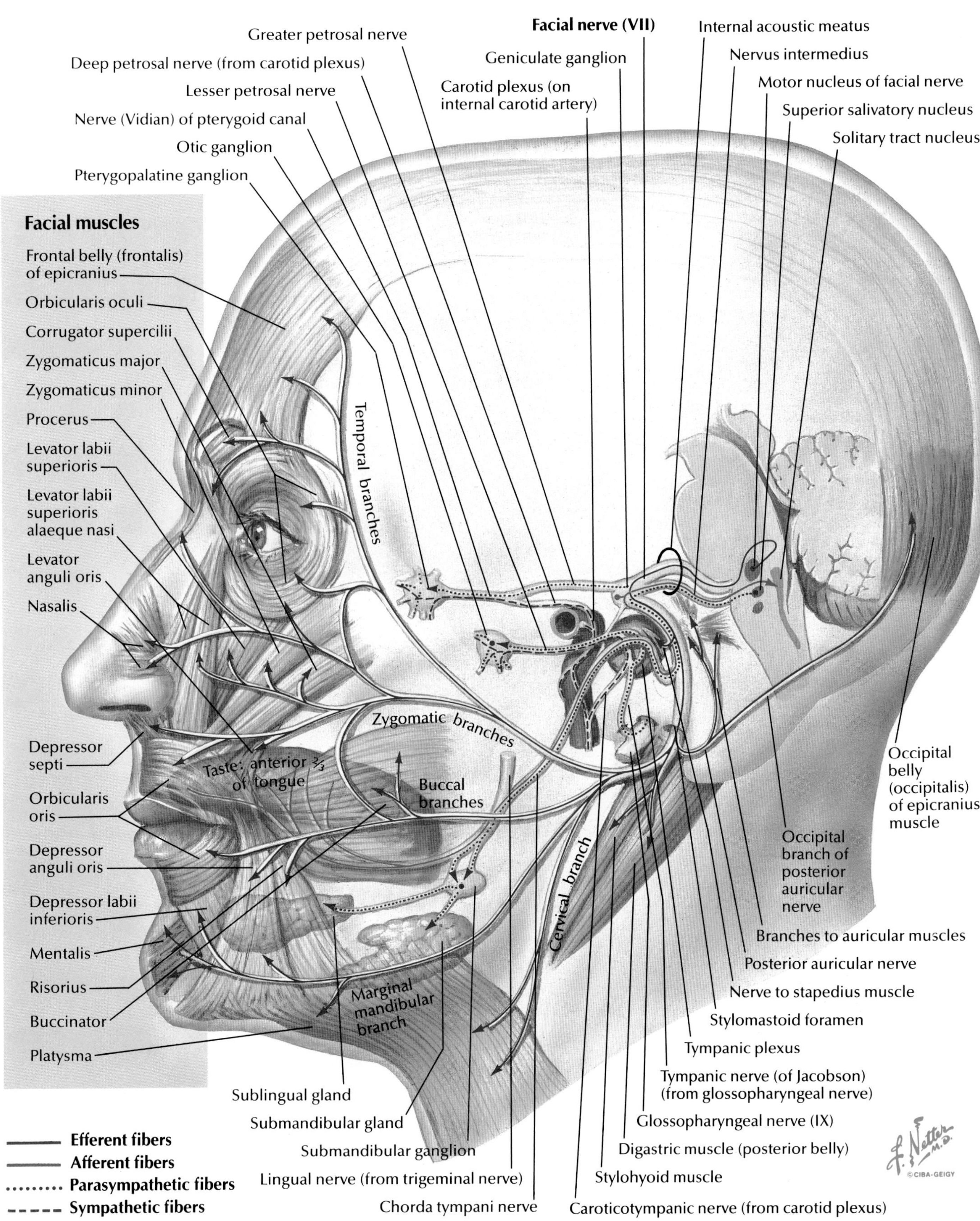

Greater petrosal nerve

Deep petrosal nerve (from carotid plexus)

Lesser petrosal nerve

Nerve (Vidian) of pterygoid canal

Otic ganglion

Pterygopalatine ganglion

Facial nerve (VII)

Geniculate ganglion

Carotid plexus (on internal carotid artery)

Internal acoustic meatus

Nervus intermedius

Motor nucleus of facial nerve

Superior salivatory nucleus

Solitary tract nucleus

Facial muscles

Frontal belly (frontalis) of epicranius

Orbicularis oculi

Corrugator supercilii

Zygomaticus major

Zygomaticus minor

Procerus

Levator labii superioris

Levator labii superioris alaeque nasi

Levator anguli oris

Nasalis

Depressor septi

Orbicularis oris

Depressor anguli oris

Depressor labii inferioris

Mentalis

Risorius

Buccinator

Platysma

Temporal branches

Zygomatic branches

Taste: anterior ⅔ of tongue

Buccal branches

Cervical branch

Marginal mandibular branch

Sublingual gland

Submandibular gland

Submandibular ganglion

Lingual nerve (from trigeminal nerve)

Chorda tympani nerve

Occipital belly (occipitalis) of epicranius muscle

Occipital branch of posterior auricular nerve

Branches to auricular muscles

Posterior auricular nerve

Nerve to stapedius muscle

Stylomastoid foramen

Tympanic plexus

Tympanic nerve (of Jacobson) (from glossopharyngeal nerve)

Glossopharyngeal nerve (IX)

Digastric muscle (posterior belly)

Stylohyoid muscle

Caroticotympanic nerve (from carotid plexus)

————— Efferent fibers

————— Afferent fibers

·········· Parasympathetic fibers

- - - - - Sympathetic fibers

Vestibulocochlear Nerve: Schema

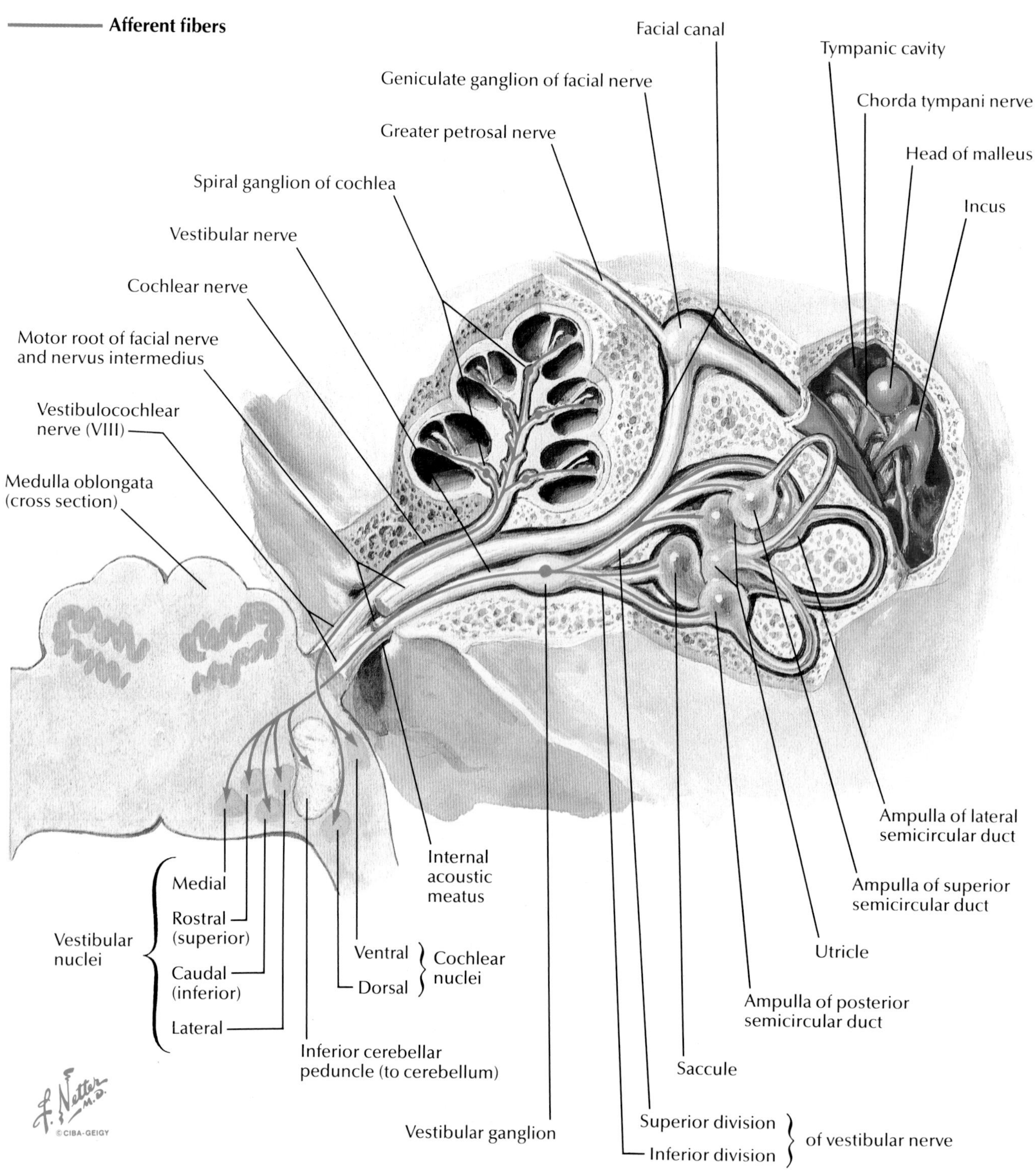

Afferent fibers

Facial canal

Tympanic cavity

Geniculate ganglion of facial nerve

Chorda tympani nerve

Greater petrosal nerve

Head of malleus

Spiral ganglion of cochlea

Incus

Vestibular nerve

Cochlear nerve

Motor root of facial nerve and nervus intermedius

Vestibulocochlear nerve (VIII)

Medulla oblongata (cross section)

Ampulla of lateral semicircular duct

Ampulla of superior semicircular duct

Internal acoustic meatus

Utricle

Medial

Rostral (superior)

Ventral } Cochlear
Dorsal } nuclei

Ampulla of posterior semicircular duct

Vestibular nuclei

Caudal (inferior)

Lateral

Inferior cerebellar peduncle (to cerebellum)

Saccule

Vestibular ganglion

Superior division } of vestibular nerve
Inferior division }

PLATE 118

HEAD AND NECK

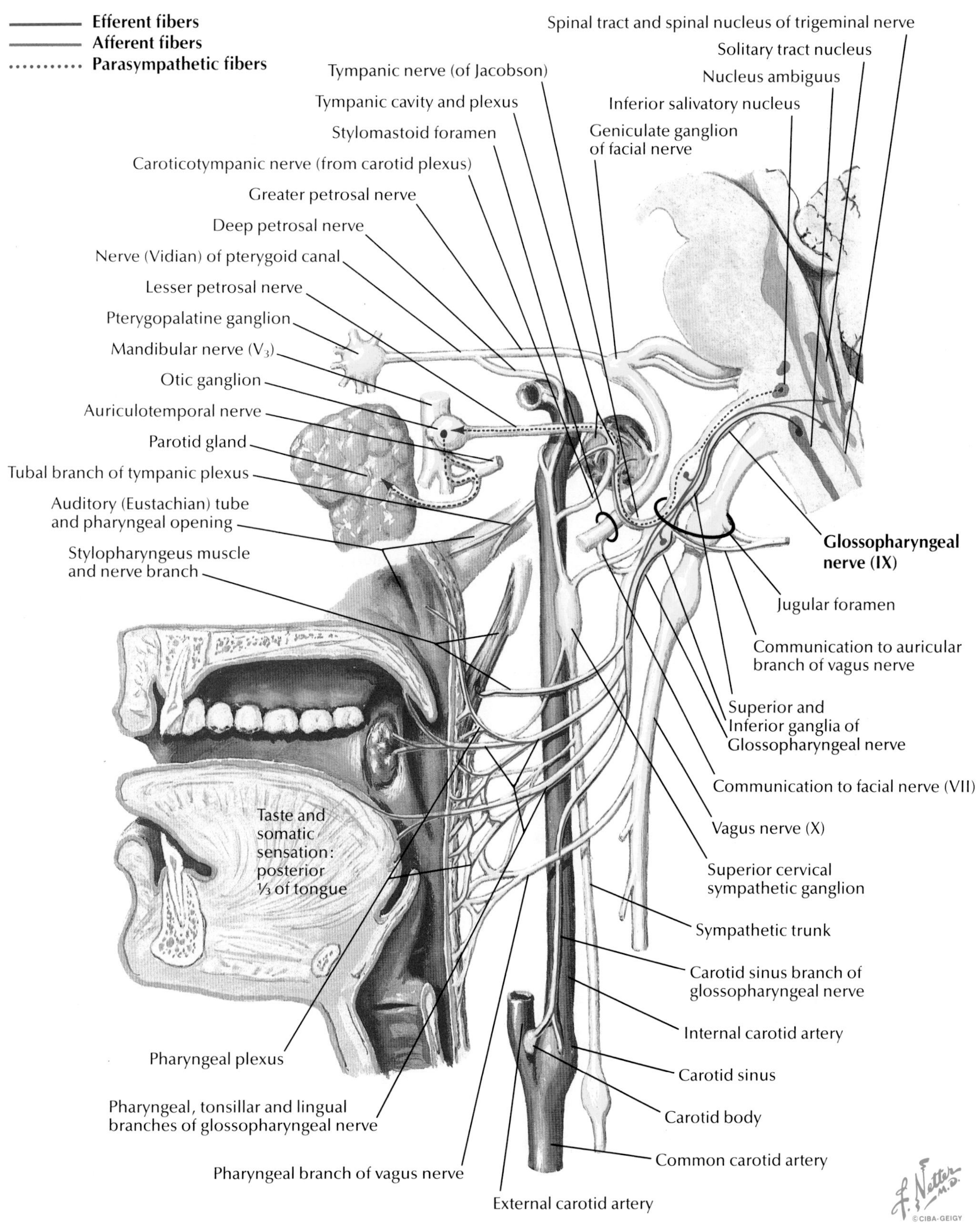

————— Efferent fibers
————— Afferent fibers
··········· Parasympathetic fibers

Tympanic nerve (of Jacobson)

Tympanic cavity and plexus

Stylomastoid foramen

Caroticotympanic nerve (from carotid plexus)

Greater petrosal nerve

Deep petrosal nerve

Nerve (Vidian) of pterygoid canal

Lesser petrosal nerve

Pterygopalatine ganglion

Mandibular nerve (V₃)

Otic ganglion

Auriculotemporal nerve

Parotid gland

Tubal branch of tympanic plexus

Auditory (Eustachian) tube and pharyngeal opening

Stylopharyngeus muscle and nerve branch

Taste and somatic sensation: posterior ⅓ of tongue

Pharyngeal plexus

Pharyngeal, tonsillar and lingual branches of glossopharyngeal nerve

Pharyngeal branch of vagus nerve

External carotid artery

Spinal tract and spinal nucleus of trigeminal nerve

Solitary tract nucleus

Nucleus ambiguus

Inferior salivatory nucleus

Geniculate ganglion of facial nerve

Glossopharyngeal nerve (IX)

Jugular foramen

Communication to auricular branch of vagus nerve

Superior and Inferior ganglia of Glossopharyngeal nerve

Communication to facial nerve (VII)

Vagus nerve (X)

Superior cervical sympathetic ganglion

Sympathetic trunk

Carotid sinus branch of glossopharyngeal nerve

Internal carotid artery

Carotid sinus

Carotid body

Common carotid artery

Vagus Nerve: Schema

SEE ALSO PLATE 153

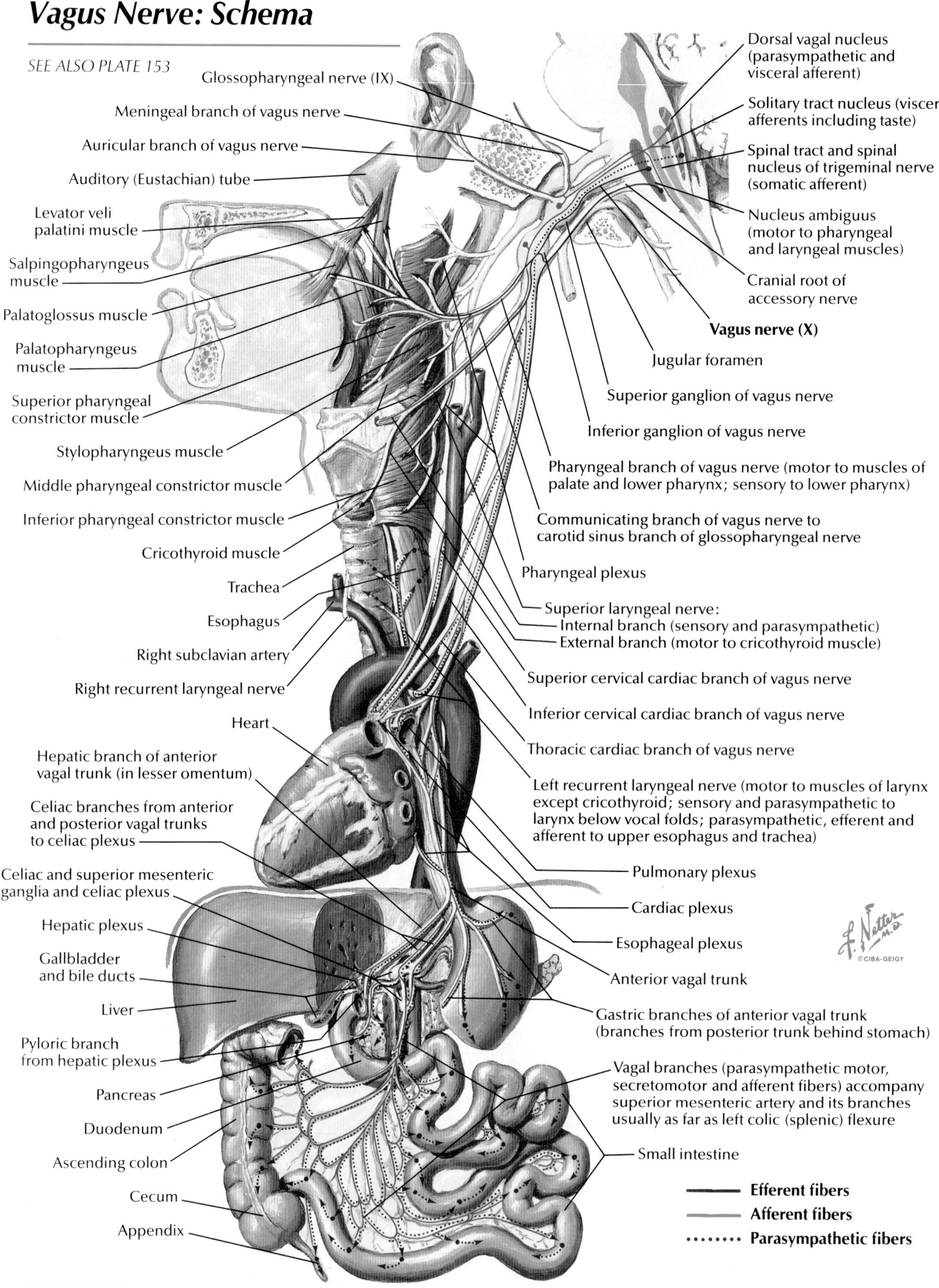

Glossopharyngeal nerve (IX)

Meningeal branch of vagus nerve

Auricular branch of vagus nerve

Auditory (Eustachian) tube

Levator veli palatini muscle

Salpingopharyngeus muscle

Palatoglossus muscle

Palatopharyngeus muscle

Superior pharyngeal constrictor muscle

Stylopharyngeus muscle

Middle pharyngeal constrictor muscle

Inferior pharyngeal constrictor muscle

Cricothyroid muscle

Trachea

Esophagus

Right subclavian artery

Right recurrent laryngeal nerve

Heart

Hepatic branch of anterior vagal trunk (in lesser omentum)

Celiac branches from anterior and posterior vagal trunks to celiac plexus

Celiac and superior mesenteric ganglia and celiac plexus

Hepatic plexus

Gallbladder and bile ducts

Liver

Pyloric branch from hepatic plexus

Pancreas

Duodenum

Ascending colon

Cecum

Appendix

Dorsal vagal nucleus (parasympathetic and visceral afferent)

Solitary tract nucleus (visceral afferents including taste)

Spinal tract and spinal nucleus of trigeminal nerve (somatic afferent)

Nucleus ambiguus (motor to pharyngeal and laryngeal muscles)

Cranial root of accessory nerve

Vagus nerve (X)

Jugular foramen

Superior ganglion of vagus nerve

Inferior ganglion of vagus nerve

Pharyngeal branch of vagus nerve (motor to muscles of palate and lower pharynx; sensory to lower pharynx)

Communicating branch of vagus nerve to carotid sinus branch of glossopharyngeal nerve

Pharyngeal plexus

Superior laryngeal nerve:
Internal branch (sensory and parasympathetic)
External branch (motor to cricothyroid muscle)

Superior cervical cardiac branch of vagus nerve

Inferior cervical cardiac branch of vagus nerve

Thoracic cardiac branch of vagus nerve

Left recurrent laryngeal nerve (motor to muscles of larynx except cricothyroid; sensory and parasympathetic to larynx below vocal folds; parasympathetic, efferent and afferent to upper esophagus and trachea)

Pulmonary plexus

Cardiac plexus

Esophageal plexus

Anterior vagal trunk

Gastric branches of anterior vagal trunk (branches from posterior trunk behind stomach)

Vagal branches (parasympathetic motor, secretomotor and afferent fibers) accompany superior mesenteric artery and its branches usually as far as left colic (splenic) flexure

Small intestine

─────── **Efferent fibers**
─────── **Afferent fibers**
·············· **Parasympathetic fibers**

PLATE 120

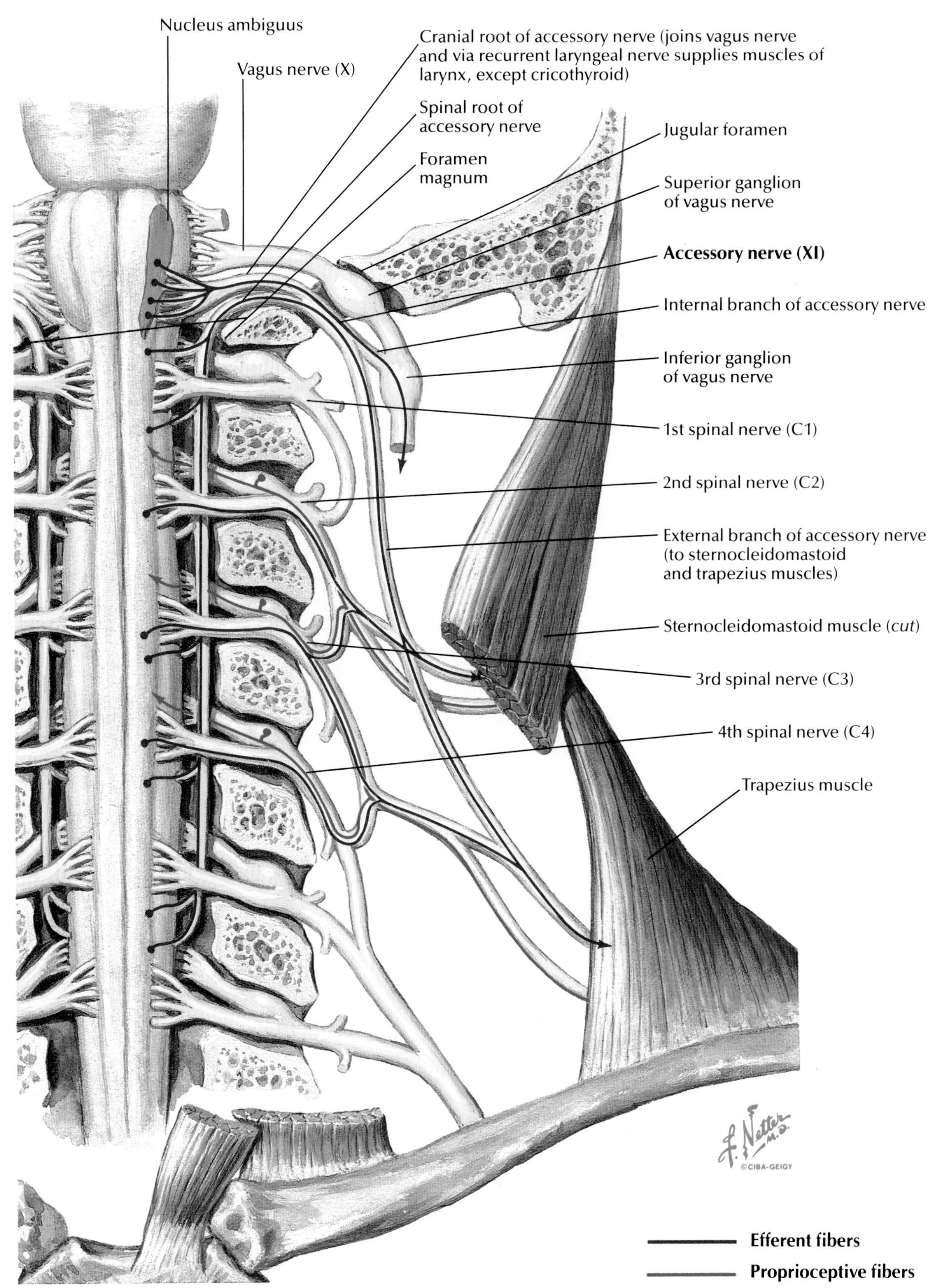

Nucleus ambiguus

Vagus nerve (X)

Cranial root of accessory nerve (joins vagus nerve and via recurrent laryngeal nerve supplies muscles of larynx, except cricothyroid)

Spinal root of accessory nerve

Foramen magnum

Jugular foramen

Superior ganglion of vagus nerve

Accessory nerve (XI)

Internal branch of accessory nerve

Inferior ganglion of vagus nerve

1st spinal nerve (C1)

2nd spinal nerve (C2)

External branch of accessory nerve (to sternocleidomastoid and trapezius muscles)

Sternocleidomastoid muscle (*cut*)

3rd spinal nerve (C3)

4th spinal nerve (C4)

Trapezius muscle

Efferent fibers

Proprioceptive fibers

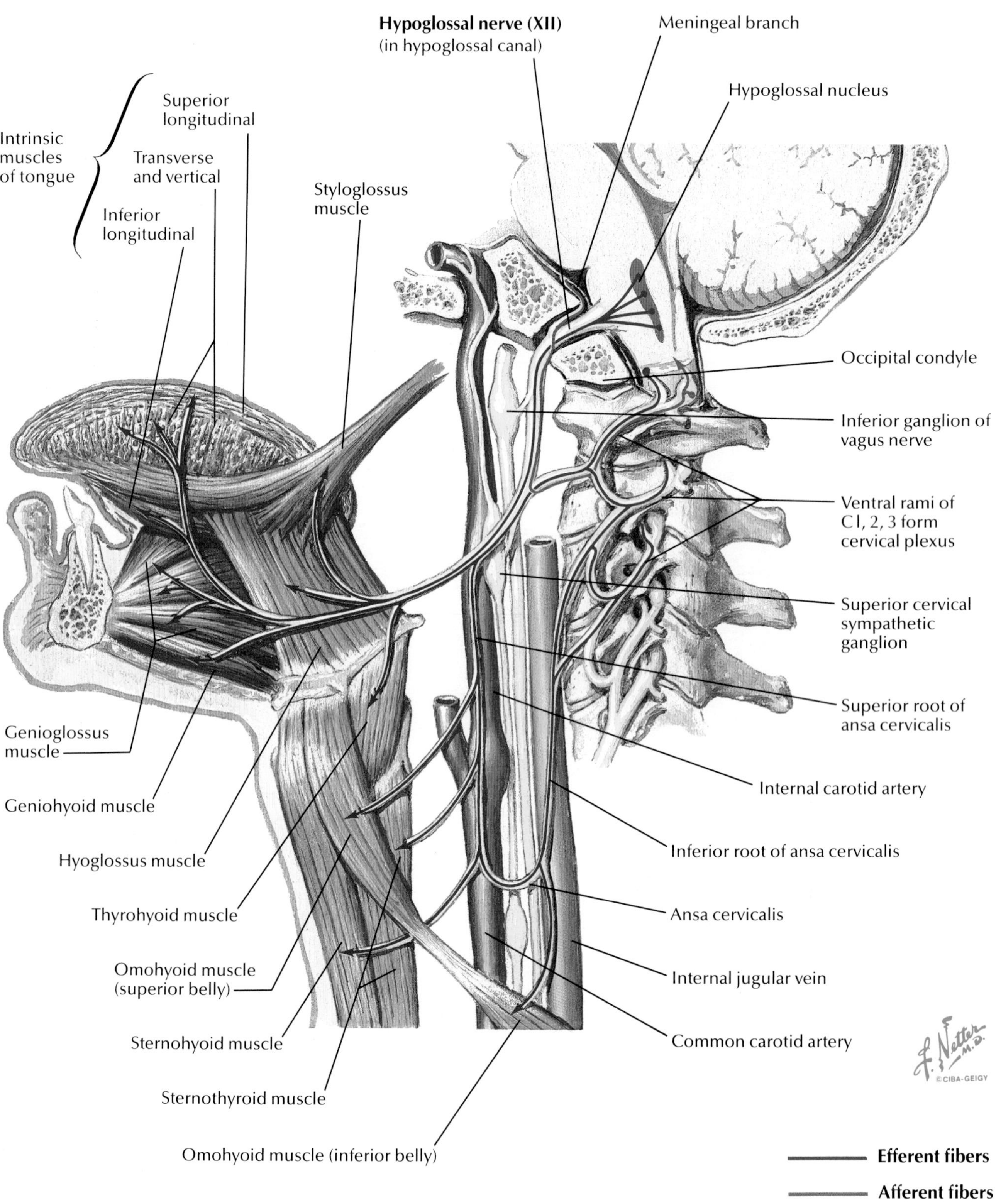

Hypoglossal nerve (XII)
(in hypoglossal canal)

Meningeal branch

Hypoglossal nucleus

Intrinsic muscles of tongue

Superior longitudinal

Transverse and vertical

Inferior longitudinal

Styloglossus muscle

Occipital condyle

Inferior ganglion of vagus nerve

Ventral rami of CI, 2, 3 form cervical plexus

Superior cervical sympathetic ganglion

Superior root of ansa cervicalis

Internal carotid artery

Inferior root of ansa cervicalis

Ansa cervicalis

Internal jugular vein

Common carotid artery

Genioglossus muscle

Geniohyoid muscle

Hyoglossus muscle

Thyrohyoid muscle

Omohyoid muscle (superior belly)

Sternohyoid muscle

Sternothyroid muscle

Omohyoid muscle (inferior belly)

———— **Efferent fibers**

———— **Afferent fibers**

PLATE 122

HEAD AND NECK

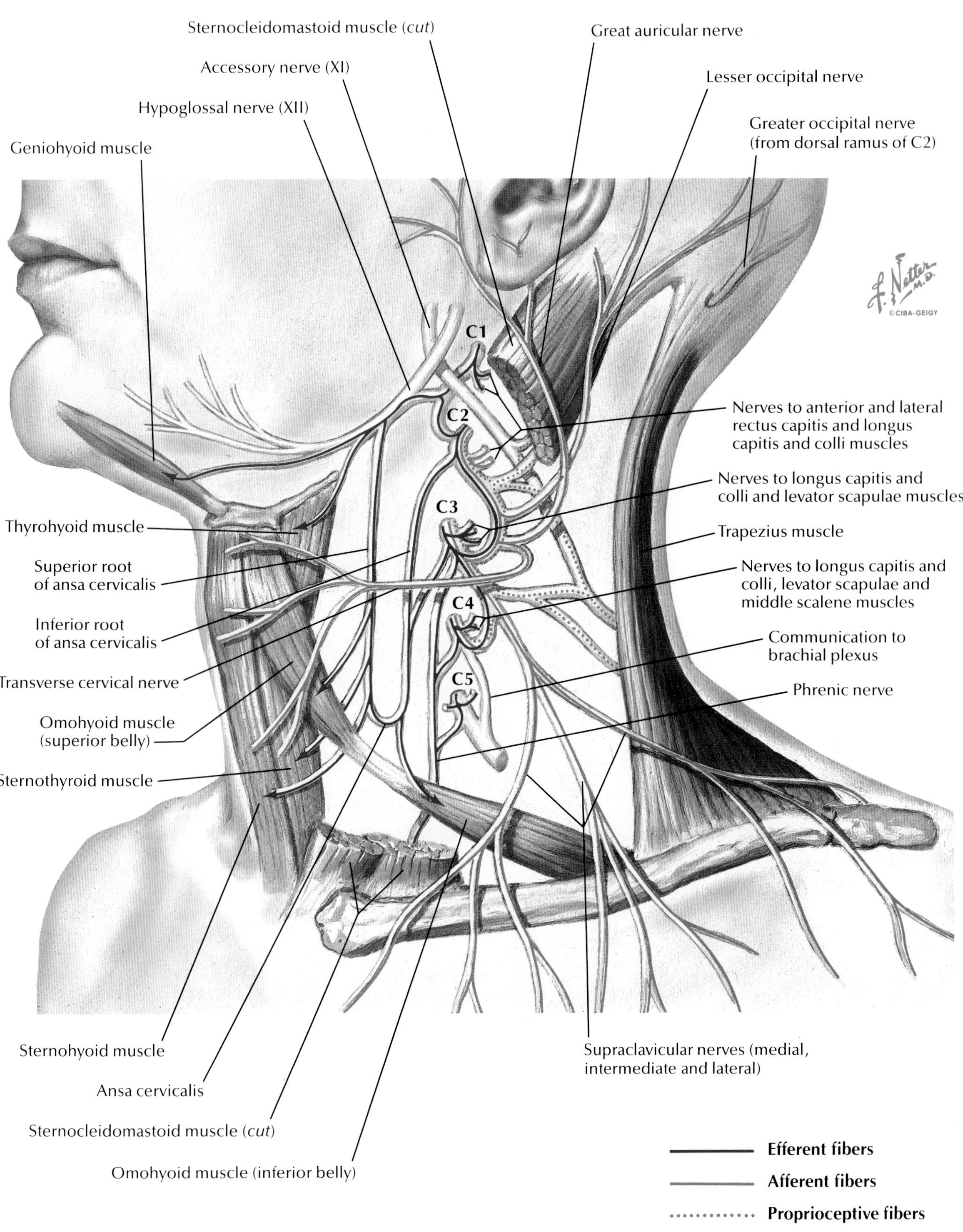

Sternocleidomastoid muscle (*cut*)

Accessory nerve (XI)

Hypoglossal nerve (XII)

Geniohyoid muscle

Great auricular nerve

Lesser occipital nerve

Greater occipital nerve (from dorsal ramus of C2)

C1

C2

C3

C4

C5

Nerves to anterior and lateral rectus capitis and longus capitis and colli muscles

Nerves to longus capitis and colli and levator scapulae muscles

Trapezius muscle

Nerves to longus capitis and colli, levator scapulae and middle scalene muscles

Communication to brachial plexus

Phrenic nerve

Thyrohyoid muscle

Superior root of ansa cervicalis

Inferior root of ansa cervicalis

Transverse cervical nerve

Omohyoid muscle (superior belly)

Sternothyroid muscle

Sternohyoid muscle

Ansa cervicalis

Sternocleidomastoid muscle (*cut*)

Omohyoid muscle (inferior belly)

Supraclavicular nerves (medial, intermediate and lateral)

——— Efferent fibers

——— Afferent fibers

·········· Proprioceptive fibers

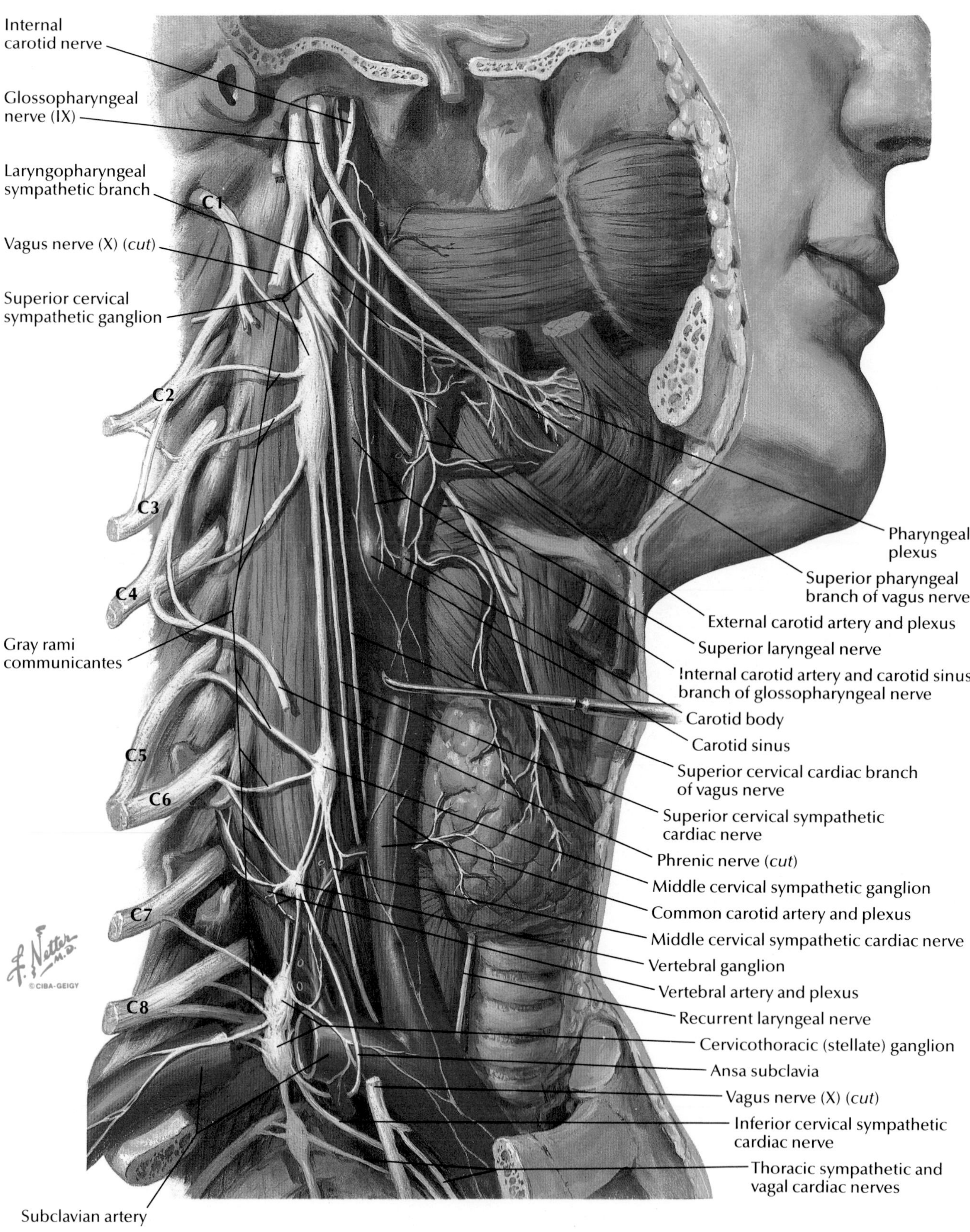

Internal carotid nerve

Glossopharyngeal nerve (IX)

Laryngopharyngeal sympathetic branch

Vagus nerve (X) (*cut*)

Superior cervical sympathetic ganglion

Gray rami communicantes

C1

C2

C3

C4

C5

C6

C7

C8

Subclavian artery

Pharyngeal plexus

Superior pharyngeal branch of vagus nerve

External carotid artery and plexus

Superior laryngeal nerve

Internal carotid artery and carotid sinus branch of glossopharyngeal nerve

Carotid body

Carotid sinus

Superior cervical cardiac branch of vagus nerve

Superior cervical sympathetic cardiac nerve

Phrenic nerve (*cut*)

Middle cervical sympathetic ganglion

Common carotid artery and plexus

Middle cervical sympathetic cardiac nerve

Vertebral ganglion

Vertebral artery and plexus

Recurrent laryngeal nerve

Cervicothoracic (stellate) ganglion

Ansa subclavia

Vagus nerve (X) (*cut*)

Inferior cervical sympathetic cardiac nerve

Thoracic sympathetic and vagal cardiac nerves

PLATE 124

HEAD AND NECK

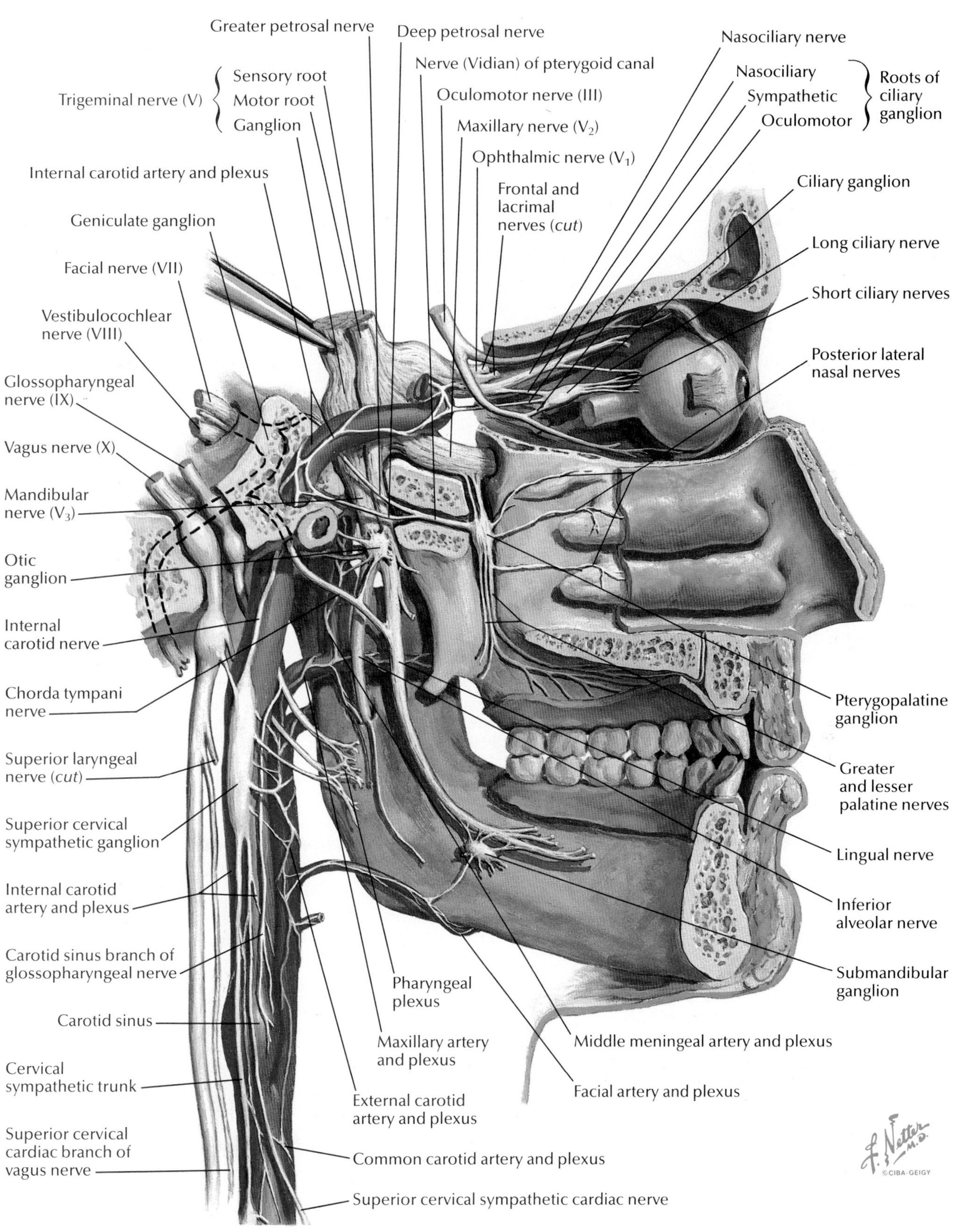

Greater petrosal nerve

Deep petrosal nerve

Nasociliary nerve

Sensory root

Motor root

Ganglion

Trigeminal nerve (V)

Nerve (Vidian) of pterygoid canal

Oculomotor nerve (III)

Maxillary nerve (V$_2$)

Ophthalmic nerve (V$_1$)

Nasociliary

Sympathetic

Oculomotor

Roots of ciliary ganglion

Internal carotid artery and plexus

Frontal and lacrimal nerves (*cut*)

Ciliary ganglion

Geniculate ganglion

Long ciliary nerve

Facial nerve (VII)

Short ciliary nerves

Vestibulocochlear nerve (VIII)

Posterior lateral nasal nerves

Glossopharyngeal nerve (IX)

Vagus nerve (X)

Mandibular nerve (V$_3$)

Otic ganglion

Internal carotid nerve

Chorda tympani nerve

Pterygopalatine ganglion

Superior laryngeal nerve (*cut*)

Greater and lesser palatine nerves

Superior cervical sympathetic ganglion

Lingual nerve

Internal carotid artery and plexus

Inferior alveolar nerve

Carotid sinus branch of glossopharyngeal nerve

Submandibular ganglion

Carotid sinus

Pharyngeal plexus

Middle meningeal artery and plexus

Cervical sympathetic trunk

Maxillary artery and plexus

Facial artery and plexus

Superior cervical cardiac branch of vagus nerve

External carotid artery and plexus

Common carotid artery and plexus

Superior cervical sympathetic cardiac nerve

Ciliary Ganglion: Schema

SEE ALSO PLATE 153

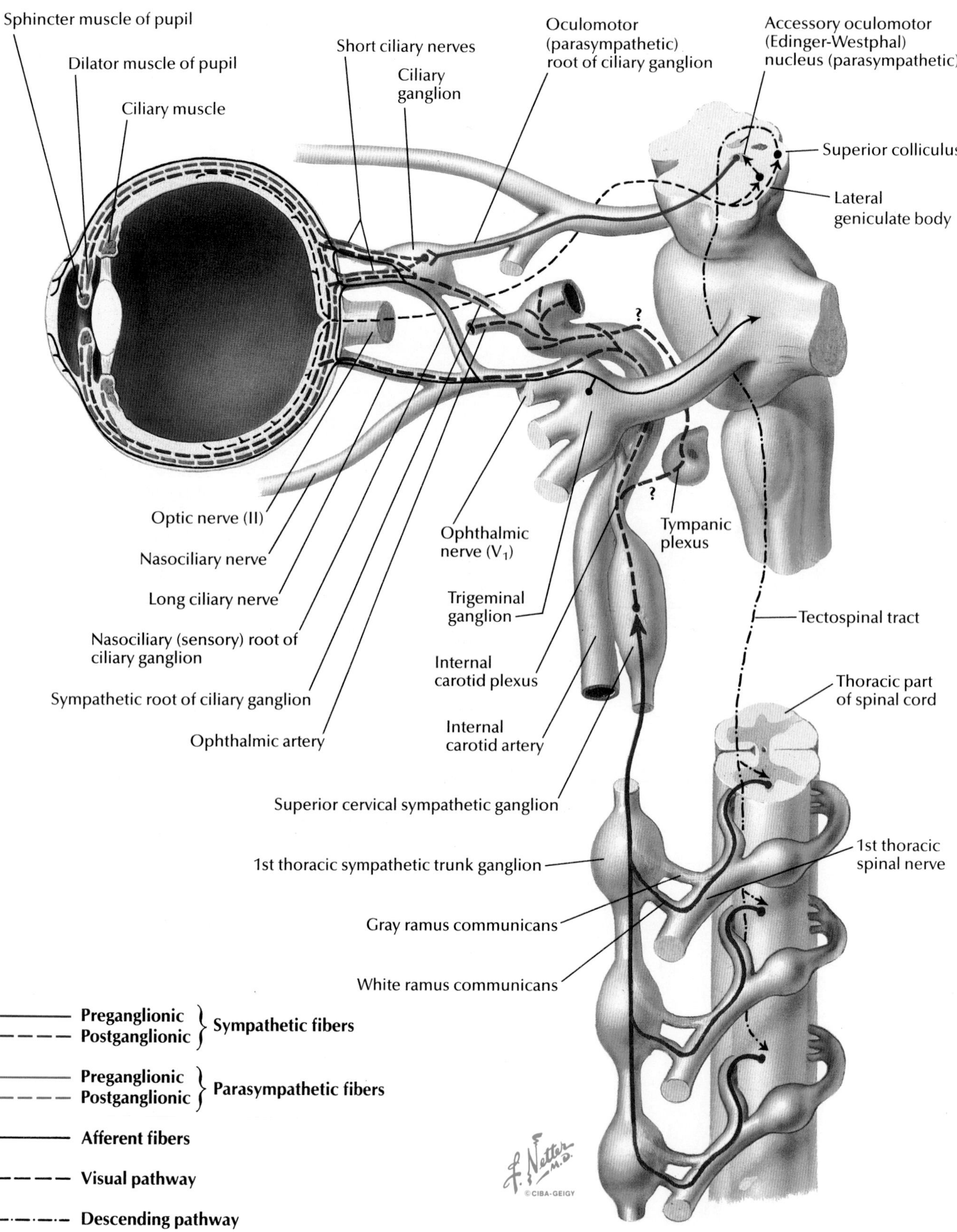

Sphincter muscle of pupil

Dilator muscle of pupil

Ciliary muscle

Short ciliary nerves

Ciliary ganglion

Oculomotor (parasympathetic) root of ciliary ganglion

Accessory oculomotor (Edinger-Westphal) nucleus (parasympathetic)

Superior colliculus

Lateral geniculate body

Optic nerve (II)

Nasociliary nerve

Long ciliary nerve

Nasociliary (sensory) root of ciliary ganglion

Sympathetic root of ciliary ganglion

Ophthalmic artery

Ophthalmic nerve (V₁)

Trigeminal ganglion

Internal carotid plexus

Internal carotid artery

Superior cervical sympathetic ganglion

1st thoracic sympathetic trunk ganglion

Gray ramus communicans

White ramus communicans

Tympanic plexus

Tectospinal tract

Thoracic part of spinal cord

1st thoracic spinal nerve

Preganglionic }
Postganglionic } Sympathetic fibers

Preganglionic }
Postganglionic } Parasympathetic fibers

Afferent fibers

Visual pathway

Descending pathway

PLATE 126

HEAD AND NECK

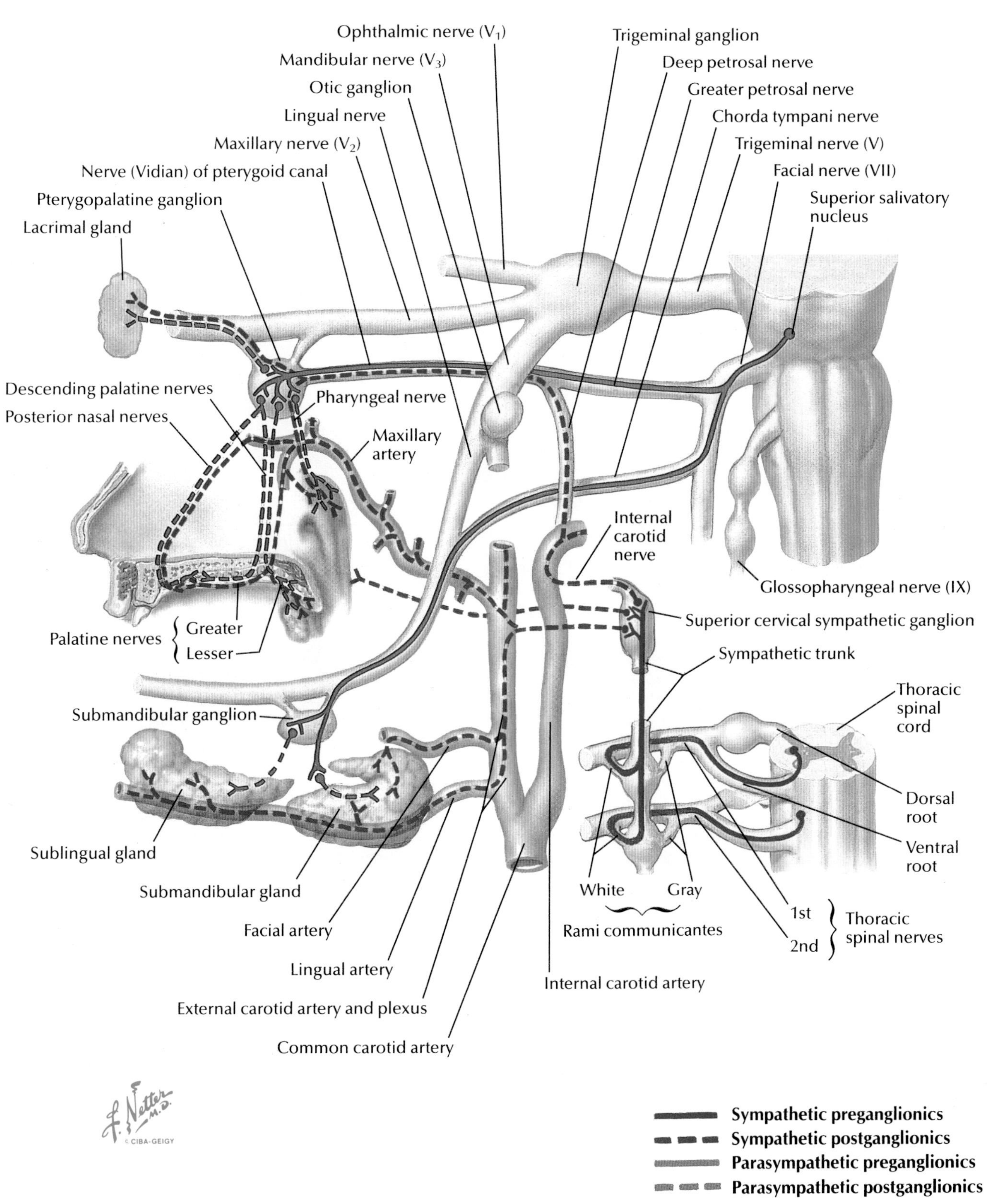

Ophthalmic nerve (V₁)

Mandibular nerve (V₃)

Otic ganglion

Lingual nerve

Maxillary nerve (V₂)

Nerve (Vidian) of pterygoid canal

Pterygopalatine ganglion

Lacrimal gland

Trigeminal ganglion

Deep petrosal nerve

Greater petrosal nerve

Chorda tympani nerve

Trigeminal nerve (V)

Facial nerve (VII)

Superior salivatory nucleus

Descending palatine nerves

Posterior nasal nerves

Pharyngeal nerve

Maxillary artery

Internal carotid nerve

Glossopharyngeal nerve (IX)

Superior cervical sympathetic ganglion

Sympathetic trunk

Palatine nerves { Greater Lesser

Thoracic spinal cord

Submandibular ganglion

Dorsal root

Ventral root

Sublingual gland

Submandibular gland

Facial artery

Lingual artery

External carotid artery and plexus

Common carotid artery

White   Gray

Rami communicantes

Internal carotid artery

1st } Thoracic
2nd } spinal nerves

━━━━━ **Sympathetic preganglionics**
╴ ╴ ╴ **Sympathetic postganglionics**
▬▬▬▬ **Parasympathetic preganglionics**
▬ ▬ ▬ **Parasympathetic postganglionics**

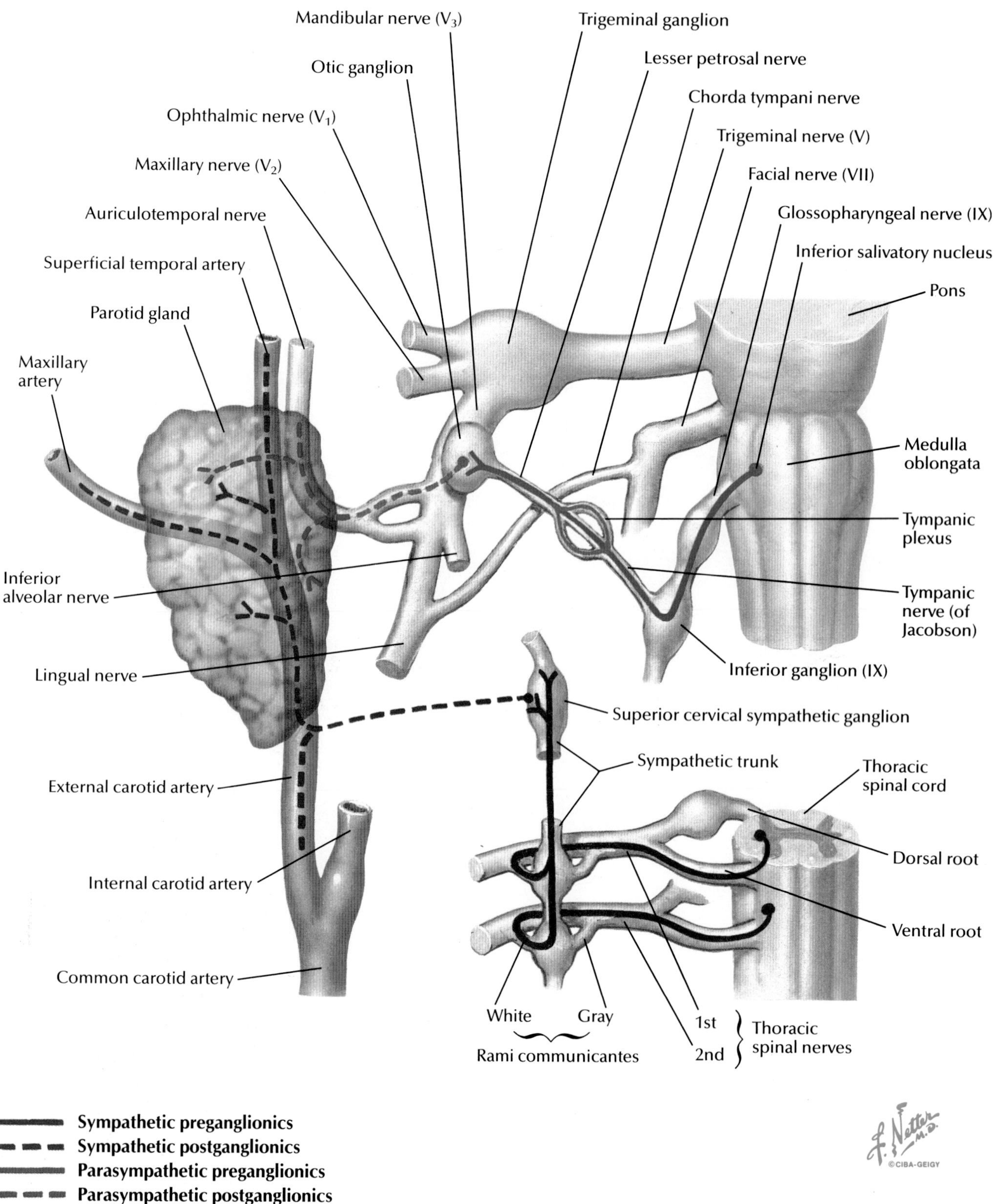

Mandibular nerve (V₃)

Otic ganglion

Ophthalmic nerve (V₁)

Maxillary nerve (V₂)

Auriculotemporal nerve

Superficial temporal artery

Parotid gland

Maxillary artery

Inferior alveolar nerve

Lingual nerve

External carotid artery

Internal carotid artery

Common carotid artery

Trigeminal ganglion

Lesser petrosal nerve

Chorda tympani nerve

Trigeminal nerve (V)

Facial nerve (VII)

Glossopharyngeal nerve (IX)

Inferior salivatory nucleus

Pons

Medulla oblongata

Tympanic plexus

Tympanic nerve (of Jacobson)

Inferior ganglion (IX)

Superior cervical sympathetic ganglion

Sympathetic trunk

Thoracic spinal cord

Dorsal root

Ventral root

White   Gray

Rami communicantes

1st
2nd } Thoracic spinal nerves

─────── Sympathetic preganglionics
– – – Sympathetic postganglionics
─────── Parasympathetic preganglionics
– – – Parasympathetic postganglionics

PLATE 128

HEAD AND NECK

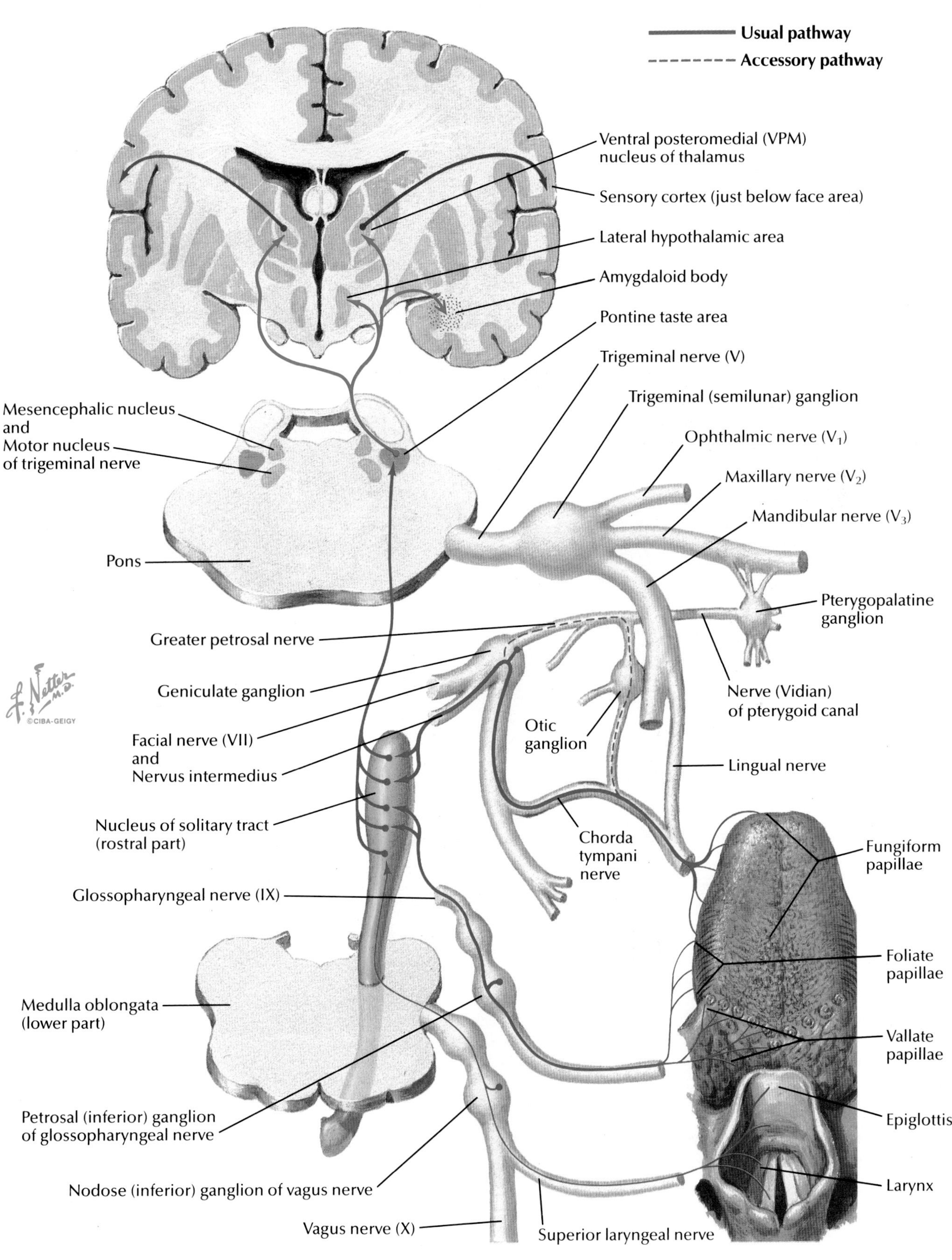

Usual pathway
- - - - - - Accessory pathway

Ventral posteromedial (VPM) nucleus of thalamus

Sensory cortex (just below face area)

Lateral hypothalamic area

Amygdaloid body

Pontine taste area

Trigeminal nerve (V)

Trigeminal (semilunar) ganglion

Ophthalmic nerve (V₁)

Maxillary nerve (V₂)

Mandibular nerve (V₃)

Pterygopalatine ganglion

Nerve (Vidian) of pterygoid canal

Lingual nerve

Fungiform papillae

Foliate papillae

Vallate papillae

Epiglottis

Larynx

Superior laryngeal nerve

Vagus nerve (X)

Nodose (inferior) ganglion of vagus nerve

Petrosal (inferior) ganglion of glossopharyngeal nerve

Medulla oblongata (lower part)

Glossopharyngeal nerve (IX)

Nucleus of solitary tract (rostral part)

Facial nerve (VII) and Nervus intermedius

Geniculate ganglion

Greater petrosal nerve

Pons

Mesencephalic nucleus and Motor nucleus of trigeminal nerve

Otic ganglion

Chorda tympani nerve

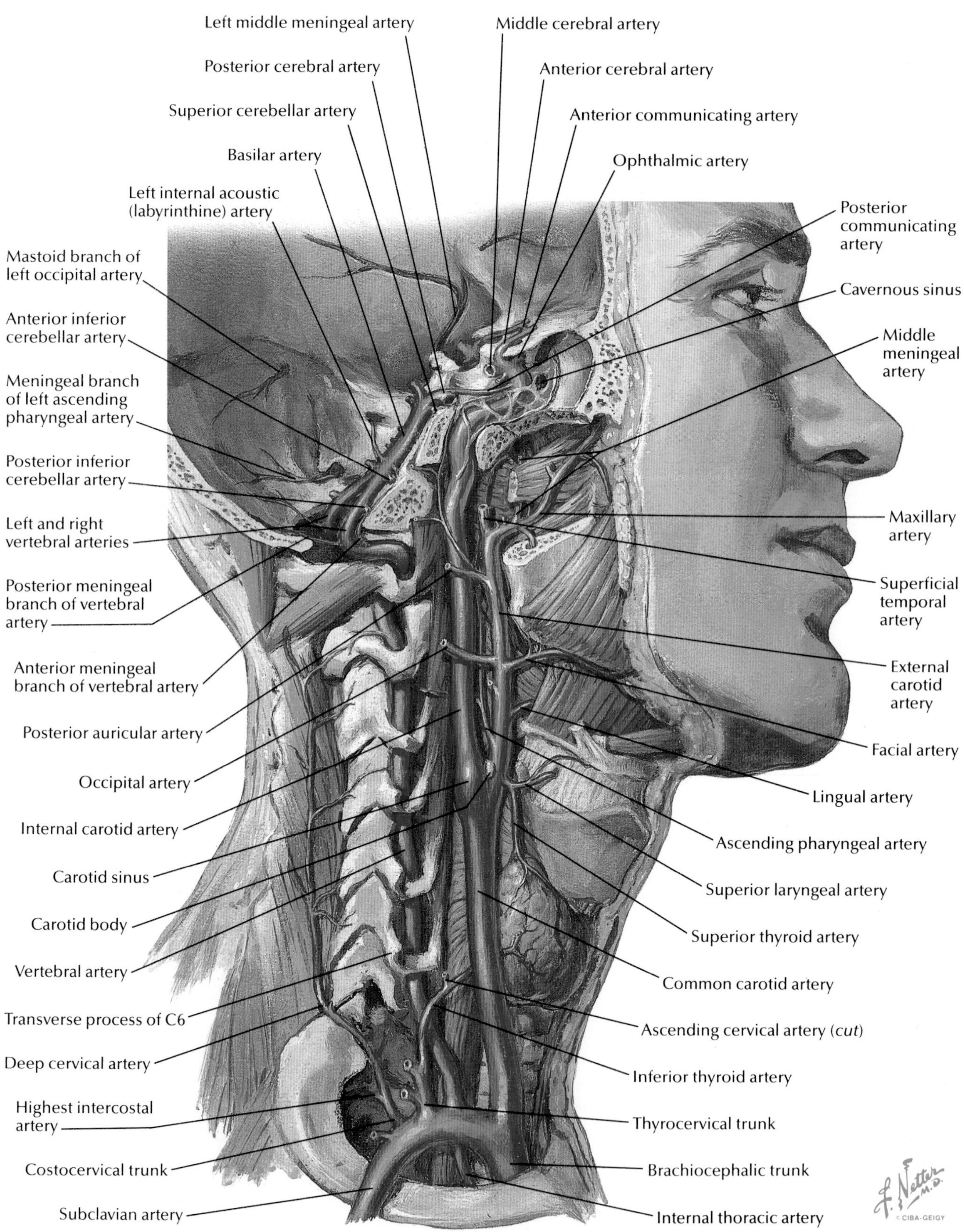

Left middle meningeal artery

Posterior cerebral artery

Superior cerebellar artery

Basilar artery

Left internal acoustic (labyrinthine) artery

Mastoid branch of left occipital artery

Anterior inferior cerebellar artery

Meningeal branch of left ascending pharyngeal artery

Posterior inferior cerebellar artery

Left and right vertebral arteries

Posterior meningeal branch of vertebral artery

Anterior meningeal branch of vertebral artery

Posterior auricular artery

Occipital artery

Internal carotid artery

Carotid sinus

Carotid body

Vertebral artery

Transverse process of C6

Deep cervical artery

Highest intercostal artery

Costocervical trunk

Subclavian artery

Middle cerebral artery

Anterior cerebral artery

Anterior communicating artery

Ophthalmic artery

Posterior communicating artery

Cavernous sinus

Middle meningeal artery

Maxillary artery

Superficial temporal artery

External carotid artery

Facial artery

Lingual artery

Ascending pharyngeal artery

Superior laryngeal artery

Superior thyroid artery

Common carotid artery

Ascending cervical artery (cut)

Inferior thyroid artery

Thyrocervical trunk

Brachiocephalic trunk

Internal thoracic artery

PLATE 130

HEAD AND NECK

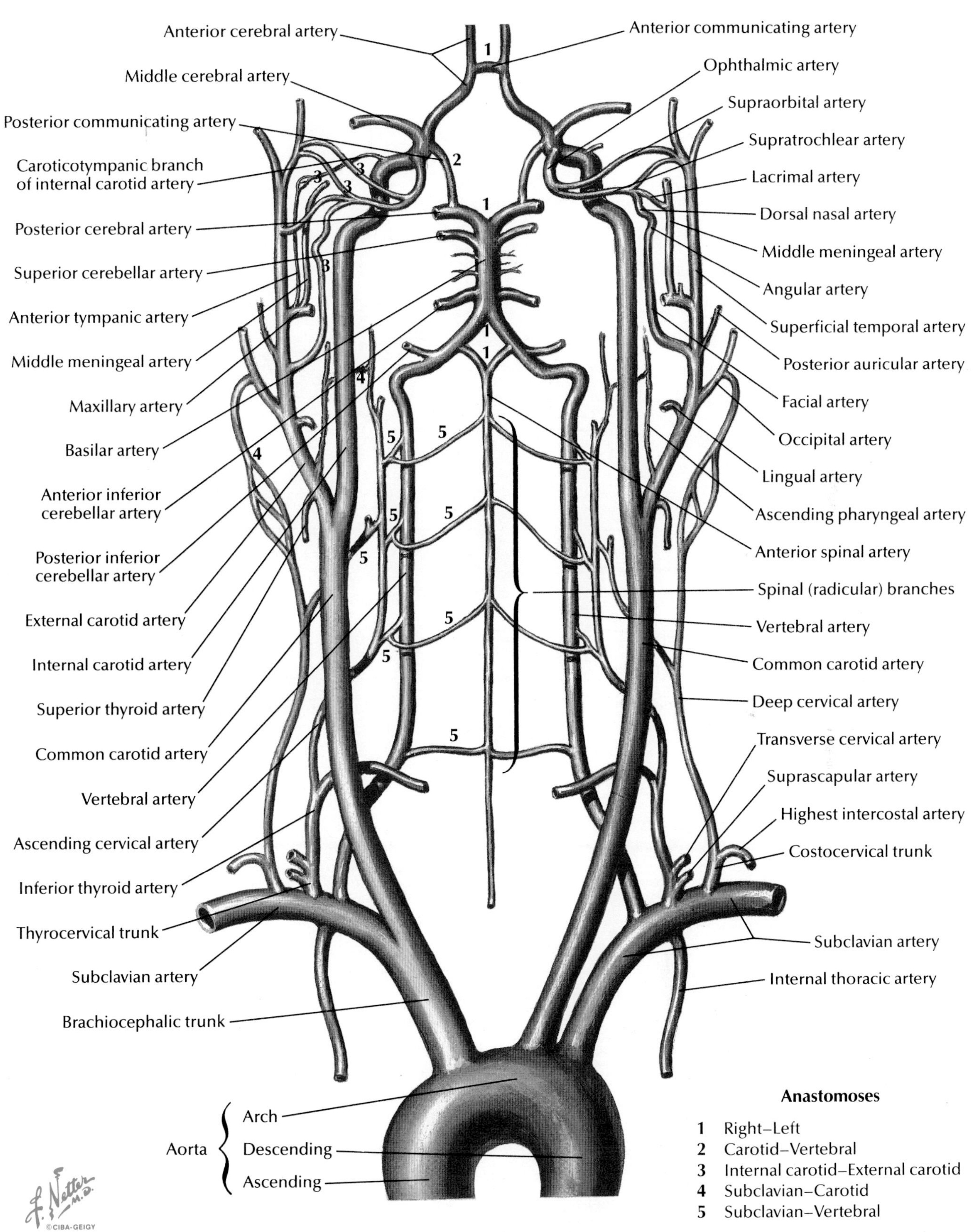

Anterior cerebral artery

Middle cerebral artery

Posterior communicating artery

Caroticotympanic branch of internal carotid artery

Posterior cerebral artery

Superior cerebellar artery

Anterior tympanic artery

Middle meningeal artery

Maxillary artery

Basilar artery

Anterior inferior cerebellar artery

Posterior inferior cerebellar artery

External carotid artery

Internal carotid artery

Superior thyroid artery

Common carotid artery

Vertebral artery

Ascending cervical artery

Inferior thyroid artery

Thyrocervical trunk

Subclavian artery

Brachiocephalic trunk

Anterior communicating artery

Ophthalmic artery

Supraorbital artery

Supratrochlear artery

Lacrimal artery

Dorsal nasal artery

Middle meningeal artery

Angular artery

Superficial temporal artery

Posterior auricular artery

Facial artery

Occipital artery

Lingual artery

Ascending pharyngeal artery

Anterior spinal artery

Spinal (radicular) branches

Vertebral artery

Common carotid artery

Deep cervical artery

Transverse cervical artery

Suprascapular artery

Highest intercostal artery

Costocervical trunk

Subclavian artery

Internal thoracic artery

Aorta { Arch, Descending, Ascending }

Anastomoses
1 Right–Left
2 Carotid–Vertebral
3 Internal carotid–External carotid
4 Subclavian–Carotid
5 Subclavian–Vertebral

CEREBRAL VASCULATURE

PLATE 131

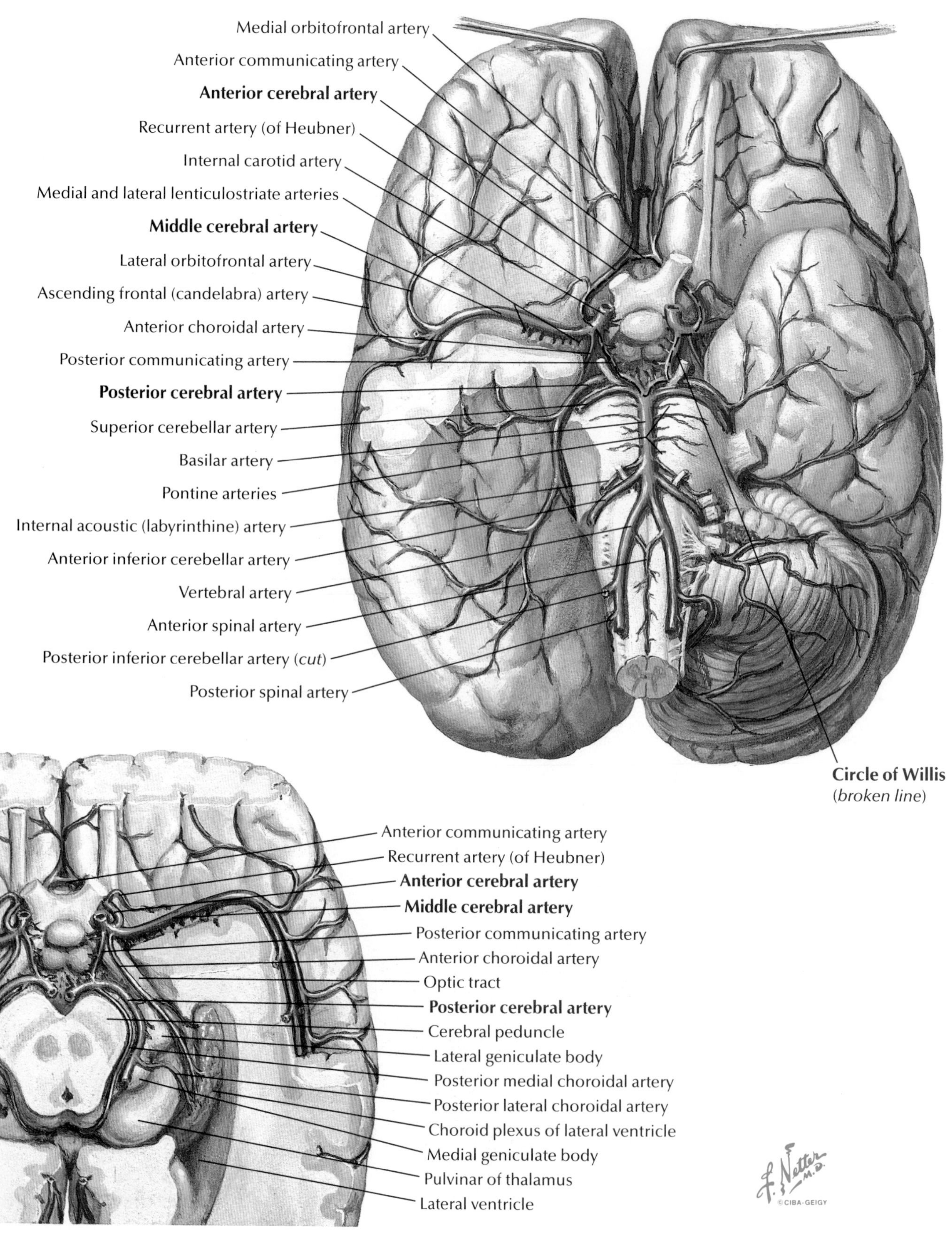

Medial orbitofrontal artery

Anterior communicating artery

Anterior cerebral artery

Recurrent artery (of Heubner)

Internal carotid artery

Medial and lateral lenticulostriate arteries

Middle cerebral artery

Lateral orbitofrontal artery

Ascending frontal (candelabra) artery

Anterior choroidal artery

Posterior communicating artery

Posterior cerebral artery

Superior cerebellar artery

Basilar artery

Pontine arteries

Internal acoustic (labyrinthine) artery

Anterior inferior cerebellar artery

Vertebral artery

Anterior spinal artery

Posterior inferior cerebellar artery (*cut*)

Posterior spinal artery

Circle of Willis
(*broken line*)

Anterior communicating artery

Recurrent artery (of Heubner)

Anterior cerebral artery

Middle cerebral artery

Posterior communicating artery

Anterior choroidal artery

Optic tract

Posterior cerebral artery

Cerebral peduncle

Lateral geniculate body

Posterior medial choroidal artery

Posterior lateral choroidal artery

Choroid plexus of lateral ventricle

Medial geniculate body

Pulvinar of thalamus

Lateral ventricle

PLATE 132

HEAD AND NECK

Vessels dissected out: inferior view

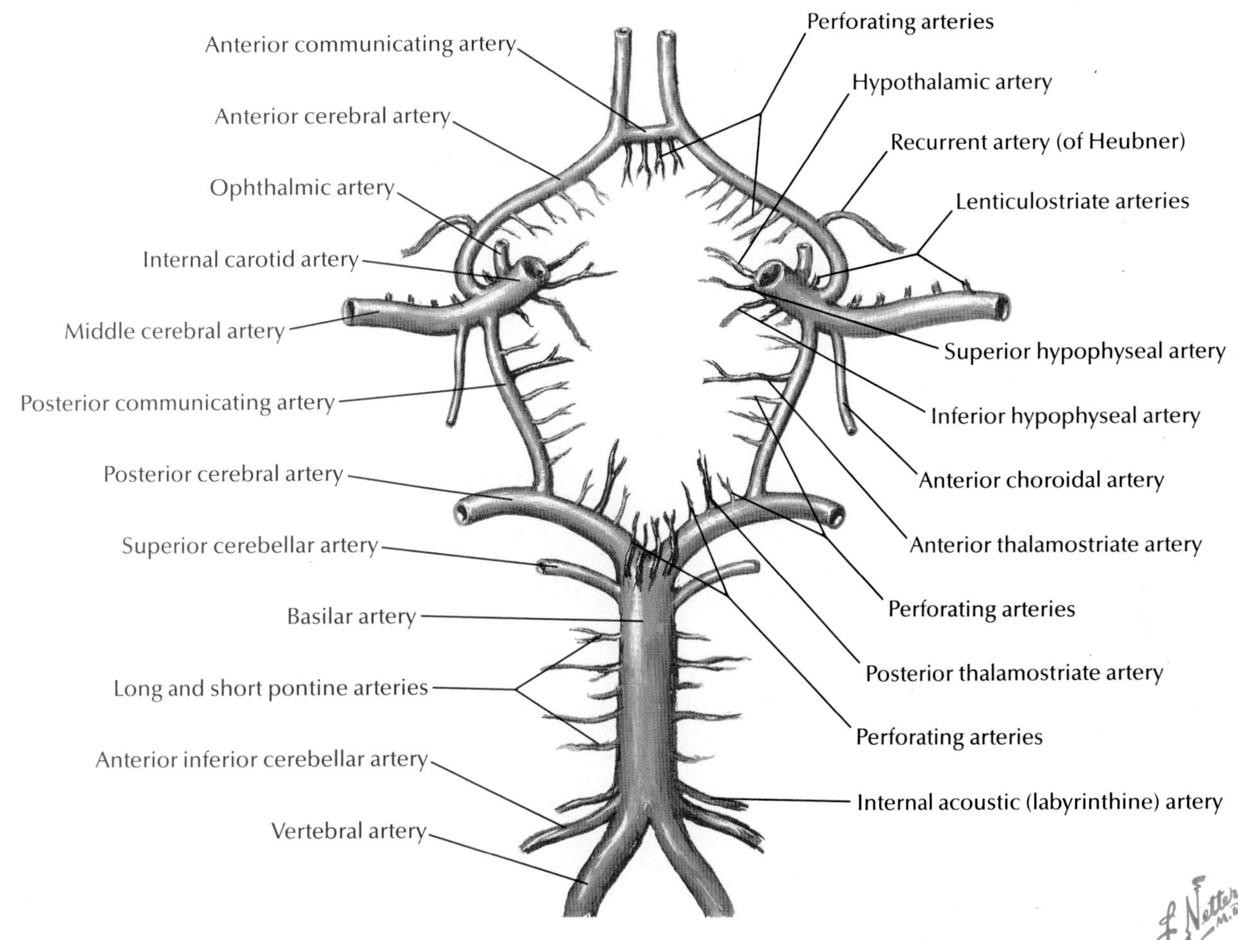

Anterior communicating artery

Anterior cerebral artery

Ophthalmic artery

Internal carotid artery

Middle cerebral artery

Posterior communicating artery

Posterior cerebral artery

Superior cerebellar artery

Basilar artery

Long and short pontine arteries

Anterior inferior cerebellar artery

Vertebral artery

Perforating arteries

Hypothalamic artery

Recurrent artery (of Heubner)

Lenticulostriate arteries

Superior hypophyseal artery

Inferior hypophyseal artery

Anterior choroidal artery

Anterior thalamostriate artery

Perforating arteries

Posterior thalamostriate artery

Perforating arteries

Internal acoustic (labyrinthine) artery

Vessels in situ: inferior view

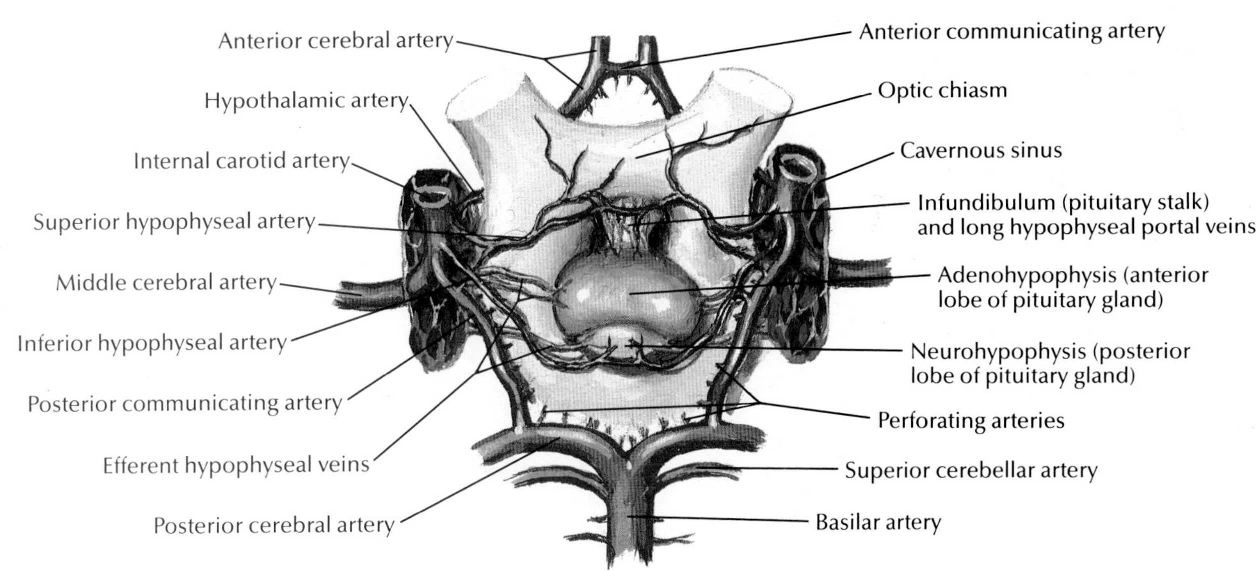

Anterior cerebral artery

Hypothalamic artery

Internal carotid artery

Superior hypophyseal artery

Middle cerebral artery

Inferior hypophyseal artery

Posterior communicating artery

Efferent hypophyseal veins

Posterior cerebral artery

Anterior communicating artery

Optic chiasm

Cavernous sinus

Infundibulum (pituitary stalk) and long hypophyseal portal veins

Adenohypophysis (anterior lobe of pituitary gland)

Neurohypophysis (posterior lobe of pituitary gland)

Perforating arteries

Superior cerebellar artery

Basilar artery

Arteries of Brain: Frontal View and Section

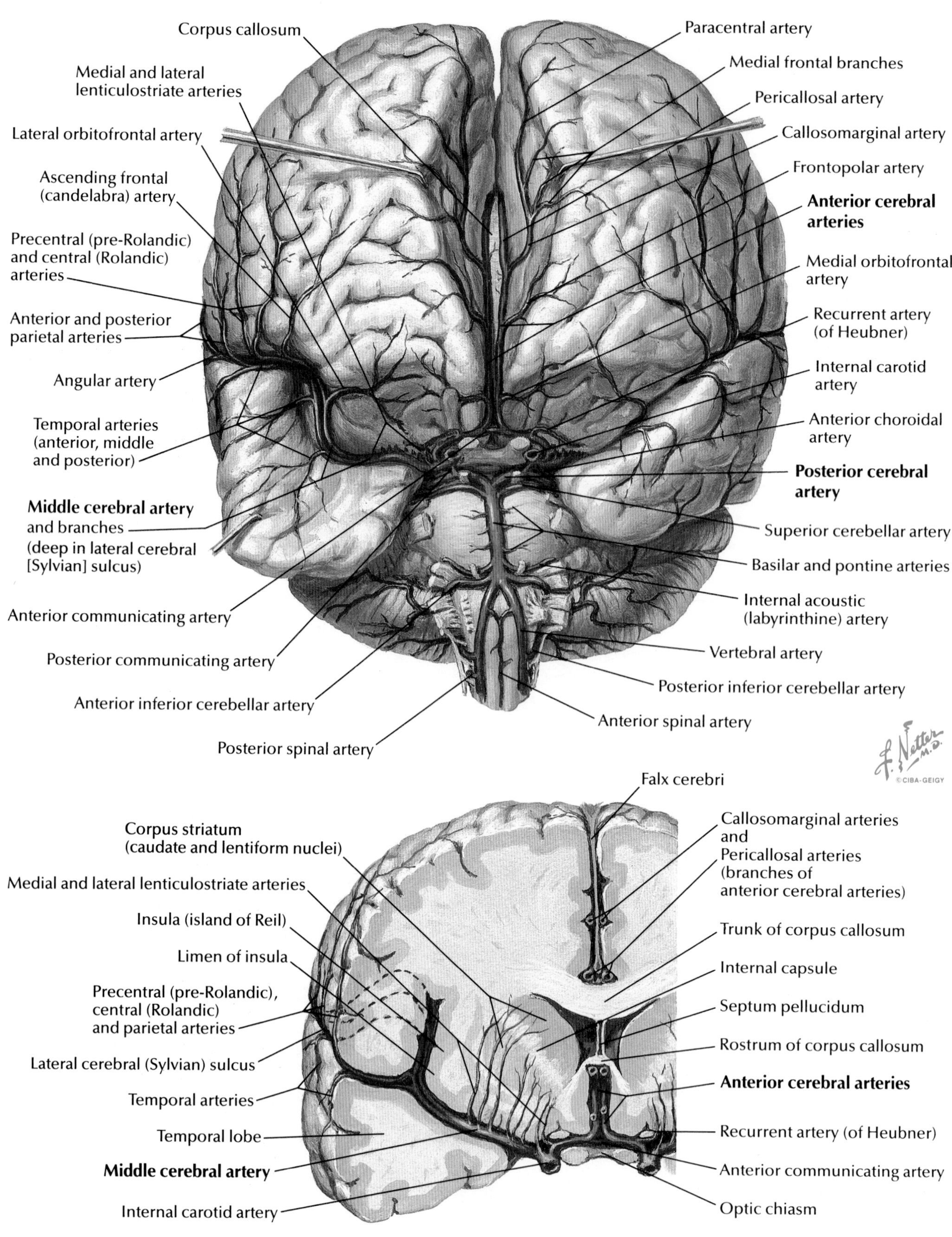

Corpus callosum

Medial and lateral lenticulostriate arteries

Lateral orbitofrontal artery

Ascending frontal (candelabra) artery

Precentral (pre-Rolandic) and central (Rolandic) arteries

Anterior and posterior parietal arteries

Angular artery

Temporal arteries (anterior, middle and posterior)

Middle cerebral artery and branches (deep in lateral cerebral [Sylvian] sulcus)

Anterior communicating artery

Posterior communicating artery

Anterior inferior cerebellar artery

Posterior spinal artery

Paracentral artery

Medial frontal branches

Pericallosal artery

Callosomarginal artery

Frontopolar artery

Anterior cerebral arteries

Medial orbitofrontal artery

Recurrent artery (of Heubner)

Internal carotid artery

Anterior choroidal artery

Posterior cerebral artery

Superior cerebellar artery

Basilar and pontine arteries

Internal acoustic (labyrinthine) artery

Vertebral artery

Posterior inferior cerebellar artery

Anterior spinal artery

Corpus striatum (caudate and lentiform nuclei)

Medial and lateral lenticulostriate arteries

Insula (island of Reil)

Limen of insula

Precentral (pre-Rolandic), central (Rolandic) and parietal arteries

Lateral cerebral (Sylvian) sulcus

Temporal arteries

Temporal lobe

Middle cerebral artery

Internal carotid artery

Falx cerebri

Callosomarginal arteries and Pericallosal arteries (branches of anterior cerebral arteries)

Trunk of corpus callosum

Internal capsule

Septum pellucidum

Rostrum of corpus callosum

Anterior cerebral arteries

Recurrent artery (of Heubner)

Anterior communicating artery

Optic chiasm

PLATE 134

HEAD AND NECK

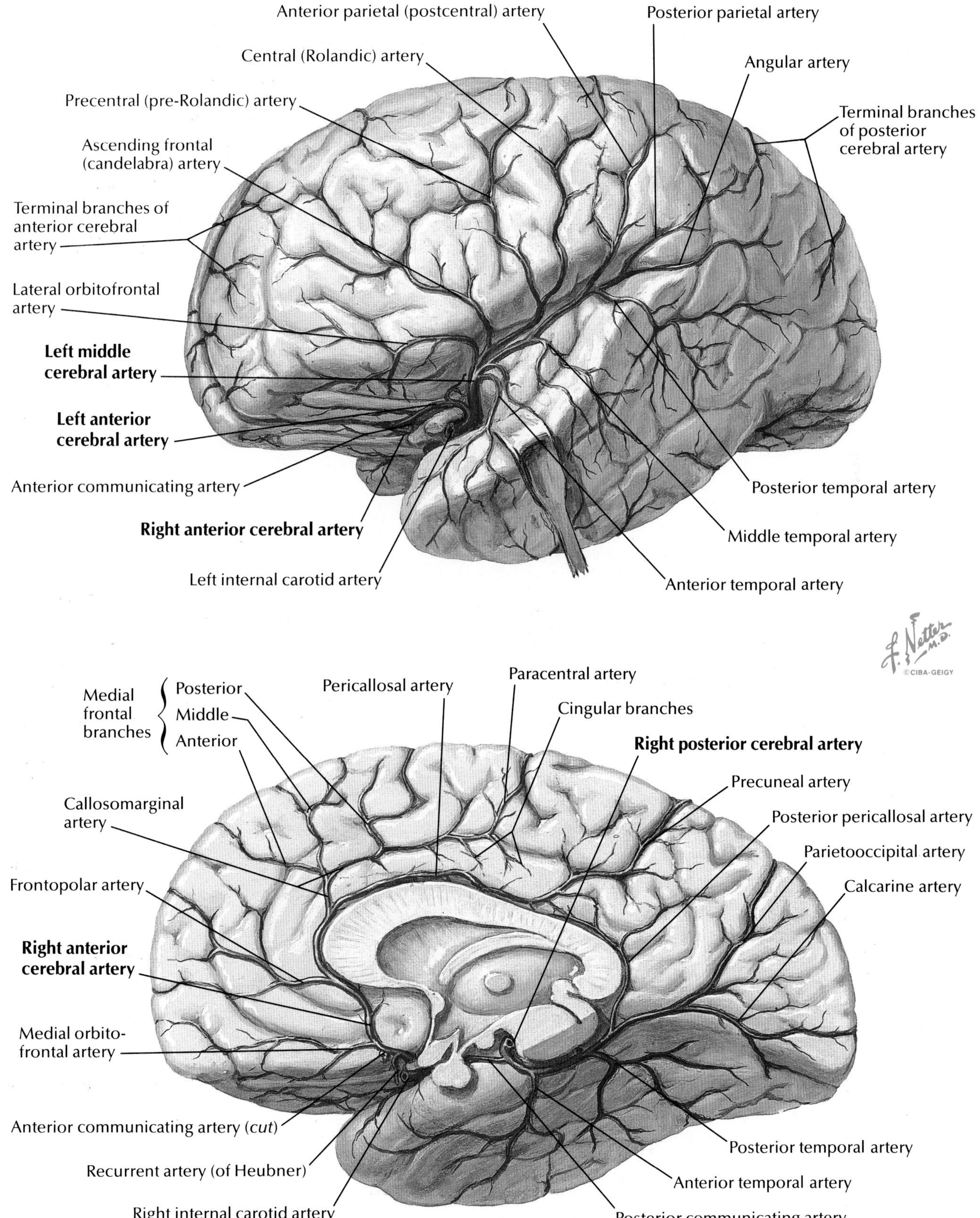

Anterior parietal (postcentral) artery

Central (Rolandic) artery

Precentral (pre-Rolandic) artery

Ascending frontal (candelabra) artery

Terminal branches of anterior cerebral artery

Lateral orbitofrontal artery

Left middle cerebral artery

Left anterior cerebral artery

Anterior communicating artery

Right anterior cerebral artery

Left internal carotid artery

Posterior parietal artery

Angular artery

Terminal branches of posterior cerebral artery

Posterior temporal artery

Middle temporal artery

Anterior temporal artery

Medial frontal branches { Posterior / Middle / Anterior

Callosomarginal artery

Frontopolar artery

Right anterior cerebral artery

Medial orbito-frontal artery

Anterior communicating artery (*cut*)

Recurrent artery (of Heubner)

Right internal carotid artery

Pericallosal artery

Paracentral artery

Cingular branches

Right posterior cerebral artery

Precuneal artery

Posterior pericallosal artery

Parietooccipital artery

Calcarine artery

Posterior temporal artery

Anterior temporal artery

Posterior communicating artery

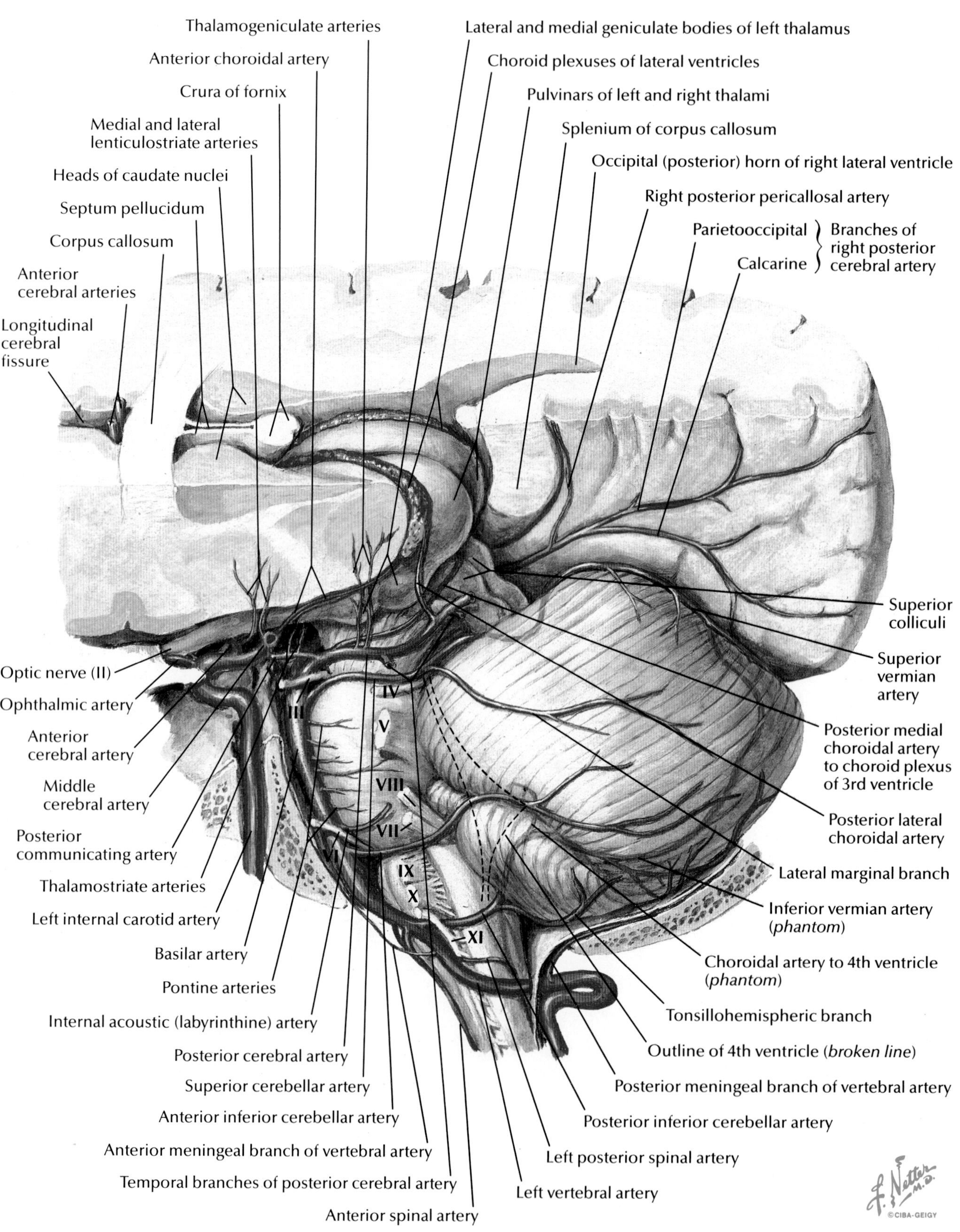

Thalamogeniculate arteries

Anterior choroidal artery

Crura of fornix

Medial and lateral
lenticulostriate arteries

Heads of caudate nuclei

Septum pellucidum

Corpus callosum

Anterior
cerebral arteries

Longitudinal
cerebral
fissure

Lateral and medial geniculate bodies of left thalamus

Choroid plexuses of lateral ventricles

Pulvinars of left and right thalami

Splenium of corpus callosum

Occipital (posterior) horn of right lateral ventricle

Right posterior pericallosal artery

Parietooccipital } Branches of
right posterior
Calcarine } cerebral artery

Optic nerve (II)

Ophthalmic artery

Anterior
cerebral artery

Middle
cerebral artery

Posterior
communicating artery

Thalamostriate arteries

Left internal carotid artery

Basilar artery

Pontine arteries

Internal acoustic (labyrinthine) artery

Posterior cerebral artery

Superior cerebellar artery

Anterior inferior cerebellar artery

Anterior meningeal branch of vertebral artery

Temporal branches of posterior cerebral artery

Anterior spinal artery

Superior
colliculi

Superior
vermian
artery

Posterior medial
choroidal artery
to choroid plexus
of 3rd ventricle

Posterior lateral
choroidal artery

Lateral marginal branch

Inferior vermian artery
(phantom)

Choroidal artery to 4th ventricle
(phantom)

Tonsillohemispheric branch

Outline of 4th ventricle (broken line)

Posterior meningeal branch of vertebral artery

Posterior inferior cerebellar artery

Left posterior spinal artery

Left vertebral artery

II IV V VIII VII VI IX X XI

PLATE 136

HEAD AND NECK

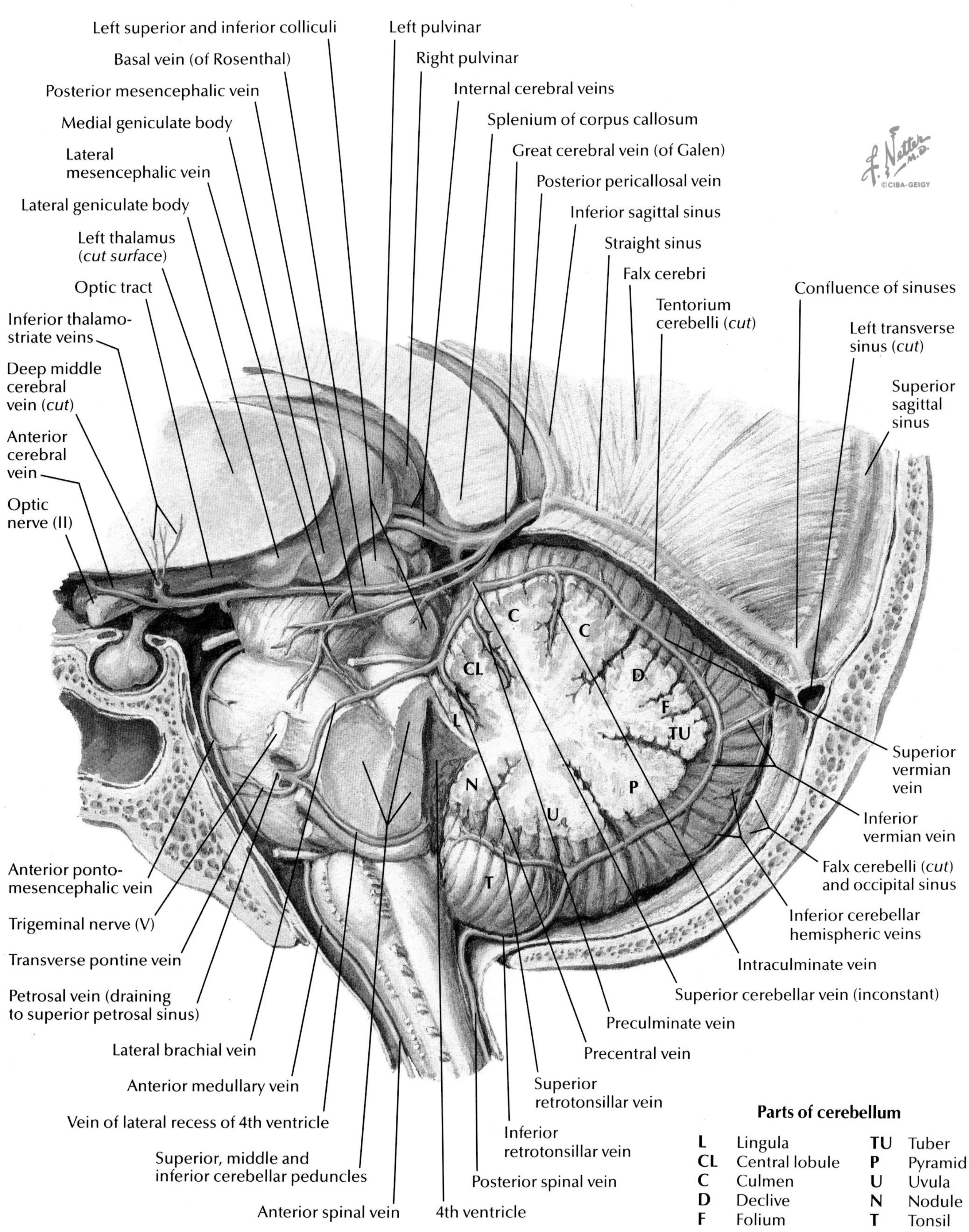

Left superior and inferior colliculi
Basal vein (of Rosenthal)
Posterior mesencephalic vein
Medial geniculate body
Lateral mesencephalic vein
Lateral geniculate body
Left thalamus (cut surface)
Optic tract
Inferior thalamo-striate veins
Deep middle cerebral vein (cut)
Anterior cerebral vein
Optic nerve (II)

Left pulvinar
Right pulvinar
Internal cerebral veins
Splenium of corpus callosum
Great cerebral vein (of Galen)
Posterior pericallosal vein
Inferior sagittal sinus
Straight sinus
Falx cerebri
Tentorium cerebelli (cut)

Confluence of sinuses
Left transverse sinus (cut)
Superior sagittal sinus

Anterior ponto-mesencephalic vein
Trigeminal nerve (V)
Transverse pontine vein
Petrosal vein (draining to superior petrosal sinus)
Lateral brachial vein
Anterior medullary vein
Vein of lateral recess of 4th ventricle
Superior, middle and inferior cerebellar peduncles
Anterior spinal vein
4th ventricle
Posterior spinal vein
Inferior retrotonsillar vein
Superior retrotonsillar vein
Precentral vein
Preculminate vein
Superior cerebellar vein (inconstant)
Intraculminate vein
Inferior cerebellar hemispheric veins
Falx cerebelli (cut) and occipital sinus
Inferior vermian vein
Superior vermian vein

Parts of cerebellum

L	Lingula	**TU**	Tuber
CL	Central lobule	**P**	Pyramid
C	Culmen	**U**	Uvula
D	Declive	**N**	Nodule
F	Folium	**T**	Tonsil

Deep Veins of Brain

FOR SUPERFICIAL VEINS OF BRAIN SEE PLATE 96

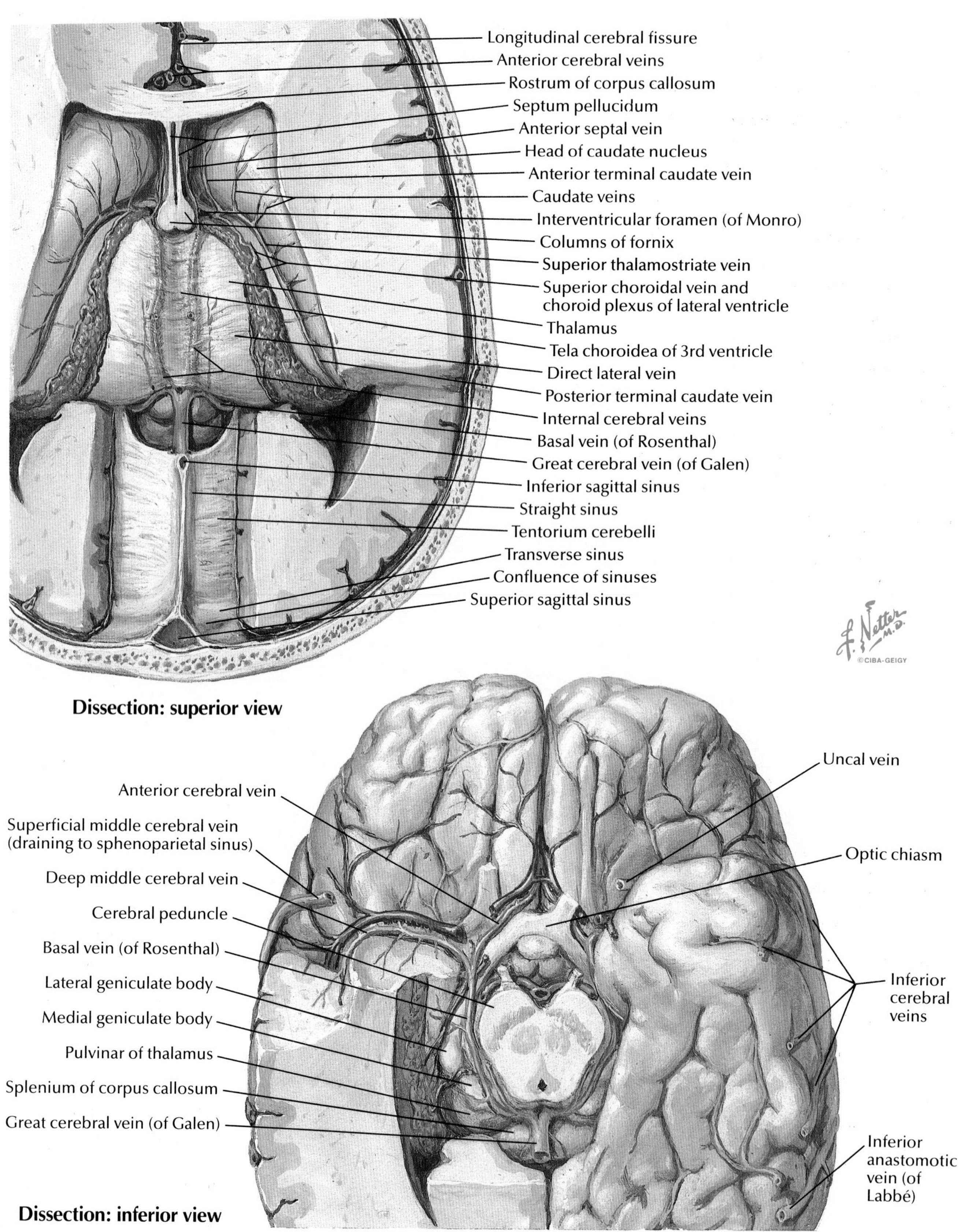

Longitudinal cerebral fissure
Anterior cerebral veins
Rostrum of corpus callosum
Septum pellucidum
Anterior septal vein
Head of caudate nucleus
Anterior terminal caudate vein
Caudate veins
Interventricular foramen (of Monro)
Columns of fornix
Superior thalamostriate vein
Superior choroidal vein and choroid plexus of lateral ventricle
Thalamus
Tela choroidea of 3rd ventricle
Direct lateral vein
Posterior terminal caudate vein
Internal cerebral veins
Basal vein (of Rosenthal)
Great cerebral vein (of Galen)
Inferior sagittal sinus
Straight sinus
Tentorium cerebelli
Transverse sinus
Confluence of sinuses
Superior sagittal sinus

Dissection: superior view

Anterior cerebral vein
Superficial middle cerebral vein (draining to sphenoparietal sinus)
Deep middle cerebral vein
Cerebral peduncle
Basal vein (of Rosenthal)
Lateral geniculate body
Medial geniculate body
Pulvinar of thalamus
Splenium of corpus callosum
Great cerebral vein (of Galen)

Uncal vein
Optic chiasm
Inferior cerebral veins
Inferior anastomotic vein (of Labbé)

Dissection: inferior view

PLATE 138

HEAD AND NECK

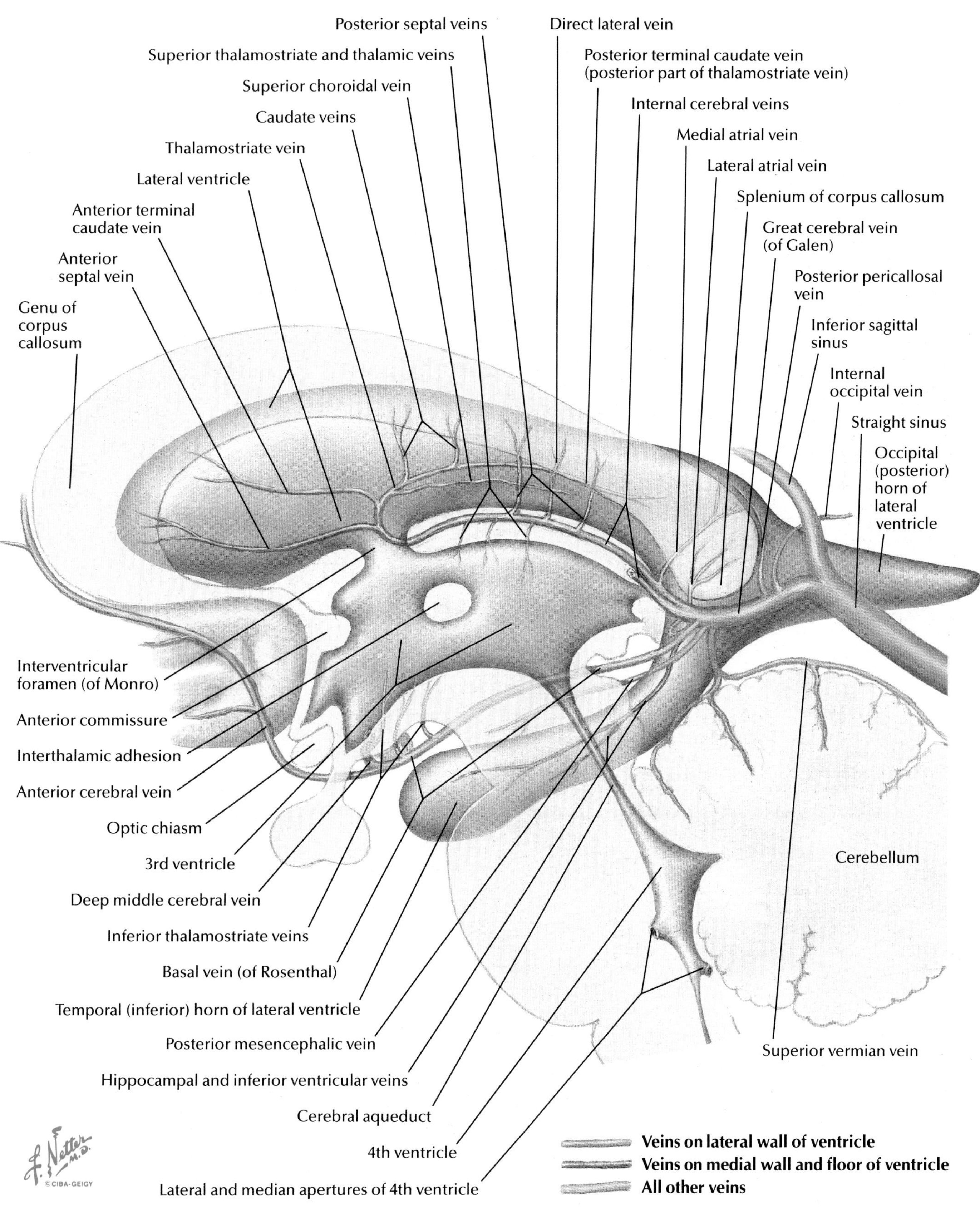

Posterior septal veins

Direct lateral vein

Superior thalamostriate and thalamic veins

Posterior terminal caudate vein
(posterior part of thalamostriate vein)

Superior choroidal vein

Internal cerebral veins

Caudate veins

Medial atrial vein

Thalamostriate vein

Lateral atrial vein

Lateral ventricle

Splenium of corpus callosum

Anterior terminal
caudate vein

Great cerebral vein
(of Galen)

Anterior
septal vein

Posterior pericallosal
vein

Genu of
corpus
callosum

Inferior sagittal
sinus

Internal
occipital vein

Straight sinus

Occipital
(posterior)
horn of
lateral
ventricle

Interventricular
foramen (of Monro)

Anterior commissure

Interthalamic adhesion

Anterior cerebral vein

Optic chiasm

3rd ventricle

Cerebellum

Deep middle cerebral vein

Inferior thalamostriate veins

Basal vein (of Rosenthal)

Temporal (inferior) horn of lateral ventricle

Posterior mesencephalic vein

Superior vermian vein

Hippocampal and inferior ventricular veins

Cerebral aqueduct

4th ventricle

Lateral and median apertures of 4th ventricle

Veins on lateral wall of ventricle
Veins on medial wall and floor of ventricle
All other veins

Hypothalamus and Hypophysis

SEE ALSO PLATES 100, 101

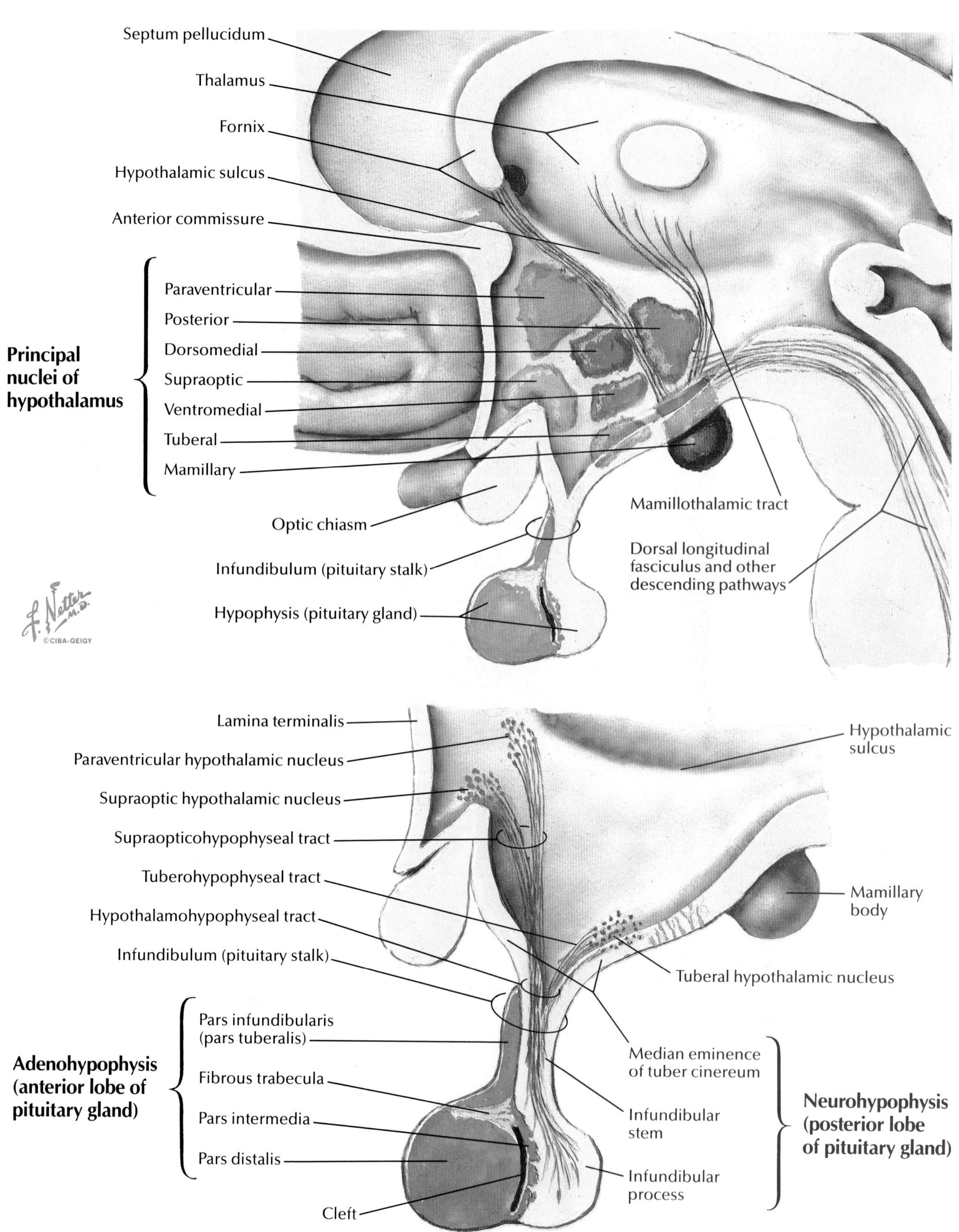

Septum pellucidum

Thalamus

Fornix

Hypothalamic sulcus

Anterior commissure

Principal nuclei of hypothalamus

Paraventricular

Posterior

Dorsomedial

Supraoptic

Ventromedial

Tuberal

Mamillary

Optic chiasm

Infundibulum (pituitary stalk)

Hypophysis (pituitary gland)

Mamillothalamic tract

Dorsal longitudinal fasciculus and other descending pathways

Lamina terminalis

Paraventricular hypothalamic nucleus

Supraoptic hypothalamic nucleus

Supraopticohypophyseal tract

Tuberohypophyseal tract

Hypothalamohypophyseal tract

Infundibulum (pituitary stalk)

Hypothalamic sulcus

Mamillary body

Tuberal hypothalamic nucleus

Median eminence of tuber cinereum

Adenohypophysis (anterior lobe of pituitary gland)

Pars infundibularis (pars tuberalis)

Fibrous trabecula

Pars intermedia

Pars distalis

Cleft

Infundibular stem

Infundibular process

Neurohypophysis (posterior lobe of pituitary gland)

PLATE 140

HEAD AND NECK

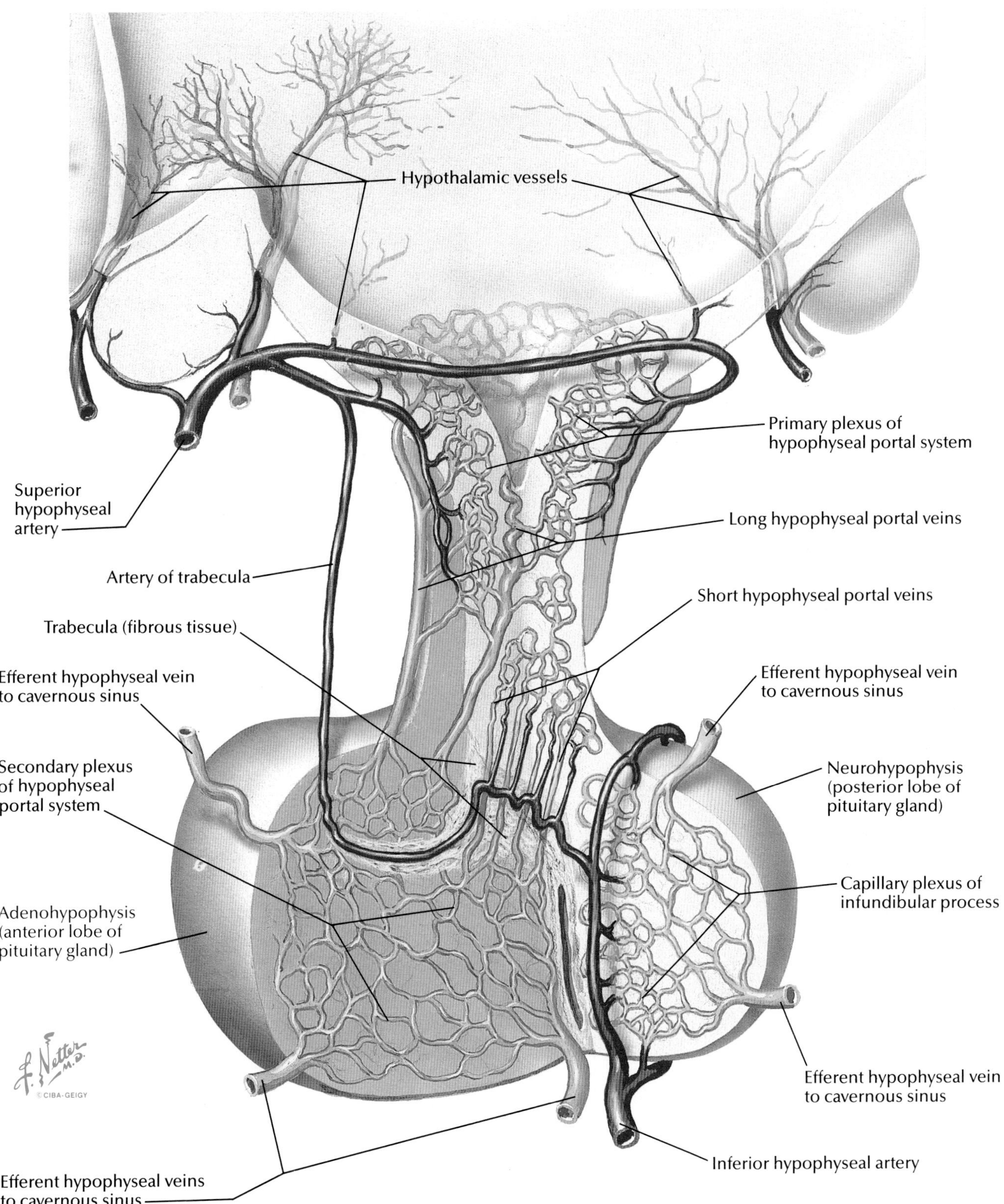

Hypothalamic vessels

Primary plexus of hypophyseal portal system

Superior hypophyseal artery

Long hypophyseal portal veins

Artery of trabecula

Short hypophyseal portal veins

Trabecula (fibrous tissue)

Efferent hypophyseal vein to cavernous sinus

Efferent hypophyseal vein to cavernous sinus

Secondary plexus of hypophyseal portal system

Neurohypophysis (posterior lobe of pituitary gland)

Adenohypophysis (anterior lobe of pituitary gland)

Capillary plexus of infundibular process

Efferent hypophyseal vein to cavernous sinus

Efferent hypophyseal veins to cavernous sinus

Inferior hypophyseal artery

Section II

BACK AND SPINAL CORD

SEE ALSO PLATES 9, 12, 13, 143, 144, 145, 170, 231

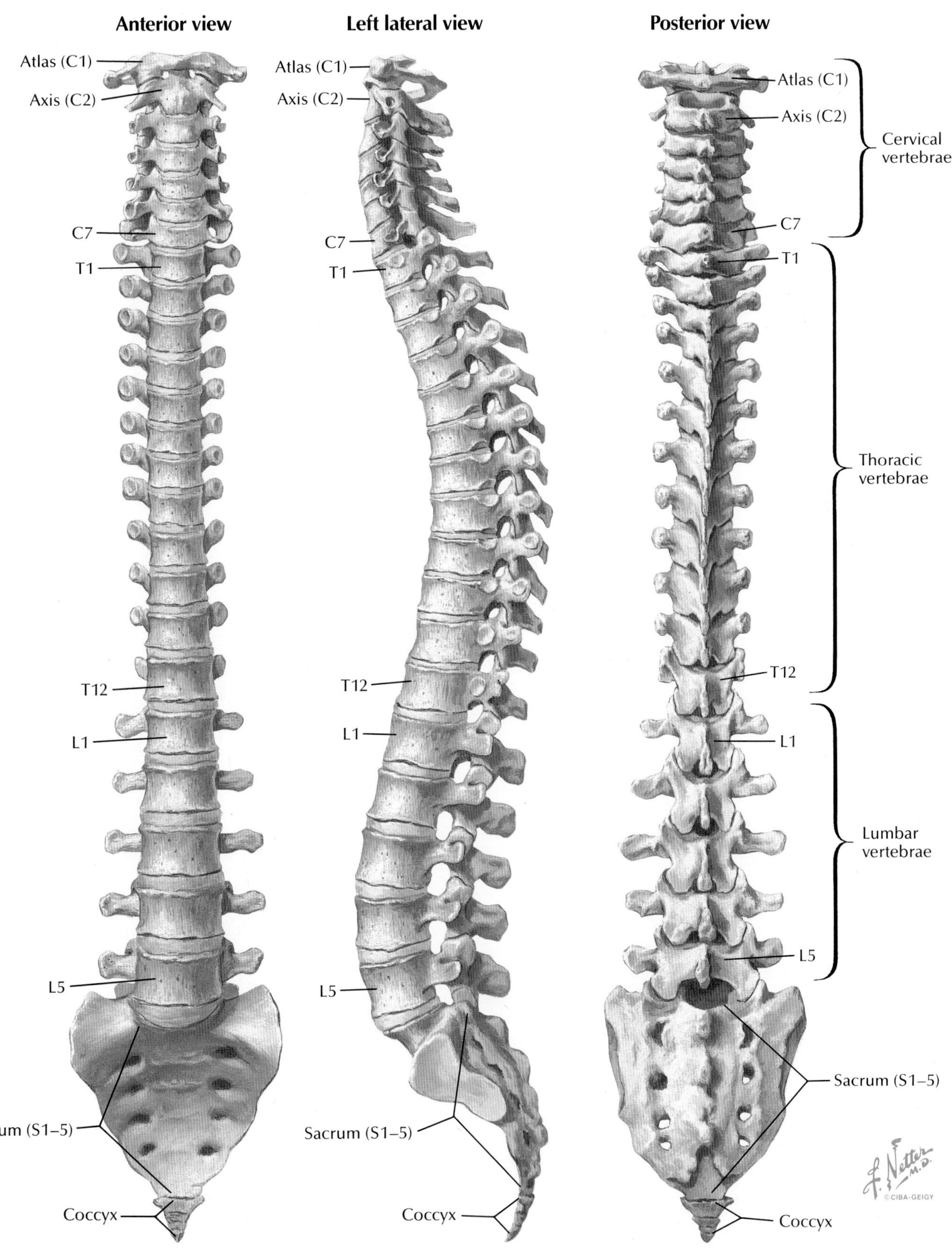

Anterior view

Atlas (C1)
Axis (C2)
C7
T1
T12
L1
L5
Sacrum (S1–5)
Coccyx

Left lateral view

Atlas (C1)
Axis (C2)
C7
T1
T12
L1
L5
Sacrum (S1–5)
Coccyx

Posterior view

Atlas (C1)
Axis (C2)
Cervical vertebrae
C7
T1
Thoracic vertebrae
T12
L1
Lumbar vertebrae
L5
Sacrum (S1–5)
Coccyx

Thoracic Vertebrae

SEE ALSO PLATE 172

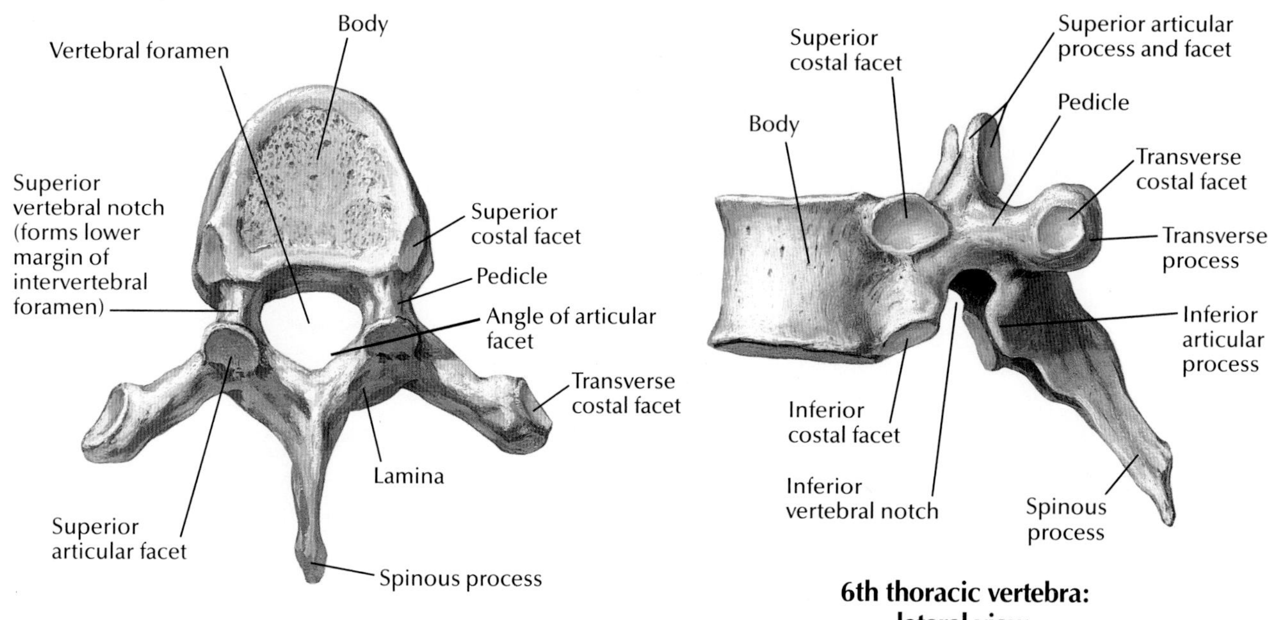

Vertebral foramen

Body

Superior vertebral notch (forms lower margin of intervertebral foramen)

Superior costal facet

Pedicle

Angle of articular facet

Transverse costal facet

Superior articular facet

Lamina

Spinous process

6th thoracic vertebra: superior view

Superior costal facet

Body

Superior articular process and facet

Pedicle

Transverse costal facet

Transverse process

Inferior articular process

Inferior costal facet

Inferior vertebral notch

Spinous process

6th thoracic vertebra: lateral view

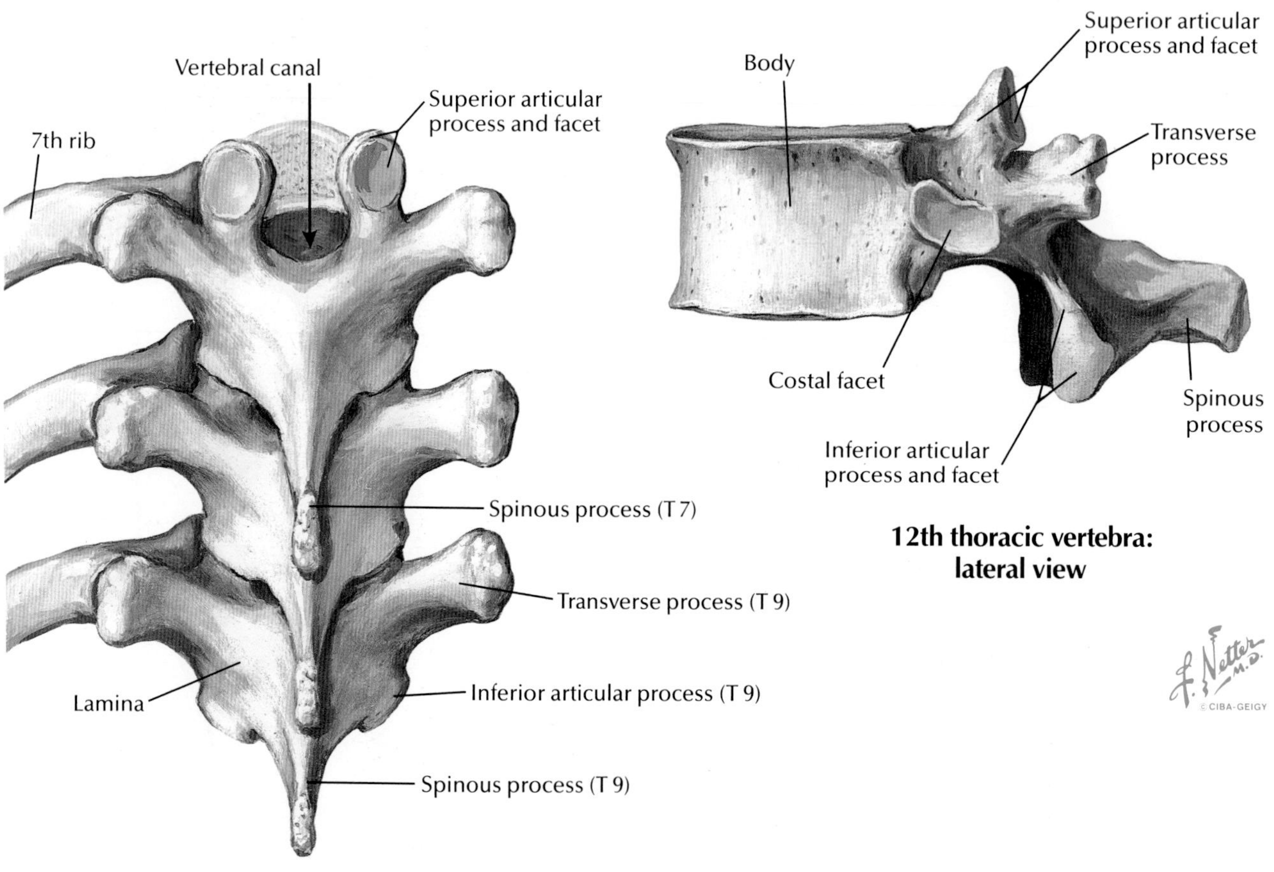

Vertebral canal

Superior articular process and facet

7th rib

Spinous process (T 7)

Transverse process (T 9)

Inferior articular process (T 9)

Lamina

Spinous process (T 9)

7th, 8th and 9th thoracic vertebrae: posterior view

Body

Superior articular process and facet

Transverse process

Costal facet

Spinous process

Inferior articular process and facet

12th thoracic vertebra: lateral view

PLATE 143

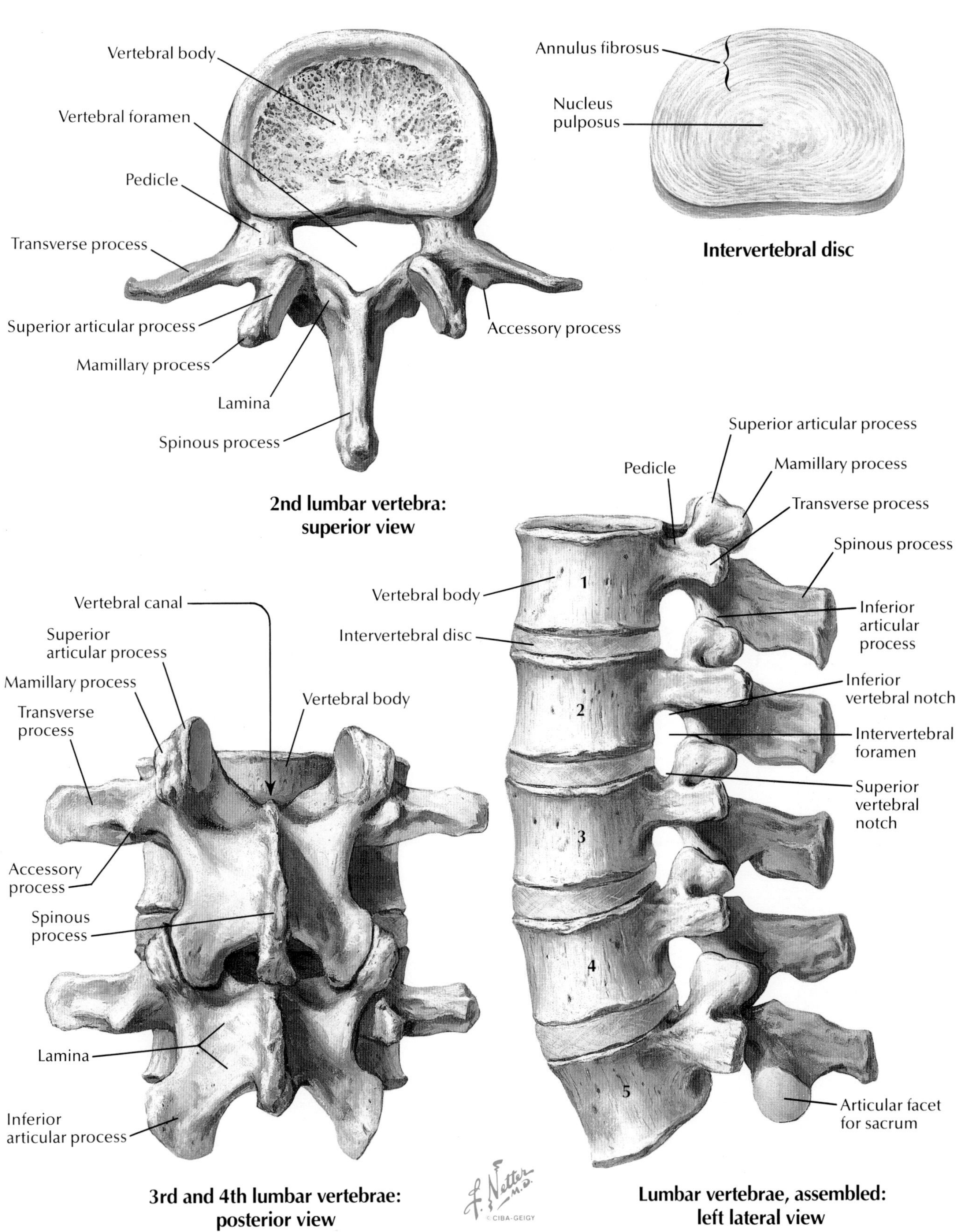

Vertebral body

Vertebral foramen

Pedicle

Transverse process

Superior articular process

Mamillary process

Lamina

Spinous process

**2nd lumbar vertebra:
superior view**

Annulus fibrosus

Nucleus
pulposus

Intervertebral disc

Vertebral canal

Superior
articular process

Mamillary process

Transverse
process

Accessory
process

Spinous
process

Lamina

Inferior
articular process

Vertebral body

**3rd and 4th lumbar vertebrae:
posterior view**

Pedicle

Superior articular process

Mamillary process

Transverse process

Spinous process

Inferior
articular
process

Inferior
vertebral notch

Intervertebral
foramen

Superior
vertebral
notch

Vertebral body

Intervertebral disc

1

2

3

4

5

Articular facet
for sacrum

**Lumbar vertebrae, assembled:
left lateral view**

Sacrum and Coccyx

SEE ALSO PLATES 142, 147, 231, 334, 335, 336

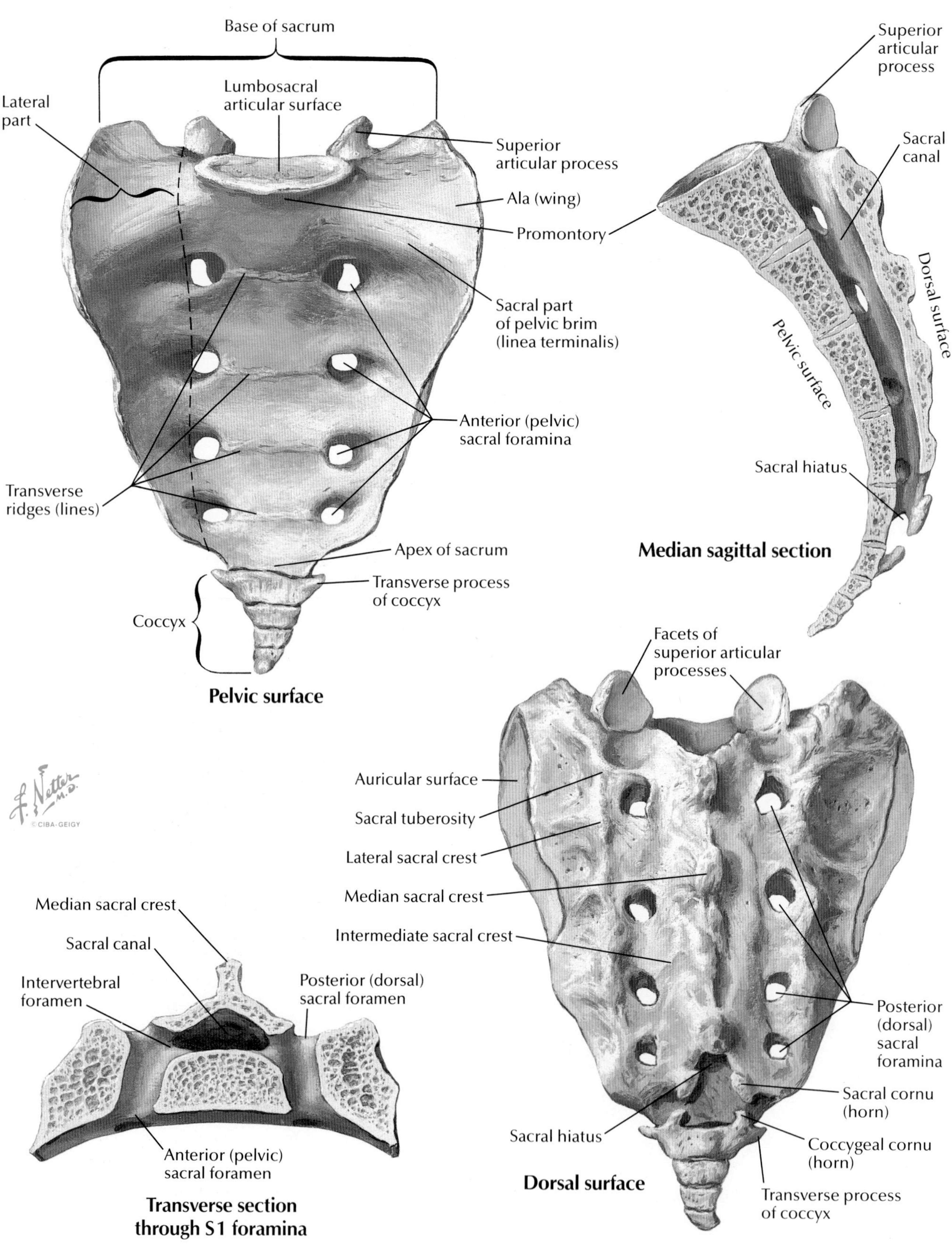

Base of sacrum

Lumbosacral articular surface

Lateral part

Superior articular process

Ala (wing)

Promontory

Sacral part of pelvic brim (linea terminalis)

Anterior (pelvic) sacral foramina

Transverse ridges (lines)

Apex of sacrum

Transverse process of coccyx

Coccyx

Pelvic surface

Superior articular process

Sacral canal

Dorsal surface

Pelvic surface

Sacral hiatus

Median sagittal section

Facets of superior articular processes

Auricular surface

Sacral tuberosity

Lateral sacral crest

Median sacral crest

Intermediate sacral crest

Posterior (dorsal) sacral foramina

Sacral cornu (horn)

Coccygeal cornu (horn)

Sacral hiatus

Transverse process of coccyx

Dorsal surface

Median sacral crest

Sacral canal

Intervertebral foramen

Posterior (dorsal) sacral foramen

Anterior (pelvic) sacral foramen

Transverse section through S1 foramina

PLATE 145

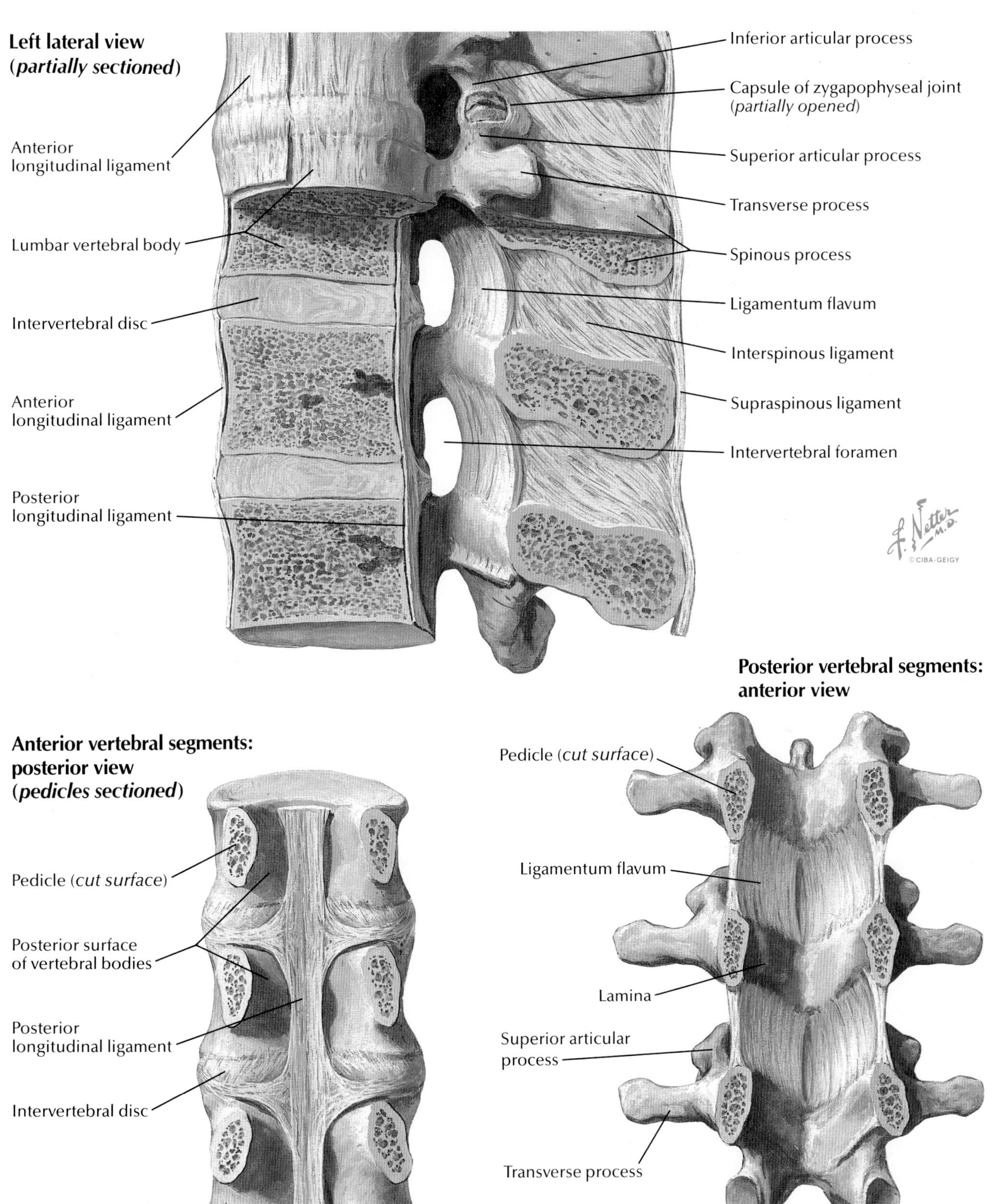

Left lateral view
(*partially sectioned*)

Anterior
longitudinal ligament

Lumbar vertebral body

Intervertebral disc

Anterior
longitudinal ligament

Posterior
longitudinal ligament

Inferior articular process

Capsule of zygapophyseal joint
(*partially opened*)

Superior articular process

Transverse process

Spinous process

Ligamentum flavum

Interspinous ligament

Supraspinous ligament

Intervertebral foramen

**Anterior vertebral segments:
posterior view**
(*pedicles sectioned*)

Pedicle (*cut surface*)

Posterior surface
of vertebral bodies

Posterior
longitudinal ligament

Intervertebral disc

**Posterior vertebral segments:
anterior view**

Pedicle (*cut surface*)

Ligamentum flavum

Lamina

Superior articular
process

Transverse process

Inferior articular facet

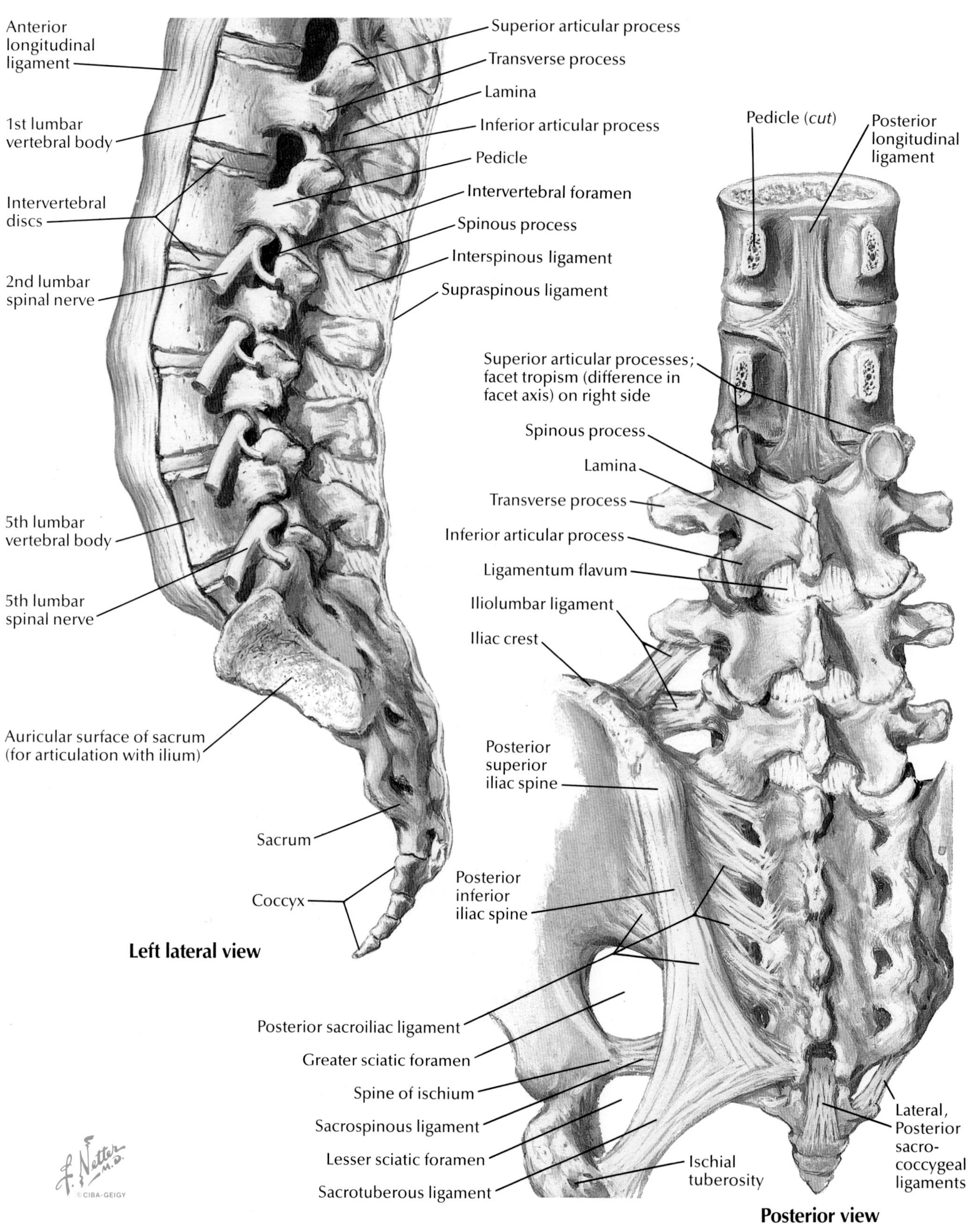

Anterior longitudinal ligament

1st lumbar vertebral body

Intervertebral discs

2nd lumbar spinal nerve

5th lumbar vertebral body

5th lumbar spinal nerve

Auricular surface of sacrum (for articulation with ilium)

Sacrum

Coccyx

Left lateral view

Superior articular process

Transverse process

Lamina

Inferior articular process

Pedicle

Intervertebral foramen

Spinous process

Interspinous ligament

Supraspinous ligament

Pedicle (*cut*)

Posterior longitudinal ligament

Superior articular processes; facet tropism (difference in facet axis) on right side

Spinous process

Lamina

Transverse process

Inferior articular process

Ligamentum flavum

Iliolumbar ligament

Iliac crest

Posterior superior iliac spine

Posterior inferior iliac spine

Posterior sacroiliac ligament

Greater sciatic foramen

Spine of ischium

Sacrospinous ligament

Lesser sciatic foramen

Sacrotuberous ligament

Ischial tuberosity

Lateral, Posterior sacro-coccygeal ligaments

Posterior view

PLATE 147

BACK AND SPINAL CORD

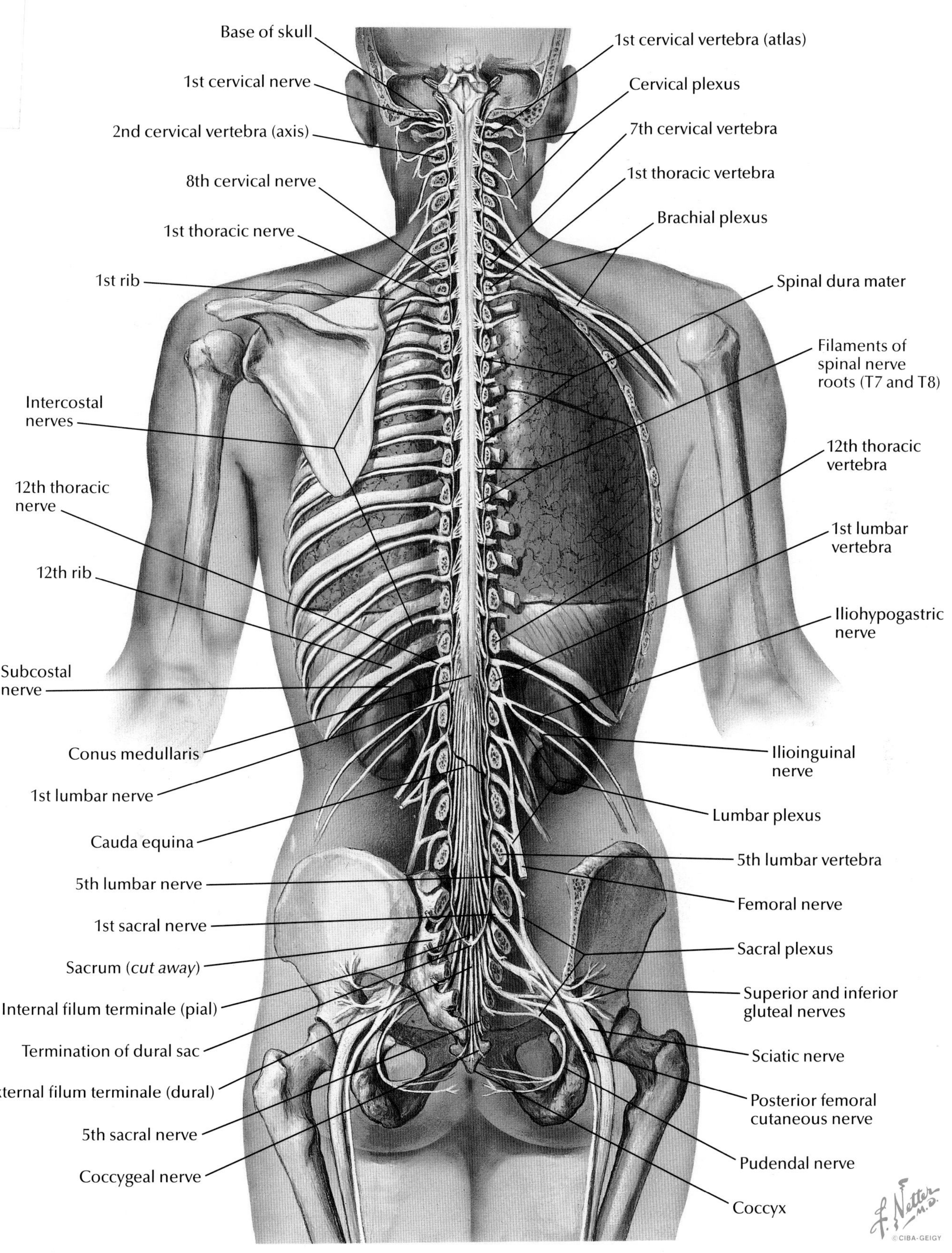

Base of skull

1st cervical nerve

2nd cervical vertebra (axis)

8th cervical nerve

1st thoracic nerve

1st rib

Intercostal nerves

12th thoracic nerve

12th rib

Subcostal nerve

Conus medullaris

1st lumbar nerve

Cauda equina

5th lumbar nerve

1st sacral nerve

Sacrum (*cut away*)

Internal filum terminale (pial)

Termination of dural sac

External filum terminale (dural)

5th sacral nerve

Coccygeal nerve

1st cervical vertebra (atlas)

Cervical plexus

7th cervical vertebra

1st thoracic vertebra

Brachial plexus

Spinal dura mater

Filaments of spinal nerve roots (T7 and T8)

12th thoracic vertebra

1st lumbar vertebra

Iliohypogastric nerve

Ilioinguinal nerve

Lumbar plexus

5th lumbar vertebra

Femoral nerve

Sacral plexus

Superior and inferior gluteal nerves

Sciatic nerve

Posterior femoral cutaneous nerve

Pudendal nerve

Coccyx

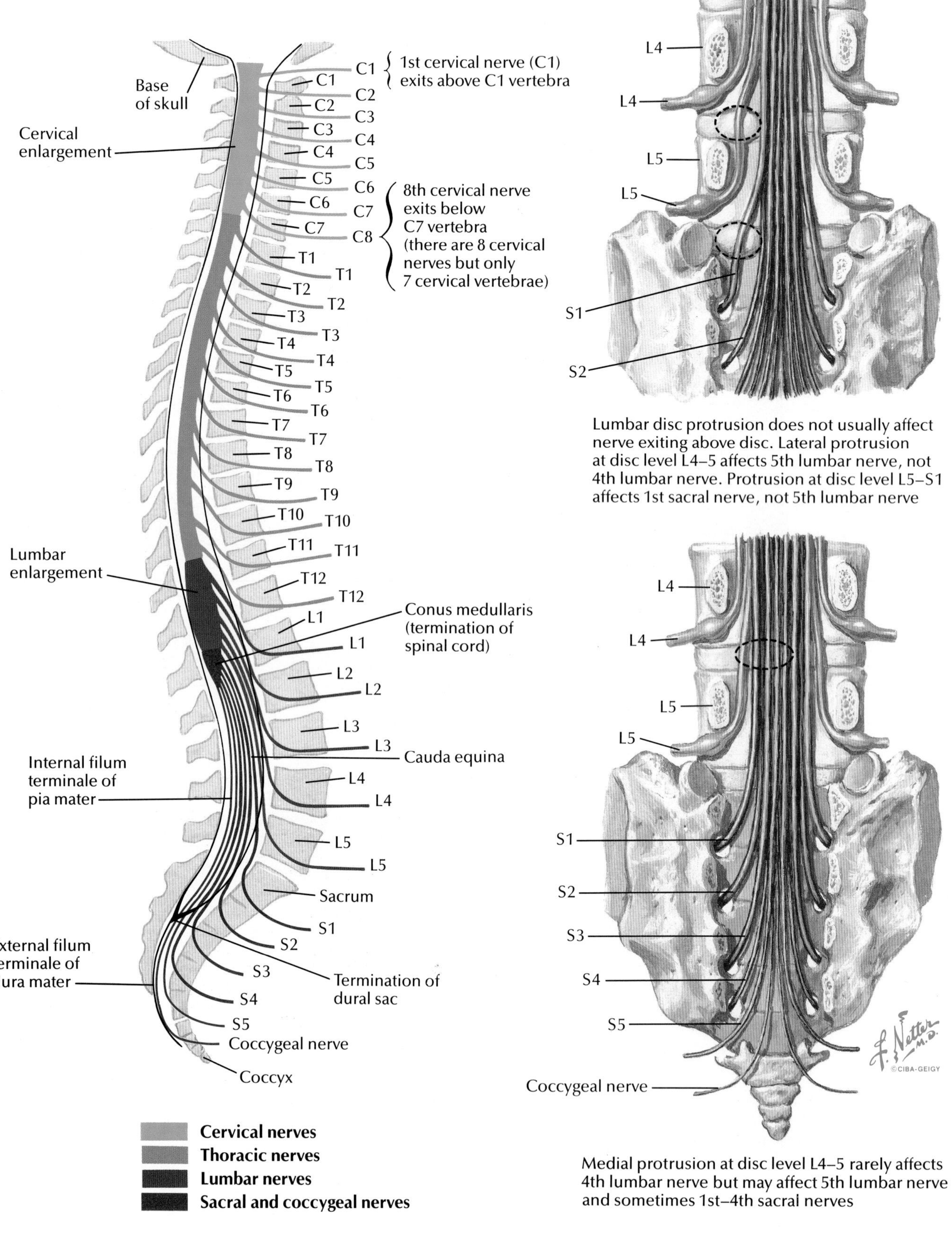

Base of skull

Cervical enlargement

C1 — 1st cervical nerve (C1) exits above C1 vertebra

C1
C2
C3
C4
C5
C6
C7
C8

8th cervical nerve exits below C7 vertebra (there are 8 cervical nerves but only 7 cervical vertebrae)

T1
T2
T3
T4
T5
T6
T7
T8
T9
T10
T11
T12

Lumbar enlargement

Conus medullaris (termination of spinal cord)

L1
L2
L3 — Cauda equina
L4
L5

Internal filum terminale of pia mater

Sacrum

S1
S2
S3 — Termination of dural sac
S4
S5

External filum terminale of dura mater

Coccygeal nerve

Coccyx

Cervical nerves
Thoracic nerves
Lumbar nerves
Sacral and coccygeal nerves

L4
L4
L5
L5
S1
S2

Lumbar disc protrusion does not usually affect nerve exiting above disc. Lateral protrusion at disc level L4–5 affects 5th lumbar nerve, not 4th lumbar nerve. Protrusion at disc level L5–S1 affects 1st sacral nerve, not 5th lumbar nerve

L4
L4
L5
L5
S1
S2
S3
S4
S5

Coccygeal nerve

Medial protrusion at disc level L4–5 rarely affects 4th lumbar nerve but may affect 5th lumbar nerve and sometimes 1st–4th sacral nerves

PLATE 149

BACK AND SPINAL CORD

SEE ALSO PLATES 455, 511; FOR MAPS OF CUTANEOUS NERVES SEE PLATES 18, 445, 447, 448, 449, 451, 454, 506–510

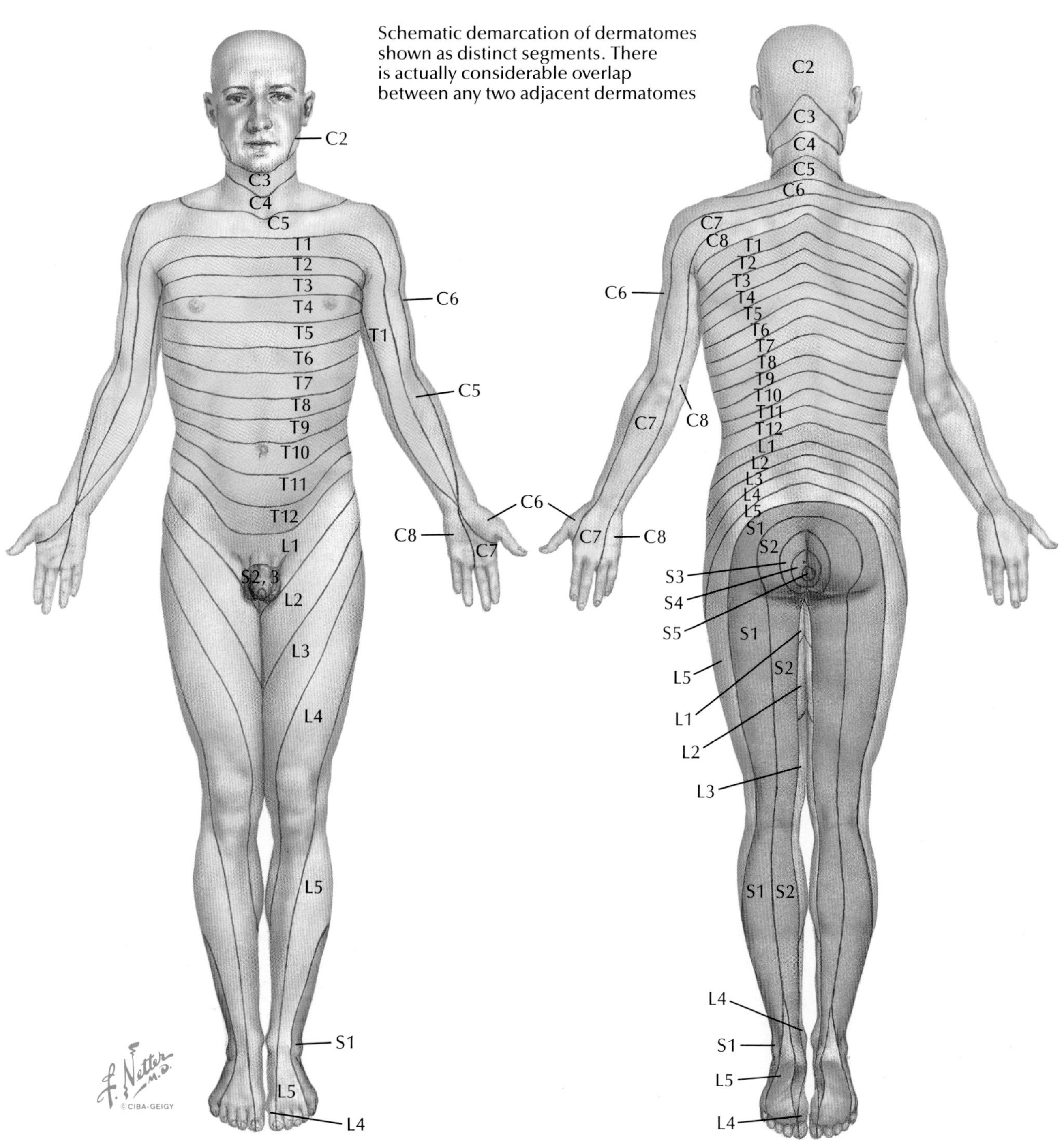

Schematic demarcation of dermatomes shown as distinct segments. There is actually considerable overlap between any two adjacent dermatomes

Levels of principal dermatomes

C5	Clavicles
C5, 6, 7	Lateral parts of upper limbs
C8, T1	Medial sides of upper limbs
C6	Thumb
C6, 7, 8	Hand
C8	Ring and little fingers
T4	Level of nipples
T10	Level of umbilicus
T12	Inguinal or groin regions
L1, 2, 3, 4	Anterior and inner surfaces of lower limbs
L4, 5, S1	Foot
L4	Medial side of great toe
S1, 2, L5	Posterior and outer surfaces of lower limbs
S1	Lateral margin of foot and little toe
S2, 3, 4	Perineum

Spinal Cord Cross Sections: Fiber Tracts

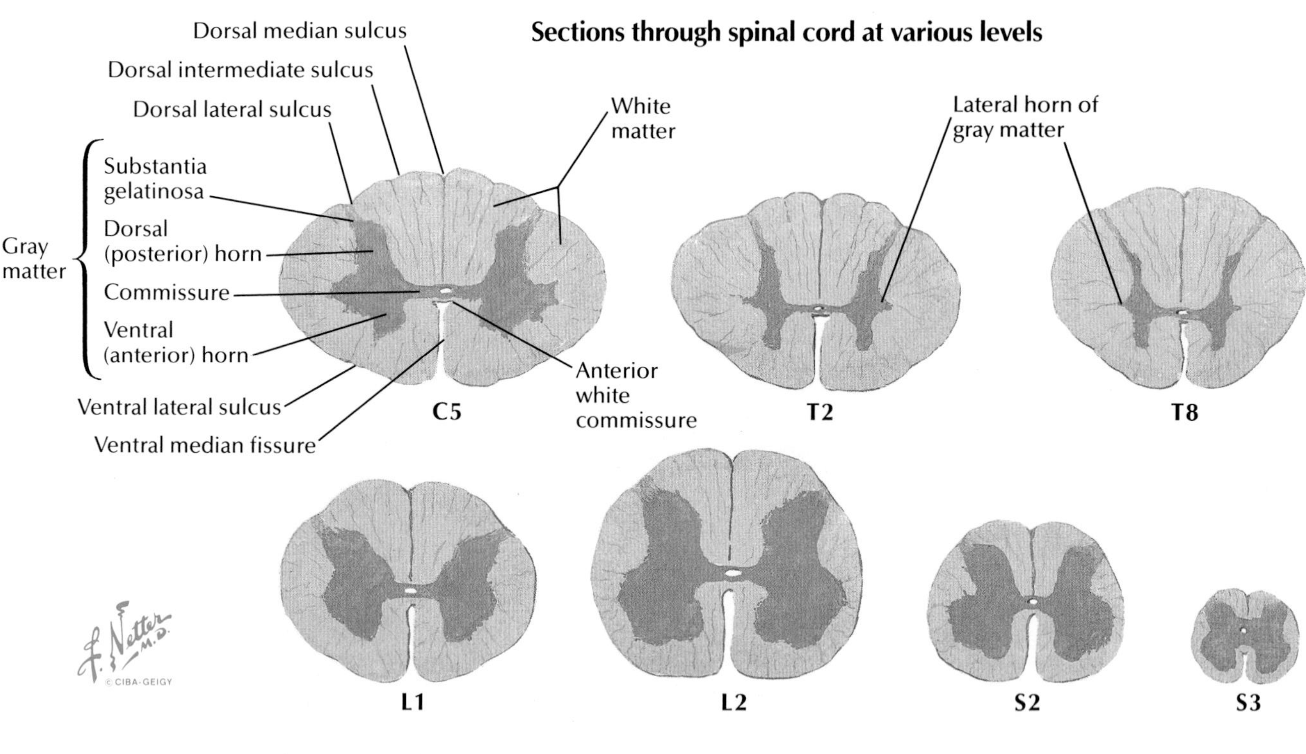

Sections through spinal cord at various levels

Dorsal median sulcus

Dorsal intermediate sulcus

Dorsal lateral sulcus

White matter

Lateral horn of gray matter

Gray matter
- Substantia gelatinosa
- Dorsal (posterior) horn
- Commissure
- Ventral (anterior) horn

Ventral lateral sulcus

Ventral median fissure

Anterior white commissure

C5

T2

T8

L1

L2

S2

S3

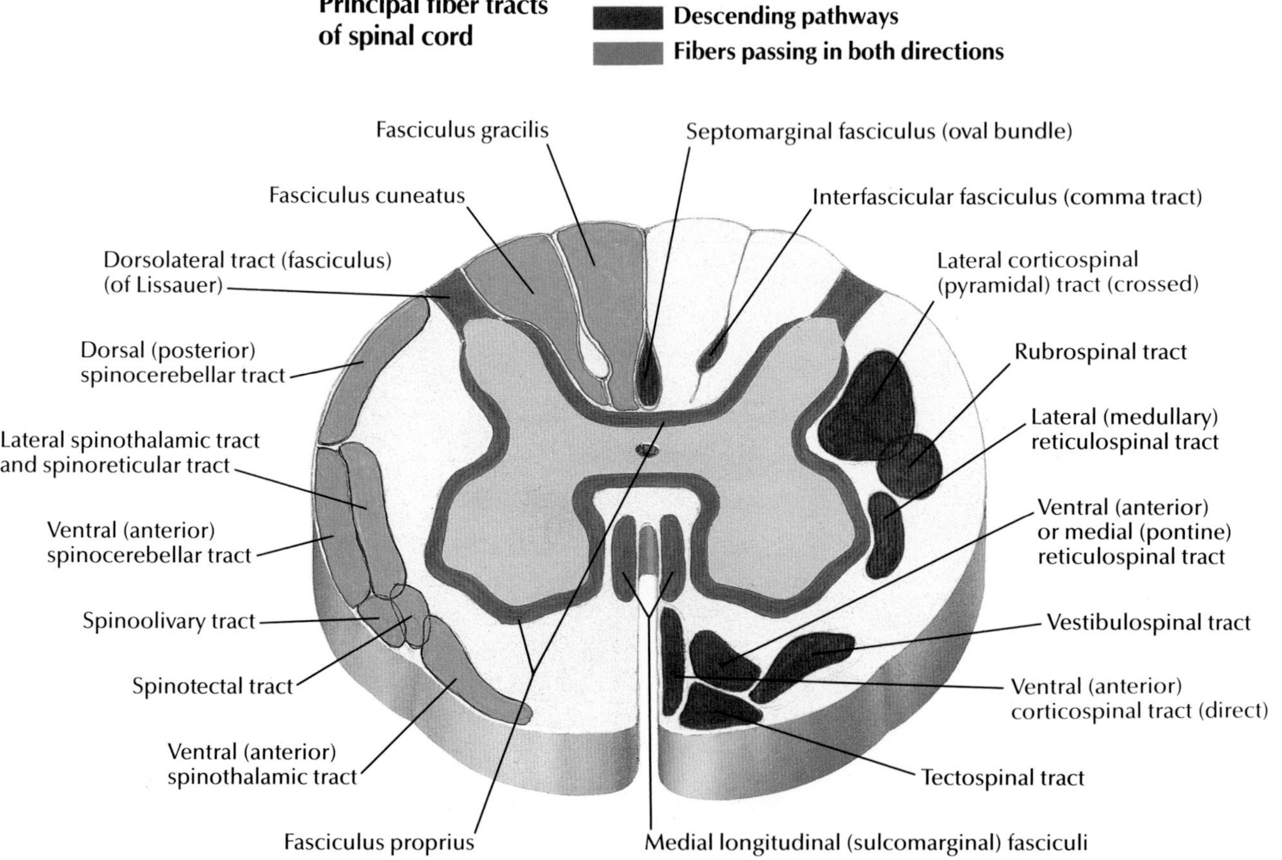

Principal fiber tracts of spinal cord

- Ascending pathways
- Descending pathways
- Fibers passing in both directions

Fasciculus gracilis

Fasciculus cuneatus

Dorsolateral tract (fasciculus) (of Lissauer)

Dorsal (posterior) spinocerebellar tract

Lateral spinothalamic tract and spinoreticular tract

Ventral (anterior) spinocerebellar tract

Spinoolivary tract

Spinotectal tract

Ventral (anterior) spinothalamic tract

Fasciculus proprius

Septomarginal fasciculus (oval bundle)

Interfascicular fasciculus (comma tract)

Lateral corticospinal (pyramidal) tract (crossed)

Rubrospinal tract

Lateral (medullary) reticulospinal tract

Ventral (anterior) or medial (pontine) reticulospinal tract

Vestibulospinal tract

Ventral (anterior) corticospinal tract (direct)

Tectospinal tract

Medial longitudinal (sulcomarginal) fasciculi

PLATE 151

BACK AND SPINAL CORD

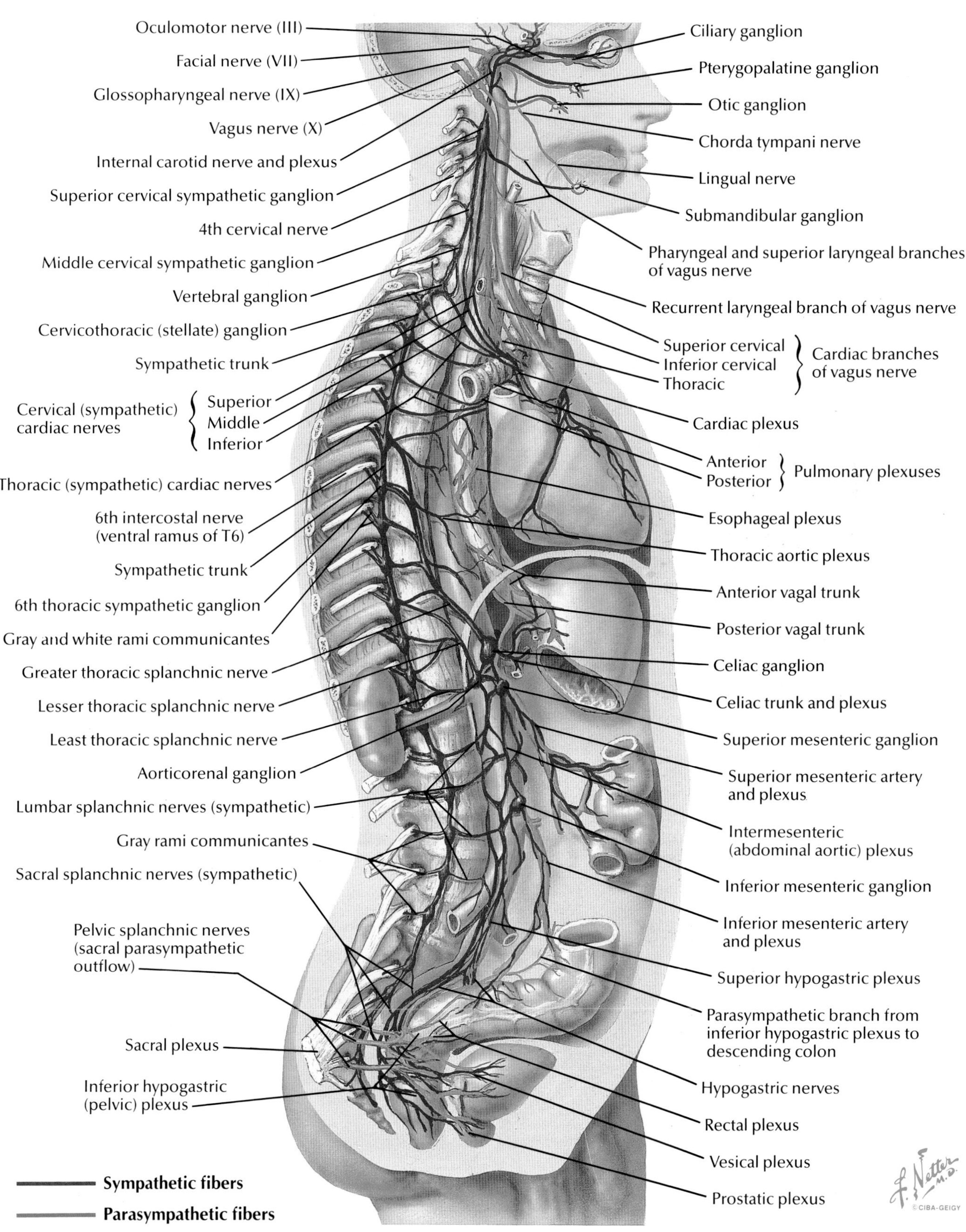

Oculomotor nerve (III)

Facial nerve (VII)

Glossopharyngeal nerve (IX)

Vagus nerve (X)

Internal carotid nerve and plexus

Superior cervical sympathetic ganglion

4th cervical nerve

Middle cervical sympathetic ganglion

Vertebral ganglion

Cervicothoracic (stellate) ganglion

Sympathetic trunk

Cervical (sympathetic) cardiac nerves { Superior / Middle / Inferior

Thoracic (sympathetic) cardiac nerves

6th intercostal nerve (ventral ramus of T6)

Sympathetic trunk

6th thoracic sympathetic ganglion

Gray and white rami communicantes

Greater thoracic splanchnic nerve

Lesser thoracic splanchnic nerve

Least thoracic splanchnic nerve

Aorticorenal ganglion

Lumbar splanchnic nerves (sympathetic)

Gray rami communicantes

Sacral splanchnic nerves (sympathetic)

Pelvic splanchnic nerves (sacral parasympathetic outflow)

Sacral plexus

Inferior hypogastric (pelvic) plexus

Ciliary ganglion

Pterygopalatine ganglion

Otic ganglion

Chorda tympani nerve

Lingual nerve

Submandibular ganglion

Pharyngeal and superior laryngeal branches of vagus nerve

Recurrent laryngeal branch of vagus nerve

Superior cervical / Inferior cervical / Thoracic } Cardiac branches of vagus nerve

Cardiac plexus

Anterior / Posterior } Pulmonary plexuses

Esophageal plexus

Thoracic aortic plexus

Anterior vagal trunk

Posterior vagal trunk

Celiac ganglion

Celiac trunk and plexus

Superior mesenteric ganglion

Superior mesenteric artery and plexus

Intermesenteric (abdominal aortic) plexus

Inferior mesenteric ganglion

Inferior mesenteric artery and plexus

Superior hypogastric plexus

Parasympathetic branch from inferior hypogastric plexus to descending colon

Hypogastric nerves

Rectal plexus

Vesical plexus

Prostatic plexus

———— **Sympathetic fibers**

———— **Parasympathetic fibers**

Autonomic Nervous System: Schema

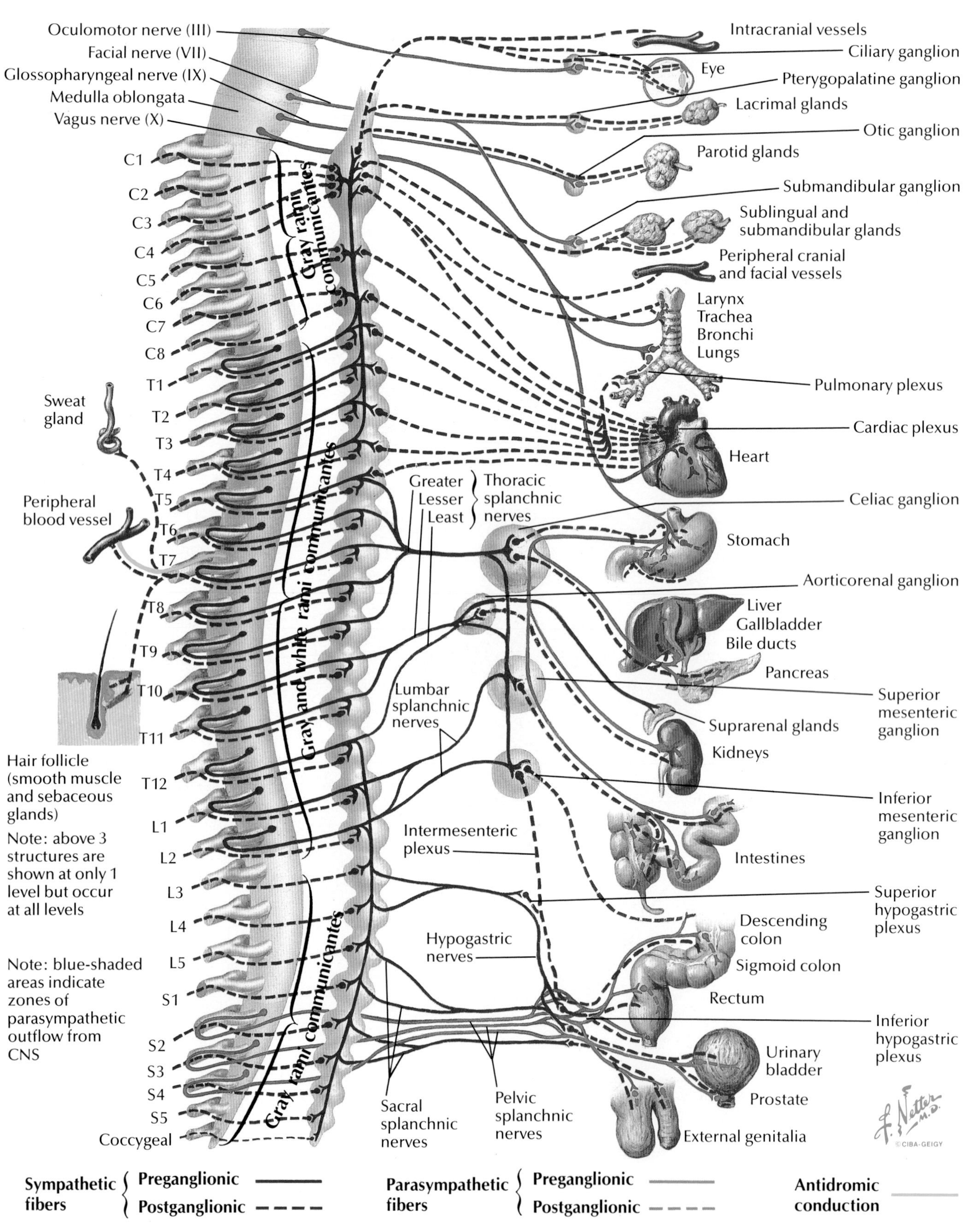

Oculomotor nerve (III)
Facial nerve (VII)
Glossopharyngeal nerve (IX)
Medulla oblongata
Vagus nerve (X)

Intracranial vessels
Ciliary ganglion
Eye
Pterygopalatine ganglion
Lacrimal glands
Otic ganglion
Parotid glands
Submandibular ganglion
Sublingual and submandibular glands
Peripheral cranial and facial vessels

C1
C2
C3
C4
C5
C6
C7
C8
T1
T2
T3
T4
T5
T6
T7
T8
T9
T10
T11
T12
L1
L2
L3
L4
L5
S1
S2
S3
S4
S5
Coccygeal

Gray rami communicantes

Gray and white rami communicantes

Gray rami communicantes

Sweat gland

Peripheral blood vessel

Hair follicle (smooth muscle and sebaceous glands)
Note: above 3 structures are shown at only 1 level but occur at all levels

Note: blue-shaded areas indicate zones of parasympathetic outflow from CNS

Greater ⎱
Lesser ⎰ Thoracic
Least splanchnic nerves

Lumbar splanchnic nerves

Intermesenteric plexus

Hypogastric nerves

Sacral splanchnic nerves

Pelvic splanchnic nerves

Larynx
Trachea
Bronchi
Lungs
Pulmonary plexus
Cardiac plexus
Heart
Celiac ganglion
Stomach
Aorticorenal ganglion
Liver
Gallbladder
Bile ducts
Pancreas
Superior mesenteric ganglion
Suprarenal glands
Kidneys
Inferior mesenteric ganglion
Intestines
Superior hypogastric plexus
Descending colon
Sigmoid colon
Rectum
Inferior hypogastric plexus
Urinary bladder
Prostate
External genitalia

Sympathetic fibers	Preganglionic ———	Parasympathetic fibers	Preganglionic ———	Antidromic conduction ———
	Postganglionic - - -		Postganglionic - - -	

PLATE 153

BACK AND SPINAL CORD

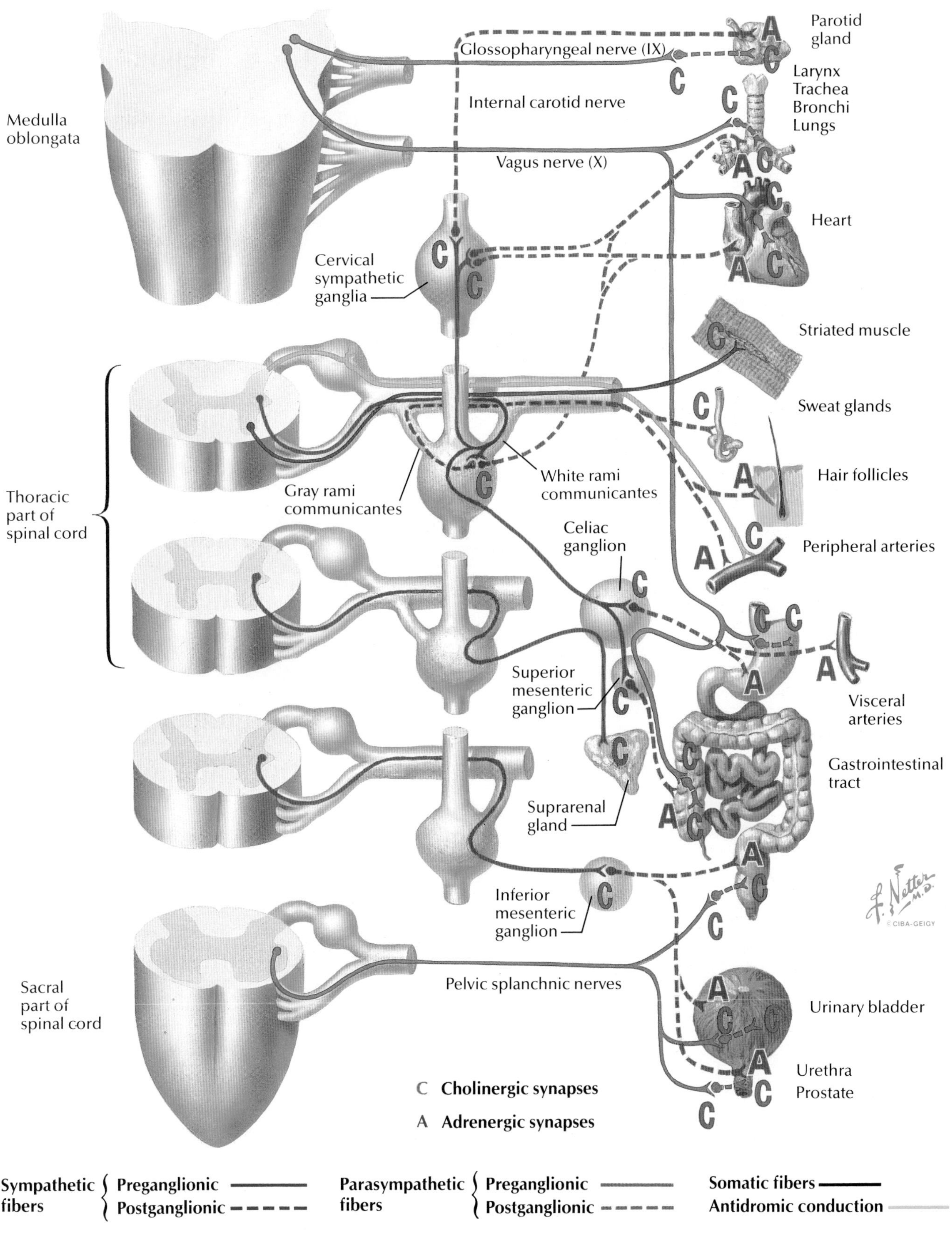

Medulla oblongata

Parotid gland

Glossopharyngeal nerve (IX)

Larynx
Trachea
Bronchi
Lungs

Internal carotid nerve

Vagus nerve (X)

Heart

Cervical sympathetic ganglia

Striated muscle

Thoracic part of spinal cord

Sweat glands

White rami communicantes

Gray rami communicantes

Hair follicles

Celiac ganglion

Peripheral arteries

Superior mesenteric ganglion

Visceral arteries

Gastrointestinal tract

Suprarenal gland

Inferior mesenteric ganglion

Sacral part of spinal cord

Pelvic splanchnic nerves

Urinary bladder

Urethra
Prostate

C Cholinergic synapses

A Adrenergic synapses

Sympathetic fibers { Preganglionic ——— Postganglionic -------

Parasympathetic fibers { Preganglionic ——— Postganglionic -------

Somatic fibers ———
Antidromic conduction ———

Spinal Membranes and Nerve Roots

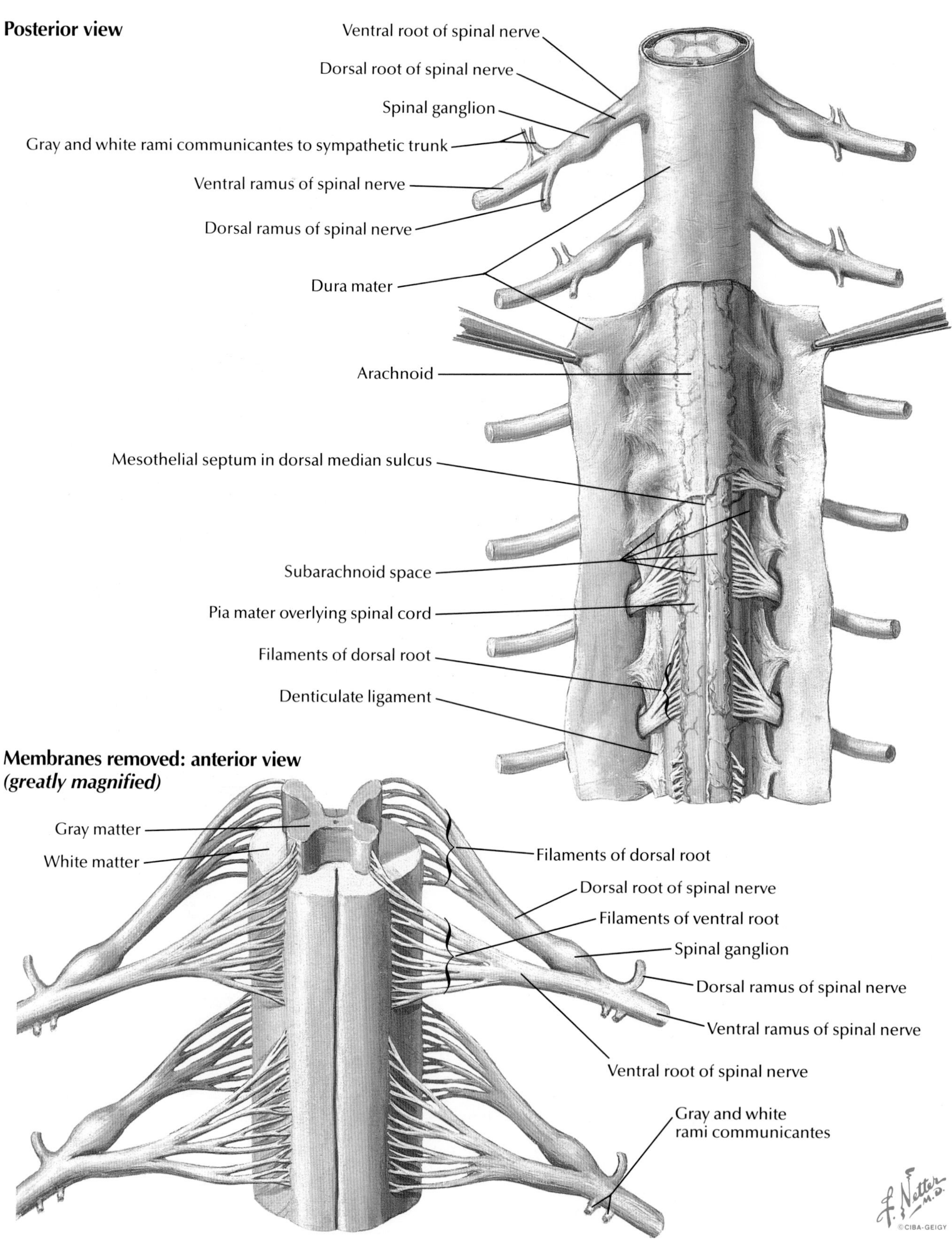

Posterior view

Ventral root of spinal nerve

Dorsal root of spinal nerve

Spinal ganglion

Gray and white rami communicantes to sympathetic trunk

Ventral ramus of spinal nerve

Dorsal ramus of spinal nerve

Dura mater

Arachnoid

Mesothelial septum in dorsal median sulcus

Subarachnoid space

Pia mater overlying spinal cord

Filaments of dorsal root

Denticulate ligament

Membranes removed: anterior view
(greatly magnified)

Gray matter

White matter

Filaments of dorsal root

Dorsal root of spinal nerve

Filaments of ventral root

Spinal ganglion

Dorsal ramus of spinal nerve

Ventral ramus of spinal nerve

Ventral root of spinal nerve

Gray and white rami communicantes

PLATE 155

BACK AND SPINAL CORD

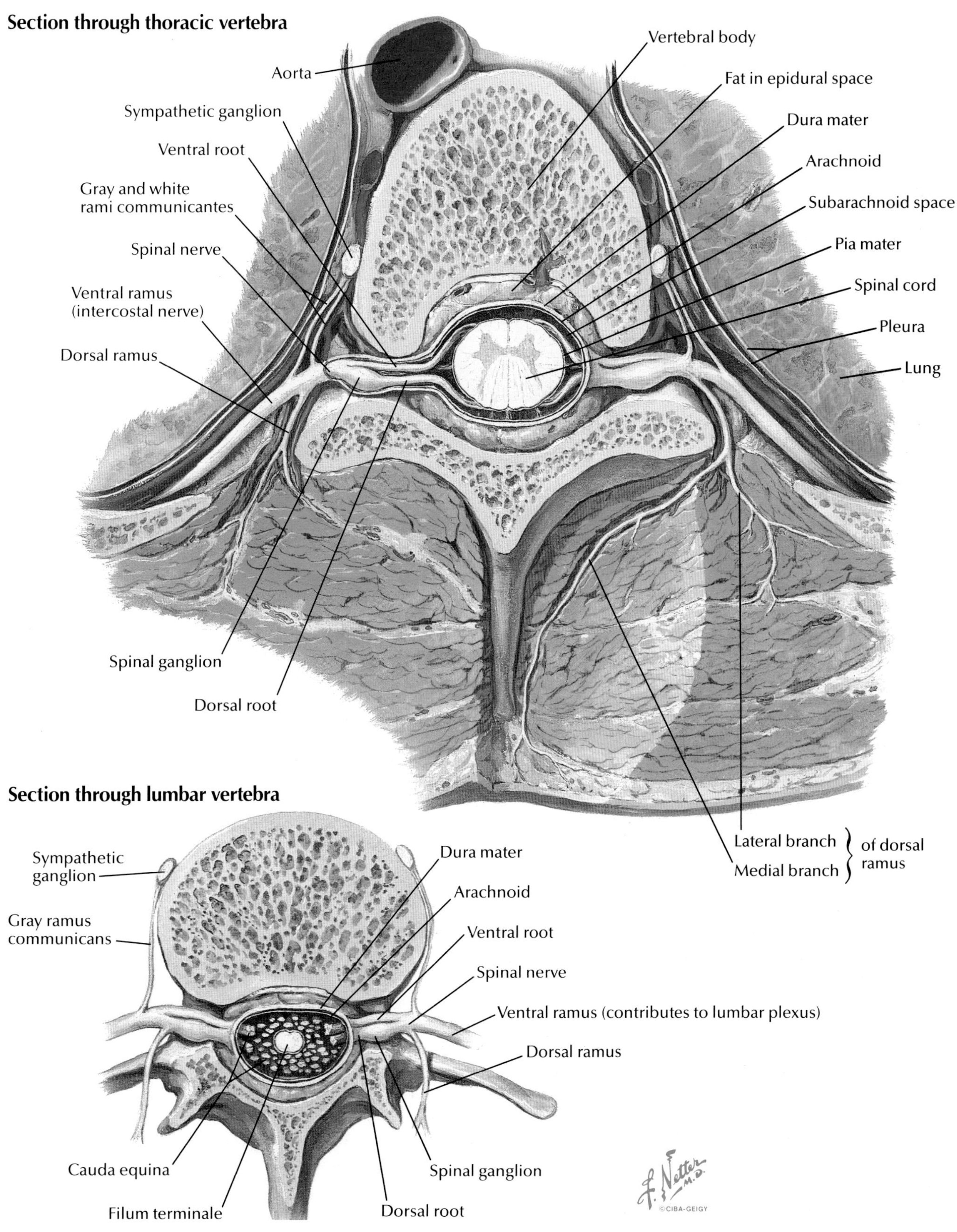

Section through thoracic vertebra

Aorta

Sympathetic ganglion

Ventral root

Gray and white rami communicantes

Spinal nerve

Ventral ramus (intercostal nerve)

Dorsal ramus

Spinal ganglion

Dorsal root

Vertebral body

Fat in epidural space

Dura mater

Arachnoid

Subarachnoid space

Pia mater

Spinal cord

Pleura

Lung

Lateral branch } of dorsal
Medial branch } ramus

Section through lumbar vertebra

Sympathetic ganglion

Gray ramus communicans

Dura mater

Arachnoid

Ventral root

Spinal nerve

Ventral ramus (contributes to lumbar plexus)

Dorsal ramus

Spinal ganglion

Dorsal root

Cauda equina

Filum terminale

Arteries of Spinal Cord: Schema

SEE ALSO PLATE 131

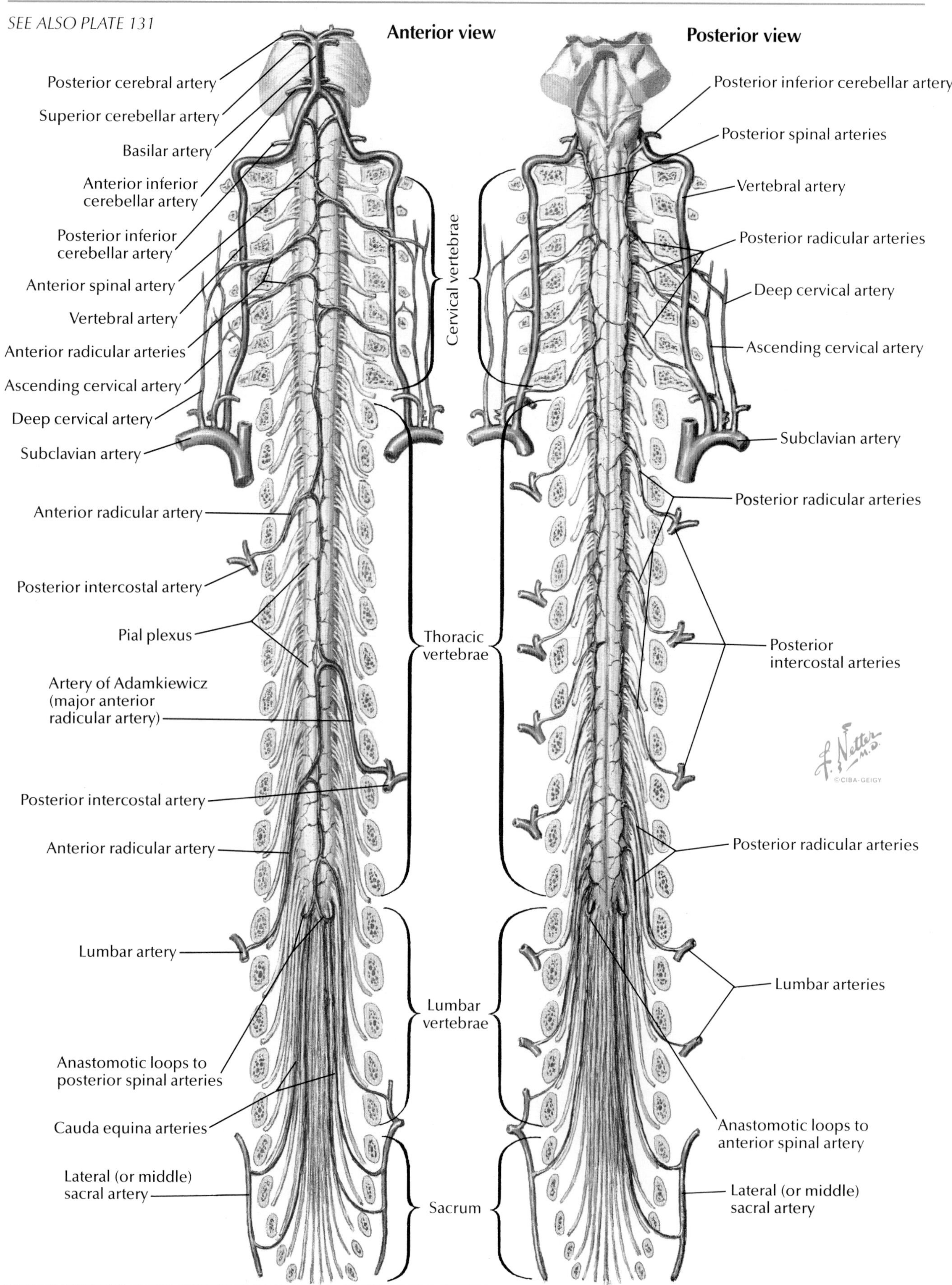

Anterior view

Posterior view

Posterior cerebral artery

Superior cerebellar artery

Basilar artery

Anterior inferior cerebellar artery

Posterior inferior cerebellar artery

Anterior spinal artery

Vertebral artery

Anterior radicular arteries

Ascending cervical artery

Deep cervical artery

Subclavian artery

Anterior radicular artery

Posterior intercostal artery

Pial plexus

Artery of Adamkiewicz (major anterior radicular artery)

Posterior intercostal artery

Anterior radicular artery

Lumbar artery

Anastomotic loops to posterior spinal arteries

Cauda equina arteries

Lateral (or middle) sacral artery

Cervical vertebrae

Thoracic vertebrae

Lumbar vertebrae

Sacrum

Posterior inferior cerebellar artery

Posterior spinal arteries

Vertebral artery

Posterior radicular arteries

Deep cervical artery

Ascending cervical artery

Subclavian artery

Posterior radicular arteries

Posterior intercostal arteries

Posterior radicular arteries

Lumbar arteries

Anastomotic loops to anterior spinal artery

Lateral (or middle) sacral artery

PLATE 157

BACK AND SPINAL CORD

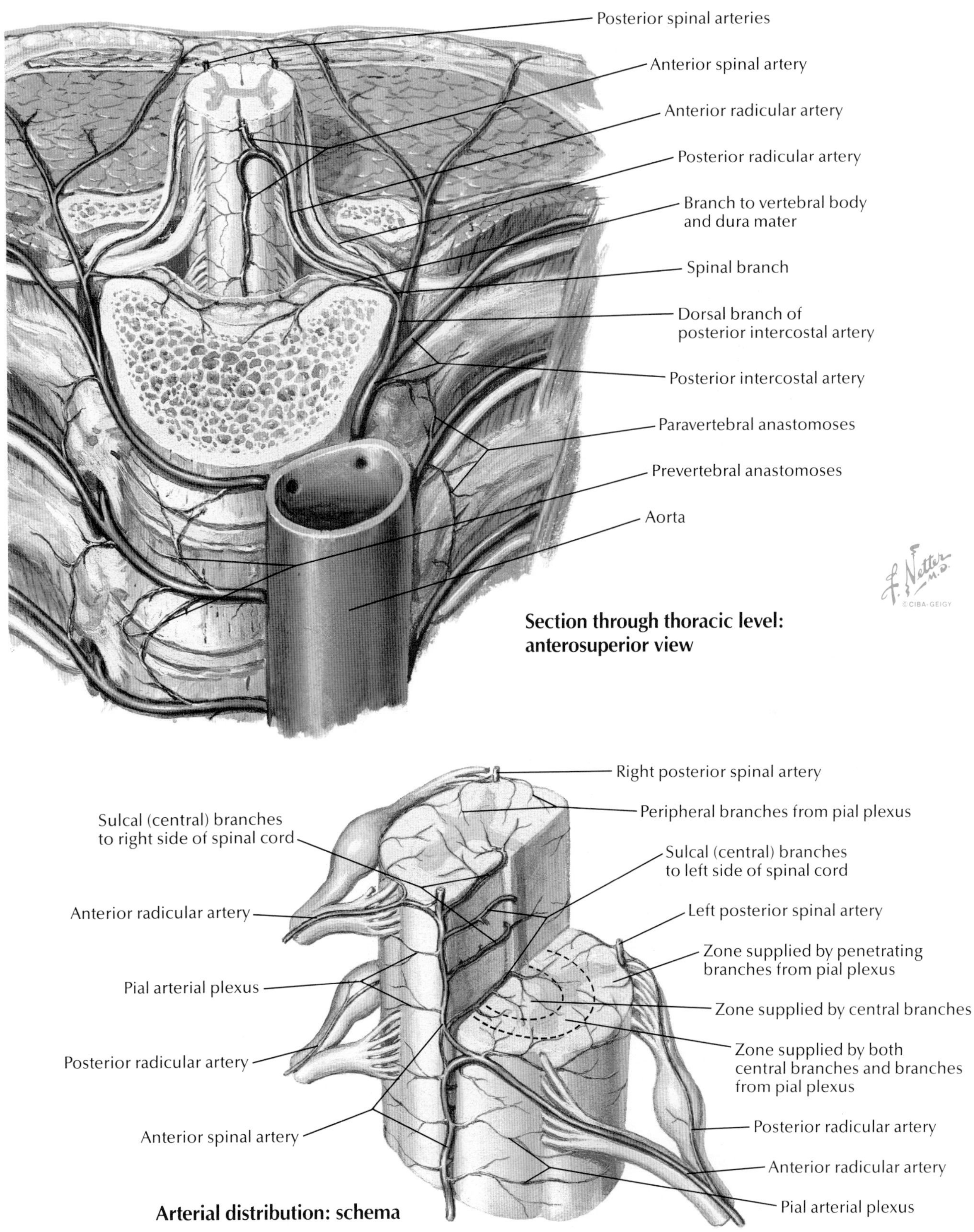

Posterior spinal arteries

Anterior spinal artery

Anterior radicular artery

Posterior radicular artery

Branch to vertebral body and dura mater

Spinal branch

Dorsal branch of posterior intercostal artery

Posterior intercostal artery

Paravertebral anastomoses

Prevertebral anastomoses

Aorta

Section through thoracic level: anterosuperior view

Right posterior spinal artery

Peripheral branches from pial plexus

Sulcal (central) branches to right side of spinal cord

Sulcal (central) branches to left side of spinal cord

Anterior radicular artery

Left posterior spinal artery

Zone supplied by penetrating branches from pial plexus

Pial arterial plexus

Zone supplied by central branches

Posterior radicular artery

Zone supplied by both central branches and branches from pial plexus

Posterior radicular artery

Anterior radicular artery

Anterior spinal artery

Pial arterial plexus

Arterial distribution: schema

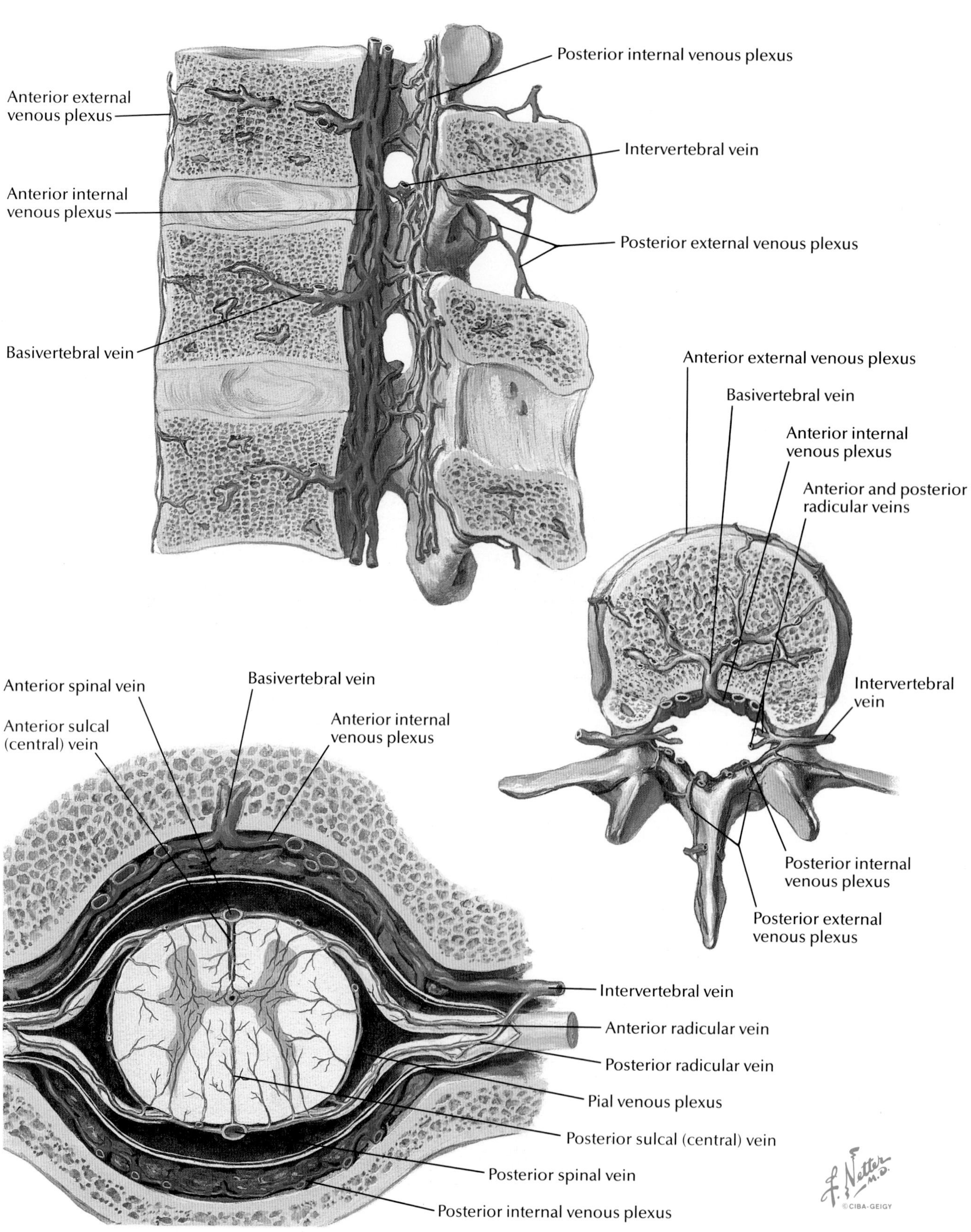

Anterior external venous plexus

Anterior internal venous plexus

Basivertebral vein

Posterior internal venous plexus

Intervertebral vein

Posterior external venous plexus

Anterior external venous plexus

Basivertebral vein

Anterior internal venous plexus

Anterior and posterior radicular veins

Intervertebral vein

Posterior internal venous plexus

Posterior external venous plexus

Anterior spinal vein

Anterior sulcal (central) vein

Basivertebral vein

Anterior internal venous plexus

Intervertebral vein

Anterior radicular vein

Posterior radicular vein

Pial venous plexus

Posterior sulcal (central) vein

Posterior spinal vein

Posterior internal venous plexus

PLATE 159

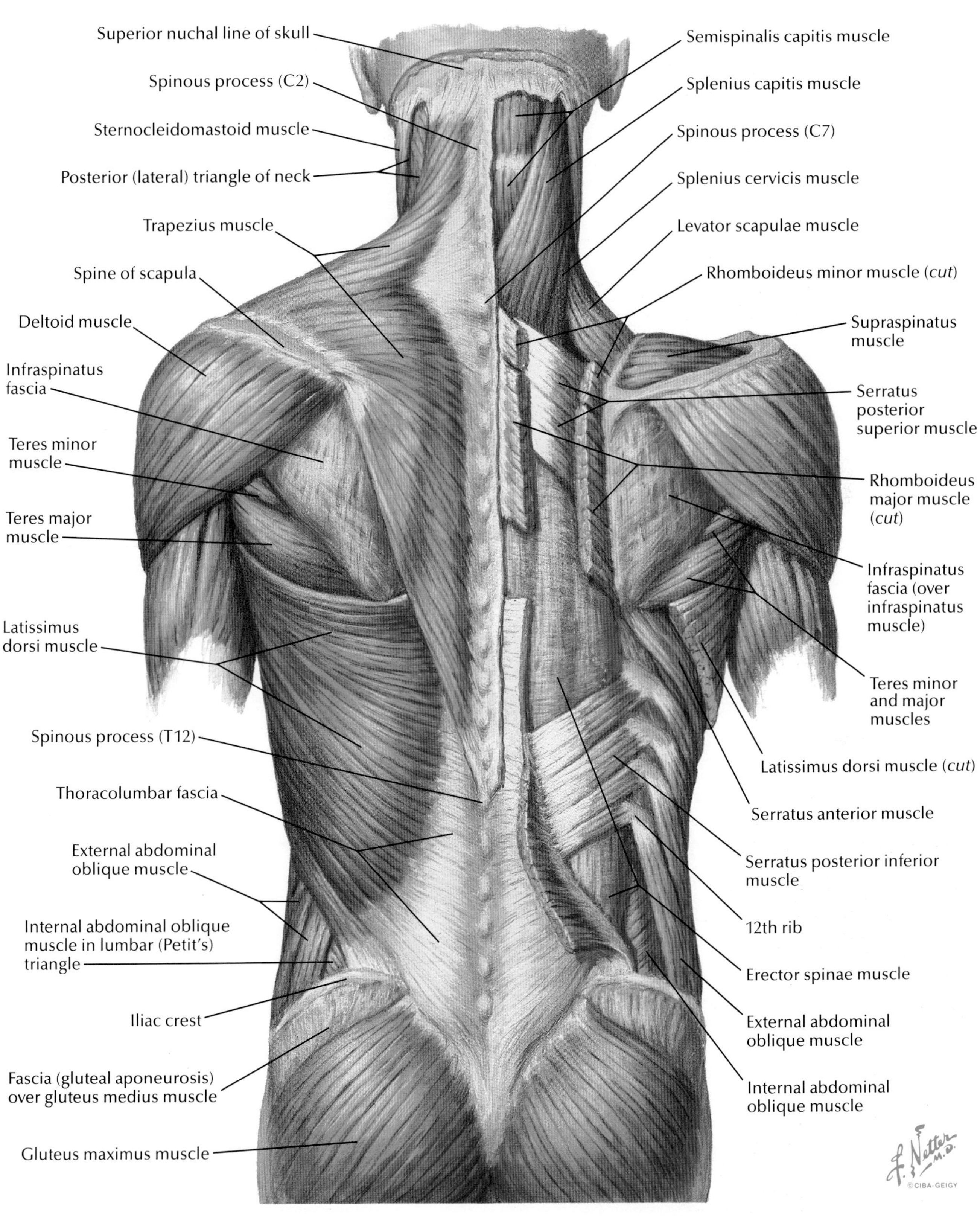

Superior nuchal line of skull

Spinous process (C2)

Sternocleidomastoid muscle

Posterior (lateral) triangle of neck

Trapezius muscle

Spine of scapula

Deltoid muscle

Infraspinatus fascia

Teres minor muscle

Teres major muscle

Latissimus dorsi muscle

Spinous process (T12)

Thoracolumbar fascia

External abdominal oblique muscle

Internal abdominal oblique muscle in lumbar (Petit's) triangle

Iliac crest

Fascia (gluteal aponeurosis) over gluteus medius muscle

Gluteus maximus muscle

Semispinalis capitis muscle

Splenius capitis muscle

Spinous process (C7)

Splenius cervicis muscle

Levator scapulae muscle

Rhomboideus minor muscle (cut)

Supraspinatus muscle

Serratus posterior superior muscle

Rhomboideus major muscle (cut)

Infraspinatus fascia (over infraspinatus muscle)

Teres minor and major muscles

Latissimus dorsi muscle (cut)

Serratus anterior muscle

Serratus posterior inferior muscle

12th rib

Erector spinae muscle

External abdominal oblique muscle

Internal abdominal oblique muscle

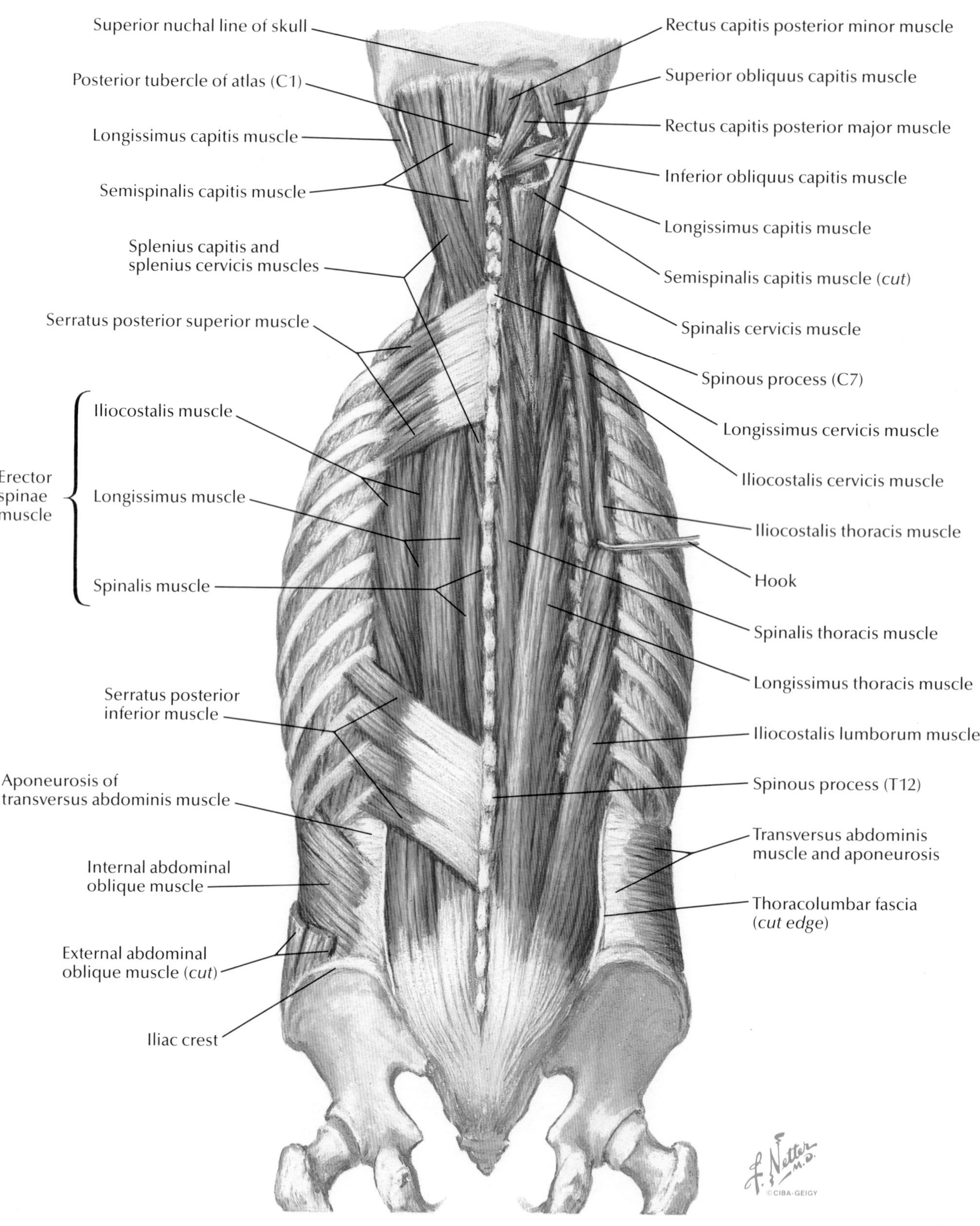

Superior nuchal line of skull

Posterior tubercle of atlas (C1)

Longissimus capitis muscle

Semispinalis capitis muscle

Splenius capitis and
splenius cervicis muscles

Serratus posterior superior muscle

Erector spinae muscle {
Iliocostalis muscle

Longissimus muscle

Spinalis muscle
}

Serratus posterior
inferior muscle

Aponeurosis of
transversus abdominis muscle

Internal abdominal
oblique muscle

External abdominal
oblique muscle (cut)

Iliac crest

Rectus capitis posterior minor muscle

Superior obliquus capitis muscle

Rectus capitis posterior major muscle

Inferior obliquus capitis muscle

Longissimus capitis muscle

Semispinalis capitis muscle (cut)

Spinalis cervicis muscle

Spinous process (C7)

Longissimus cervicis muscle

Iliocostalis cervicis muscle

Iliocostalis thoracis muscle

Hook

Spinalis thoracis muscle

Longissimus thoracis muscle

Iliocostalis lumborum muscle

Spinous process (T12)

Transversus abdominis
muscle and aponeurosis

Thoracolumbar fascia
(cut edge)

PLATE 161

BACK AND SPINAL CORD

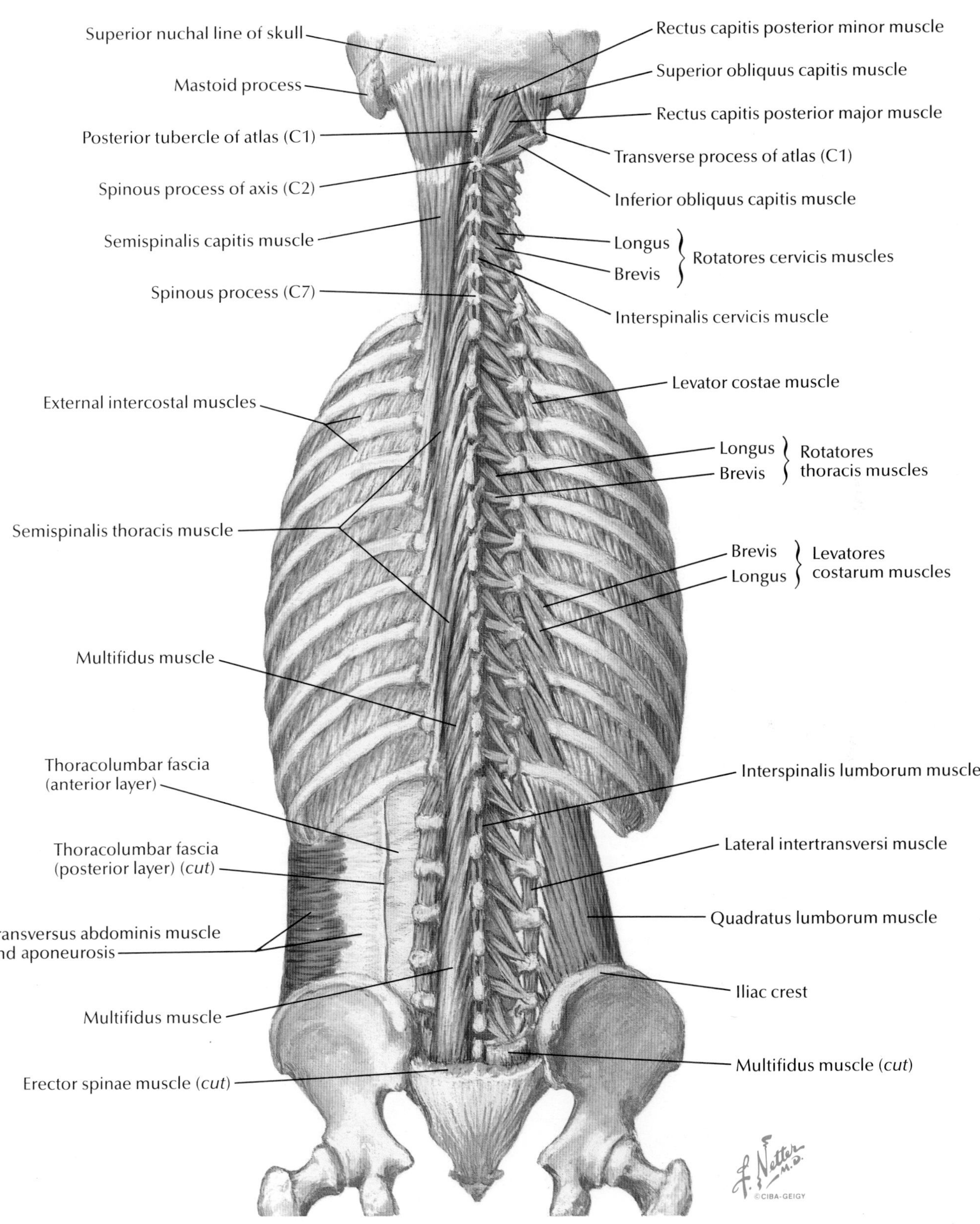

Superior nuchal line of skull

Mastoid process

Posterior tubercle of atlas (C1)

Spinous process of axis (C2)

Semispinalis capitis muscle

Spinous process (C7)

External intercostal muscles

Semispinalis thoracis muscle

Multifidus muscle

Thoracolumbar fascia (anterior layer)

Thoracolumbar fascia (posterior layer) (*cut*)

Transversus abdominis muscle and aponeurosis

Multifidus muscle

Erector spinae muscle (*cut*)

Rectus capitis posterior minor muscle

Superior obliquus capitis muscle

Rectus capitis posterior major muscle

Transverse process of atlas (C1)

Inferior obliquus capitis muscle

Longus
Brevis } Rotatores cervicis muscles

Interspinalis cervicis muscle

Levator costae muscle

Longus } Rotatores
Brevis } thoracis muscles

Brevis } Levatores
Longus } costarum muscles

Interspinalis lumborum muscle

Lateral intertransversi muscle

Quadratus lumborum muscle

Iliac crest

Multifidus muscle (*cut*)

Nerves of Back

SEE ALSO PLATES 166, 179, 237, 241

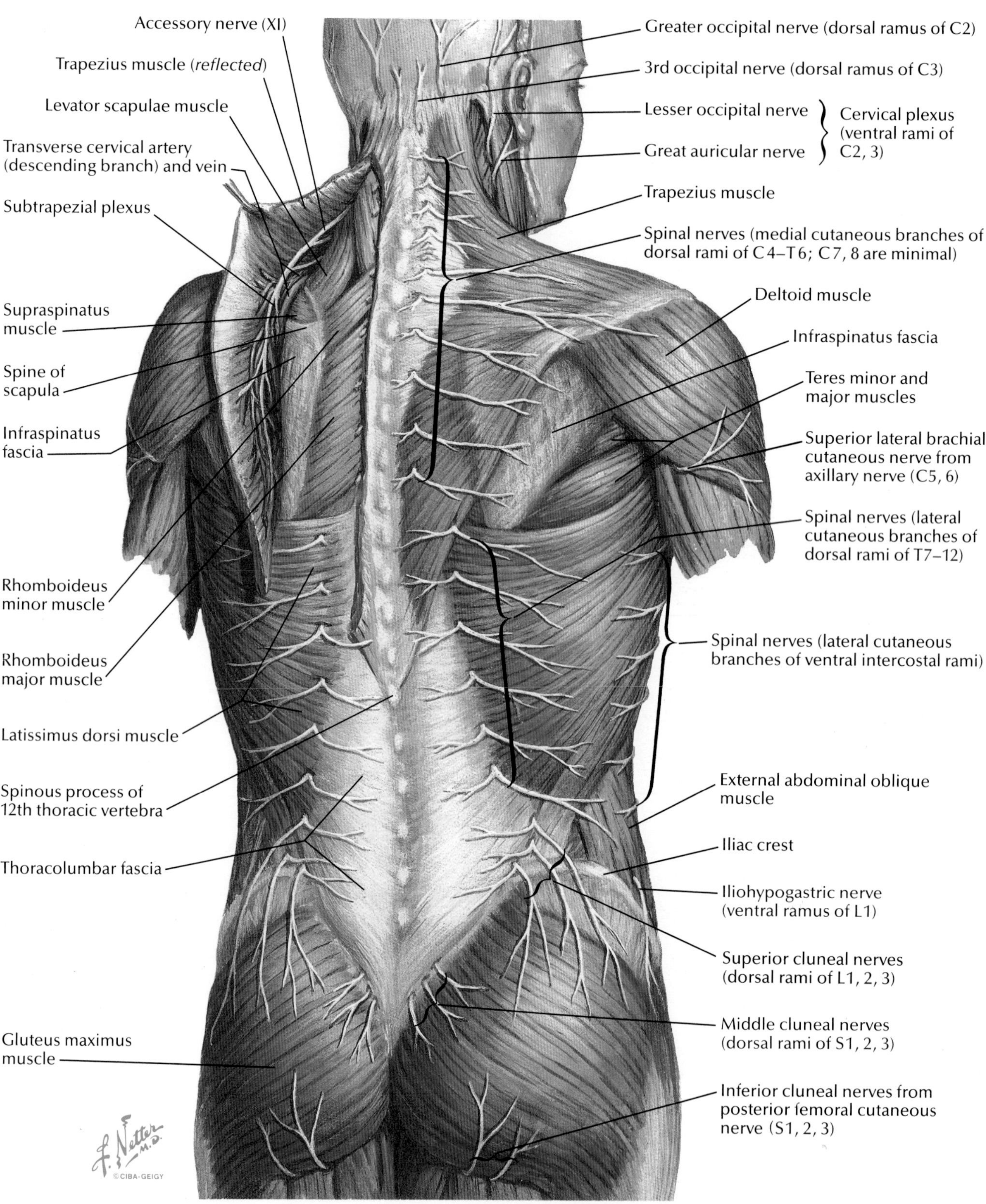

Accessory nerve (XI)

Trapezius muscle (*reflected*)

Levator scapulae muscle

Transverse cervical artery (descending branch) and vein

Subtrapezial plexus

Supraspinatus muscle

Spine of scapula

Infraspinatus fascia

Rhomboideus minor muscle

Rhomboideus major muscle

Latissimus dorsi muscle

Spinous process of 12th thoracic vertebra

Thoracolumbar fascia

Gluteus maximus muscle

Greater occipital nerve (dorsal ramus of C2)

3rd occipital nerve (dorsal ramus of C3)

Lesser occipital nerve }
Great auricular nerve } Cervical plexus (ventral rami of C2, 3)

Trapezius muscle

Spinal nerves (medial cutaneous branches of dorsal rami of C4–T6; C7, 8 are minimal)

Deltoid muscle

Infraspinatus fascia

Teres minor and major muscles

Superior lateral brachial cutaneous nerve from axillary nerve (C5, 6)

Spinal nerves (lateral cutaneous branches of dorsal rami of T7–12)

Spinal nerves (lateral cutaneous branches of ventral intercostal rami)

External abdominal oblique muscle

Iliac crest

Iliohypogastric nerve (ventral ramus of L1)

Superior cluneal nerves (dorsal rami of L1, 2, 3)

Middle cluneal nerves (dorsal rami of S1, 2, 3)

Inferior cluneal nerves from posterior femoral cutaneous nerve (S1, 2, 3)

PLATE 163

BACK AND SPINAL CORD

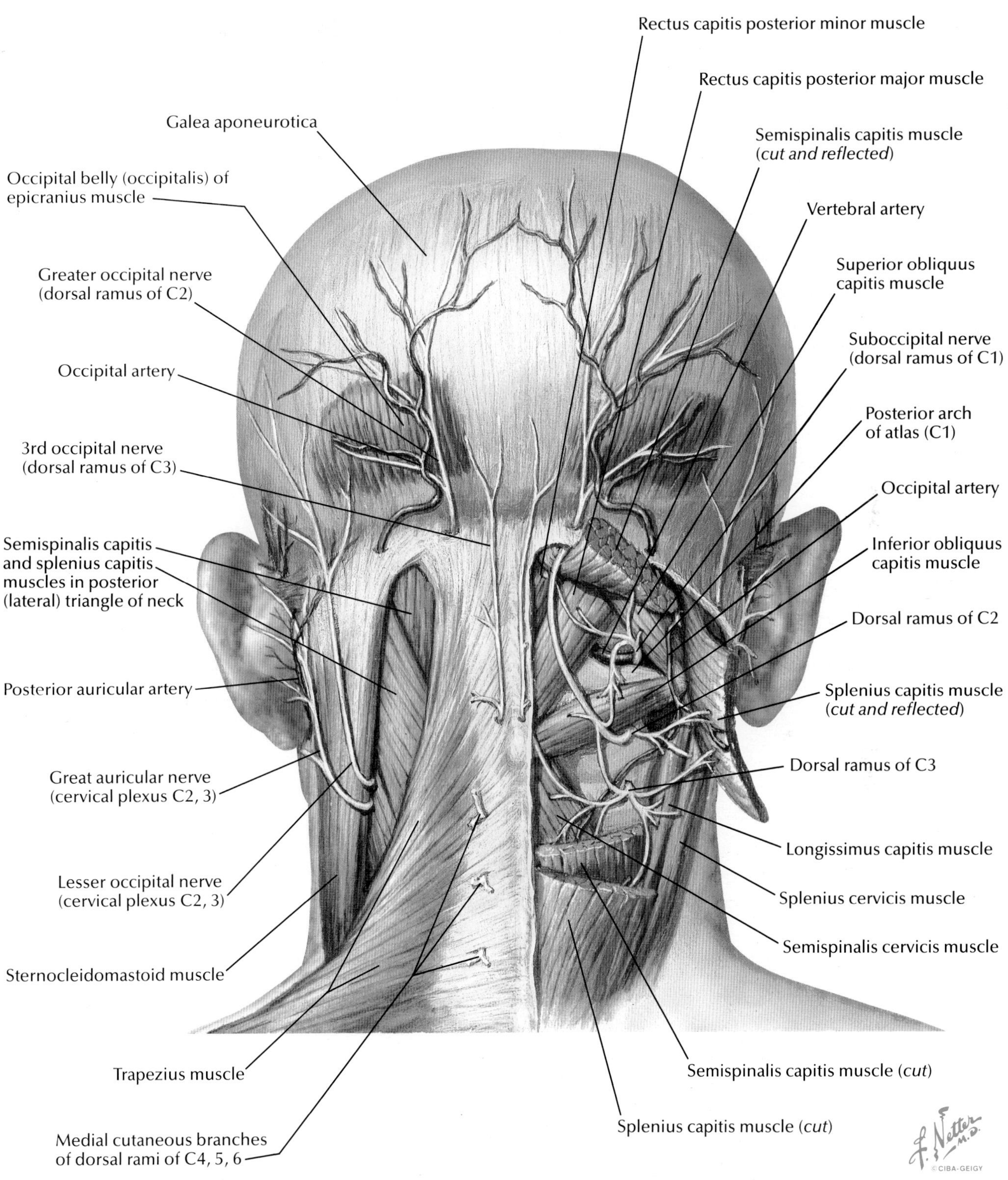

Rectus capitis posterior minor muscle

Rectus capitis posterior major muscle

Semispinalis capitis muscle
(*cut and reflected*)

Vertebral artery

Superior obliquus
capitis muscle

Suboccipital nerve
(dorsal ramus of C1)

Posterior arch
of atlas (C1)

Occipital artery

Inferior obliquus
capitis muscle

Dorsal ramus of C2

Splenius capitis muscle
(*cut and reflected*)

Dorsal ramus of C3

Longissimus capitis muscle

Splenius cervicis muscle

Semispinalis cervicis muscle

Semispinalis capitis muscle (*cut*)

Splenius capitis muscle (*cut*)

Galea aponeurotica

Occipital belly (occipitalis) of
epicranius muscle

Greater occipital nerve
(dorsal ramus of C2)

Occipital artery

3rd occipital nerve
(dorsal ramus of C3)

Semispinalis capitis
and splenius capitis
muscles in posterior
(lateral) triangle of neck

Posterior auricular artery

Great auricular nerve
(cervical plexus C2, 3)

Lesser occipital nerve
(cervical plexus C2, 3)

Sternocleidomastoid muscle

Trapezius muscle

Medial cutaneous branches
of dorsal rami of C4, 5, 6

MUSCLES AND NERVES

PLATE 164

Lumbar Region of Back: Cross Section

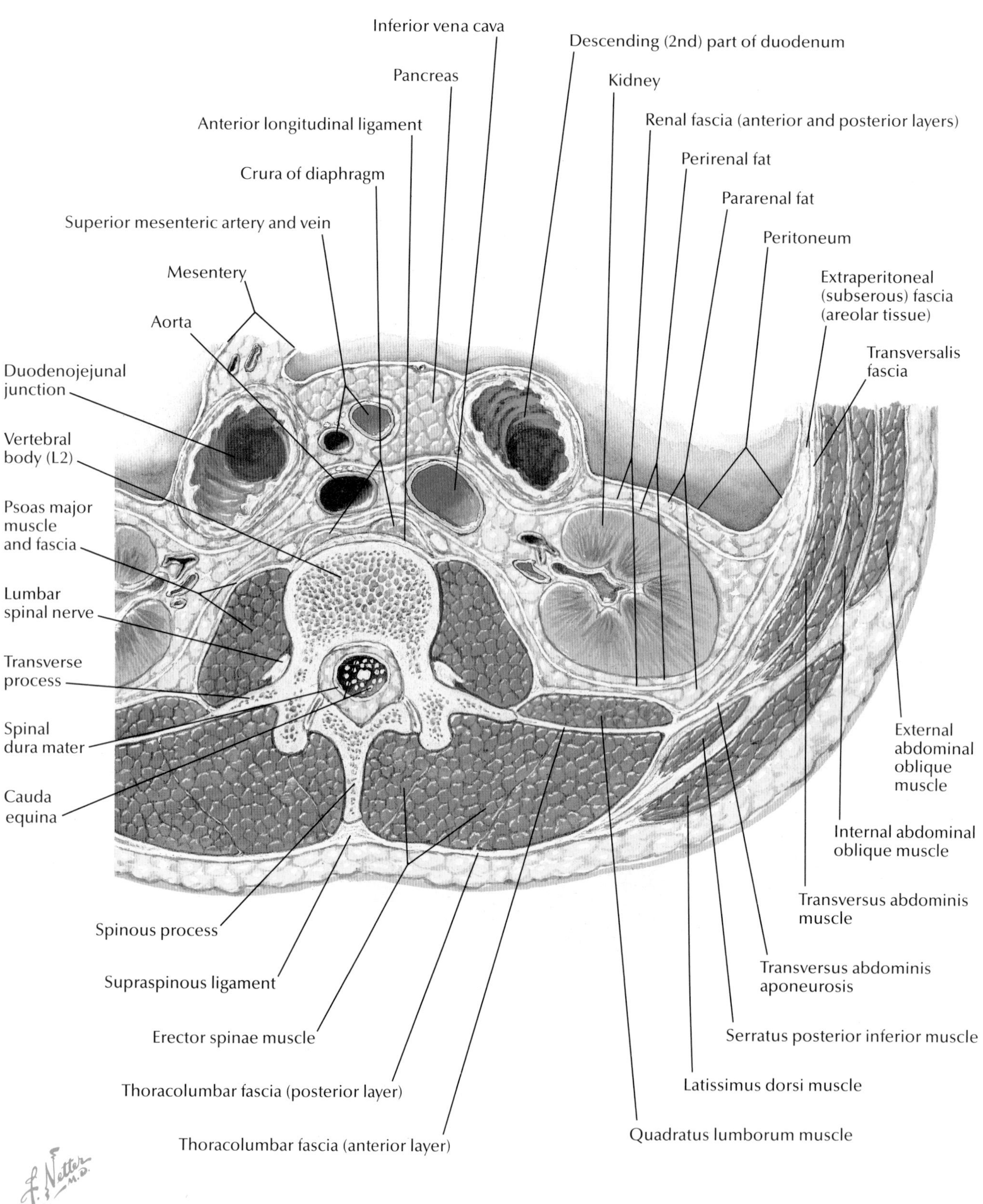

Inferior vena cava

Pancreas

Anterior longitudinal ligament

Crura of diaphragm

Superior mesenteric artery and vein

Mesentery

Aorta

Duodenojejunal junction

Vertebral body (L2)

Psoas major muscle and fascia

Lumbar spinal nerve

Transverse process

Spinal dura mater

Cauda equina

Descending (2nd) part of duodenum

Kidney

Renal fascia (anterior and posterior layers)

Perirenal fat

Pararenal fat

Peritoneum

Extraperitoneal (subserous) fascia (areolar tissue)

Transversalis fascia

External abdominal oblique muscle

Internal abdominal oblique muscle

Transversus abdominis muscle

Transversus abdominis aponeurosis

Serratus posterior inferior muscle

Latissimus dorsi muscle

Quadratus lumborum muscle

Spinous process

Supraspinous ligament

Erector spinae muscle

Thoracolumbar fascia (posterior layer)

Thoracolumbar fascia (anterior layer)

PLATE 165

BACK AND SPINAL CORD

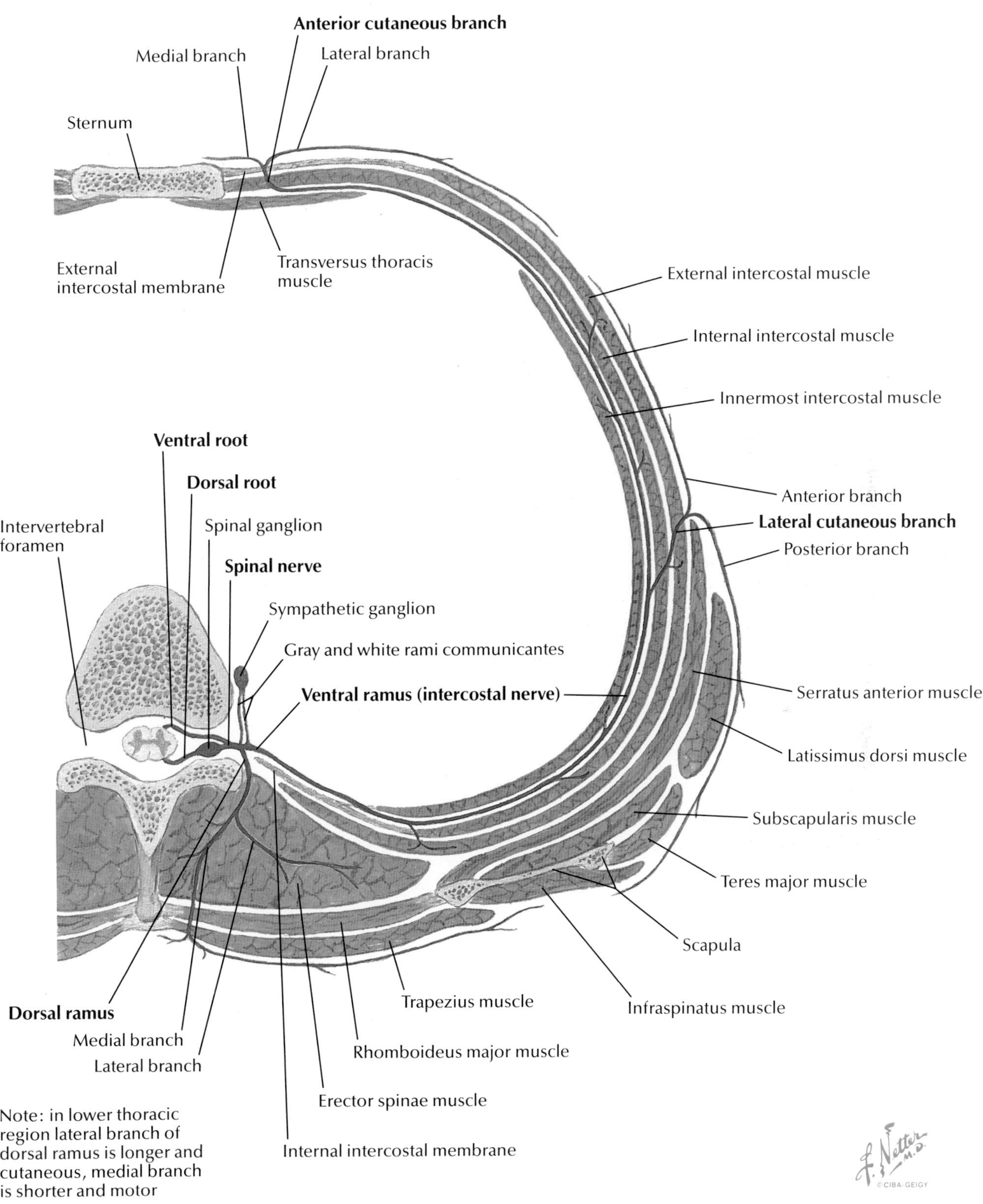

Anterior cutaneous branch

Lateral branch

Medial branch

Sternum

External intercostal membrane

Transversus thoracis muscle

External intercostal muscle

Internal intercostal muscle

Innermost intercostal muscle

Ventral root

Dorsal root

Spinal ganglion

Anterior branch

Lateral cutaneous branch

Posterior branch

Intervertebral foramen

Spinal nerve

Sympathetic ganglion

Gray and white rami communicantes

Ventral ramus (intercostal nerve)

Serratus anterior muscle

Latissimus dorsi muscle

Subscapularis muscle

Teres major muscle

Scapula

Infraspinatus muscle

Dorsal ramus

Medial branch

Lateral branch

Trapezius muscle

Rhomboideus major muscle

Erector spinae muscle

Internal intercostal membrane

Note: in lower thoracic region lateral branch of dorsal ramus is longer and cutaneous, medial branch is shorter and motor

Section III

THORAX

HEART
Plates 200—217

MEDIASTINUM
Plates 218—230

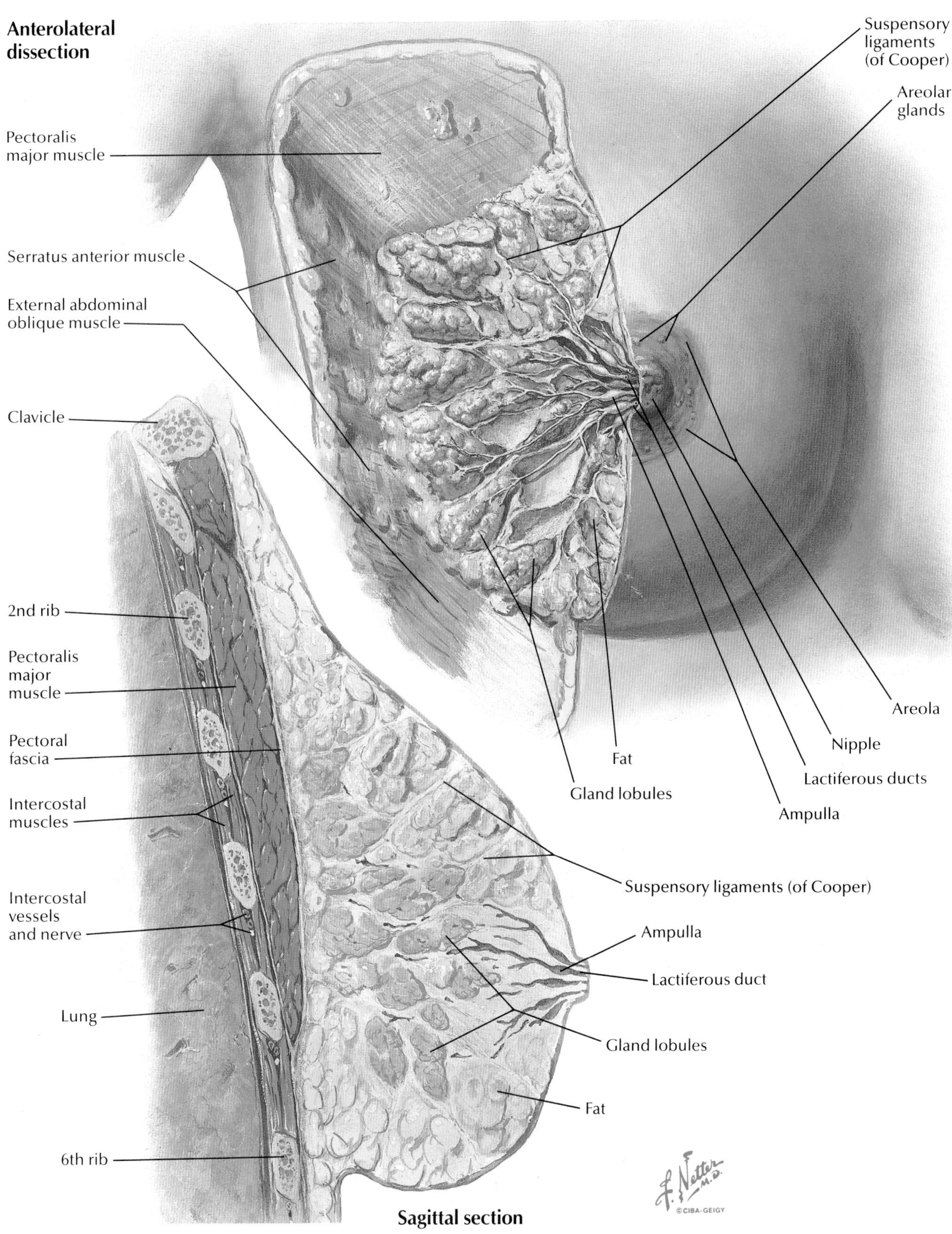

Anterolateral dissection

Pectoralis major muscle

Serratus anterior muscle

External abdominal oblique muscle

Clavicle

2nd rib

Pectoralis major muscle

Pectoral fascia

Intercostal muscles

Intercostal vessels and nerve

Lung

6th rib

Suspensory ligaments (of Cooper)

Areolar glands

Areola

Nipple

Lactiferous ducts

Ampulla

Fat

Gland lobules

Suspensory ligaments (of Cooper)

Ampulla

Lactiferous duct

Gland lobules

Fat

Sagittal section

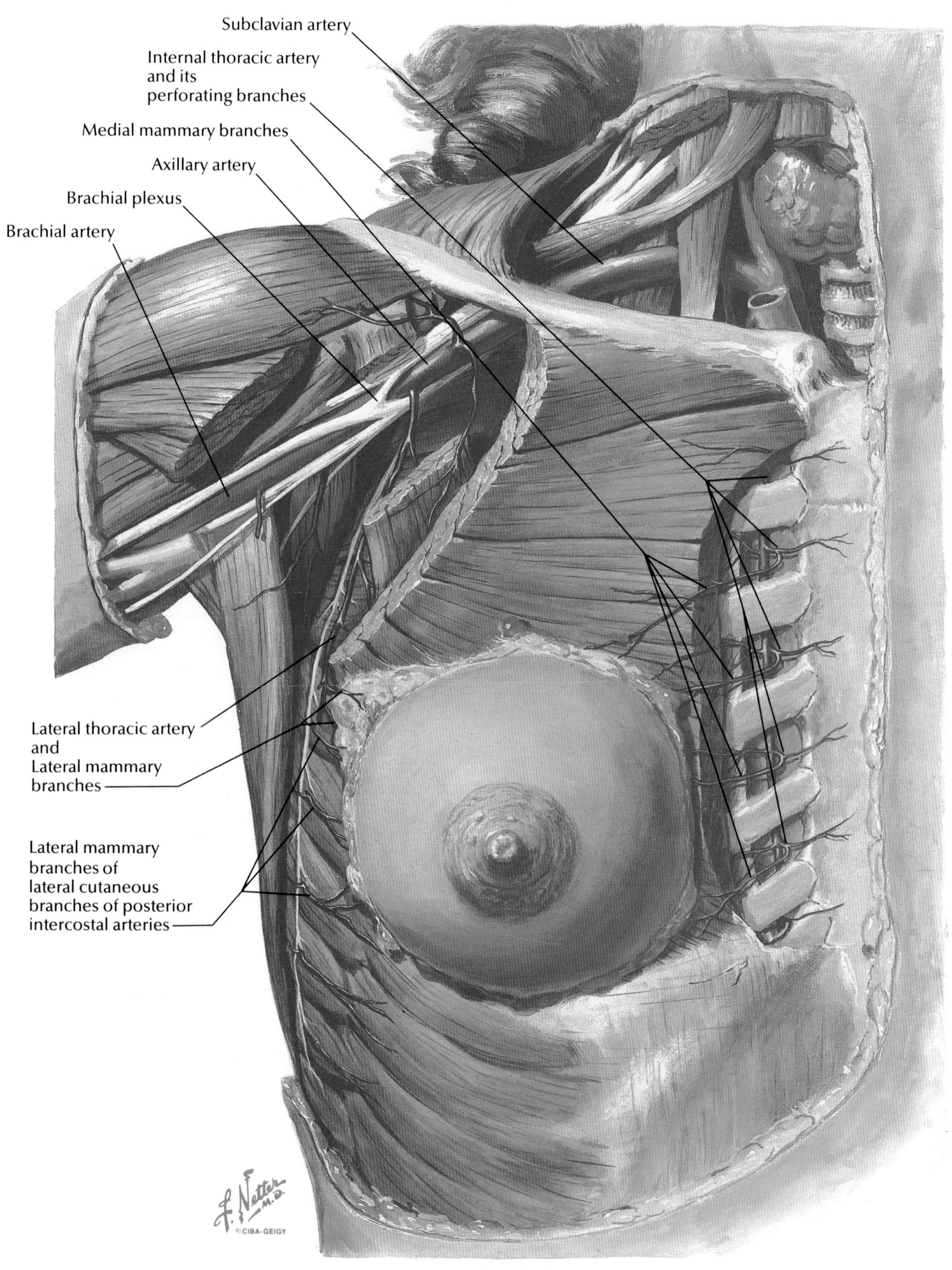

Subclavian artery

Internal thoracic artery
and its
perforating branches

Medial mammary branches

Axillary artery

Brachial plexus

Brachial artery

Lateral thoracic artery
and
Lateral mammary
branches

Lateral mammary
branches of
lateral cutaneous
branches of posterior
intercostal arteries

PLATE 168

THORAX

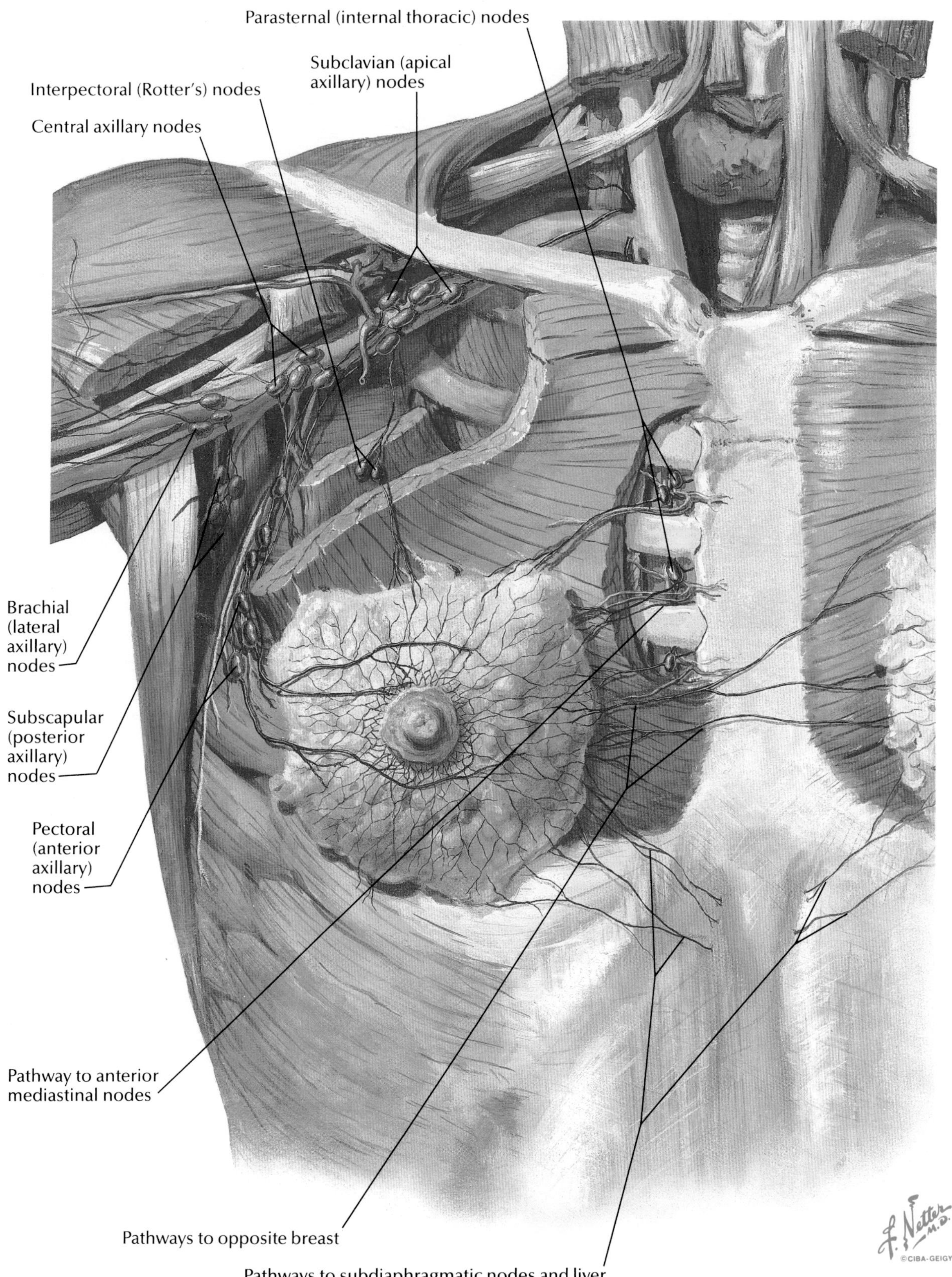

Parasternal (internal thoracic) nodes

Subclavian (apical axillary) nodes

Interpectoral (Rotter's) nodes

Central axillary nodes

Brachial (lateral axillary) nodes

Subscapular (posterior axillary) nodes

Pectoral (anterior axillary) nodes

Pathway to anterior mediastinal nodes

Pathways to opposite breast

Pathways to subdiaphragmatic nodes and liver

Bony Framework of Thorax

SEE ALSO PLATE 231

Anterior view

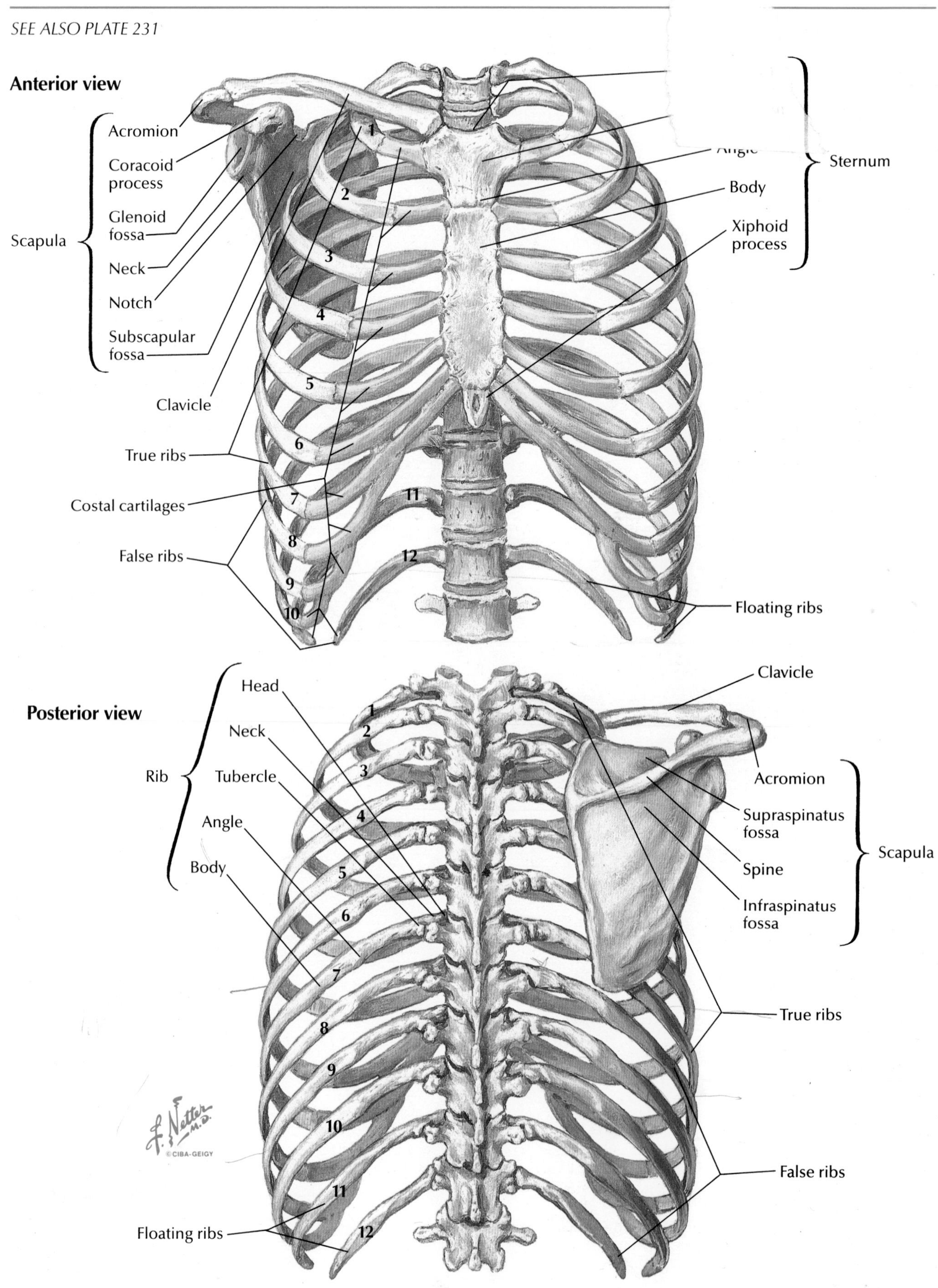

Scapula
- Acromion
- Coracoid process
- Glenoid fossa
- Neck
- Notch
- Subscapular fossa

Clavicle

True ribs

Costal cartilages

False ribs

Angle

Body

Xiphoid process

Sternum

Floating ribs

Posterior view

Rib
- Head
- Neck
- Tubercle
- Angle
- Body

Clavicle

Acromion

Supraspinatus fossa

Spine

Infraspinatus fossa

Scapula

True ribs

False ribs

Floating ribs

PLATE 170

THORAX

Ribs and Sternocostal Joints

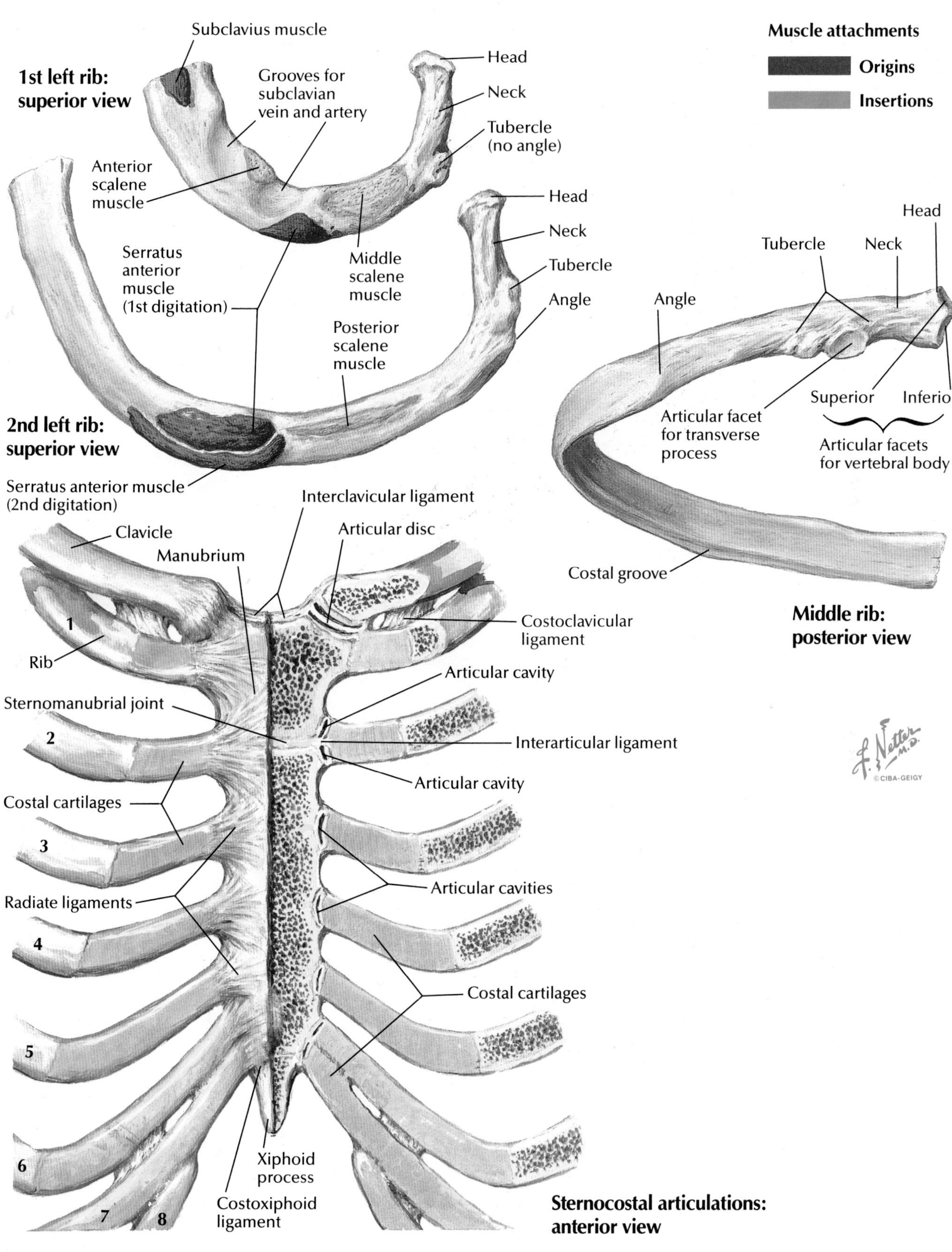

Muscle attachments

- ■ Origins
- ■ Insertions

1st left rib: superior view

- Subclavius muscle
- Grooves for subclavian vein and artery
- Head
- Neck
- Tubercle (no angle)
- Anterior scalene muscle
- Serratus anterior muscle (1st digitation)
- Middle scalene muscle
- Posterior scalene muscle
- Head
- Neck
- Tubercle
- Angle

2nd left rib: superior view

- Serratus anterior muscle (2nd digitation)

Middle rib: posterior view

- Tubercle
- Neck
- Head
- Angle
- Articular facet for transverse process
- Superior
- Inferior
- Articular facets for vertebral body
- Costal groove

Sternocostal articulations: anterior view

- Clavicle
- Manubrium
- Interclavicular ligament
- Articular disc
- 1
- Rib
- Costoclavicular ligament
- Sternomanubrial joint
- 2
- Articular cavity
- Interarticular ligament
- Articular cavity
- Costal cartilages
- 3
- Radiate ligaments
- 4
- Articular cavities
- Costal cartilages
- 5
- 6
- 7
- 8
- Xiphoid process
- Costoxiphoid ligament

BODY WALL

PLATE 171

Costovertebral Joints

SEE ALSO PLATE 143

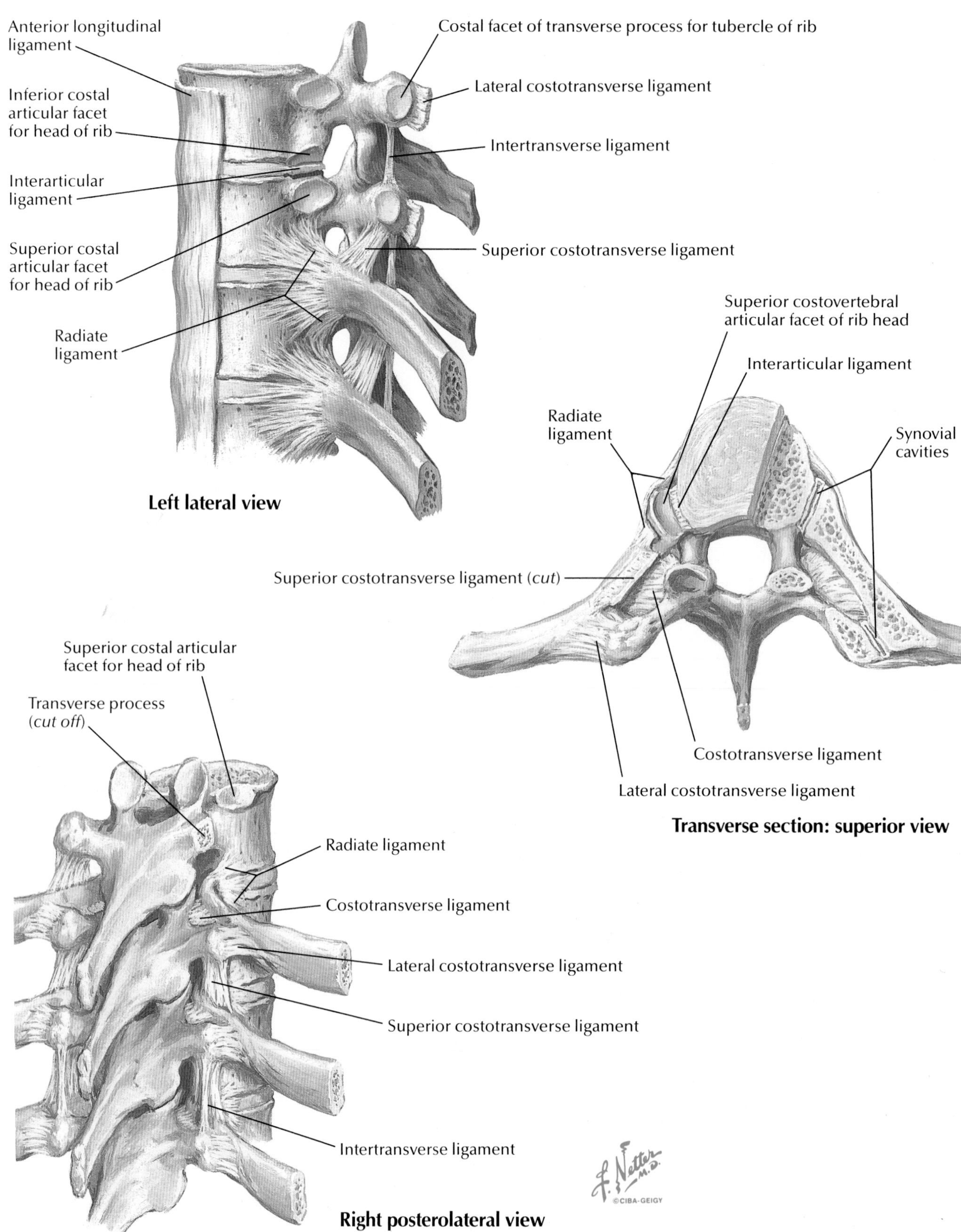

Anterior longitudinal ligament

Inferior costal articular facet for head of rib

Interarticular ligament

Superior costal articular facet for head of rib

Radiate ligament

Costal facet of transverse process for tubercle of rib

Lateral costotransverse ligament

Intertransverse ligament

Superior costotransverse ligament

Left lateral view

Superior costovertebral articular facet of rib head

Interarticular ligament

Radiate ligament

Synovial cavities

Superior costotransverse ligament (*cut*)

Costotransverse ligament

Lateral costotransverse ligament

Transverse section: superior view

Superior costal articular facet for head of rib

Transverse process (*cut off*)

Radiate ligament

Costotransverse ligament

Lateral costotransverse ligament

Superior costotransverse ligament

Intertransverse ligament

Right posterolateral view

PLATE 172

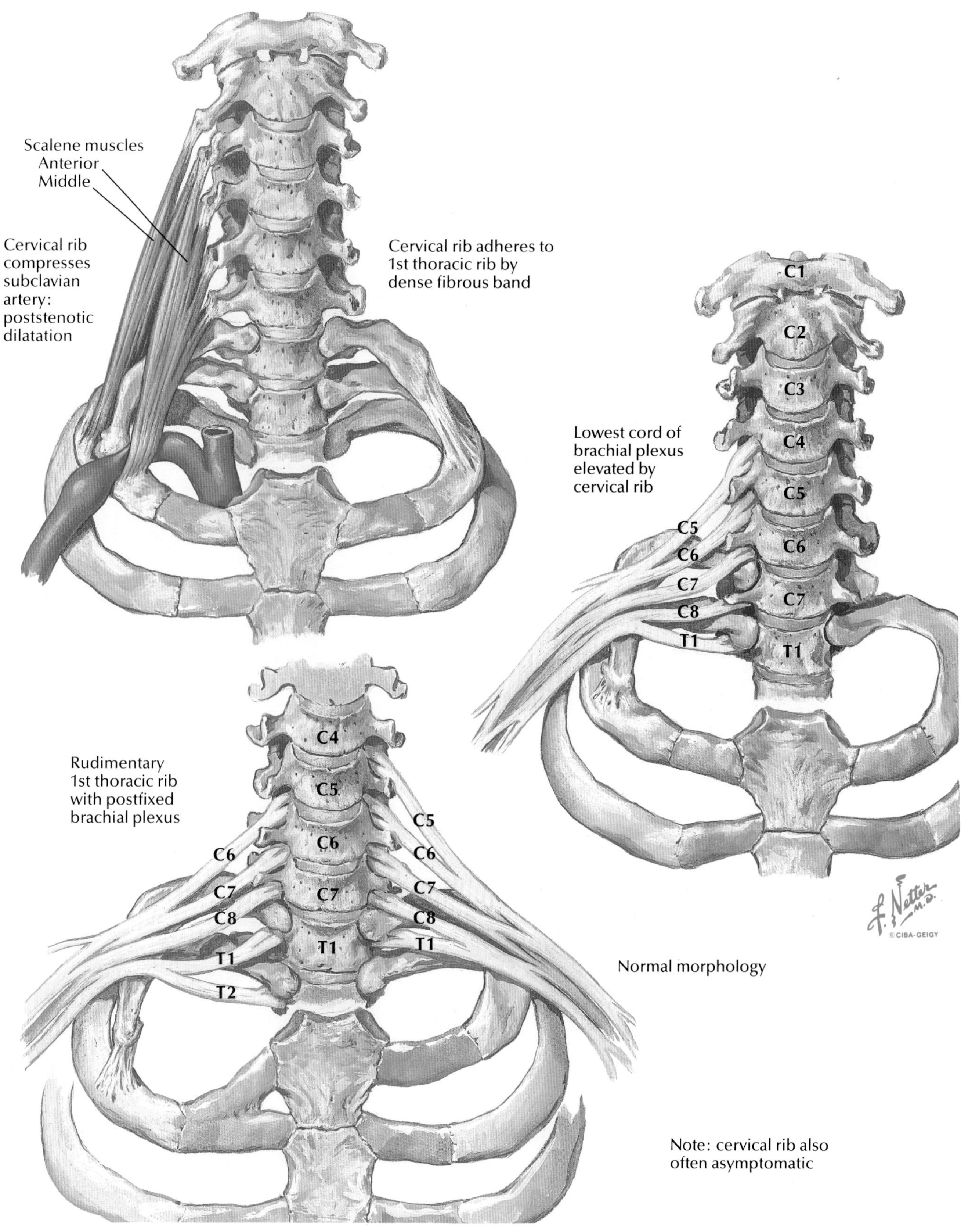

Scalene muscles
Anterior
Middle

Cervical rib
compresses
subclavian
artery:
poststenotic
dilatation

Cervical rib adheres to
1st thoracic rib by
dense fibrous band

Lowest cord of
brachial plexus
elevated by
cervical rib

C1
C2
C3
C4
C5
C6
C7
T1

C5
C6
C7
C8
T1

Rudimentary
1st thoracic rib
with postfixed
brachial plexus

C4
C5
C6
C7
T1

C6
C7
C8
T1
T2

C5
C6
C7
C8
T1

Normal morphology

Note: cervical rib also
often asymptomatic

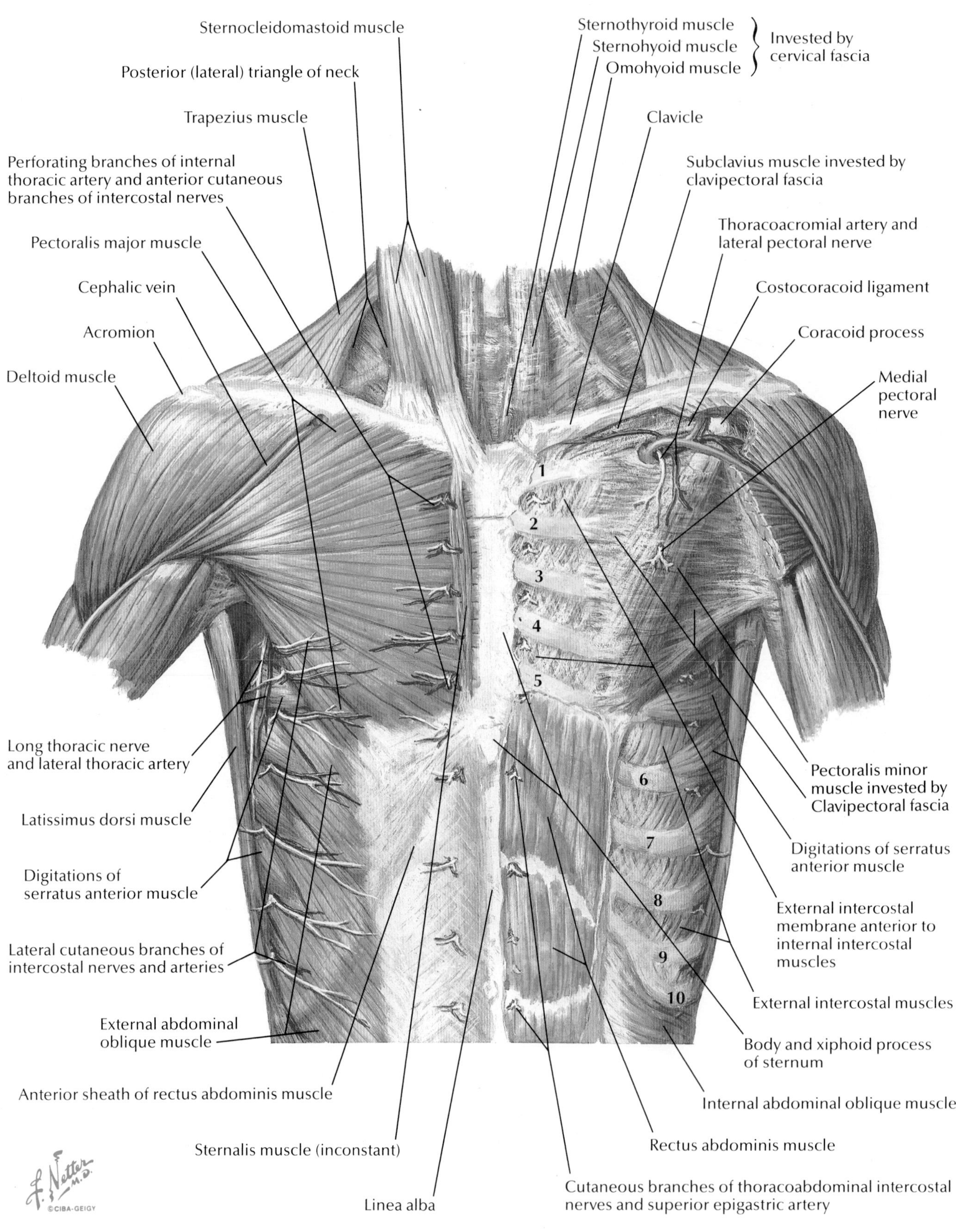

Sternocleidomastoid muscle

Posterior (lateral) triangle of neck

Trapezius muscle

Perforating branches of internal
thoracic artery and anterior cutaneous
branches of intercostal nerves

Pectoralis major muscle

Cephalic vein

Acromion

Deltoid muscle

Sternothyroid muscle
Sternohyoid muscle } Invested by
Omohyoid muscle } cervical fascia

Clavicle

Subclavius muscle invested by
clavipectoral fascia

Thoracoacromial artery and
lateral pectoral nerve

Costocoracoid ligament

Coracoid process

Medial
pectoral
nerve

Long thoracic nerve
and lateral thoracic artery

Latissimus dorsi muscle

Digitations of
serratus anterior muscle

Lateral cutaneous branches of
intercostal nerves and arteries

External abdominal
oblique muscle

Anterior sheath of rectus abdominis muscle

Sternalis muscle (inconstant)

Linea alba

Pectoralis minor
muscle invested by
Clavipectoral fascia

Digitations of serratus
anterior muscle

External intercostal
membrane anterior to
internal intercostal
muscles

External intercostal muscles

Body and xiphoid process
of sternum

Internal abdominal oblique muscle

Rectus abdominis muscle

Cutaneous branches of thoracoabdominal intercostal
nerves and superior epigastric artery

PLATE 174

THORAX

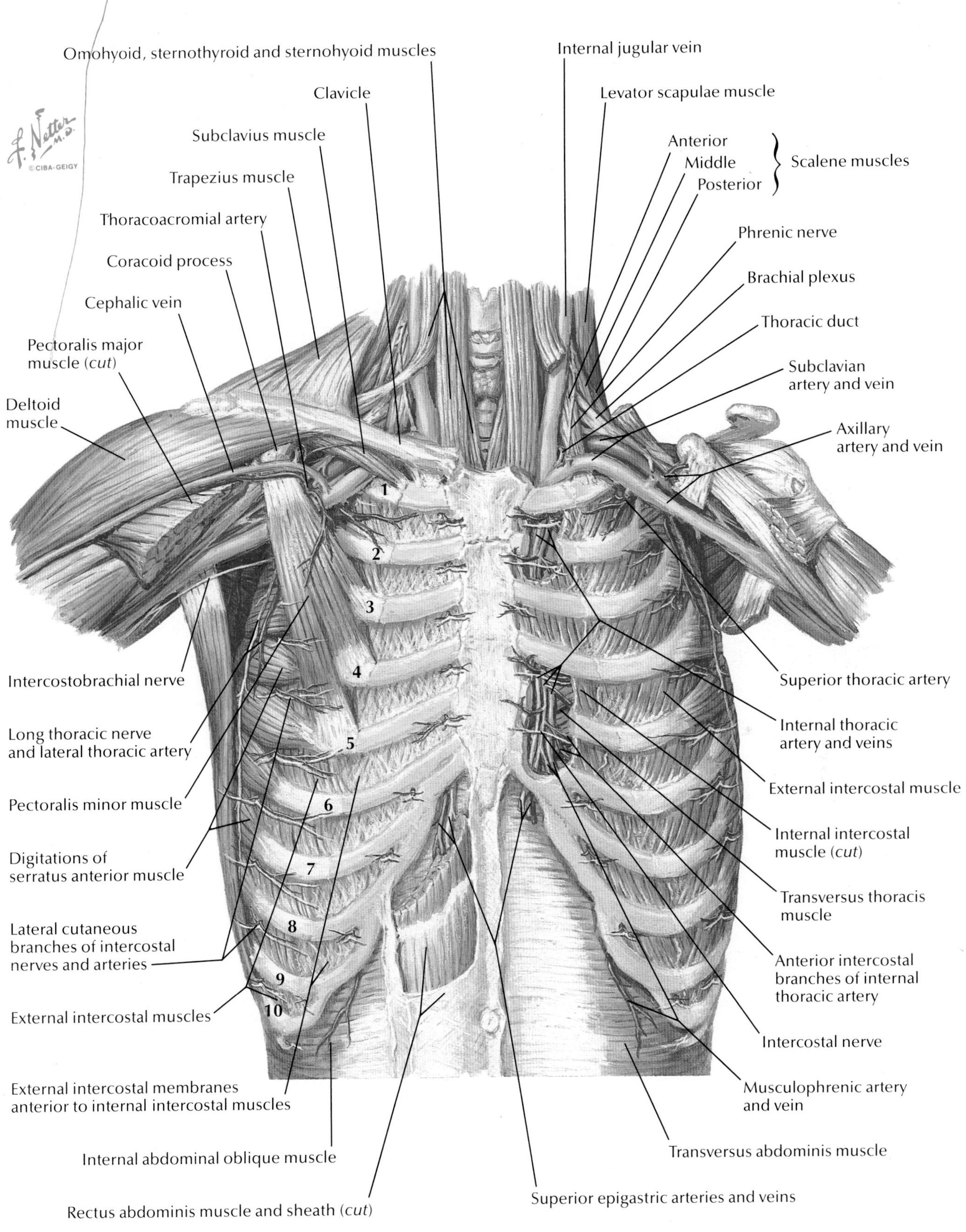

Omohyoid, sternothyroid and sternohyoid muscles

Clavicle

Subclavius muscle

Trapezius muscle

Thoracoacromial artery

Coracoid process

Cephalic vein

Pectoralis major muscle (*cut*)

Deltoid muscle

Internal jugular vein

Levator scapulae muscle

Anterior
Middle
Posterior } Scalene muscles

Phrenic nerve

Brachial plexus

Thoracic duct

Subclavian artery and vein

Axillary artery and vein

Superior thoracic artery

Internal thoracic artery and veins

External intercostal muscle

Internal intercostal muscle (*cut*)

Transversus thoracis muscle

Anterior intercostal branches of internal thoracic artery

Intercostal nerve

Musculophrenic artery and vein

Transversus abdominis muscle

Superior epigastric arteries and veins

Intercostobrachial nerve

Long thoracic nerve and lateral thoracic artery

Pectoralis minor muscle

Digitations of serratus anterior muscle

Lateral cutaneous branches of intercostal nerves and arteries

External intercostal muscles

External intercostal membranes anterior to internal intercostal muscles

Internal abdominal oblique muscle

Rectus abdominis muscle and sheath (*cut*)

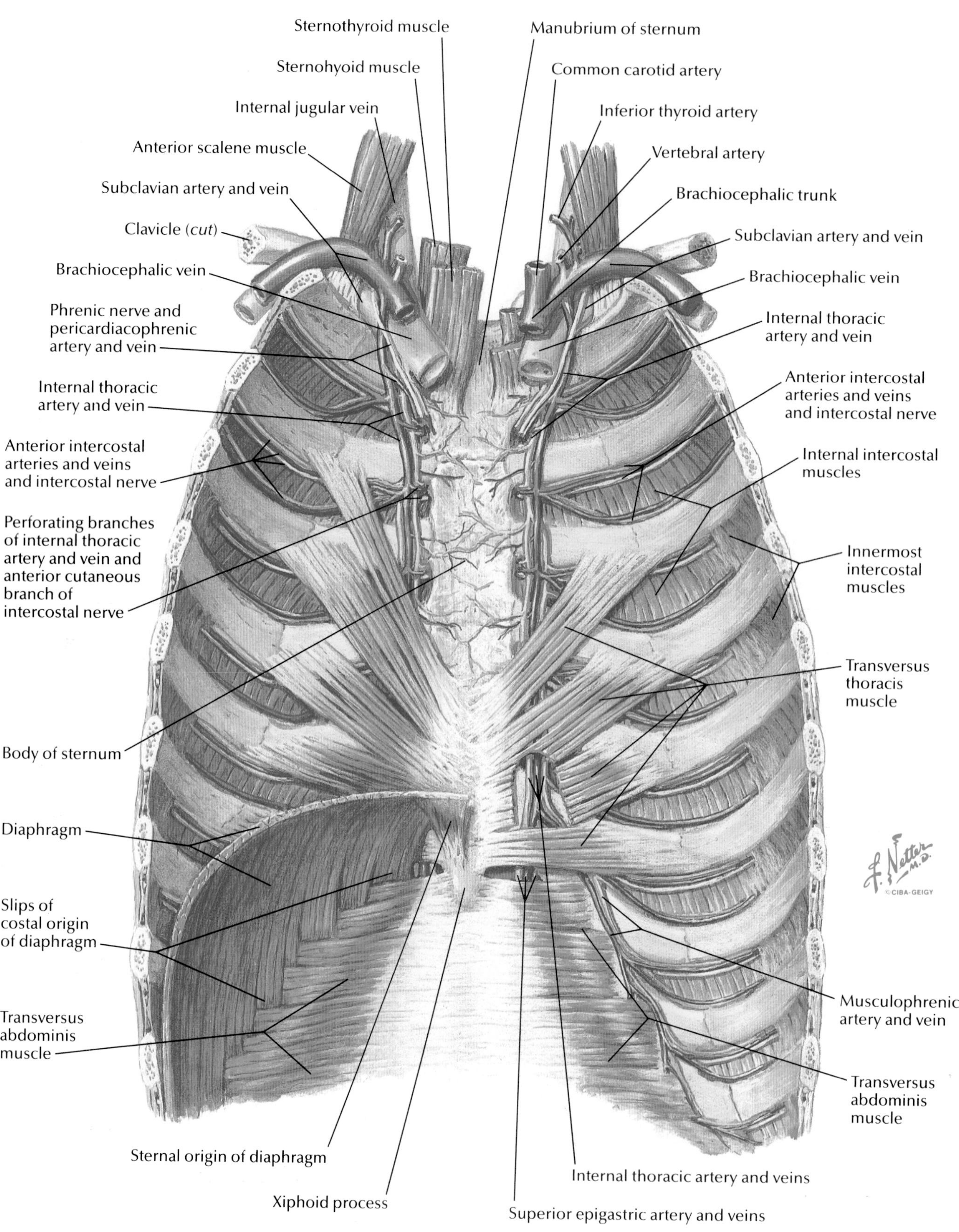

Sternothyroid muscle

Sternohyoid muscle

Internal jugular vein

Anterior scalene muscle

Subclavian artery and vein

Clavicle (cut)

Brachiocephalic vein

Phrenic nerve and pericardiacophrenic artery and vein

Internal thoracic artery and vein

Anterior intercostal arteries and veins and intercostal nerve

Perforating branches of internal thoracic artery and vein and anterior cutaneous branch of intercostal nerve

Body of sternum

Diaphragm

Slips of costal origin of diaphragm

Transversus abdominis muscle

Manubrium of sternum

Common carotid artery

Inferior thyroid artery

Vertebral artery

Brachiocephalic trunk

Subclavian artery and vein

Brachiocephalic vein

Internal thoracic artery and vein

Anterior intercostal arteries and veins and intercostal nerve

Internal intercostal muscles

Innermost intercostal muscles

Transversus thoracis muscle

Musculophrenic artery and vein

Transversus abdominis muscle

Sternal origin of diaphragm

Xiphoid process

Internal thoracic artery and veins

Superior epigastric artery and veins

PLATE 176

THORAX

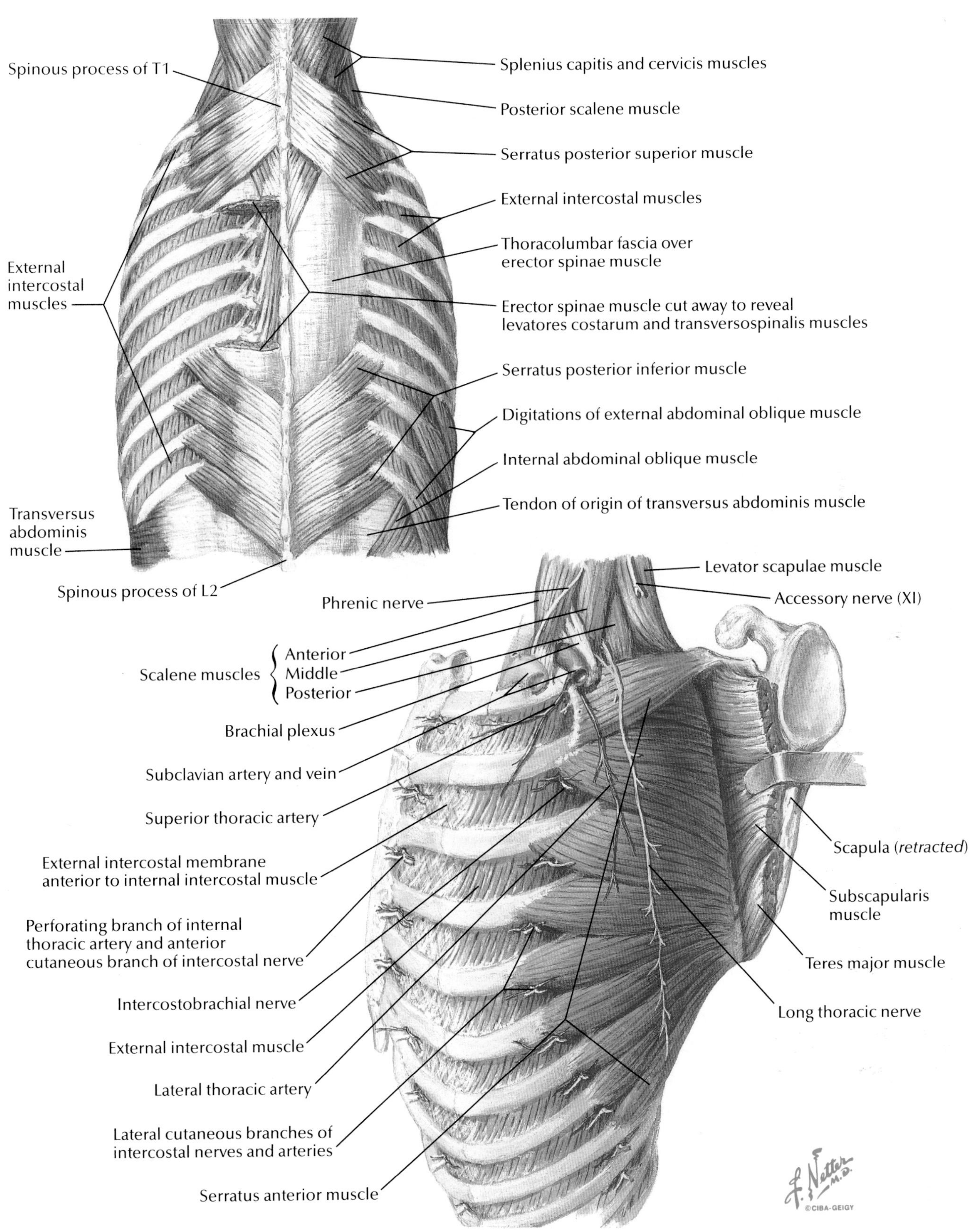

Spinous process of T1

Splenius capitis and cervicis muscles

Posterior scalene muscle

Serratus posterior superior muscle

External intercostal muscles

Thoracolumbar fascia over erector spinae muscle

External intercostal muscles

Erector spinae muscle cut away to reveal levatores costarum and transversospinalis muscles

Serratus posterior inferior muscle

Digitations of external abdominal oblique muscle

Internal abdominal oblique muscle

Transversus abdominis muscle

Tendon of origin of transversus abdominis muscle

Spinous process of L2

Levator scapulae muscle

Phrenic nerve

Accessory nerve (XI)

Scalene muscles { Anterior / Middle / Posterior

Brachial plexus

Subclavian artery and vein

Superior thoracic artery

Scapula (*retracted*)

External intercostal membrane anterior to internal intercostal muscle

Subscapularis muscle

Perforating branch of internal thoracic artery and anterior cutaneous branch of intercostal nerve

Teres major muscle

Intercostobrachial nerve

Long thoracic nerve

External intercostal muscle

Lateral thoracic artery

Lateral cutaneous branches of intercostal nerves and arteries

Serratus anterior muscle

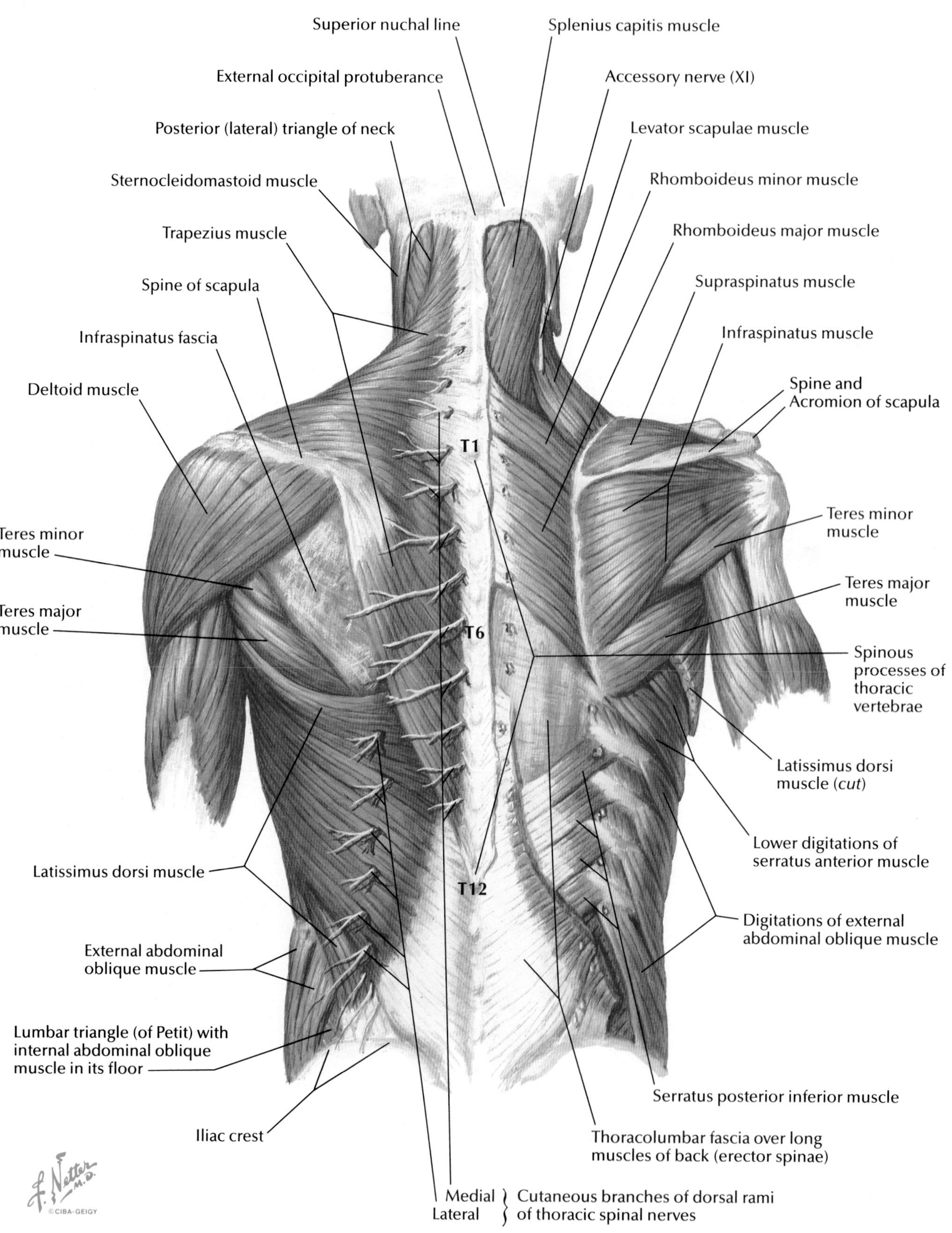

Superior nuchal line

Splenius capitis muscle

External occipital protuberance

Accessory nerve (XI)

Posterior (lateral) triangle of neck

Levator scapulae muscle

Sternocleidomastoid muscle

Rhomboideus minor muscle

Trapezius muscle

Rhomboideus major muscle

Spine of scapula

Supraspinatus muscle

Infraspinatus fascia

Infraspinatus muscle

Deltoid muscle

Spine and Acromion of scapula

T1

Teres minor muscle

Teres minor muscle

Teres major muscle

T6

Teres major muscle

Spinous processes of thoracic vertebrae

Latissimus dorsi muscle (cut)

Lower digitations of serratus anterior muscle

Latissimus dorsi muscle

T12

Digitations of external abdominal oblique muscle

External abdominal oblique muscle

Lumbar triangle (of Petit) with internal abdominal oblique muscle in its floor

Serratus posterior inferior muscle

Iliac crest

Thoracolumbar fascia over long muscles of back (erector spinae)

Medial } Lateral } Cutaneous branches of dorsal rami of thoracic spinal nerves

PLATE 178

THORAX

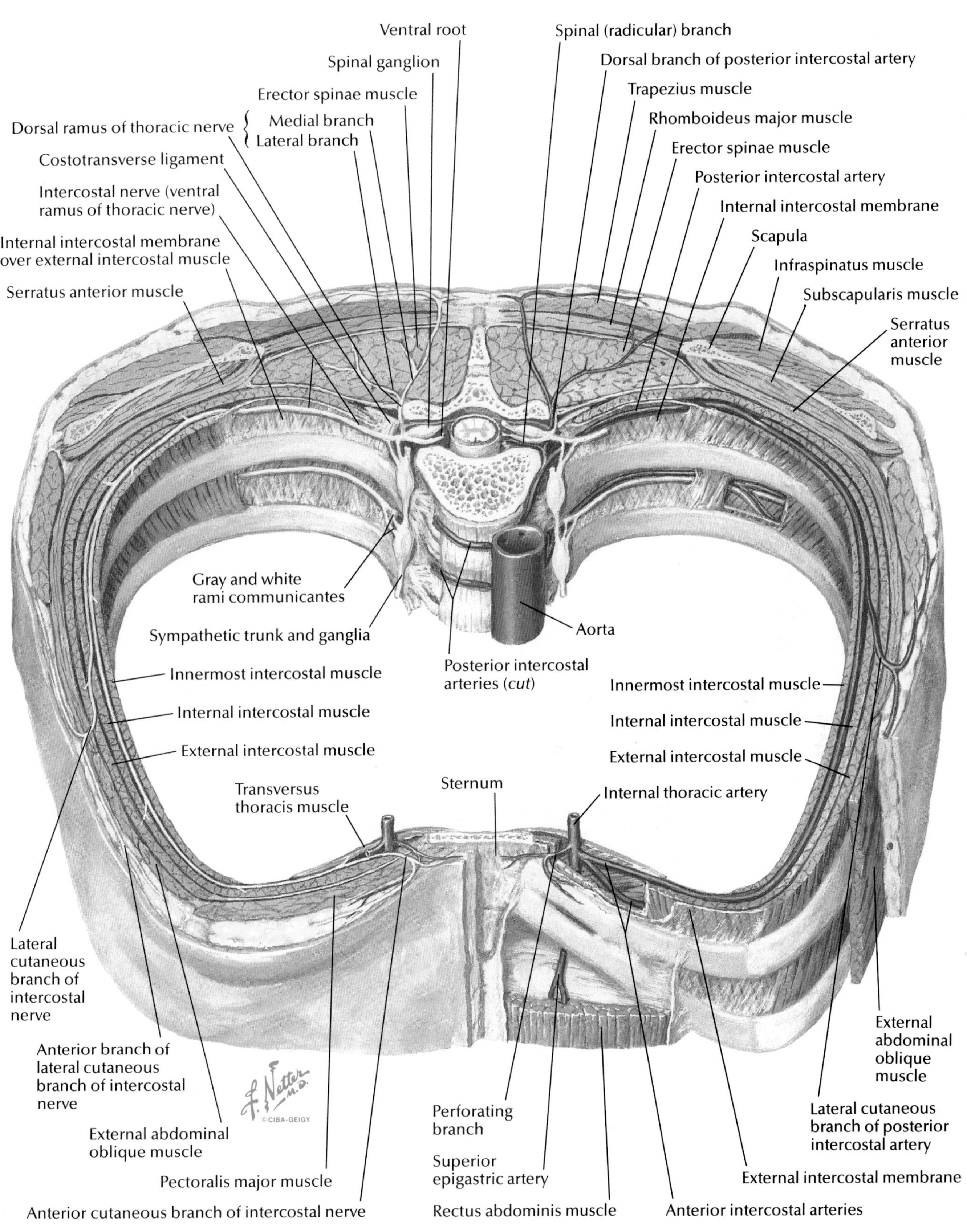

Ventral root
Spinal ganglion
Erector spinae muscle
Medial branch
Lateral branch
Spinal (radicular) branch
Dorsal branch of posterior intercostal artery
Trapezius muscle
Rhomboideus major muscle
Erector spinae muscle
Posterior intercostal artery
Internal intercostal membrane
Scapula
Infraspinatus muscle
Subscapularis muscle
Serratus anterior muscle

Dorsal ramus of thoracic nerve
Costotransverse ligament
Intercostal nerve (ventral ramus of thoracic nerve)
Internal intercostal membrane over external intercostal muscle
Serratus anterior muscle

Gray and white rami communicantes
Sympathetic trunk and ganglia
Innermost intercostal muscle
Internal intercostal muscle
External intercostal muscle

Aorta
Posterior intercostal arteries (cut)

Innermost intercostal muscle
Internal intercostal muscle
External intercostal muscle
Internal thoracic artery

Transversus thoracis muscle
Sternum

Lateral cutaneous branch of intercostal nerve

Anterior branch of lateral cutaneous branch of intercostal nerve

External abdominal oblique muscle

Pectoralis major muscle

Anterior cutaneous branch of intercostal nerve

Perforating branch
Superior epigastric artery
Rectus abdominis muscle

External abdominal oblique muscle

Lateral cutaneous branch of posterior intercostal artery

External intercostal membrane

Anterior intercostal arteries

f. Netter
©CIBA-GEIGY

Diaphragm: Thoracic Surface

SEE ALSO PLATES 218, 219

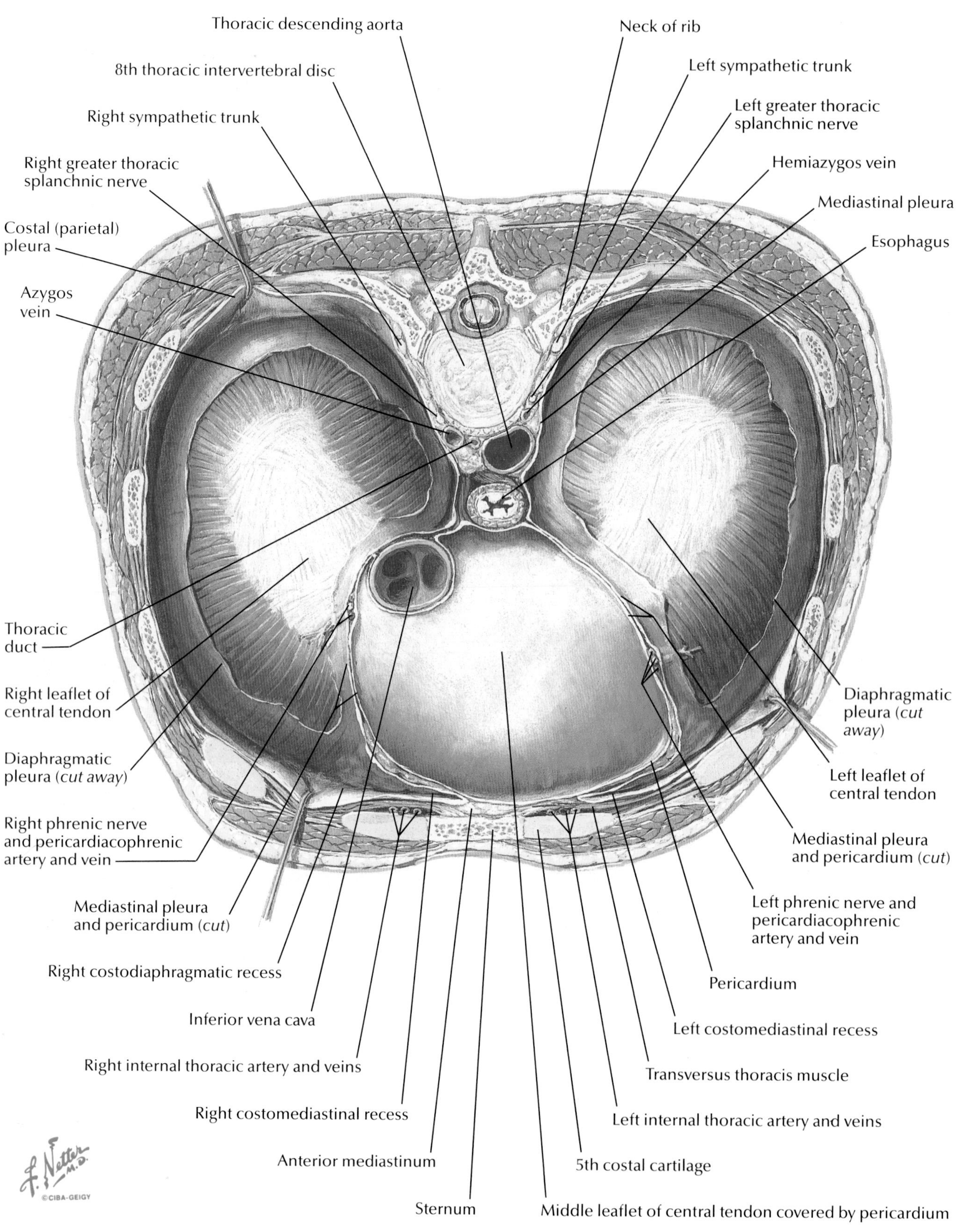

Thoracic descending aorta

Neck of rib

8th thoracic intervertebral disc

Left sympathetic trunk

Right sympathetic trunk

Left greater thoracic splanchnic nerve

Right greater thoracic splanchnic nerve

Hemiazygos vein

Mediastinal pleura

Costal (parietal) pleura

Esophagus

Azygos vein

Thoracic duct

Right leaflet of central tendon

Diaphragmatic pleura (cut away)

Diaphragmatic pleura (cut away)

Left leaflet of central tendon

Right phrenic nerve and pericardiacophrenic artery and vein

Mediastinal pleura and pericardium (cut)

Mediastinal pleura and pericardium (cut)

Right costodiaphragmatic recess

Left phrenic nerve and pericardiacophrenic artery and vein

Inferior vena cava

Pericardium

Right internal thoracic artery and veins

Left costomediastinal recess

Right costomediastinal recess

Transversus thoracis muscle

Anterior mediastinum

Left internal thoracic artery and veins

Sternum

5th costal cartilage

Middle leaflet of central tendon covered by pericardium

PLATE 180

THORAX

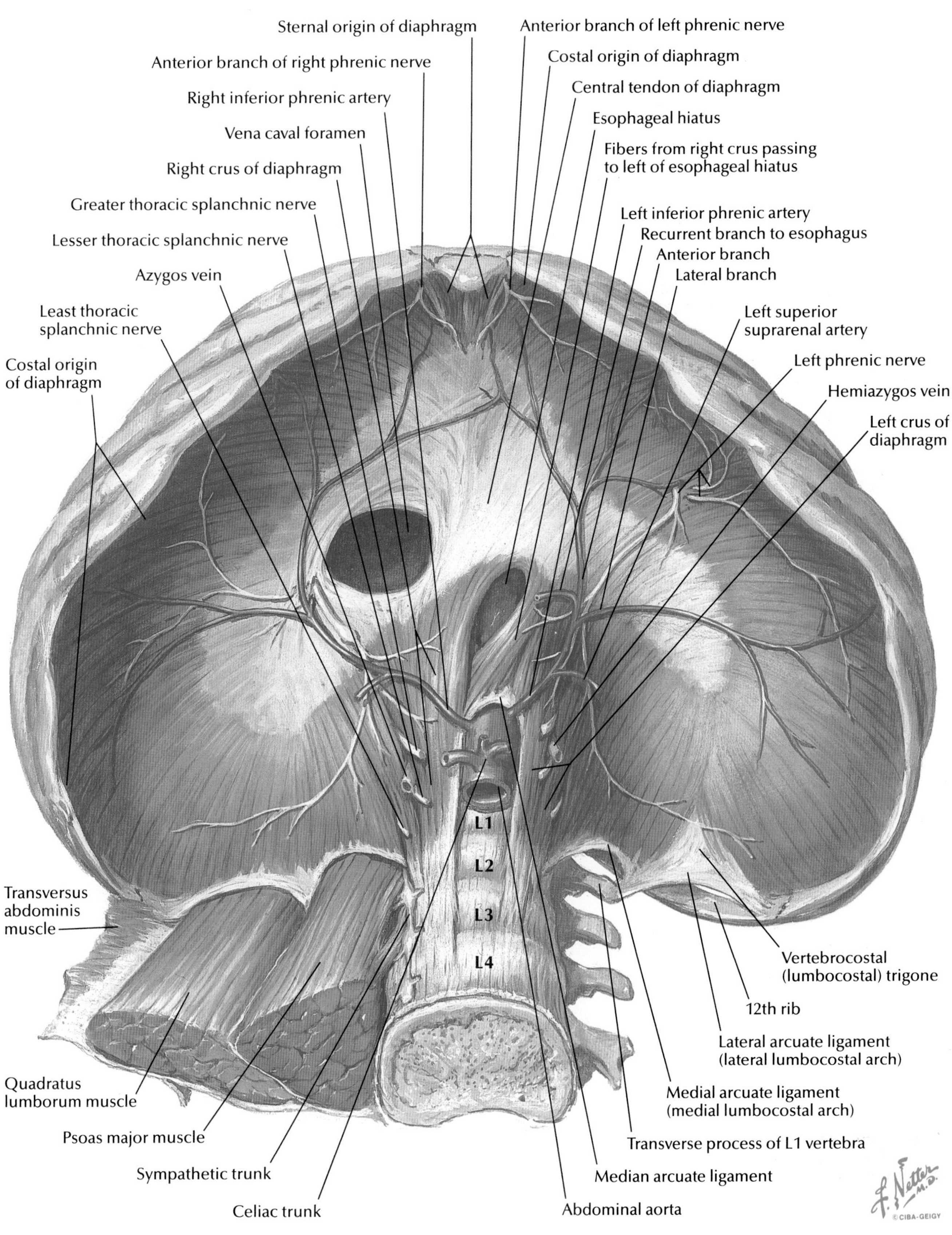

Sternal origin of diaphragm

Anterior branch of right phrenic nerve

Right inferior phrenic artery

Vena caval foramen

Right crus of diaphragm

Greater thoracic splanchnic nerve

Lesser thoracic splanchnic nerve

Azygos vein

Least thoracic splanchnic nerve

Costal origin of diaphragm

Anterior branch of left phrenic nerve

Costal origin of diaphragm

Central tendon of diaphragm

Esophageal hiatus

Fibers from right crus passing to left of esophageal hiatus

Left inferior phrenic artery

Recurrent branch to esophagus

Anterior branch

Lateral branch

Left superior suprarenal artery

Left phrenic nerve

Hemiazygos vein

Left crus of diaphragm

Transversus abdominis muscle

Quadratus lumborum muscle

Psoas major muscle

Sympathetic trunk

Celiac trunk

L1

L2

L3

L4

Vertebrocostal (lumbocostal) trigone

12th rib

Lateral arcuate ligament (lateral lumbocostal arch)

Medial arcuate ligament (medial lumbocostal arch)

Transverse process of L1 vertebra

Median arcuate ligament

Abdominal aorta

Phrenic Nerve

SEE ALSO PLATES 27, 123

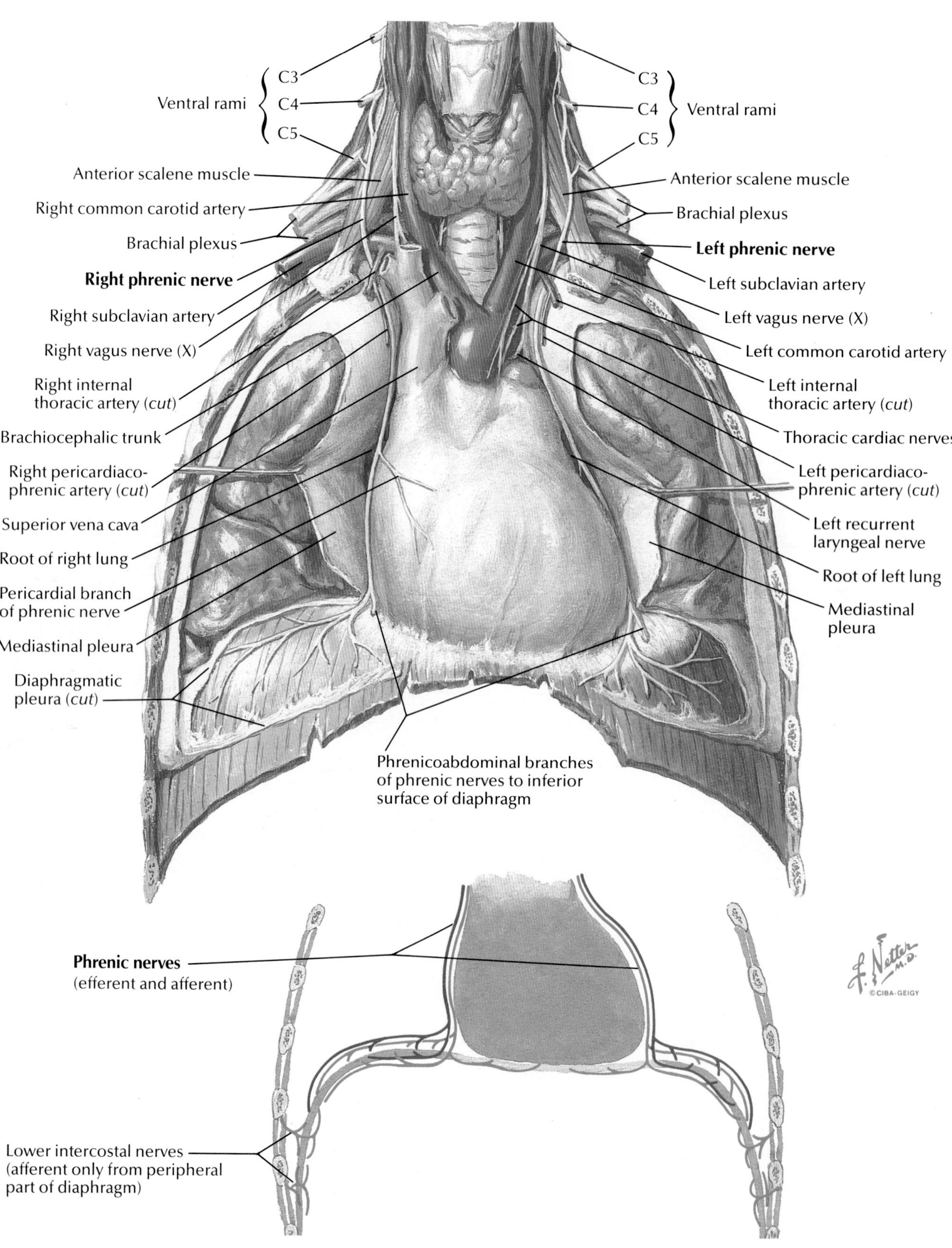

Ventral rami { C3
C4
C5

C3 } Ventral rami
C4
C5

Anterior scalene muscle

Right common carotid artery

Brachial plexus

Right phrenic nerve

Right subclavian artery

Right vagus nerve (X)

Right internal thoracic artery (*cut*)

Brachiocephalic trunk

Right pericardiaco-phrenic artery (*cut*)

Superior vena cava

Root of right lung

Pericardial branch of phrenic nerve

Mediastinal pleura

Diaphragmatic pleura (*cut*)

Anterior scalene muscle

Brachial plexus

Left phrenic nerve

Left subclavian artery

Left vagus nerve (X)

Left common carotid artery

Left internal thoracic artery (*cut*)

Thoracic cardiac nerves

Left pericardiaco-phrenic artery (*cut*)

Left recurrent laryngeal nerve

Root of left lung

Mediastinal pleura

Phrenicoabdominal branches of phrenic nerves to inferior surface of diaphragm

Phrenic nerves (efferent and afferent)

Lower intercostal nerves (afferent only from peripheral part of diaphragm)

PLATE 182

THORAX

Muscles of inspiration

Accessory

Sternocleidomastoid
(elevates sternum)

Scalenes
  Anterior
  Middle
  Posterior
(elevate and fix
upper ribs)

Principal

External intercostals
(elevate ribs, thus
increasing width of
thoracic cavity)

Interchondral part
of internal intercostals
(also elevates ribs)

Diaphragm
(domes descend, thus
increasing longitudinal
dimension of thoracic
cavity; also elevates
lower ribs)

Muscles of expiration

Quiet breathing

Expiration results from
passive recoil of lungs

Active breathing

Internal intercostals,
except interchondral
part

Abdominal muscles
(depress lower ribs,
compress abdominal
contents, thus pushing
up diaphragm)
Rectus abdominis
External oblique
Internal oblique
Transversus abdominis

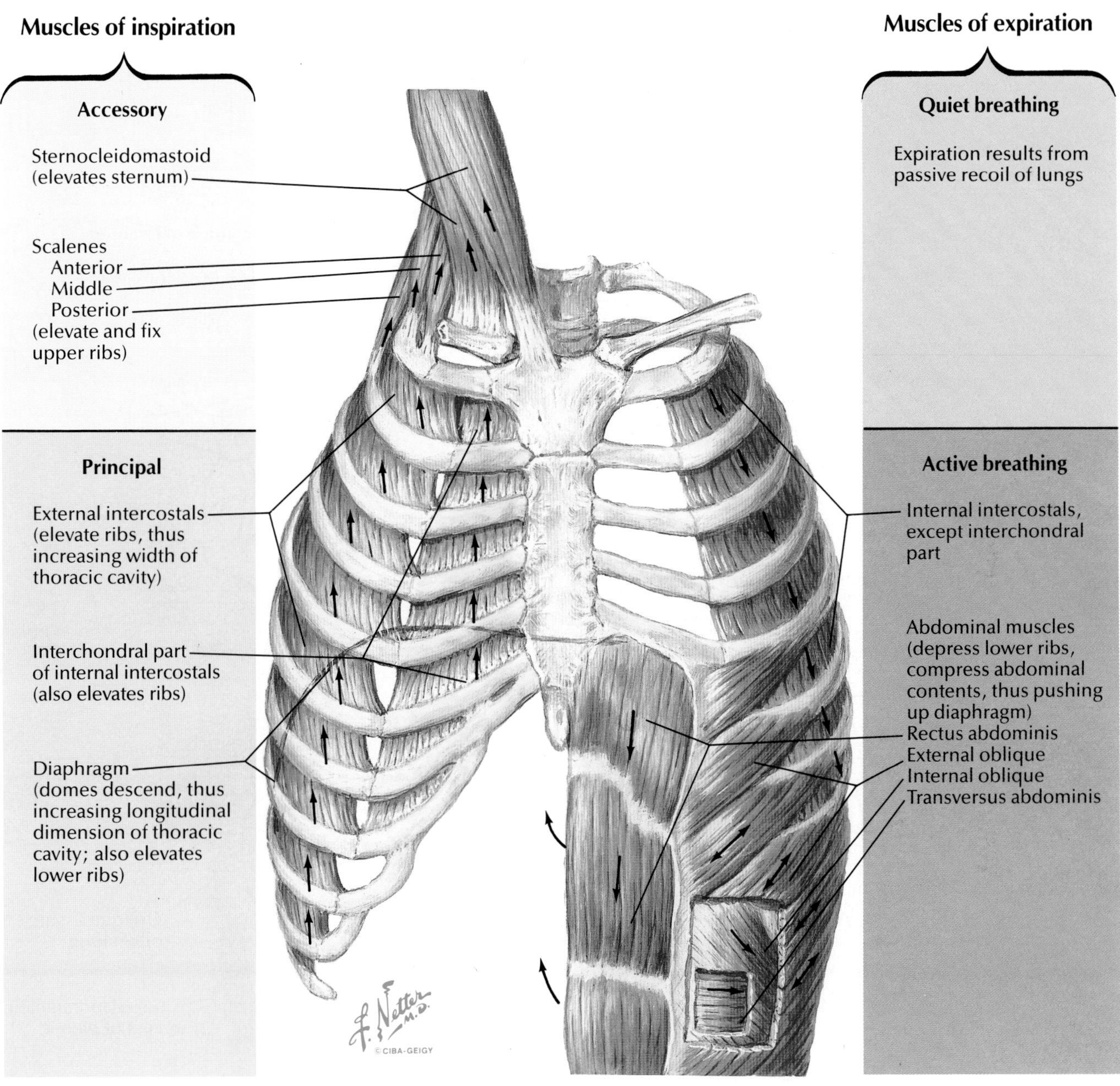

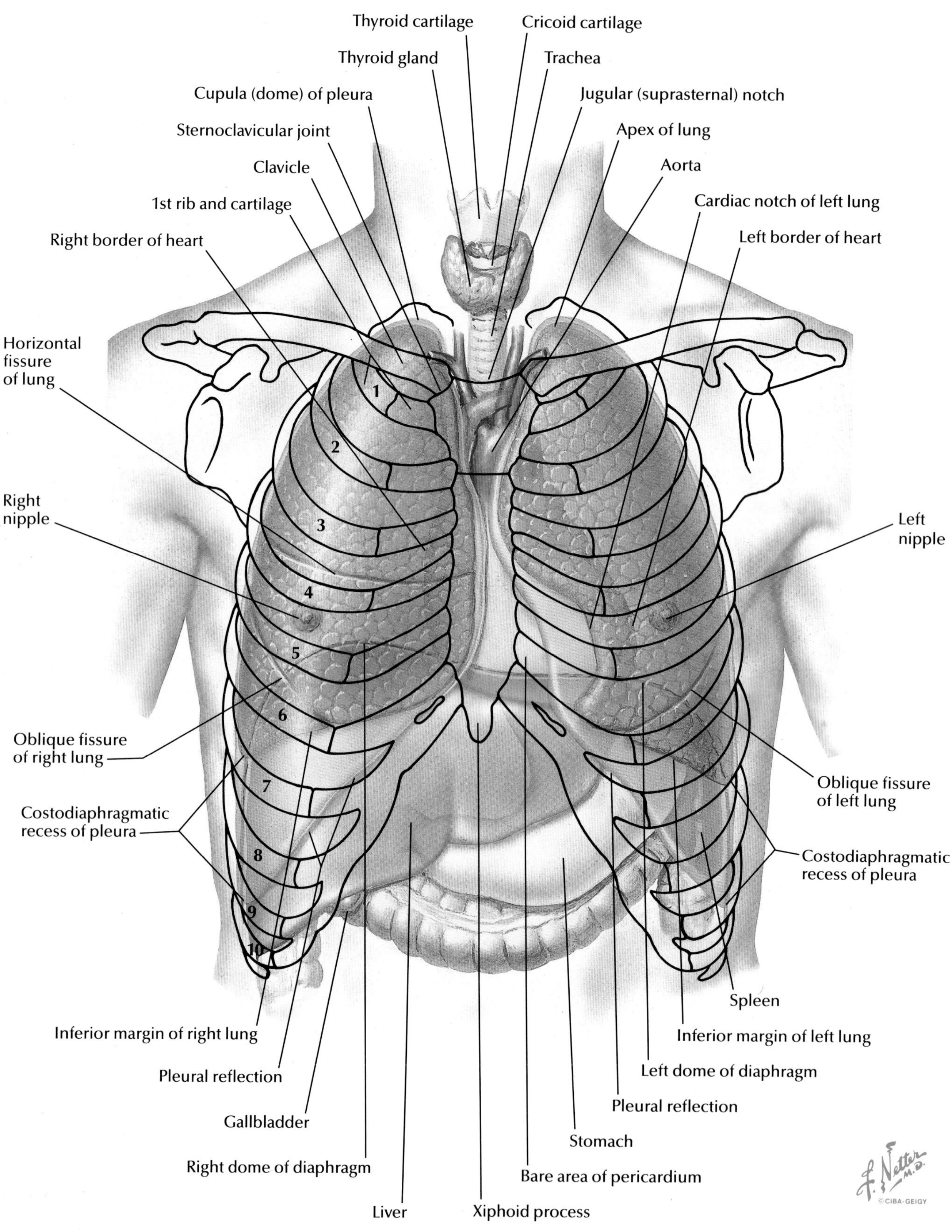

Thyroid cartilage

Cricoid cartilage

Thyroid gland

Trachea

Cupula (dome) of pleura

Jugular (suprasternal) notch

Sternoclavicular joint

Apex of lung

Clavicle

Aorta

1st rib and cartilage

Cardiac notch of left lung

Right border of heart

Left border of heart

Horizontal fissure of lung

Right nipple

Left nipple

Oblique fissure of right lung

Oblique fissure of left lung

Costodiaphragmatic recess of pleura

Costodiaphragmatic recess of pleura

Spleen

Inferior margin of right lung

Inferior margin of left lung

Pleural reflection

Left dome of diaphragm

Gallbladder

Pleural reflection

Right dome of diaphragm

Stomach

Liver

Xiphoid process

Bare area of pericardium

PLATE 184

THORAX

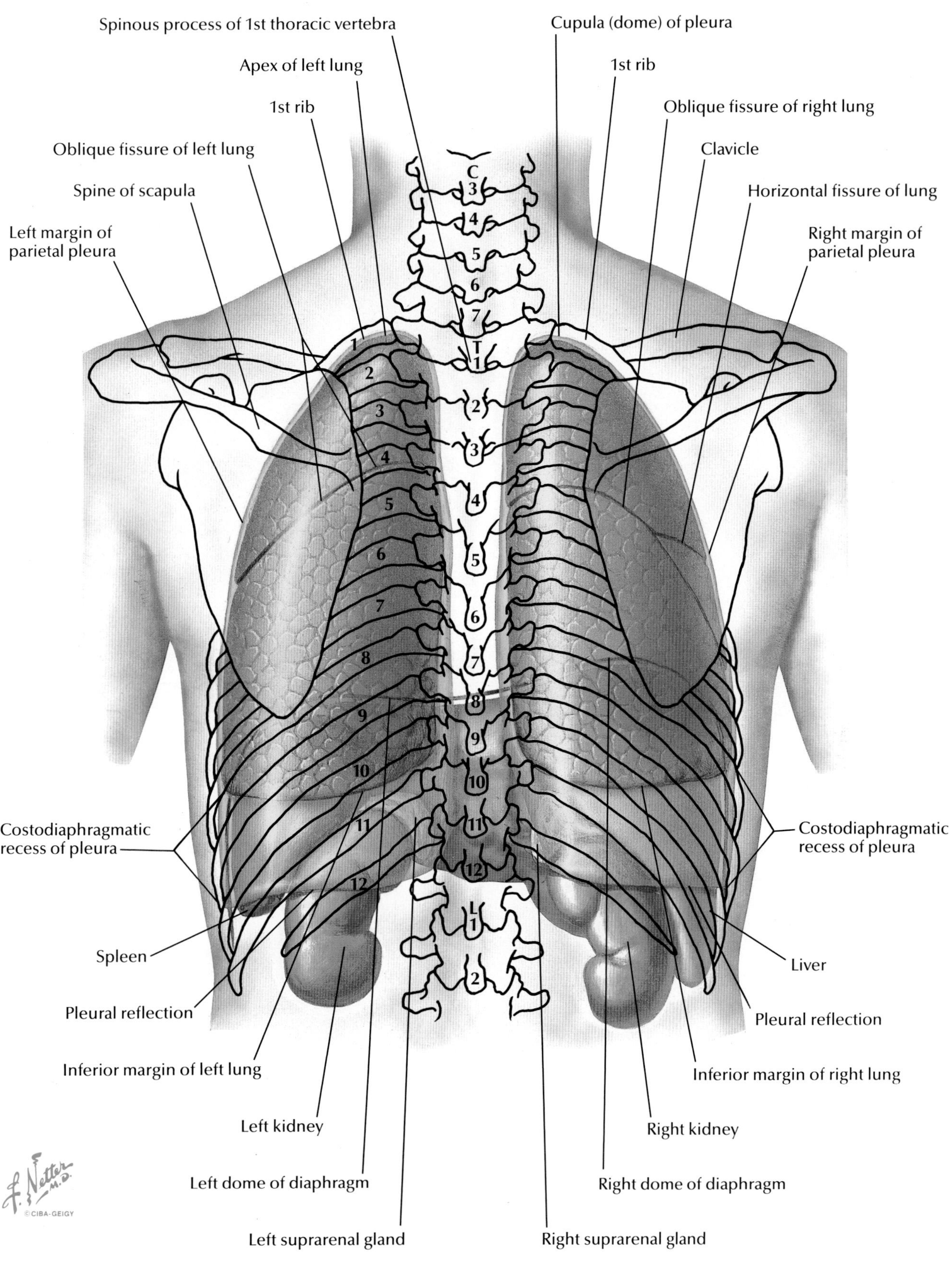

Spinous process of 1st thoracic vertebra

Apex of left lung

1st rib

Oblique fissure of left lung

Spine of scapula

Left margin of parietal pleura

Cupula (dome) of pleura

1st rib

Oblique fissure of right lung

Clavicle

Horizontal fissure of lung

Right margin of parietal pleura

Costodiaphragmatic recess of pleura

Spleen

Pleural reflection

Inferior margin of left lung

Left kidney

Left dome of diaphragm

Left suprarenal gland

Costodiaphragmatic recess of pleura

Liver

Pleural reflection

Inferior margin of right lung

Right kidney

Right dome of diaphragm

Right suprarenal gland

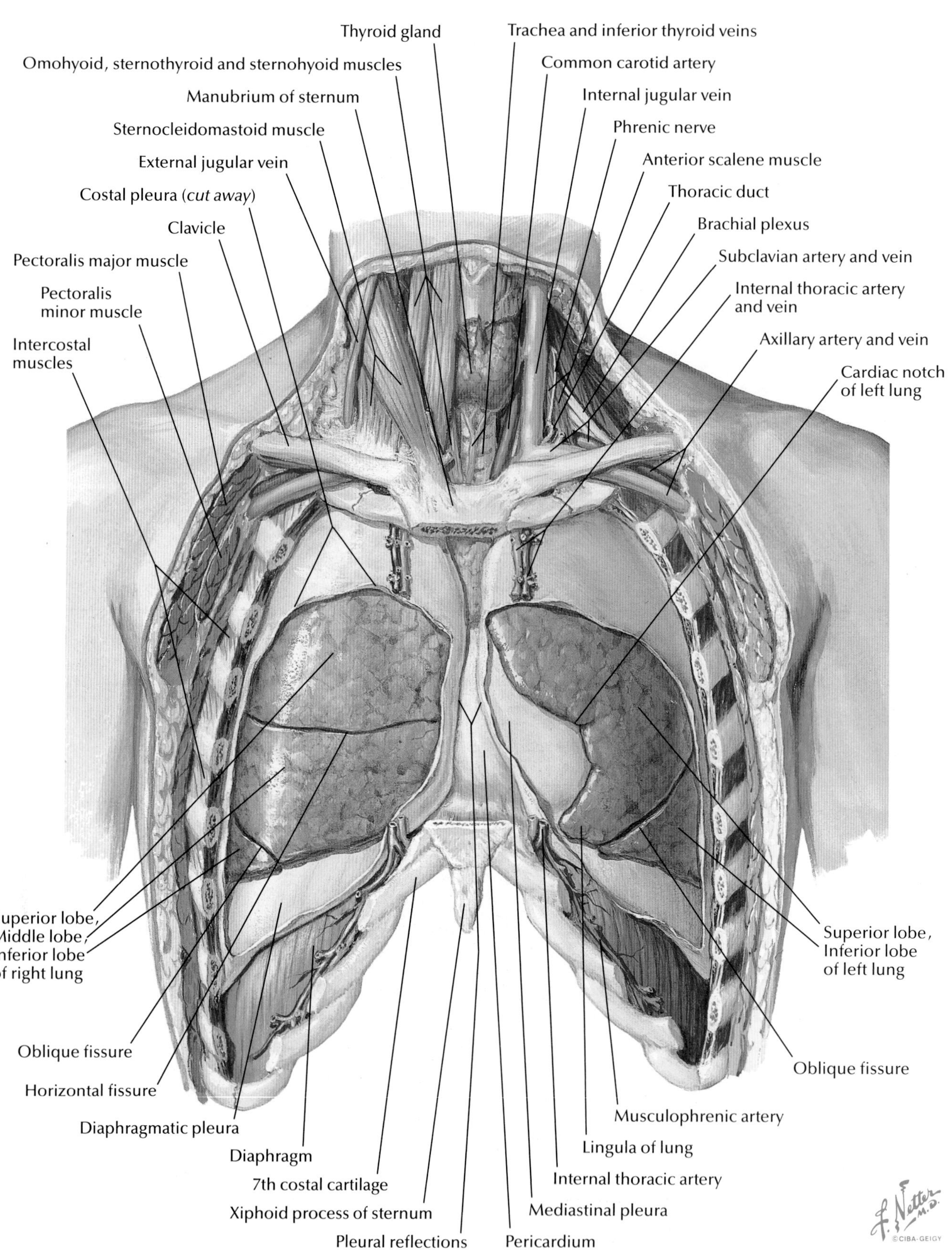

Thyroid gland

Omohyoid, sternothyroid and sternohyoid muscles

Manubrium of sternum

Sternocleidomastoid muscle

External jugular vein

Costal pleura (*cut away*)

Clavicle

Pectoralis major muscle

Pectoralis minor muscle

Intercostal muscles

Trachea and inferior thyroid veins

Common carotid artery

Internal jugular vein

Phrenic nerve

Anterior scalene muscle

Thoracic duct

Brachial plexus

Subclavian artery and vein

Internal thoracic artery and vein

Axillary artery and vein

Cardiac notch of left lung

Superior lobe, Middle lobe, Inferior lobe of right lung

Oblique fissure

Horizontal fissure

Diaphragmatic pleura

Diaphragm

7th costal cartilage

Xiphoid process of sternum

Pleural reflections

Superior lobe, Inferior lobe of left lung

Oblique fissure

Musculophrenic artery

Lingula of lung

Internal thoracic artery

Mediastinal pleura

Pericardium

PLATE 186

THORAX

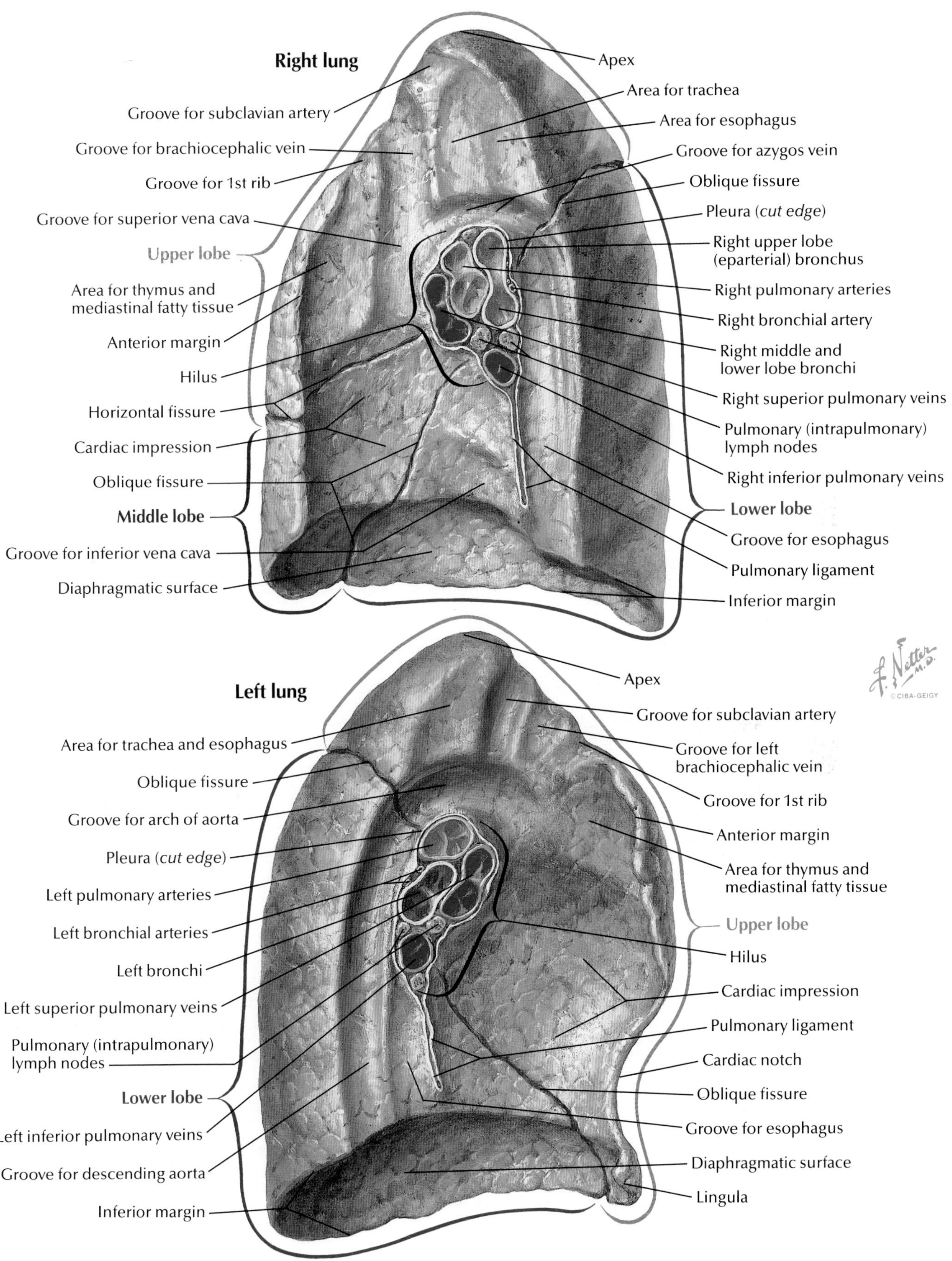

Right lung

- Groove for subclavian artery
- Groove for brachiocephalic vein
- Groove for 1st rib
- Groove for superior vena cava
- Upper lobe
- Area for thymus and mediastinal fatty tissue
- Anterior margin
- Hilus
- Horizontal fissure
- Cardiac impression
- Oblique fissure
- Middle lobe
- Groove for inferior vena cava
- Diaphragmatic surface

- Apex
- Area for trachea
- Area for esophagus
- Groove for azygos vein
- Oblique fissure
- Pleura (*cut edge*)
- Right upper lobe (eparterial) bronchus
- Right pulmonary arteries
- Right bronchial artery
- Right middle and lower lobe bronchi
- Right superior pulmonary veins
- Pulmonary (intrapulmonary) lymph nodes
- Right inferior pulmonary veins
- Lower lobe
- Groove for esophagus
- Pulmonary ligament
- Inferior margin

Left lung

- Area for trachea and esophagus
- Oblique fissure
- Groove for arch of aorta
- Pleura (*cut edge*)
- Left pulmonary arteries
- Left bronchial arteries
- Left bronchi
- Left superior pulmonary veins
- Pulmonary (intrapulmonary) lymph nodes
- Lower lobe
- Left inferior pulmonary veins
- Groove for descending aorta
- Inferior margin

- Apex
- Groove for subclavian artery
- Groove for left brachiocephalic vein
- Groove for 1st rib
- Anterior margin
- Area for thymus and mediastinal fatty tissue
- Upper lobe
- Hilus
- Cardiac impression
- Pulmonary ligament
- Cardiac notch
- Oblique fissure
- Groove for esophagus
- Diaphragmatic surface
- Lingula

Bronchopulmonary Segments

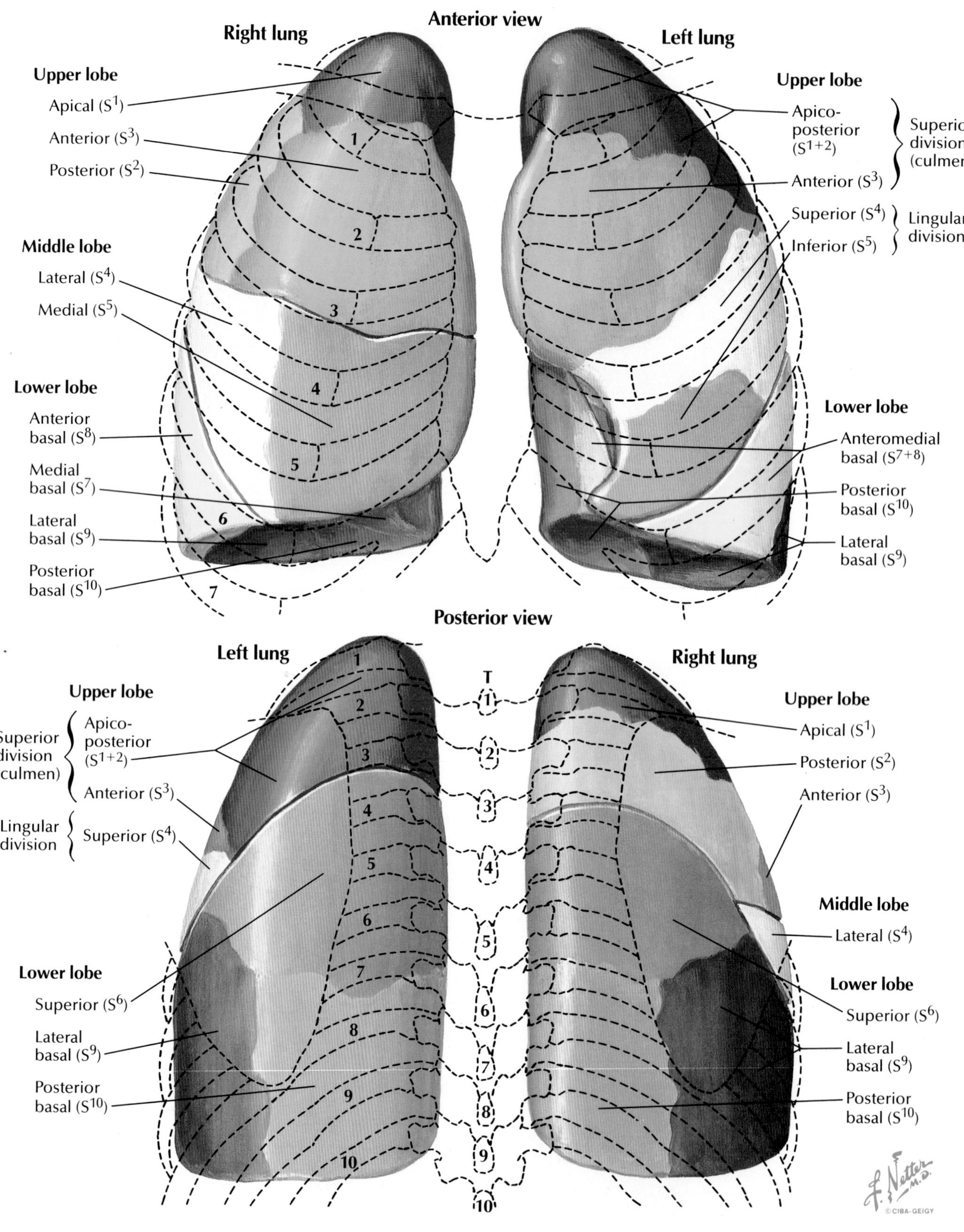

Anterior view

Right lung

Left lung

Upper lobe

Apical (S^1)
Anterior (S^3)
Posterior (S^2)

Middle lobe

Lateral (S^4)
Medial (S^5)

Lower lobe

Anterior basal (S^8)
Medial basal (S^7)
Lateral basal (S^9)
Posterior basal (S^{10})

Upper lobe

Apico-posterior (S^{1+2}) } Superior division (culmen)
Anterior (S^3) }
Superior (S^4) } Lingular division
Inferior (S^5) }

Lower lobe

Anteromedial basal (S^{7+8})
Posterior basal (S^{10})
Lateral basal (S^9)

Posterior view

Left lung

Right lung

Upper lobe

Superior division (culmen) { Apico-posterior (S^{1+2})
Anterior (S^3)
Lingular division { Superior (S^4)

Lower lobe

Superior (S^6)
Lateral basal (S^9)
Posterior basal (S^{10})

Upper lobe

Apical (S^1)
Posterior (S^2)
Anterior (S^3)

Middle lobe

Lateral (S^4)

Lower lobe

Superior (S^6)
Lateral basal (S^9)
Posterior basal (S^{10})

PLATE 188

THORAX

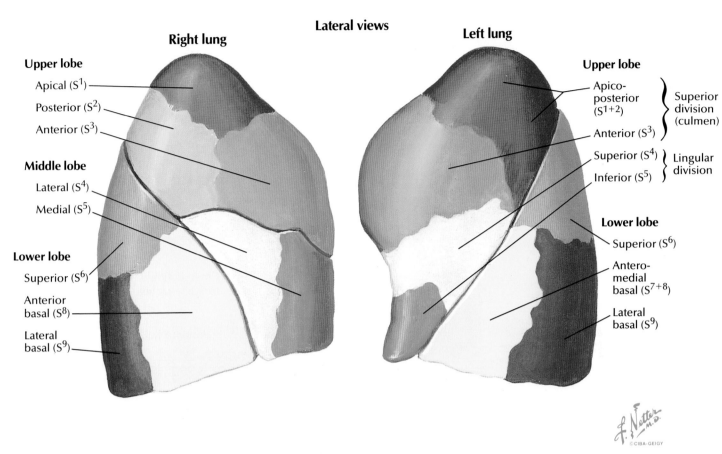

Lateral views

Right lung

Left lung

Upper lobe
Apical (S¹)
Posterior (S²)
Anterior (S³)

Middle lobe
Lateral (S⁴)
Medial (S⁵)

Lower lobe
Superior (S⁶)
Anterior basal (S⁸)
Lateral basal (S⁹)

Upper lobe
Apicoposterior (S¹⁺²) } Superior division (culmen)
Anterior (S³)
Superior (S⁴) } Lingular division
Inferior (S⁵)

Lower lobe
Superior (S⁶)
Anteromedial basal (S⁷⁺⁸)
Lateral basal (S⁹)

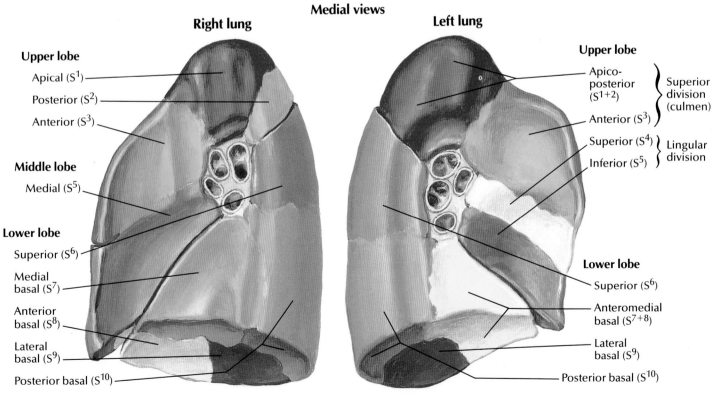

Medial views

Right lung

Left lung

Upper lobe
Apical (S¹)
Posterior (S²)
Anterior (S³)

Middle lobe
Medial (S⁵)

Lower lobe
Superior (S⁶)
Medial basal (S⁷)
Anterior basal (S⁸)
Lateral basal (S⁹)
Posterior basal (S¹⁰)

Upper lobe
Apicoposterior (S¹⁺²) } Superior division (culmen)
Anterior (S³)
Superior (S⁴) } Lingular division
Inferior (S⁵)

Lower lobe
Superior (S⁶)
Anteromedial basal (S⁷⁺⁸)
Lateral basal (S⁹)
Posterior basal (S¹⁰)

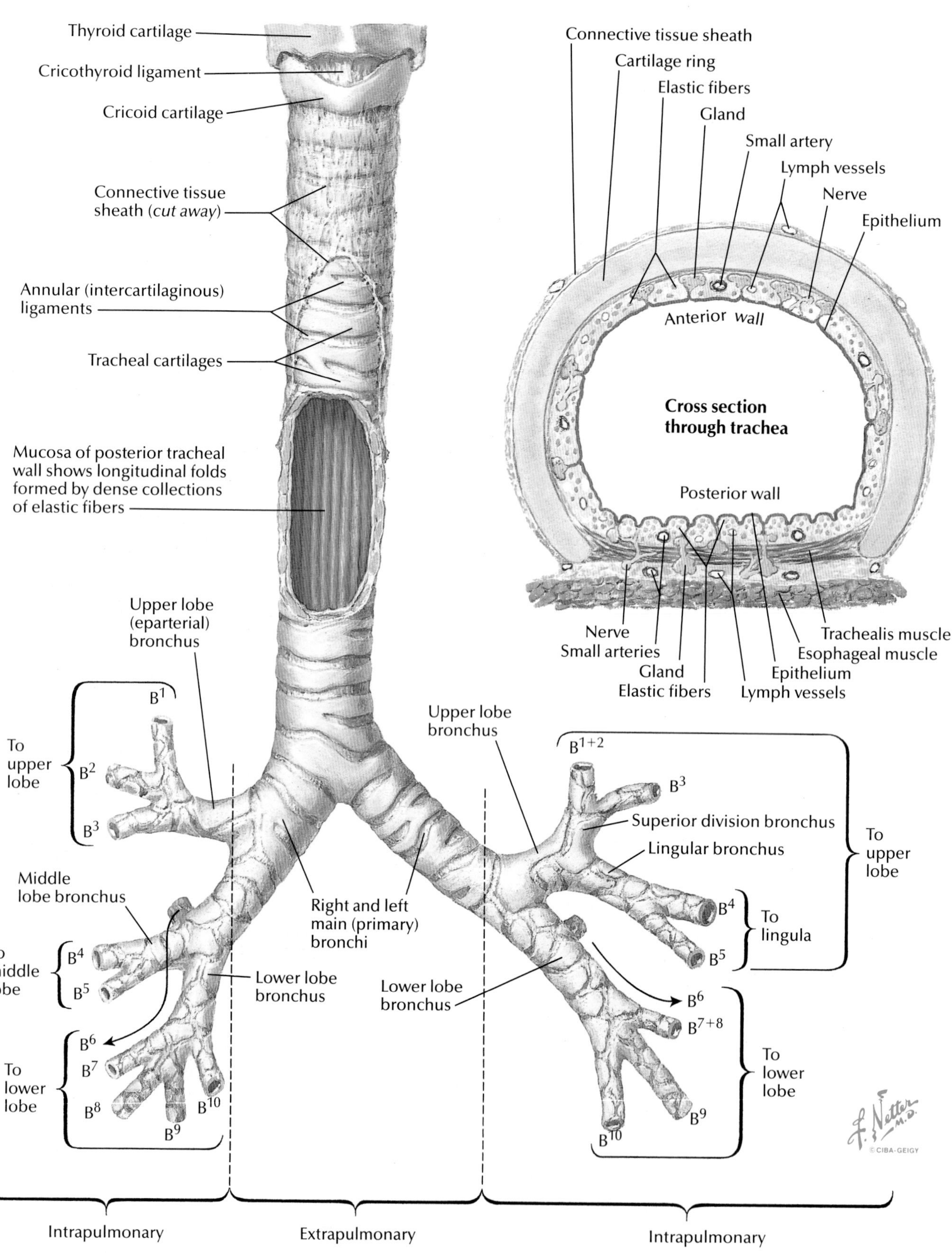

Thyroid cartilage

Cricothyroid ligament

Cricoid cartilage

Connective tissue sheath (*cut away*)

Annular (intercartilaginous) ligaments

Tracheal cartilages

Mucosa of posterior tracheal wall shows longitudinal folds formed by dense collections of elastic fibers

Connective tissue sheath

Cartilage ring

Elastic fibers

Gland

Small artery

Lymph vessels

Nerve

Epithelium

Anterior *wall*

Cross section through trachea

Posterior wall

Nerve
Small arteries
Gland
Elastic fibers

Trachealis muscle
Esophageal muscle
Epithelium
Lymph vessels

Upper lobe (eparterial) bronchus

B^1

To upper lobe

B^2

B^3

Middle lobe bronchus

To middle lobe

B^4

B^5

Right and left main (primary) bronchi

Lower lobe bronchus

To lower lobe

B^6

B^7

B^8

B^{10}

B^9

Upper lobe bronchus

B^{1+2}

B^3

Superior division bronchus

Lingular bronchus

To upper lobe

B^4

To lingula

B^5

Lower lobe bronchus

B^6

B^{7+8}

To lower lobe

B^9

B^{10}

Intrapulmonary

Extrapulmonary

Intrapulmonary

PLATE 190

THORAX

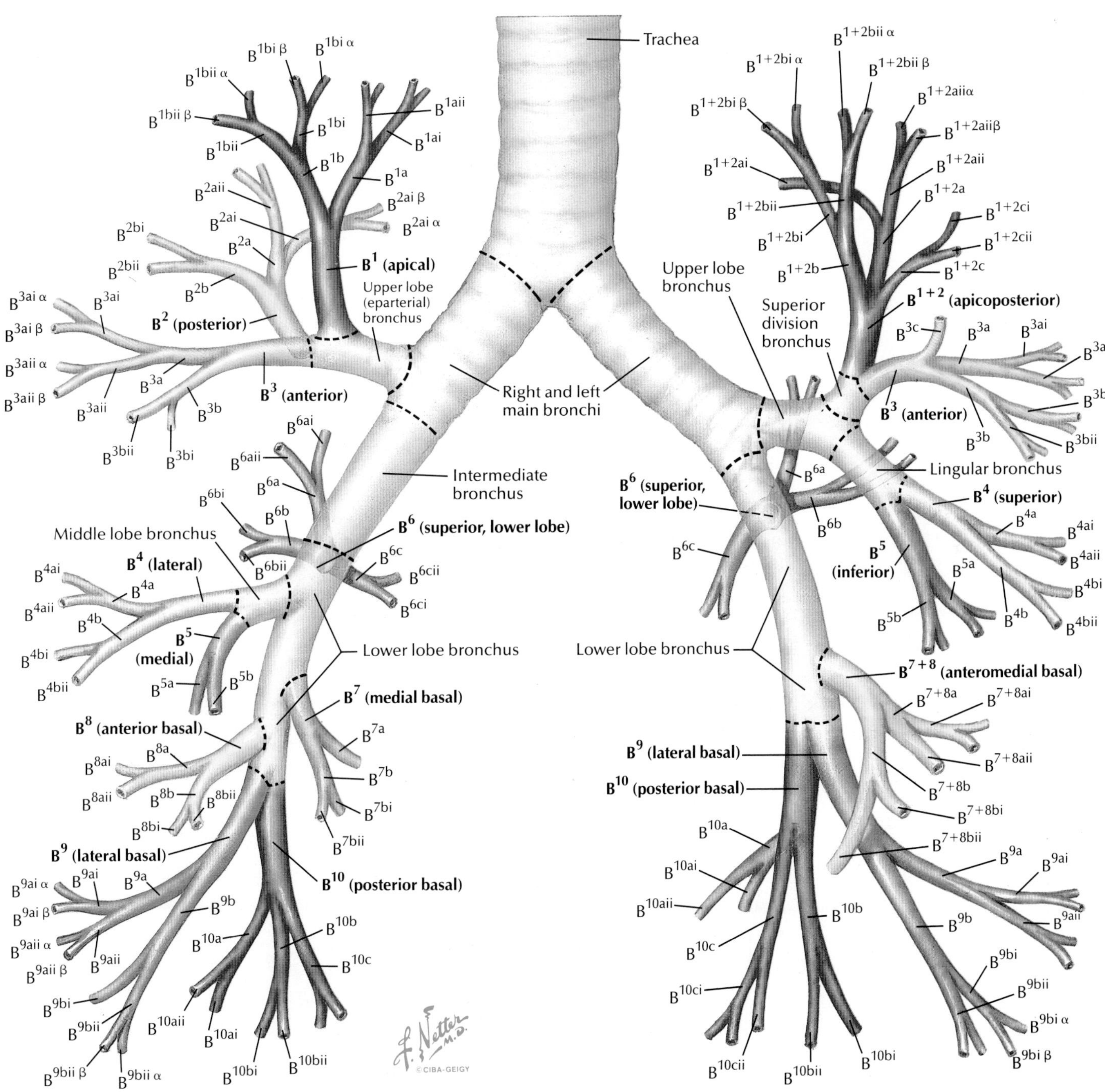

Nomenclature in common usage for bronchopulmonary segments (Plates 188 and 189) is that of Jackson and Huber, and segmental bronchi are named accordingly. Ikeda proposed nomenclature (as demonstrated here) for bronchial subdivisions as far as 6th generation. For simplification in this illustration, only some bronchial subdivisions are labeled as far as 5th or 6th generation. Segmental bronchi (B) are numbered from 1 to 10 in each lung, corresponding to pulmonary segments. In left lung, B^1

and B^2 are combined as are B^7 and B^8. Subsegmental, or 4th order, bronchi are indicated by addition of lower case letters a, b or c when an additional branch is present. Fifth order bronchi are designated by Roman numerals i (anterior) or ii (posterior), and 6th order bronchi by Greek letters α or β. Several texts use alternate numbers (as proposed by Boyden) for segmental bronchi.

Variations of standard bronchial pattern shown here are common, especially in peripheral airways

Intrapulmonary Airways: Schema

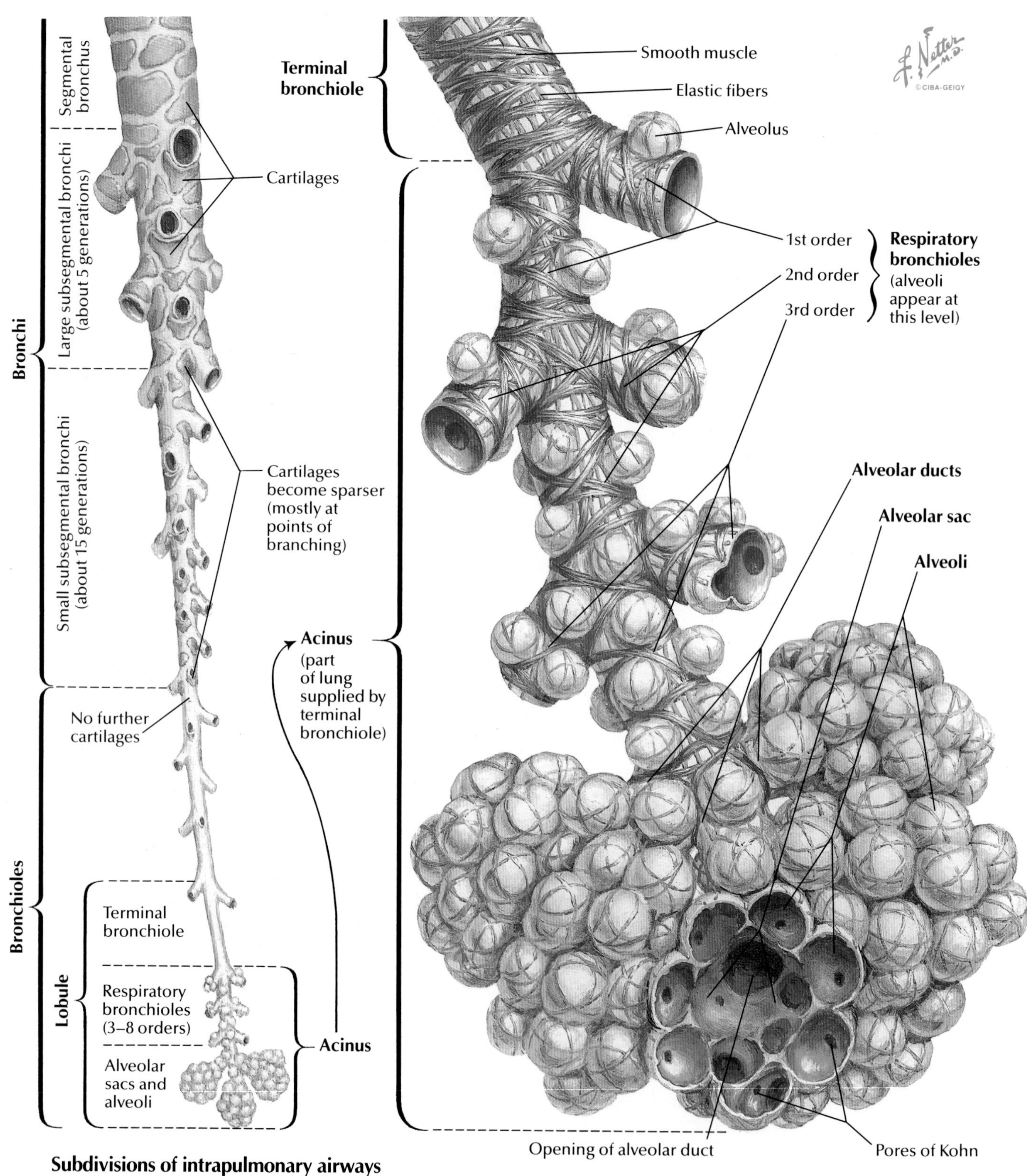

Terminal bronchiole

Segmental bronchus

Large subsegmental bronchi (about 5 generations)

Cartilages

Small subsegmental bronchi (about 15 generations)

Cartilages become sparser (mostly at points of branching)

Bronchi

No further cartilages

Acinus (part of lung supplied by terminal bronchiole)

Bronchioles

Lobule

Terminal bronchiole

Respiratory bronchioles (3–8 orders)

Alveolar sacs and alveoli

Acinus

Subdivisions of intrapulmonary airways

Smooth muscle

Elastic fibers

Alveolus

1st order

2nd order

3rd order

Respiratory bronchioles (alveoli appear at this level)

Alveolar ducts

Alveolar sac

Alveoli

Opening of alveolar duct

Pores of Kohn

Structure of intrapulmonary airways

PLATE 192

THORAX

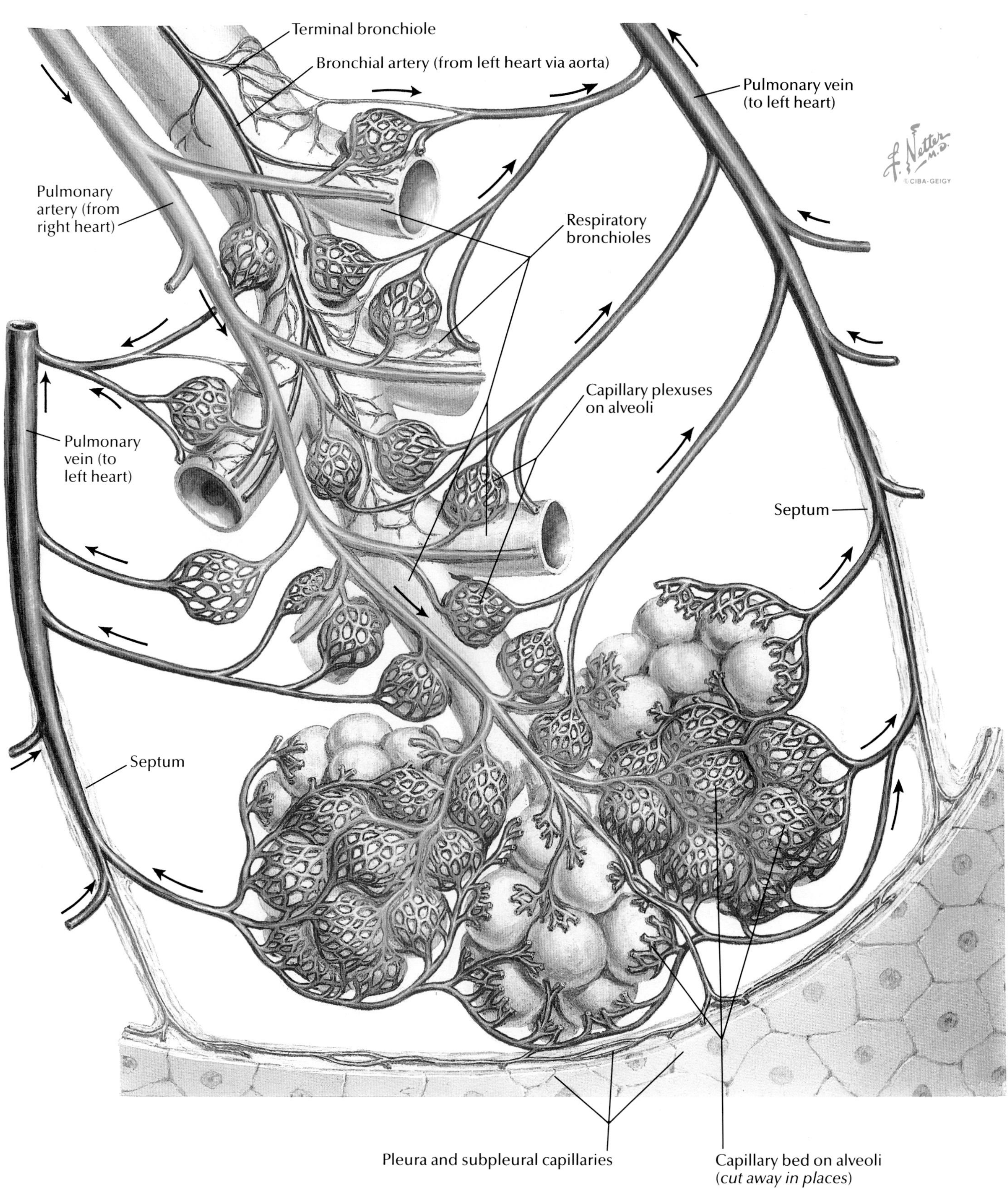

Terminal bronchiole

Bronchial artery (from left heart via aorta)

Pulmonary vein (to left heart)

Pulmonary artery (from right heart)

Respiratory bronchioles

Pulmonary vein (to left heart)

Capillary plexuses on alveoli

Septum

Septum

Pleura and subpleural capillaries

Capillary bed on alveoli (*cut away in places*)

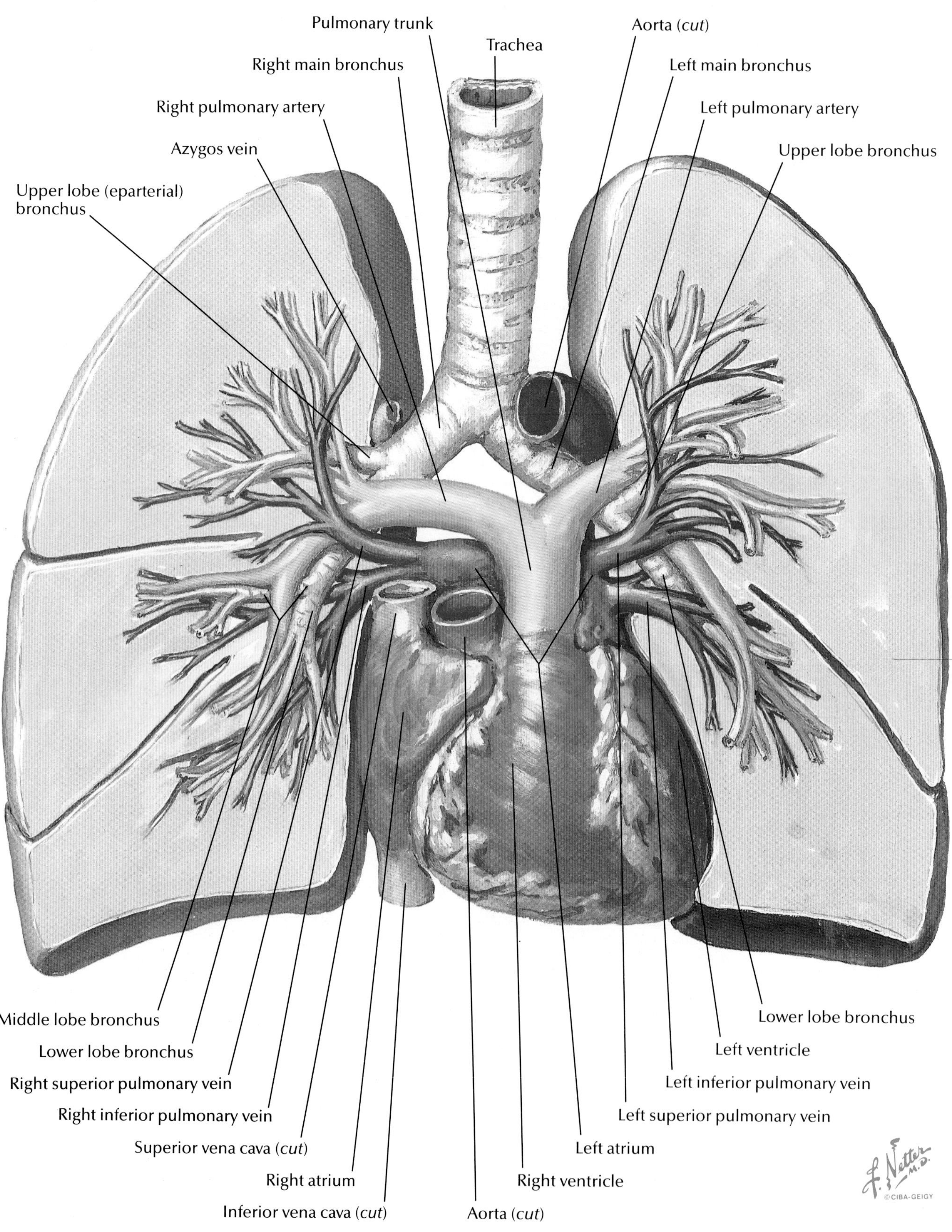

Pulmonary trunk

Trachea

Aorta (*cut*)

Right main bronchus

Left main bronchus

Right pulmonary artery

Left pulmonary artery

Azygos vein

Upper lobe bronchus

Upper lobe (eparterial) bronchus

Middle lobe bronchus

Lower lobe bronchus

Lower lobe bronchus

Right superior pulmonary vein

Left ventricle

Right inferior pulmonary vein

Left inferior pulmonary vein

Superior vena cava (*cut*)

Left superior pulmonary vein

Right atrium

Left atrium

Inferior vena cava (*cut*)

Right ventricle

Aorta (*cut*)

PLATE 194

THORAX

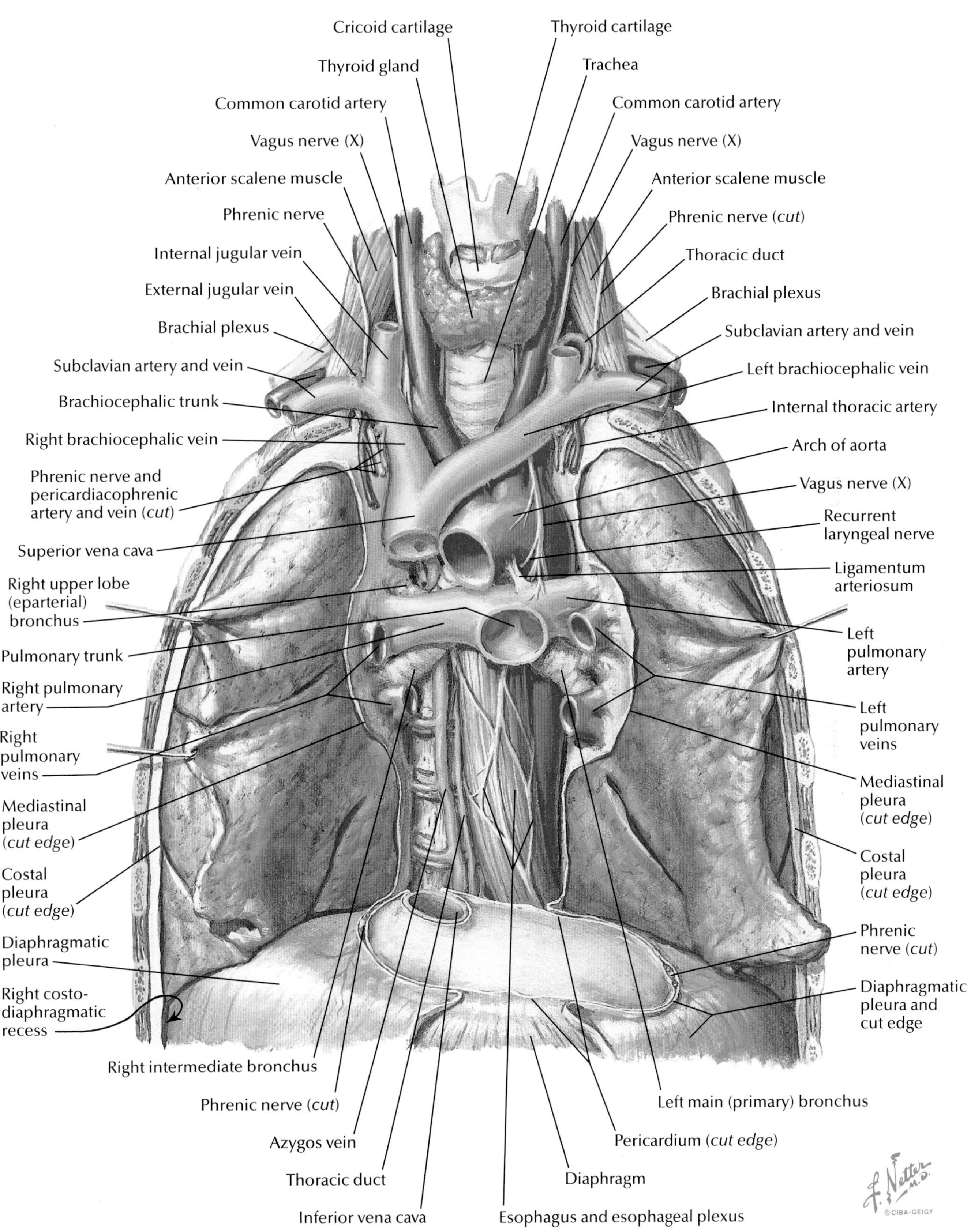

Cricoid cartilage

Thyroid cartilage

Thyroid gland

Trachea

Common carotid artery

Common carotid artery

Vagus nerve (X)

Vagus nerve (X)

Anterior scalene muscle

Anterior scalene muscle

Phrenic nerve

Phrenic nerve (*cut*)

Internal jugular vein

Thoracic duct

External jugular vein

Brachial plexus

Brachial plexus

Subclavian artery and vein

Subclavian artery and vein

Left brachiocephalic vein

Brachiocephalic trunk

Internal thoracic artery

Right brachiocephalic vein

Arch of aorta

Phrenic nerve and pericardiacophrenic artery and vein (*cut*)

Vagus nerve (X)

Recurrent laryngeal nerve

Superior vena cava

Ligamentum arteriosum

Right upper lobe (eparterial) bronchus

Left pulmonary artery

Pulmonary trunk

Left pulmonary veins

Right pulmonary artery

Right pulmonary veins

Mediastinal pleura (*cut edge*)

Mediastinal pleura (*cut edge*)

Costal pleura (*cut edge*)

Costal pleura (*cut edge*)

Diaphragmatic pleura

Phrenic nerve (*cut*)

Right costo-diaphragmatic recess

Diaphragmatic pleura and cut edge

Right intermediate bronchus

Phrenic nerve (*cut*)

Left main (primary) bronchus

Azygos vein

Pericardium (*cut edge*)

Thoracic duct

Diaphragm

Inferior vena cava

Esophagus and esophageal plexus

f. Netter M.D.

©CIBA-GEIGY

Bronchial Arteries and Veins

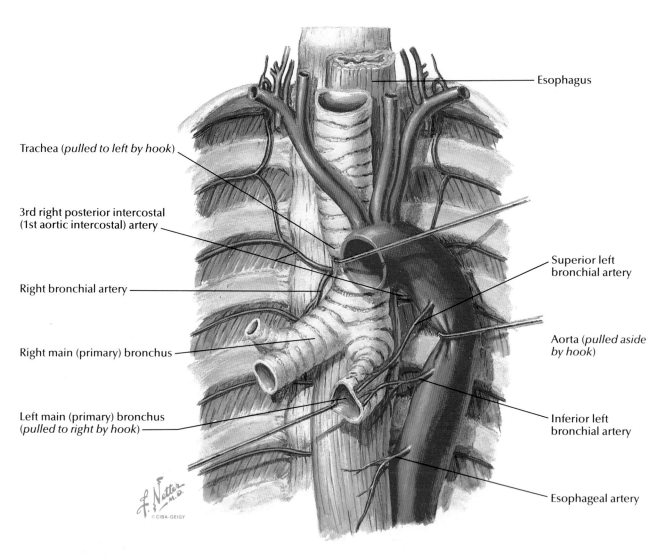

Trachea (*pulled to left by hook*)

3rd right posterior intercostal (1st aortic intercostal) artery

Right bronchial artery

Right main (primary) bronchus

Left main (primary) bronchus (*pulled to right by hook*)

Esophagus

Superior left bronchial artery

Aorta (*pulled aside by hook*)

Inferior left bronchial artery

Esophageal artery

Variations in bronchial arteries

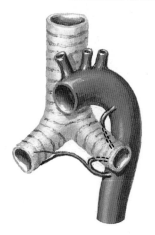

Right and left bronchial arteries originating from aorta by single stem

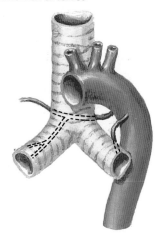

Only single bronchial artery to each bronchus (normally, two to left bronchus)

Bronchial veins

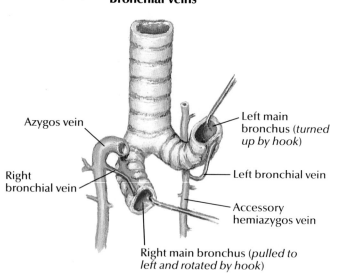

Azygos vein

Right bronchial vein

Left main bronchus (*turned up by hook*)

Left bronchial vein

Accessory hemiazygos vein

Right main bronchus (*pulled to left and rotated by hook*)

PLATE 196

THORAX

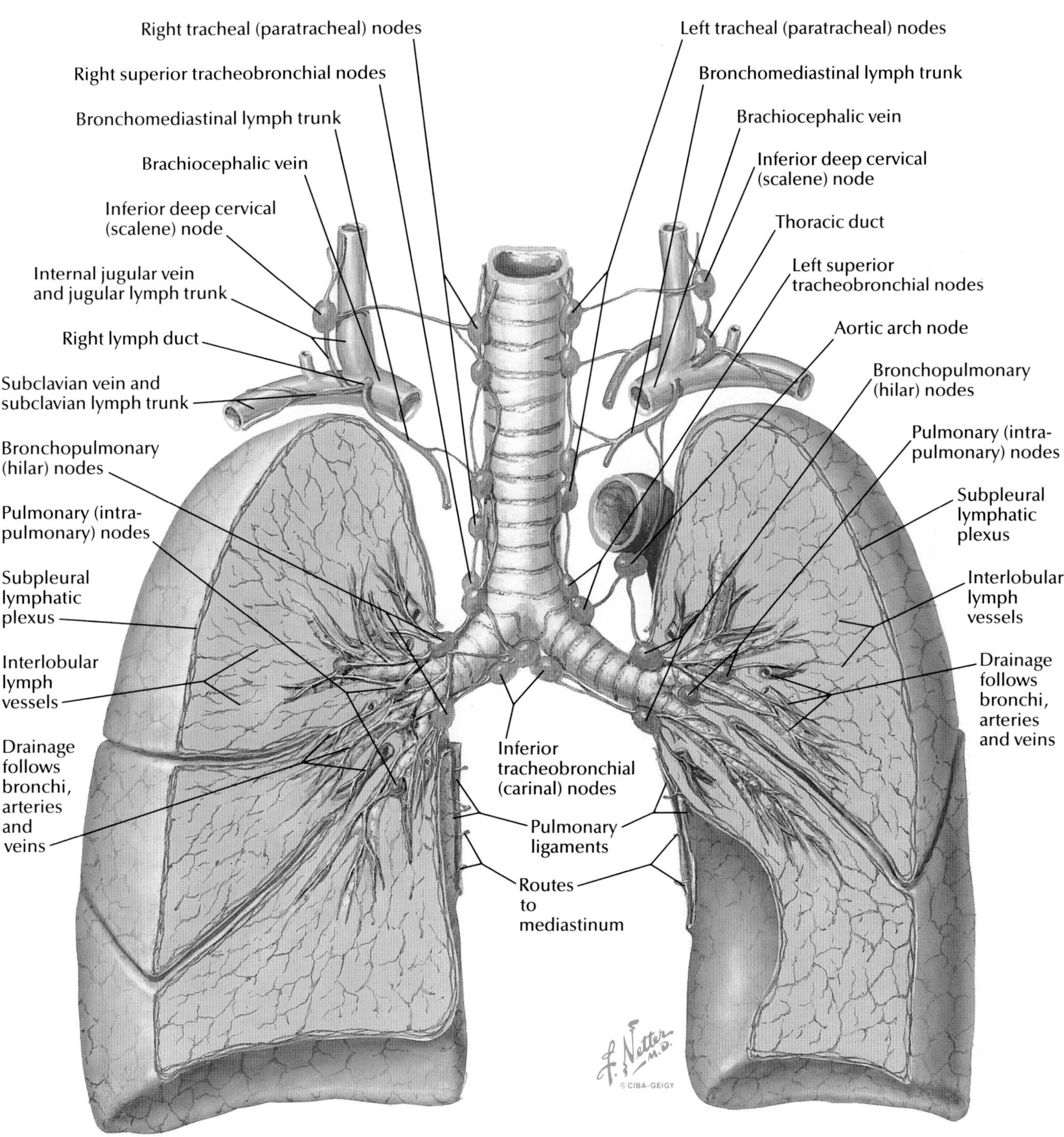

Right tracheal (paratracheal) nodes

Right superior tracheobronchial nodes

Bronchomediastinal lymph trunk

Brachiocephalic vein

Inferior deep cervical (scalene) node

Internal jugular vein and jugular lymph trunk

Right lymph duct

Subclavian vein and subclavian lymph trunk

Bronchopulmonary (hilar) nodes

Pulmonary (intra-pulmonary) nodes

Subpleural lymphatic plexus

Interlobular lymph vessels

Drainage follows bronchi, arteries and veins

Left tracheal (paratracheal) nodes

Bronchomediastinal lymph trunk

Brachiocephalic vein

Inferior deep cervical (scalene) node

Thoracic duct

Left superior tracheobronchial nodes

Aortic arch node

Bronchopulmonary (hilar) nodes

Pulmonary (intra-pulmonary) nodes

Subpleural lymphatic plexus

Interlobular lymph vessels

Drainage follows bronchi, arteries and veins

Inferior tracheobronchial (carinal) nodes

Pulmonary ligaments

Routes to mediastinum

Drainage routes

Right lung: All lobes drain to intrapulmonary and broncho-pulmonary (hilar) nodes, then to inferior tracheobronchial (carinal) nodes, right superior tracheobronchial nodes and to right tracheal nodes on way to brachiocephalic vein via bronchomediastinal lymph trunk and/or scalene node.
Left lung: Upper lobe drains to pulmonary and hilar nodes, carinal nodes, left superior tracheobronchial nodes, left tracheal nodes and/or aortic arch node, then to brachio-cephalic vein via left bronchomediastinal trunk and thoracic duct. Left lower lobe drains also to pulmonary and hilar nodes and to carinal nodes, but then mostly to right superior tracheobronchial nodes, where it follows same route as lymph from right lung

SEE ALSO PLATES 124, 125, 152, 304

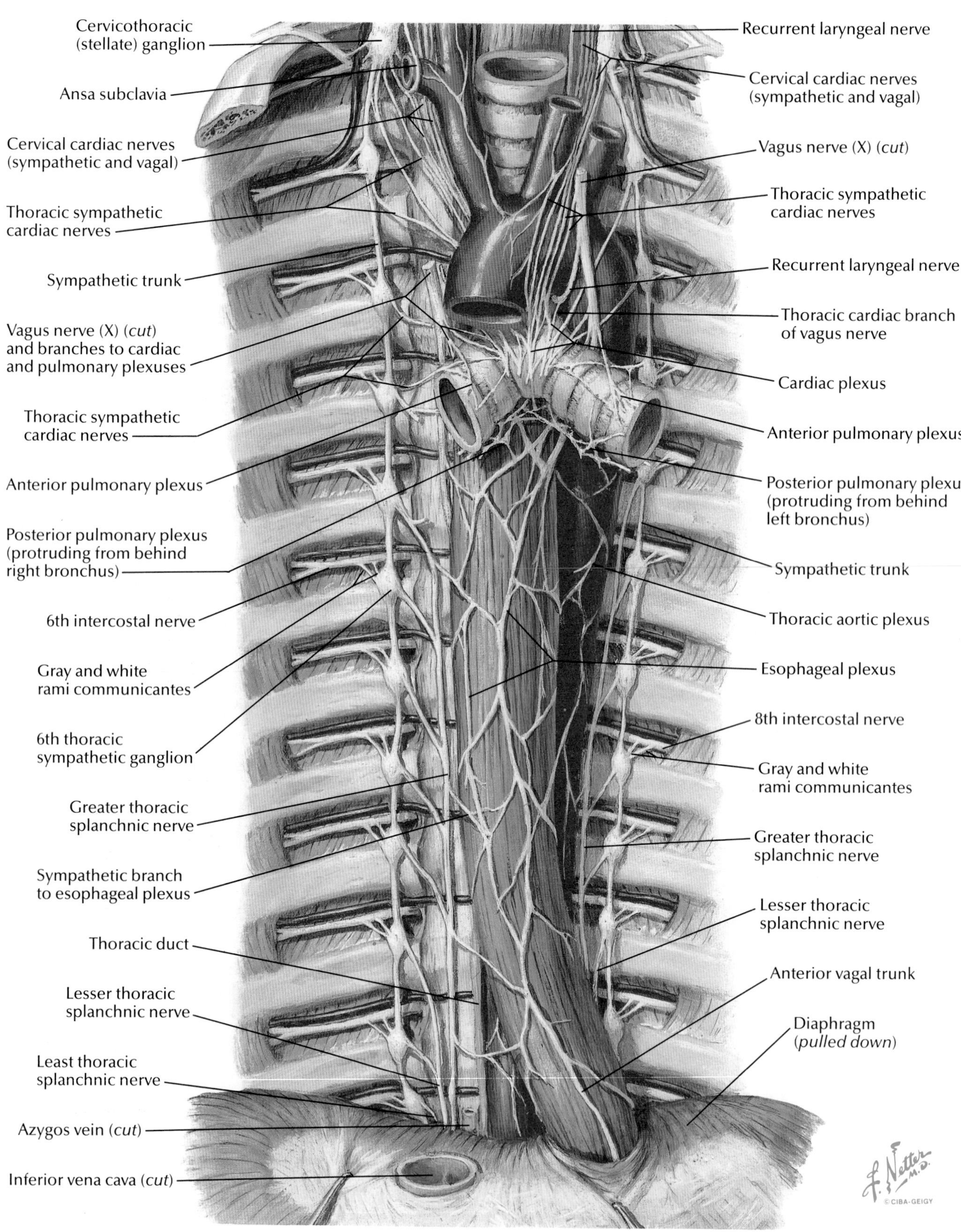

Cervicothoracic (stellate) ganglion

Ansa subclavia

Cervical cardiac nerves (sympathetic and vagal)

Thoracic sympathetic cardiac nerves

Sympathetic trunk

Vagus nerve (X) (cut) and branches to cardiac and pulmonary plexuses

Thoracic sympathetic cardiac nerves

Anterior pulmonary plexus

Posterior pulmonary plexus (protruding from behind right bronchus)

6th intercostal nerve

Gray and white rami communicantes

6th thoracic sympathetic ganglion

Greater thoracic splanchnic nerve

Sympathetic branch to esophageal plexus

Thoracic duct

Lesser thoracic splanchnic nerve

Least thoracic splanchnic nerve

Azygos vein (cut)

Inferior vena cava (cut)

Recurrent laryngeal nerve

Cervical cardiac nerves (sympathetic and vagal)

Vagus nerve (X) (cut)

Thoracic sympathetic cardiac nerves

Recurrent laryngeal nerve

Thoracic cardiac branch of vagus nerve

Cardiac plexus

Anterior pulmonary plexus

Posterior pulmonary plexus (protruding from behind left bronchus)

Sympathetic trunk

Thoracic aortic plexus

Esophageal plexus

8th intercostal nerve

Gray and white rami communicantes

Greater thoracic splanchnic nerve

Lesser thoracic splanchnic nerve

Anterior vagal trunk

Diaphragm (pulled down)

© CIBA-GEIGY

PLATE 198

THORAX

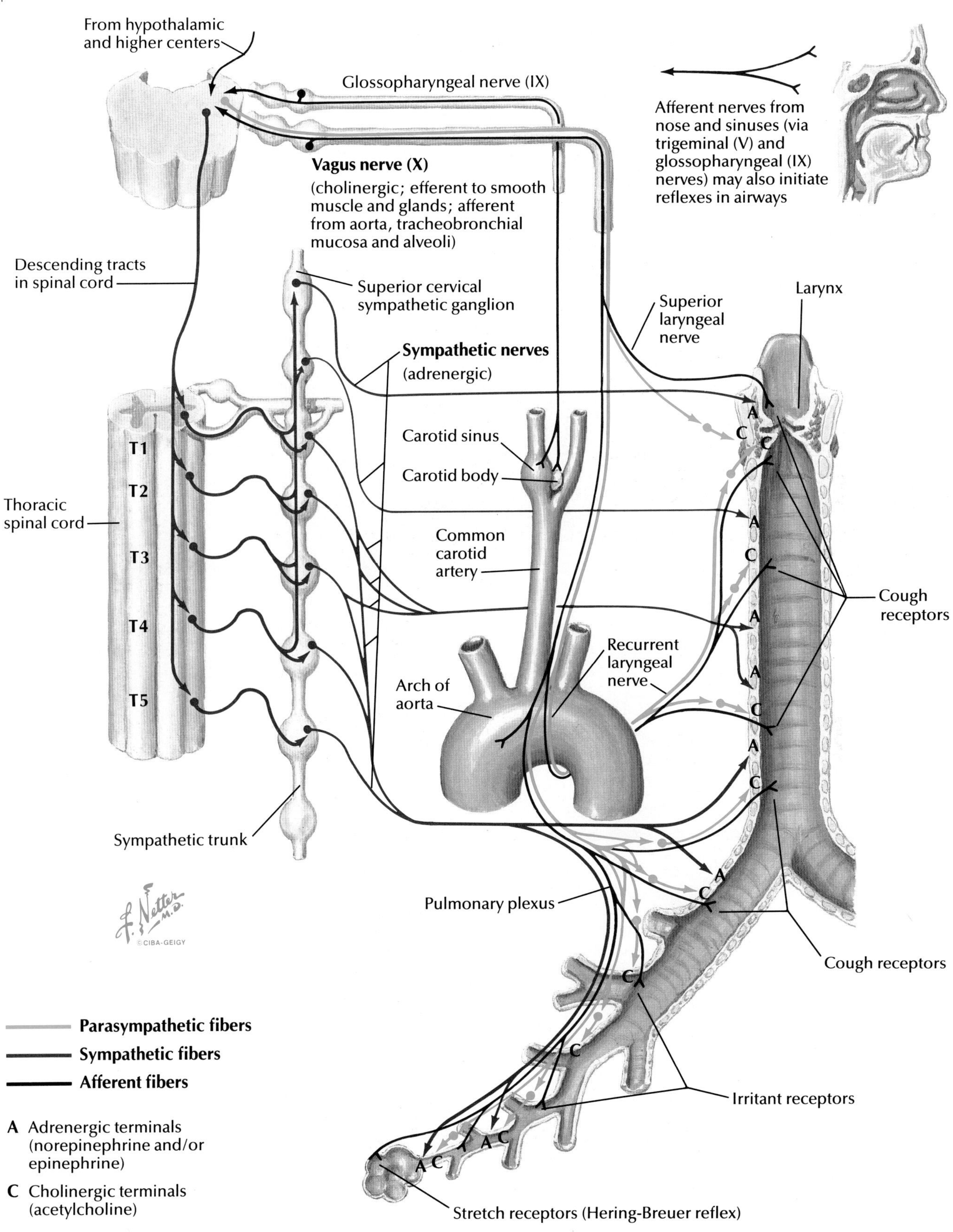

From hypothalamic and higher centers

Glossopharyngeal nerve (IX)

Afferent nerves from nose and sinuses (via trigeminal (V) and glossopharyngeal (IX) nerves) may also initiate reflexes in airways

Vagus nerve (X)
(cholinergic; efferent to smooth muscle and glands; afferent from aorta, tracheobronchial mucosa and alveoli)

Descending tracts in spinal cord

Superior cervical sympathetic ganglion

Superior laryngeal nerve

Larynx

Sympathetic nerves
(adrenergic)

Carotid sinus

Carotid body

T1

T2

Thoracic spinal cord

T3

Common carotid artery

Cough receptors

T4

Recurrent laryngeal nerve

Arch of aorta

T5

Sympathetic trunk

Pulmonary plexus

Cough receptors

f. Netter M.D.
©CIBA-GEIGY

Irritant receptors

——— **Parasympathetic fibers**

——— **Sympathetic fibers**

——— **Afferent fibers**

A Adrenergic terminals (norepinephrine and/or epinephrine)

C Cholinergic terminals (acetylcholine)

Stretch receptors (Hering-Breuer reflex)

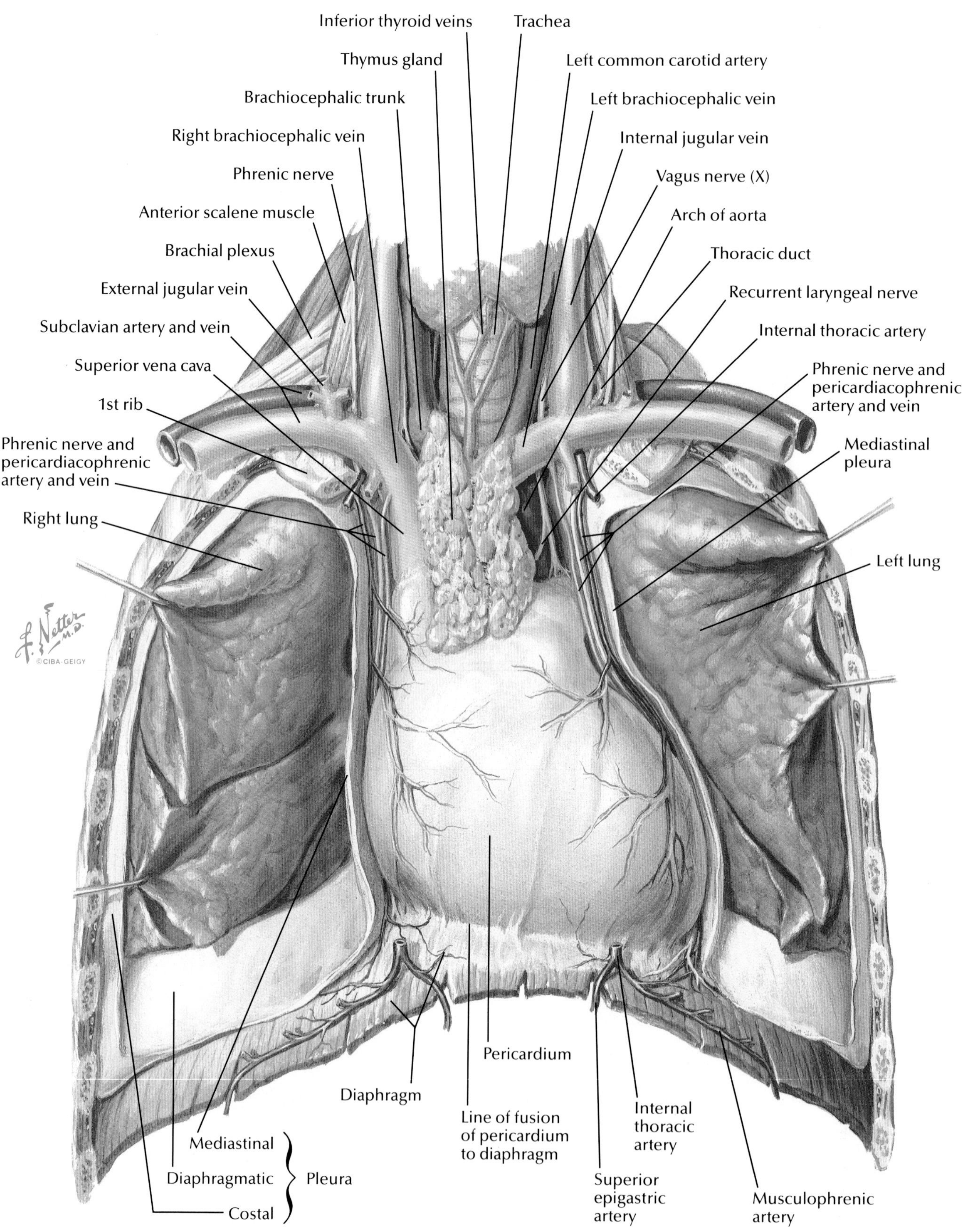

Inferior thyroid veins

Thymus gland

Brachiocephalic trunk

Right brachiocephalic vein

Phrenic nerve

Anterior scalene muscle

Brachial plexus

External jugular vein

Subclavian artery and vein

Superior vena cava

1st rib

Phrenic nerve and pericardiacophrenic artery and vein

Right lung

Trachea

Left common carotid artery

Left brachiocephalic vein

Internal jugular vein

Vagus nerve (X)

Arch of aorta

Thoracic duct

Recurrent laryngeal nerve

Internal thoracic artery

Phrenic nerve and pericardiacophrenic artery and vein

Mediastinal pleura

Left lung

Pericardium

Diaphragm

Line of fusion of pericardium to diaphragm

Internal thoracic artery

Superior epigastric artery

Musculophrenic artery

Mediastinal

Diaphragmatic } Pleura

Costal

PLATE 200

THORAX

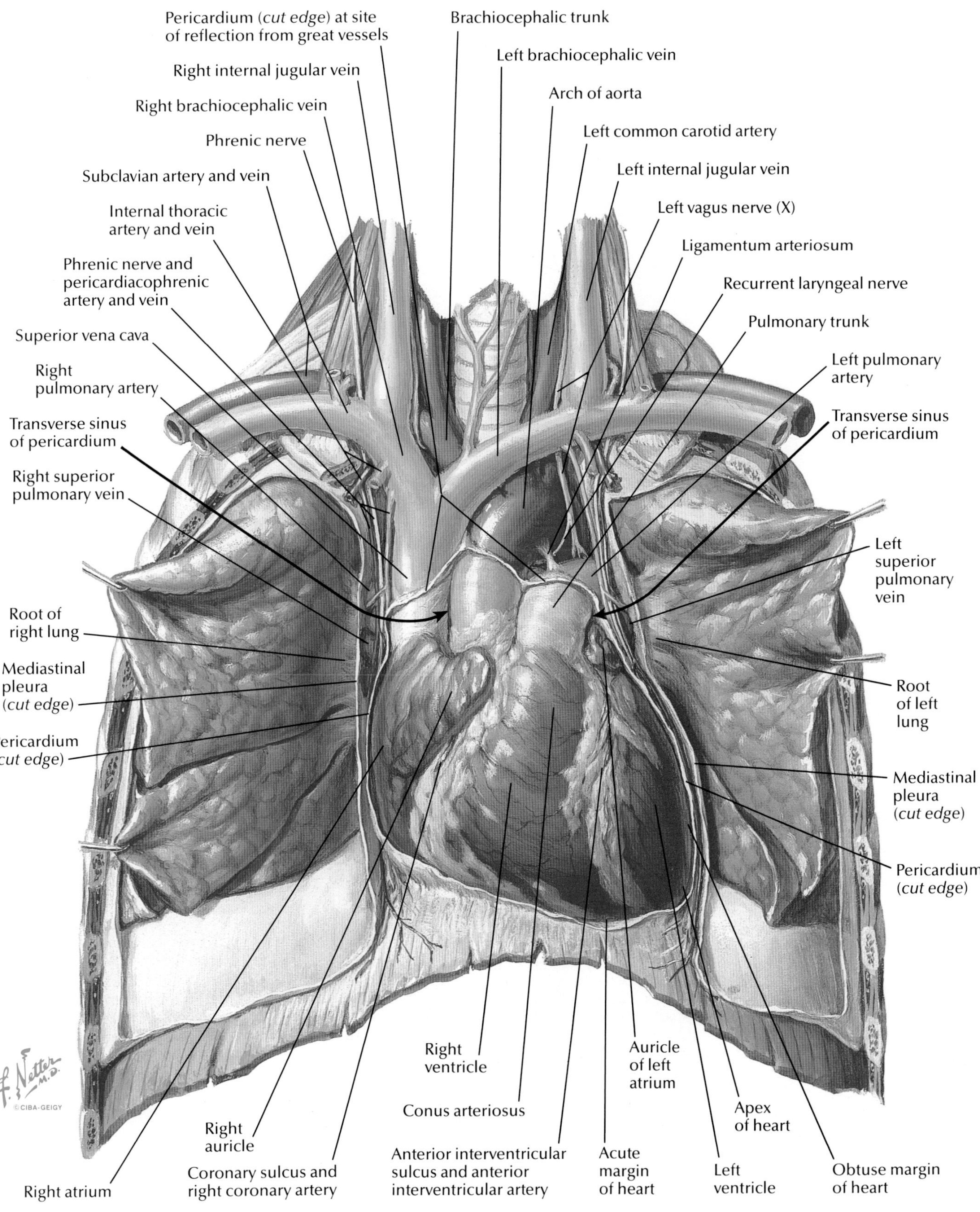

Pericardium (*cut edge*) at site of reflection from great vessels

Right internal jugular vein

Right brachiocephalic vein

Phrenic nerve

Subclavian artery and vein

Internal thoracic artery and vein

Phrenic nerve and pericardiacophrenic artery and vein

Superior vena cava

Right pulmonary artery

Transverse sinus of pericardium

Right superior pulmonary vein

Root of right lung

Mediastinal pleura (*cut edge*)

Pericardium (*cut edge*)

Right atrium

Right auricle

Coronary sulcus and right coronary artery

Right ventricle

Conus arteriosus

Anterior interventricular sulcus and anterior interventricular artery

Brachiocephalic trunk

Left brachiocephalic vein

Arch of aorta

Left common carotid artery

Left internal jugular vein

Left vagus nerve (X)

Ligamentum arteriosum

Recurrent laryngeal nerve

Pulmonary trunk

Left pulmonary artery

Transverse sinus of pericardium

Left superior pulmonary vein

Root of left lung

Mediastinal pleura (*cut edge*)

Pericardium (*cut edge*)

Auricle of left atrium

Apex of heart

Acute margin of heart

Left ventricle

Obtuse margin of heart

f. Netter
©CIBA-GEIGY

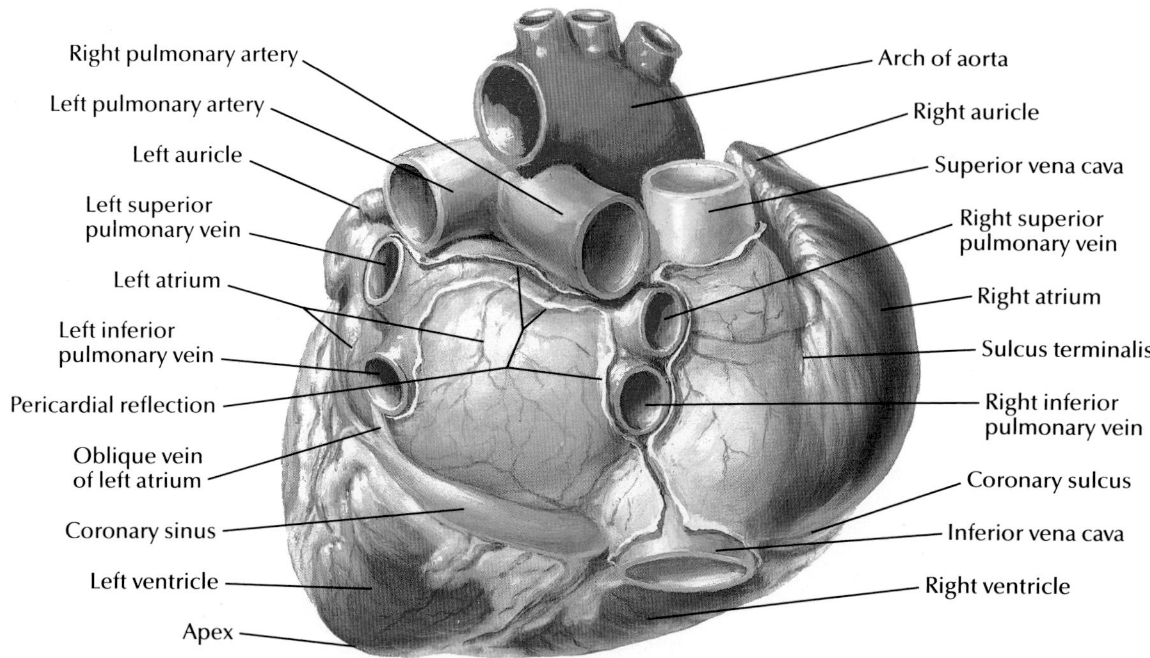

Right pulmonary artery

Left pulmonary artery

Left auricle

Left superior pulmonary vein

Left atrium

Left inferior pulmonary vein

Pericardial reflection

Oblique vein of left atrium

Coronary sinus

Left ventricle

Apex

Arch of aorta

Right auricle

Superior vena cava

Right superior pulmonary vein

Right atrium

Sulcus terminalis

Right inferior pulmonary vein

Coronary sulcus

Inferior vena cava

Right ventricle

Base of heart: posterior view

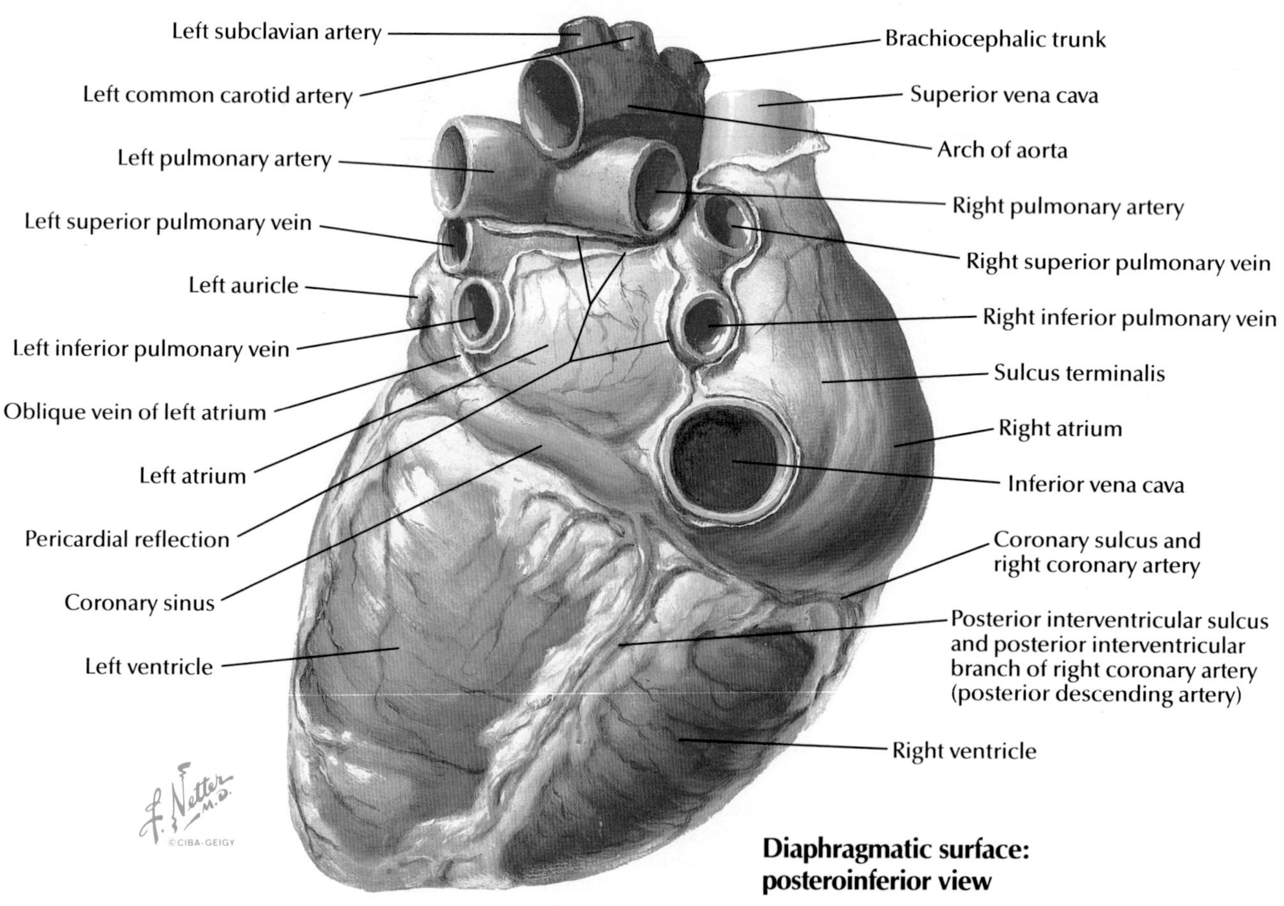

Left subclavian artery

Left common carotid artery

Left pulmonary artery

Left superior pulmonary vein

Left auricle

Left inferior pulmonary vein

Oblique vein of left atrium

Left atrium

Pericardial reflection

Coronary sinus

Left ventricle

Brachiocephalic trunk

Superior vena cava

Arch of aorta

Right pulmonary artery

Right superior pulmonary vein

Right inferior pulmonary vein

Sulcus terminalis

Right atrium

Inferior vena cava

Coronary sulcus and right coronary artery

Posterior interventricular sulcus and posterior interventricular branch of right coronary artery (posterior descending artery)

Right ventricle

Diaphragmatic surface: posteroinferior view

PLATE 202

THORAX

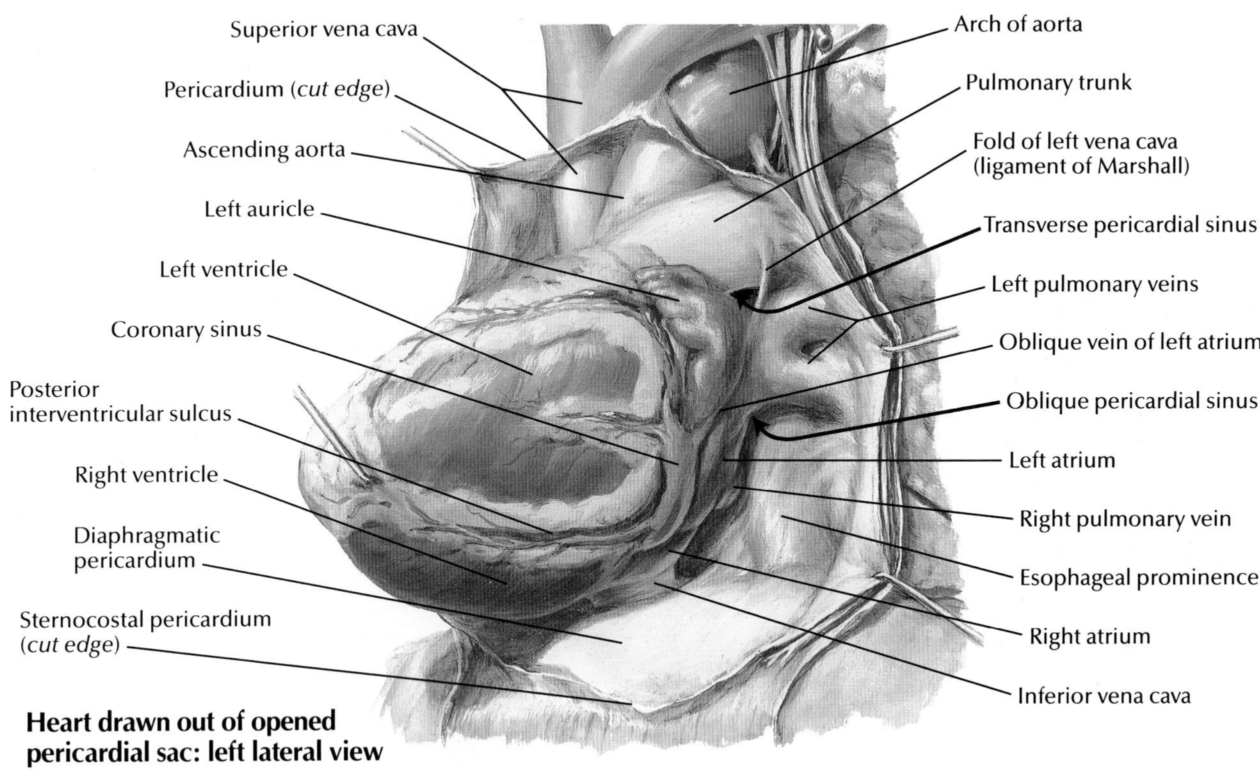

Superior vena cava

Pericardium (*cut edge*)

Ascending aorta

Left auricle

Left ventricle

Coronary sinus

Posterior interventricular sulcus

Right ventricle

Diaphragmatic pericardium

Sternocostal pericardium (*cut edge*)

Arch of aorta

Pulmonary trunk

Fold of left vena cava (ligament of Marshall)

Transverse pericardial sinus

Left pulmonary veins

Oblique vein of left atrium

Oblique pericardial sinus

Left atrium

Right pulmonary vein

Esophageal prominence

Right atrium

Inferior vena cava

Heart drawn out of opened pericardial sac: left lateral view

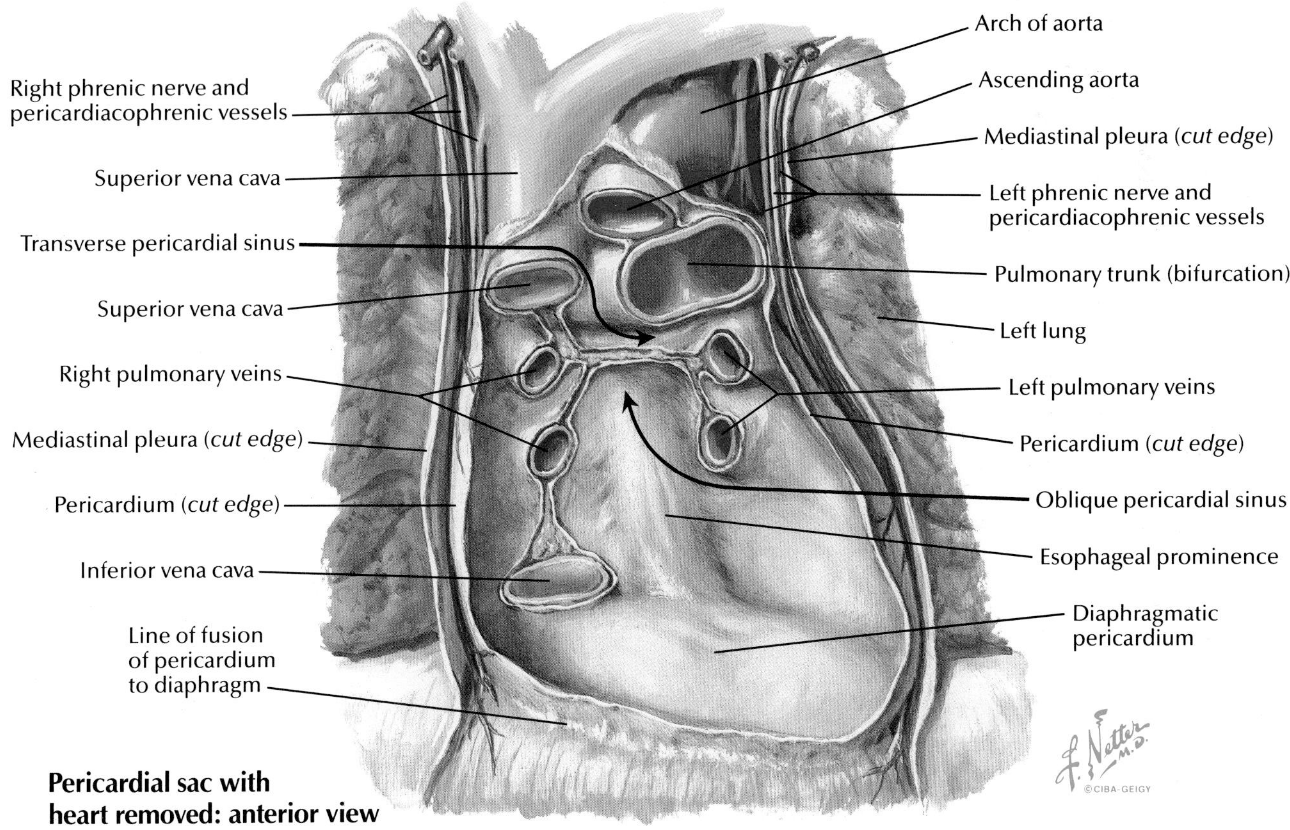

Right phrenic nerve and pericardiacophrenic vessels

Superior vena cava

Transverse pericardial sinus

Superior vena cava

Right pulmonary veins

Mediastinal pleura (*cut edge*)

Pericardium (*cut edge*)

Inferior vena cava

Line of fusion of pericardium to diaphragm

Arch of aorta

Ascending aorta

Mediastinal pleura (*cut edge*)

Left phrenic nerve and pericardiacophrenic vessels

Pulmonary trunk (bifurcation)

Left lung

Left pulmonary veins

Pericardium (*cut edge*)

Oblique pericardial sinus

Esophageal prominence

Diaphragmatic pericardium

Pericardial sac with heart removed: anterior view

PLATE 203

Coronary Arteries and Cardiac Veins

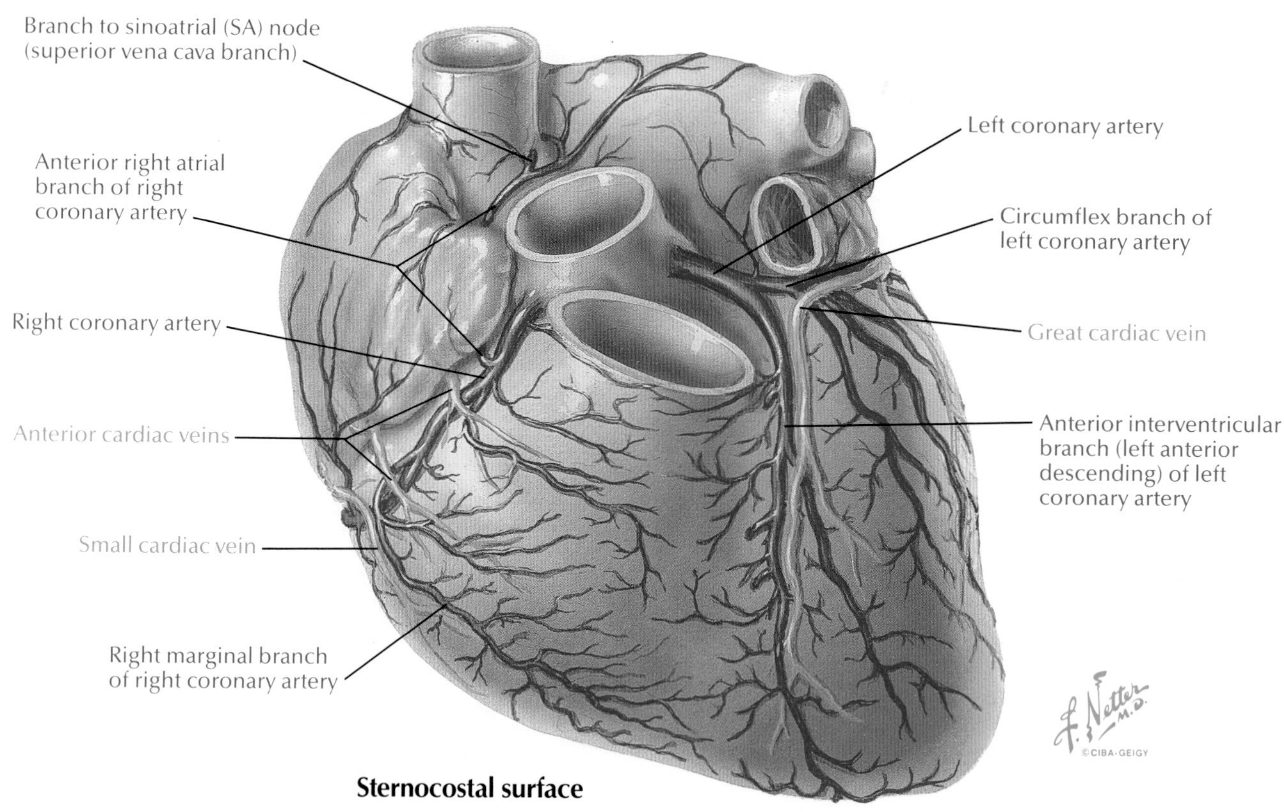

Branch to sinoatrial (SA) node (superior vena cava branch)

Anterior right atrial branch of right coronary artery

Right coronary artery

Anterior cardiac veins

Small cardiac vein

Right marginal branch of right coronary artery

Left coronary artery

Circumflex branch of left coronary artery

Great cardiac vein

Anterior interventricular branch (left anterior descending) of left coronary artery

Sternocostal surface

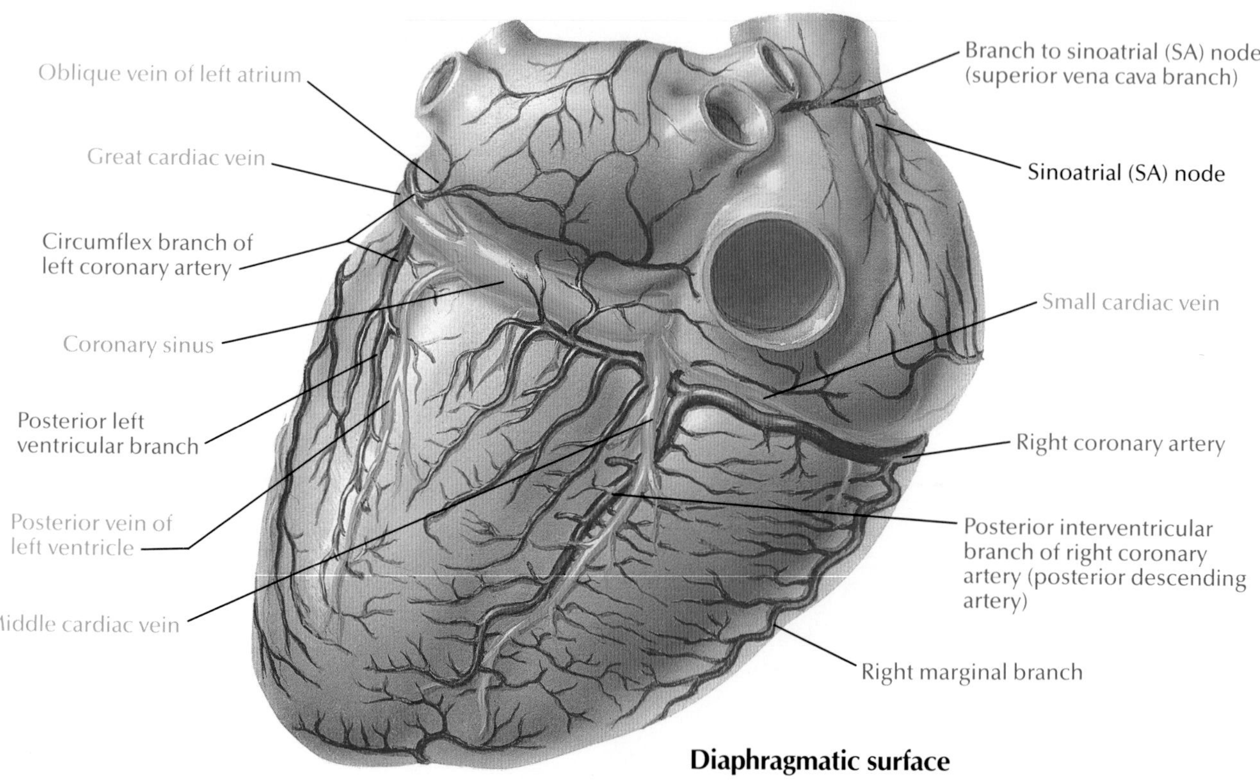

Oblique vein of left atrium

Great cardiac vein

Circumflex branch of left coronary artery

Coronary sinus

Posterior left ventricular branch

Posterior vein of left ventricle

Middle cardiac vein

Branch to sinoatrial (SA) node (superior vena cava branch)

Sinoatrial (SA) node

Small cardiac vein

Right coronary artery

Posterior interventricular branch of right coronary artery (posterior descending artery)

Right marginal branch

Diaphragmatic surface

PLATE 204

THORAX

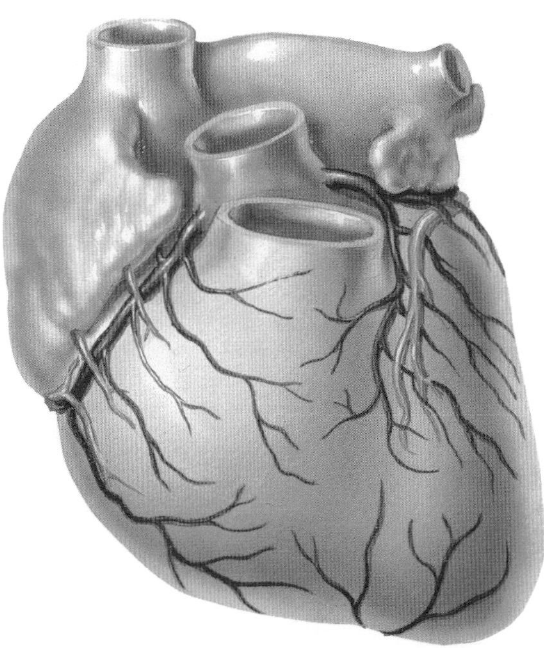

Anterior interventricular (left anterior descending) branch of left coronary artery very short. Apical part of sternocostal surface supplied by branches from posterior interventricular (posterior descending) branch of right coronary artery curving around apex

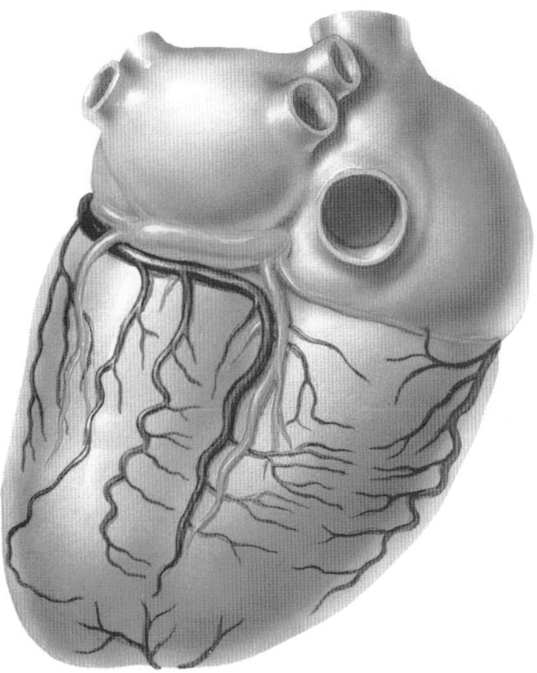

Posterior interventricular (posterior descending) branch derived from circumflex branch of left coronary artery instead of from right coronary artery

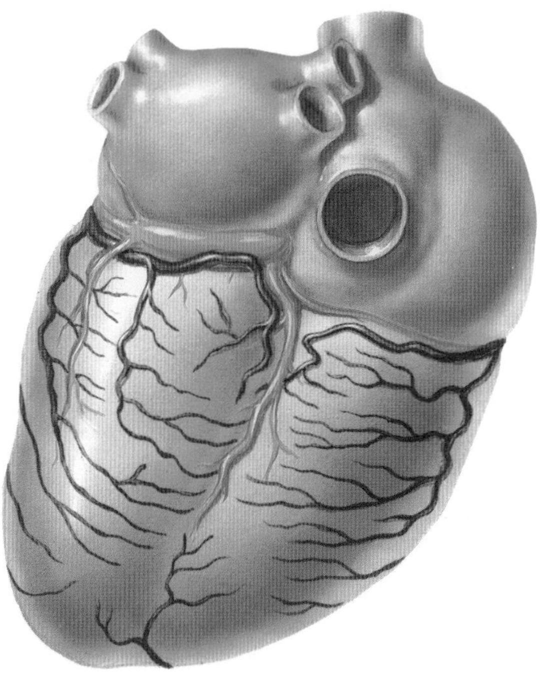

Posterior interventricular (posterior descending) branch absent. Area supplied chiefly by small branches from circumflex branch of left coronary artery and from right coronary artery

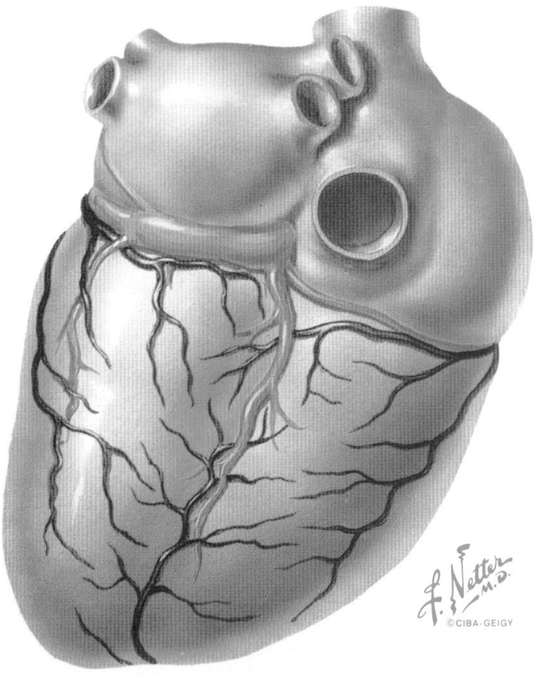

Posterior interventricular (posterior descending) branch absent. Area supplied chiefly by elongated anterior interventricular (left anterior descending) branch curving around apex

Right coronary artery: left anterior oblique view

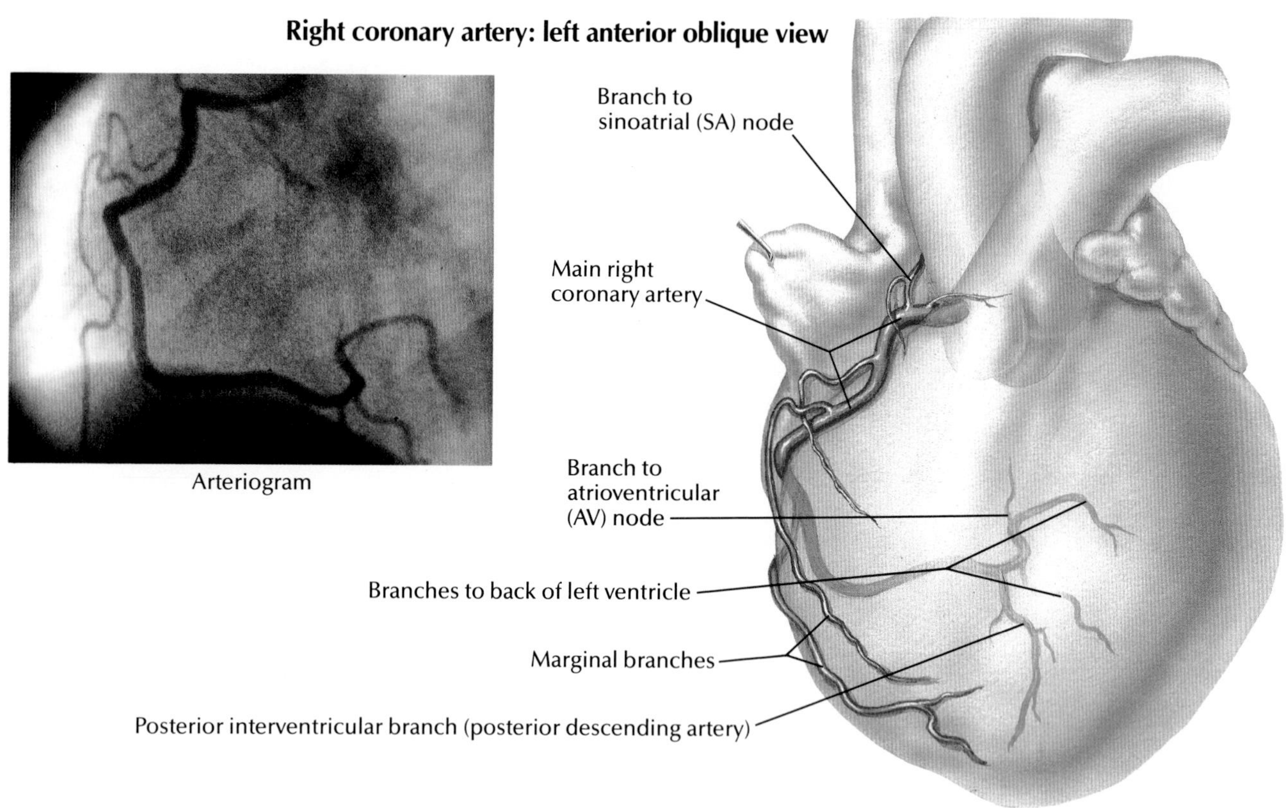

Arteriogram

Branch to sinoatrial (SA) node

Main right coronary artery

Branch to atrioventricular (AV) node

Branches to back of left ventricle

Marginal branches

Posterior interventricular branch (posterior descending artery)

Right coronary artery: right anterior oblique view

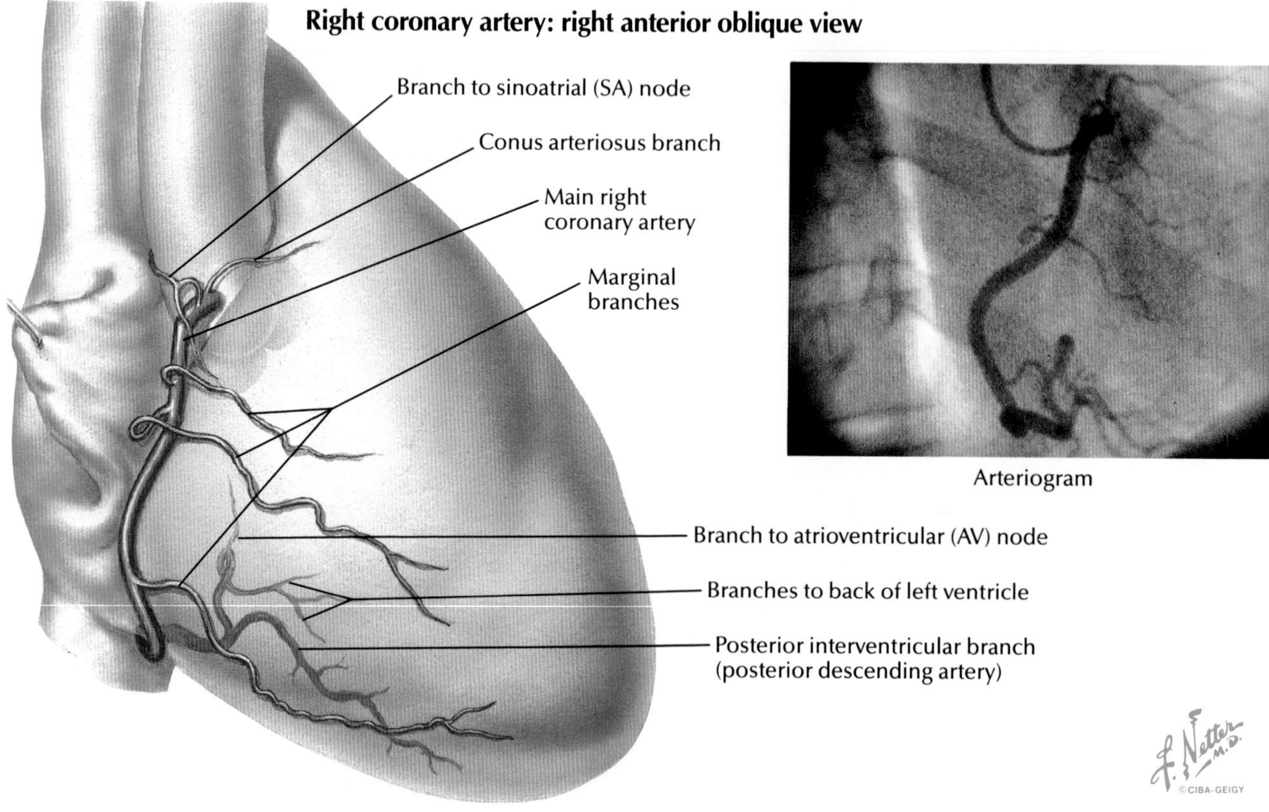

Branch to sinoatrial (SA) node

Conus arteriosus branch

Main right coronary artery

Marginal branches

Arteriogram

Branch to atrioventricular (AV) node

Branches to back of left ventricle

Posterior interventricular branch (posterior descending artery)

PLATE 206

THORAX

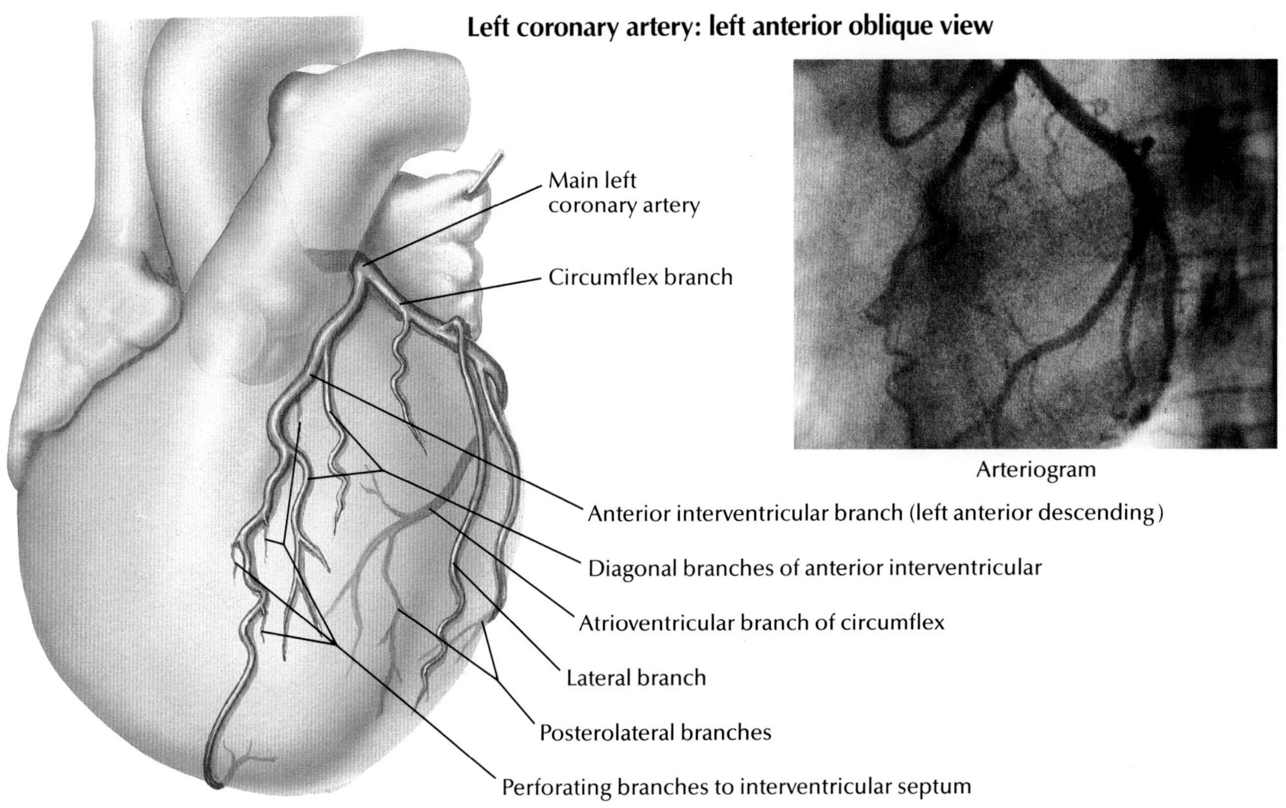

Left coronary artery: left anterior oblique view

Main left coronary artery

Circumflex branch

Arteriogram

Anterior interventricular branch (left anterior descending)

Diagonal branches of anterior interventricular

Atrioventricular branch of circumflex

Lateral branch

Posterolateral branches

Perforating branches to interventricular septum

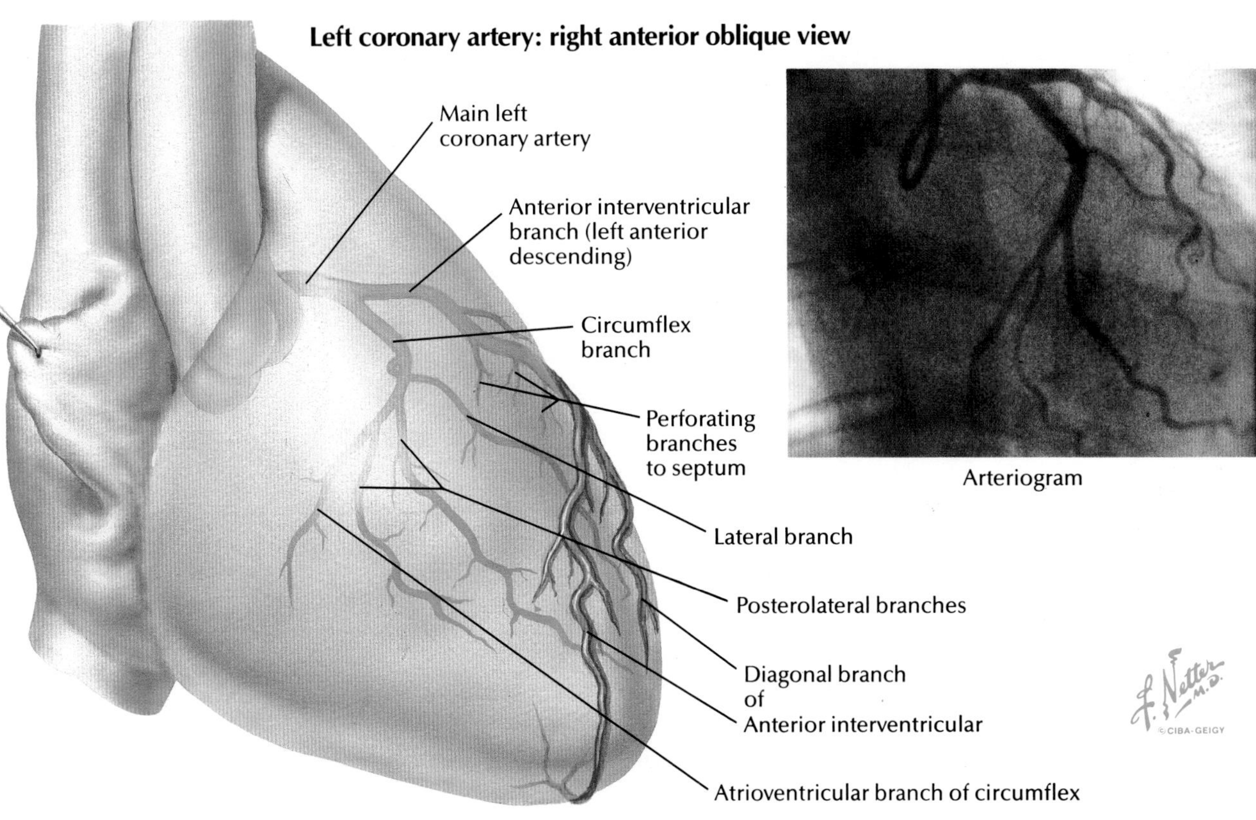

Left coronary artery: right anterior oblique view

Main left coronary artery

Anterior interventricular branch (left anterior descending)

Circumflex branch

Perforating branches to septum

Arteriogram

Lateral branch

Posterolateral branches

Diagonal branch of Anterior interventricular

Atrioventricular branch of circumflex

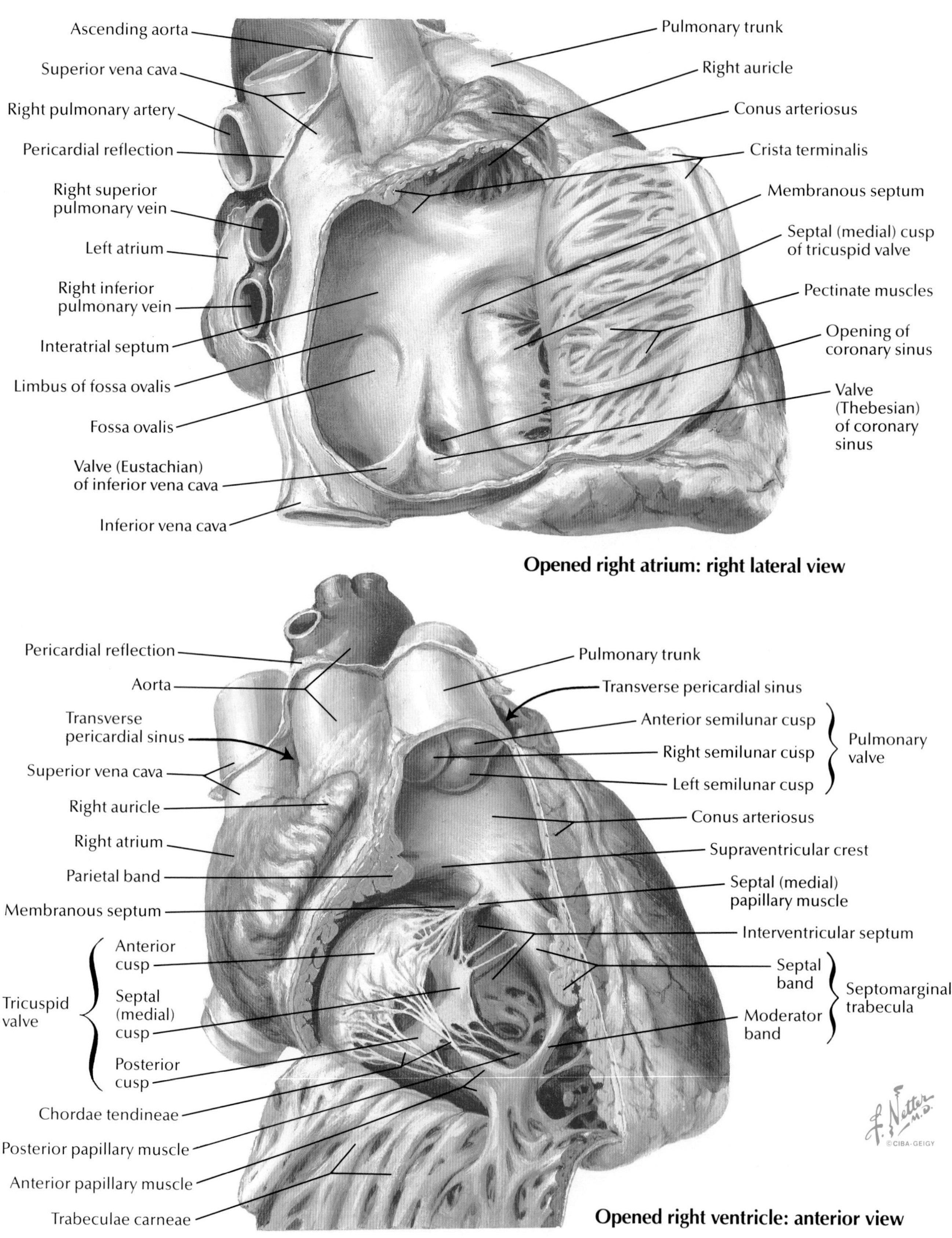

Ascending aorta

Superior vena cava

Right pulmonary artery

Pericardial reflection

Right superior pulmonary vein

Left atrium

Right inferior pulmonary vein

Interatrial septum

Limbus of fossa ovalis

Fossa ovalis

Valve (Eustachian) of inferior vena cava

Inferior vena cava

Pulmonary trunk

Right auricle

Conus arteriosus

Crista terminalis

Membranous septum

Septal (medial) cusp of tricuspid valve

Pectinate muscles

Opening of coronary sinus

Valve (Thebesian) of coronary sinus

Opened right atrium: right lateral view

Pericardial reflection

Aorta

Transverse pericardial sinus

Superior vena cava

Right auricle

Right atrium

Parietal band

Membranous septum

Tricuspid valve
- Anterior cusp
- Septal (medial) cusp
- Posterior cusp

Chordae tendineae

Posterior papillary muscle

Anterior papillary muscle

Trabeculae carneae

Pulmonary trunk

Transverse pericardial sinus

Anterior semilunar cusp

Right semilunar cusp — Pulmonary valve

Left semilunar cusp

Conus arteriosus

Supraventricular crest

Septal (medial) papillary muscle

Interventricular septum

Septal band — Septomarginal trabecula

Moderator band

Opened right ventricle: anterior view

PLATE 208

THORAX

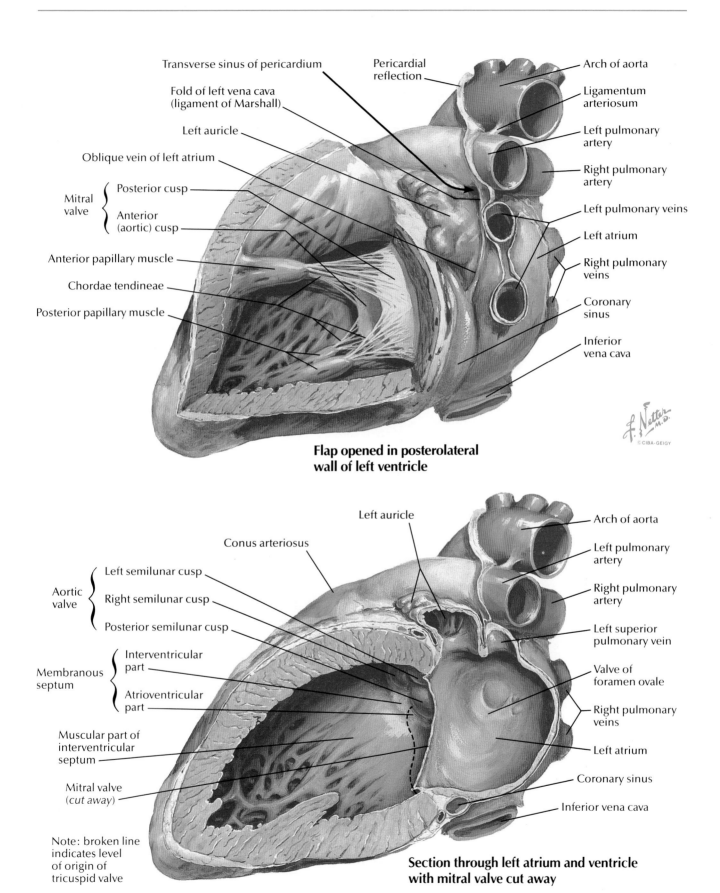

Transverse sinus of pericardium

Pericardial reflection

Arch of aorta

Ligamentum arteriosum

Fold of left vena cava (ligament of Marshall)

Left pulmonary artery

Left auricle

Right pulmonary artery

Oblique vein of left atrium

Left pulmonary veins

Mitral valve { Posterior cusp

Anterior (aortic) cusp

Left atrium

Right pulmonary veins

Anterior papillary muscle

Coronary sinus

Chordae tendineae

Posterior papillary muscle

Inferior vena cava

Flap opened in posterolateral wall of left ventricle

Left auricle

Arch of aorta

Conus arteriosus

Left pulmonary artery

Right pulmonary artery

Aortic valve { Left semilunar cusp

Right semilunar cusp

Posterior semilunar cusp

Left superior pulmonary vein

Valve of foramen ovale

Membranous septum { Interventricular part

Atrioventricular part

Right pulmonary veins

Muscular part of interventricular septum

Left atrium

Mitral valve (*cut away*)

Coronary sinus

Inferior vena cava

Note: broken line indicates level of origin of tricuspid valve

Section through left atrium and ventricle with mitral valve cut away

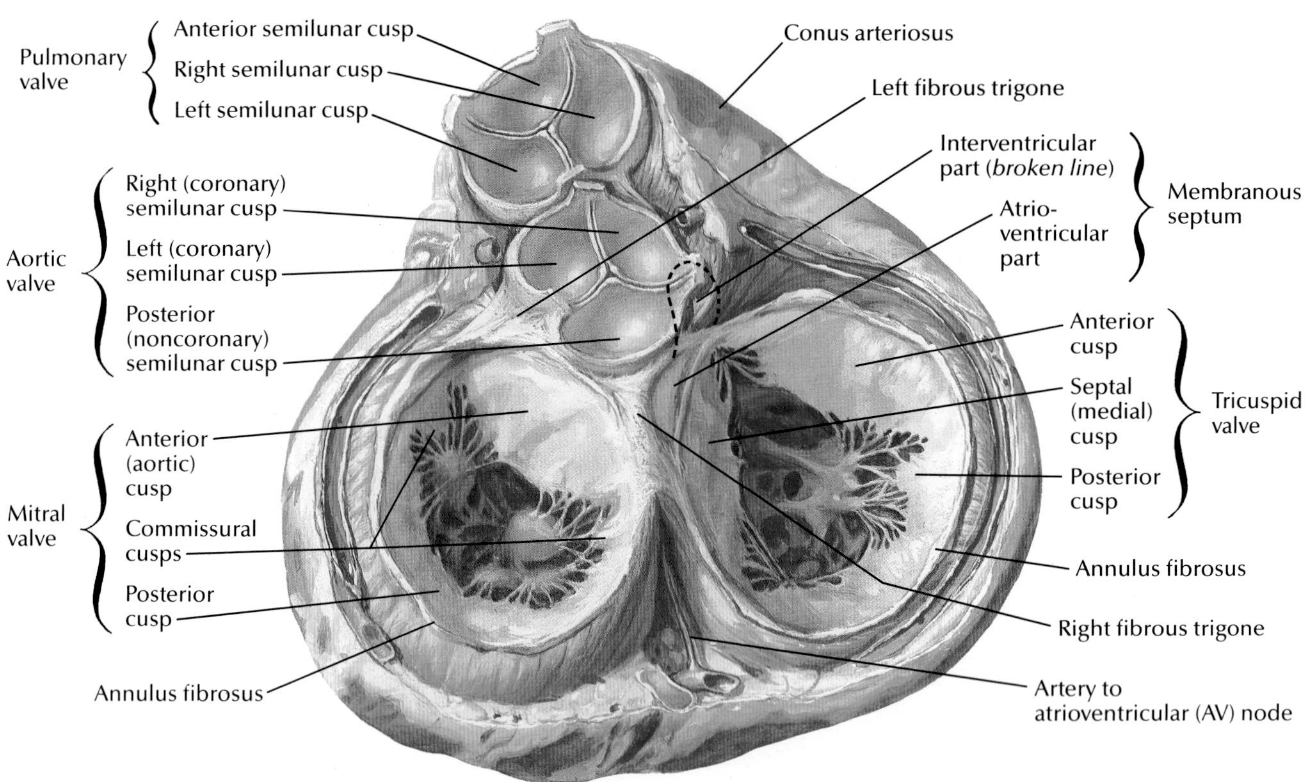

Pulmonary valve
- Anterior semilunar cusp
- Right semilunar cusp
- Left semilunar cusp

Aortic valve
- Right (coronary) semilunar cusp
- Left (coronary) semilunar cusp
- Posterior (noncoronary) semilunar cusp

Mitral valve
- Anterior (aortic) cusp
- Commissural cusps
- Posterior cusp

Annulus fibrosus

Conus arteriosus

Left fibrous trigone

Membranous septum
- Interventricular part (*broken line*)
- Atrio-ventricular part

Tricuspid valve
- Anterior cusp
- Septal (medial) cusp
- Posterior cusp

Annulus fibrosus

Right fibrous trigone

Artery to atrioventricular (AV) node

**Heart in diastole:
viewed from base with atria removed**

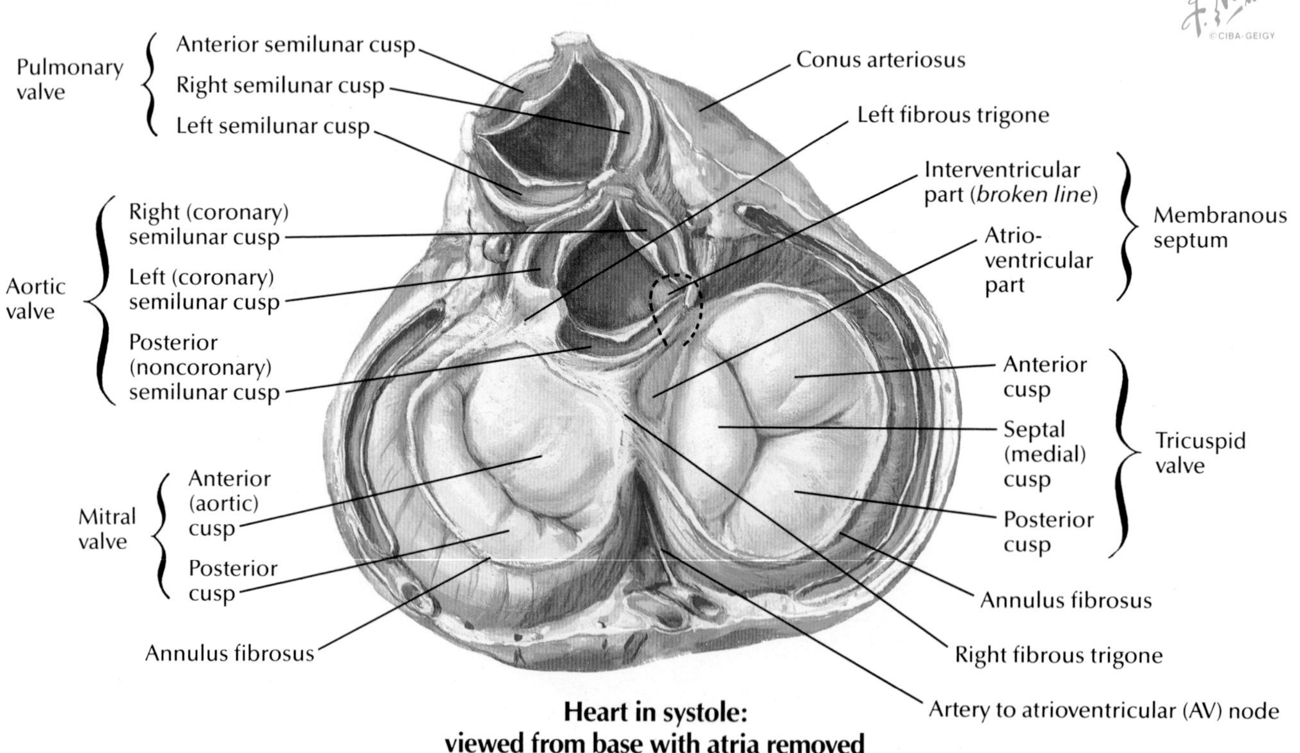

Pulmonary valve
- Anterior semilunar cusp
- Right semilunar cusp
- Left semilunar cusp

Aortic valve
- Right (coronary) semilunar cusp
- Left (coronary) semilunar cusp
- Posterior (noncoronary) semilunar cusp

Mitral valve
- Anterior (aortic) cusp
- Posterior cusp

Annulus fibrosus

Conus arteriosus

Left fibrous trigone

Membranous septum
- Interventricular part (*broken line*)
- Atrio-ventricular part

Tricuspid valve
- Anterior cusp
- Septal (medial) cusp
- Posterior cusp

Annulus fibrosus

Right fibrous trigone

Artery to atrioventricular (AV) node

**Heart in systole:
viewed from base with atria removed**

PLATE 210

THORAX

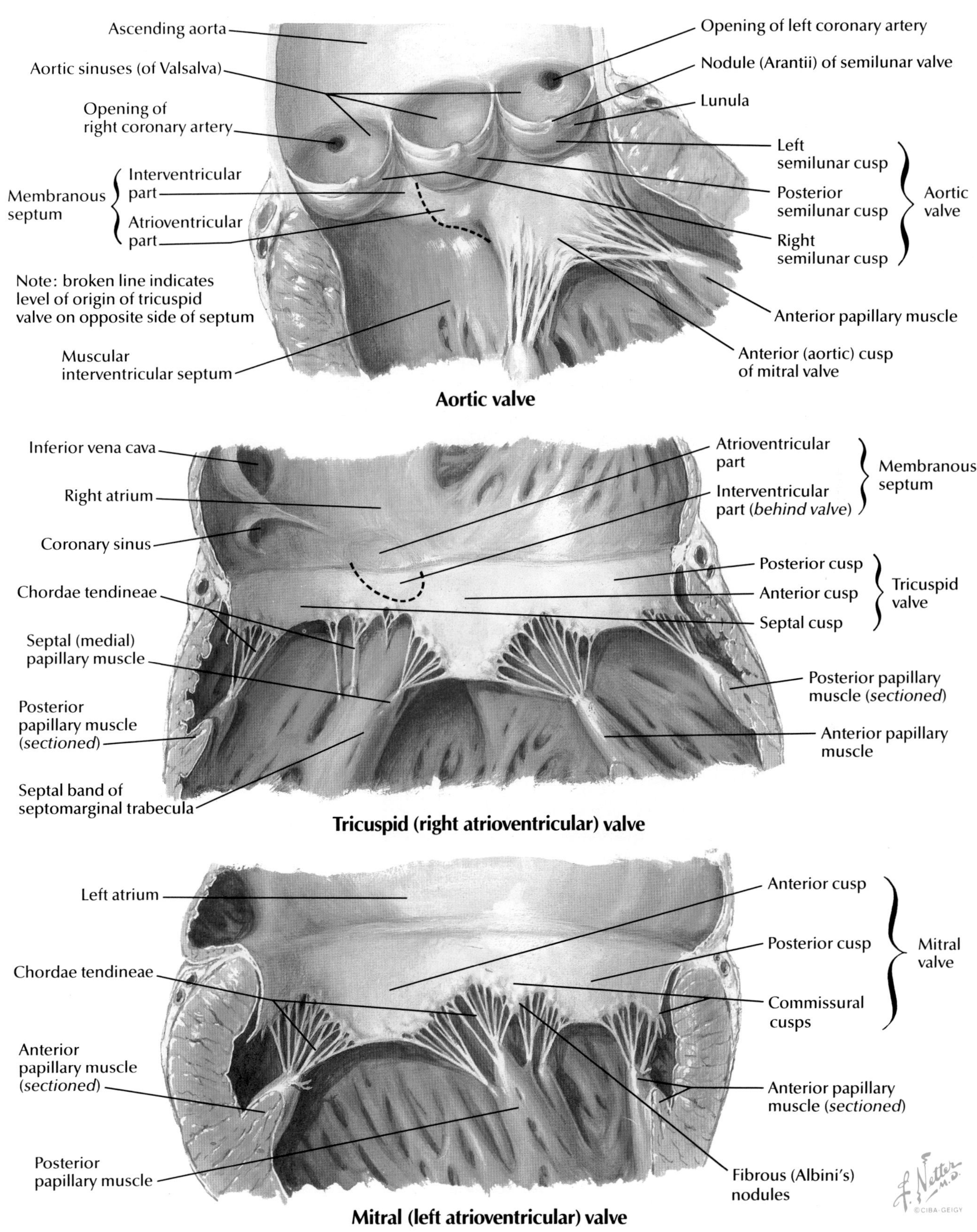

Ascending aorta

Aortic sinuses (of Valsalva)

Opening of right coronary artery

Membranous septum { Interventricular part / Atrioventricular part

Note: broken line indicates level of origin of tricuspid valve on opposite side of septum

Muscular interventricular septum

Opening of left coronary artery

Nodule (Arantii) of semilunar valve

Lunula

Left semilunar cusp

Posterior semilunar cusp } Aortic valve

Right semilunar cusp

Anterior papillary muscle

Anterior (aortic) cusp of mitral valve

Aortic valve

Inferior vena cava

Right atrium

Coronary sinus

Chordae tendineae

Septal (medial) papillary muscle

Posterior papillary muscle (*sectioned*)

Septal band of septomarginal trabecula

Atrioventricular part

Interventricular part (*behind valve*) } Membranous septum

Posterior cusp

Anterior cusp } Tricuspid valve

Septal cusp

Posterior papillary muscle (*sectioned*)

Anterior papillary muscle

Tricuspid (right atrioventricular) valve

Left atrium

Chordae tendineae

Anterior papillary muscle (*sectioned*)

Posterior papillary muscle

Anterior cusp

Posterior cusp } Mitral valve

Commissural cusps

Anterior papillary muscle (*sectioned*)

Fibrous (Albini's) nodules

Mitral (left atrioventricular) valve

Atria, Ventricles and Interventricular Septum

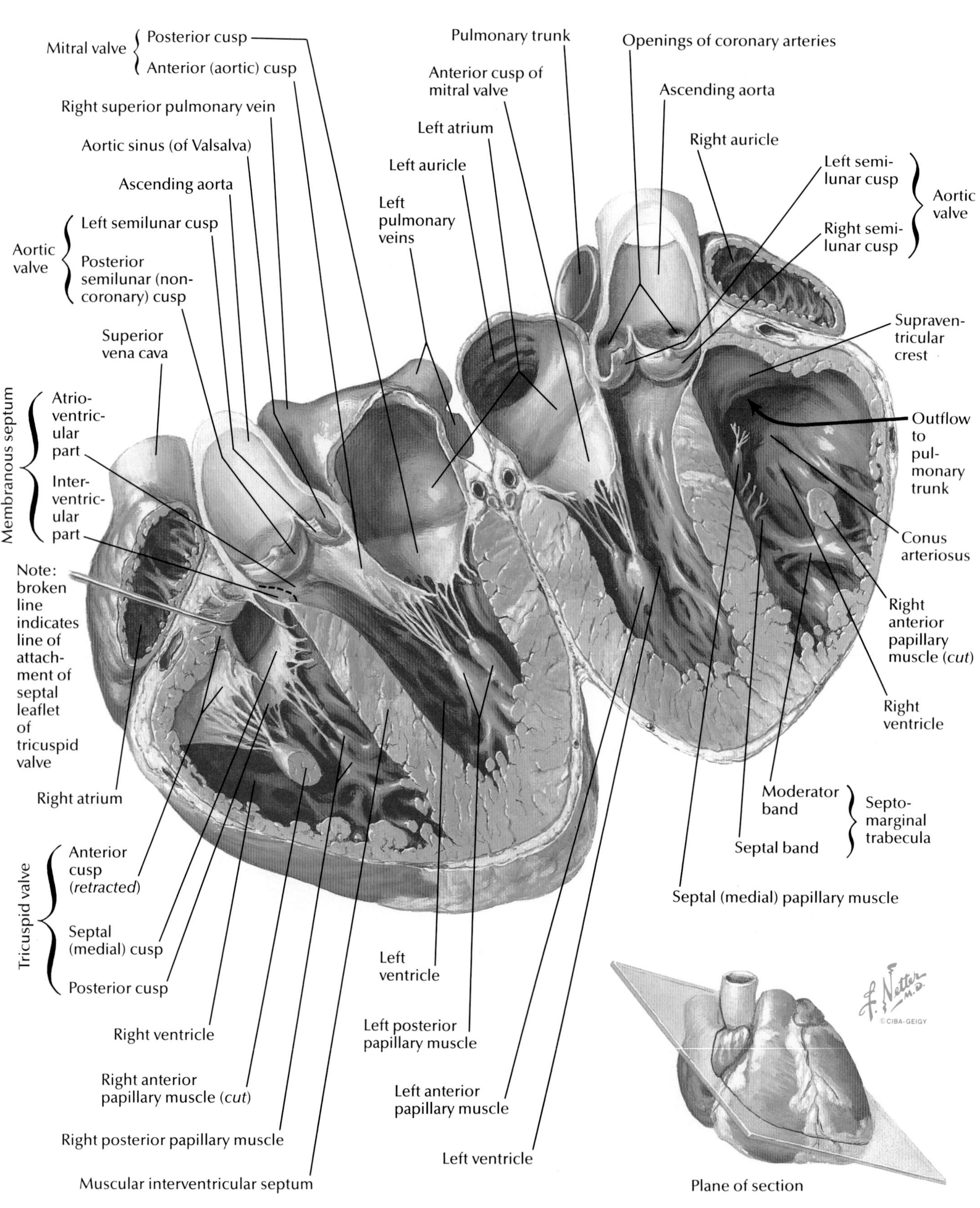

Mitral valve {
Posterior cusp
Anterior (aortic) cusp

Right superior pulmonary vein

Aortic sinus (of Valsalva)

Ascending aorta

Aortic valve {
Left semilunar cusp
Posterior semilunar (non-coronary) cusp

Superior vena cava

Membranous septum {
Atrio-ventricular part
Inter-ventricular part

Note: broken line indicates line of attachment of septal leaflet of tricuspid valve

Right atrium

Tricuspid valve {
Anterior cusp (retracted)
Septal (medial) cusp
Posterior cusp

Right ventricle

Right anterior papillary muscle (cut)

Right posterior papillary muscle

Muscular interventricular septum

Pulmonary trunk

Anterior cusp of mitral valve

Left atrium

Left auricle

Left pulmonary veins

Left ventricle

Left posterior papillary muscle

Left anterior papillary muscle

Left ventricle

Openings of coronary arteries

Ascending aorta

Right auricle

Left semilunar cusp

Right semilunar cusp

Aortic valve }

Supraventricular crest

Outflow to pulmonary trunk

Conus arteriosus

Right anterior papillary muscle (cut)

Right ventricle

Moderator band

Septal band

Septo-marginal trabecula }

Septal (medial) papillary muscle

Plane of section

PLATE 212

THORAX

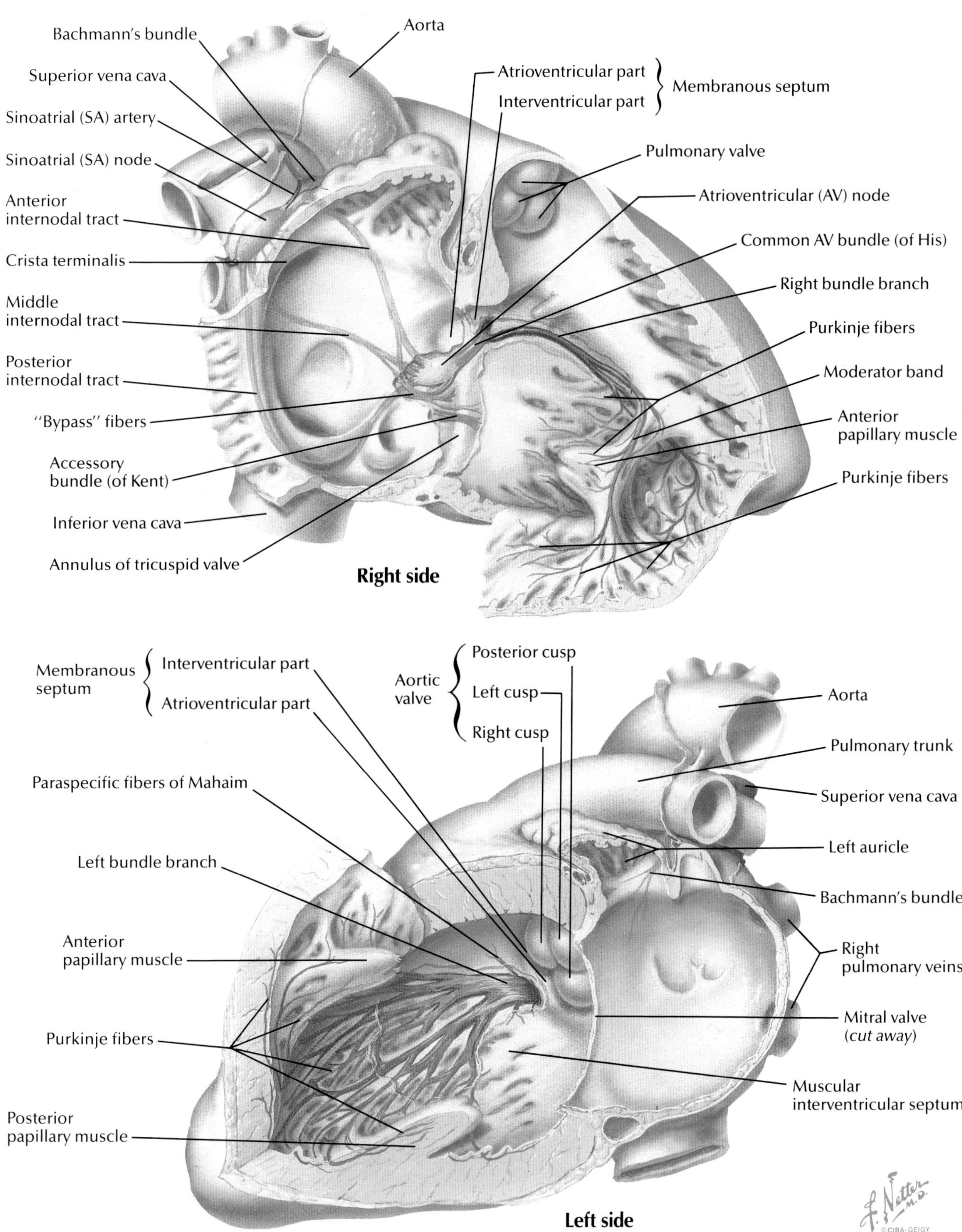

Bachmann's bundle

Aorta

Superior vena cava

Sinoatrial (SA) artery

Sinoatrial (SA) node

Atrioventricular part
Interventricular part
} Membranous septum

Anterior
internodal tract

Pulmonary valve

Atrioventricular (AV) node

Crista terminalis

Common AV bundle (of His)

Middle
internodal tract

Right bundle branch

Purkinje fibers

Posterior
internodal tract

Moderator band

"Bypass" fibers

Anterior
papillary muscle

Accessory
bundle (of Kent)

Purkinje fibers

Inferior vena cava

Annulus of tricuspid valve

Right side

Membranous
septum
{ Interventricular part
Atrioventricular part

Aortic
valve
{ Posterior cusp
Left cusp
Right cusp

Aorta

Pulmonary trunk

Superior vena cava

Paraspecific fibers of Mahaim

Left auricle

Left bundle branch

Bachmann's bundle

Anterior
papillary muscle

Right
pulmonary veins

Mitral valve
(*cut away*)

Purkinje fibers

Posterior
papillary muscle

Muscular
interventricular septum

Left side

SEE ALSO PLATES 124, 152, 198

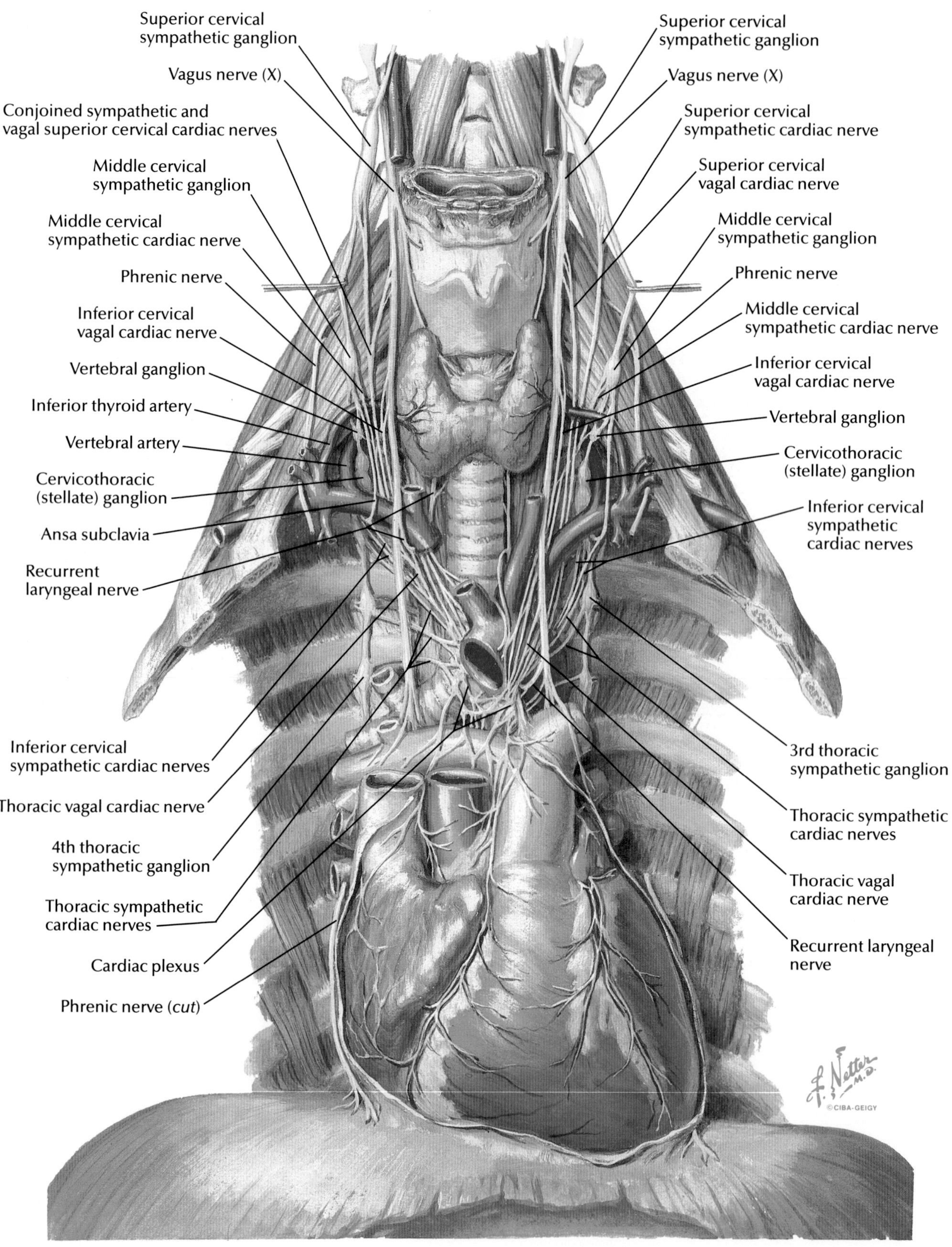

Superior cervical sympathetic ganglion

Vagus nerve (X)

Conjoined sympathetic and vagal superior cervical cardiac nerves

Middle cervical sympathetic ganglion

Middle cervical sympathetic cardiac nerve

Phrenic nerve

Inferior cervical vagal cardiac nerve

Vertebral ganglion

Inferior thyroid artery

Vertebral artery

Cervicothoracic (stellate) ganglion

Ansa subclavia

Recurrent laryngeal nerve

Inferior cervical sympathetic cardiac nerves

Thoracic vagal cardiac nerve

4th thoracic sympathetic ganglion

Thoracic sympathetic cardiac nerves

Cardiac plexus

Phrenic nerve (*cut*)

Superior cervical sympathetic ganglion

Vagus nerve (X)

Superior cervical sympathetic cardiac nerve

Superior cervical vagal cardiac nerve

Middle cervical sympathetic ganglion

Phrenic nerve

Middle cervical sympathetic cardiac nerve

Inferior cervical vagal cardiac nerve

Vertebral ganglion

Cervicothoracic (stellate) ganglion

Inferior cervical sympathetic cardiac nerves

3rd thoracic sympathetic ganglion

Thoracic sympathetic cardiac nerves

Thoracic vagal cardiac nerve

Recurrent laryngeal nerve

PLATE 214

THORAX

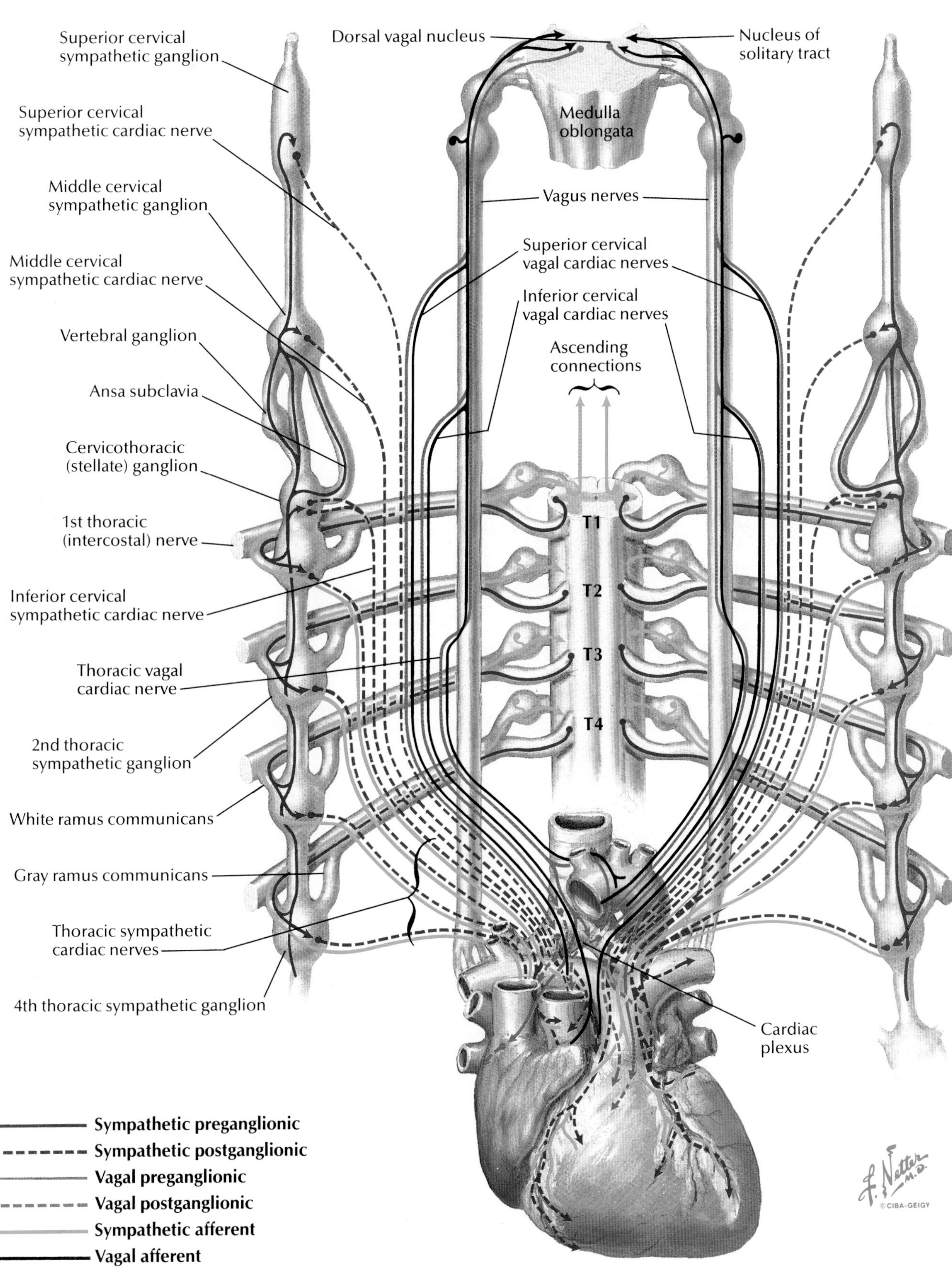

Superior cervical sympathetic ganglion

Superior cervical sympathetic cardiac nerve

Middle cervical sympathetic ganglion

Middle cervical sympathetic cardiac nerve

Vertebral ganglion

Ansa subclavia

Cervicothoracic (stellate) ganglion

1st thoracic (intercostal) nerve

Inferior cervical sympathetic cardiac nerve

Thoracic vagal cardiac nerve

2nd thoracic sympathetic ganglion

White ramus communicans

Gray ramus communicans

Thoracic sympathetic cardiac nerves

4th thoracic sympathetic ganglion

Dorsal vagal nucleus

Nucleus of solitary tract

Medulla oblongata

Vagus nerves

Superior cervical vagal cardiac nerves

Inferior cervical vagal cardiac nerves

Ascending connections

T1

T2

T3

T4

Cardiac plexus

—————— Sympathetic preganglionic
- - - - - - Sympathetic postganglionic
—————— Vagal preganglionic
- · - · - · Vagal postganglionic
—————— Sympathetic afferent
—————— Vagal afferent

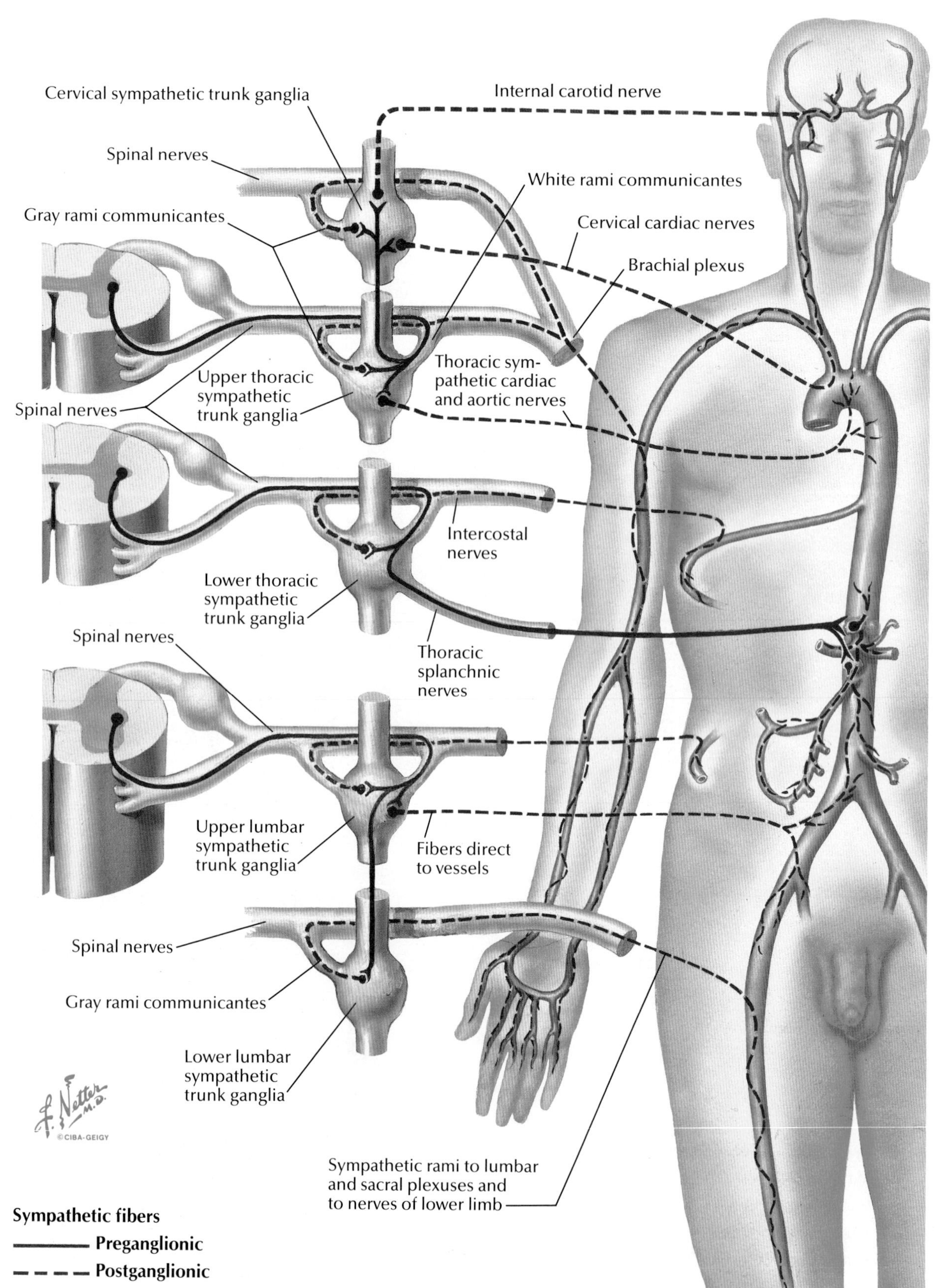

Cervical sympathetic trunk ganglia

Spinal nerves

Gray rami communicantes

Spinal nerves

Upper thoracic sympathetic trunk ganglia

Lower thoracic sympathetic trunk ganglia

Spinal nerves

Upper lumbar sympathetic trunk ganglia

Spinal nerves

Gray rami communicantes

Lower lumbar sympathetic trunk ganglia

Internal carotid nerve

White rami communicantes

Cervical cardiac nerves

Brachial plexus

Thoracic sympathetic cardiac and aortic nerves

Intercostal nerves

Thoracic splanchnic nerves

Fibers direct to vessels

Sympathetic rami to lumbar and sacral plexuses and to nerves of lower limb

Sympathetic fibers

——— **Preganglionic**

— — — **Postganglionic**

PLATE 216

THORAX

FOR OBLITERATED UMBILICAL VESSELS SEE PLATE 236

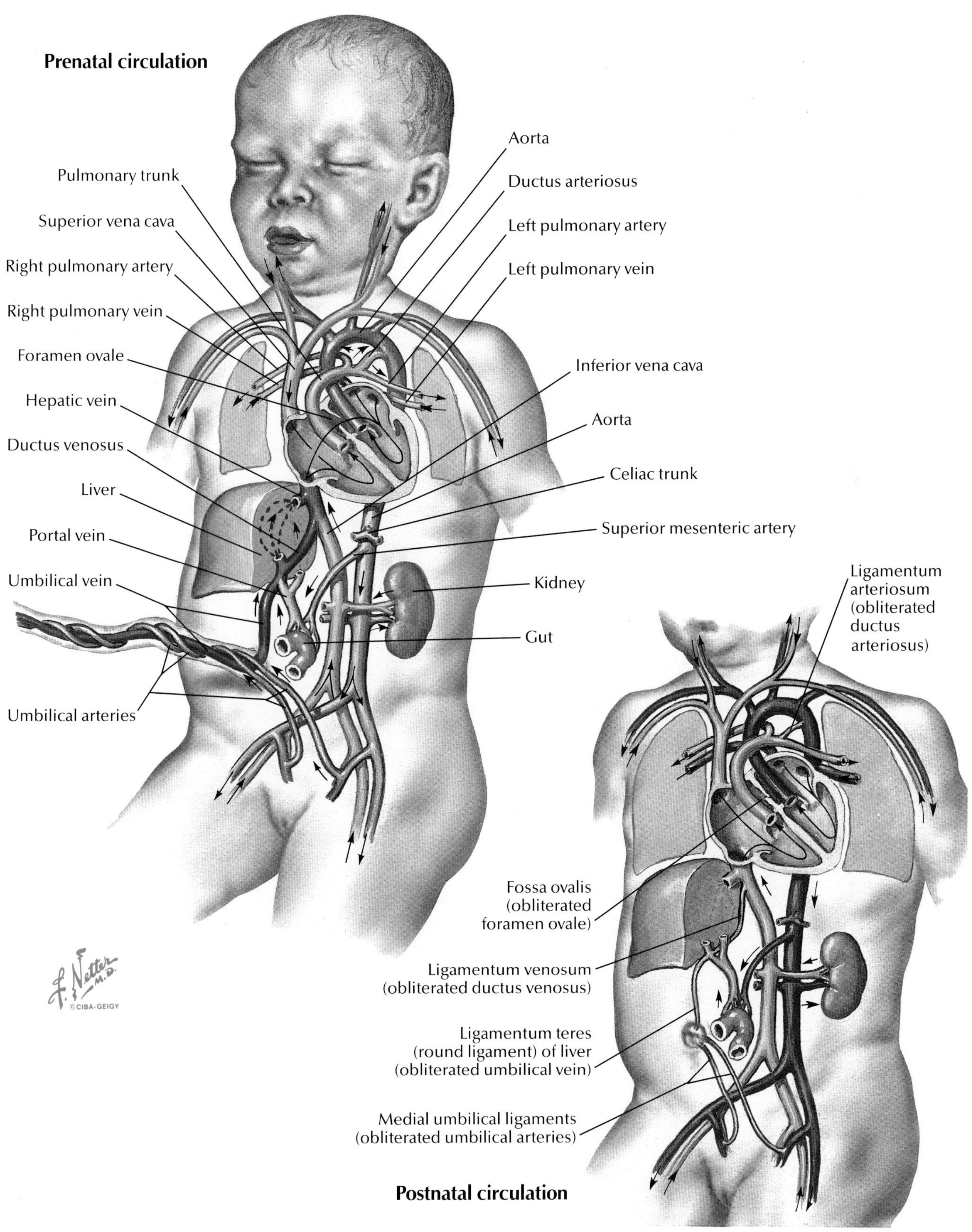

Prenatal circulation

Pulmonary trunk

Superior vena cava

Right pulmonary artery

Right pulmonary vein

Foramen ovale

Hepatic vein

Ductus venosus

Liver

Portal vein

Umbilical vein

Umbilical arteries

Aorta

Ductus arteriosus

Left pulmonary artery

Left pulmonary vein

Inferior vena cava

Aorta

Celiac trunk

Superior mesenteric artery

Kidney

Gut

Ligamentum arteriosum (obliterated ductus arteriosus)

Fossa ovalis (obliterated foramen ovale)

Ligamentum venosum (obliterated ductus venosus)

Ligamentum teres (round ligament) of liver (obliterated umbilical vein)

Medial umbilical ligaments (obliterated umbilical arteries)

Postnatal circulation

HEART

PLATE 217

Mediastinum: Right Lateral View

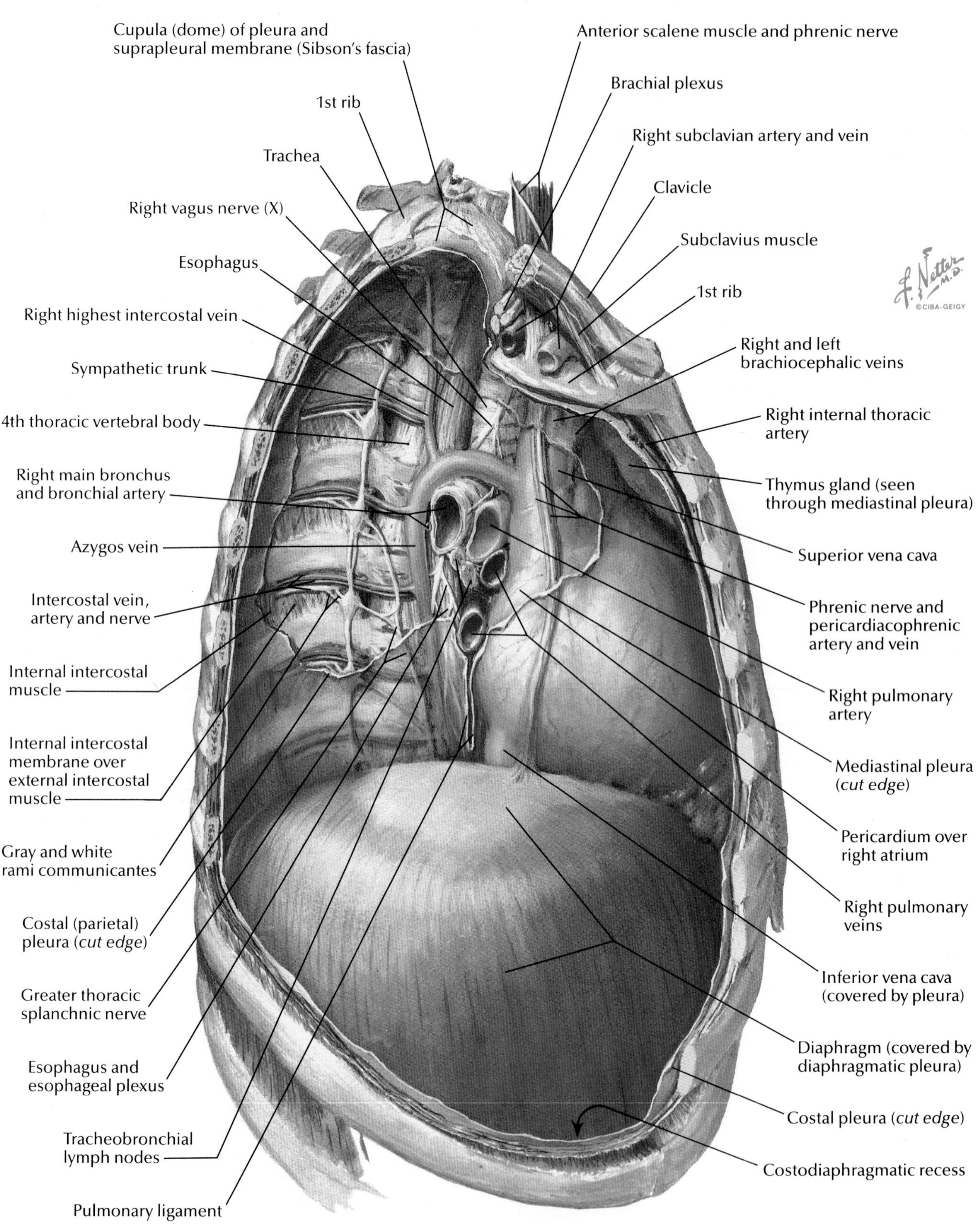

Cupula (dome) of pleura and suprapleural membrane (Sibson's fascia)

1st rib

Trachea

Right vagus nerve (X)

Esophagus

Right highest intercostal vein

Sympathetic trunk

4th thoracic vertebral body

Right main bronchus and bronchial artery

Azygos vein

Intercostal vein, artery and nerve

Internal intercostal muscle

Internal intercostal membrane over external intercostal muscle

Gray and white rami communicantes

Costal (parietal) pleura (cut edge)

Greater thoracic splanchnic nerve

Esophagus and esophageal plexus

Tracheobronchial lymph nodes

Pulmonary ligament

Anterior scalene muscle and phrenic nerve

Brachial plexus

Right subclavian artery and vein

Clavicle

Subclavius muscle

1st rib

Right and left brachiocephalic veins

Right internal thoracic artery

Thymus gland (seen through mediastinal pleura)

Superior vena cava

Phrenic nerve and pericardiacophrenic artery and vein

Right pulmonary artery

Mediastinal pleura (cut edge)

Pericardium over right atrium

Right pulmonary veins

Inferior vena cava (covered by pleura)

Diaphragm (covered by diaphragmatic pleura)

Costal pleura (cut edge)

Costodiaphragmatic recess

PLATE 218

THORAX

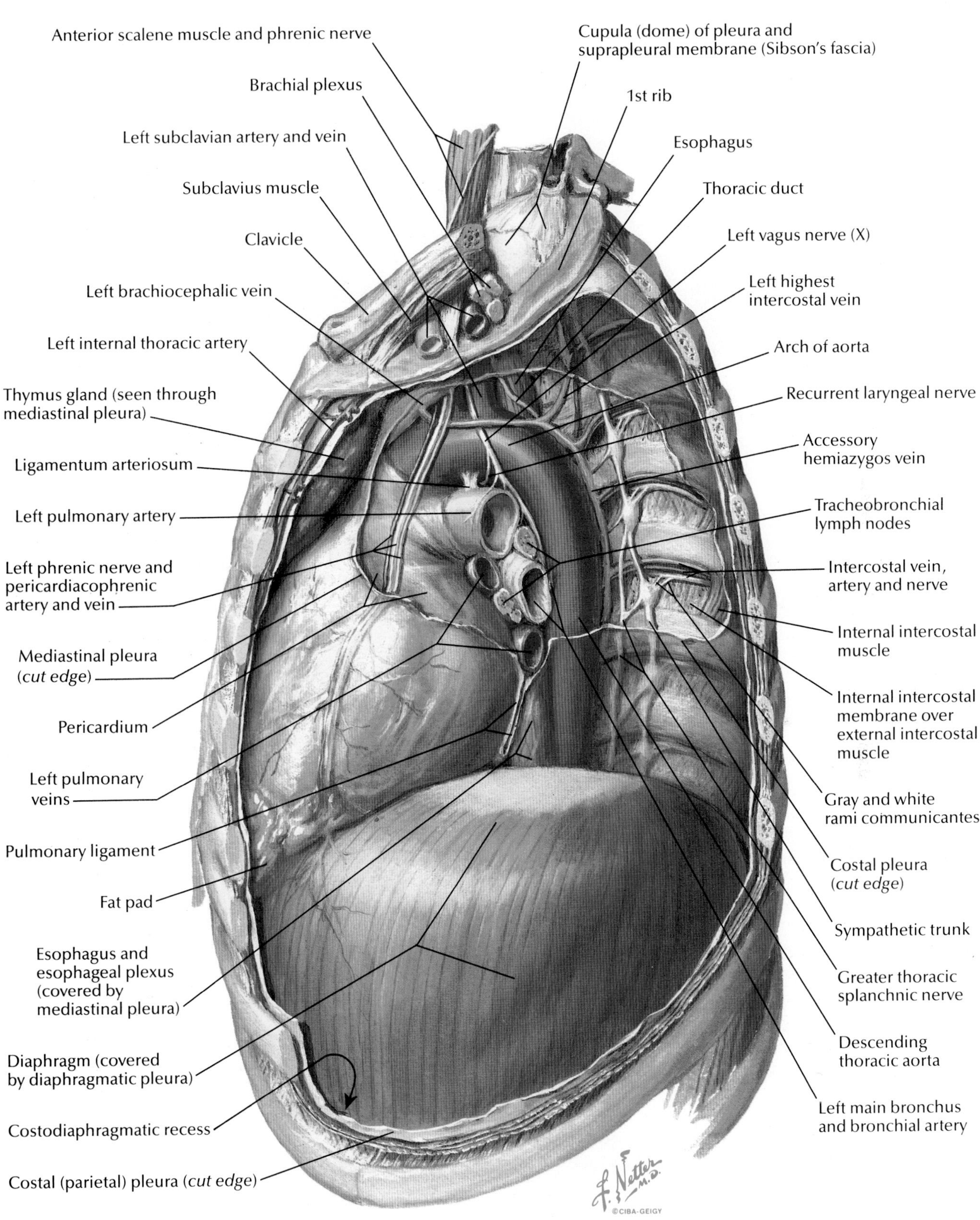

Anterior scalene muscle and phrenic nerve

Brachial plexus

Left subclavian artery and vein

Subclavius muscle

Clavicle

Left brachiocephalic vein

Left internal thoracic artery

Thymus gland (seen through mediastinal pleura)

Ligamentum arteriosum

Left pulmonary artery

Left phrenic nerve and pericardiacophrenic artery and vein

Mediastinal pleura (*cut edge*)

Pericardium

Left pulmonary veins

Pulmonary ligament

Fat pad

Esophagus and esophageal plexus (covered by mediastinal pleura)

Diaphragm (covered by diaphragmatic pleura)

Costodiaphragmatic recess

Costal (parietal) pleura (*cut edge*)

Cupula (dome) of pleura and suprapleural membrane (Sibson's fascia)

1st rib

Esophagus

Thoracic duct

Left vagus nerve (X)

Left highest intercostal vein

Arch of aorta

Recurrent laryngeal nerve

Accessory hemiazygos vein

Tracheobronchial lymph nodes

Intercostal vein, artery and nerve

Internal intercostal muscle

Internal intercostal membrane over external intercostal muscle

Gray and white rami communicantes

Costal pleura (*cut edge*)

Sympathetic trunk

Greater thoracic splanchnic nerve

Descending thoracic aorta

Left main bronchus and bronchial artery

Esophagus In Situ

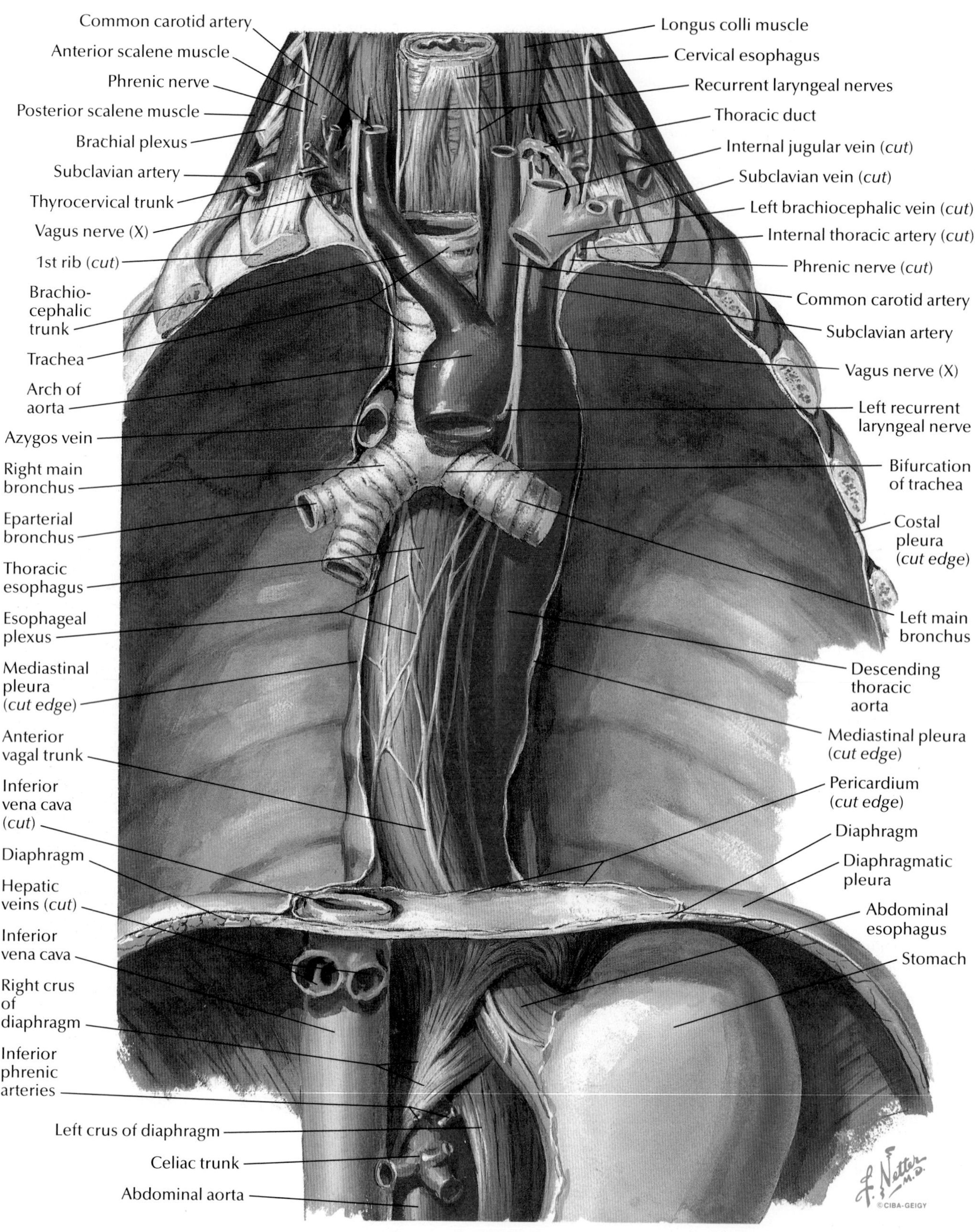

Common carotid artery

Anterior scalene muscle

Phrenic nerve

Posterior scalene muscle

Brachial plexus

Subclavian artery

Thyrocervical trunk

Vagus nerve (X)

1st rib (*cut*)

Brachio-cephalic trunk

Trachea

Arch of aorta

Azygos vein

Right main bronchus

Eparterial bronchus

Thoracic esophagus

Esophageal plexus

Mediastinal pleura (*cut edge*)

Anterior vagal trunk

Inferior vena cava (*cut*)

Diaphragm

Hepatic veins (*cut*)

Inferior vena cava

Right crus of diaphragm

Inferior phrenic arteries

Left crus of diaphragm

Celiac trunk

Abdominal aorta

Longus colli muscle

Cervical esophagus

Recurrent laryngeal nerves

Thoracic duct

Internal jugular vein (*cut*)

Subclavian vein (*cut*)

Left brachiocephalic vein (*cut*)

Internal thoracic artery (*cut*)

Phrenic nerve (*cut*)

Common carotid artery

Subclavian artery

Vagus nerve (X)

Left recurrent laryngeal nerve

Bifurcation of trachea

Costal pleura (*cut edge*)

Left main bronchus

Descending thoracic aorta

Mediastinal pleura (*cut edge*)

Pericardium (*cut edge*)

Diaphragm

Diaphragmatic pleura

Abdominal esophagus

Stomach

PLATE 220

THORAX

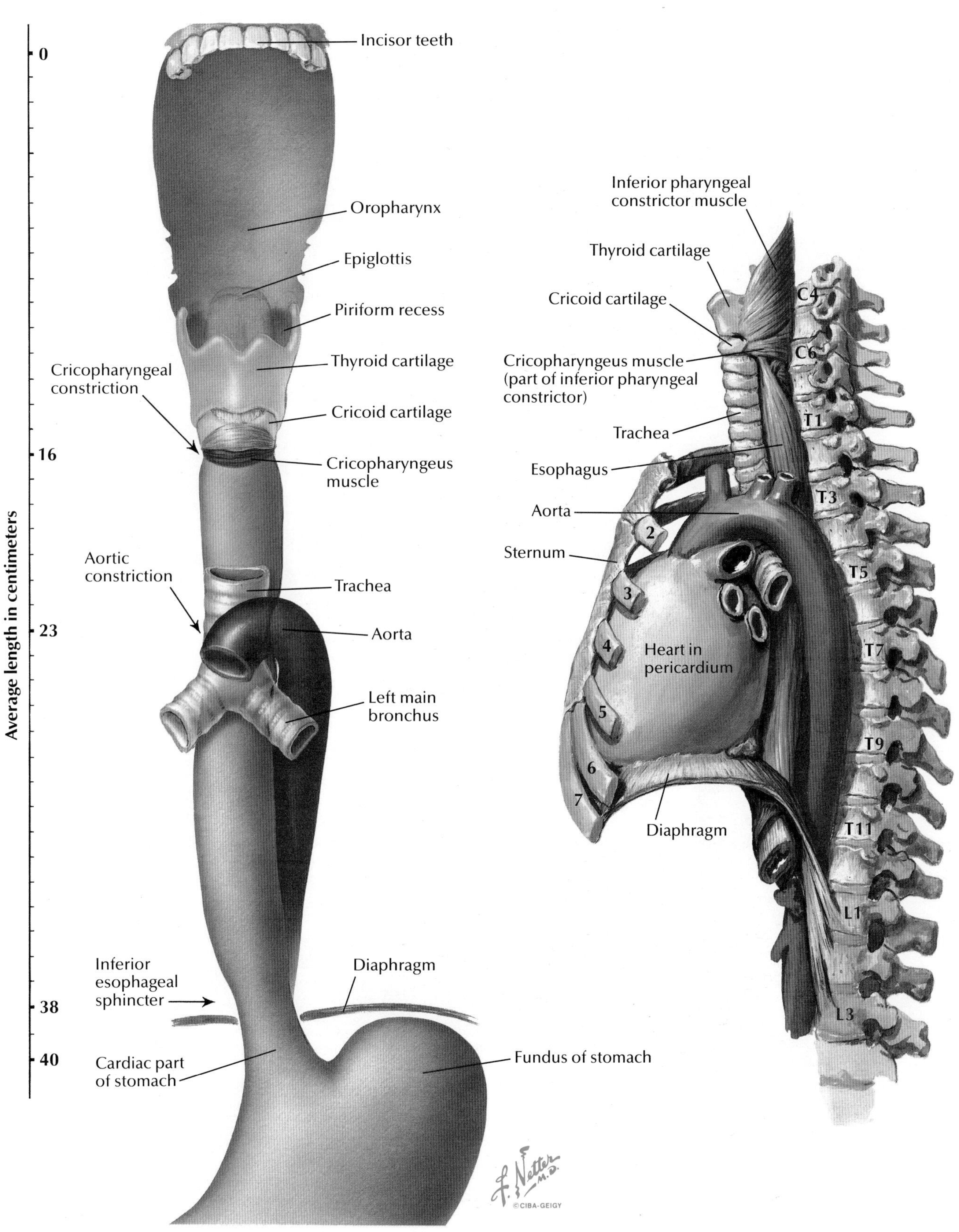

Incisor teeth

Oropharynx

Epiglottis

Piriform recess

Thyroid cartilage

Cricopharyngeal constriction

Cricoid cartilage

Cricopharyngeus muscle

Aortic constriction

Trachea

Aorta

Left main bronchus

Inferior esophageal sphincter

Diaphragm

Cardiac part of stomach

Fundus of stomach

Average length in centimeters

0

16

23

38

40

Inferior pharyngeal constrictor muscle

Thyroid cartilage

Cricoid cartilage

Cricopharyngeus muscle (part of inferior pharyngeal constrictor)

Trachea

Esophagus

Aorta

Sternum

Heart in pericardium

Diaphragm

C4

C6

T1

T3

T5

T7

T9

T11

L1

L3

2

3

4

5

6

7

Musculature of Esophagus

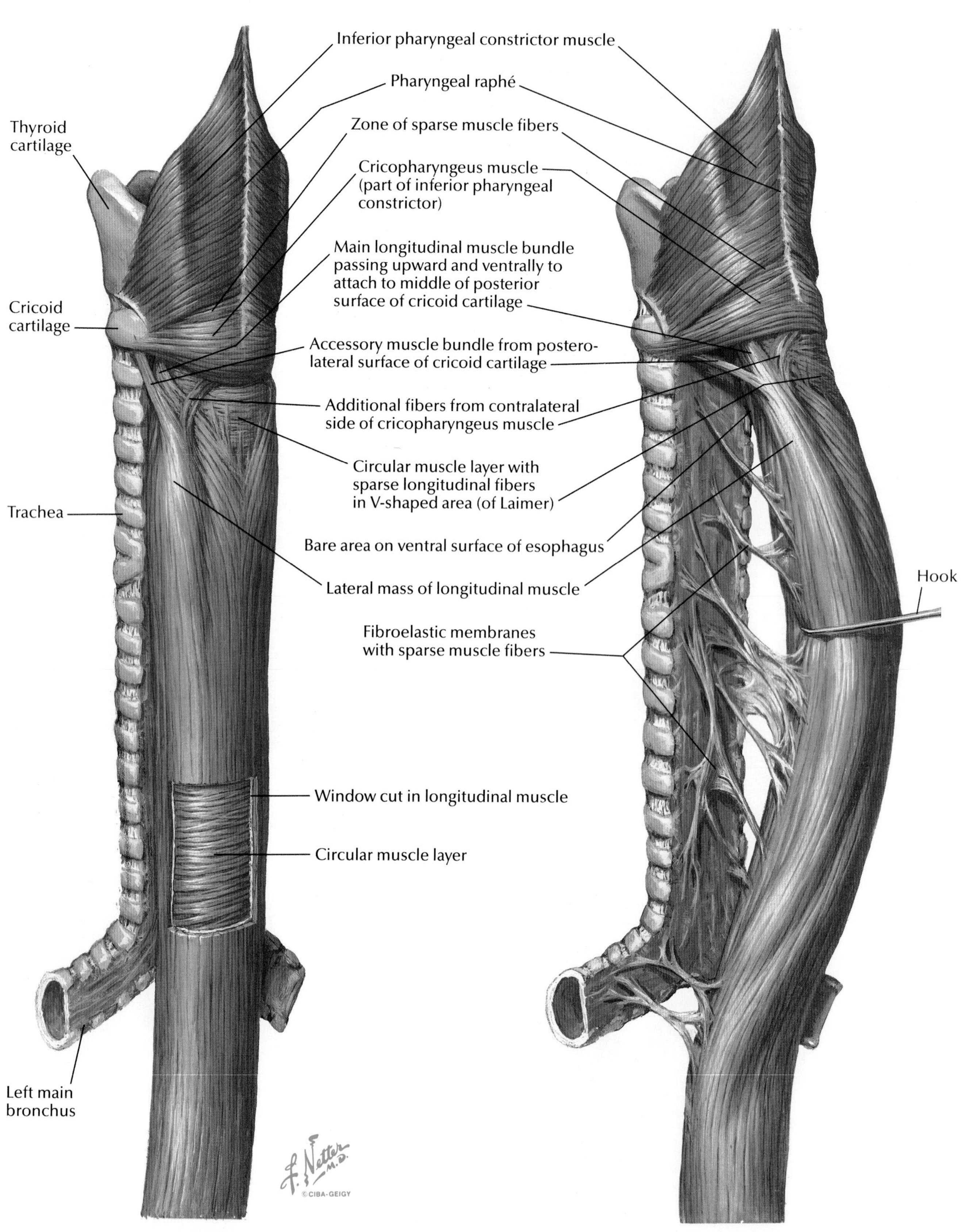

Inferior pharyngeal constrictor muscle

Pharyngeal raphé

Zone of sparse muscle fibers

Thyroid cartilage

Cricopharyngeus muscle (part of inferior pharyngeal constrictor)

Main longitudinal muscle bundle passing upward and ventrally to attach to middle of posterior surface of cricoid cartilage

Cricoid cartilage

Accessory muscle bundle from postero-lateral surface of cricoid cartilage

Additional fibers from contralateral side of cricopharyngeus muscle

Circular muscle layer with sparse longitudinal fibers in V-shaped area (of Laimer)

Bare area on ventral surface of esophagus

Trachea

Lateral mass of longitudinal muscle

Fibroelastic membranes with sparse muscle fibers

Hook

Window cut in longitudinal muscle

Circular muscle layer

Left main bronchus

PLATE 222

THORAX

SEE ALSO PLATE 61

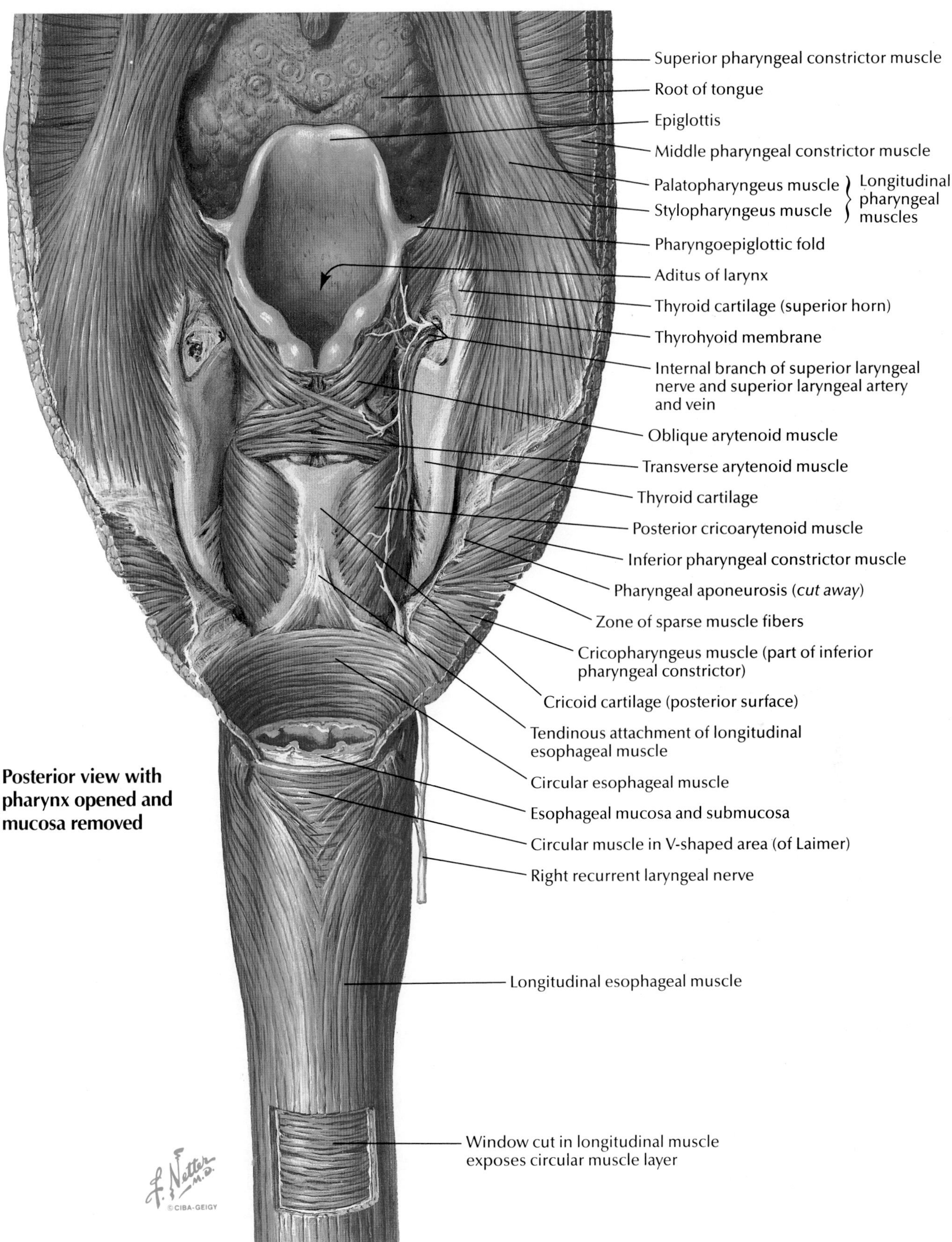

Superior pharyngeal constrictor muscle

Root of tongue

Epiglottis

Middle pharyngeal constrictor muscle

Palatopharyngeus muscle ⎫ Longitudinal
Stylopharyngeus muscle ⎬ pharyngeal
　　　　　　　　　　　⎭ muscles

Pharyngoepiglottic fold

Aditus of larynx

Thyroid cartilage (superior horn)

Thyrohyoid membrane

Internal branch of superior laryngeal nerve and superior laryngeal artery and vein

Oblique arytenoid muscle

Transverse arytenoid muscle

Thyroid cartilage

Posterior cricoarytenoid muscle

Inferior pharyngeal constrictor muscle

Pharyngeal aponeurosis (*cut away*)

Zone of sparse muscle fibers

Cricopharyngeus muscle (part of inferior pharyngeal constrictor)

Cricoid cartilage (posterior surface)

Tendinous attachment of longitudinal esophageal muscle

Circular esophageal muscle

Esophageal mucosa and submucosa

Circular muscle in V-shaped area (of Laimer)

Right recurrent laryngeal nerve

Longitudinal esophageal muscle

Window cut in longitudinal muscle exposes circular muscle layer

Posterior view with pharynx opened and mucosa removed

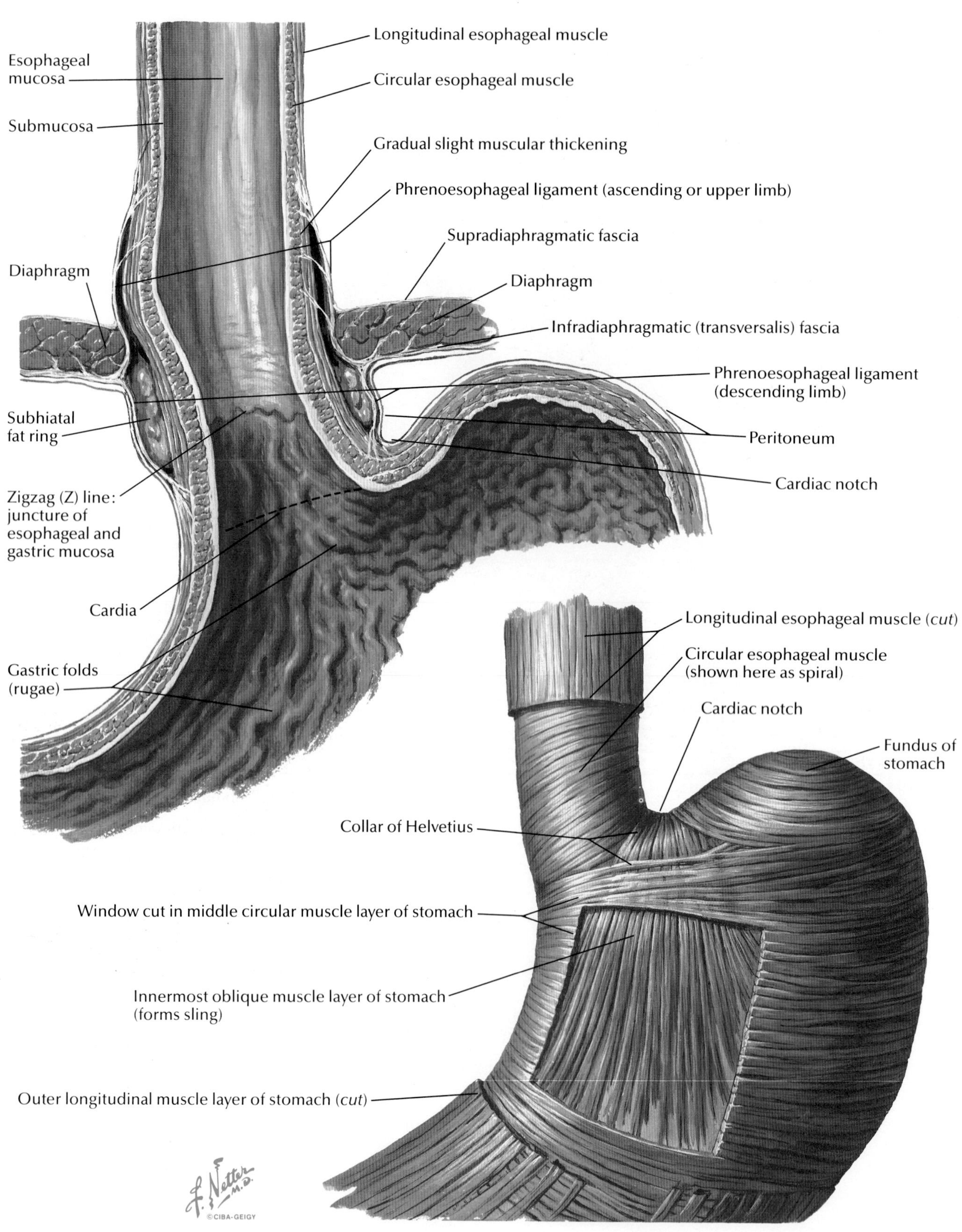

Esophageal mucosa

Submucosa

Diaphragm

Subhiatal fat ring

Zigzag (Z) line: juncture of esophageal and gastric mucosa

Cardia

Gastric folds (rugae)

Longitudinal esophageal muscle

Circular esophageal muscle

Gradual slight muscular thickening

Phrenoesophageal ligament (ascending or upper limb)

Supradiaphragmatic fascia

Diaphragm

Infradiaphragmatic (transversalis) fascia

Phrenoesophageal ligament (descending limb)

Peritoneum

Cardiac notch

Longitudinal esophageal muscle (*cut*)

Circular esophageal muscle (shown here as spiral)

Cardiac notch

Fundus of stomach

Collar of Helvetius

Window cut in middle circular muscle layer of stomach

Innermost oblique muscle layer of stomach (forms sling)

Outer longitudinal muscle layer of stomach (*cut*)

PLATE 224

THORAX

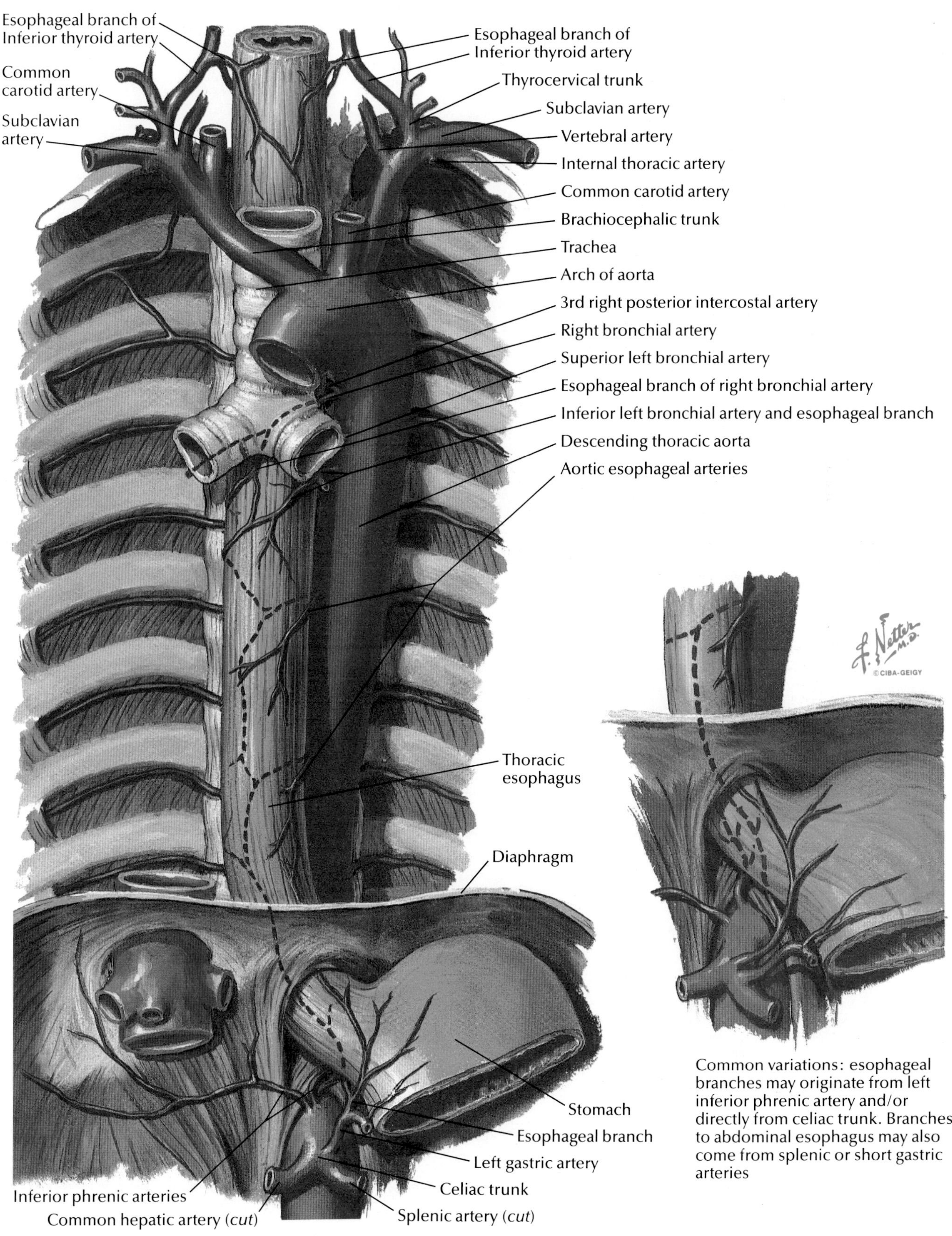

Esophageal branch of
Inferior thyroid artery

Common
carotid artery

Subclavian
artery

Esophageal branch of
Inferior thyroid artery

Thyrocervical trunk

Subclavian artery

Vertebral artery

Internal thoracic artery

Common carotid artery

Brachiocephalic trunk

Trachea

Arch of aorta

3rd right posterior intercostal artery

Right bronchial artery

Superior left bronchial artery

Esophageal branch of right bronchial artery

Inferior left bronchial artery and esophageal branch

Descending thoracic aorta

Aortic esophageal arteries

Thoracic
esophagus

Diaphragm

Stomach

Esophageal branch

Left gastric artery

Celiac trunk

Splenic artery (*cut*)

Inferior phrenic arteries

Common hepatic artery (*cut*)

Common variations: esophageal
branches may originate from left
inferior phrenic artery and/or
directly from celiac trunk. Branches
to abdominal esophagus may also
come from splenic or short gastric
arteries

SEE ALSO PLATE 297

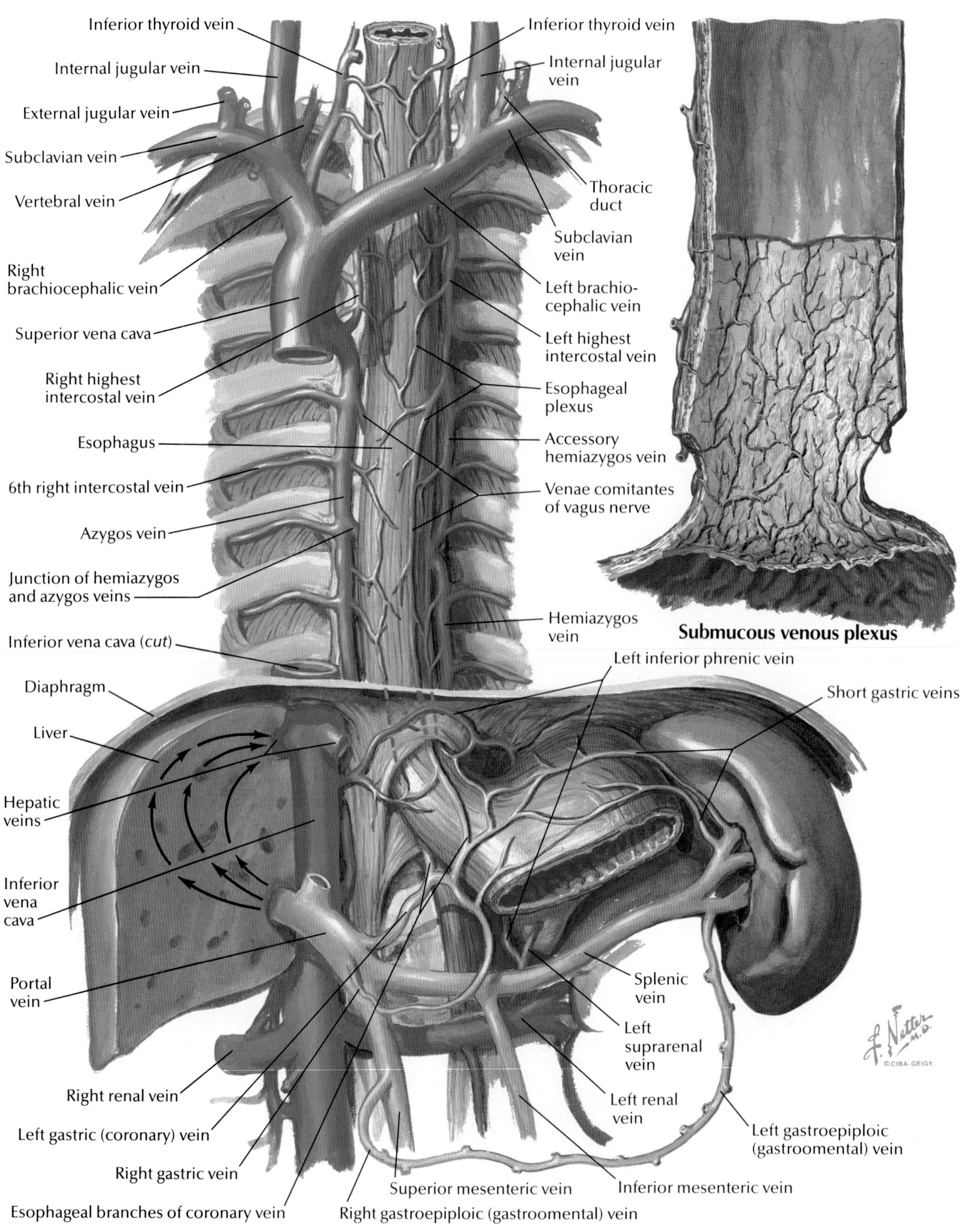

Inferior thyroid vein

Internal jugular vein

External jugular vein

Subclavian vein

Vertebral vein

Right brachiocephalic vein

Superior vena cava

Right highest intercostal vein

Esophagus

6th right intercostal vein

Azygos vein

Junction of hemiazygos and azygos veins

Inferior vena cava (cut)

Diaphragm

Liver

Hepatic veins

Inferior vena cava

Portal vein

Right renal vein

Left gastric (coronary) vein

Right gastric vein

Esophageal branches of coronary vein

Inferior thyroid vein

Internal jugular vein

Thoracic duct

Subclavian vein

Left brachio-cephalic vein

Left highest intercostal vein

Esophageal plexus

Accessory hemiazygos vein

Venae comitantes of vagus nerve

Hemiazygos vein

Submucous venous plexus

Left inferior phrenic vein

Short gastric veins

Splenic vein

Left suprarenal vein

Left renal vein

Left gastroepiploic (gastroomental) vein

Superior mesenteric vein

Right gastroepiploic (gastroomental) vein

Inferior mesenteric vein

PLATE 226

THORAX

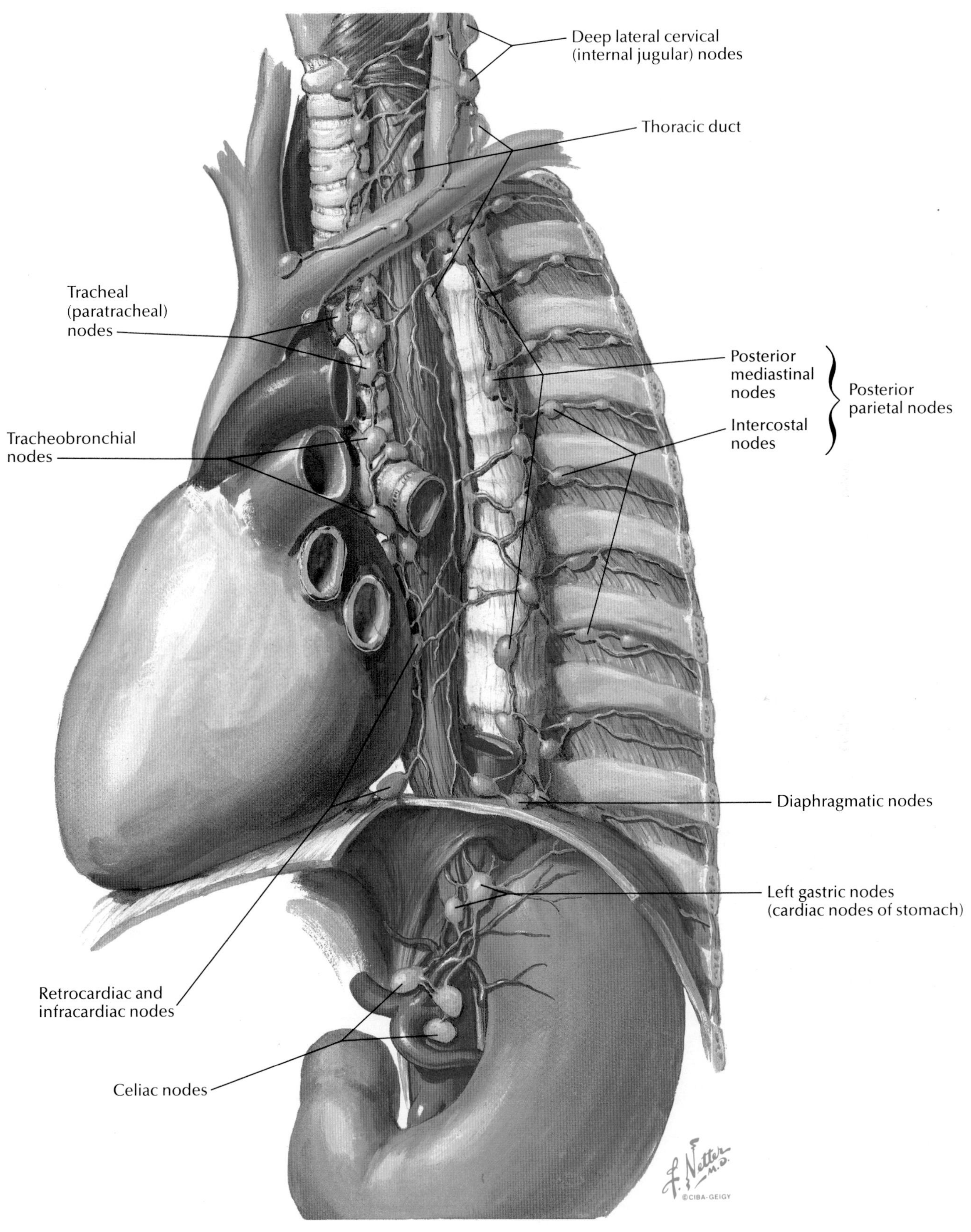

Deep lateral cervical (internal jugular) nodes

Thoracic duct

Tracheal (paratracheal) nodes

Tracheobronchial nodes

Posterior mediastinal nodes

Intercostal nodes

Posterior parietal nodes

Diaphragmatic nodes

Left gastric nodes (cardiac nodes of stomach)

Retrocardiac and infracardiac nodes

Celiac nodes

Nerves of Esophagus

SEE ALSO PLATES 152, 198

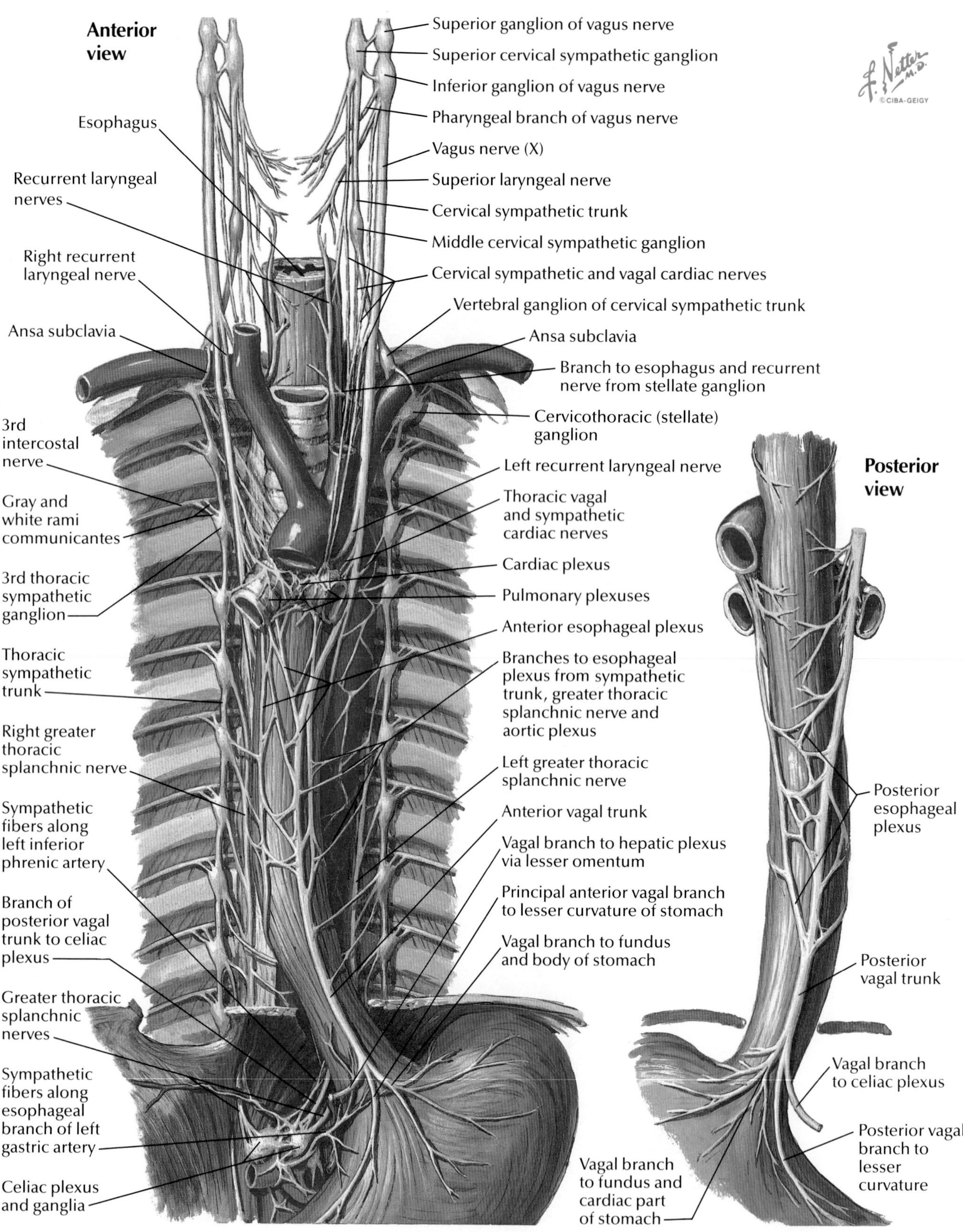

Anterior view

Esophagus

Recurrent laryngeal nerves

Right recurrent laryngeal nerve

Ansa subclavia

3rd intercostal nerve

Gray and white rami communicantes

3rd thoracic sympathetic ganglion

Thoracic sympathetic trunk

Right greater thoracic splanchnic nerve

Sympathetic fibers along left inferior phrenic artery

Branch of posterior vagal trunk to celiac plexus

Greater thoracic splanchnic nerves

Sympathetic fibers along esophageal branch of left gastric artery

Celiac plexus and ganglia

Superior ganglion of vagus nerve

Superior cervical sympathetic ganglion

Inferior ganglion of vagus nerve

Pharyngeal branch of vagus nerve

Vagus nerve (X)

Superior laryngeal nerve

Cervical sympathetic trunk

Middle cervical sympathetic ganglion

Cervical sympathetic and vagal cardiac nerves

Vertebral ganglion of cervical sympathetic trunk

Ansa subclavia

Branch to esophagus and recurrent nerve from stellate ganglion

Cervicothoracic (stellate) ganglion

Left recurrent laryngeal nerve

Thoracic vagal and sympathetic cardiac nerves

Cardiac plexus

Pulmonary plexuses

Anterior esophageal plexus

Branches to esophageal plexus from sympathetic trunk, greater thoracic splanchnic nerve and aortic plexus

Left greater thoracic splanchnic nerve

Anterior vagal trunk

Vagal branch to hepatic plexus via lesser omentum

Principal anterior vagal branch to lesser curvature of stomach

Vagal branch to fundus and body of stomach

Vagal branch to fundus and cardiac part of stomach

Posterior view

Posterior esophageal plexus

Posterior vagal trunk

Vagal branch to celiac plexus

Posterior vagal branch to lesser curvature

PLATE 228

THORAX

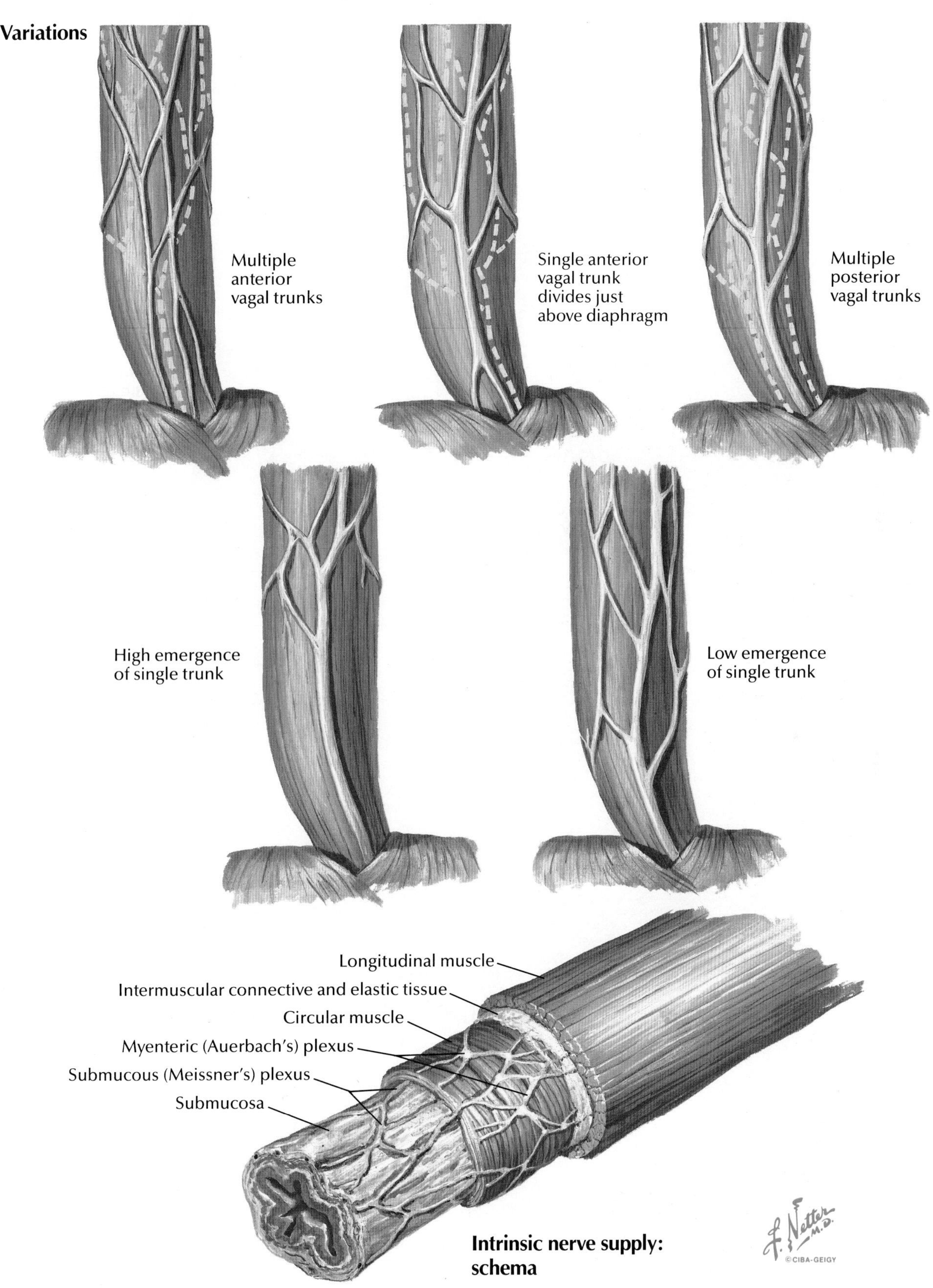

Variations

Multiple anterior vagal trunks

Single anterior vagal trunk divides just above diaphragm

Multiple posterior vagal trunks

High emergence of single trunk

Low emergence of single trunk

Longitudinal muscle

Intermuscular connective and elastic tissue

Circular muscle

Myenteric (Auerbach's) plexus

Submucous (Meissner's) plexus

Submucosa

Intrinsic nerve supply: schema

Mediastinum: Cross Section

Superior view

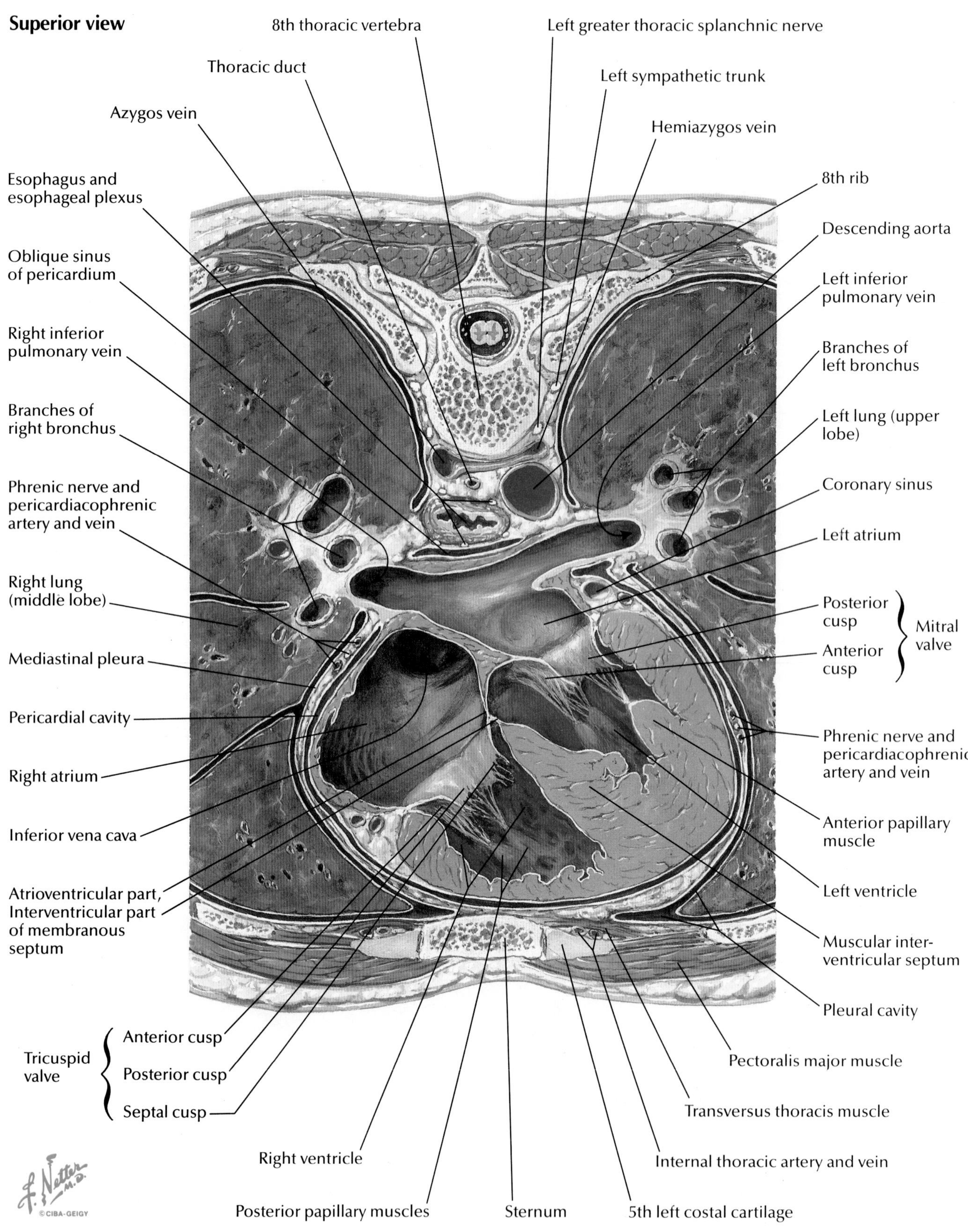

8th thoracic vertebra

Thoracic duct

Azygos vein

Esophagus and esophageal plexus

Oblique sinus of pericardium

Right inferior pulmonary vein

Branches of right bronchus

Phrenic nerve and pericardiacophrenic artery and vein

Right lung (middle lobe)

Mediastinal pleura

Pericardial cavity

Right atrium

Inferior vena cava

Atrioventricular part, Interventricular part of membranous septum

Left greater thoracic splanchnic nerve

Left sympathetic trunk

Hemiazygos vein

8th rib

Descending aorta

Left inferior pulmonary vein

Branches of left bronchus

Left lung (upper lobe)

Coronary sinus

Left atrium

Posterior cusp } Mitral valve
Anterior cusp }

Phrenic nerve and pericardiacophrenic artery and vein

Anterior papillary muscle

Left ventricle

Muscular inter-ventricular septum

Pleural cavity

Pectoralis major muscle

Transversus thoracis muscle

Internal thoracic artery and vein

Tricuspid valve {
Anterior cusp
Posterior cusp
Septal cusp

Right ventricle

Posterior papillary muscles

Sternum

5th left costal cartilage

PLATE 230

THORAX

Section IV

ABDOMEN

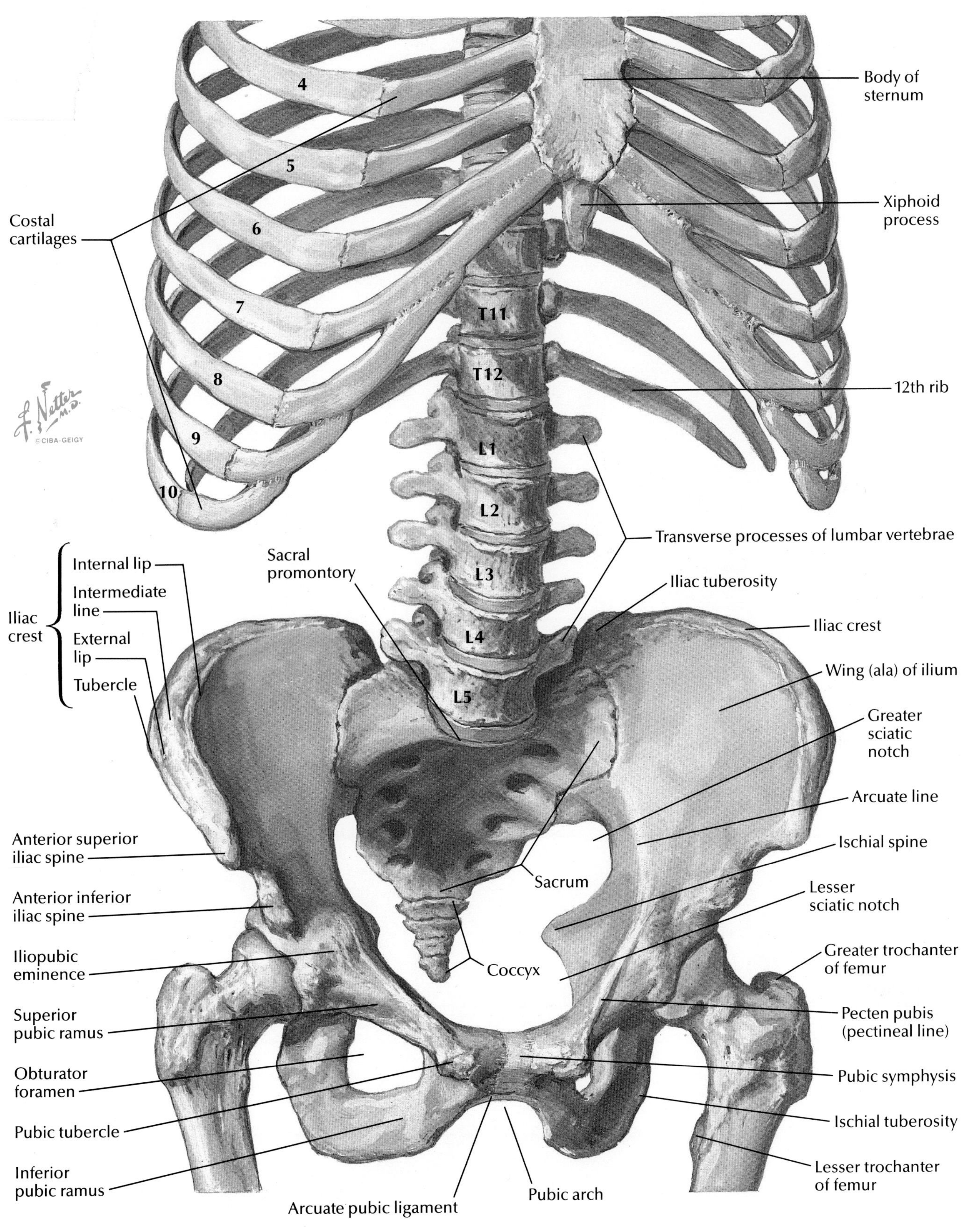

Body of sternum

Xiphoid process

12th rib

Transverse processes of lumbar vertebrae

Iliac tuberosity

Iliac crest

Wing (ala) of ilium

Greater sciatic notch

Arcuate line

Ischial spine

Lesser sciatic notch

Greater trochanter of femur

Pecten pubis (pectineal line)

Pubic symphysis

Ischial tuberosity

Lesser trochanter of femur

Costal cartilages

Iliac crest { Internal lip / Intermediate line / External lip / Tubercle }

Sacral promontory

Anterior superior iliac spine

Anterior inferior iliac spine

Iliopubic eminence

Superior pubic ramus

Obturator foramen

Pubic tubercle

Inferior pubic ramus

Arcuate pubic ligament

Sacrum

Coccyx

Pubic arch

T11

T12

L1

L2

L3

L4

L5

4

5

6

7

8

9

10

Anterior Abdominal Wall: Superficial Dissection

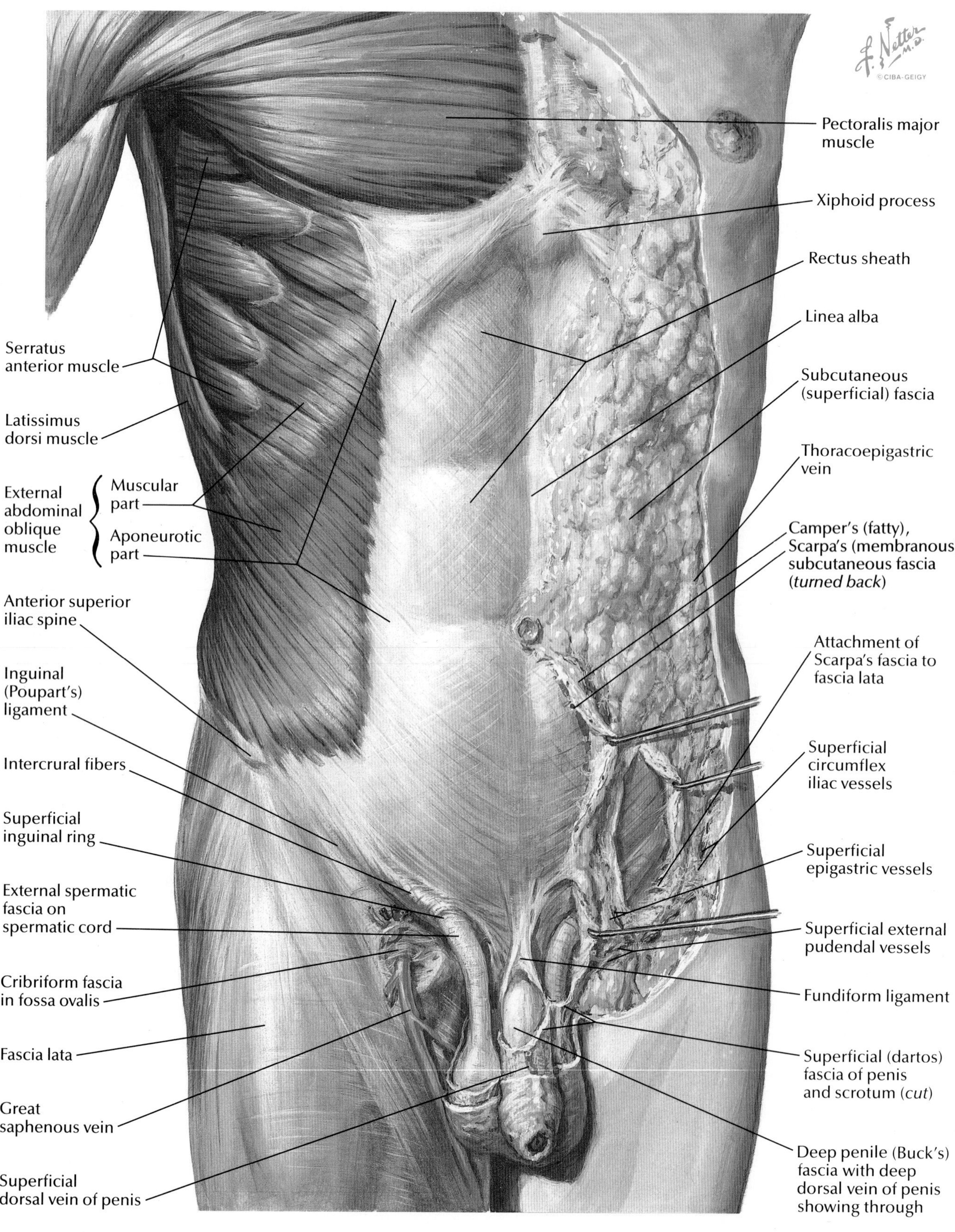

Pectoralis major muscle

Xiphoid process

Rectus sheath

Linea alba

Subcutaneous (superficial) fascia

Thoracoepigastric vein

Camper's (fatty), Scarpa's (membranous) subcutaneous fascia (*turned back*)

Attachment of Scarpa's fascia to fascia lata

Superficial circumflex iliac vessels

Superficial epigastric vessels

Superficial external pudendal vessels

Fundiform ligament

Superficial (dartos) fascia of penis and scrotum (*cut*)

Deep penile (Buck's) fascia with deep dorsal vein of penis showing through

Serratus anterior muscle

Latissimus dorsi muscle

External abdominal oblique muscle { Muscular part / Aponeurotic part }

Anterior superior iliac spine

Inguinal (Poupart's) ligament

Intercrural fibers

Superficial inguinal ring

External spermatic fascia on spermatic cord

Cribriform fascia in fossa ovalis

Fascia lata

Great saphenous vein

Superficial dorsal vein of penis

PLATE 232

ABDOMEN

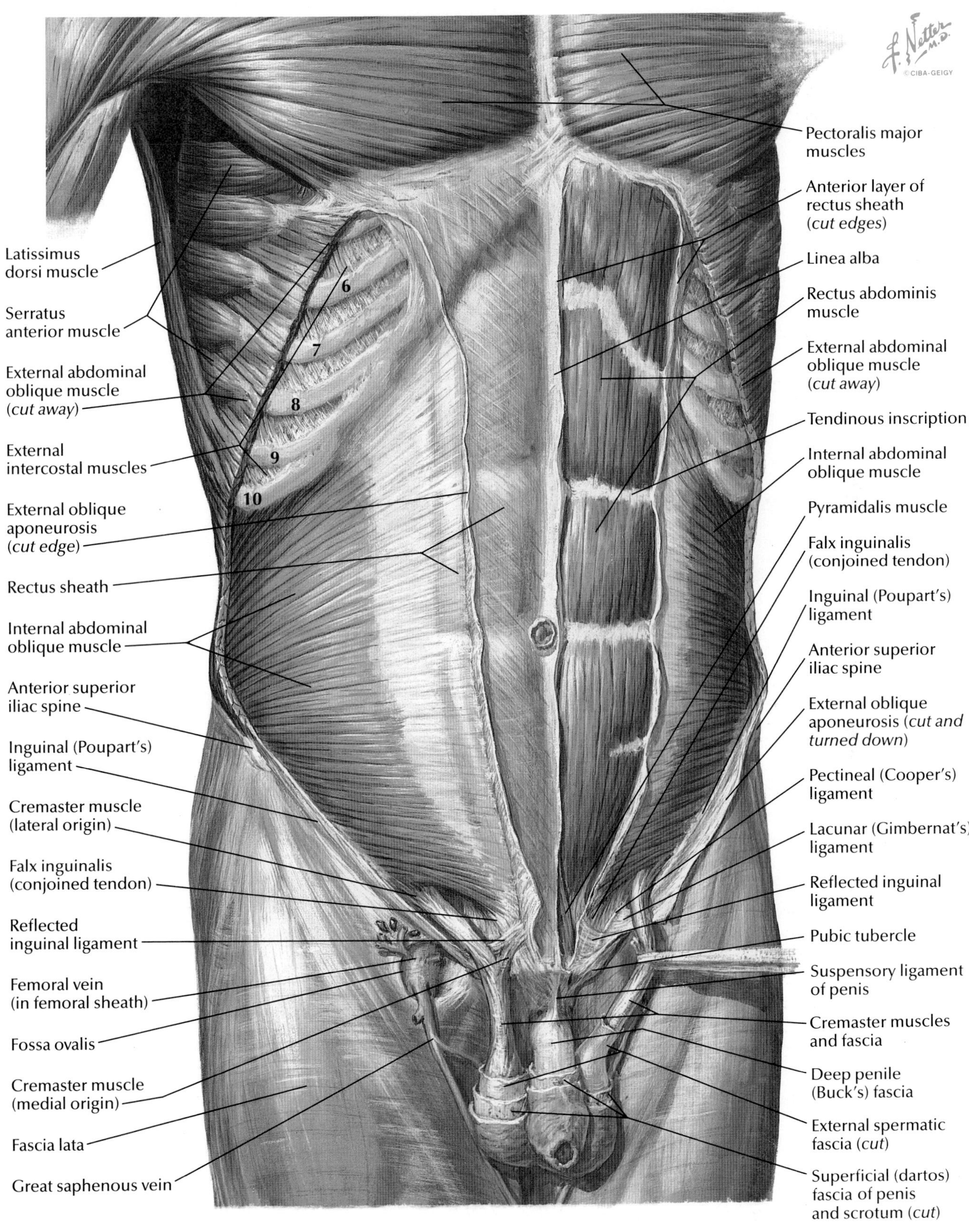

Latissimus
dorsi muscle

Serratus
anterior muscle

External abdominal
oblique muscle
(*cut away*)

External
intercostal muscles

External oblique
aponeurosis
(*cut edge*)

Rectus sheath

Internal abdominal
oblique muscle

Anterior superior
iliac spine

Inguinal (Poupart's)
ligament

Cremaster muscle
(lateral origin)

Falx inguinalis
(conjoined tendon)

Reflected
inguinal ligament

Femoral vein
(in femoral sheath)

Fossa ovalis

Cremaster muscle
(medial origin)

Fascia lata

Great saphenous vein

Pectoralis major
muscles

Anterior layer of
rectus sheath
(*cut edges*)

Linea alba

Rectus abdominis
muscle

External abdominal
oblique muscle
(*cut away*)

Tendinous inscription

Internal abdominal
oblique muscle

Pyramidalis muscle

Falx inguinalis
(conjoined tendon)

Inguinal (Poupart's)
ligament

Anterior superior
iliac spine

External oblique
aponeurosis (*cut and
turned down*)

Pectineal (Cooper's)
ligament

Lacunar (Gimbernat's)
ligament

Reflected inguinal
ligament

Pubic tubercle

Suspensory ligament
of penis

Cremaster muscles
and fascia

Deep penile
(Buck's) fascia

External spermatic
fascia (*cut*)

Superficial (dartos)
fascia of penis
and scrotum (*cut*)

6
7
8
9
10

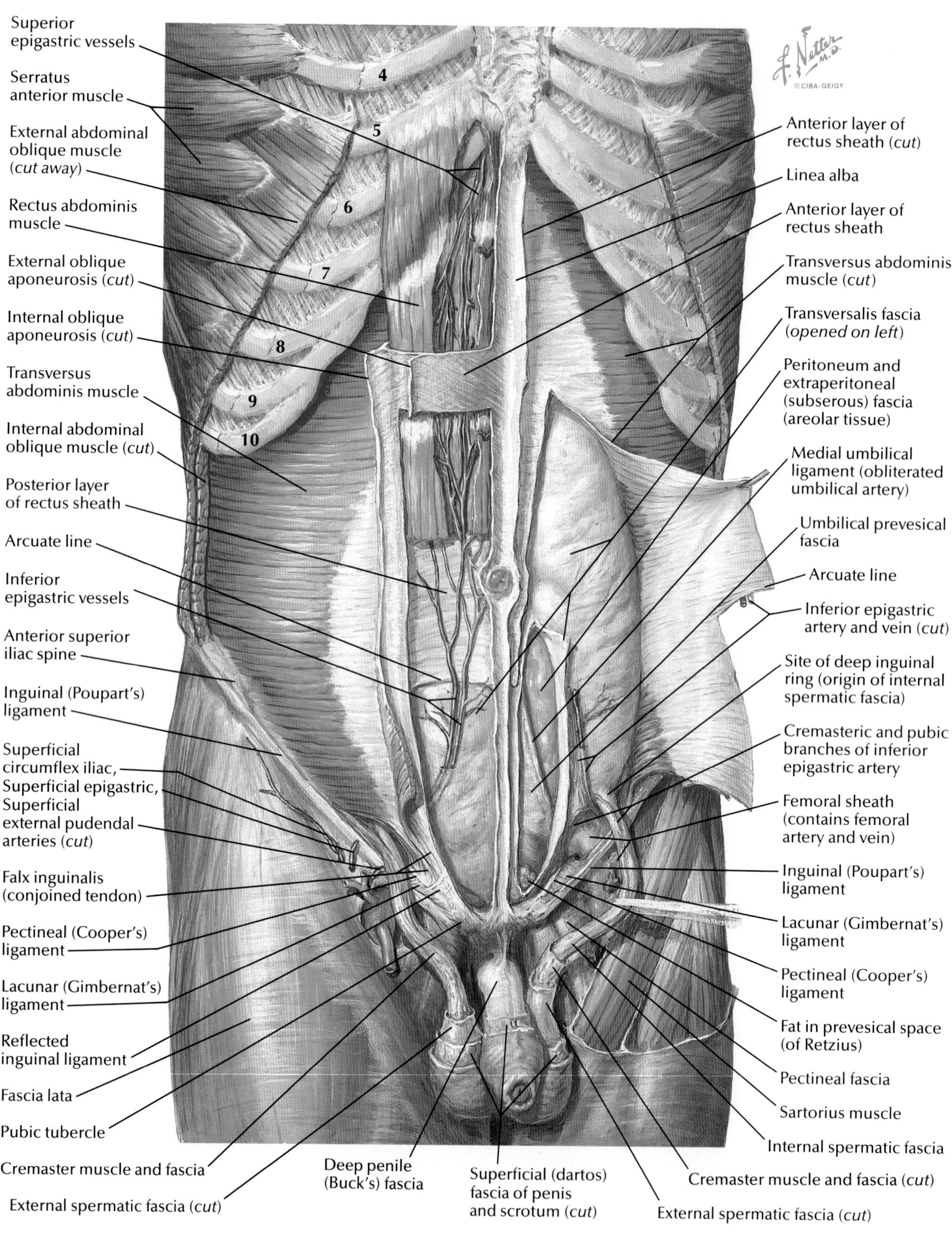

Superior epigastric vessels

Serratus anterior muscle

External abdominal oblique muscle (cut away)

Rectus abdominis muscle

External oblique aponeurosis (cut)

Internal oblique aponeurosis (cut)

Transversus abdominis muscle

Internal abdominal oblique muscle (cut)

Posterior layer of rectus sheath

Arcuate line

Inferior epigastric vessels

Anterior superior iliac spine

Inguinal (Poupart's) ligament

Superficial circumflex iliac, Superficial epigastric, Superficial external pudendal arteries (cut)

Falx inguinalis (conjoined tendon)

Pectineal (Cooper's) ligament

Lacunar (Gimbernat's) ligament

Reflected inguinal ligament

Fascia lata

Pubic tubercle

Cremaster muscle and fascia

External spermatic fascia (cut)

Deep penile (Buck's) fascia

Superficial (dartos) fascia of penis and scrotum (cut)

Anterior layer of rectus sheath (cut)

Linea alba

Anterior layer of rectus sheath

Transversus abdominis muscle (cut)

Transversalis fascia (opened on left)

Peritoneum and extraperitoneal (subserous) fascia (areolar tissue)

Medial umbilical ligament (obliterated umbilical artery)

Umbilical prevesical fascia

Arcuate line

Inferior epigastric artery and vein (cut)

Site of deep inguinal ring (origin of internal spermatic fascia)

Cremasteric and pubic branches of inferior epigastric artery

Femoral sheath (contains femoral artery and vein)

Inguinal (Poupart's) ligament

Lacunar (Gimbernat's) ligament

Pectineal (Cooper's) ligament

Fat in prevesical space (of Retzius)

Pectineal fascia

Sartorius muscle

Internal spermatic fascia

Cremaster muscle and fascia (cut)

External spermatic fascia (cut)

PLATE 234

Section above arcuate line

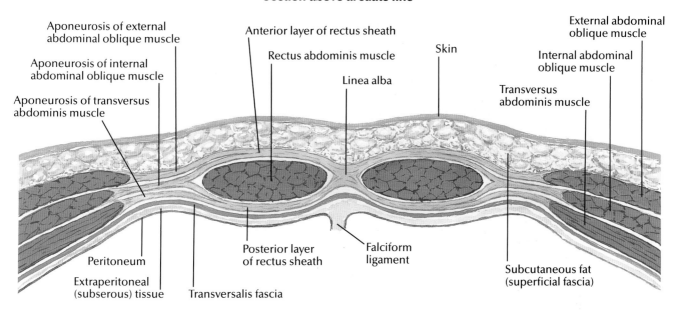

Aponeurosis of external abdominal oblique muscle

Aponeurosis of internal abdominal oblique muscle

Aponeurosis of transversus abdominis muscle

Anterior layer of rectus sheath

Rectus abdominis muscle

Linea alba

Skin

External abdominal oblique muscle

Internal abdominal oblique muscle

Transversus abdominis muscle

Peritoneum

Extraperitoneal (subserous) tissue

Transversalis fascia

Posterior layer of rectus sheath

Falciform ligament

Subcutaneous fat (superficial fascia)

Aponeurosis of internal abdominal oblique muscle splits to form anterior and posterior layers of rectus sheath. Aponeurosis of external abdominal oblique muscle joins anterior layer of sheath; aponeurosis of transversus abdominis muscle joins posterior layer. Anterior and posterior layers of rectus sheath unite medially to form linea alba

Section below arcuate line

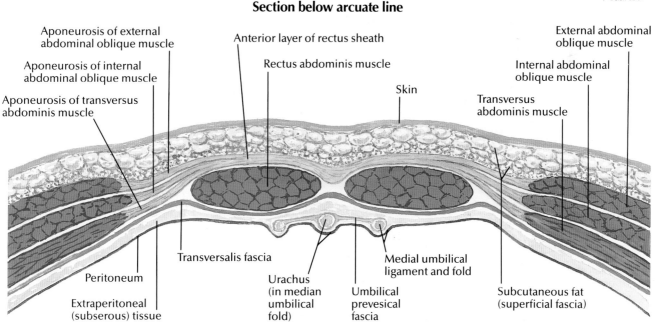

Aponeurosis of external abdominal oblique muscle

Aponeurosis of internal abdominal oblique muscle

Aponeurosis of transversus abdominis muscle

Anterior layer of rectus sheath

Rectus abdominis muscle

Skin

External abdominal oblique muscle

Internal abdominal oblique muscle

Transversus abdominis muscle

Transversalis fascia

Peritoneum

Extraperitoneal (subserous) tissue

Urachus (in median umbilical fold)

Umbilical prevesical fascia

Medial umbilical ligament and fold

Subcutaneous fat (superficial fascia)

Aponeurosis of internal abdominal oblique muscle does not split at this level but passes completely anterior to rectus abdominis muscle and is fused there with both aponeurosis of external abdominal oblique muscle and that of transversus abdominis muscle. Thus posterior wall of rectus sheath is absent below arcuate line and rectus abdominis muscle lies on transversalis fascia

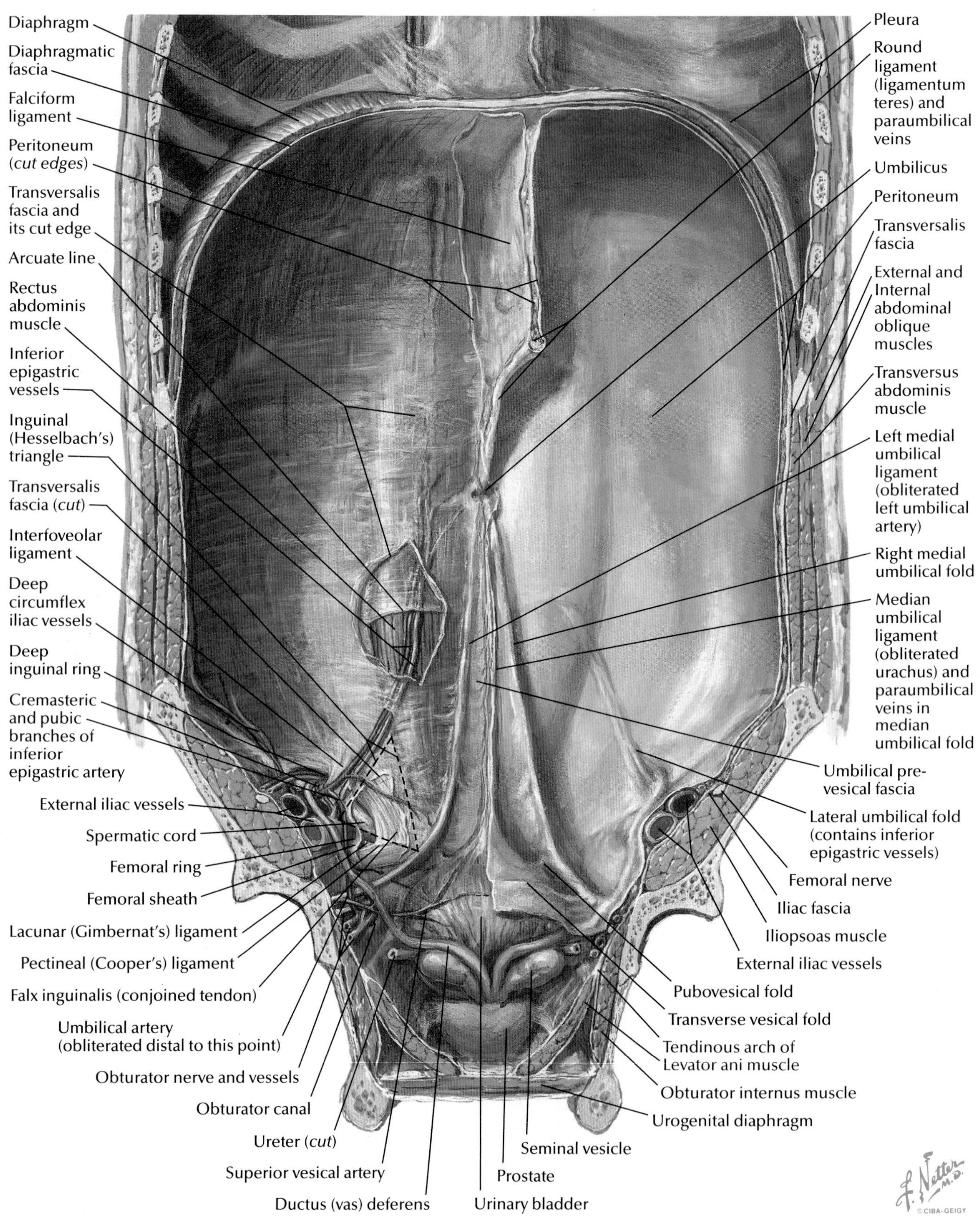

Diaphragm

Diaphragmatic fascia

Falciform ligament

Peritoneum (*cut edges*)

Transversalis fascia and its cut edge

Arcuate line

Rectus abdominis muscle

Inferior epigastric vessels

Inguinal (Hesselbach's) triangle

Transversalis fascia (*cut*)

Interfoveolar ligament

Deep circumflex iliac vessels

Deep inguinal ring

Cremasteric and pubic branches of inferior epigastric artery

External iliac vessels

Spermatic cord

Femoral ring

Femoral sheath

Lacunar (Gimbernat's) ligament

Pectineal (Cooper's) ligament

Falx inguinalis (conjoined tendon)

Umbilical artery (obliterated distal to this point)

Obturator nerve and vessels

Obturator canal

Ureter (*cut*)

Superior vesical artery

Ductus (vas) deferens

Pleura

Round ligament (ligamentum teres) and paraumbilical veins

Umbilicus

Peritoneum

Transversalis fascia

External and Internal abdominal oblique muscles

Transversus abdominis muscle

Left medial umbilical ligament (obliterated left umbilical artery)

Right medial umbilical fold

Median umbilical ligament (obliterated urachus) and paraumbilical veins in median umbilical fold

Umbilical prevesical fascia

Lateral umbilical fold (contains inferior epigastric vessels)

Femoral nerve

Iliac fascia

Iliopsoas muscle

External iliac vessels

Pubovesical fold

Transverse vesical fold

Tendinous arch of Levator ani muscle

Obturator internus muscle

Urogenital diaphragm

Seminal vesicle

Prostate

Urinary bladder

PLATE 236

ABDOMEN

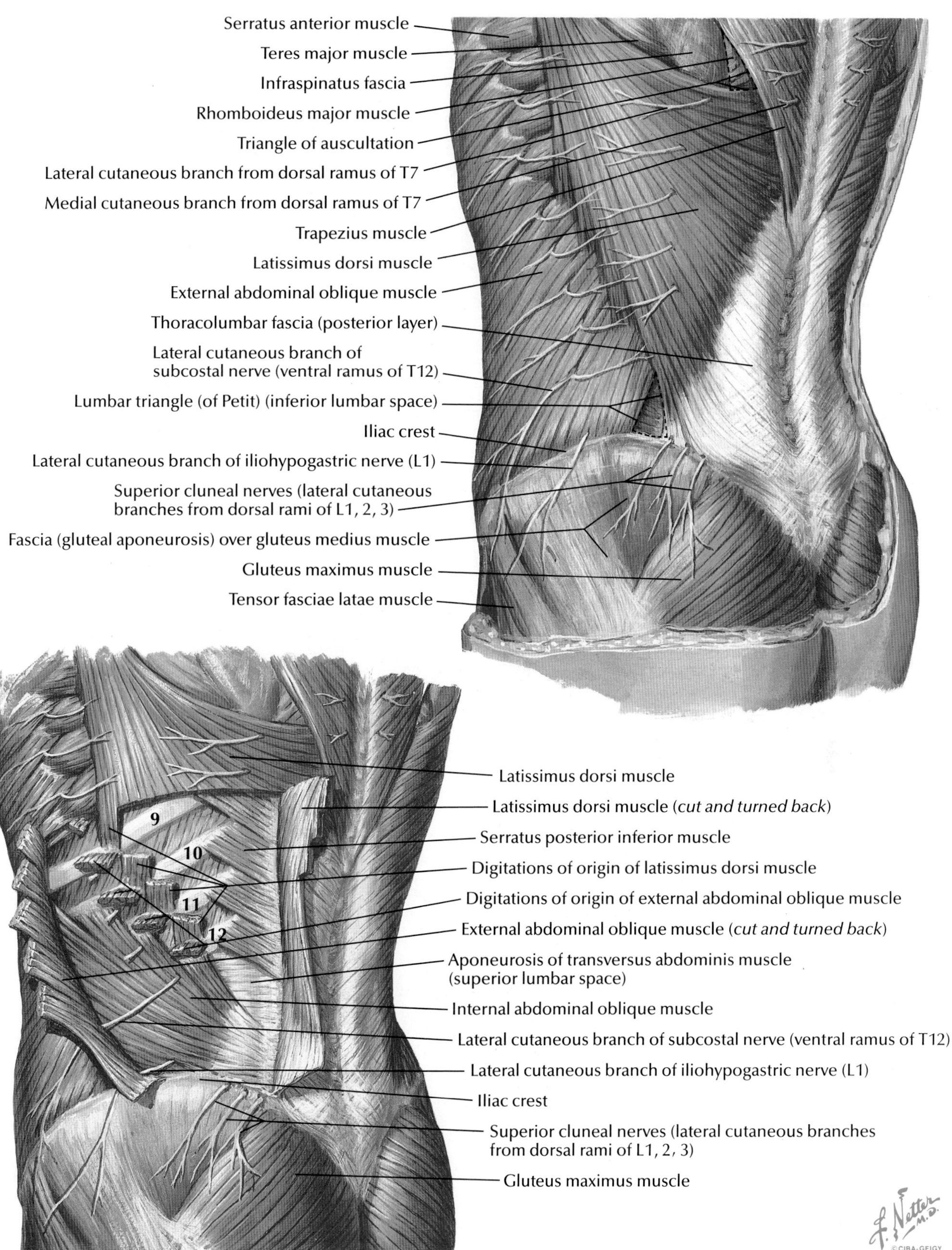

Serratus anterior muscle

Teres major muscle

Infraspinatus fascia

Rhomboideus major muscle

Triangle of auscultation

Lateral cutaneous branch from dorsal ramus of T7

Medial cutaneous branch from dorsal ramus of T7

Trapezius muscle

Latissimus dorsi muscle

External abdominal oblique muscle

Thoracolumbar fascia (posterior layer)

Lateral cutaneous branch of subcostal nerve (ventral ramus of T12)

Lumbar triangle (of Petit) (inferior lumbar space)

Iliac crest

Lateral cutaneous branch of iliohypogastric nerve (L1)

Superior cluneal nerves (lateral cutaneous branches from dorsal rami of L1, 2, 3)

Fascia (gluteal aponeurosis) over gluteus medius muscle

Gluteus maximus muscle

Tensor fasciae latae muscle

Latissimus dorsi muscle

Latissimus dorsi muscle (*cut and turned back*)

Serratus posterior inferior muscle

Digitations of origin of latissimus dorsi muscle

Digitations of origin of external abdominal oblique muscle

External abdominal oblique muscle (*cut and turned back*)

Aponeurosis of transversus abdominis muscle (superior lumbar space)

Internal abdominal oblique muscle

Lateral cutaneous branch of subcostal nerve (ventral ramus of T12)

Lateral cutaneous branch of iliohypogastric nerve (L1)

Iliac crest

Superior cluneal nerves (lateral cutaneous branches from dorsal rami of L1, 2, 3)

Gluteus maximus muscle

BODY WALL

PLATE 237

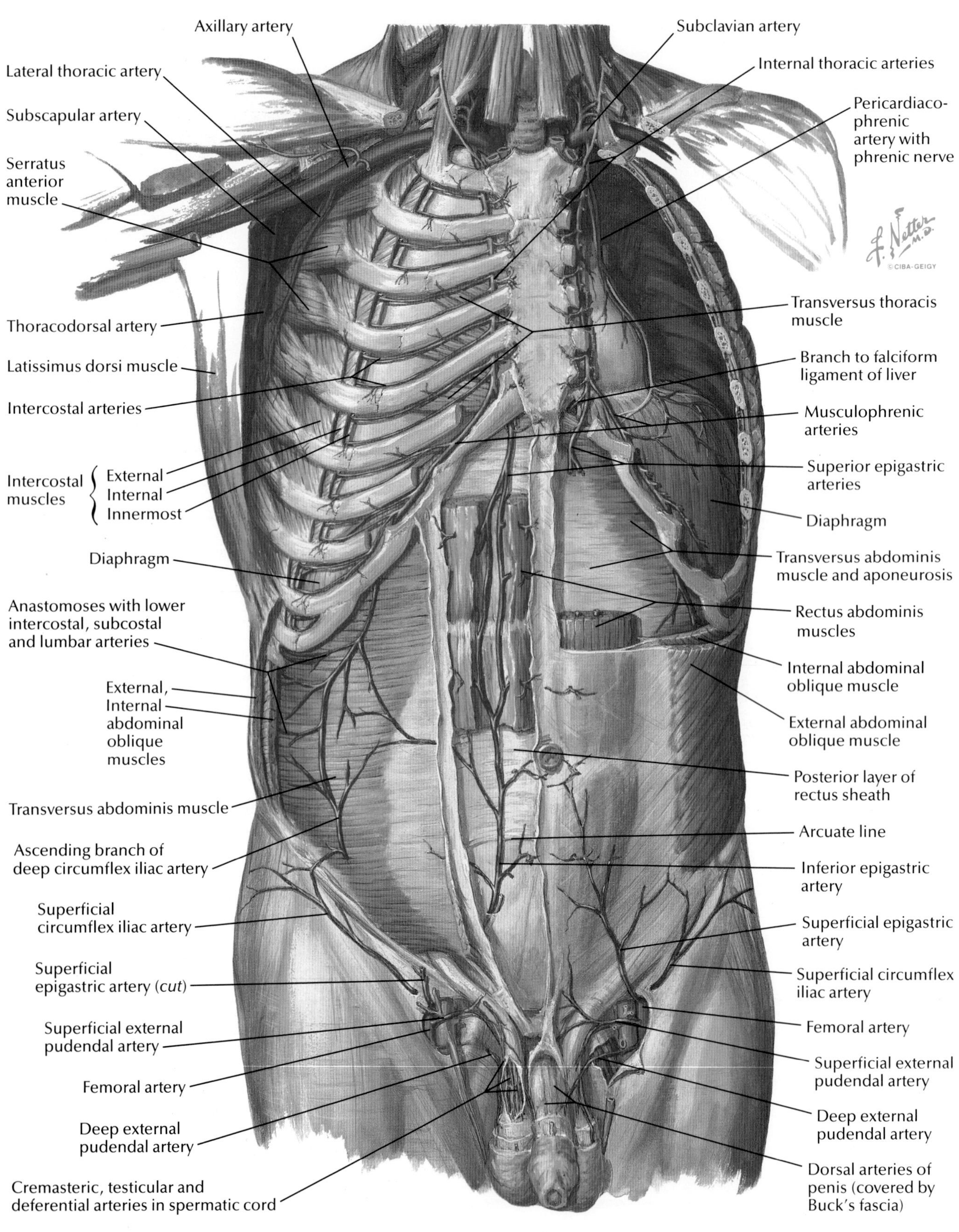

Axillary artery

Lateral thoracic artery

Subscapular artery

Serratus anterior muscle

Thoracodorsal artery

Latissimus dorsi muscle

Intercostal arteries

Intercostal muscles { External
Internal
Innermost

Diaphragm

Anastomoses with lower intercostal, subcostal and lumbar arteries

External,
Internal
abdominal
oblique
muscles

Transversus abdominis muscle

Ascending branch of deep circumflex iliac artery

Superficial circumflex iliac artery

Superficial epigastric artery (cut)

Superficial external pudendal artery

Femoral artery

Deep external pudendal artery

Cremasteric, testicular and deferential arteries in spermatic cord

Subclavian artery

Internal thoracic arteries

Pericardiaco-phrenic artery with phrenic nerve

Transversus thoracis muscle

Branch to falciform ligament of liver

Musculophrenic arteries

Superior epigastric arteries

Diaphragm

Transversus abdominis muscle and aponeurosis

Rectus abdominis muscles

Internal abdominal oblique muscle

External abdominal oblique muscle

Posterior layer of rectus sheath

Arcuate line

Inferior epigastric artery

Superficial epigastric artery

Superficial circumflex iliac artery

Femoral artery

Superficial external pudendal artery

Deep external pudendal artery

Dorsal arteries of penis (covered by Buck's fascia)

PLATE 238

ABDOMEN

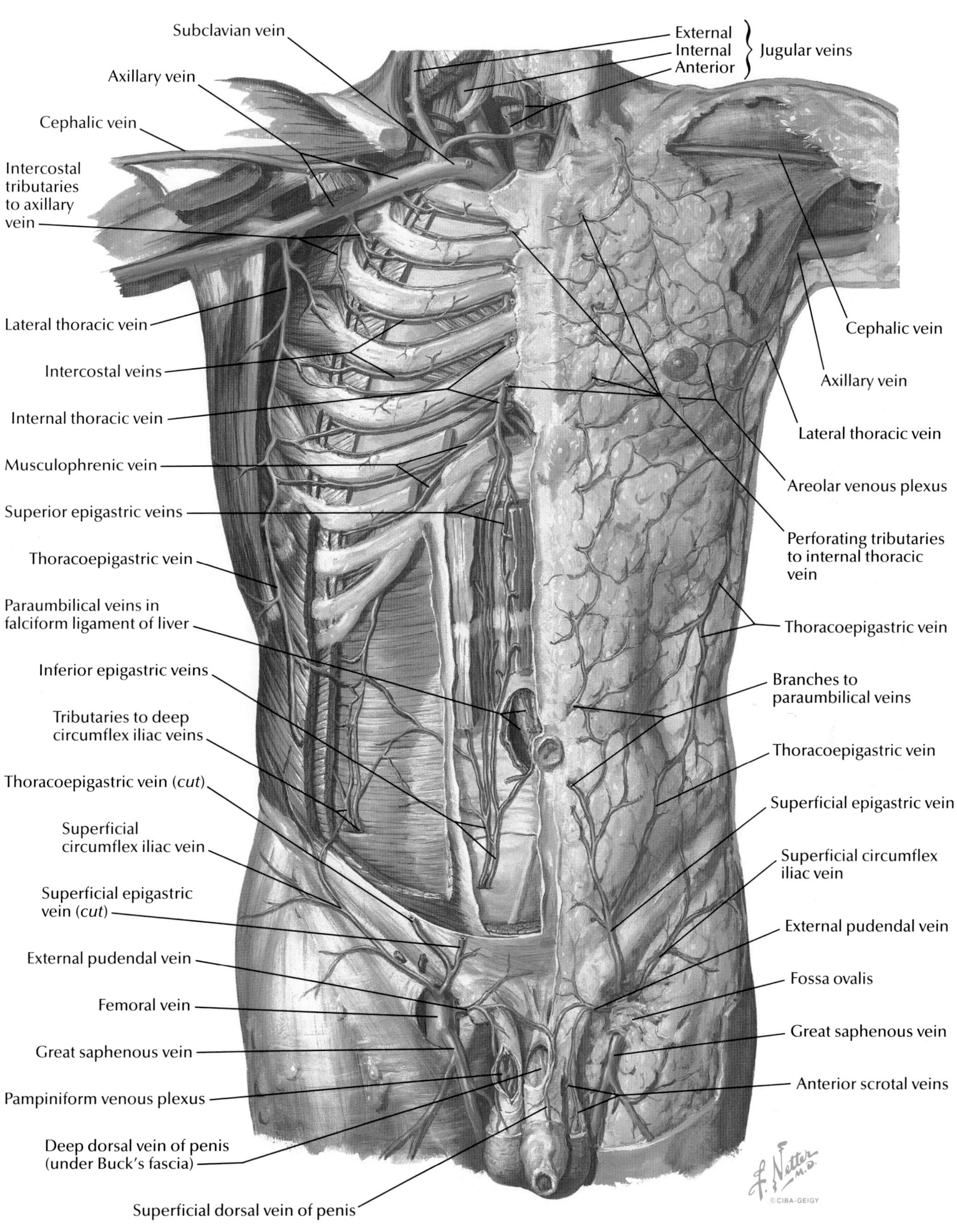

Subclavian vein

Axillary vein

Cephalic vein

Intercostal tributaries to axillary vein

Lateral thoracic vein

Intercostal veins

Internal thoracic vein

Musculophrenic vein

Superior epigastric veins

Thoracoepigastric vein

Paraumbilical veins in falciform ligament of liver

Inferior epigastric veins

Tributaries to deep circumflex iliac veins

Thoracoepigastric vein (cut)

Superficial circumflex iliac vein

Superficial epigastric vein (cut)

External pudendal vein

Femoral vein

Great saphenous vein

Pampiniform venous plexus

Deep dorsal vein of penis (under Buck's fascia)

Superficial dorsal vein of penis

External } Internal } Jugular veins Anterior }

Cephalic vein

Axillary vein

Lateral thoracic vein

Areolar venous plexus

Perforating tributaries to internal thoracic vein

Thoracoepigastric vein

Branches to paraumbilical veins

Thoracoepigastric vein

Superficial epigastric vein

Superficial circumflex iliac vein

External pudendal vein

Fossa ovalis

Great saphenous vein

Anterior scrotal veins

Nerves of Anterior Abdominal Wall

SEE ALSO PLATES 163, 237, 250, 468

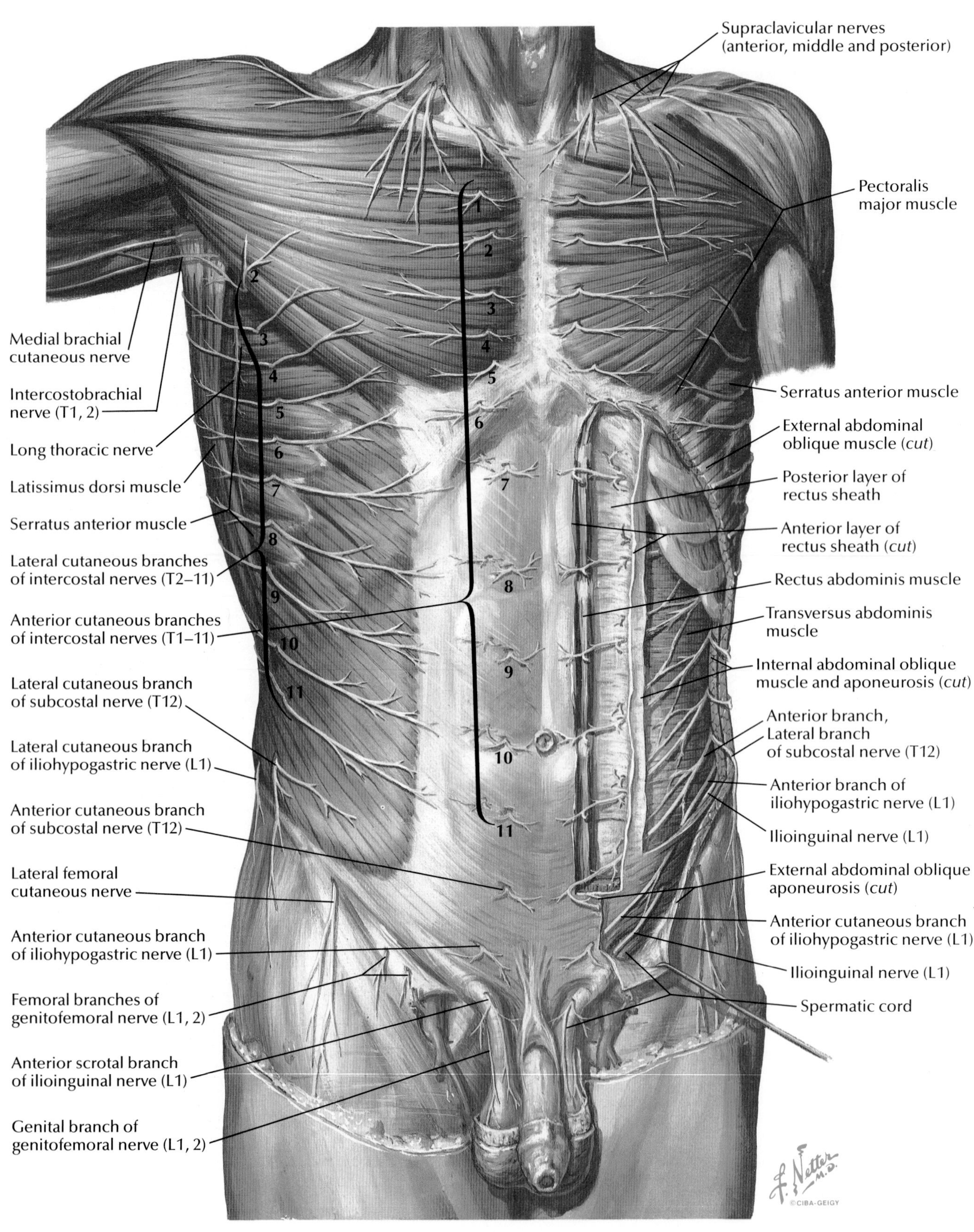

Supraclavicular nerves
(anterior, middle and posterior)

Pectoralis
major muscle

Medial brachial
cutaneous nerve

Intercostobrachial
nerve (T1, 2)

Long thoracic nerve

Latissimus dorsi muscle

Serratus anterior muscle

Lateral cutaneous branches
of intercostal nerves (T2–11)

Anterior cutaneous branches
of intercostal nerves (T1–11)

Lateral cutaneous branch
of subcostal nerve (T12)

Lateral cutaneous branch
of iliohypogastric nerve (L1)

Anterior cutaneous branch
of subcostal nerve (T12)

Lateral femoral
cutaneous nerve

Anterior cutaneous branch
of iliohypogastric nerve (L1)

Femoral branches of
genitofemoral nerve (L1, 2)

Anterior scrotal branch
of ilioinguinal nerve (L1)

Genital branch of
genitofemoral nerve (L1, 2)

Serratus anterior muscle

External abdominal
oblique muscle (cut)

Posterior layer of
rectus sheath

Anterior layer of
rectus sheath (cut)

Rectus abdominis muscle

Transversus abdominis
muscle

Internal abdominal oblique
muscle and aponeurosis (cut)

Anterior branch,
Lateral branch
of subcostal nerve (T12)

Anterior branch of
iliohypogastric nerve (L1)

Ilioinguinal nerve (L1)

External abdominal oblique
aponeurosis (cut)

Anterior cutaneous branch
of iliohypogastric nerve (L1)

Ilioinguinal nerve (L1)

Spermatic cord

PLATE 240

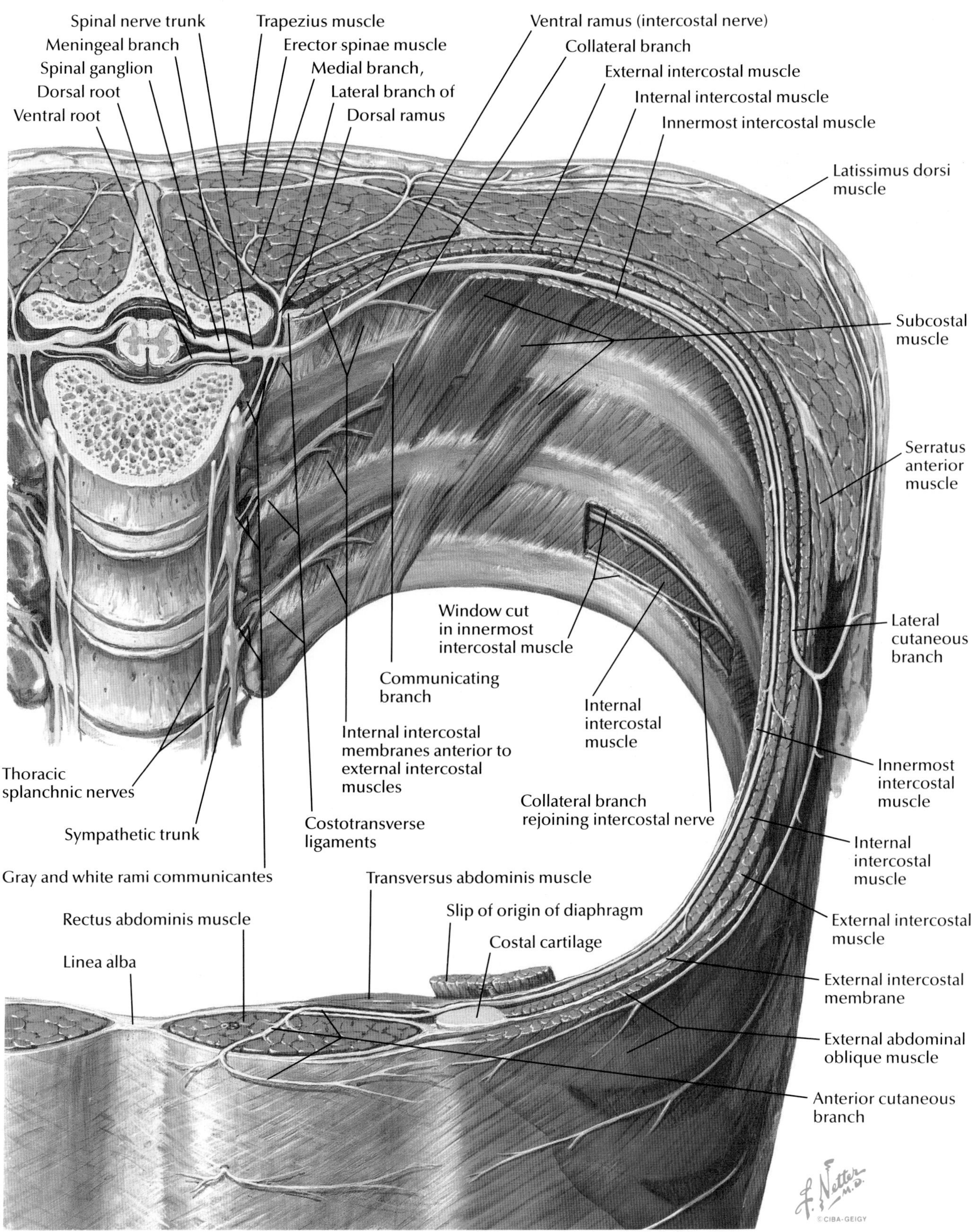

Spinal nerve trunk
Meningeal branch
Spinal ganglion
Dorsal root
Ventral root

Trapezius muscle
Erector spinae muscle
Medial branch,
Lateral branch of
Dorsal ramus

Ventral ramus (intercostal nerve)
Collateral branch
External intercostal muscle
Internal intercostal muscle
Innermost intercostal muscle

Latissimus dorsi muscle

Subcostal muscle

Serratus anterior muscle

Window cut in innermost intercostal muscle

Communicating branch

Internal intercostal membranes anterior to external intercostal muscles

Internal intercostal muscle

Lateral cutaneous branch

Thoracic splanchnic nerves

Collateral branch rejoining intercostal nerve

Innermost intercostal muscle

Internal intercostal muscle

Sympathetic trunk

Costotransverse ligaments

External intercostal muscle

Gray and white rami communicantes

Transversus abdominis muscle

External intercostal membrane

Rectus abdominis muscle

Slip of origin of diaphragm

External abdominal oblique muscle

Linea alba

Costal cartilage

Anterior cutaneous branch

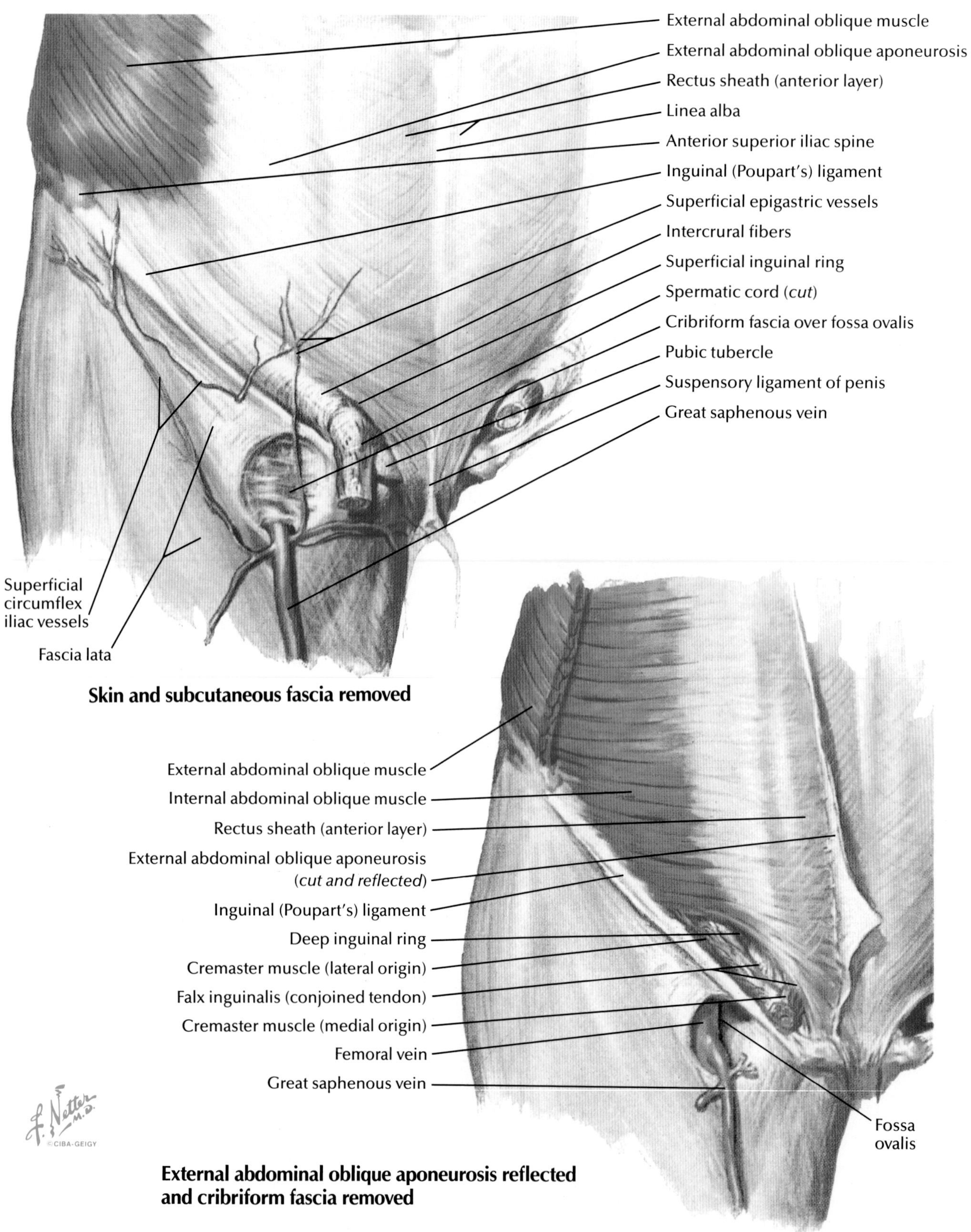

External abdominal oblique muscle
External abdominal oblique aponeurosis
Rectus sheath (anterior layer)
Linea alba
Anterior superior iliac spine
Inguinal (Poupart's) ligament
Superficial epigastric vessels
Intercrural fibers
Superficial inguinal ring
Spermatic cord (*cut*)
Cribriform fascia over fossa ovalis
Pubic tubercle
Suspensory ligament of penis
Great saphenous vein

Superficial
circumflex
iliac vessels

Fascia lata

Skin and subcutaneous fascia removed

External abdominal oblique muscle
Internal abdominal oblique muscle
Rectus sheath (anterior layer)
External abdominal oblique aponeurosis
(*cut and reflected*)
Inguinal (Poupart's) ligament
Deep inguinal ring
Cremaster muscle (lateral origin)
Falx inguinalis (conjoined tendon)
Cremaster muscle (medial origin)
Femoral vein
Great saphenous vein

Fossa
ovalis

**External abdominal oblique aponeurosis reflected
and cribriform fascia removed**

PLATE 242

ABDOMEN

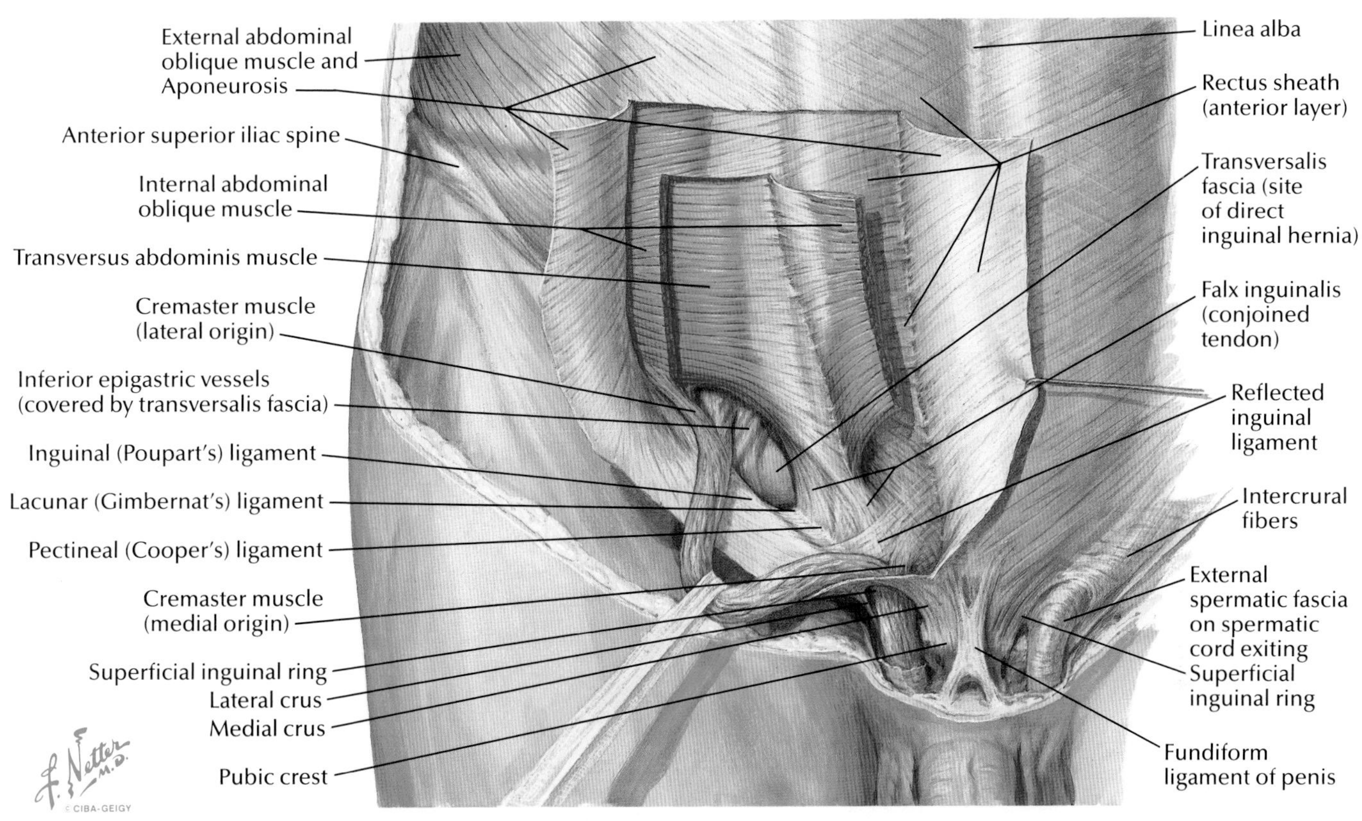

External abdominal oblique muscle and Aponeurosis

Anterior superior iliac spine

Internal abdominal oblique muscle

Transversus abdominis muscle

Cremaster muscle (lateral origin)

Inferior epigastric vessels (covered by transversalis fascia)

Inguinal (Poupart's) ligament

Lacunar (Gimbernat's) ligament

Pectineal (Cooper's) ligament

Cremaster muscle (medial origin)

Superficial inguinal ring

Lateral crus

Medial crus

Pubic crest

Linea alba

Rectus sheath (anterior layer)

Transversalis fascia (site of direct inguinal hernia)

Falx inguinalis (conjoined tendon)

Reflected inguinal ligament

Intercrural fibers

External spermatic fascia on spermatic cord exiting Superficial inguinal ring

Fundiform ligament of penis

Anterior view

Posterior (internal) view

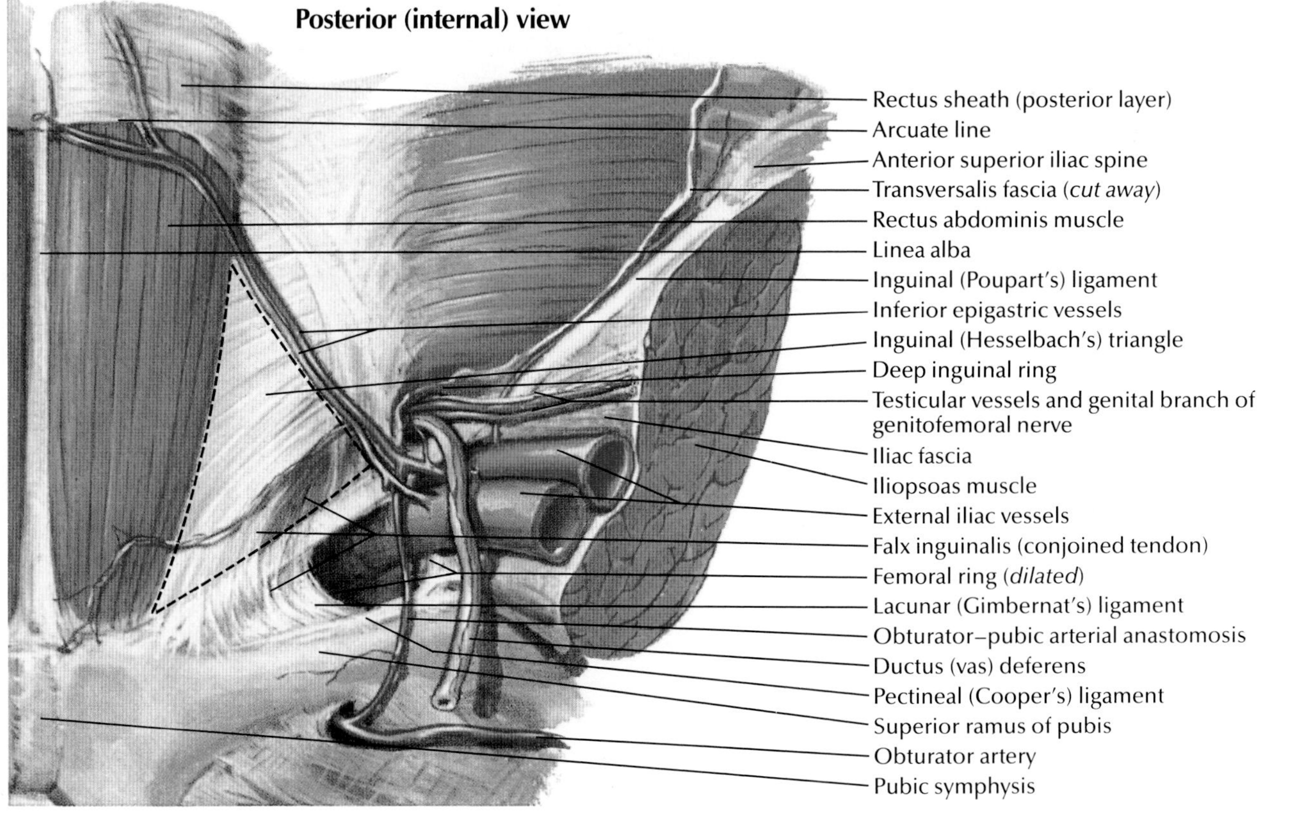

Rectus sheath (posterior layer)

Arcuate line

Anterior superior iliac spine

Transversalis fascia (*cut away*)

Rectus abdominis muscle

Linea alba

Inguinal (Poupart's) ligament

Inferior epigastric vessels

Inguinal (Hesselbach's) triangle

Deep inguinal ring

Testicular vessels and genital branch of genitofemoral nerve

Iliac fascia

Iliopsoas muscle

External iliac vessels

Falx inguinalis (conjoined tendon)

Femoral ring (*dilated*)

Lacunar (Gimbernat's) ligament

Obturator–pubic arterial anastomosis

Ductus (vas) deferens

Pectineal (Cooper's) ligament

Superior ramus of pubis

Obturator artery

Pubic symphysis

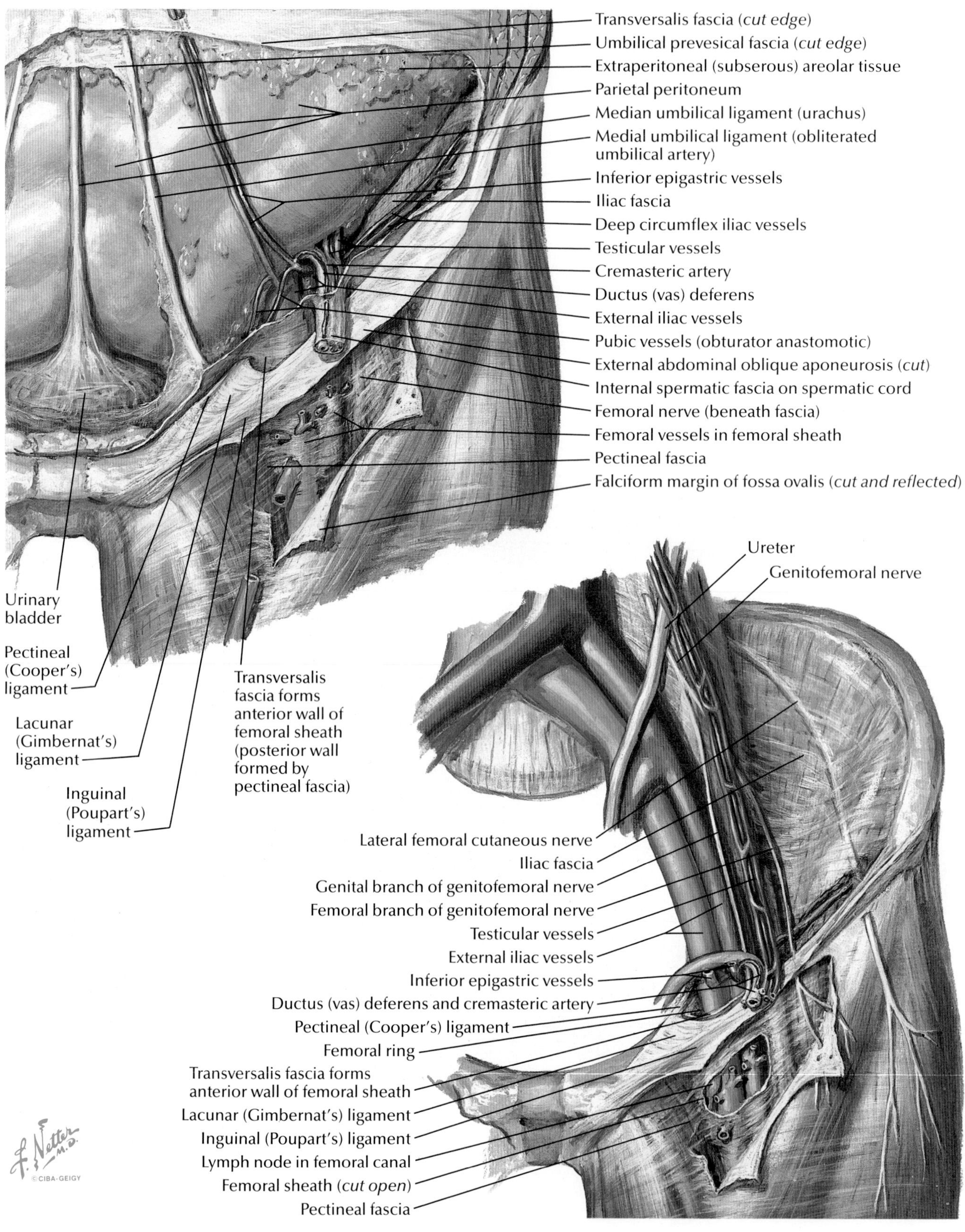

Transversalis fascia (*cut edge*)

Umbilical prevesical fascia (*cut edge*)

Extraperitoneal (subserous) areolar tissue

Parietal peritoneum

Median umbilical ligament (urachus)

Medial umbilical ligament (obliterated umbilical artery)

Inferior epigastric vessels

Iliac fascia

Deep circumflex iliac vessels

Testicular vessels

Cremasteric artery

Ductus (vas) deferens

External iliac vessels

Pubic vessels (obturator anastomotic)

External abdominal oblique aponeurosis (*cut*)

Internal spermatic fascia on spermatic cord

Femoral nerve (beneath fascia)

Femoral vessels in femoral sheath

Pectineal fascia

Falciform margin of fossa ovalis (*cut and reflected*)

Urinary bladder

Pectineal (Cooper's) ligament

Lacunar (Gimbernat's) ligament

Inguinal (Poupart's) ligament

Transversalis fascia forms anterior wall of femoral sheath (posterior wall formed by pectineal fascia)

Ureter

Genitofemoral nerve

Lateral femoral cutaneous nerve

Iliac fascia

Genital branch of genitofemoral nerve

Femoral branch of genitofemoral nerve

Testicular vessels

External iliac vessels

Inferior epigastric vessels

Ductus (vas) deferens and cremasteric artery

Pectineal (Cooper's) ligament

Femoral ring

Transversalis fascia forms anterior wall of femoral sheath

Lacunar (Gimbernat's) ligament

Inguinal (Poupart's) ligament

Lymph node in femoral canal

Femoral sheath (*cut open*)

Pectineal fascia

PLATE 244

ABDOMEN

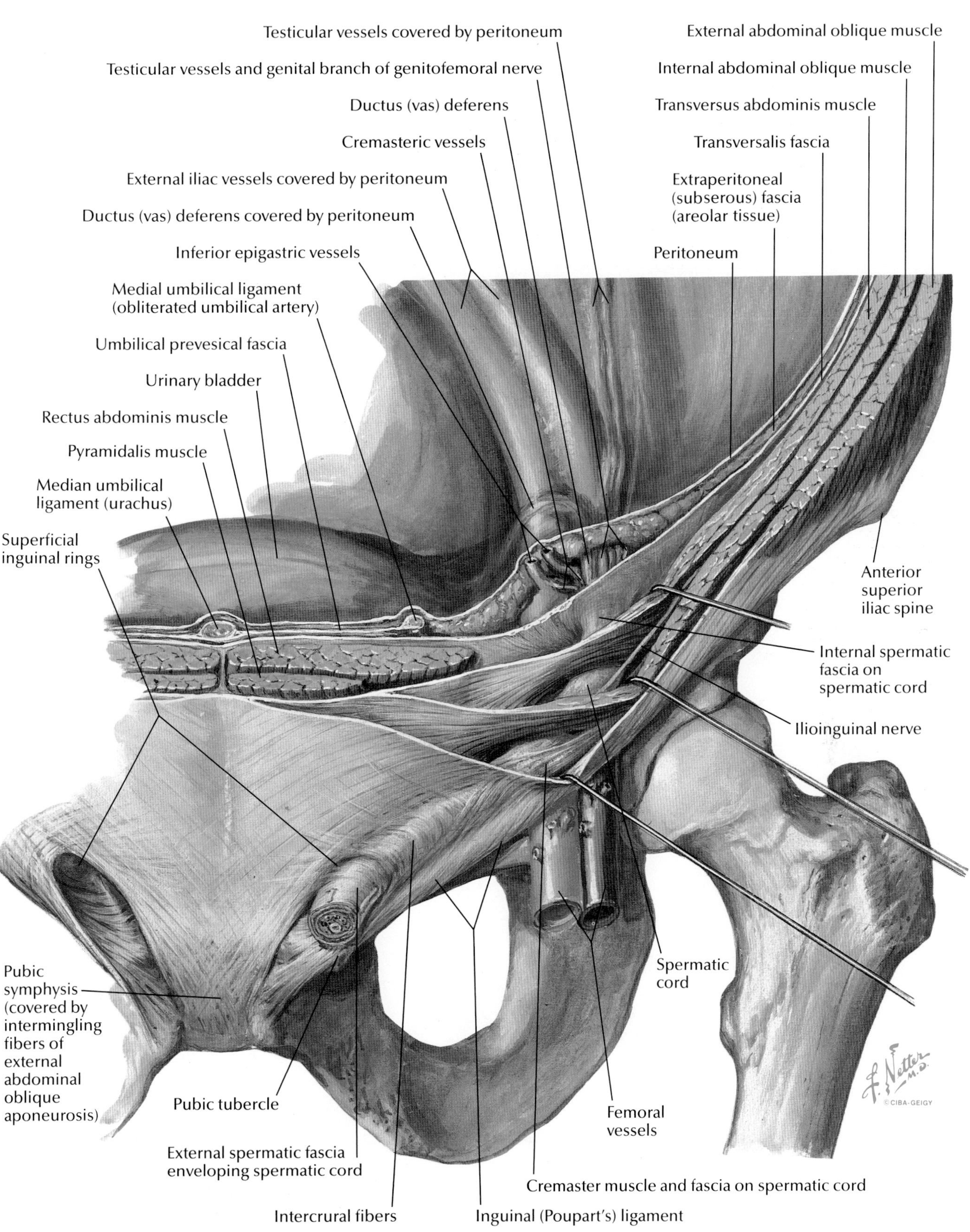

Testicular vessels covered by peritoneum

Testicular vessels and genital branch of genitofemoral nerve

Ductus (vas) deferens

Cremasteric vessels

External iliac vessels covered by peritoneum

Ductus (vas) deferens covered by peritoneum

Inferior epigastric vessels

Medial umbilical ligament (obliterated umbilical artery)

Umbilical prevesical fascia

Urinary bladder

Rectus abdominis muscle

Pyramidalis muscle

Median umbilical ligament (urachus)

Superficial inguinal rings

Pubic symphysis (covered by intermingling fibers of external abdominal oblique aponeurosis)

Pubic tubercle

External spermatic fascia enveloping spermatic cord

Intercrural fibers

Inguinal (Poupart's) ligament

External abdominal oblique muscle

Internal abdominal oblique muscle

Transversus abdominis muscle

Transversalis fascia

Extraperitoneal (subserous) fascia (areolar tissue)

Peritoneum

Anterior superior iliac spine

Internal spermatic fascia on spermatic cord

Ilioinguinal nerve

Spermatic cord

Femoral vessels

Cremaster muscle and fascia on spermatic cord

Posterior Abdominal Wall: Internal View

FOR DIAPHRAGM SEE ALSO PLATE 181

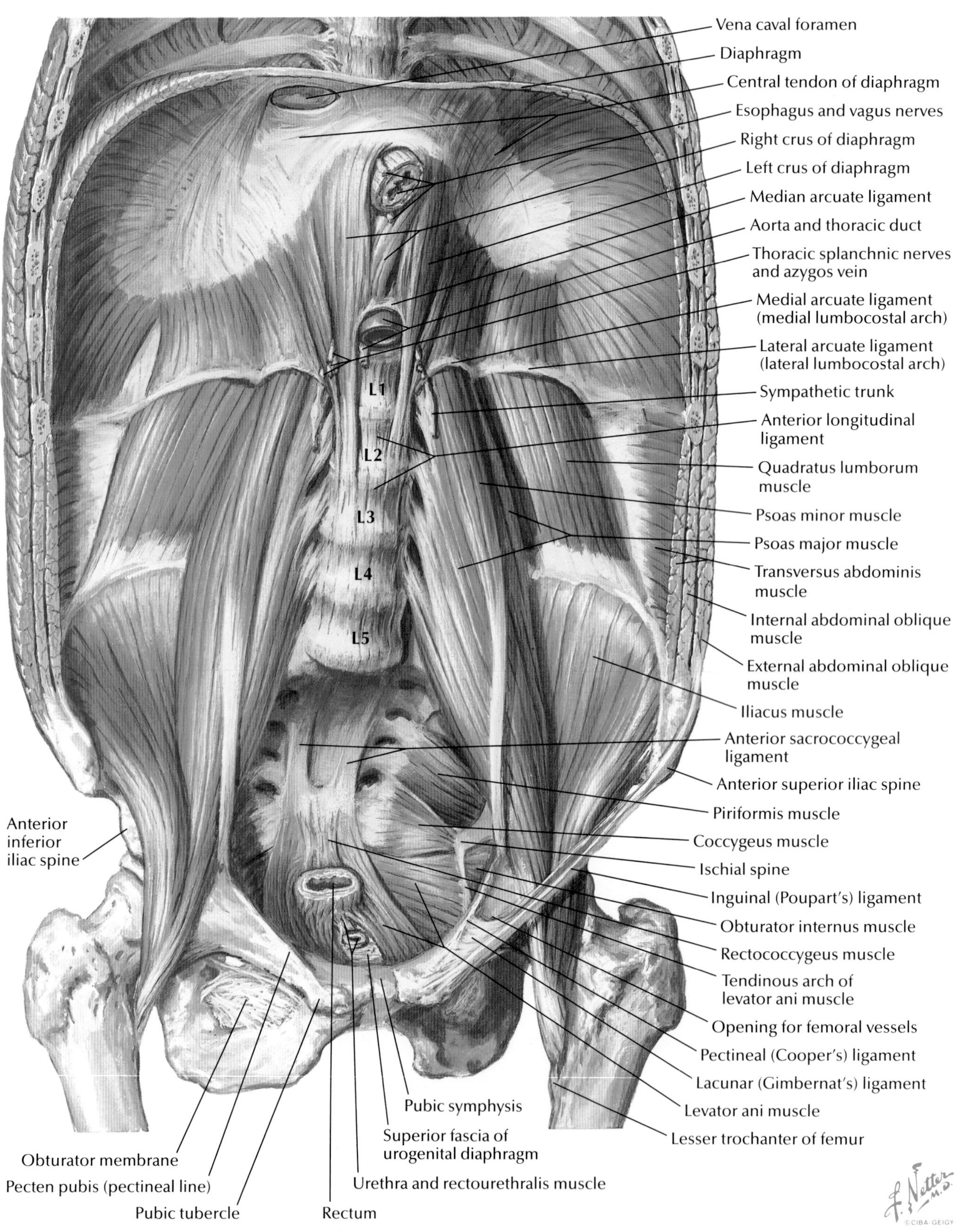

Vena caval foramen

Diaphragm

Central tendon of diaphragm

Esophagus and vagus nerves

Right crus of diaphragm

Left crus of diaphragm

Median arcuate ligament

Aorta and thoracic duct

Thoracic splanchnic nerves and azygos vein

Medial arcuate ligament (medial lumbocostal arch)

Lateral arcuate ligament (lateral lumbocostal arch)

Sympathetic trunk

Anterior longitudinal ligament

Quadratus lumborum muscle

Psoas minor muscle

Psoas major muscle

Transversus abdominis muscle

Internal abdominal oblique muscle

External abdominal oblique muscle

Iliacus muscle

Anterior sacrococcygeal ligament

Anterior superior iliac spine

Piriformis muscle

Coccygeus muscle

Ischial spine

Inguinal (Poupart's) ligament

Obturator internus muscle

Rectococcygeus muscle

Tendinous arch of levator ani muscle

Opening for femoral vessels

Pectineal (Cooper's) ligament

Lacunar (Gimbernat's) ligament

Levator ani muscle

Lesser trochanter of femur

L1

L2

L3

L4

L5

Anterior inferior iliac spine

Obturator membrane

Pecten pubis (pectineal line)

Pubic tubercle

Rectum

Pubic symphysis

Superior fascia of urogenital diaphragm

Urethra and rectourethralis muscle

PLATE 246

ABDOMEN

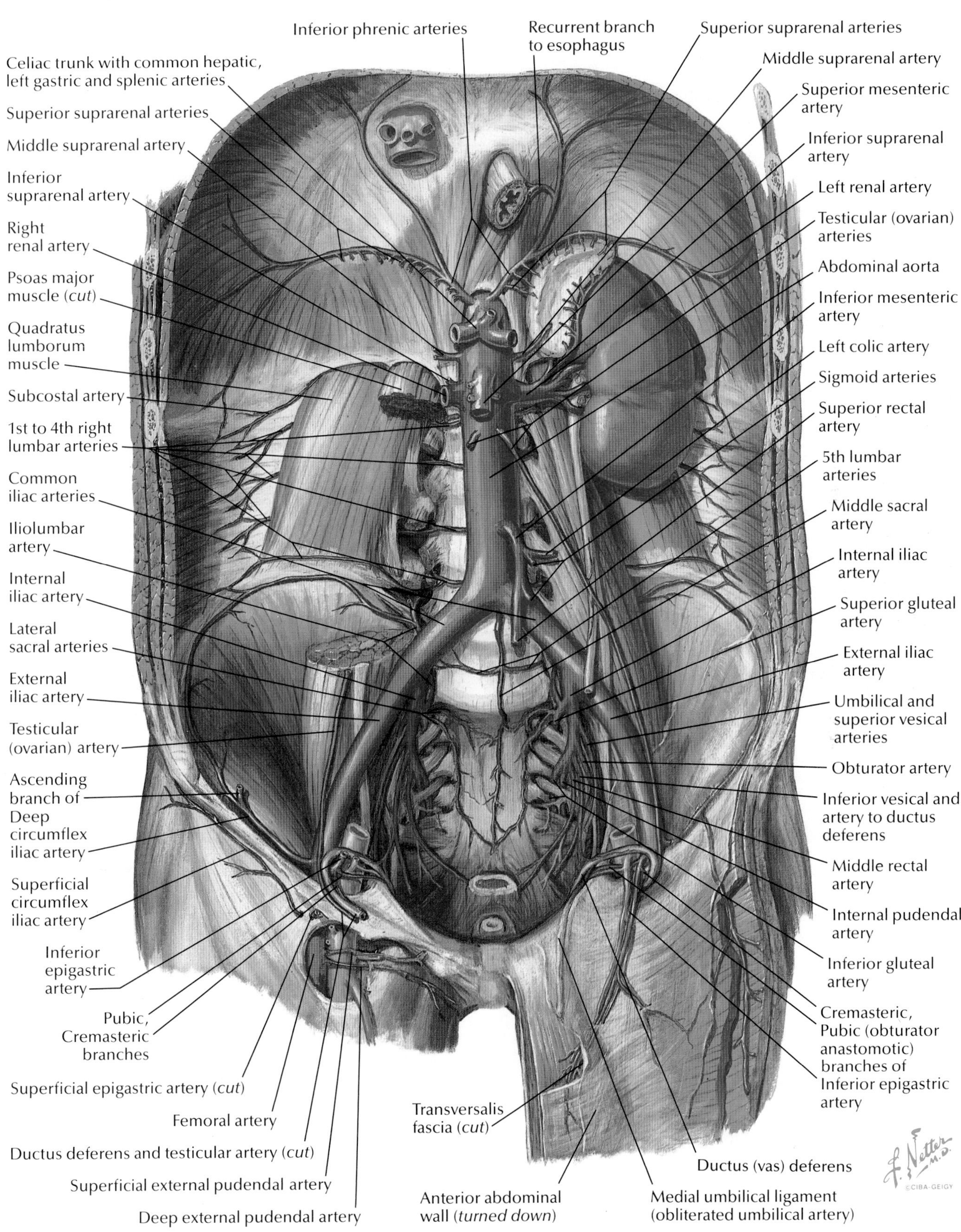

Inferior phrenic arteries

Recurrent branch to esophagus

Superior suprarenal arteries

Celiac trunk with common hepatic, left gastric and splenic arteries

Superior suprarenal arteries

Middle suprarenal artery

Inferior suprarenal artery

Right renal artery

Psoas major muscle (cut)

Quadratus lumborum muscle

Subcostal artery

1st to 4th right lumbar arteries

Common iliac arteries

Iliolumbar artery

Internal iliac artery

Lateral sacral arteries

External iliac artery

Testicular (ovarian) artery

Ascending branch of Deep circumflex iliac artery

Superficial circumflex iliac artery

Inferior epigastric artery

Pubic, Cremasteric branches

Superficial epigastric artery (cut)

Femoral artery

Ductus deferens and testicular artery (cut)

Superficial external pudendal artery

Deep external pudendal artery

Middle suprarenal artery

Superior mesenteric artery

Inferior suprarenal artery

Left renal artery

Testicular (ovarian) arteries

Abdominal aorta

Inferior mesenteric artery

Left colic artery

Sigmoid arteries

Superior rectal artery

5th lumbar arteries

Middle sacral artery

Internal iliac artery

Superior gluteal artery

External iliac artery

Umbilical and superior vesical arteries

Obturator artery

Inferior vesical and artery to ductus deferens

Middle rectal artery

Internal pudendal artery

Inferior gluteal artery

Cremasteric, Pubic (obturator anastomotic) branches of Inferior epigastric artery

Ductus (vas) deferens

Medial umbilical ligament (obliterated umbilical artery)

Transversalis fascia (cut)

Anterior abdominal wall (turned down)

Veins of Posterior Abdominal Wall

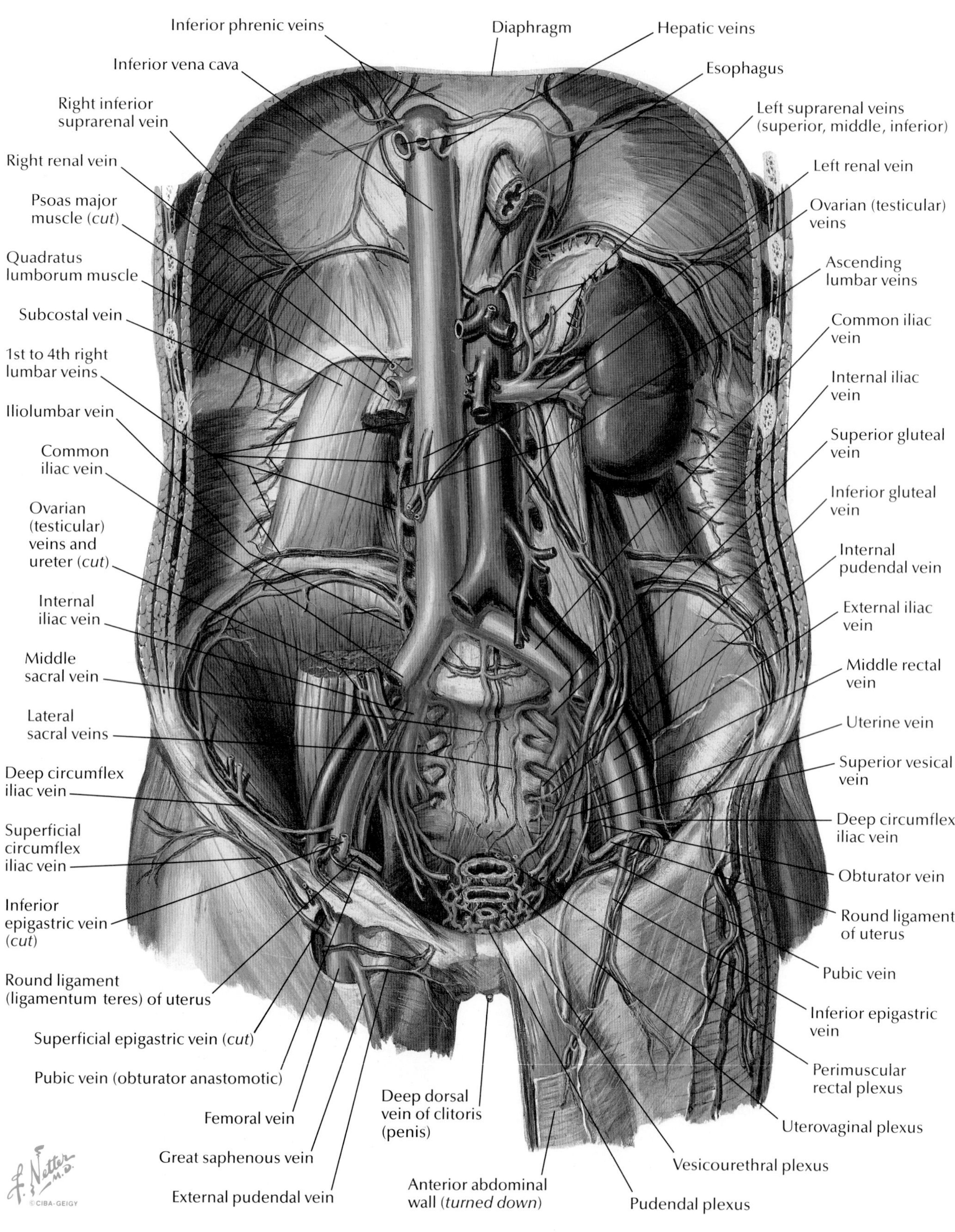

Inferior phrenic veins

Diaphragm

Hepatic veins

Inferior vena cava

Esophagus

Right inferior suprarenal vein

Left suprarenal veins (superior, middle, inferior)

Right renal vein

Left renal vein

Psoas major muscle (cut)

Ovarian (testicular) veins

Quadratus lumborum muscle

Ascending lumbar veins

Subcostal vein

Common iliac vein

1st to 4th right lumbar veins

Internal iliac vein

Iliolumbar vein

Superior gluteal vein

Common iliac vein

Inferior gluteal vein

Ovarian (testicular) veins and ureter (cut)

Internal pudendal vein

Internal iliac vein

External iliac vein

Middle sacral vein

Middle rectal vein

Lateral sacral veins

Uterine vein

Deep circumflex iliac vein

Superior vesical vein

Superficial circumflex iliac vein

Deep circumflex iliac vein

Inferior epigastric vein (cut)

Obturator vein

Round ligament of uterus

Round ligament (ligamentum teres) of uterus

Pubic vein

Superficial epigastric vein (cut)

Inferior epigastric vein

Pubic vein (obturator anastomotic)

Perimuscular rectal plexus

Femoral vein

Deep dorsal vein of clitoris (penis)

Uterovaginal plexus

Great saphenous vein

Vesicourethral plexus

External pudendal vein

Anterior abdominal wall (turned down)

Pudendal plexus

PLATE 248

ABDOMEN

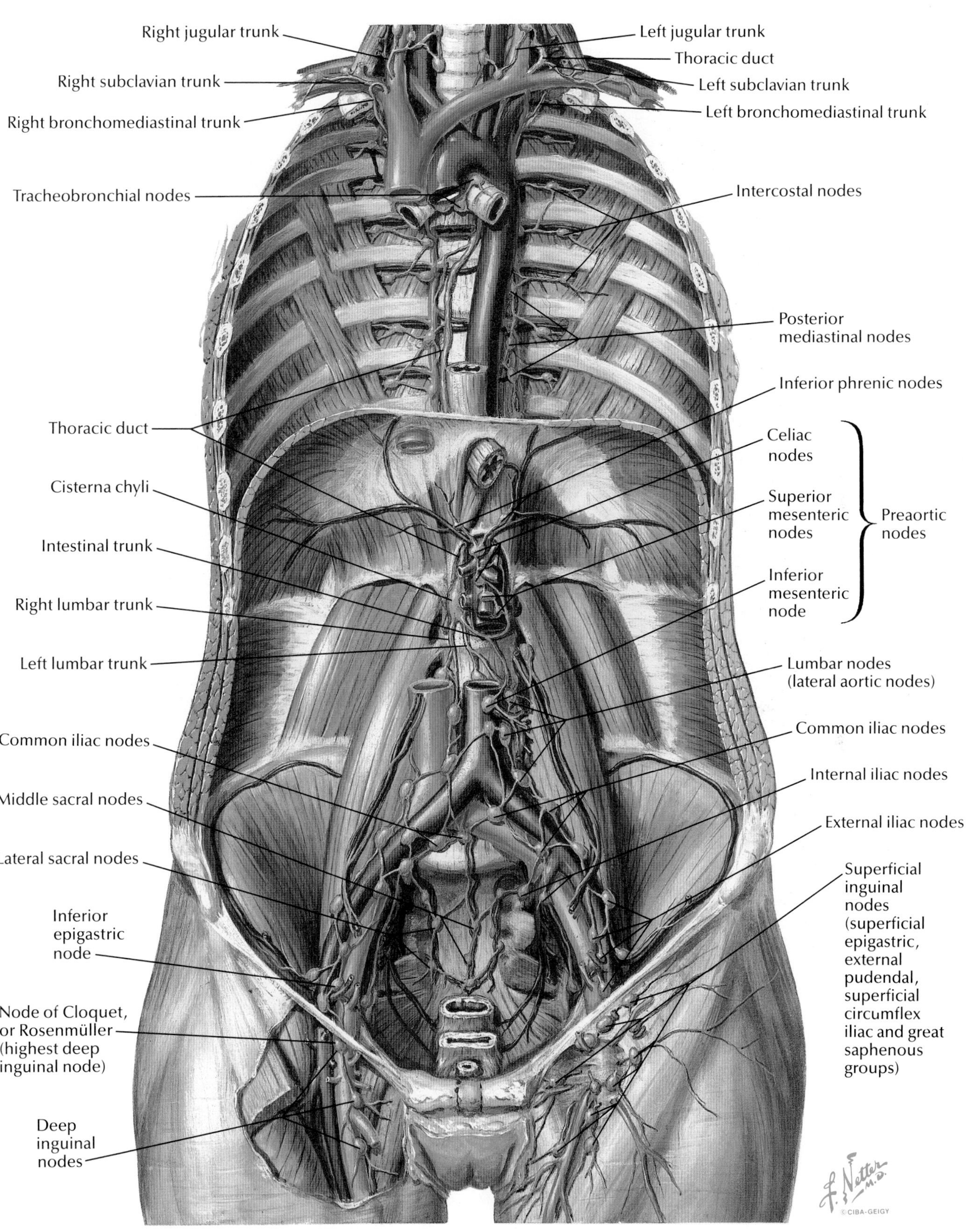

Right jugular trunk

Right subclavian trunk

Right bronchomediastinal trunk

Tracheobronchial nodes

Thoracic duct

Cisterna chyli

Intestinal trunk

Right lumbar trunk

Left lumbar trunk

Common iliac nodes

Middle sacral nodes

Lateral sacral nodes

Inferior epigastric node

Node of Cloquet, or Rosenmüller (highest deep inguinal node)

Deep inguinal nodes

Left jugular trunk

Thoracic duct

Left subclavian trunk

Left bronchomediastinal trunk

Intercostal nodes

Posterior mediastinal nodes

Inferior phrenic nodes

Celiac nodes

Superior mesenteric nodes

Preaortic nodes

Inferior mesenteric node

Lumbar nodes (lateral aortic nodes)

Common iliac nodes

Internal iliac nodes

External iliac nodes

Superficial inguinal nodes (superficial epigastric, external pudendal, superficial circumflex iliac and great saphenous groups)

Nerves of Posterior Abdominal Wall

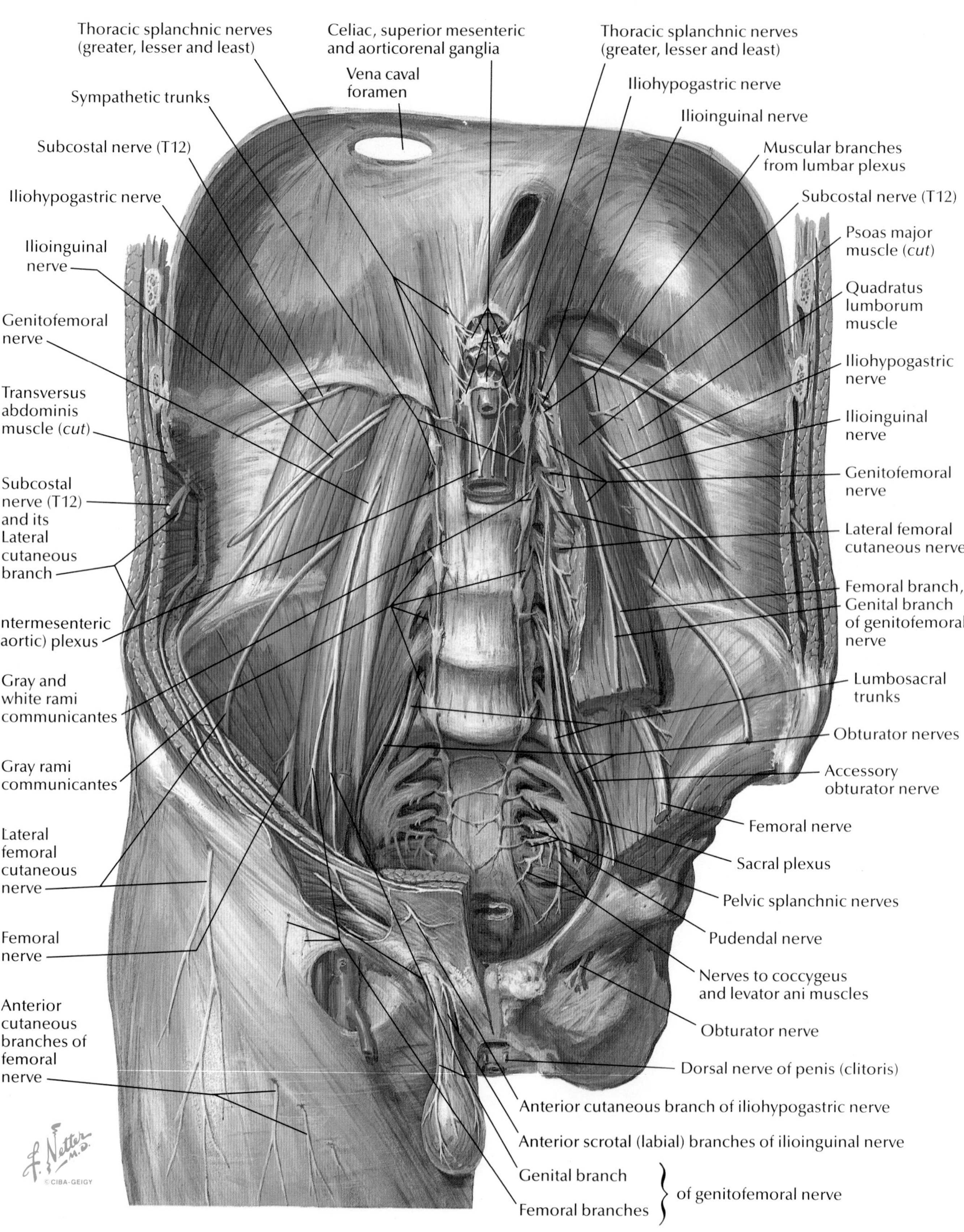

Thoracic splanchnic nerves (greater, lesser and least)

Celiac, superior mesenteric and aorticorenal ganglia

Vena caval foramen

Thoracic splanchnic nerves (greater, lesser and least)

Iliohypogastric nerve

Ilioinguinal nerve

Sympathetic trunks

Muscular branches from lumbar plexus

Subcostal nerve (T12)

Subcostal nerve (T12)

Iliohypogastric nerve

Psoas major muscle (cut)

Ilioinguinal nerve

Quadratus lumborum muscle

Genitofemoral nerve

Iliohypogastric nerve

Transversus abdominis muscle (cut)

Ilioinguinal nerve

Genitofemoral nerve

Subcostal nerve (T12) and its Lateral cutaneous branch

Lateral femoral cutaneous nerve

Femoral branch, Genital branch of genitofemoral nerve

Intermesenteric (aortic) plexus

Gray and white rami communicantes

Lumbosacral trunks

Gray rami communicantes

Obturator nerves

Accessory obturator nerve

Lateral femoral cutaneous nerve

Femoral nerve

Femoral nerve

Sacral plexus

Pelvic splanchnic nerves

Pudendal nerve

Anterior cutaneous branches of femoral nerve

Nerves to coccygeus and levator ani muscles

Obturator nerve

Dorsal nerve of penis (clitoris)

Anterior cutaneous branch of iliohypogastric nerve

Anterior scrotal (labial) branches of ilioinguinal nerve

Genital branch

Femoral branches
} of genitofemoral nerve

PLATE 250

ABDOMEN

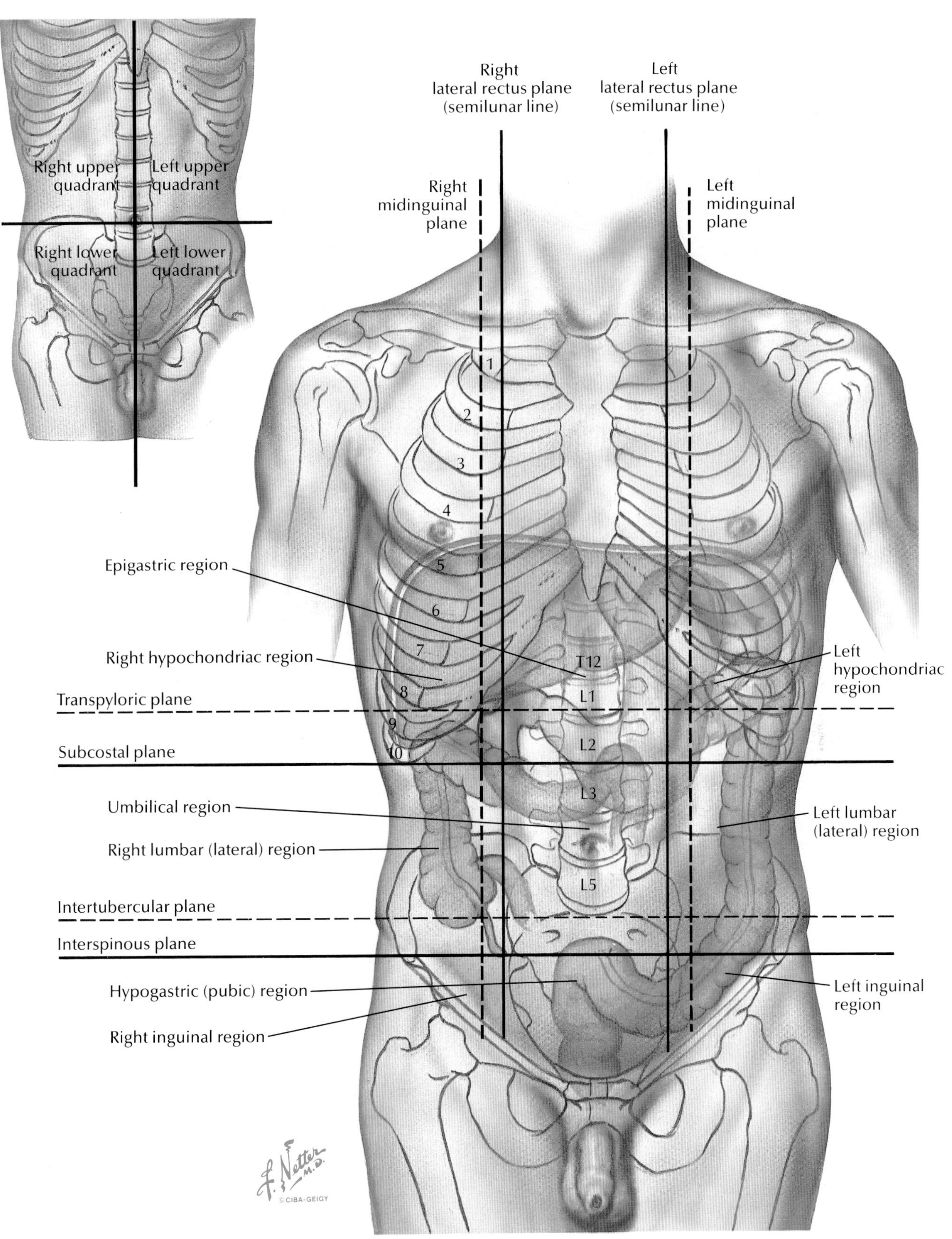

Right upper quadrant

Left upper quadrant

Right lower quadrant

Left lower quadrant

Right lateral rectus plane (semilunar line)

Left lateral rectus plane (semilunar line)

Right midinguinal plane

Left midinguinal plane

Epigastric region

Right hypochondriac region

Transpyloric plane

Subcostal plane

Umbilical region

Right lumbar (lateral) region

Intertubercular plane

Interspinous plane

Hypogastric (pubic) region

Right inguinal region

Left hypochondriac region

Left lumbar (lateral) region

Left inguinal region

T12
L1
L2
L3
L5

Greater Omentum and Abdominal Viscera

SEE ALSO PLATES 258, 332, 333

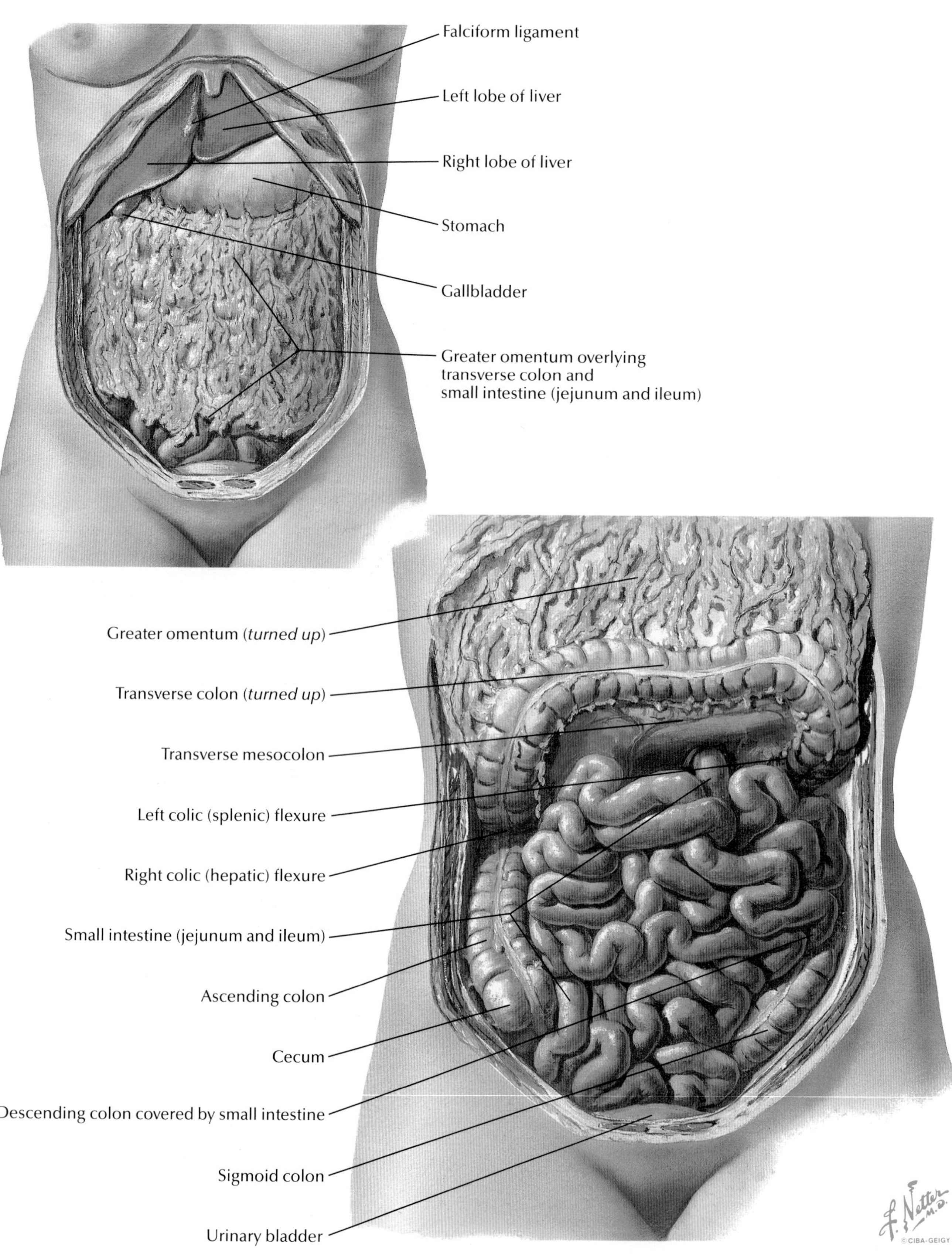

Falciform ligament

Left lobe of liver

Right lobe of liver

Stomach

Gallbladder

Greater omentum overlying
transverse colon and
small intestine (jejunum and ileum)

Greater omentum (*turned up*)

Transverse colon (*turned up*)

Transverse mesocolon

Left colic (splenic) flexure

Right colic (hepatic) flexure

Small intestine (jejunum and ileum)

Ascending colon

Cecum

Descending colon covered by small intestine

Sigmoid colon

Urinary bladder

PLATE 252

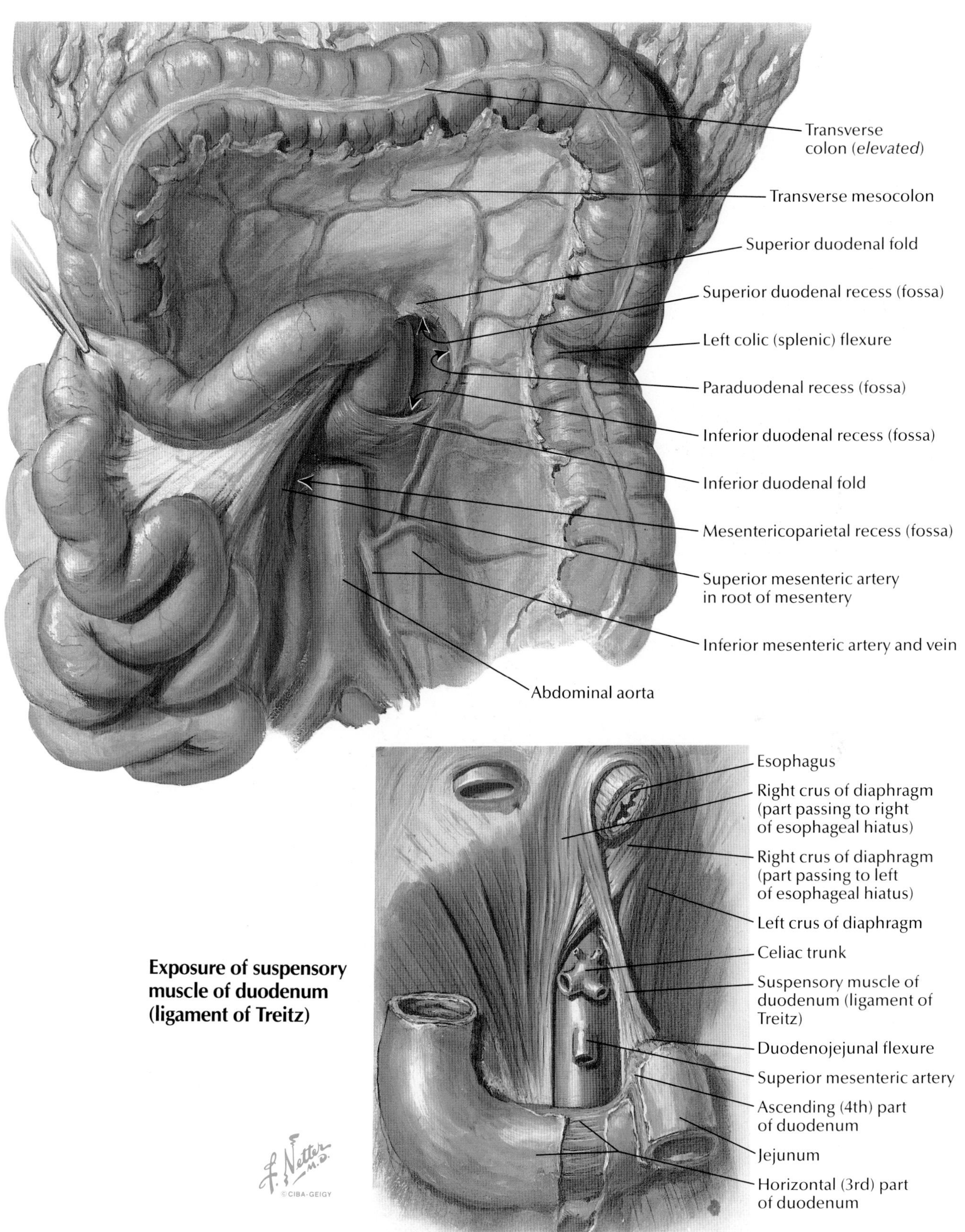

Transverse colon (*elevated*)

Transverse mesocolon

Superior duodenal fold

Superior duodenal recess (fossa)

Left colic (splenic) flexure

Paraduodenal recess (fossa)

Inferior duodenal recess (fossa)

Inferior duodenal fold

Mesentericoparietal recess (fossa)

Superior mesenteric artery in root of mesentery

Inferior mesenteric artery and vein

Abdominal aorta

Esophagus

Right crus of diaphragm (part passing to right of esophageal hiatus)

Right crus of diaphragm (part passing to left of esophageal hiatus)

Left crus of diaphragm

Celiac trunk

Suspensory muscle of duodenum (ligament of Treitz)

Duodenojejunal flexure

Superior mesenteric artery

Ascending (4th) part of duodenum

Jejunum

Horizontal (3rd) part of duodenum

Exposure of suspensory muscle of duodenum (ligament of Treitz)

Mesenteric Relations of Intestines (continued)

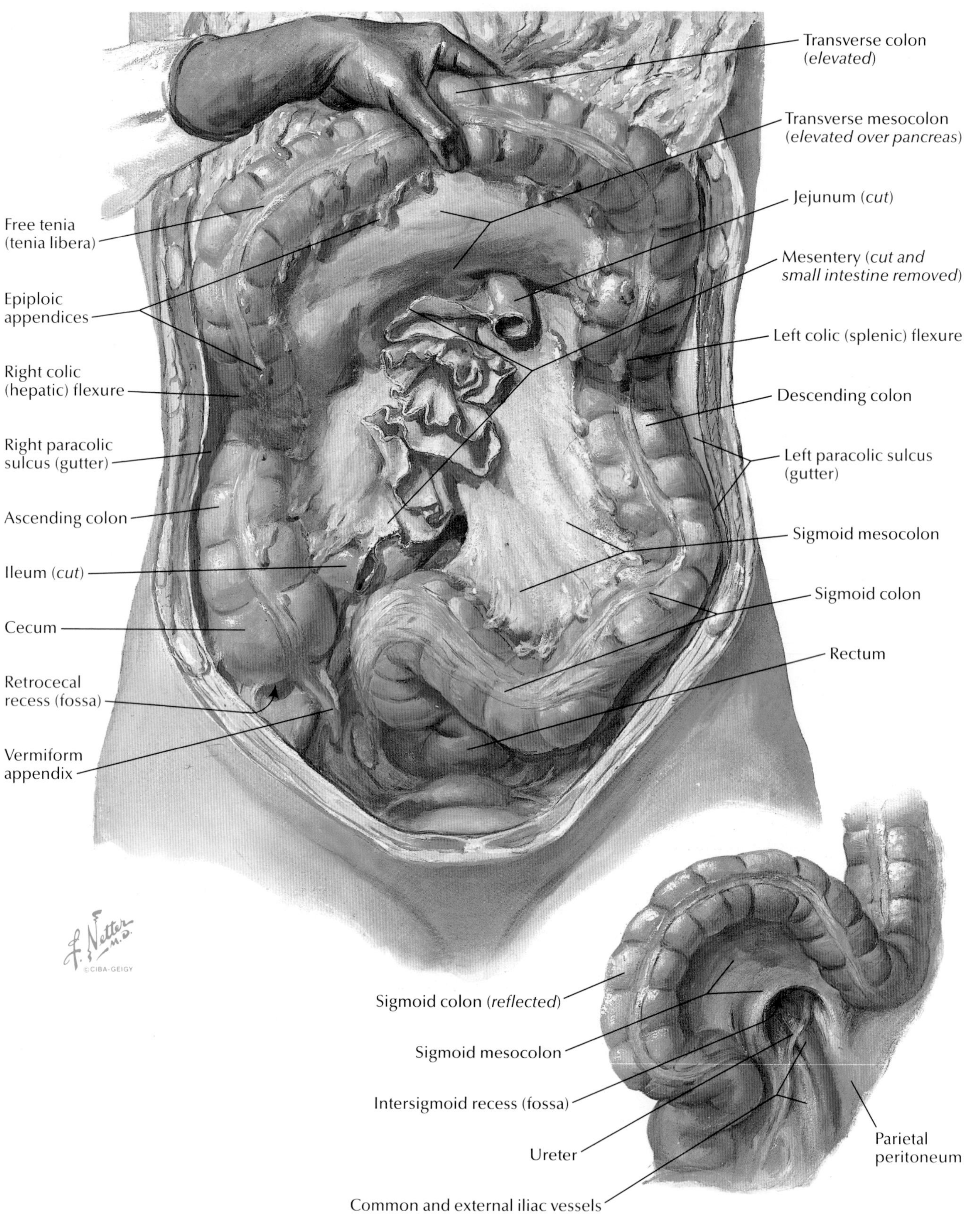

Transverse colon (*elevated*)

Transverse mesocolon (*elevated over pancreas*)

Jejunum (*cut*)

Mesentery (*cut and small intestine removed*)

Left colic (splenic) flexure

Descending colon

Left paracolic sulcus (gutter)

Sigmoid mesocolon

Sigmoid colon

Rectum

Free tenia (tenia libera)

Epiploic appendices

Right colic (hepatic) flexure

Right paracolic sulcus (gutter)

Ascending colon

Ileum (*cut*)

Cecum

Retrocecal recess (fossa)

Vermiform appendix

Sigmoid colon (*reflected*)

Sigmoid mesocolon

Intersigmoid recess (fossa)

Ureter

Common and external iliac vessels

Parietal peritoneum

PLATE 254

ABDOMEN

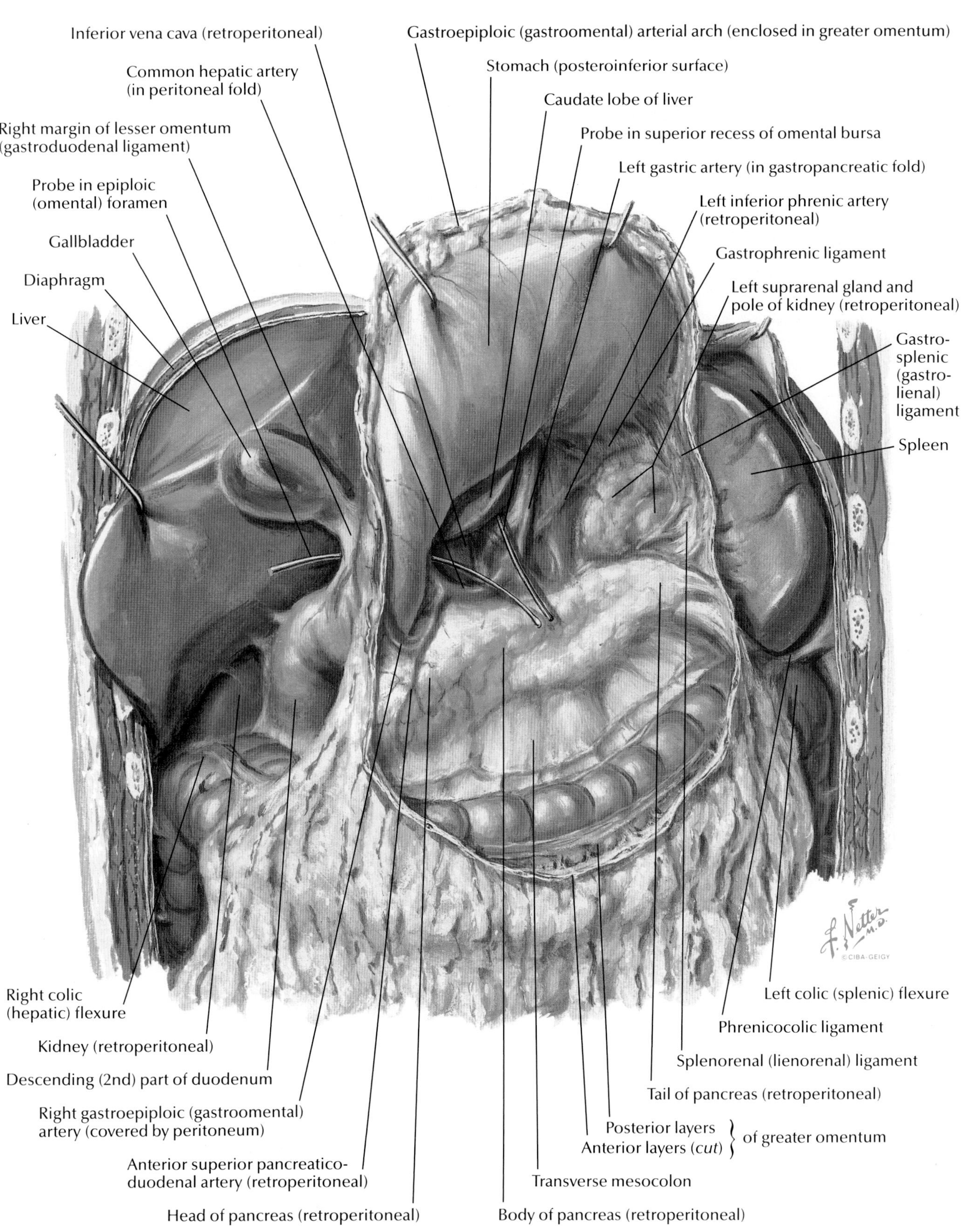

Inferior vena cava (retroperitoneal)

Common hepatic artery (in peritoneal fold)

Right margin of lesser omentum (gastroduodenal ligament)

Probe in epiploic (omental) foramen

Gallbladder

Diaphragm

Liver

Gastroepiploic (gastroomental) arterial arch (enclosed in greater omentum)

Stomach (posteroinferior surface)

Caudate lobe of liver

Probe in superior recess of omental bursa

Left gastric artery (in gastropancreatic fold)

Left inferior phrenic artery (retroperitoneal)

Gastrophrenic ligament

Left suprarenal gland and pole of kidney (retroperitoneal)

Gastro-splenic (gastro-lienal) ligament

Spleen

Right colic (hepatic) flexure

Kidney (retroperitoneal)

Descending (2nd) part of duodenum

Right gastroepiploic (gastroomental) artery (covered by peritoneum)

Anterior superior pancreatico-duodenal artery (retroperitoneal)

Head of pancreas (retroperitoneal)

Left colic (splenic) flexure

Phrenicocolic ligament

Splenorenal (lienorenal) ligament

Tail of pancreas (retroperitoneal)

Posterior layers } of greater omentum
Anterior layers (cut) }

Transverse mesocolon

Body of pancreas (retroperitoneal)

Omental Bursa: Cross Section

SEE ALSO PLATE 331

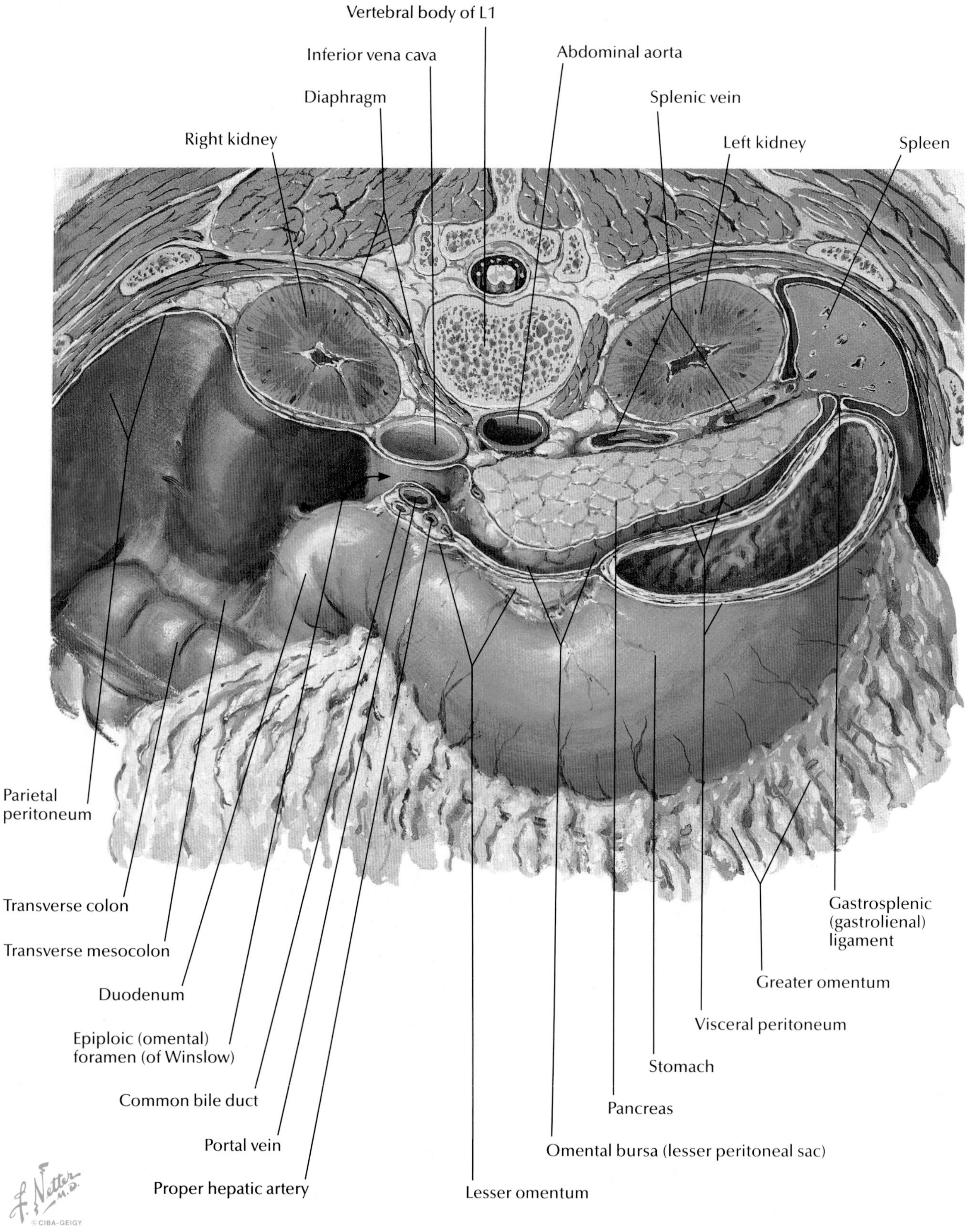

Vertebral body of L1

Inferior vena cava

Abdominal aorta

Diaphragm

Splenic vein

Right kidney

Left kidney

Spleen

Parietal
peritoneum

Transverse colon

Transverse mesocolon

Duodenum

Epiploic (omental)
foramen (of Winslow)

Common bile duct

Portal vein

Proper hepatic artery

Lesser omentum

Omental bursa (lesser peritoneal sac)

Pancreas

Stomach

Visceral peritoneum

Greater omentum

Gastrosplenic
(gastrolienal)
ligament

PLATE 256

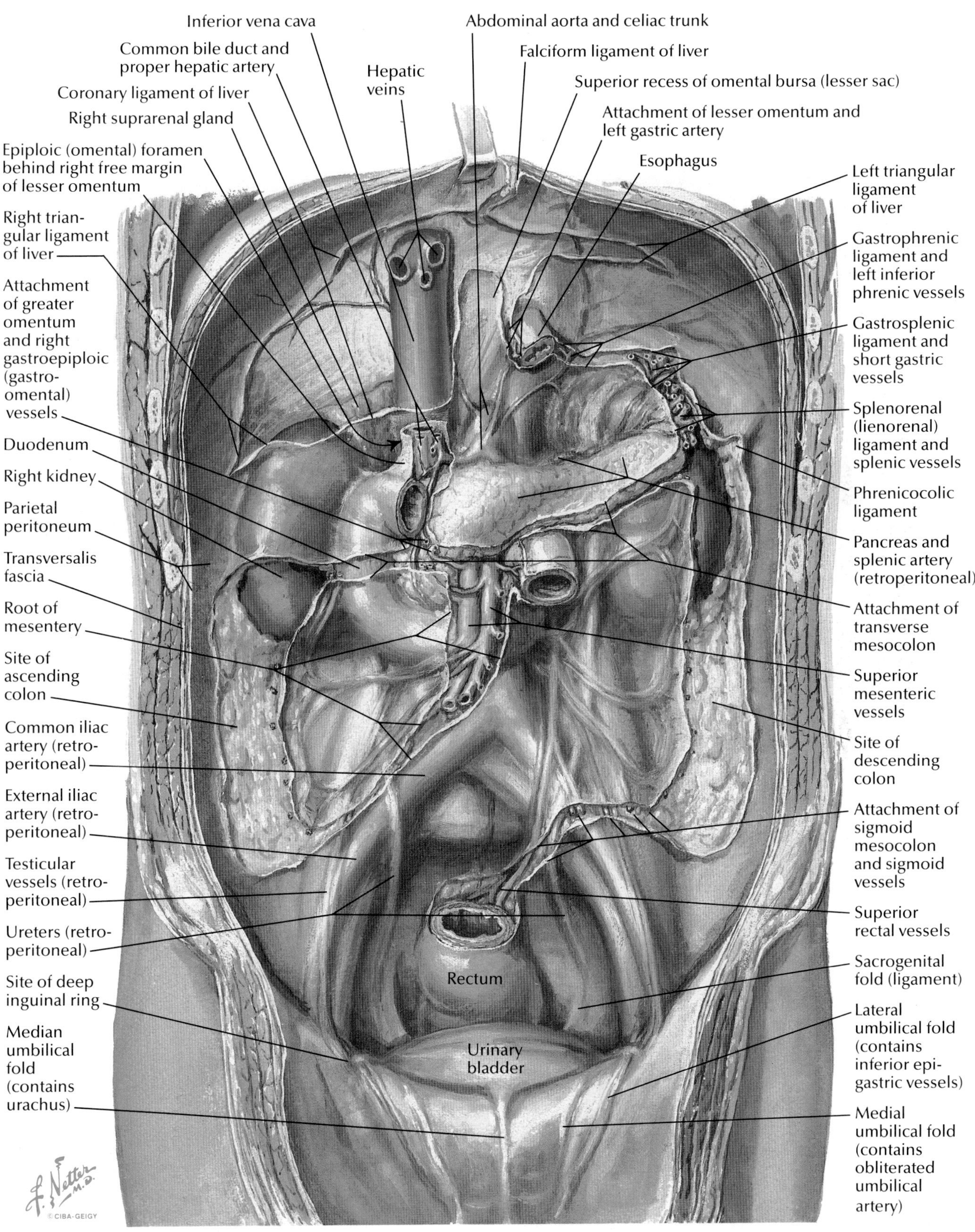

Inferior vena cava

Common bile duct and proper hepatic artery

Coronary ligament of liver

Right suprarenal gland

Epiploic (omental) foramen behind right free margin of lesser omentum

Right triangular ligament of liver

Attachment of greater omentum and right gastroepiploic (gastro-omental) vessels

Duodenum

Right kidney

Parietal peritoneum

Transversalis fascia

Root of mesentery

Site of ascending colon

Common iliac artery (retro-peritoneal)

External iliac artery (retro-peritoneal)

Testicular vessels (retro-peritoneal)

Ureters (retro-peritoneal)

Site of deep inguinal ring

Median umbilical fold (contains urachus)

Hepatic veins

Abdominal aorta and celiac trunk

Falciform ligament of liver

Superior recess of omental bursa (lesser sac)

Attachment of lesser omentum and left gastric artery

Esophagus

Left triangular ligament of liver

Gastrophrenic ligament and left inferior phrenic vessels

Gastrosplenic ligament and short gastric vessels

Splenorenal (lienorenal) ligament and splenic vessels

Phrenicocolic ligament

Pancreas and splenic artery (retroperitoneal)

Attachment of transverse mesocolon

Superior mesenteric vessels

Site of descending colon

Attachment of sigmoid mesocolon and sigmoid vessels

Superior rectal vessels

Sacrogenital fold (ligament)

Lateral umbilical fold (contains inferior epigastric vessels)

Medial umbilical fold (contains obliterated umbilical artery)

Rectum

Urinary bladder

Stomach In Situ

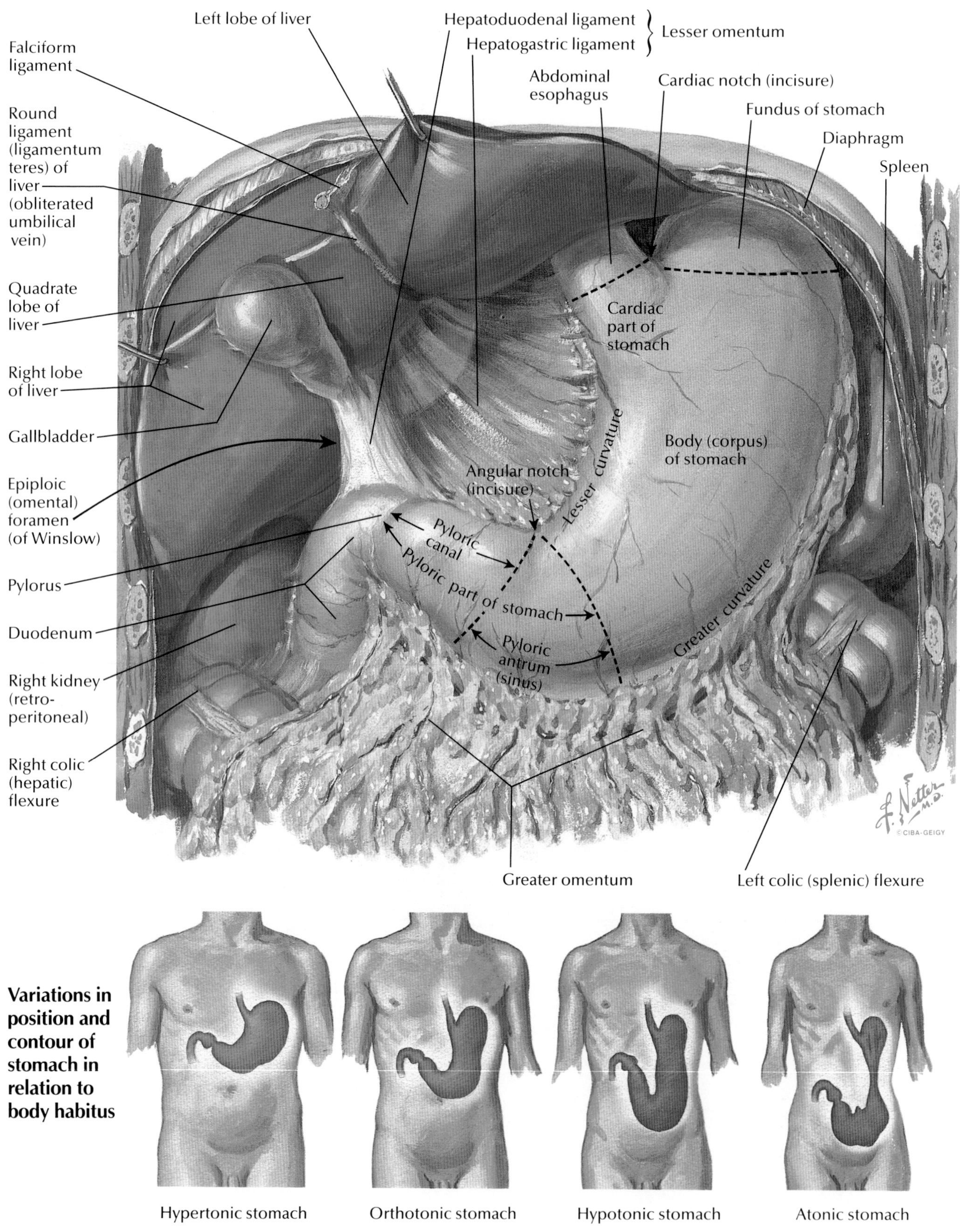

Falciform ligament

Round ligament (ligamentum teres) of liver (obliterated umbilical vein)

Quadrate lobe of liver

Right lobe of liver

Gallbladder

Epiploic (omental) foramen (of Winslow)

Pylorus

Duodenum

Right kidney (retro-peritoneal)

Right colic (hepatic) flexure

Left lobe of liver

Hepatoduodenal ligament
Hepatogastric ligament } Lesser omentum

Abdominal esophagus

Cardiac notch (incisure)

Fundus of stomach

Diaphragm

Spleen

Cardiac part of stomach

Body (corpus) of stomach

Lesser curvature

Greater curvature

Angular notch (incisure)

Pyloric canal

Pyloric part of stomach

Pyloric antrum (sinus)

Greater omentum

Left colic (splenic) flexure

F. Netter M.D.
©CIBA-GEIGY

Variations in position and contour of stomach in relation to body habitus

Hypertonic stomach

Orthotonic stomach

Hypotonic stomach

Atonic stomach

PLATE 258

ABDOMEN

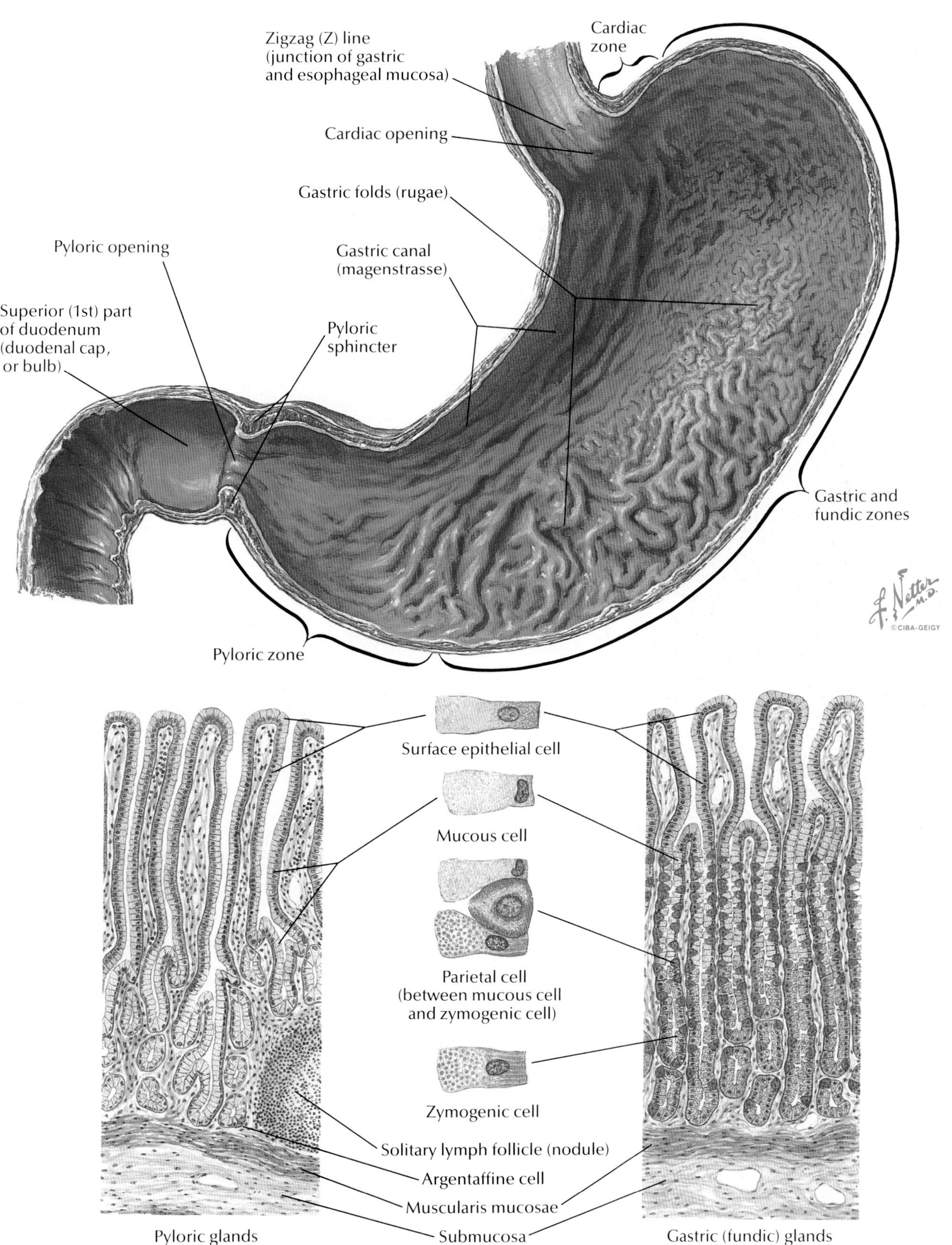

Zigzag (Z) line
(junction of gastric
and esophageal mucosa)

Cardiac
zone

Cardiac opening

Gastric folds (rugae)

Pyloric opening

Gastric canal
(magenstrasse)

Superior (1st) part
of duodenum
(duodenal cap,
or bulb)

Pyloric
sphincter

Gastric and
fundic zones

Pyloric zone

Surface epithelial cell

Mucous cell

Parietal cell
(between mucous cell
and zymogenic cell)

Zymogenic cell

Solitary lymph follicle (nodule)

Argentaffine cell

Muscularis mucosae

Pyloric glands

Submucosa

Gastric (fundic) glands

Musculature of Stomach

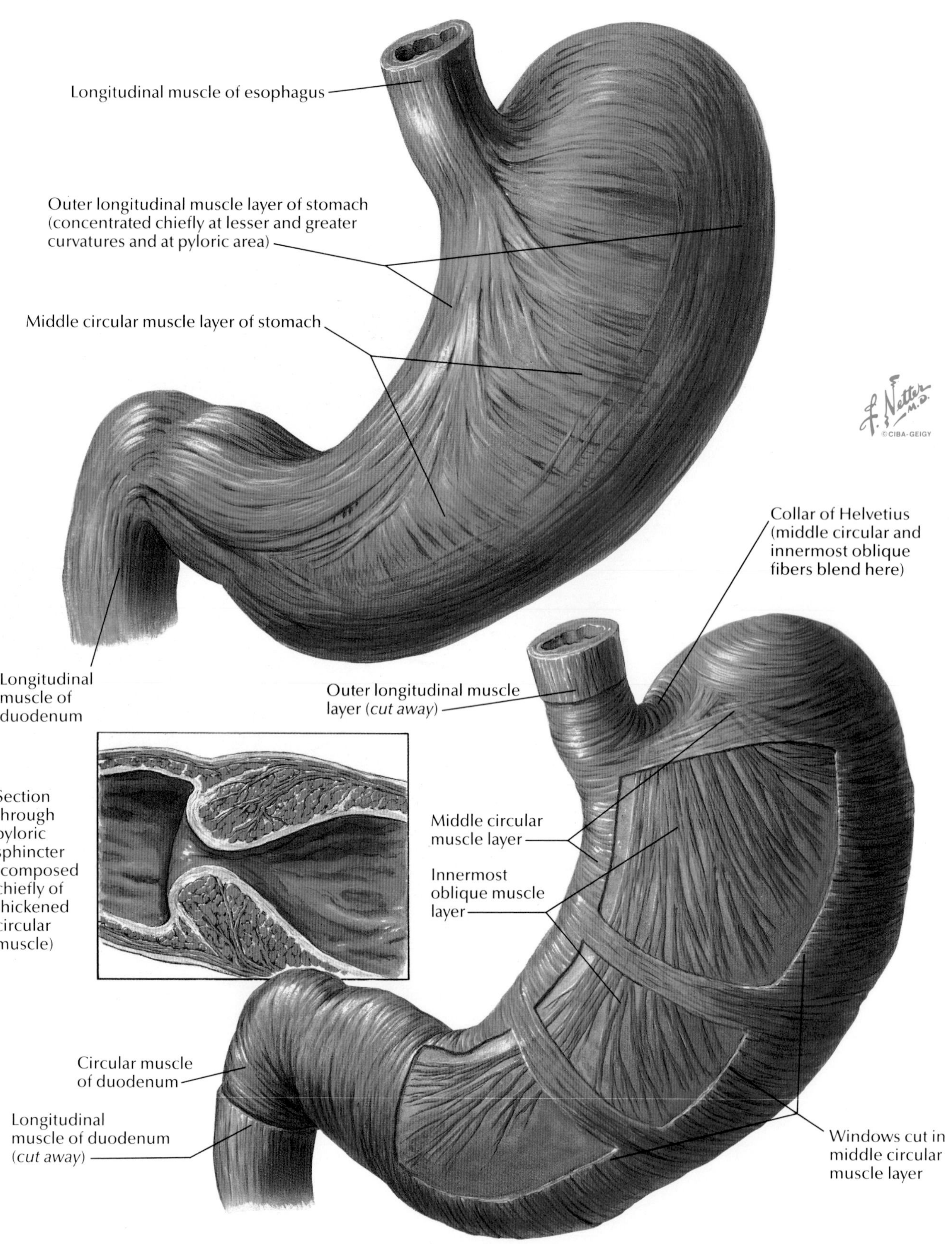

Longitudinal muscle of esophagus

Outer longitudinal muscle layer of stomach (concentrated chiefly at lesser and greater curvatures and at pyloric area)

Middle circular muscle layer of stomach

Longitudinal muscle of duodenum

Section through pyloric sphincter (composed chiefly of thickened circular muscle)

Collar of Helvetius (middle circular and innermost oblique fibers blend here)

Outer longitudinal muscle layer (*cut away*)

Middle circular muscle layer

Innermost oblique muscle layer

Circular muscle of duodenum

Longitudinal muscle of duodenum (*cut away*)

Windows cut in middle circular muscle layer

PLATE 260

ABDOMEN

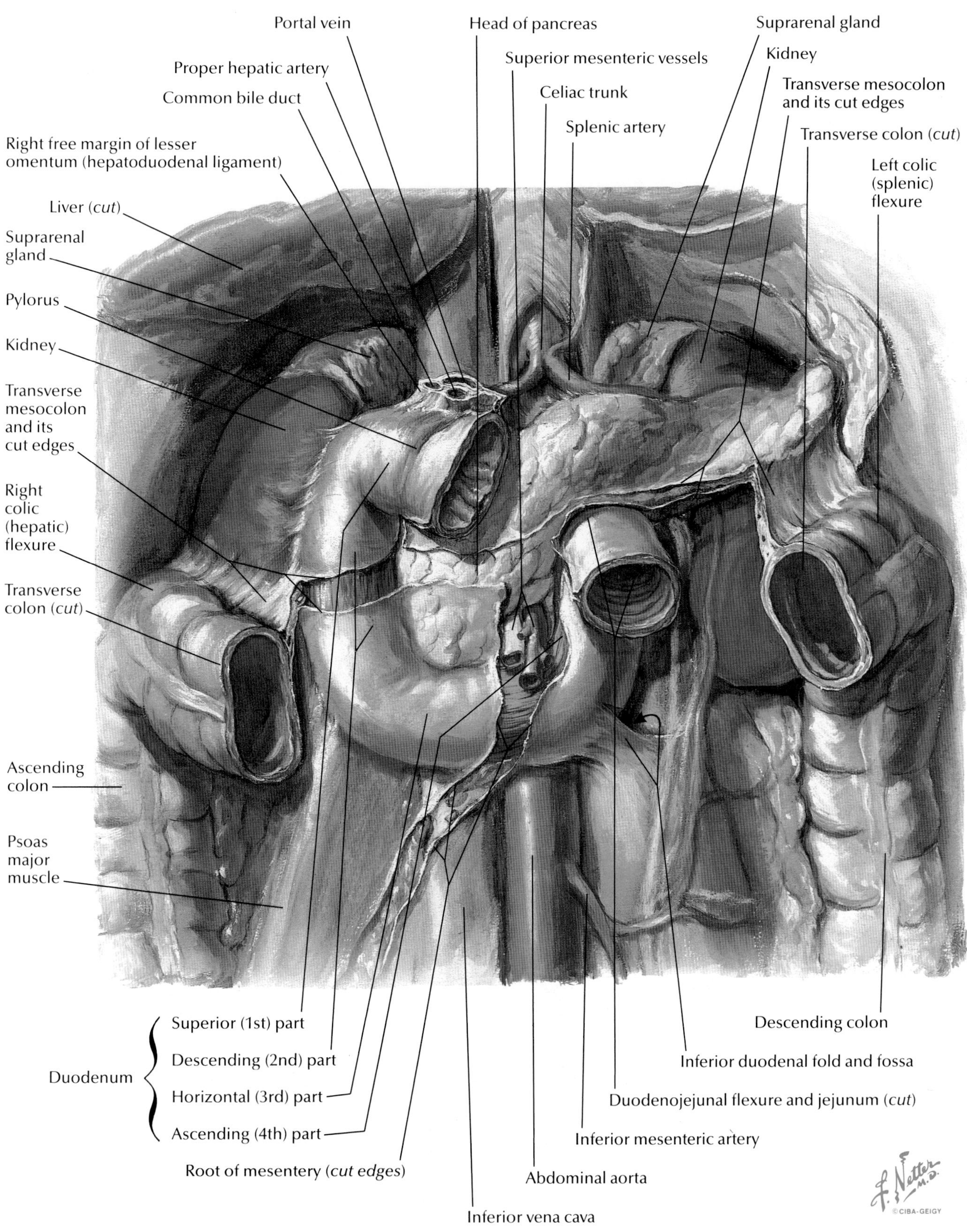

Portal vein

Proper hepatic artery

Common bile duct

Right free margin of lesser
omentum (hepatoduodenal ligament)

Liver (*cut*)

Suprarenal
gland

Pylorus

Kidney

Transverse
mesocolon
and its
cut edges

Right
colic
(hepatic)
flexure

Transverse
colon (*cut*)

Ascending
colon

Psoas
major
muscle

Head of pancreas

Superior mesenteric vessels

Celiac trunk

Splenic artery

Suprarenal gland

Kidney

Transverse mesocolon
and its cut edges

Transverse colon (*cut*)

Left colic
(splenic)
flexure

Descending colon

Inferior duodenal fold and fossa

Duodenojejunal flexure and jejunum (*cut*)

Inferior mesenteric artery

Abdominal aorta

Inferior vena cava

Duodenum

Superior (1st) part

Descending (2nd) part

Horizontal (3rd) part

Ascending (4th) part

Root of mesentery (*cut edges*)

Mucosa and Musculature of Duodenum

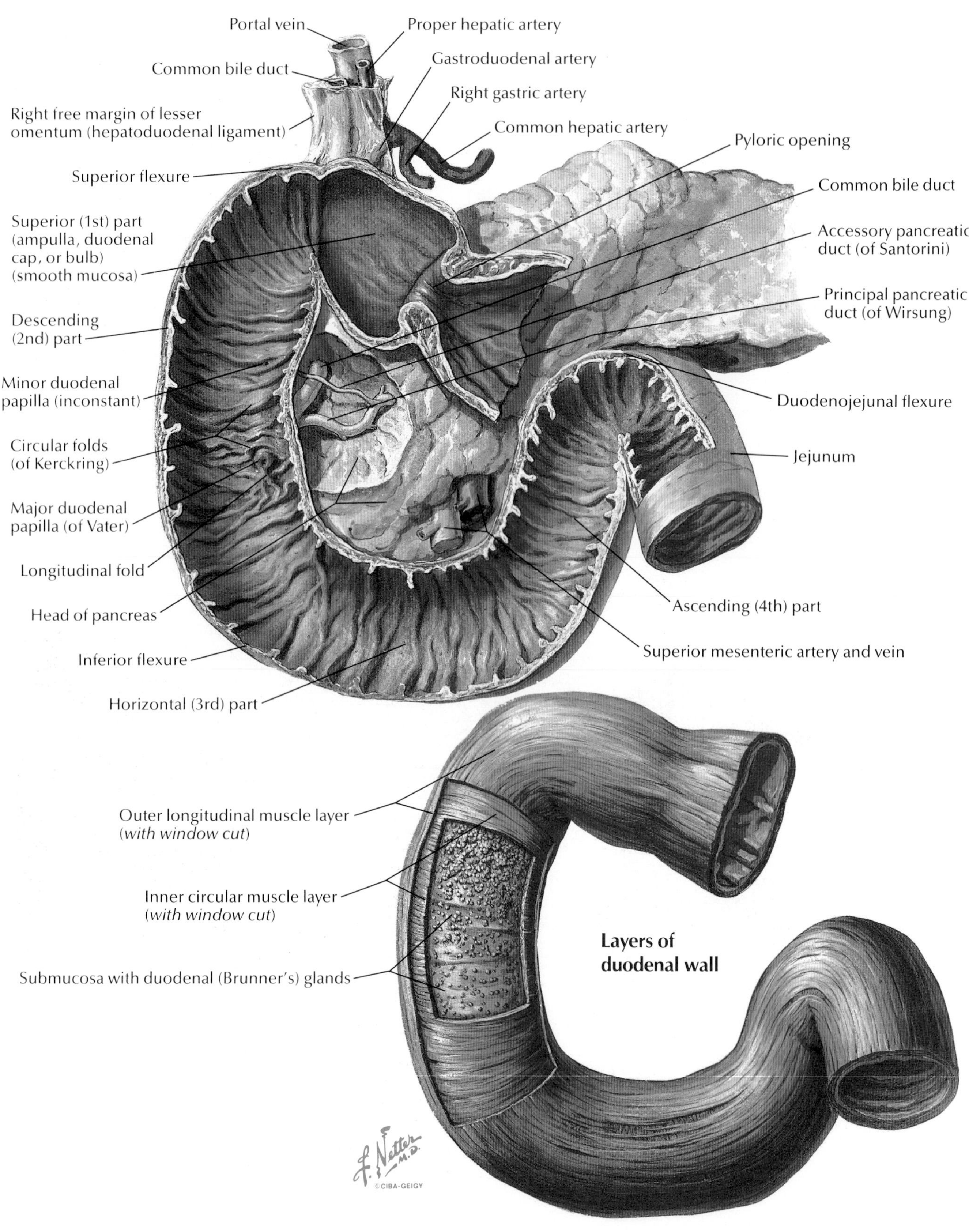

Portal vein

Proper hepatic artery

Common bile duct

Gastroduodenal artery

Right gastric artery

Right free margin of lesser omentum (hepatoduodenal ligament)

Common hepatic artery

Pyloric opening

Superior flexure

Common bile duct

Superior (1st) part (ampulla, duodenal cap, or bulb) (smooth mucosa)

Accessory pancreatic duct (of Santorini)

Principal pancreatic duct (of Wirsung)

Descending (2nd) part

Minor duodenal papilla (inconstant)

Duodenojejunal flexure

Circular folds (of Kerckring)

Jejunum

Major duodenal papilla (of Vater)

Longitudinal fold

Head of pancreas

Ascending (4th) part

Inferior flexure

Superior mesenteric artery and vein

Horizontal (3rd) part

Outer longitudinal muscle layer (*with window cut*)

Inner circular muscle layer (*with window cut*)

Layers of duodenal wall

Submucosa with duodenal (Brunner's) glands

PLATE 262

ABDOMEN

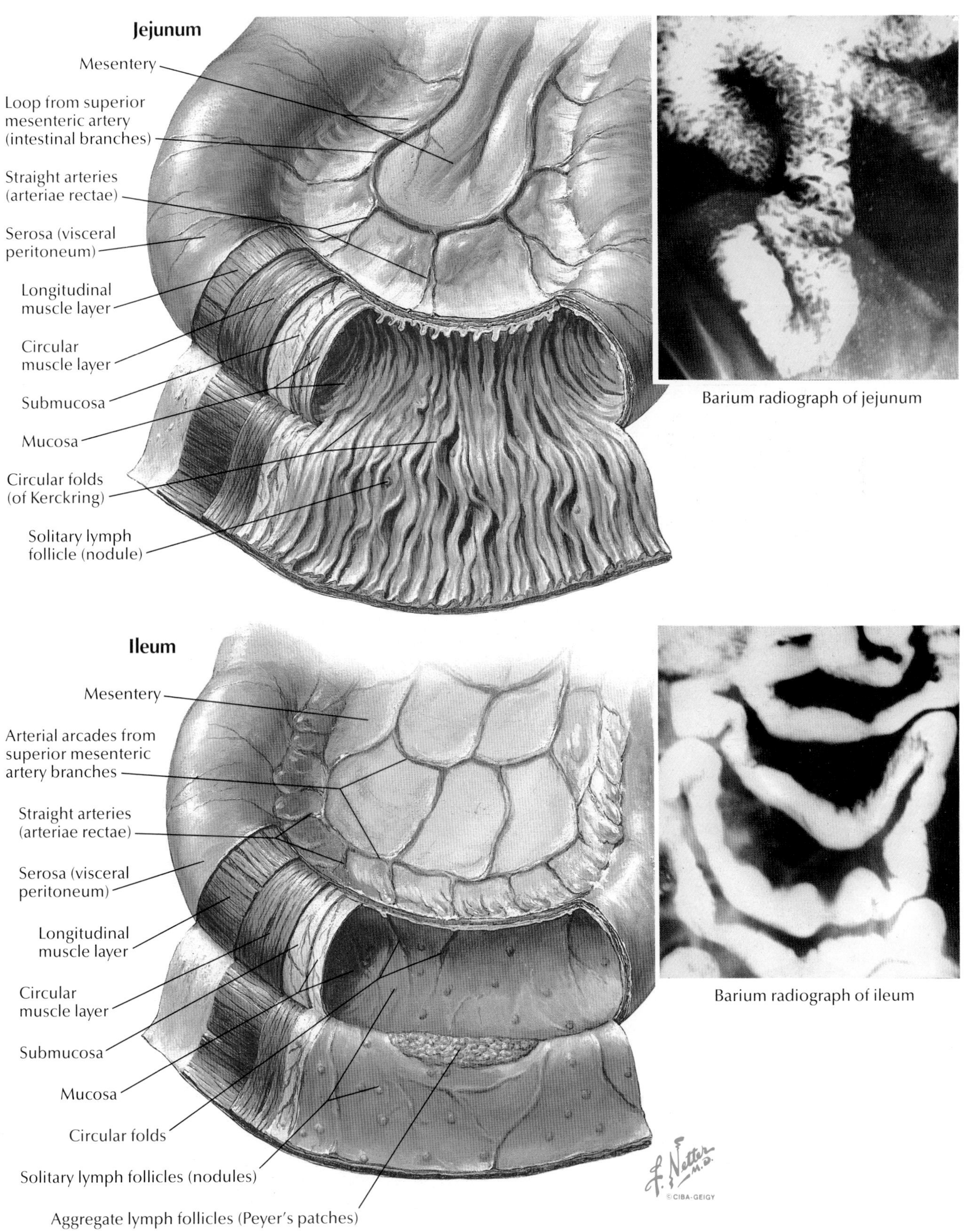

Jejunum

- Mesentery
- Loop from superior mesenteric artery (intestinal branches)
- Straight arteries (arteriae rectae)
- Serosa (visceral peritoneum)
- Longitudinal muscle layer
- Circular muscle layer
- Submucosa
- Mucosa
- Circular folds (of Kerckring)
- Solitary lymph follicle (nodule)

Barium radiograph of jejunum

Ileum

- Mesentery
- Arterial arcades from superior mesenteric artery branches
- Straight arteries (arteriae rectae)
- Serosa (visceral peritoneum)
- Longitudinal muscle layer
- Circular muscle layer
- Submucosa
- Mucosa
- Circular folds
- Solitary lymph follicles (nodules)
- Aggregate lymph follicles (Peyer's patches)

Barium radiograph of ileum

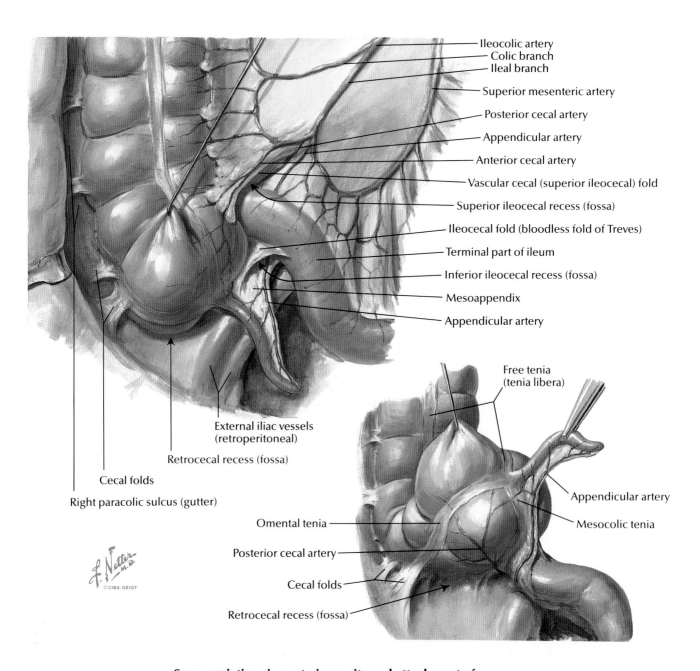

Ileocolic artery
Colic branch
Ileal branch
Superior mesenteric artery
Posterior cecal artery
Appendicular artery
Anterior cecal artery
Vascular cecal (superior ileocecal) fold
Superior ileocecal recess (fossa)
Ileocecal fold (bloodless fold of Treves)
Terminal part of ileum
Inferior ileocecal recess (fossa)
Mesoappendix
Appendicular artery

External iliac vessels (retroperitoneal)
Retrocecal recess (fossa)
Cecal folds
Right paracolic sulcus (gutter)

Free tenia (tenia libera)
Appendicular artery
Mesocolic tenia
Omental tenia
Posterior cecal artery
Cecal folds
Retrocecal recess (fossa)

Some variations in posterior peritoneal attachment of cecum

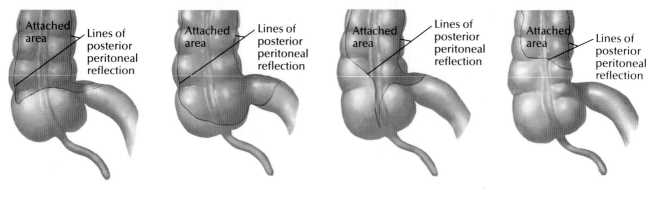

Attached area — Lines of posterior peritoneal reflection

Attached area — Lines of posterior peritoneal reflection

Attached area — Lines of posterior peritoneal reflection

Attached area — Lines of posterior peritoneal reflection

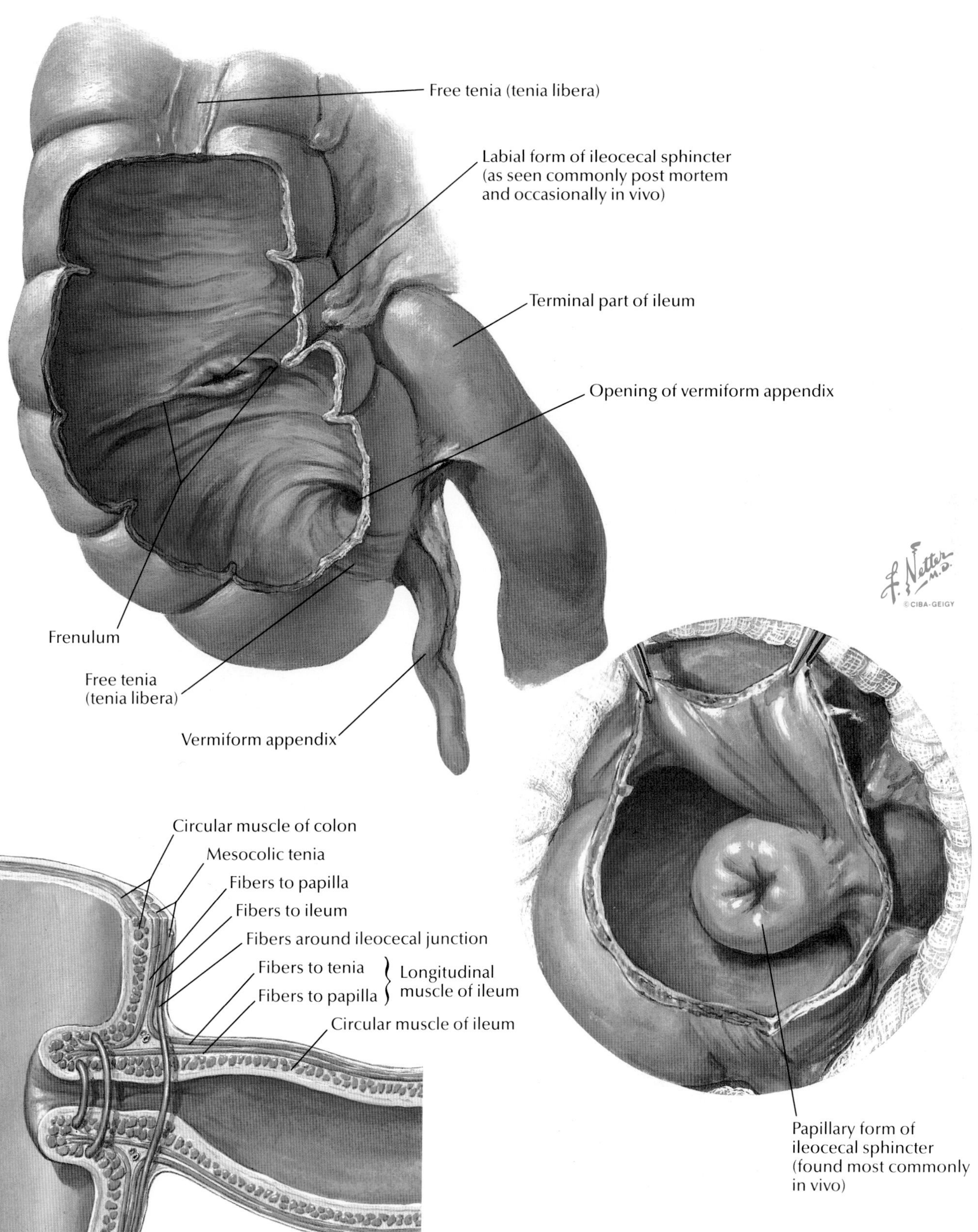

Free tenia (tenia libera)

Labial form of ileocecal sphincter
(as seen commonly post mortem
and occasionally in vivo)

Terminal part of ileum

Opening of vermiform appendix

Frenulum

Free tenia
(tenia libera)

Vermiform appendix

Circular muscle of colon
Mesocolic tenia
Fibers to papilla
Fibers to ileum
Fibers around ileocecal junction
Fibers to tenia } Longitudinal
Fibers to papilla } muscle of ileum
Circular muscle of ileum

Papillary form of
ileocecal sphincter
(found most commonly
in vivo)

Schema of muscle fibers at ileocecal sphincter

Vermiform Appendix

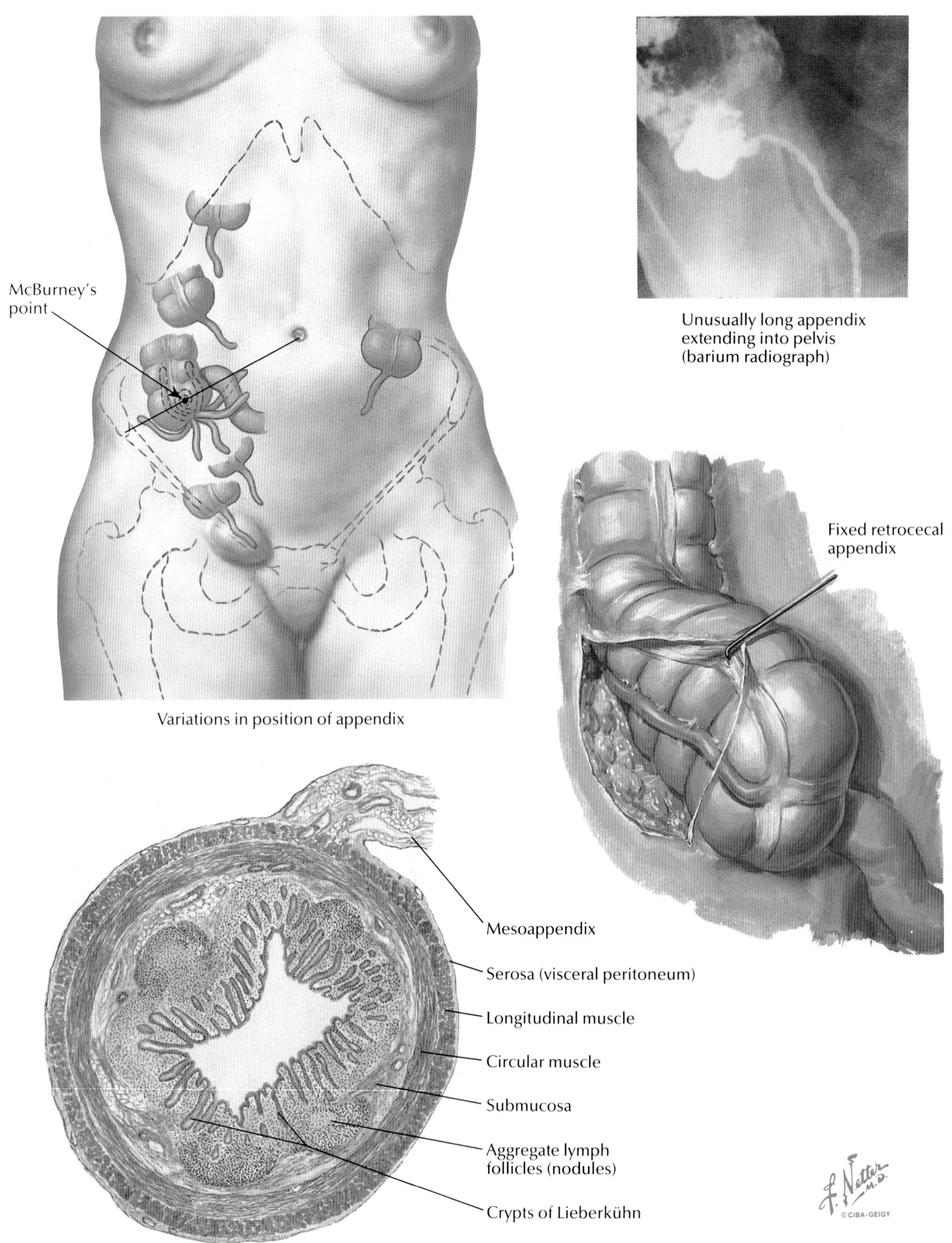

McBurney's point

Variations in position of appendix

Unusually long appendix extending into pelvis (barium radiograph)

Fixed retrocecal appendix

Mesoappendix

Serosa (visceral peritoneum)

Longitudinal muscle

Circular muscle

Submucosa

Aggregate lymph follicles (nodules)

Crypts of Lieberkühn

PLATE 266

ABDOMEN

FOR RECTUM AND ANAL CANAL SEE PLATES 367–372

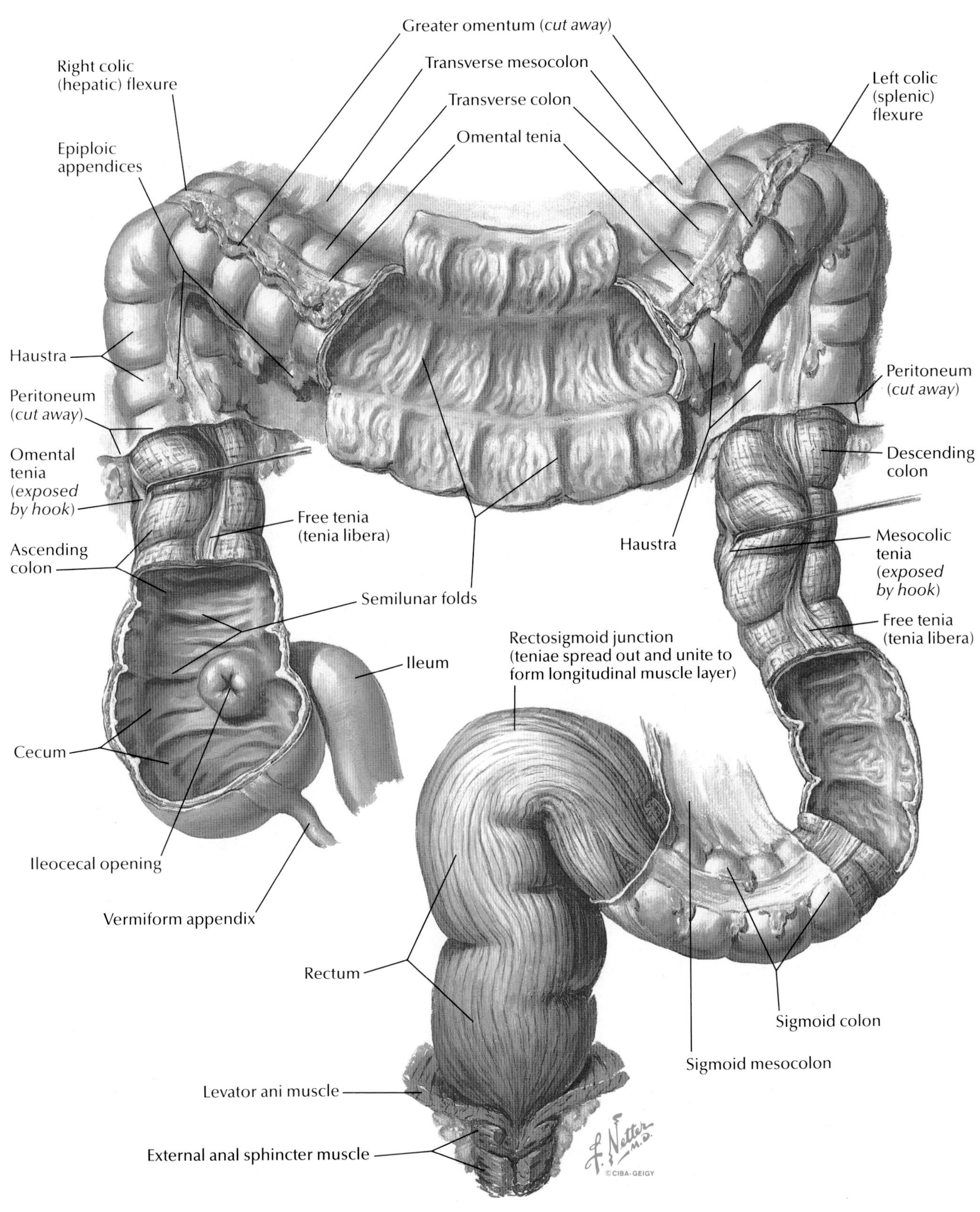

Greater omentum (*cut away*)

Transverse mesocolon

Transverse colon

Omental tenia

Right colic (hepatic) flexure

Epiploic appendices

Left colic (splenic) flexure

Haustra

Peritoneum (*cut away*)

Omental tenia (*exposed by hook*)

Ascending colon

Free tenia (tenia libera)

Semilunar folds

Peritoneum (*cut away*)

Descending colon

Haustra

Mesocolic tenia (*exposed by hook*)

Free tenia (tenia libera)

Ileum

Rectosigmoid junction (teniae spread out and unite to form longitudinal muscle layer)

Cecum

Ileocecal opening

Vermiform appendix

Rectum

Sigmoid colon

Sigmoid mesocolon

Levator ani muscle

External anal sphincter muscle

Sigmoid Colon: Variations in Position

FOR RECTUM SEE PLATES 341, 342, 367, 368, 369, 370

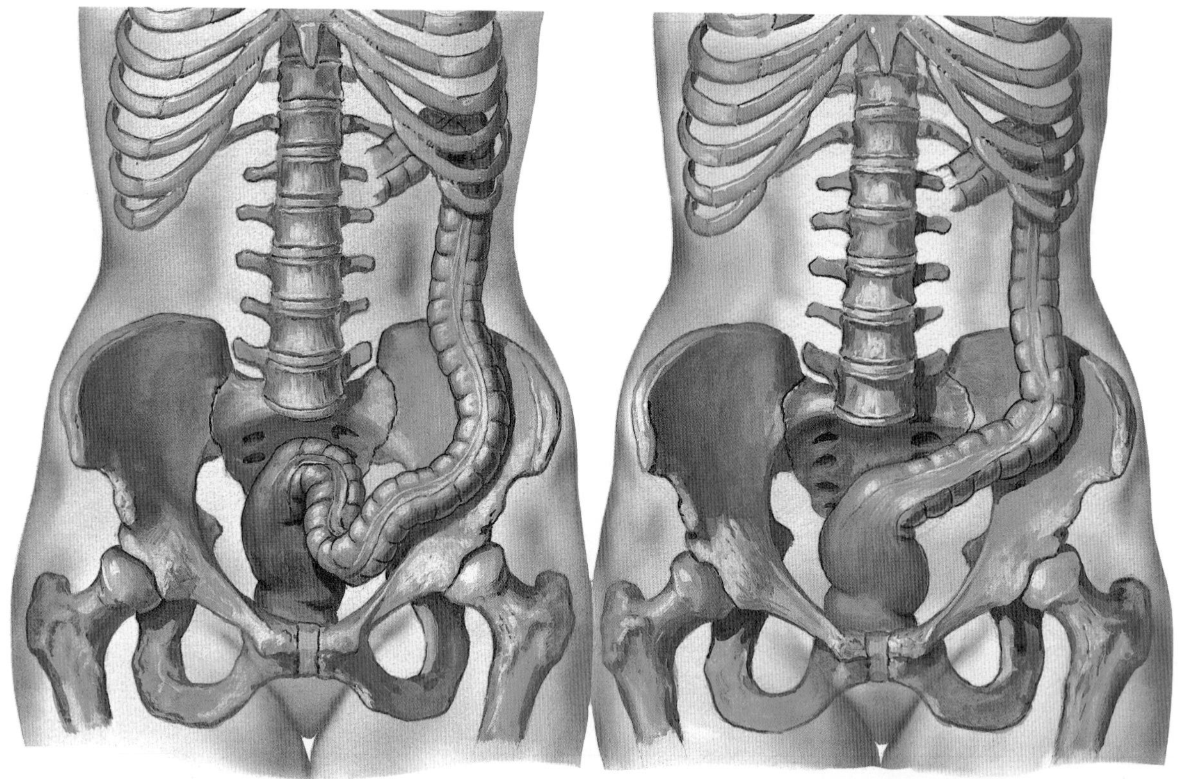

Typical

Short, straight, obliquely into pelvis

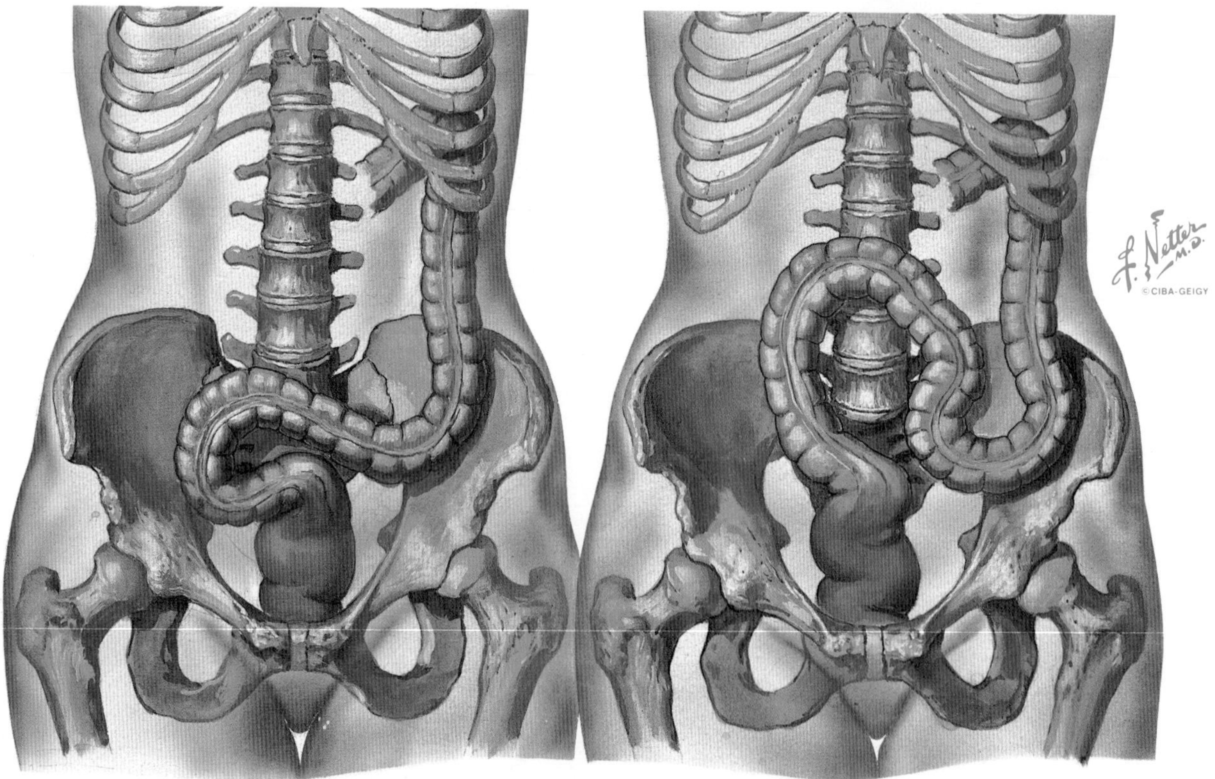

Looping to right side

Ascending high into abdomen

PLATE 268

ABDOMEN

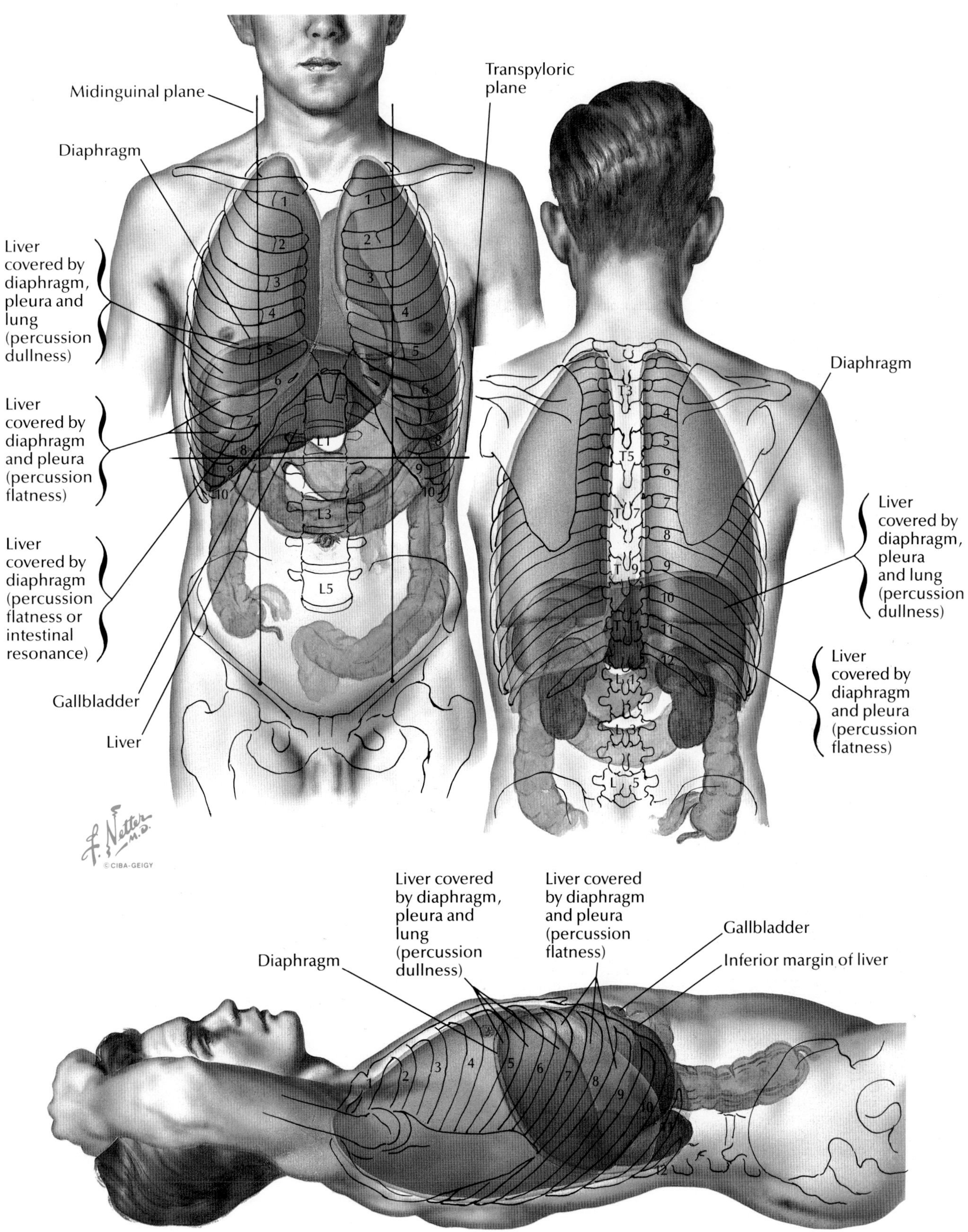

Midinguinal plane

Transpyloric plane

Diaphragm

Liver covered by diaphragm, pleura and lung (percussion dullness)

Liver covered by diaphragm and pleura (percussion flatness)

Liver covered by diaphragm (percussion flatness or intestinal resonance)

Gallbladder

Liver

Diaphragm

Liver covered by diaphragm, pleura and lung (percussion dullness)

Liver covered by diaphragm and pleura (percussion flatness)

Liver covered by diaphragm, pleura and lung (percussion dullness)

Liver covered by diaphragm and pleura (percussion flatness)

Diaphragm

Gallbladder

Inferior margin of liver

Surfaces and Bed of Liver

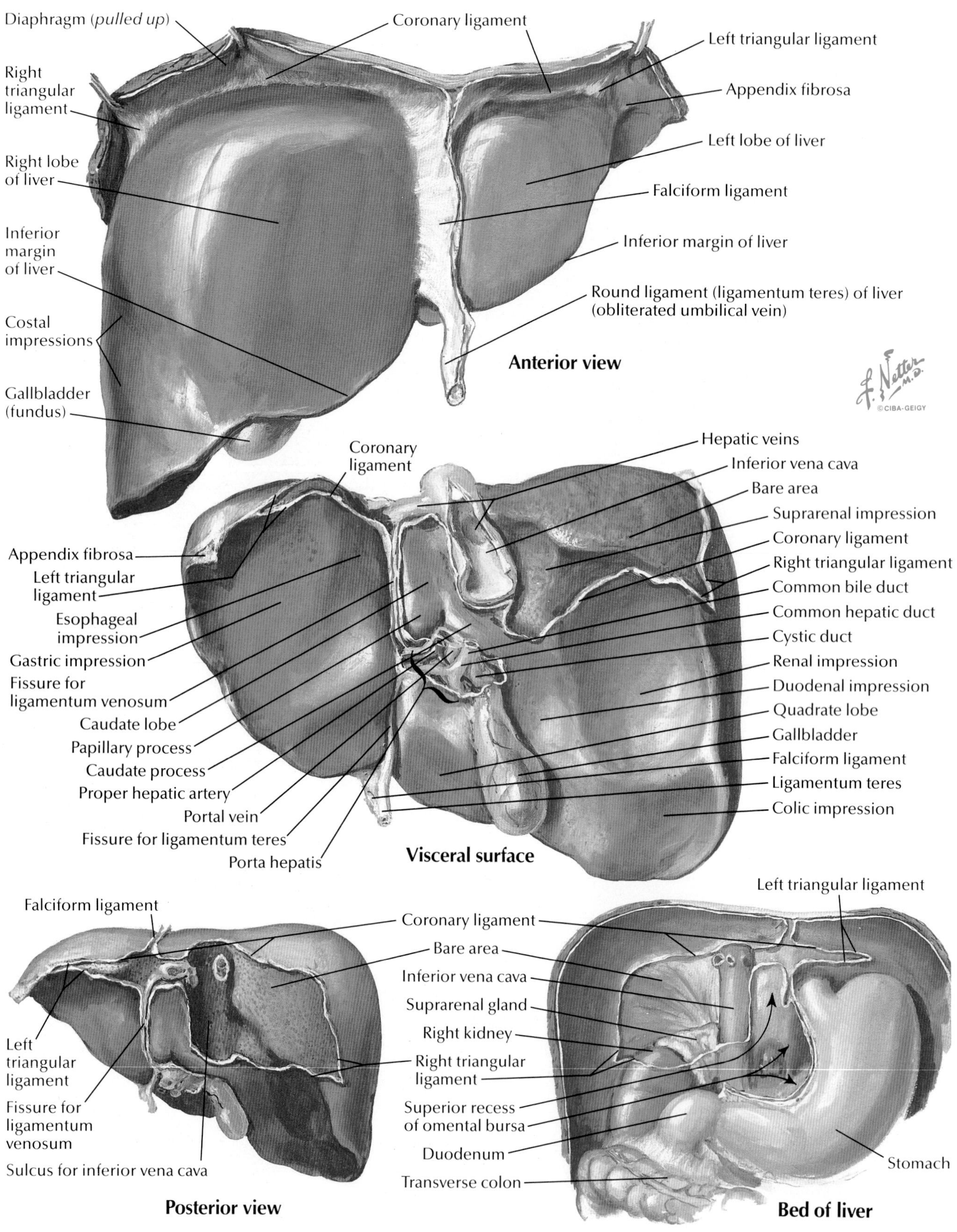

Diaphragm (*pulled up*)

Coronary ligament

Left triangular ligament

Right triangular ligament

Appendix fibrosa

Left lobe of liver

Right lobe of liver

Falciform ligament

Inferior margin of liver

Inferior margin of liver

Costal impressions

Round ligament (ligamentum teres) of liver (obliterated umbilical vein)

Gallbladder (fundus)

Anterior view

Coronary ligament

Hepatic veins

Inferior vena cava

Bare area

Suprarenal impression

Coronary ligament

Appendix fibrosa

Right triangular ligament

Left triangular ligament

Common bile duct

Esophageal impression

Common hepatic duct

Gastric impression

Cystic duct

Fissure for ligamentum venosum

Renal impression

Caudate lobe

Duodenal impression

Papillary process

Quadrate lobe

Caudate process

Gallbladder

Proper hepatic artery

Falciform ligament

Portal vein

Ligamentum teres

Fissure for ligamentum teres

Colic impression

Porta hepatis

Visceral surface

Falciform ligament

Left triangular ligament

Coronary ligament

Bare area

Inferior vena cava

Suprarenal gland

Right kidney

Left triangular ligament

Right triangular ligament

Fissure for ligamentum venosum

Superior recess of omental bursa

Sulcus for inferior vena cava

Duodenum

Transverse colon

Stomach

Posterior view

Bed of liver

PLATE 270

ABDOMEN

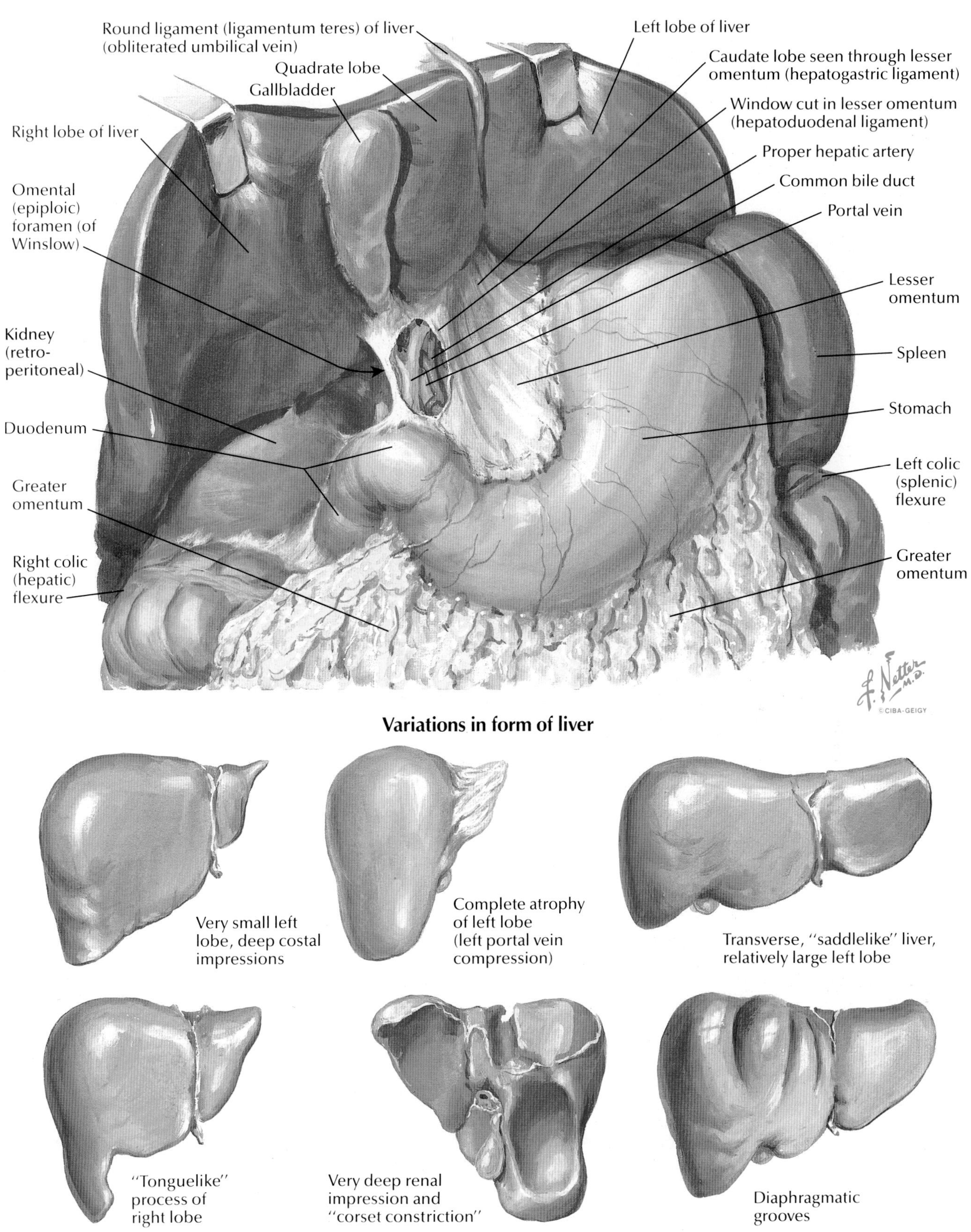

Round ligament (ligamentum teres) of liver (obliterated umbilical vein)

Quadrate lobe

Gallbladder

Right lobe of liver

Omental (epiploic) foramen (of Winslow)

Kidney (retro-peritoneal)

Duodenum

Greater omentum

Right colic (hepatic) flexure

Left lobe of liver

Caudate lobe seen through lesser omentum (hepatogastric ligament)

Window cut in lesser omentum (hepatoduodenal ligament)

Proper hepatic artery

Common bile duct

Portal vein

Lesser omentum

Spleen

Stomach

Left colic (splenic) flexure

Greater omentum

Variations in form of liver

Very small left lobe, deep costal impressions

Complete atrophy of left lobe (left portal vein compression)

Transverse, "saddlelike" liver, relatively large left lobe

"Tonguelike" process of right lobe

Very deep renal impression and "corset constriction"

Diaphragmatic grooves

Liver Segments and Lobules: Vessel and Duct Distribution

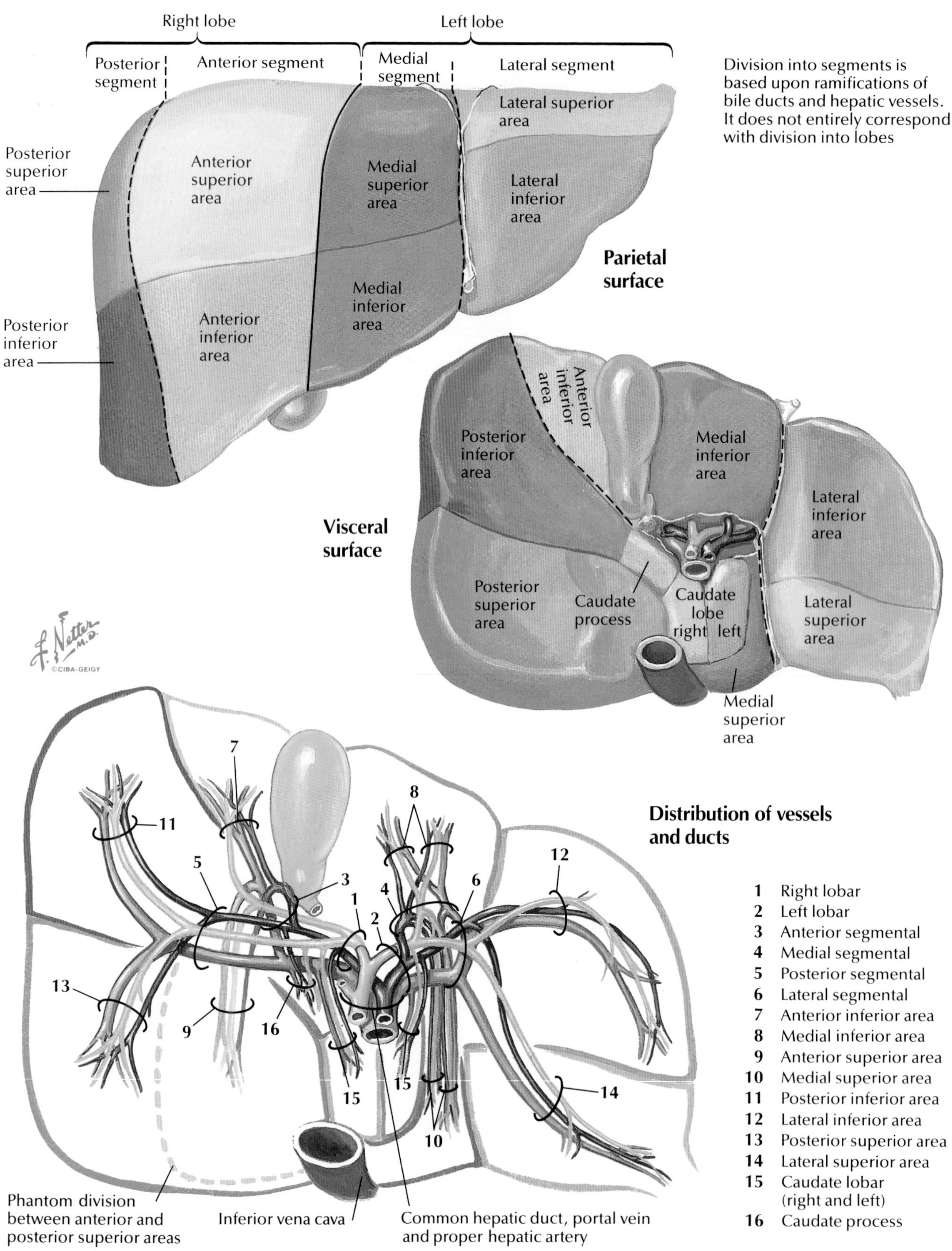

Right lobe

Left lobe

Posterior segment | Anterior segment | Medial segment | Lateral segment

Lateral superior area

Posterior superior area

Anterior superior area

Medial superior area

Lateral inferior area

Posterior inferior area

Anterior inferior area

Medial inferior area

Parietal surface

Division into segments is based upon ramifications of bile ducts and hepatic vessels. It does not entirely correspond with division into lobes

Visceral surface

Anterior inferior area

Posterior inferior area

Medial inferior area

Lateral inferior area

Posterior superior area

Caudate process

Caudate lobe right | left

Lateral superior area

Medial superior area

Phantom division between anterior and posterior superior areas

Inferior vena cava

Common hepatic duct, portal vein and proper hepatic artery

Distribution of vessels and ducts

1 Right lobar
2 Left lobar
3 Anterior segmental
4 Medial segmental
5 Posterior segmental
6 Lateral segmental
7 Anterior inferior area
8 Medial inferior area
9 Anterior superior area
10 Medial superior area
11 Posterior inferior area
12 Lateral inferior area
13 Posterior superior area
14 Lateral superior area
15 Caudate lobar (right and left)
16 Caudate process

PLATE 272

ABDOMEN

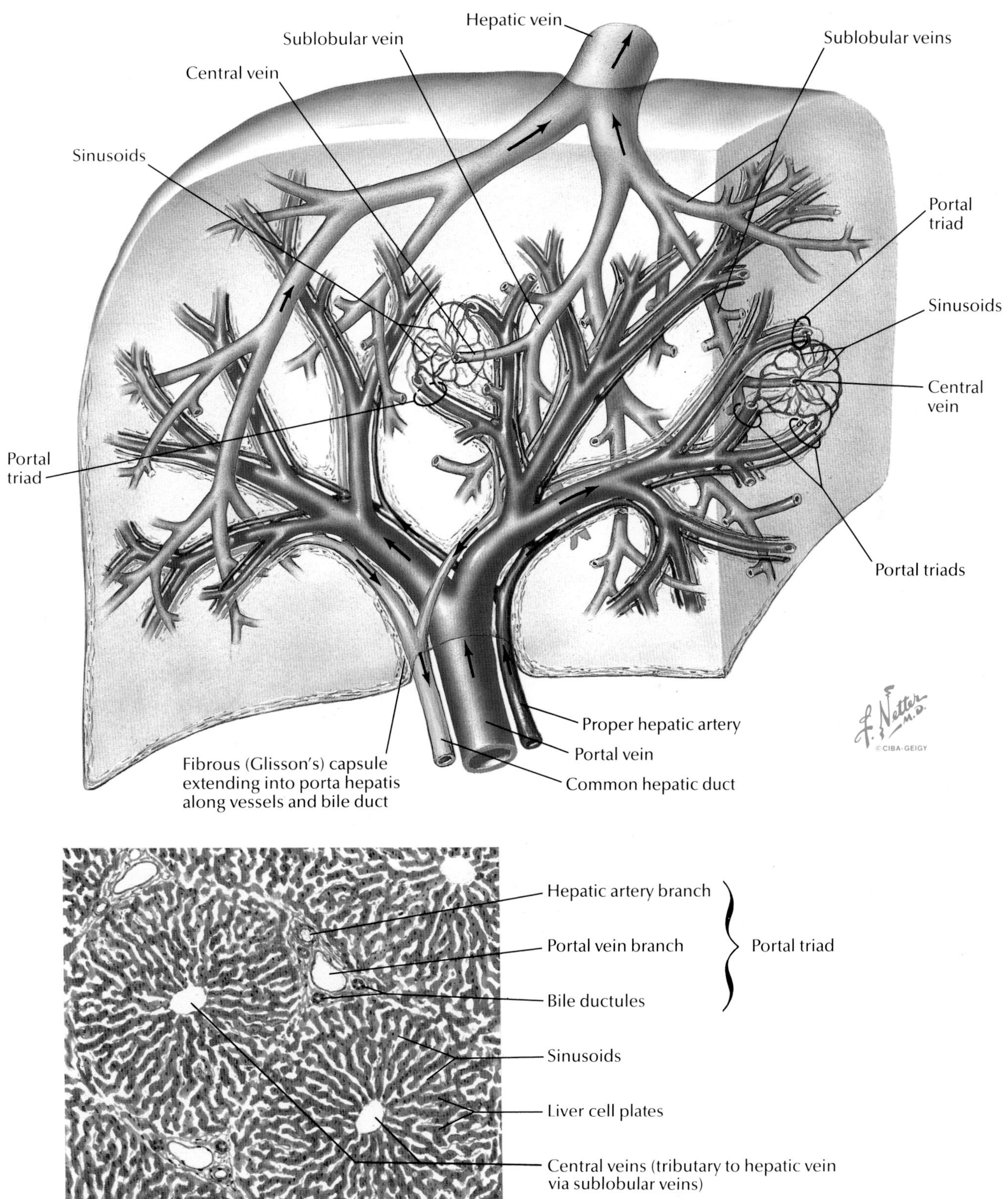

Hepatic vein

Sublobular vein

Central vein

Sinusoids

Portal triad

Sublobular veins

Portal triad

Sinusoids

Central vein

Portal triads

Proper hepatic artery

Portal vein

Common hepatic duct

Fibrous (Glisson's) capsule extending into porta hepatis along vessels and bile duct

Hepatic artery branch

Portal vein branch

Bile ductules

Portal triad

Sinusoids

Liver cell plates

Central veins (tributary to hepatic vein via sublobular veins)

Normal lobular pattern of liver

Liver Structure: Schema

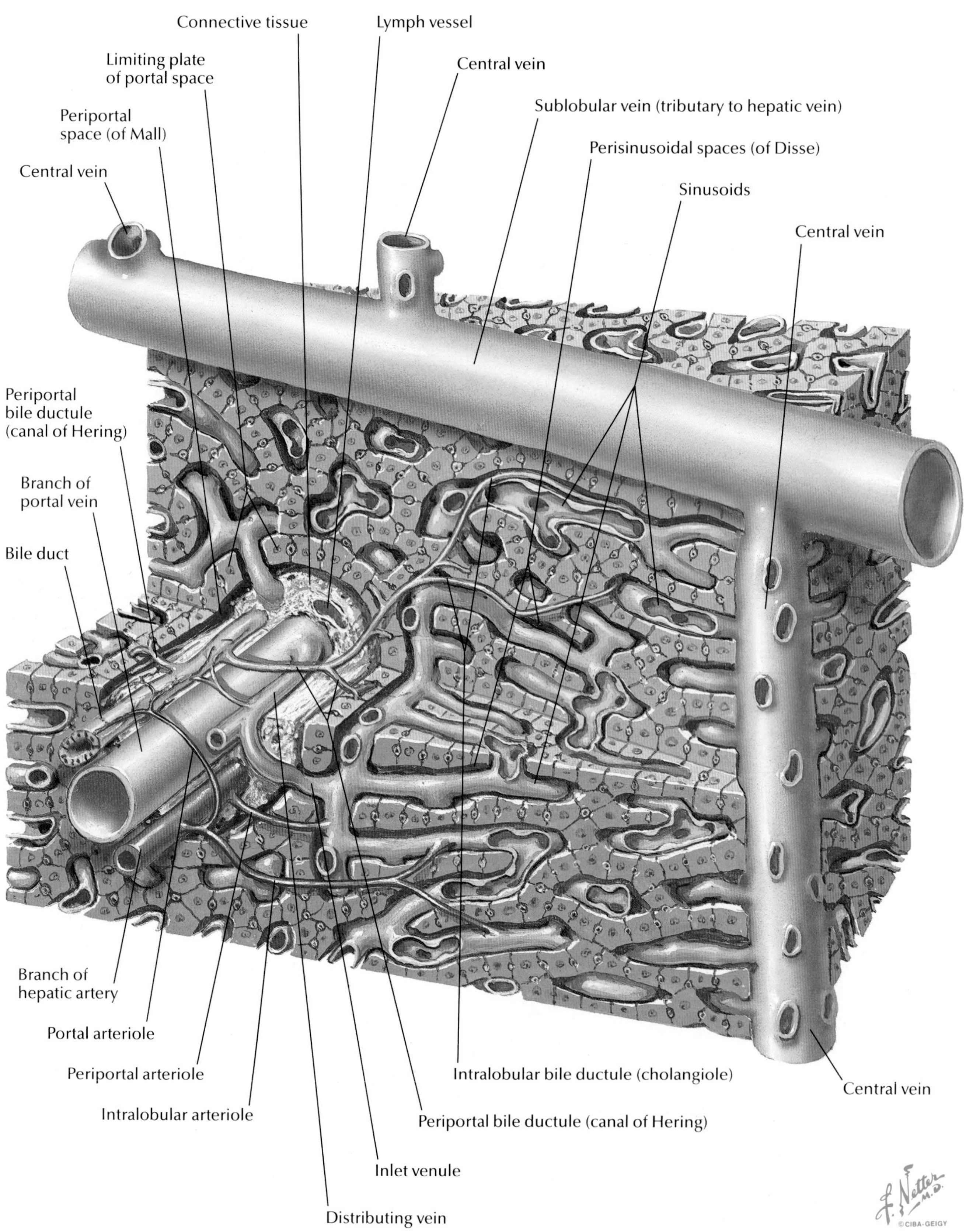

Connective tissue

Lymph vessel

Limiting plate
of portal space

Central vein

Sublobular vein (tributary to hepatic vein)

Periportal
space (of Mall)

Perisinusoidal spaces (of Disse)

Central vein

Sinusoids

Central vein

Periportal
bile ductule
(canal of Hering)

Branch of
portal vein

Bile duct

Branch of
hepatic artery

Portal arteriole

Periportal arteriole

Intralobular bile ductule (cholangiole)

Intralobular arteriole

Central vein

Periportal bile ductule (canal of Hering)

Inlet venule

Distributing vein

PLATE 274

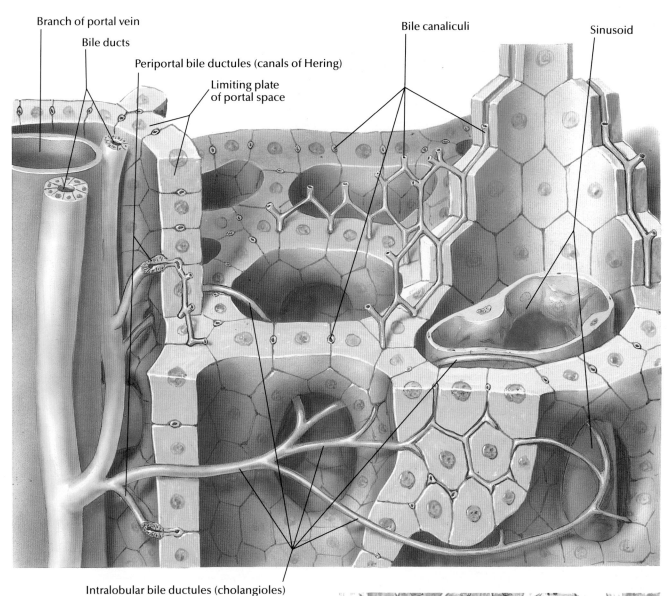

Branch of portal vein

Bile ducts

Periportal bile ductules (canals of Hering)

Limiting plate of portal space

Bile canaliculi

Sinusoid

Intralobular bile ductules (cholangioles)

Note: in above illustration, bile canaliculi appear as structures with walls of their own. However, as shown in histologic section at right, boundaries of canaliculi are actually a specialization of surface membranes of adjoining liver parenchymal cells

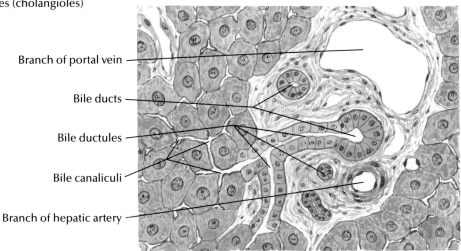

Branch of portal vein

Bile ducts

Bile ductules

Bile canaliculi

Branch of hepatic artery

Low-power section of liver

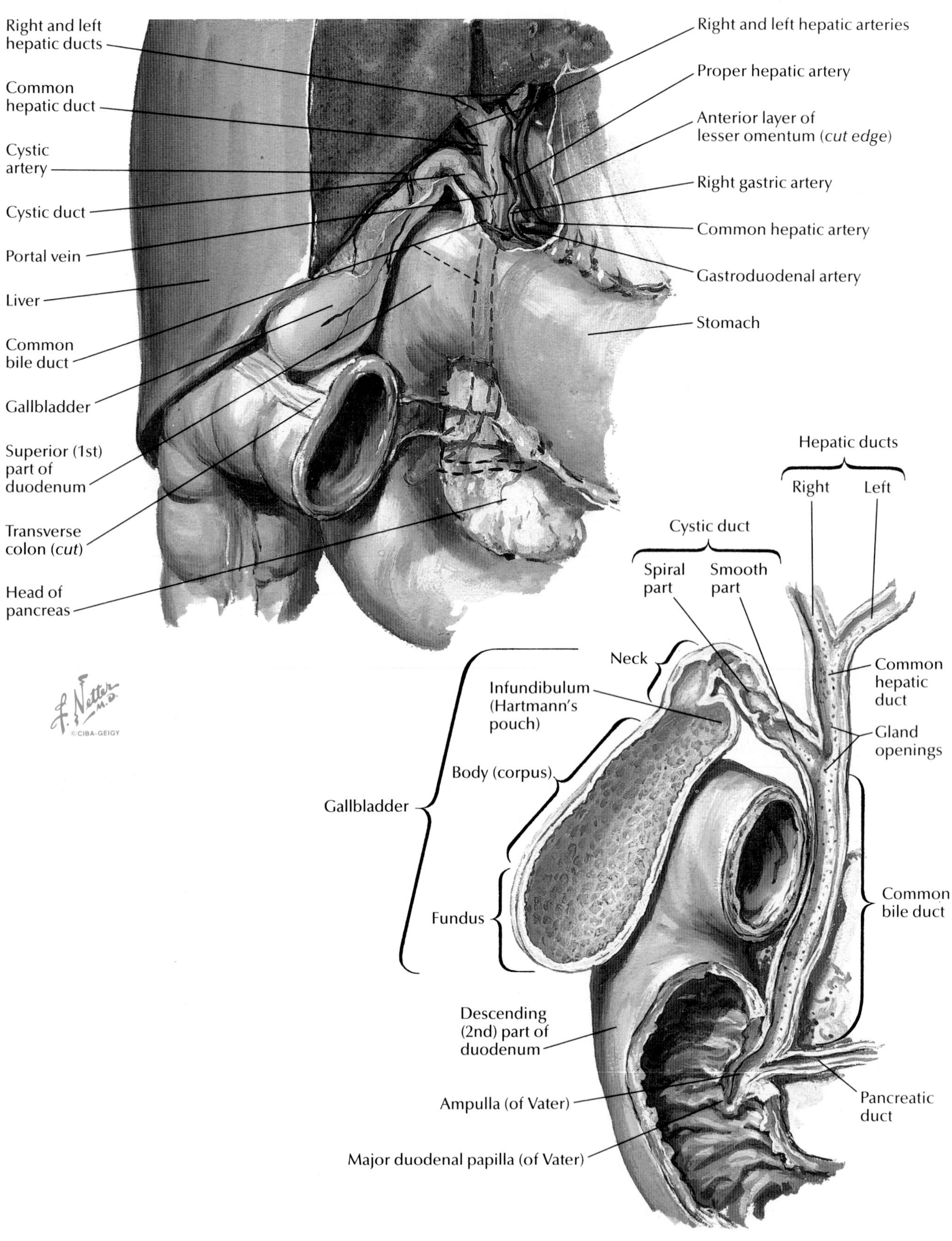

Right and left hepatic ducts

Common hepatic duct

Cystic artery

Cystic duct

Portal vein

Liver

Common bile duct

Gallbladder

Superior (1st) part of duodenum

Transverse colon (*cut*)

Head of pancreas

Right and left hepatic arteries

Proper hepatic artery

Anterior layer of lesser omentum (*cut edge*)

Right gastric artery

Common hepatic artery

Gastroduodenal artery

Stomach

Hepatic ducts

Right   Left

Cystic duct

Spiral part   Smooth part

Neck

Infundibulum (Hartmann's pouch)

Body (corpus)

Gallbladder

Fundus

Common hepatic duct

Gland openings

Common bile duct

Descending (2nd) part of duodenum

Ampulla (of Vater)

Major duodenal papilla (of Vater)

Pancreatic duct

PLATE 276

ABDOMEN

Variations in cystic duct

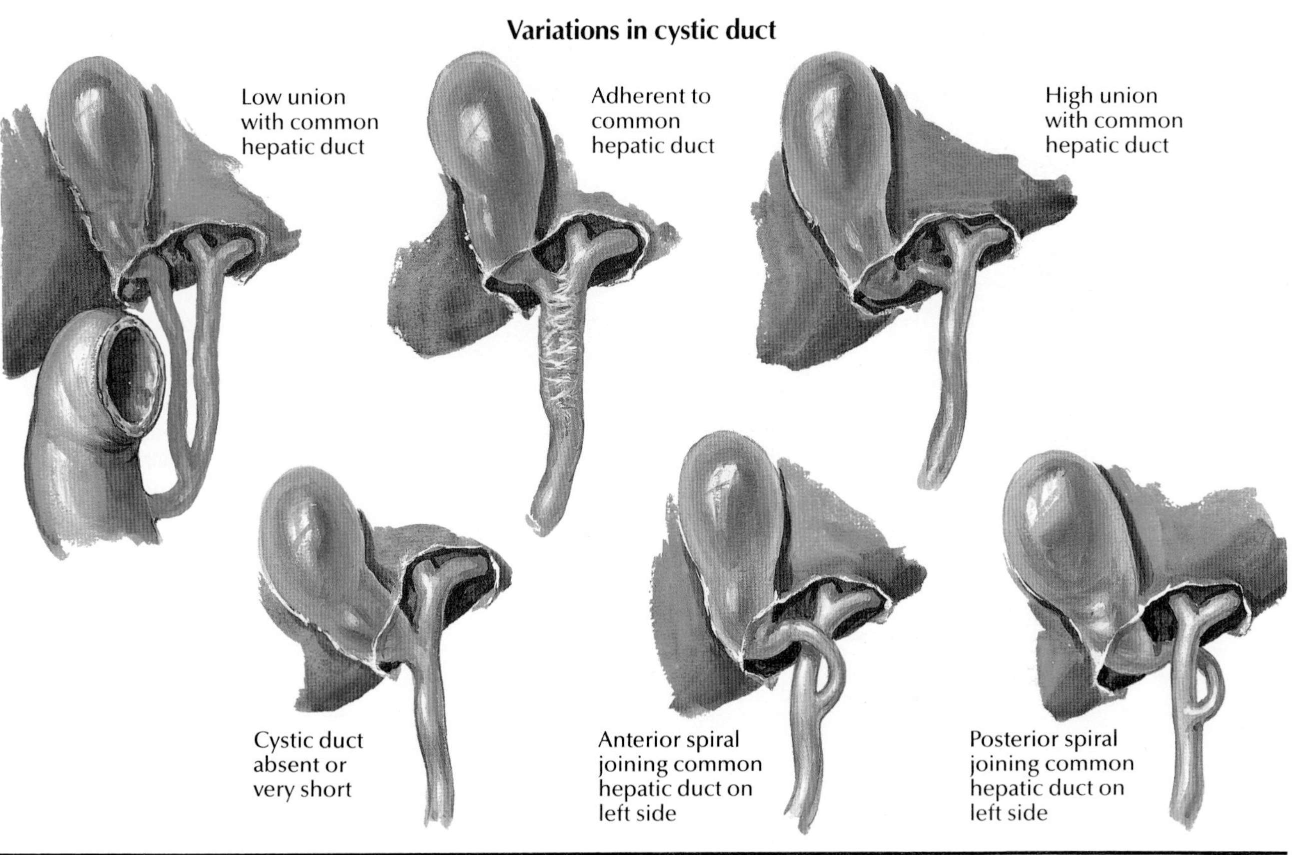

Low union
with common
hepatic duct

Adherent to
common
hepatic duct

High union
with common
hepatic duct

Cystic duct
absent or
very short

Anterior spiral
joining common
hepatic duct on
left side

Posterior spiral
joining common
hepatic duct on
left side

Accessory (aberrant) hepatic ducts

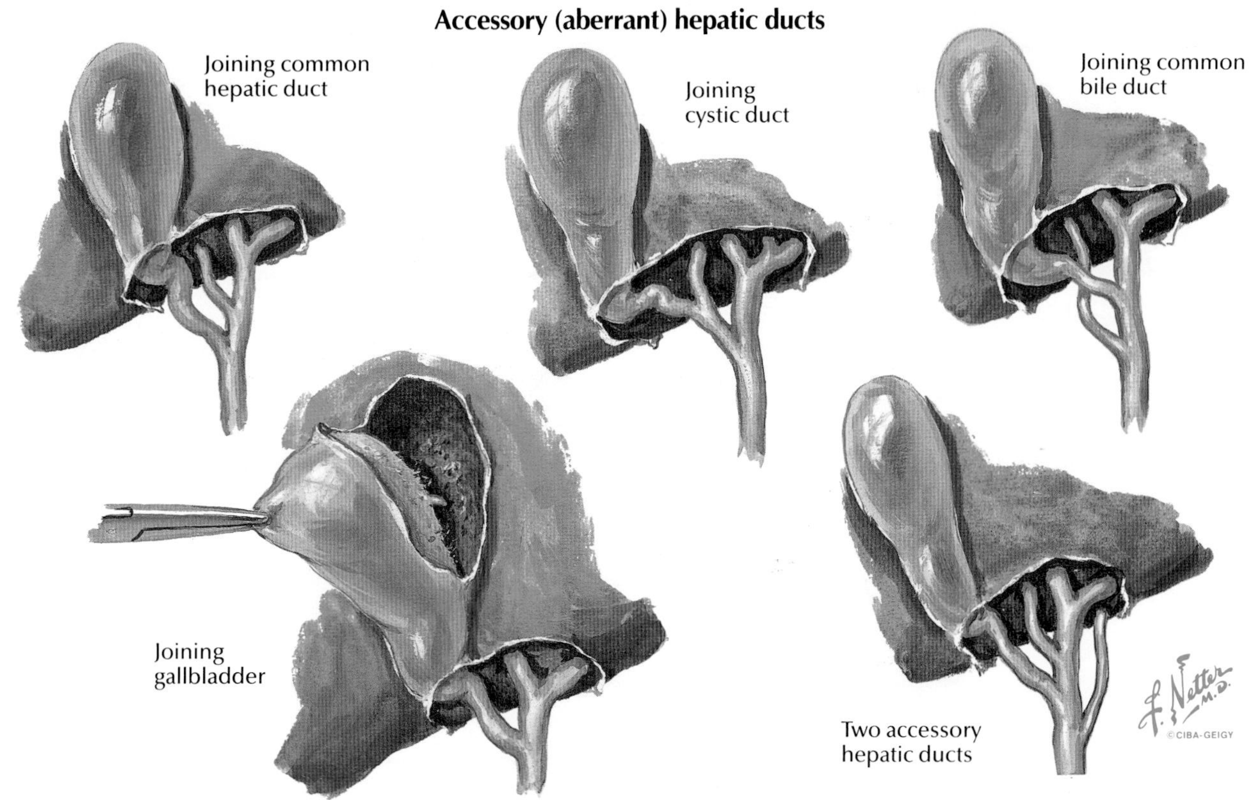

Joining common
hepatic duct

Joining
cystic duct

Joining common
bile duct

Joining
gallbladder

Two accessory
hepatic ducts

Choledochoduodenal Junction

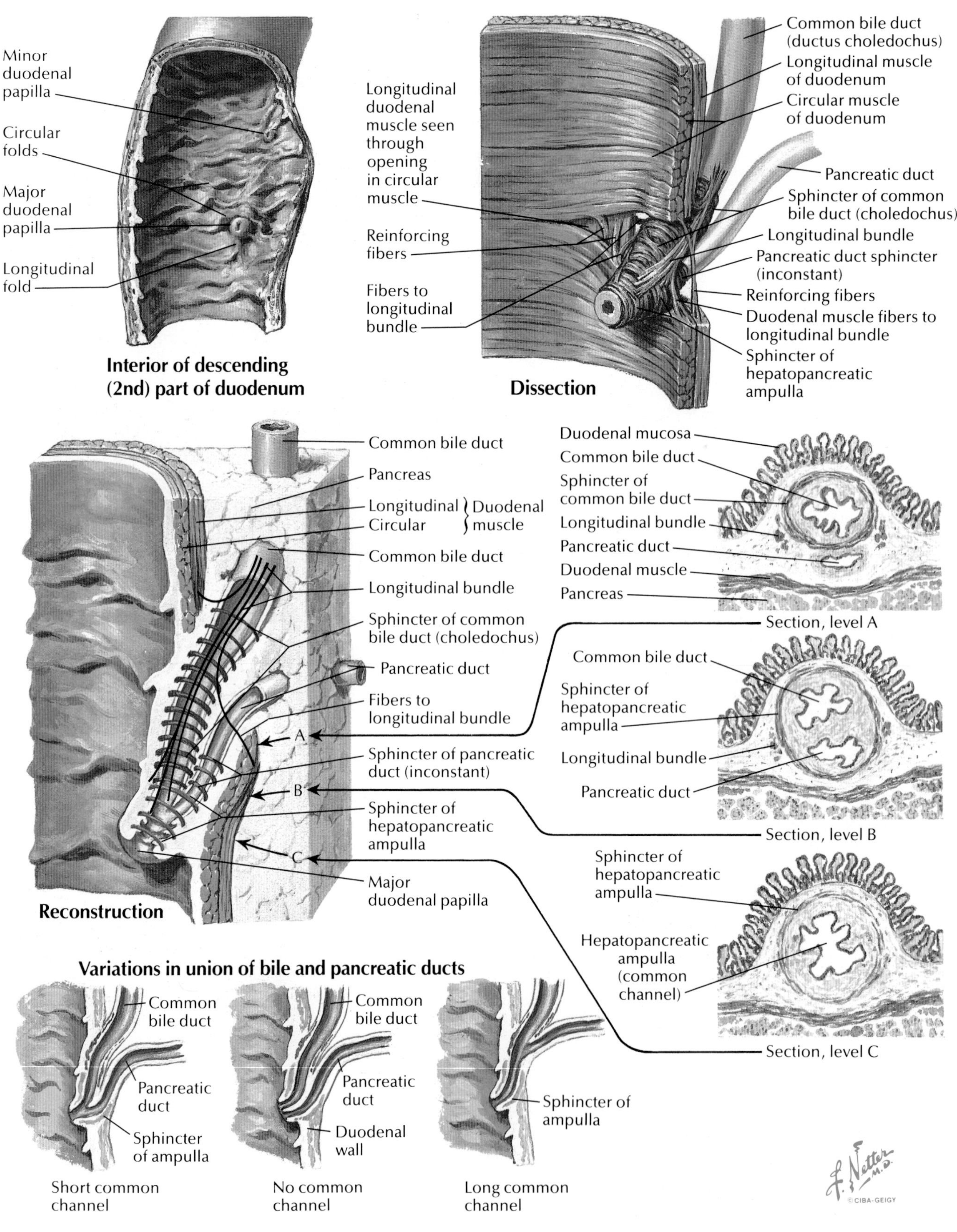

Minor duodenal papilla

Circular folds

Major duodenal papilla

Longitudinal fold

Interior of descending (2nd) part of duodenum

Longitudinal duodenal muscle seen through opening in circular muscle

Reinforcing fibers

Fibers to longitudinal bundle

Dissection

Common bile duct (ductus choledochus)

Longitudinal muscle of duodenum

Circular muscle of duodenum

Pancreatic duct

Sphincter of common bile duct (choledochus)

Longitudinal bundle

Pancreatic duct sphincter (inconstant)

Reinforcing fibers

Duodenal muscle fibers to longitudinal bundle

Sphincter of hepatopancreatic ampulla

Common bile duct

Pancreas

Longitudinal ⎫ Duodenal

Circular ⎬ muscle

Common bile duct

Longitudinal bundle

Sphincter of common bile duct (choledochus)

Pancreatic duct

Fibers to longitudinal bundle

Sphincter of pancreatic duct (inconstant)

Sphincter of hepatopancreatic ampulla

Major duodenal papilla

Reconstruction

Duodenal mucosa

Common bile duct

Sphincter of common bile duct

Longitudinal bundle

Pancreatic duct

Duodenal muscle

Pancreas

Section, level A

Common bile duct

Sphincter of hepatopancreatic ampulla

Longitudinal bundle

Pancreatic duct

Section, level B

Sphincter of hepatopancreatic ampulla

Hepatopancreatic ampulla (common channel)

Section, level C

Variations in union of bile and pancreatic ducts

Common bile duct

Pancreatic duct

Sphincter of ampulla

Short common channel

Common bile duct

Pancreatic duct

Duodenal wall

No common channel

Sphincter of ampulla

Long common channel

PLATE 278

ABDOMEN

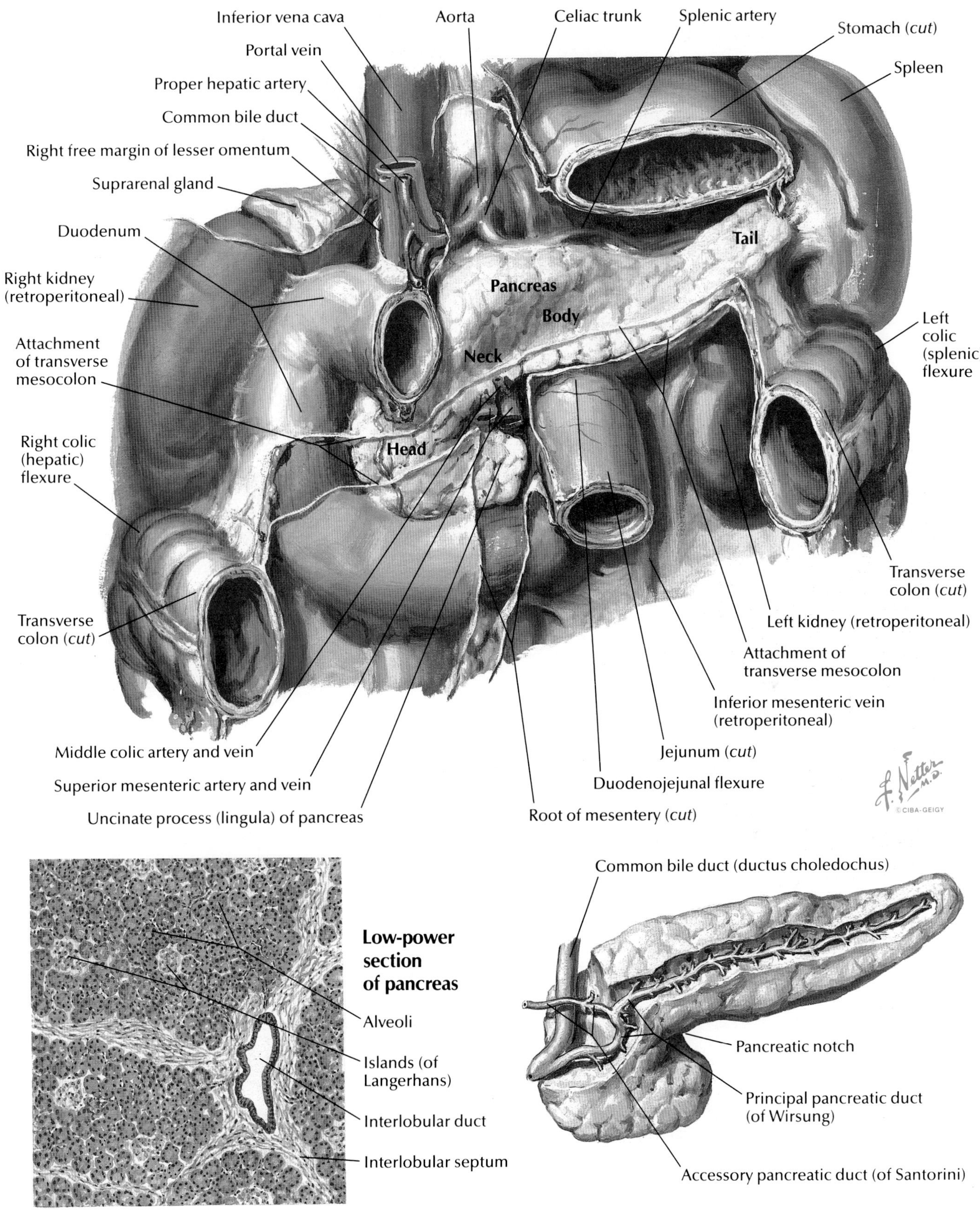

Inferior vena cava

Portal vein

Proper hepatic artery

Common bile duct

Right free margin of lesser omentum

Suprarenal gland

Duodenum

Right kidney (retroperitoneal)

Attachment of transverse mesocolon

Right colic (hepatic) flexure

Transverse colon (*cut*)

Middle colic artery and vein

Superior mesenteric artery and vein

Uncinate process (lingula) of pancreas

Aorta

Celiac trunk

Splenic artery

Stomach (*cut*)

Spleen

Tail

Pancreas

Body

Neck

Head

Left colic (splenic) flexure

Transverse colon (*cut*)

Left kidney (retroperitoneal)

Attachment of transverse mesocolon

Inferior mesenteric vein (retroperitoneal)

Jejunum (*cut*)

Duodenojejunal flexure

Root of mesentery (*cut*)

Low-power section of pancreas

Alveoli

Islands (of Langerhans)

Interlobular duct

Interlobular septum

Common bile duct (ductus choledochus)

Pancreatic notch

Principal pancreatic duct (of Wirsung)

Accessory pancreatic duct (of Santorini)

Variations in Pancreatic Ducts

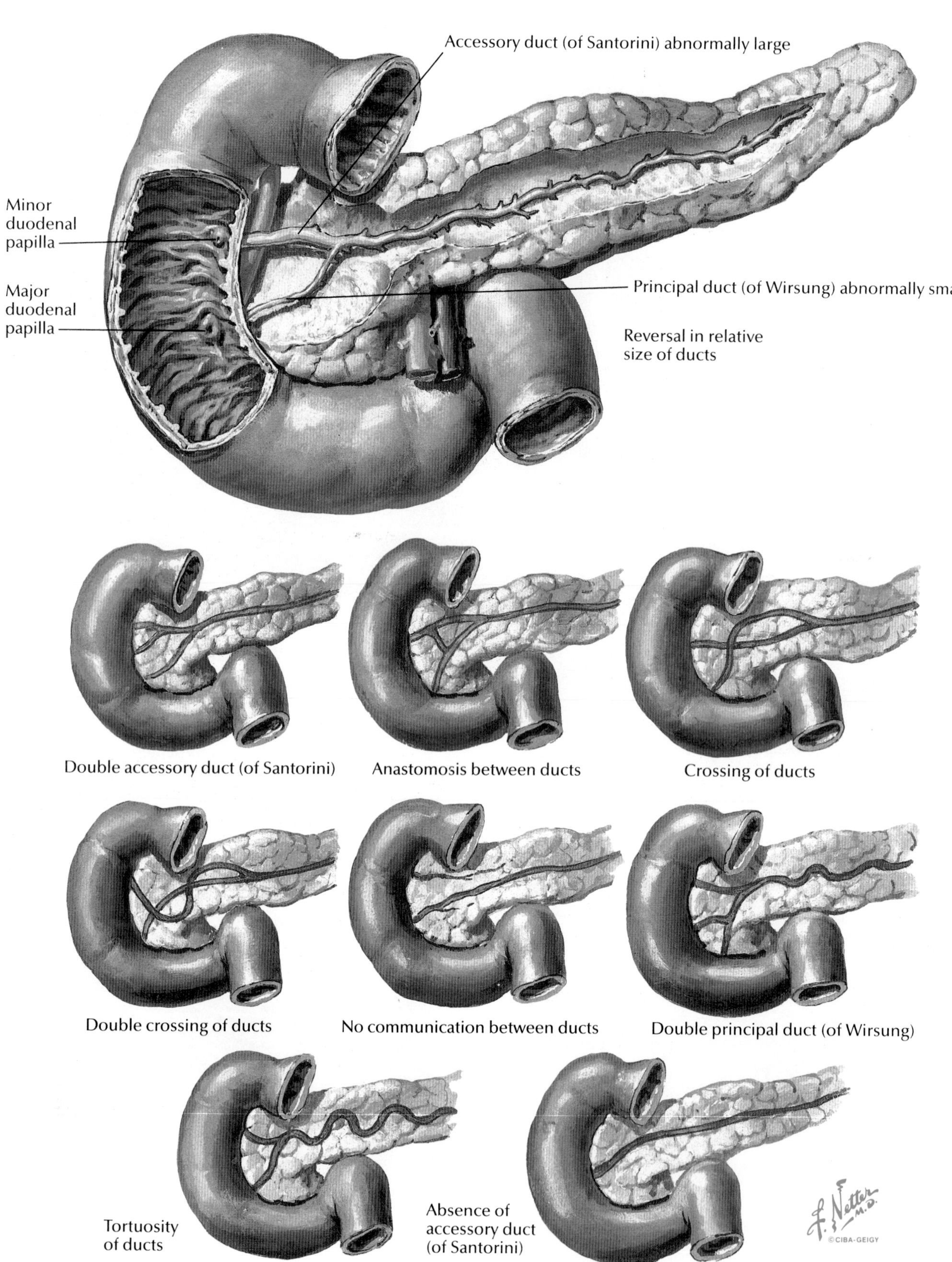

Accessory duct (of Santorini) abnormally large

Minor duodenal papilla

Major duodenal papilla

Principal duct (of Wirsung) abnormally small

Reversal in relative size of ducts

Double accessory duct (of Santorini)

Anastomosis between ducts

Crossing of ducts

Double crossing of ducts

No communication between ducts

Double principal duct (of Wirsung)

Tortuosity of ducts

Absence of accessory duct (of Santorini)

PLATE 280

ABDOMEN

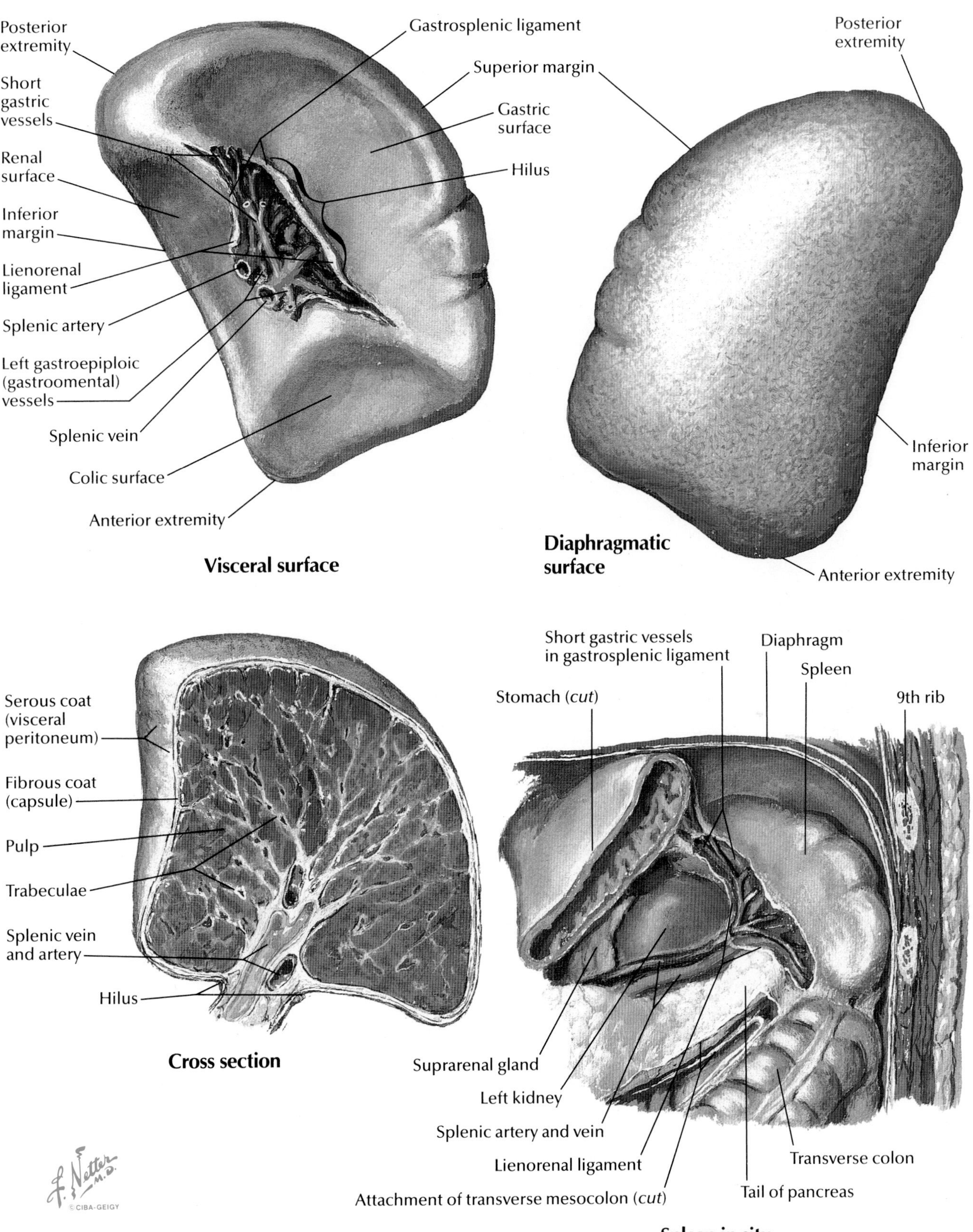

Posterior extremity

Short gastric vessels

Renal surface

Inferior margin

Lienorenal ligament

Splenic artery

Left gastroepiploic (gastroomental) vessels

Splenic vein

Colic surface

Anterior extremity

Gastrosplenic ligament

Superior margin

Gastric surface

Hilus

Visceral surface

Posterior extremity

Inferior margin

Anterior extremity

Diaphragmatic surface

Serous coat (visceral peritoneum)

Fibrous coat (capsule)

Pulp

Trabeculae

Splenic vein and artery

Hilus

Cross section

Short gastric vessels in gastrosplenic ligament

Stomach (*cut*)

Diaphragm

Spleen

9th rib

Suprarenal gland

Left kidney

Splenic artery and vein

Lienorenal ligament

Attachment of transverse mesocolon (*cut*)

Tail of pancreas

Transverse colon

Spleen in situ

Arteries of Stomach, Liver and Spleen

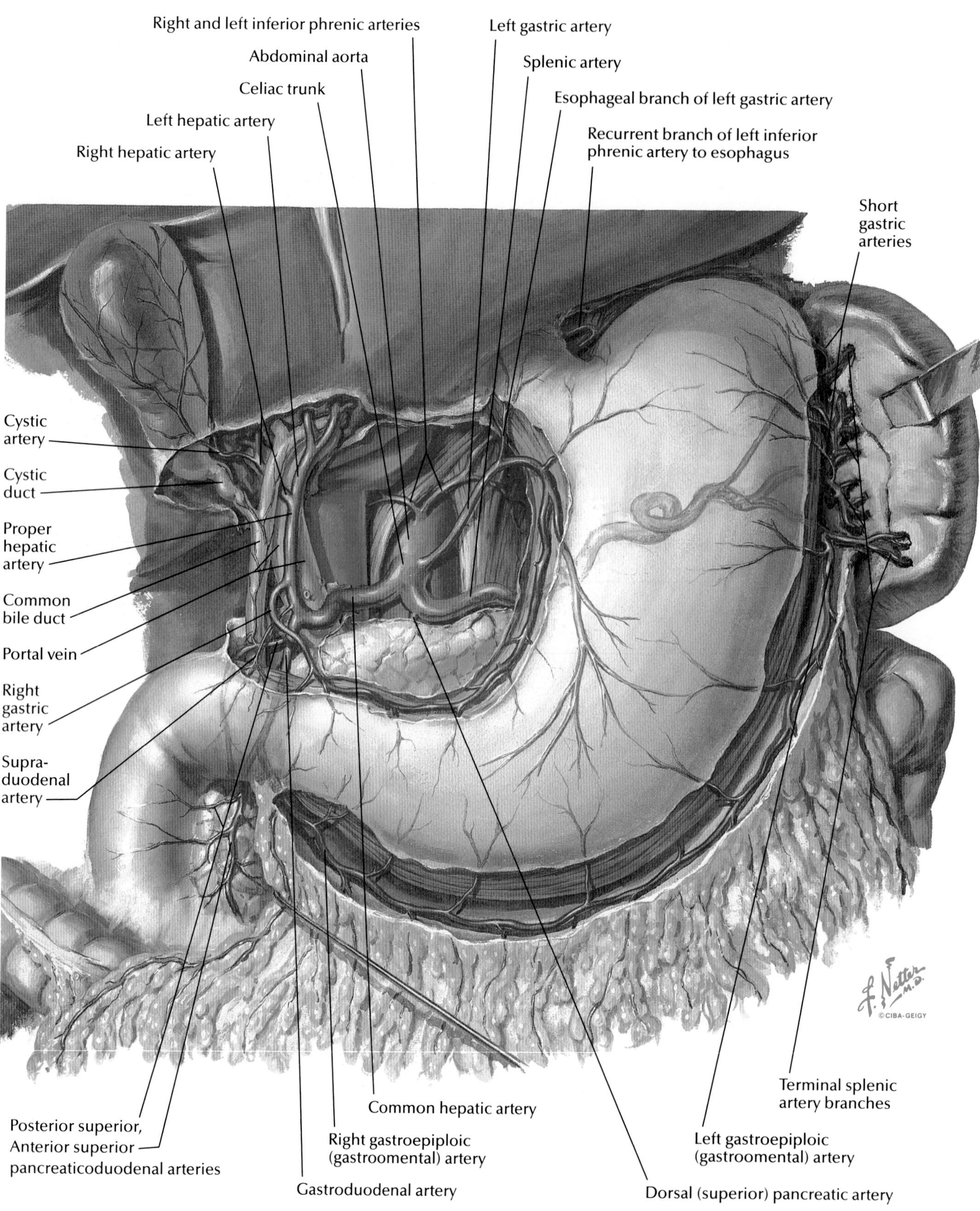

Right and left inferior phrenic arteries

Left gastric artery

Abdominal aorta

Splenic artery

Celiac trunk

Esophageal branch of left gastric artery

Left hepatic artery

Recurrent branch of left inferior phrenic artery to esophagus

Right hepatic artery

Short gastric arteries

Cystic artery

Cystic duct

Proper hepatic artery

Common bile duct

Portal vein

Right gastric artery

Supra-duodenal artery

Posterior superior, Anterior superior pancreaticoduodenal arteries

Right gastroepiploic (gastroomental) artery

Gastroduodenal artery

Common hepatic artery

Dorsal (superior) pancreatic artery

Left gastroepiploic (gastroomental) artery

Terminal splenic artery branches

PLATE 282

ABDOMEN

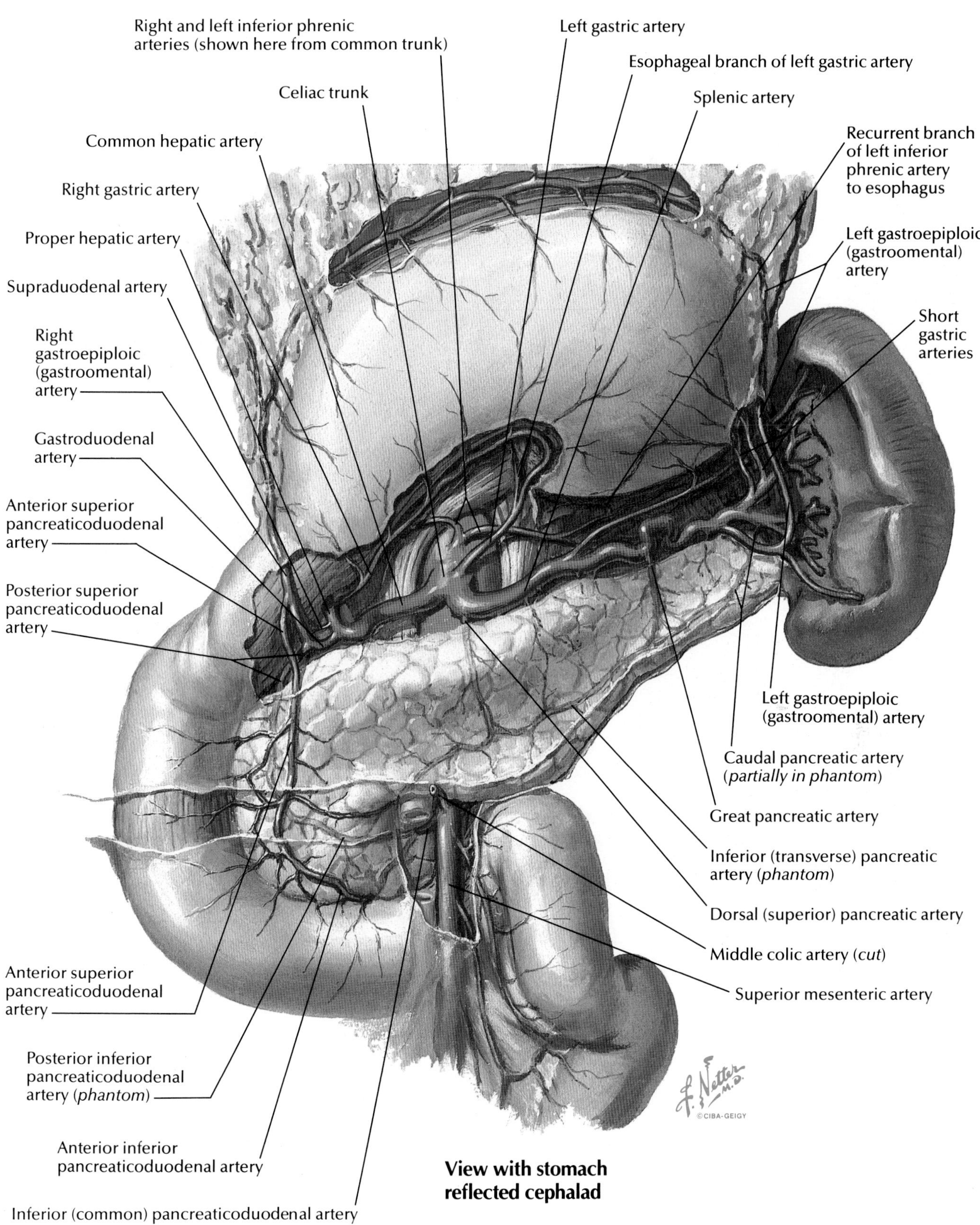

Right and left inferior phrenic arteries (shown here from common trunk)

Left gastric artery

Esophageal branch of left gastric artery

Celiac trunk

Splenic artery

Common hepatic artery

Recurrent branch of left inferior phrenic artery to esophagus

Right gastric artery

Proper hepatic artery

Left gastroepiploic (gastroomental) artery

Supraduodenal artery

Short gastric arteries

Right gastroepiploic (gastroomental) artery

Gastroduodenal artery

Anterior superior pancreaticoduodenal artery

Posterior superior pancreaticoduodenal artery

Left gastroepiploic (gastroomental) artery

Caudal pancreatic artery (*partially in phantom*)

Great pancreatic artery

Inferior (transverse) pancreatic artery (*phantom*)

Dorsal (superior) pancreatic artery

Middle colic artery (*cut*)

Anterior superior pancreaticoduodenal artery

Superior mesenteric artery

Posterior inferior pancreaticoduodenal artery (*phantom*)

Anterior inferior pancreaticoduodenal artery

View with stomach reflected cephalad

Inferior (common) pancreaticoduodenal artery

Arteries of Liver, Pancreas, Duodenum and Spleen

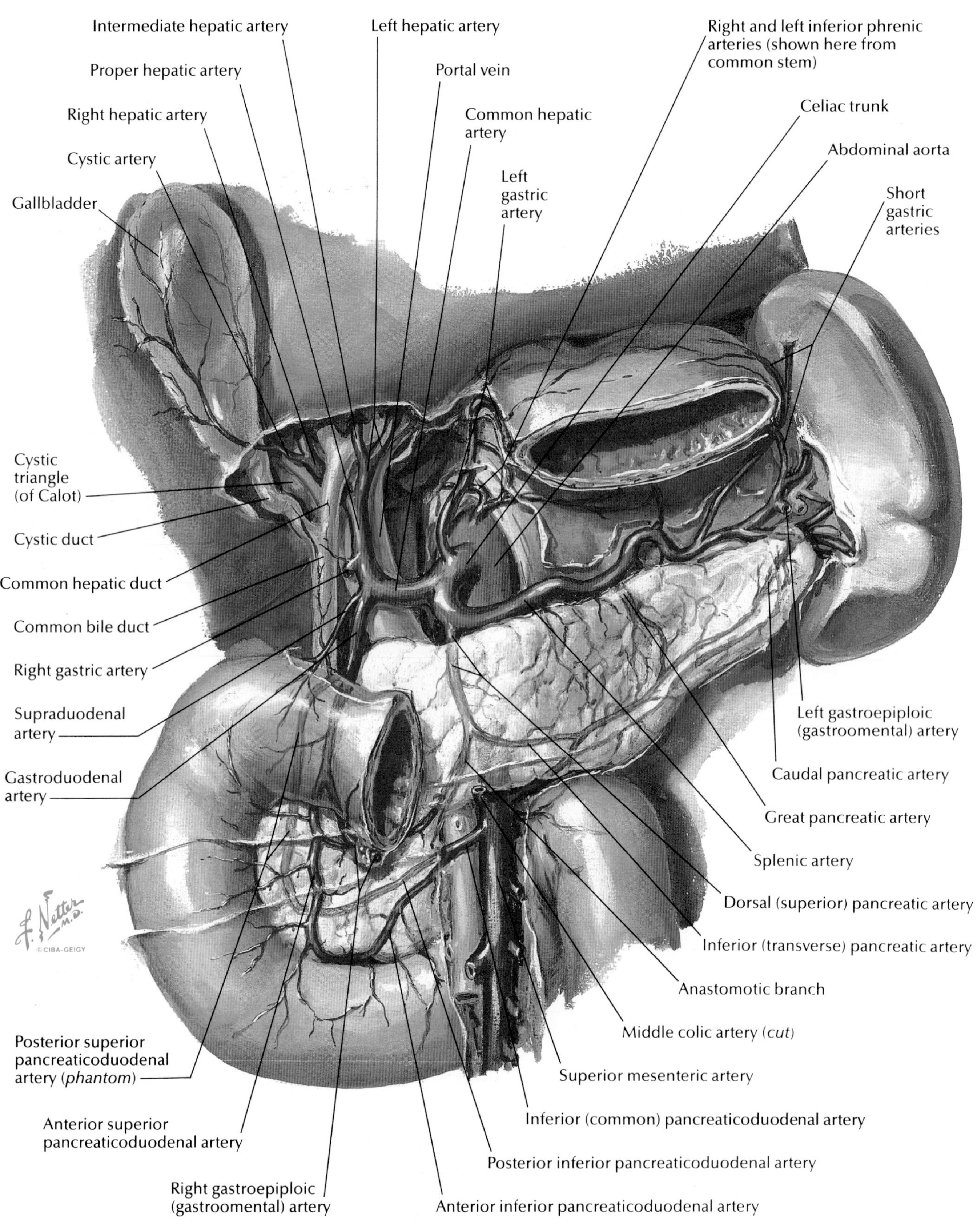

Intermediate hepatic artery

Proper hepatic artery

Right hepatic artery

Cystic artery

Gallbladder

Left hepatic artery

Portal vein

Common hepatic artery

Left gastric artery

Right and left inferior phrenic arteries (shown here from common stem)

Celiac trunk

Abdominal aorta

Short gastric arteries

Cystic triangle (of Calot)

Cystic duct

Common hepatic duct

Common bile duct

Right gastric artery

Supraduodenal artery

Gastroduodenal artery

Left gastroepiploic (gastroomental) artery

Caudal pancreatic artery

Great pancreatic artery

Splenic artery

Dorsal (superior) pancreatic artery

Inferior (transverse) pancreatic artery

Anastomotic branch

Middle colic artery (cut)

Superior mesenteric artery

Inferior (common) pancreaticoduodenal artery

Posterior inferior pancreaticoduodenal artery

Anterior inferior pancreaticoduodenal artery

Posterior superior pancreaticoduodenal artery (phantom)

Anterior superior pancreaticoduodenal artery

Right gastroepiploic (gastroomental) artery

PLATE 284

ABDOMEN

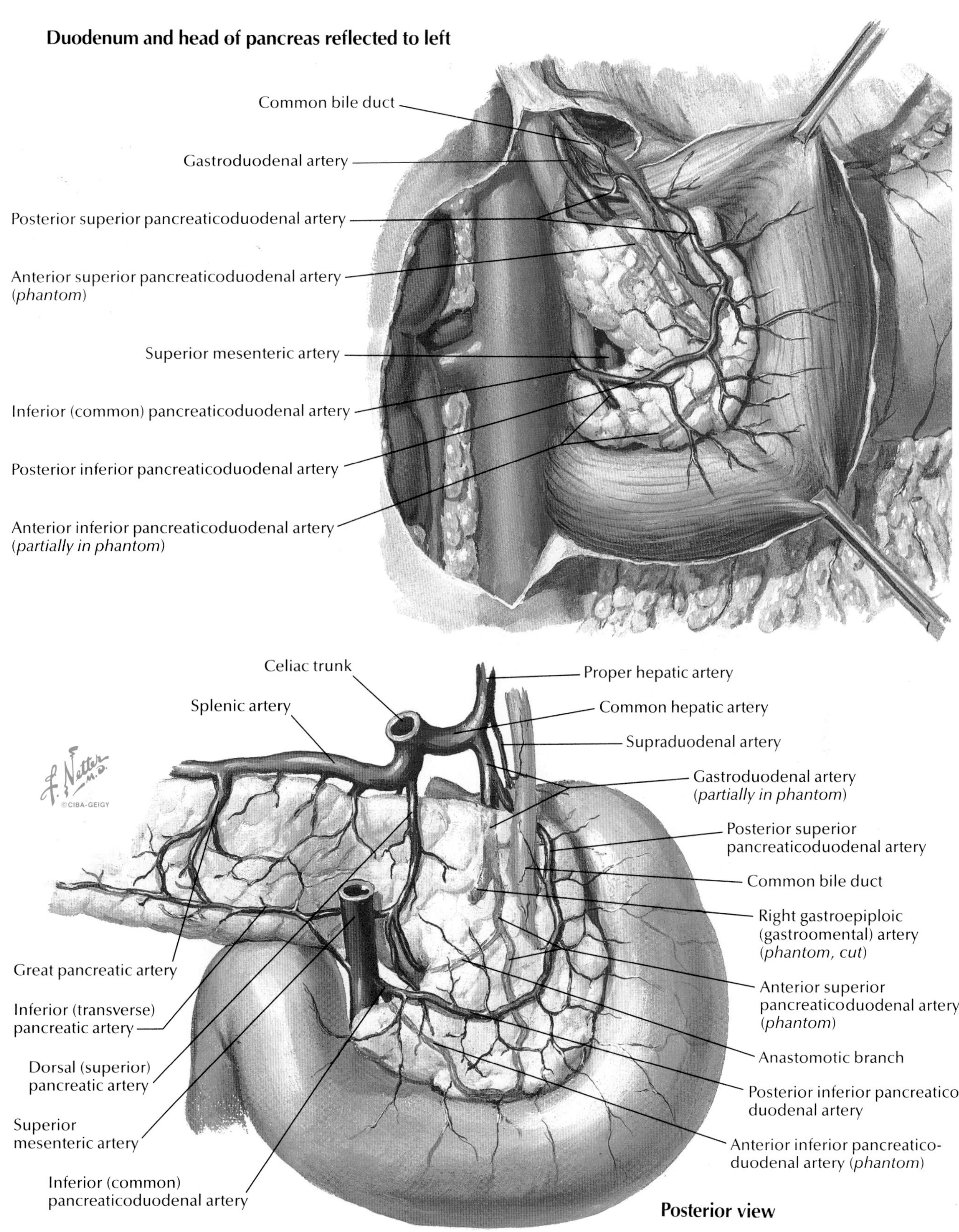

Duodenum and head of pancreas reflected to left

Common bile duct

Gastroduodenal artery

Posterior superior pancreaticoduodenal artery

Anterior superior pancreaticoduodenal artery
(*phantom*)

Superior mesenteric artery

Inferior (common) pancreaticoduodenal artery

Posterior inferior pancreaticoduodenal artery

Anterior inferior pancreaticoduodenal artery
(*partially in phantom*)

Celiac trunk

Splenic artery

Proper hepatic artery

Common hepatic artery

Supraduodenal artery

Gastroduodenal artery
(*partially in phantom*)

Posterior superior
pancreaticoduodenal artery

Common bile duct

Right gastroepiploic
(gastroomental) artery
(*phantom, cut*)

Anterior superior
pancreaticoduodenal artery
(*phantom*)

Anastomotic branch

Posterior inferior pancreaticoduodenal artery

Anterior inferior pancreaticoduodenal artery (*phantom*)

Great pancreatic artery

Inferior (transverse)
pancreatic artery

Dorsal (superior)
pancreatic artery

Superior
mesenteric artery

Inferior (common)
pancreaticoduodenal artery

Posterior view

Arteries of Small Intestine

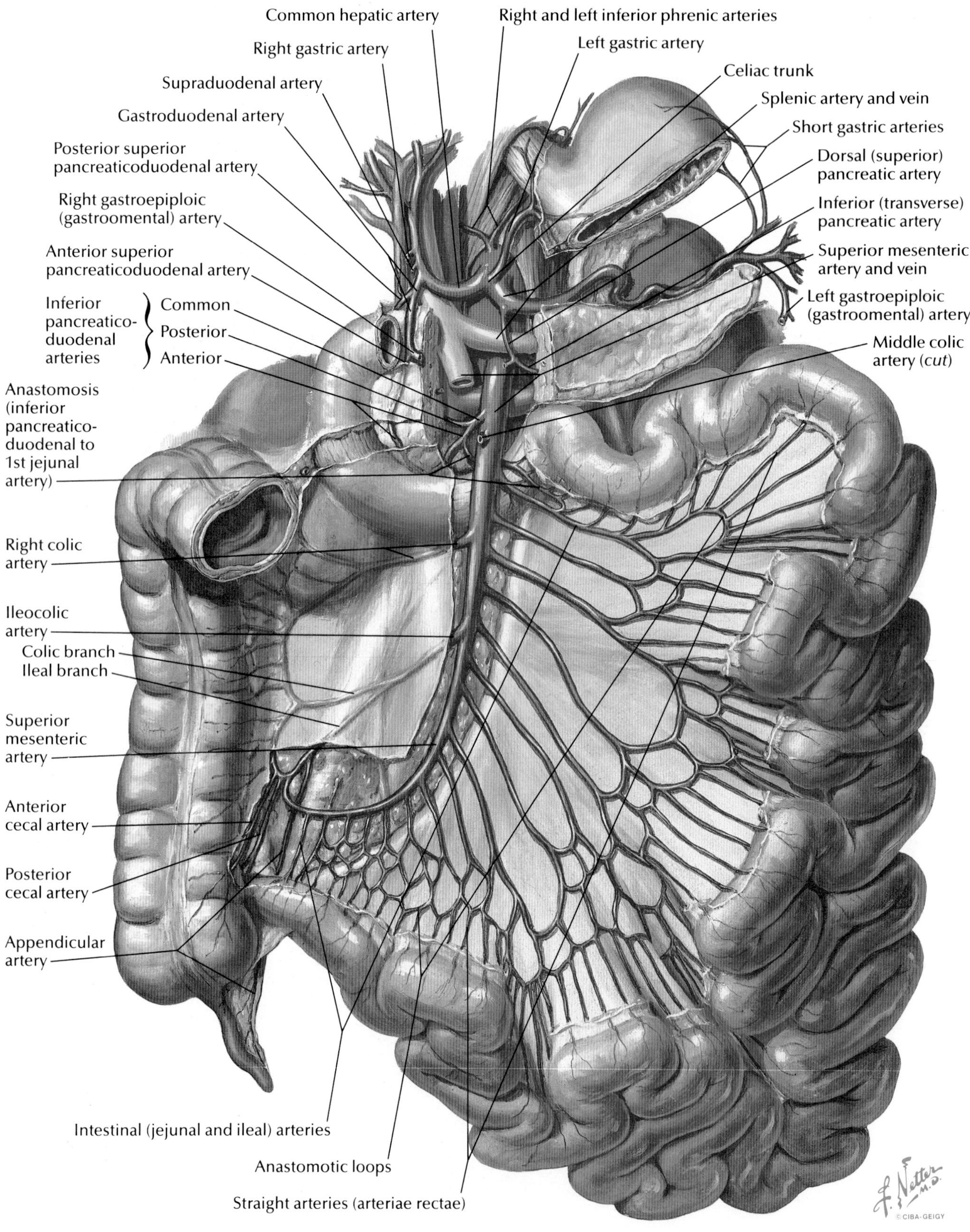

Common hepatic artery

Right gastric artery

Supraduodenal artery

Gastroduodenal artery

Posterior superior pancreaticoduodenal artery

Right gastroepiploic (gastroomental) artery

Anterior superior pancreaticoduodenal artery

Inferior pancreatico- duodenal arteries
{ Common
Posterior
Anterior

Anastomosis (inferior pancreatico- duodenal to 1st jejunal artery)

Right colic artery

Ileocolic artery

Colic branch
Ileal branch

Superior mesenteric artery

Anterior cecal artery

Posterior cecal artery

Appendicular artery

Right and left inferior phrenic arteries

Left gastric artery

Celiac trunk

Splenic artery and vein

Short gastric arteries

Dorsal (superior) pancreatic artery

Inferior (transverse) pancreatic artery

Superior mesenteric artery and vein

Left gastroepiploic (gastroomental) artery

Middle colic artery (cut)

Intestinal (jejunal and ileal) arteries

Anastomotic loops

Straight arteries (arteriae rectae)

PLATE 286

ABDOMEN

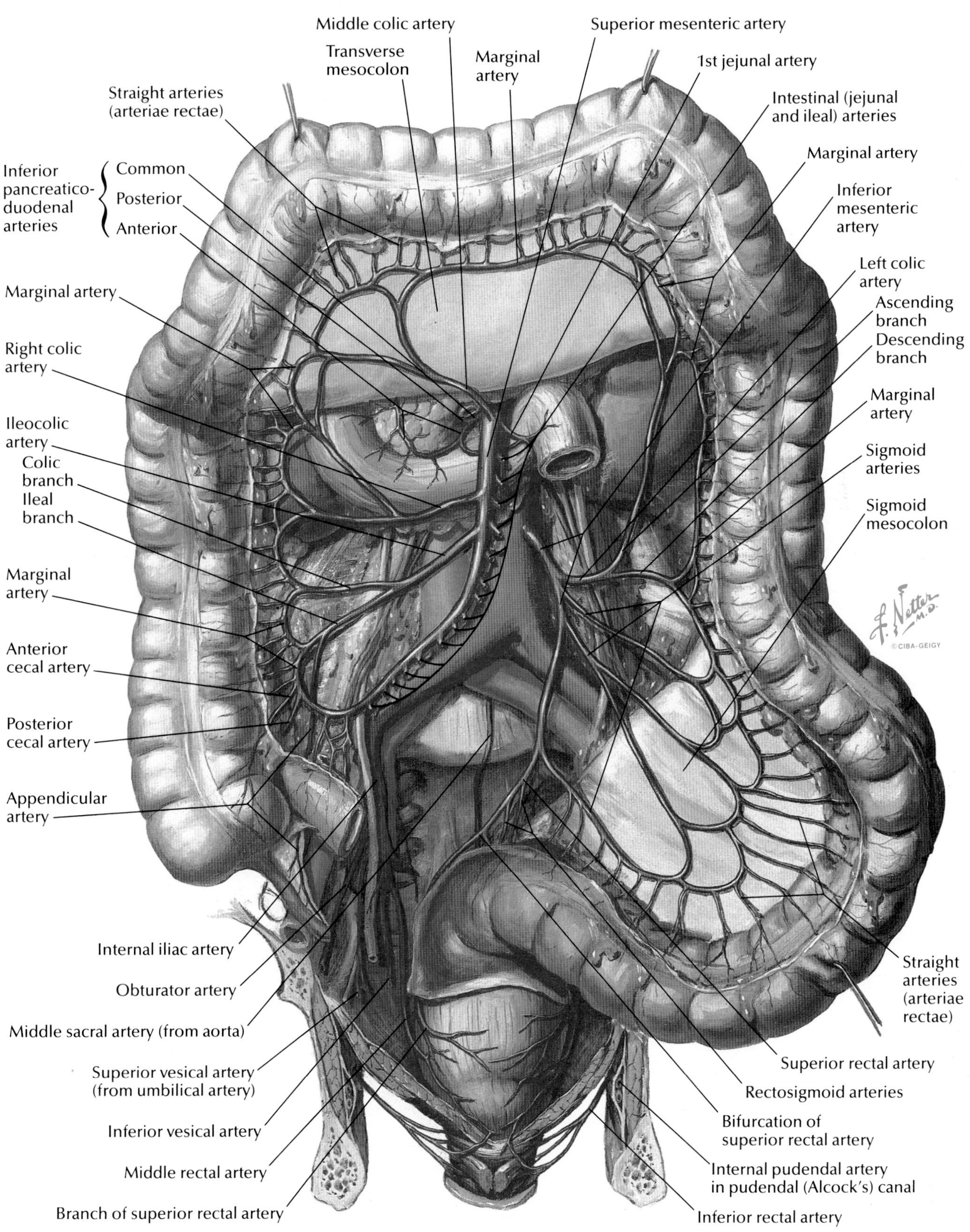

Middle colic artery

Transverse mesocolon

Marginal artery

Superior mesenteric artery

1st jejunal artery

Intestinal (jejunal and ileal) arteries

Marginal artery

Inferior mesenteric artery

Left colic artery

Ascending branch

Descending branch

Marginal artery

Sigmoid arteries

Sigmoid mesocolon

Straight arteries (arteriae rectae)

Inferior pancreatico-duodenal arteries { Common, Posterior, Anterior

Marginal artery

Right colic artery

Ileocolic artery

Colic branch

Ileal branch

Marginal artery

Anterior cecal artery

Posterior cecal artery

Appendicular artery

Internal iliac artery

Obturator artery

Middle sacral artery (from aorta)

Superior vesical artery (from umbilical artery)

Inferior vesical artery

Middle rectal artery

Branch of superior rectal artery

Straight arteries (arteriae rectae)

Superior rectal artery

Rectosigmoid arteries

Bifurcation of superior rectal artery

Internal pudendal artery in pudendal (Alcock's) canal

Inferior rectal artery

Variations in Celiac Trunk

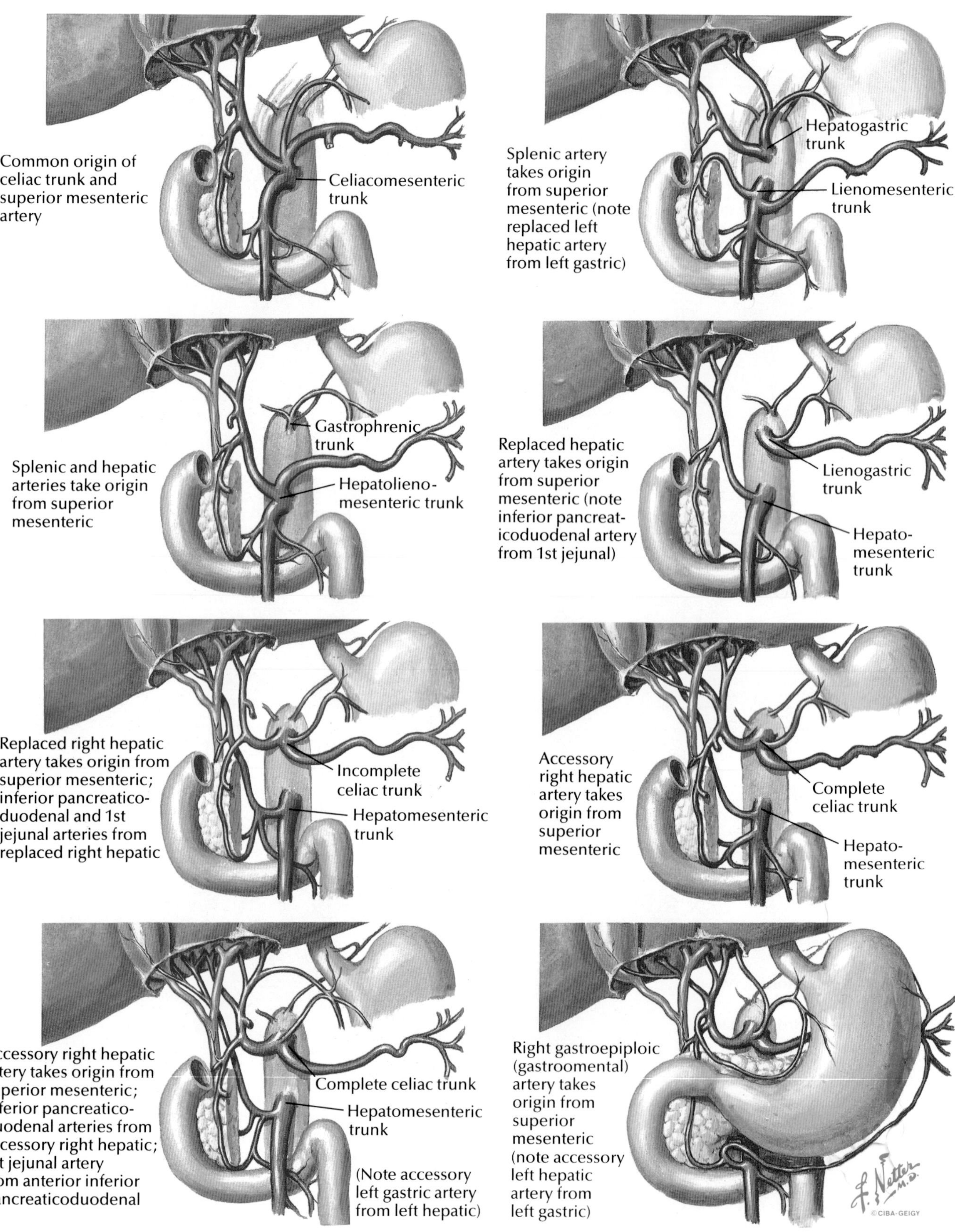

Common origin of celiac trunk and superior mesenteric artery

Celiacomesenteric trunk

Splenic artery takes origin from superior mesenteric (note replaced left hepatic artery from left gastric)

Hepatogastric trunk

Lienomesenteric trunk

Splenic and hepatic arteries take origin from superior mesenteric

Gastrophrenic trunk

Hepatolieno-mesenteric trunk

Replaced hepatic artery takes origin from superior mesenteric (note inferior pancreaticoduodenal artery from 1st jejunal)

Lienogastric trunk

Hepato-mesenteric trunk

Replaced right hepatic artery takes origin from superior mesenteric; inferior pancreaticoduodenal and 1st jejunal arteries from replaced right hepatic

Incomplete celiac trunk

Hepatomesenteric trunk

Accessory right hepatic artery takes origin from superior mesenteric

Complete celiac trunk

Hepato-mesenteric trunk

Accessory right hepatic artery takes origin from superior mesenteric; inferior pancreaticoduodenal arteries from accessory right hepatic; 1st jejunal artery from anterior inferior pancreaticoduodenal

Complete celiac trunk

Hepatomesenteric trunk

(Note accessory left gastric artery from left hepatic)

Right gastroepiploic (gastroomental) artery takes origin from superior mesenteric (note accessory left hepatic artery from left gastric)

PLATE 288

ABDOMEN

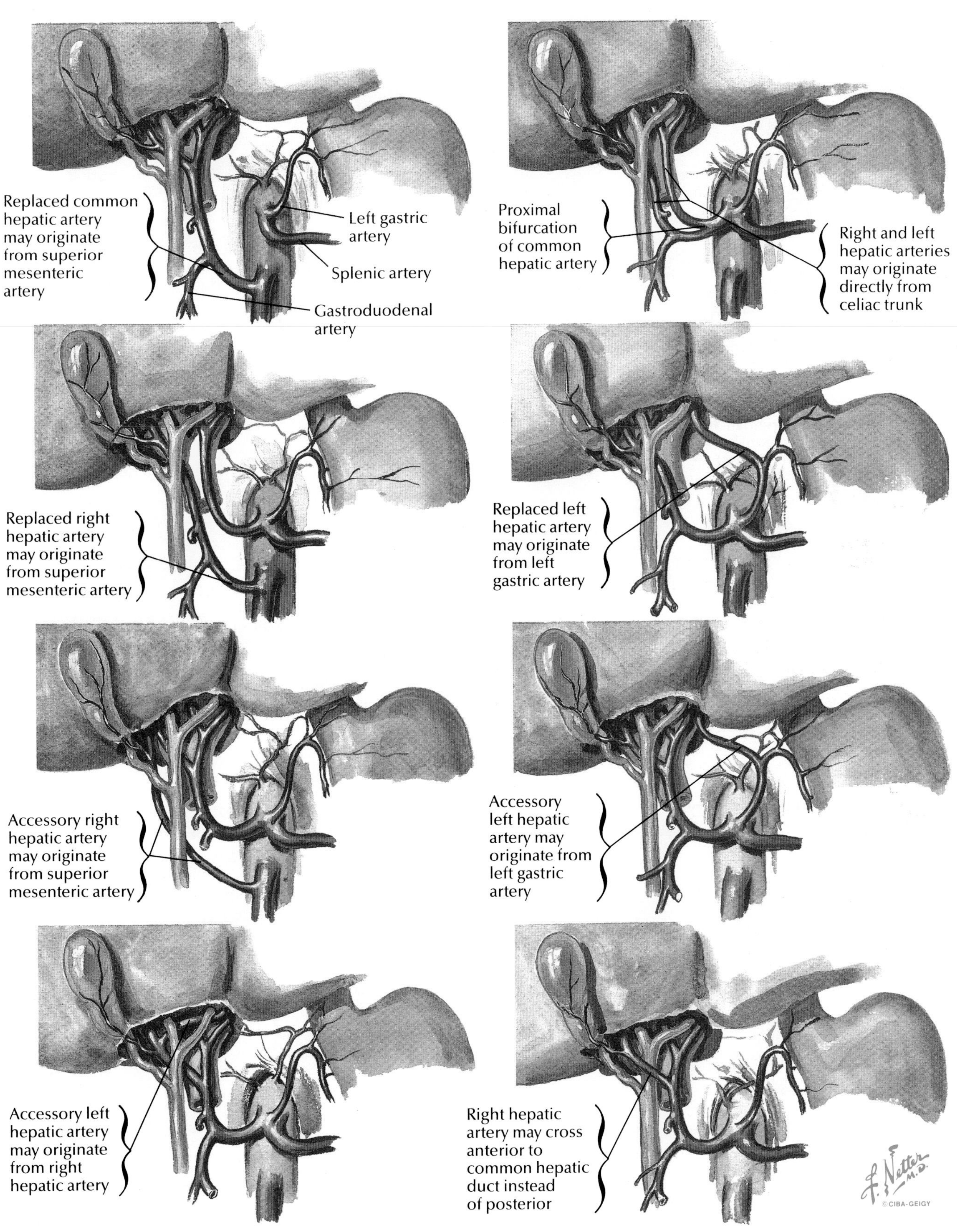

Replaced common hepatic artery may originate from superior mesenteric artery

Left gastric artery

Splenic artery

Gastroduodenal artery

Proximal bifurcation of common hepatic artery

Right and left hepatic arteries may originate directly from celiac trunk

Replaced right hepatic artery may originate from superior mesenteric artery

Replaced left hepatic artery may originate from left gastric artery

Accessory right hepatic artery may originate from superior mesenteric artery

Accessory left hepatic artery may originate from left gastric artery

Accessory left hepatic artery may originate from right hepatic artery

Right hepatic artery may cross anterior to common hepatic duct instead of posterior

Variations in Cystic Artery

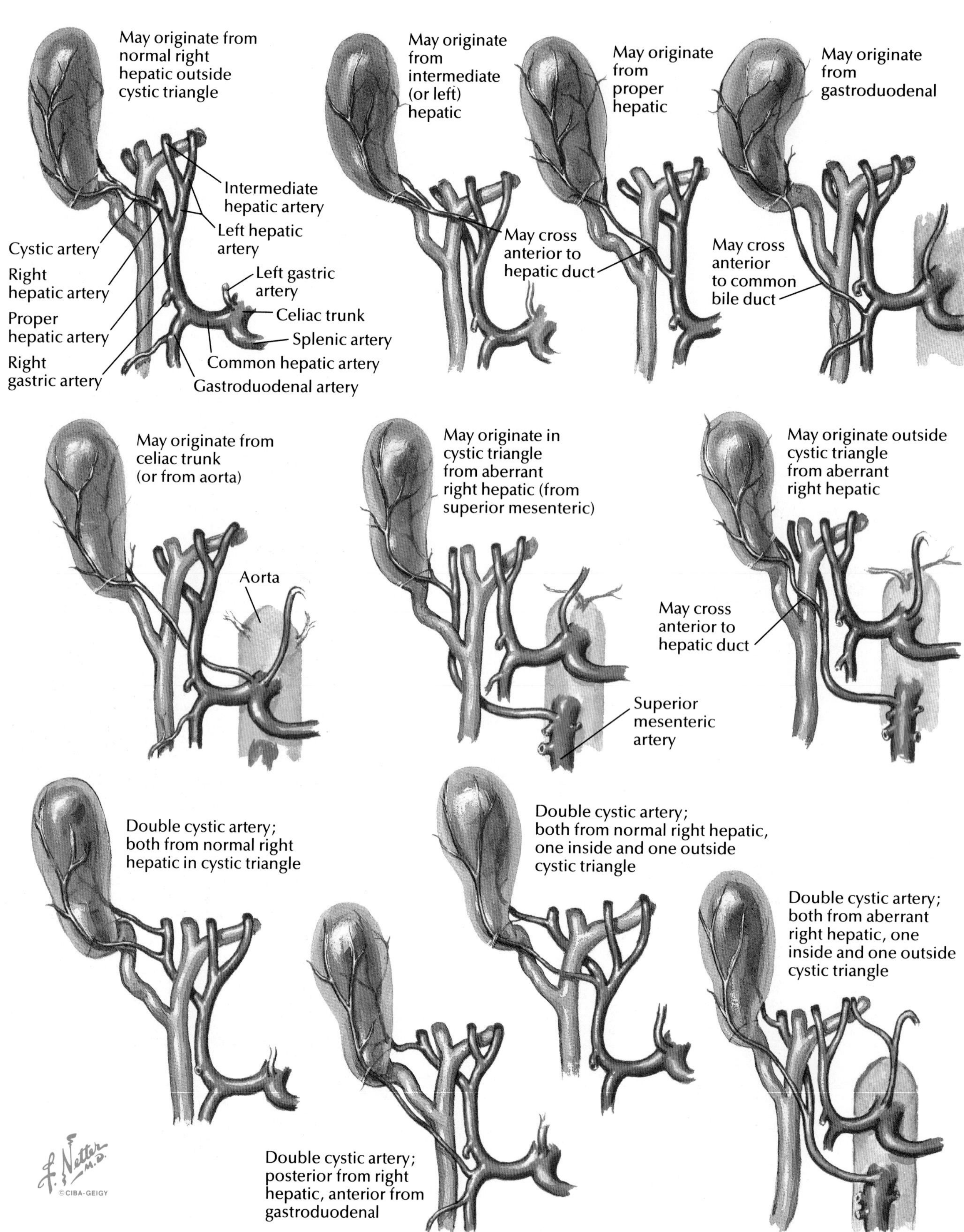

May originate from normal right hepatic outside cystic triangle

Intermediate hepatic artery

Left hepatic artery

Cystic artery

Right hepatic artery

Left gastric artery

Proper hepatic artery

Celiac trunk

Splenic artery

Right gastric artery

Common hepatic artery

Gastroduodenal artery

May originate from intermediate (or left) hepatic

May cross anterior to hepatic duct

May originate from proper hepatic

May originate from gastroduodenal

May cross anterior to common bile duct

May originate from celiac trunk (or from aorta)

Aorta

May originate in cystic triangle from aberrant right hepatic (from superior mesenteric)

Superior mesenteric artery

May originate outside cystic triangle from aberrant right hepatic

May cross anterior to hepatic duct

Double cystic artery; both from normal right hepatic in cystic triangle

Double cystic artery; both from normal right hepatic, one inside and one outside cystic triangle

Double cystic artery; both from aberrant right hepatic, one inside and one outside cystic triangle

Double cystic artery; posterior from right hepatic, anterior from gastroduodenal

PLATE 290

ABDOMEN

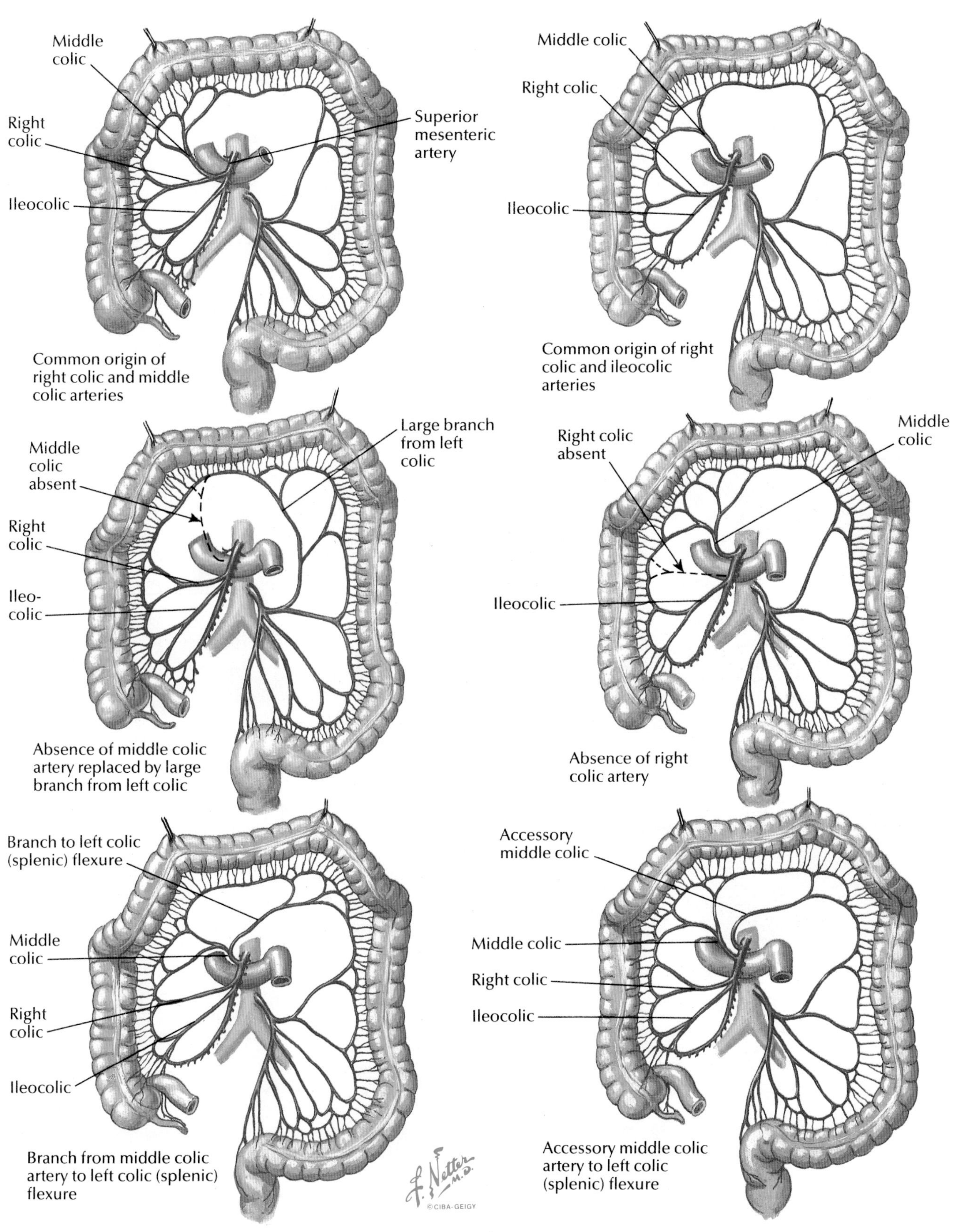

Middle colic

Right colic

Ileocolic

Superior mesenteric artery

Common origin of right colic and middle colic arteries

Middle colic

Right colic

Ileocolic

Common origin of right colic and ileocolic arteries

Middle colic absent

Right colic

Ileo-colic

Large branch from left colic

Absence of middle colic artery replaced by large branch from left colic

Right colic absent

Ileocolic

Middle colic

Absence of right colic artery

Branch to left colic (splenic) flexure

Middle colic

Right colic

Ileocolic

Branch from middle colic artery to left colic (splenic) flexure

Accessory middle colic

Middle colic

Right colic

Ileocolic

Accessory middle colic artery to left colic (splenic) flexure

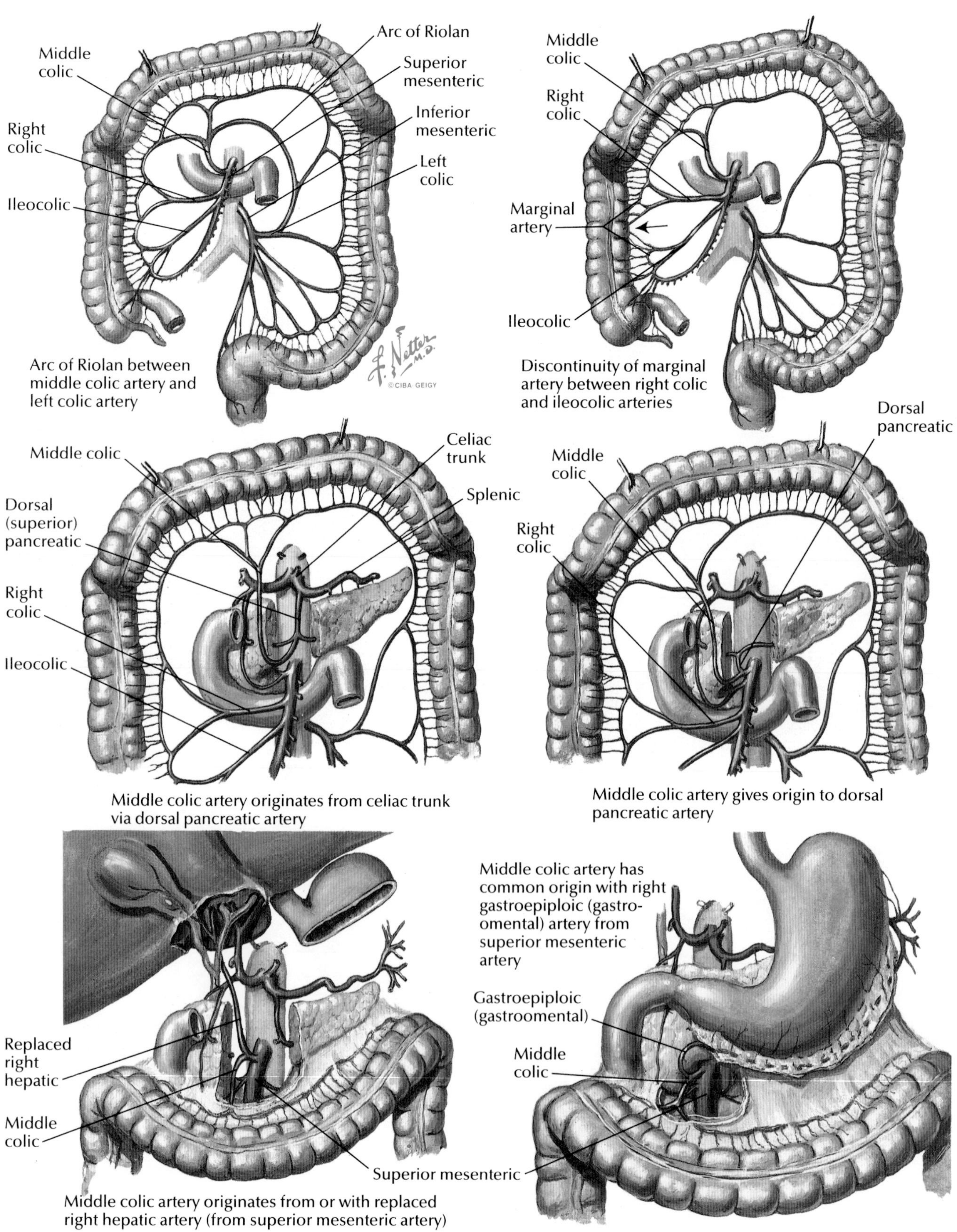

Arc of Riolan

Middle colic

Superior mesenteric

Inferior mesenteric

Right colic

Left colic

Ileocolic

Arc of Riolan between middle colic artery and left colic artery

Middle colic

Right colic

Marginal artery

Ileocolic

Discontinuity of marginal artery between right colic and ileocolic arteries

Middle colic

Celiac trunk

Dorsal (superior) pancreatic

Splenic

Right colic

Ileocolic

Middle colic artery originates from celiac trunk via dorsal pancreatic artery

Dorsal pancreatic

Middle colic

Right colic

Middle colic artery gives origin to dorsal pancreatic artery

Replaced right hepatic

Middle colic

Superior mesenteric

Middle colic artery originates from or with replaced right hepatic artery (from superior mesenteric artery)

Middle colic artery has common origin with right gastroepiploic (gastro-omental) artery from superior mesenteric artery

Gastroepiploic (gastroomental)

Middle colic

PLATE 292

ABDOMEN

Variations in Cecal and Appendicular Arteries

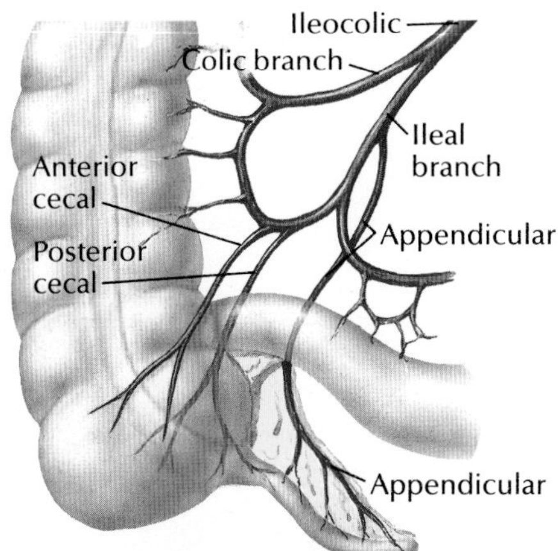

Anterior cecal and posterior cecal arteries originate from arcade between colic and ileal branches of ileocolic; appendicular artery from ileal branch

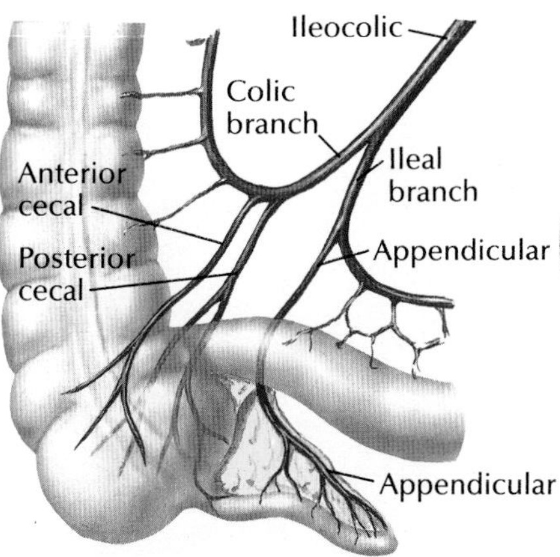

Anterior cecal and posterior cecal arteries originate from colic branch; appendicular artery from ileal branch of ileocolic artery

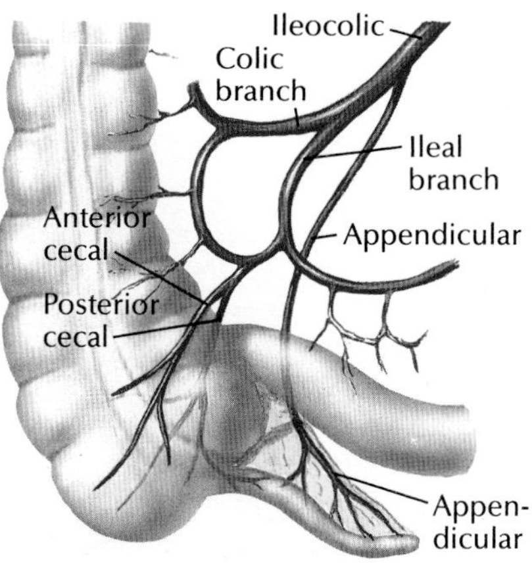

Anterior cecal and posterior cecal arteries have common origin from arcade; appendicular artery from ileocolic artery proper

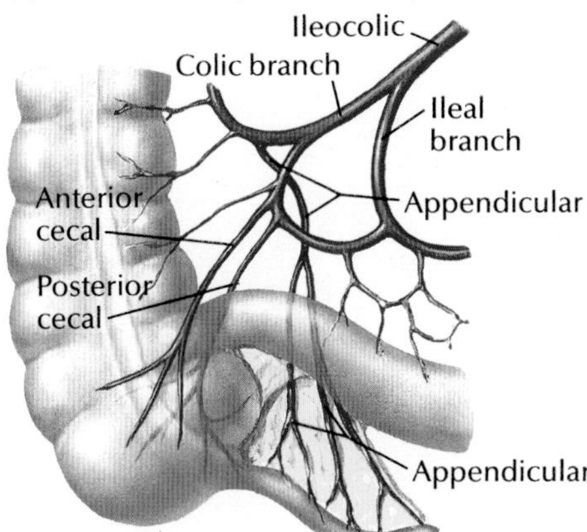

Anterior cecal and posterior cecal arteries originate from arcade between colic and ileal branches of ileocolic artery; appendicular artery from colic branch bifurcates high

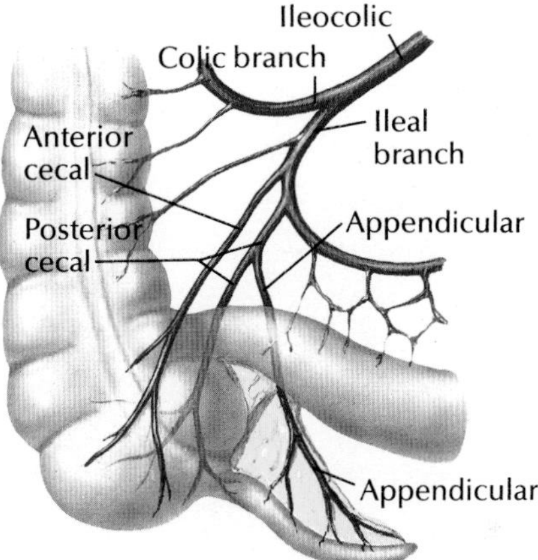

Anterior cecal and posterior cecal arteries originate from ileal branch of ileocolic artery; appendicular artery from posterior cecal artery

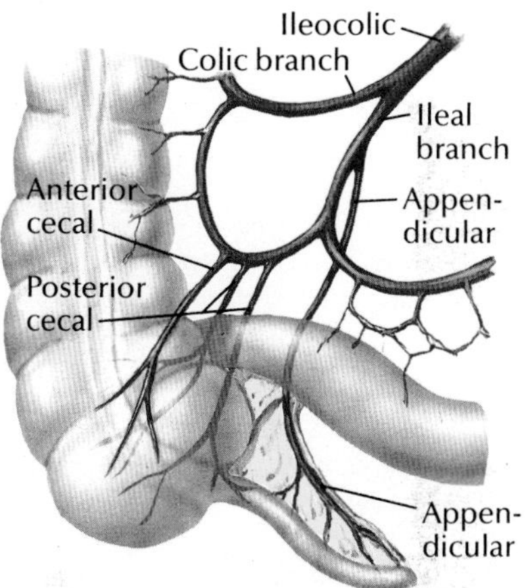

Anterior cecal and two posterior cecal arteries originate from arcade; appendicular artery from ileal branch of ileocolic artery

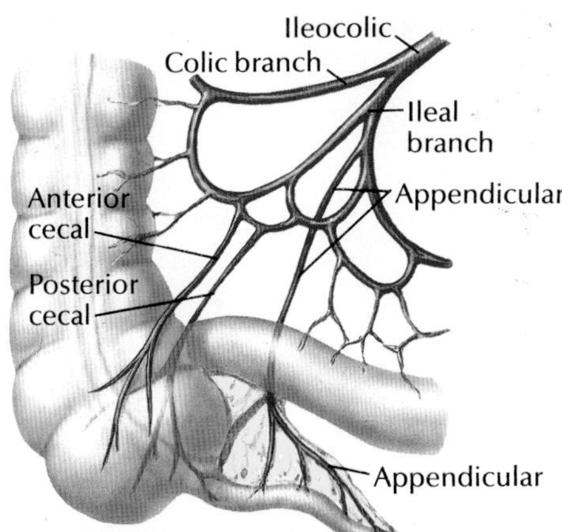

Multiple arcades between ileal branch and colic branch of ileocolic artery; anterior cecal and posterior cecal arteries originate from these arcades; appendicular artery from ileal branch of ileocolic artery

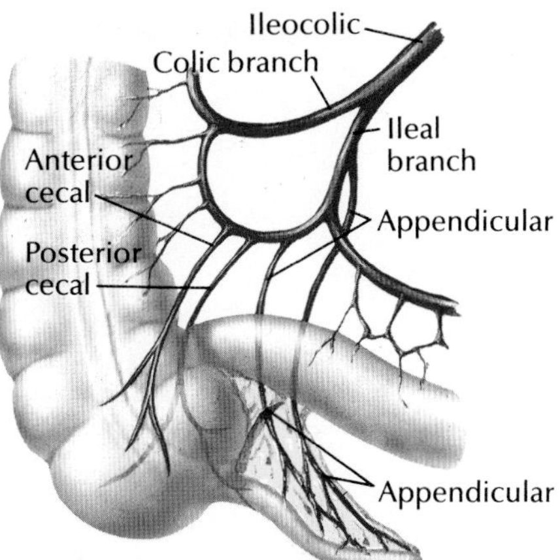

Anterior cecal and posterior cecal arteries originate from arcade between colic and ileal branches of ileocolic artery; two appendicular arteries, one from arcade, one from ileal branch of ileocolic artery

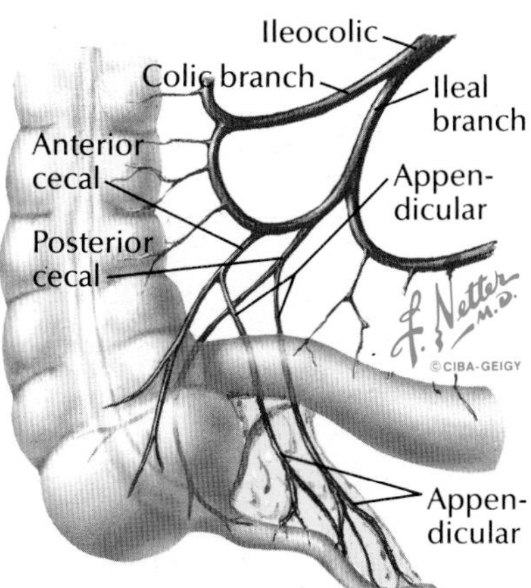

Anterior cecal and posterior cecal arteries originate from arcade; two appendicular arteries, one from anterior cecal, other from posterior cecal artery

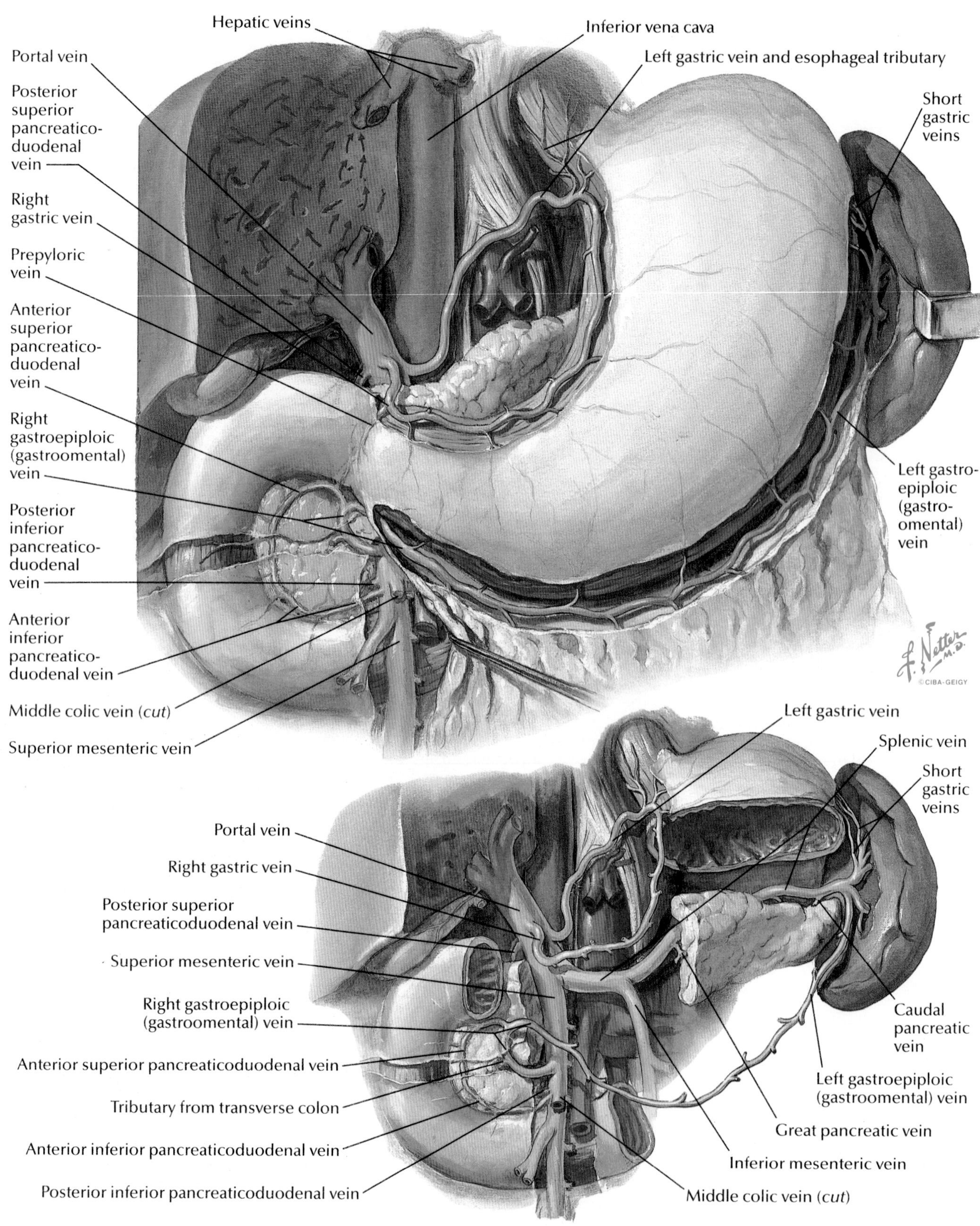

Hepatic veins

Inferior vena cava

Portal vein

Left gastric vein and esophageal tributary

Posterior superior pancreatico-duodenal vein

Short gastric veins

Right gastric vein

Prepyloric vein

Anterior superior pancreatico-duodenal vein

Right gastroepiploic (gastroomental) vein

Posterior inferior pancreatico-duodenal vein

Anterior inferior pancreatico-duodenal vein

Left gastro-epiploic (gastro-omental) vein

Middle colic vein (cut)

Superior mesenteric vein

Left gastric vein

Splenic vein

Short gastric veins

Portal vein

Right gastric vein

Posterior superior pancreaticoduodenal vein

Superior mesenteric vein

Right gastroepiploic (gastroomental) vein

Anterior superior pancreaticoduodenal vein

Tributary from transverse colon

Anterior inferior pancreaticoduodenal vein

Posterior inferior pancreaticoduodenal vein

Caudal pancreatic vein

Left gastroepiploic (gastroomental) vein

Great pancreatic vein

Inferior mesenteric vein

Middle colic vein (cut)

PLATE 294

ABDOMEN

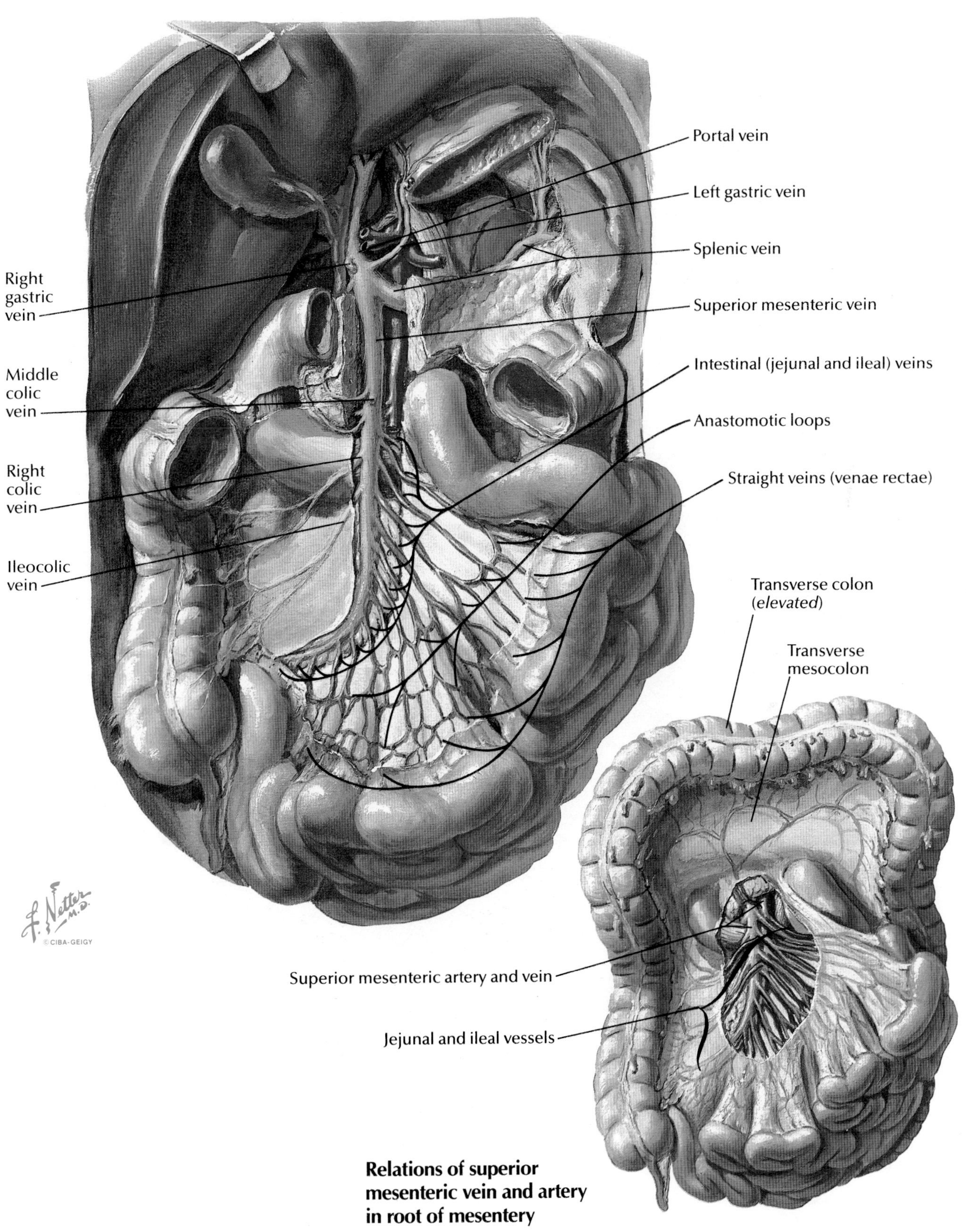

Portal vein

Left gastric vein

Splenic vein

Superior mesenteric vein

Intestinal (jejunal and ileal) veins

Anastomotic loops

Straight veins (venae rectae)

Right gastric vein

Middle colic vein

Right colic vein

Ileocolic vein

Transverse colon (*elevated*)

Transverse mesocolon

Superior mesenteric artery and vein

Jejunal and ileal vessels

Relations of superior mesenteric vein and artery in root of mesentery

Veins of Small and Large Intestines

FOR VEINS OF RECTUM SEE ALSO PLATE 374

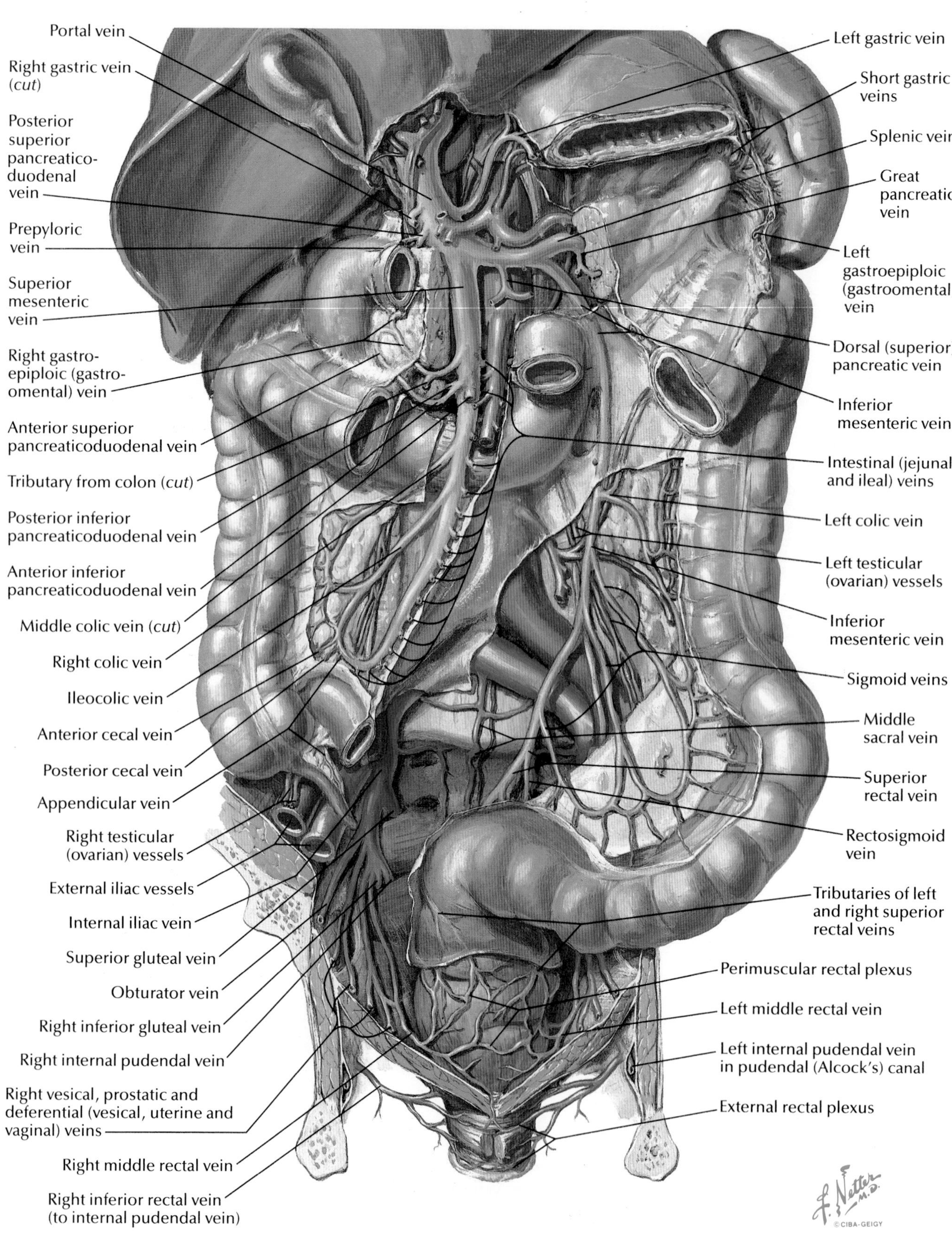

Portal vein

Right gastric vein (*cut*)

Posterior superior pancreatico-duodenal vein

Prepyloric vein

Superior mesenteric vein

Right gastro-epiploic (gastro-omental) vein

Anterior superior pancreaticoduodenal vein

Tributary from colon (*cut*)

Posterior inferior pancreaticoduodenal vein

Anterior inferior pancreaticoduodenal vein

Middle colic vein (*cut*)

Right colic vein

Ileocolic vein

Anterior cecal vein

Posterior cecal vein

Appendicular vein

Right testicular (ovarian) vessels

External iliac vessels

Internal iliac vein

Superior gluteal vein

Obturator vein

Right inferior gluteal vein

Right internal pudendal vein

Right vesical, prostatic and deferential (vesical, uterine and vaginal) veins

Right middle rectal vein

Right inferior rectal vein (to internal pudendal vein)

Left gastric vein

Short gastric veins

Splenic vein

Great pancreatic vein

Left gastroepiploic (gastroomental) vein

Dorsal (superior) pancreatic vein

Inferior mesenteric vein

Intestinal (jejunal and ileal) veins

Left colic vein

Left testicular (ovarian) vessels

Inferior mesenteric vein

Sigmoid veins

Middle sacral vein

Superior rectal vein

Rectosigmoid vein

Tributaries of left and right superior rectal veins

Perimuscular rectal plexus

Left middle rectal vein

Left internal pudendal vein in pudendal (Alcock's) canal

External rectal plexus

PLATE 296

ABDOMEN

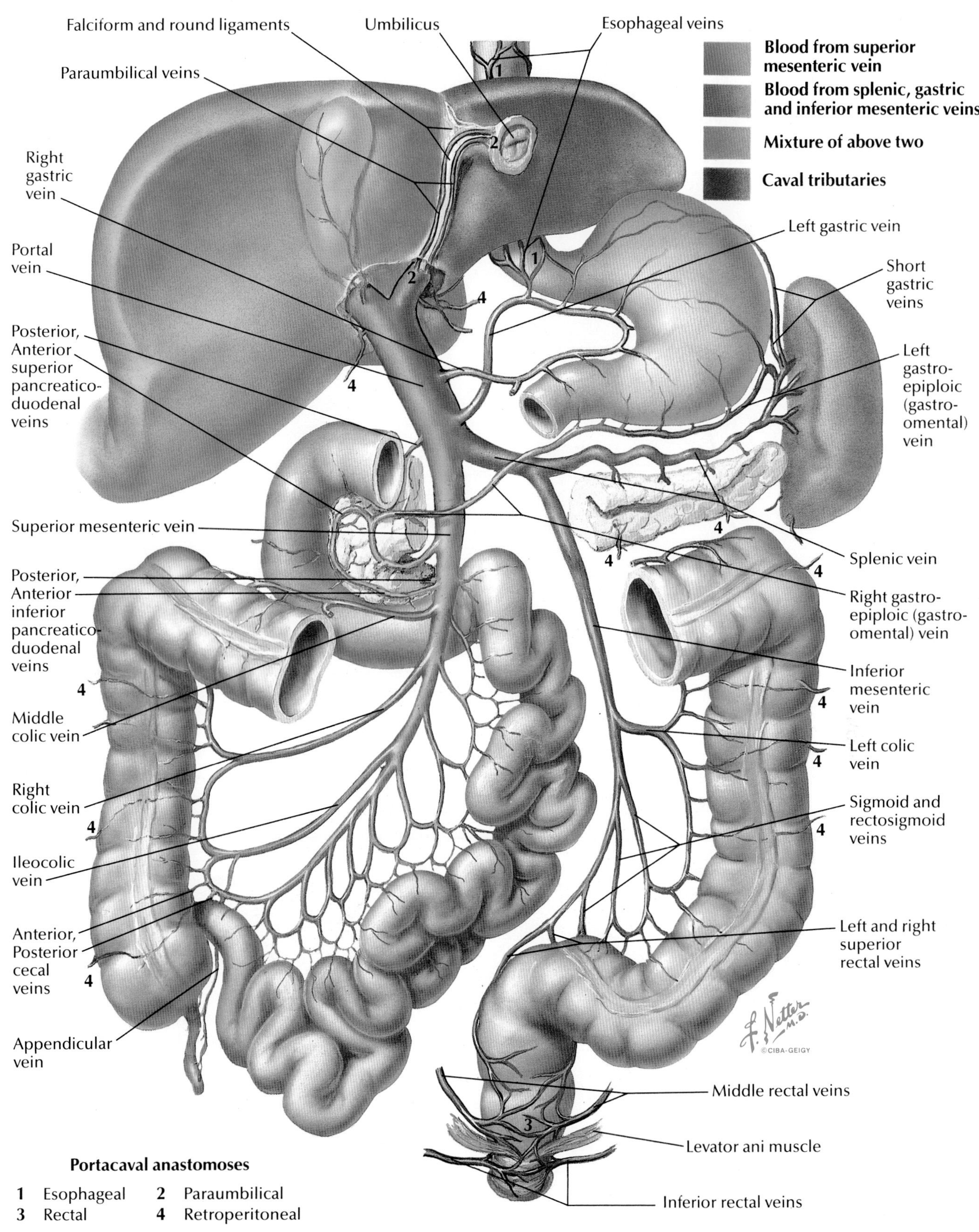

Falciform and round ligaments

Umbilicus

Esophageal veins

Blood from superior mesenteric vein

Blood from splenic, gastric and inferior mesenteric veins

Mixture of above two

Caval tributaries

Paraumbilical veins

Right gastric vein

Portal vein

Posterior, Anterior superior pancreatico-duodenal veins

Superior mesenteric vein

Posterior, Anterior inferior pancreatico-duodenal veins

Middle colic vein

Right colic vein

Ileocolic vein

Anterior, Posterior cecal veins

Appendicular vein

Left gastric vein

Short gastric veins

Left gastro-epiploic (gastro-omental) vein

Splenic vein

Right gastro-epiploic (gastro-omental) vein

Inferior mesenteric vein

Left colic vein

Sigmoid and rectosigmoid veins

Left and right superior rectal veins

Middle rectal veins

Levator ani muscle

Inferior rectal veins

Portacaval anastomoses

| 1 | Esophageal | 2 | Paraumbilical |
| 3 | Rectal | 4 | Retroperitoneal |

Variations and Anomalies of Portal Vein

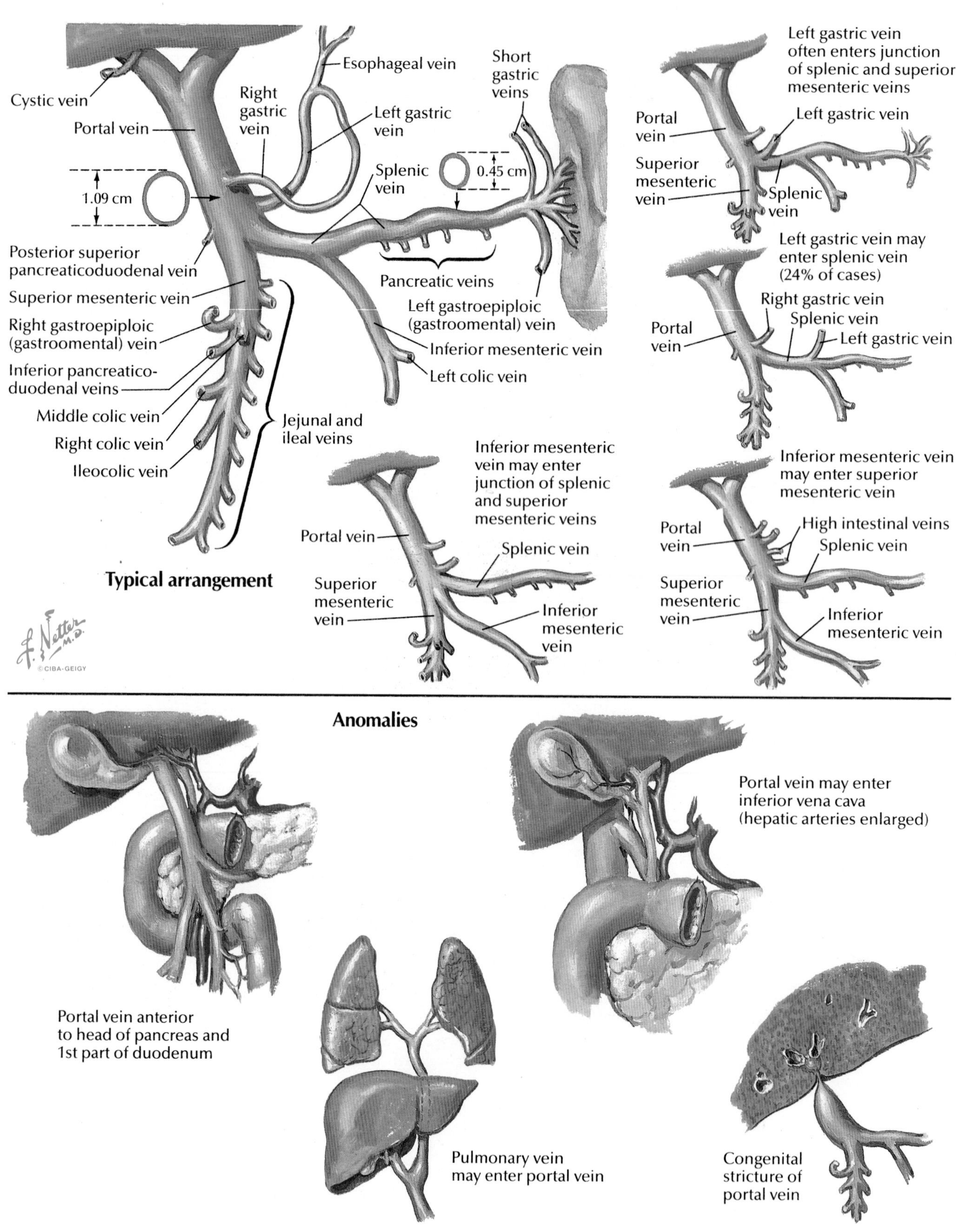

Cystic vein

Portal vein

Right gastric vein

Esophageal vein

Short gastric veins

Left gastric vein

1.09 cm

Splenic vein

0.45 cm

Posterior superior pancreaticoduodenal vein

Superior mesenteric vein

Right gastroepiploic (gastroomental) vein

Inferior pancreatico-duodenal veins

Middle colic vein

Right colic vein

Ileocolic vein

Pancreatic veins

Left gastroepiploic (gastroomental) vein

Inferior mesenteric vein

Left colic vein

Jejunal and ileal veins

Typical arrangement

Left gastric vein often enters junction of splenic and superior mesenteric veins

Portal vein

Superior mesenteric vein

Left gastric vein

Splenic vein

Left gastric vein may enter splenic vein (24% of cases)

Portal vein

Right gastric vein

Splenic vein

Left gastric vein

Inferior mesenteric vein may enter junction of splenic and superior mesenteric veins

Portal vein

Splenic vein

Superior mesenteric vein

Inferior mesenteric vein

Inferior mesenteric vein may enter superior mesenteric vein

Portal vein

High intestinal veins

Splenic vein

Superior mesenteric vein

Inferior mesenteric vein

Anomalies

Portal vein anterior to head of pancreas and 1st part of duodenum

Portal vein may enter inferior vena cava (hepatic arteries enlarged)

Pulmonary vein may enter portal vein

Congenital stricture of portal vein

PLATE 298

ABDOMEN

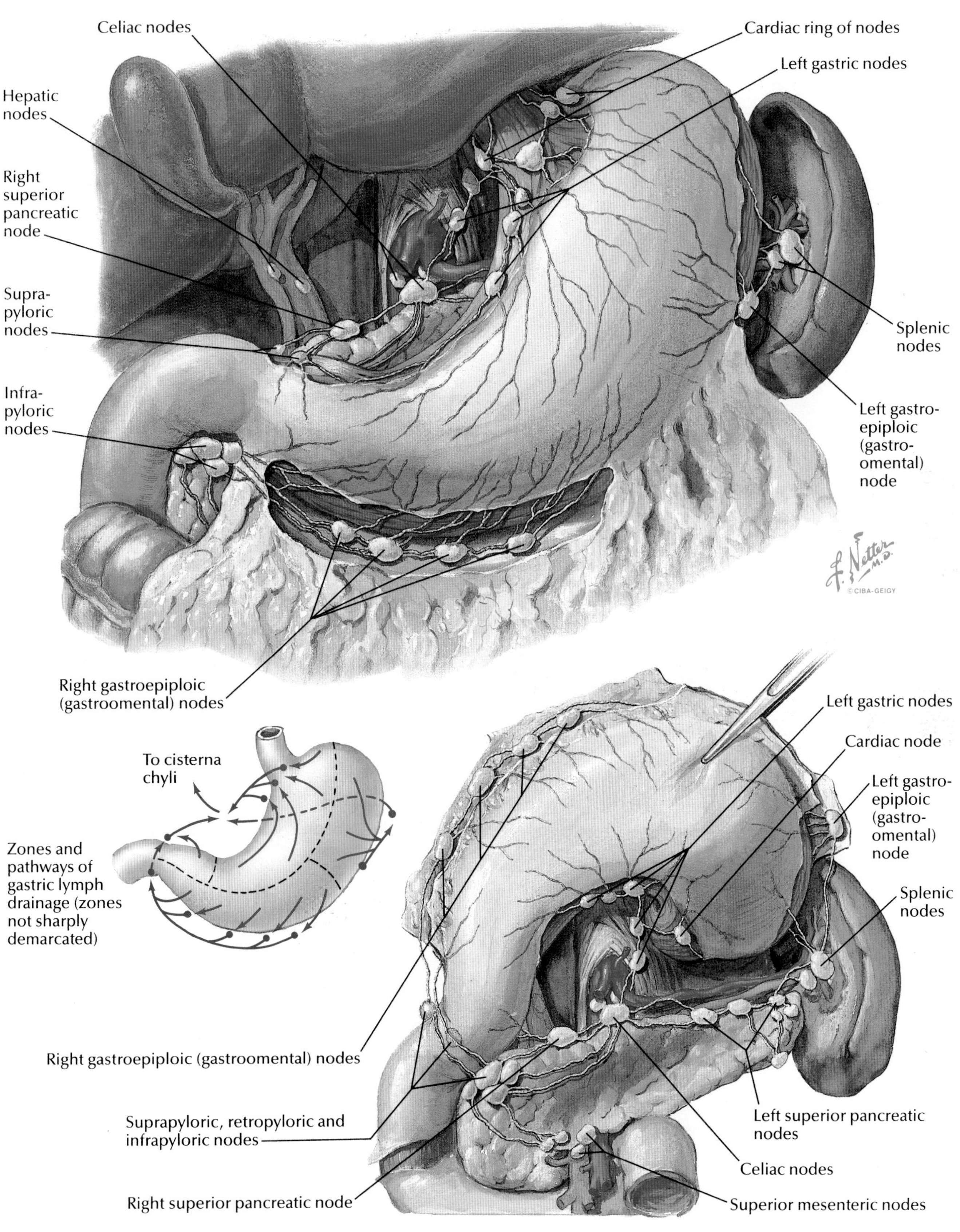

Celiac nodes

Cardiac ring of nodes

Left gastric nodes

Hepatic nodes

Right superior pancreatic node

Supra-pyloric nodes

Infra-pyloric nodes

Splenic nodes

Left gastro-epiploic (gastro-omental) node

Right gastroepiploic (gastroomental) nodes

To cisterna chyli

Zones and pathways of gastric lymph drainage (zones not sharply demarcated)

Left gastric nodes

Cardiac node

Left gastro-epiploic (gastro-omental) node

Splenic nodes

Right gastroepiploic (gastroomental) nodes

Suprapyloric, retropyloric and infrapyloric nodes

Left superior pancreatic nodes

Celiac nodes

Right superior pancreatic node

Superior mesenteric nodes

Lymph Vessels and Nodes of Small Intestine

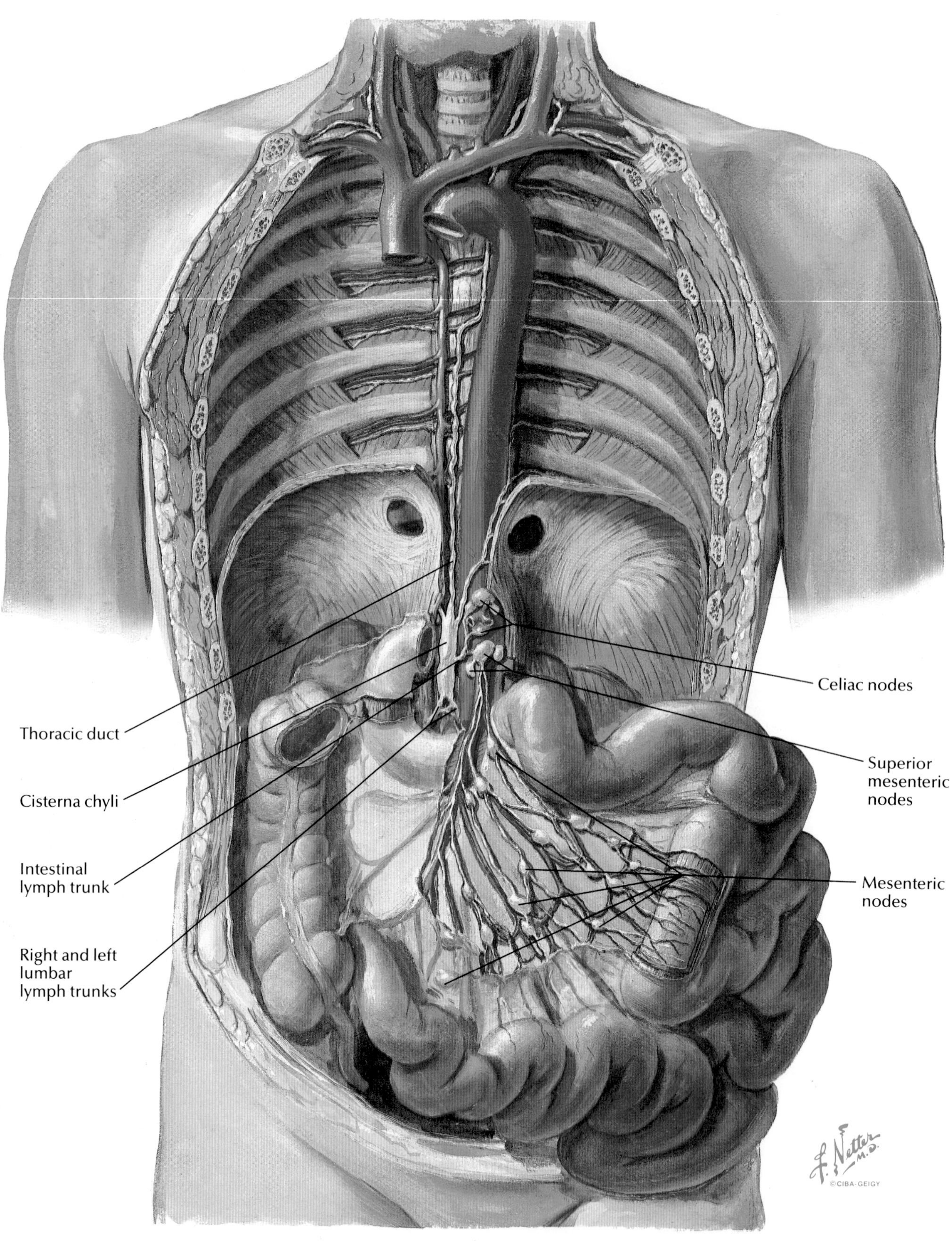

Celiac nodes

Superior mesenteric nodes

Mesenteric nodes

Thoracic duct

Cisterna chyli

Intestinal lymph trunk

Right and left lumbar lymph trunks

PLATE 300

ABDOMEN

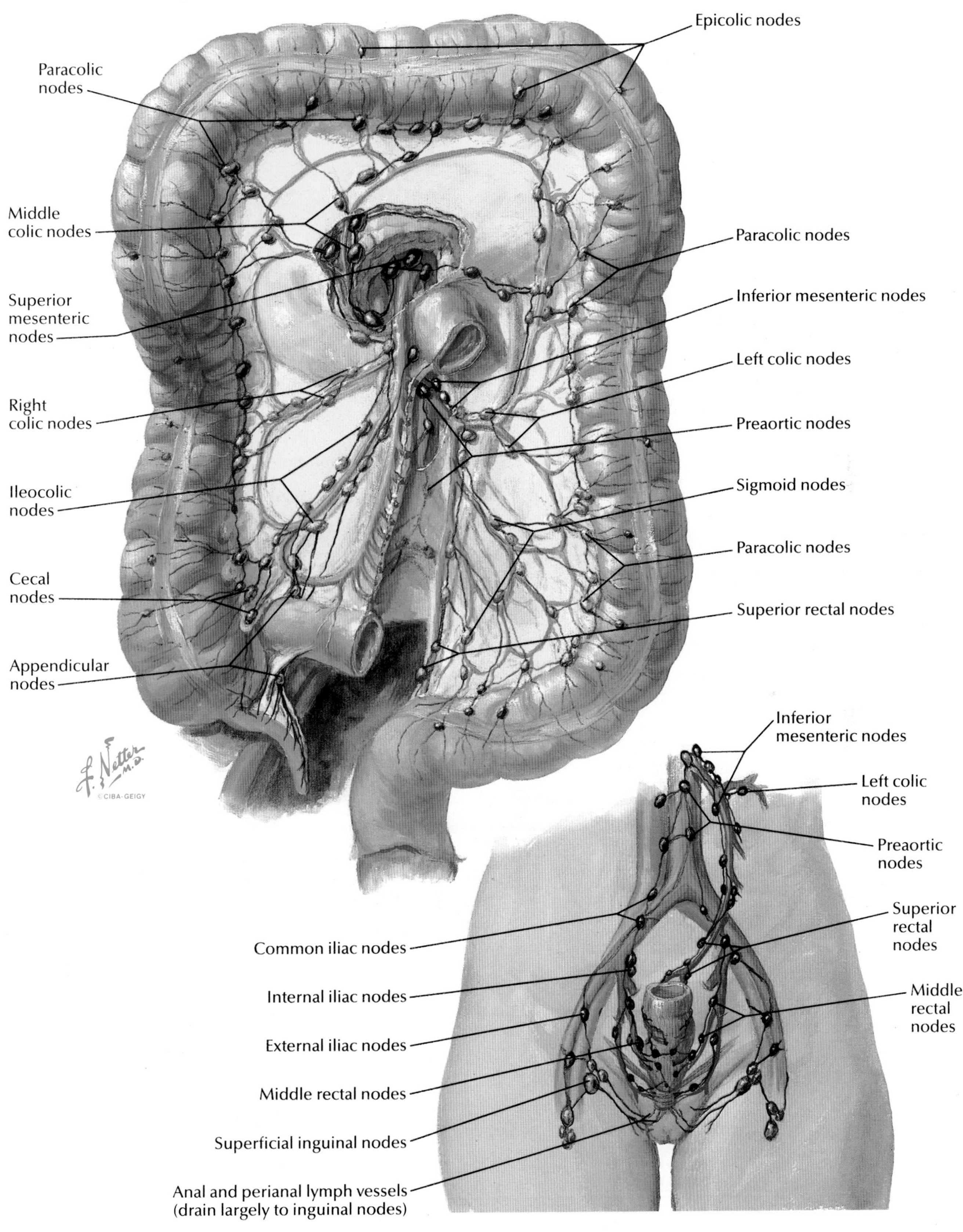

Epicolic nodes

Paracolic nodes

Middle colic nodes

Superior mesenteric nodes

Right colic nodes

Ileocolic nodes

Cecal nodes

Appendicular nodes

Paracolic nodes

Inferior mesenteric nodes

Left colic nodes

Preaortic nodes

Sigmoid nodes

Paracolic nodes

Superior rectal nodes

Inferior mesenteric nodes

Left colic nodes

Preaortic nodes

Superior rectal nodes

Middle rectal nodes

Common iliac nodes

Internal iliac nodes

External iliac nodes

Middle rectal nodes

Superficial inguinal nodes

Anal and perianal lymph vessels
(drain largely to inguinal nodes)

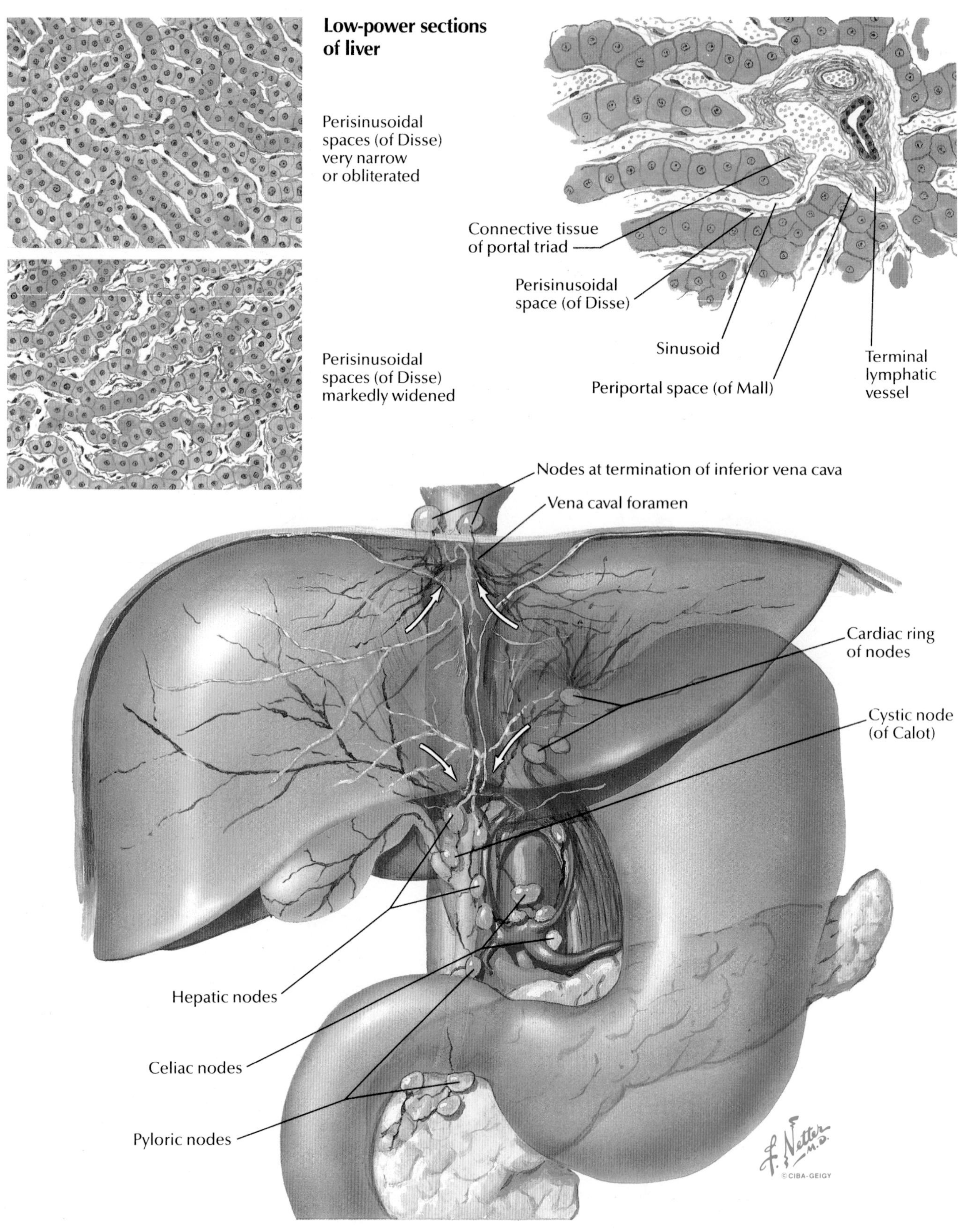

Low-power sections of liver

Perisinusoidal spaces (of Disse) very narrow or obliterated

Perisinusoidal spaces (of Disse) markedly widened

Connective tissue of portal triad

Perisinusoidal space (of Disse)

Sinusoid

Periportal space (of Mall)

Terminal lymphatic vessel

Nodes at termination of inferior vena cava

Vena caval foramen

Cardiac ring of nodes

Cystic node (of Calot)

Hepatic nodes

Celiac nodes

Pyloric nodes

PLATE 302

ABDOMEN

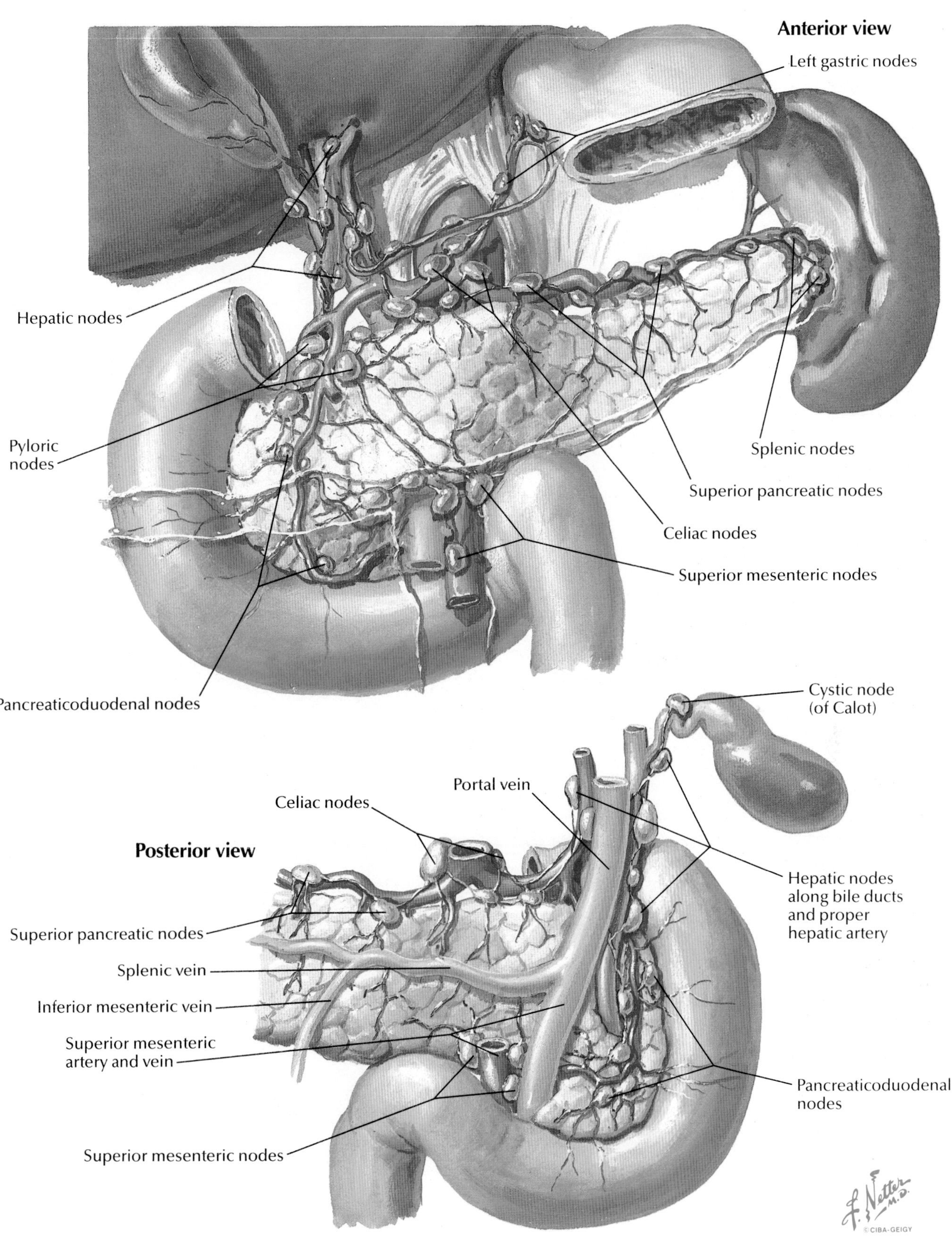

Anterior view

Left gastric nodes

Hepatic nodes

Pyloric nodes

Pancreaticoduodenal nodes

Splenic nodes

Superior pancreatic nodes

Celiac nodes

Superior mesenteric nodes

Cystic node (of Calot)

Celiac nodes

Portal vein

Posterior view

Superior pancreatic nodes

Splenic vein

Inferior mesenteric vein

Superior mesenteric artery and vein

Superior mesenteric nodes

Hepatic nodes along bile ducts and proper hepatic artery

Pancreaticoduodenal nodes

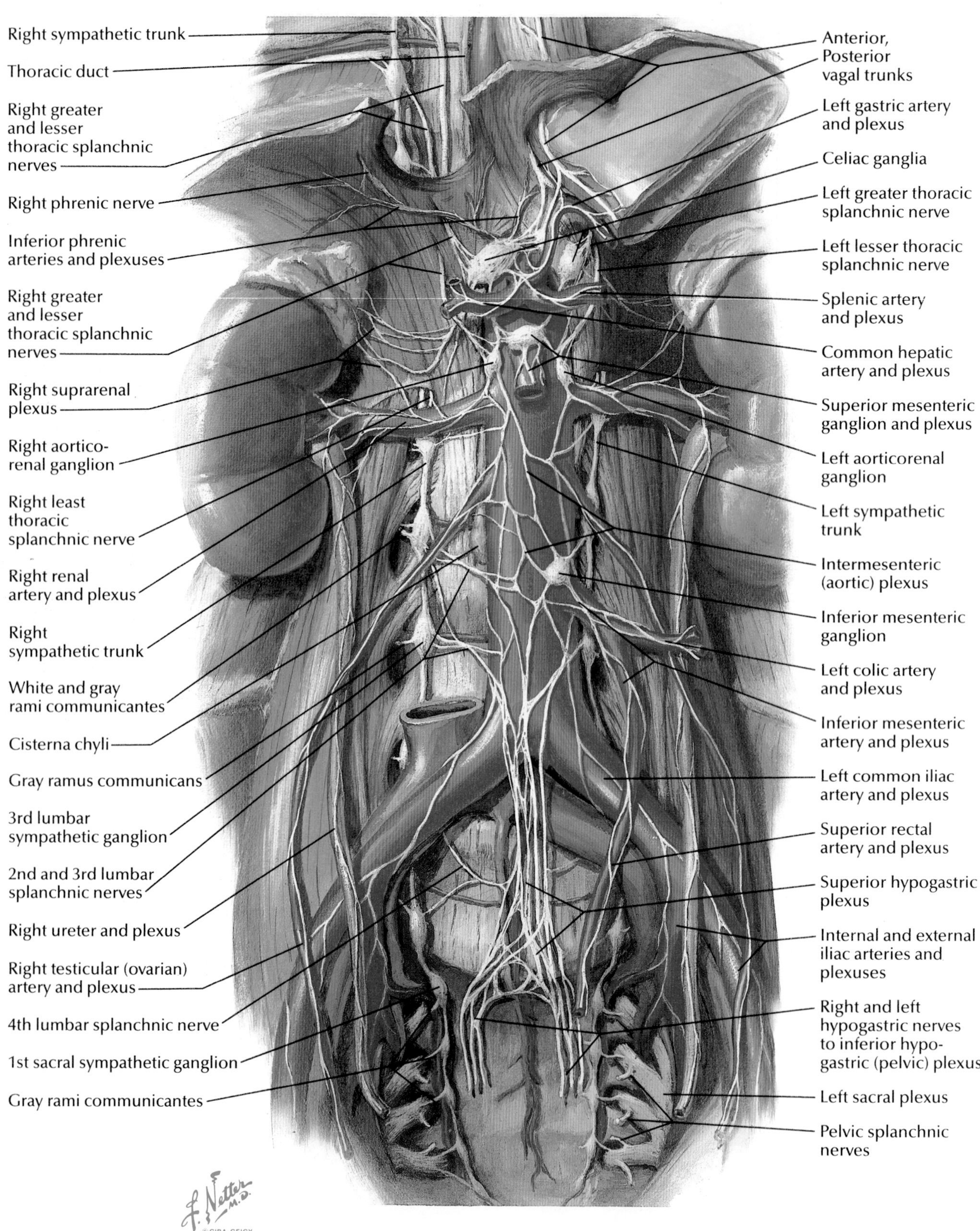

Right sympathetic trunk

Thoracic duct

Right greater and lesser thoracic splanchnic nerves

Right phrenic nerve

Inferior phrenic arteries and plexuses

Right greater and lesser thoracic splanchnic nerves

Right suprarenal plexus

Right aortico-renal ganglion

Right least thoracic splanchnic nerve

Right renal artery and plexus

Right sympathetic trunk

White and gray rami communicantes

Cisterna chyli

Gray ramus communicans

3rd lumbar sympathetic ganglion

2nd and 3rd lumbar splanchnic nerves

Right ureter and plexus

Right testicular (ovarian) artery and plexus

4th lumbar splanchnic nerve

1st sacral sympathetic ganglion

Gray rami communicantes

Anterior, Posterior vagal trunks

Left gastric artery and plexus

Celiac ganglia

Left greater thoracic splanchnic nerve

Left lesser thoracic splanchnic nerve

Splenic artery and plexus

Common hepatic artery and plexus

Superior mesenteric ganglion and plexus

Left aorticorenal ganglion

Left sympathetic trunk

Intermesenteric (aortic) plexus

Inferior mesenteric ganglion

Left colic artery and plexus

Inferior mesenteric artery and plexus

Left common iliac artery and plexus

Superior rectal artery and plexus

Superior hypogastric plexus

Internal and external iliac arteries and plexuses

Right and left hypogastric nerves to inferior hypo-gastric (pelvic) plexus

Left sacral plexus

Pelvic splanchnic nerves

PLATE 304

ABDOMEN

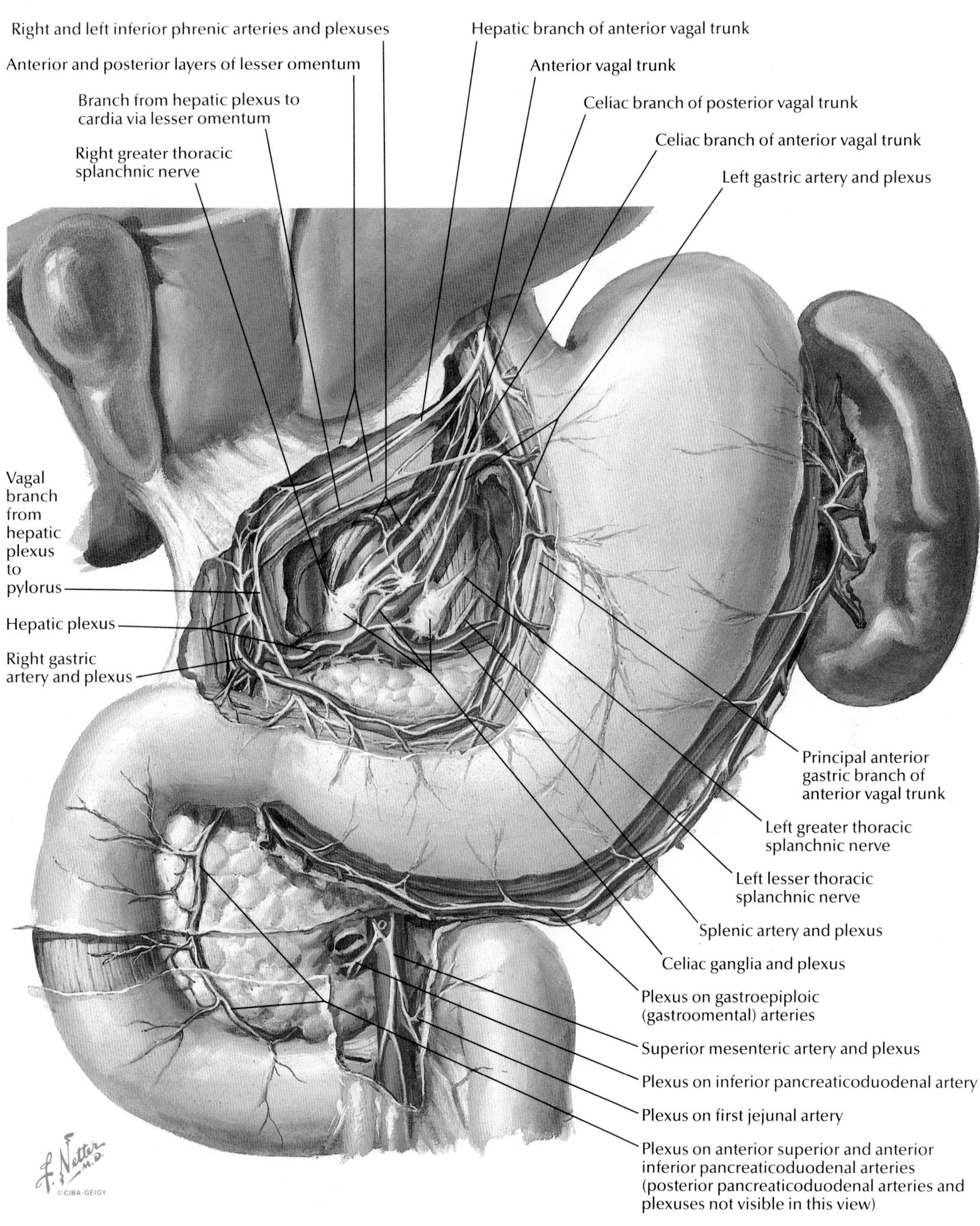

Right and left inferior phrenic arteries and plexuses

Anterior and posterior layers of lesser omentum

Branch from hepatic plexus to cardia via lesser omentum

Right greater thoracic splanchnic nerve

Vagal branch from hepatic plexus to pylorus

Hepatic plexus

Right gastric artery and plexus

Hepatic branch of anterior vagal trunk

Anterior vagal trunk

Celiac branch of posterior vagal trunk

Celiac branch of anterior vagal trunk

Left gastric artery and plexus

Principal anterior gastric branch of anterior vagal trunk

Left greater thoracic splanchnic nerve

Left lesser thoracic splanchnic nerve

Splenic artery and plexus

Celiac ganglia and plexus

Plexus on gastroepiploic (gastroomental) arteries

Superior mesenteric artery and plexus

Plexus on inferior pancreaticoduodenal artery

Plexus on first jejunal artery

Plexus on anterior superior and anterior inferior pancreaticoduodenal arteries (posterior pancreaticoduodenal arteries and plexuses not visible in this view)

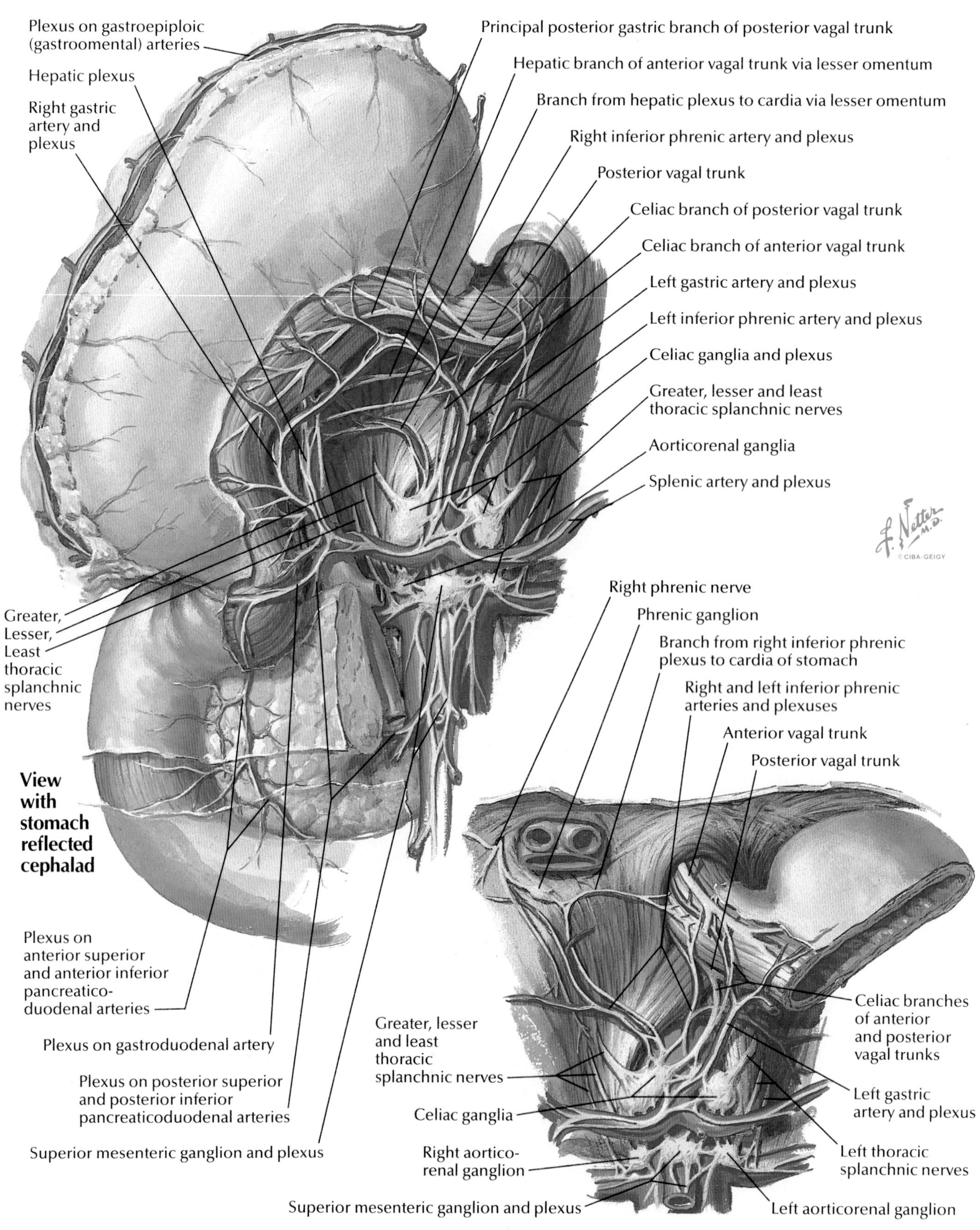

Plexus on gastroepiploic (gastroomental) arteries

Hepatic plexus

Right gastric artery and plexus

Principal posterior gastric branch of posterior vagal trunk

Hepatic branch of anterior vagal trunk via lesser omentum

Branch from hepatic plexus to cardia via lesser omentum

Right inferior phrenic artery and plexus

Posterior vagal trunk

Celiac branch of posterior vagal trunk

Celiac branch of anterior vagal trunk

Left gastric artery and plexus

Left inferior phrenic artery and plexus

Celiac ganglia and plexus

Greater, lesser and least thoracic splanchnic nerves

Aorticorenal ganglia

Splenic artery and plexus

Greater, Lesser, Least thoracic splanchnic nerves

View with stomach reflected cephalad

Plexus on anterior superior and anterior inferior pancreaticoduodenal arteries

Plexus on gastroduodenal artery

Plexus on posterior superior and posterior inferior pancreaticoduodenal arteries

Superior mesenteric ganglion and plexus

Greater, lesser and least thoracic splanchnic nerves

Celiac ganglia

Right aortico-renal ganglion

Superior mesenteric ganglion and plexus

Right phrenic nerve

Phrenic ganglion

Branch from right inferior phrenic plexus to cardia of stomach

Right and left inferior phrenic arteries and plexuses

Anterior vagal trunk

Posterior vagal trunk

Celiac branches of anterior and posterior vagal trunks

Left gastric artery and plexus

Left thoracic splanchnic nerves

Left aorticorenal ganglion

PLATE 306

ABDOMEN

Innervation of Stomach and Duodenum: Schema

SEE ALSO PLATE 153

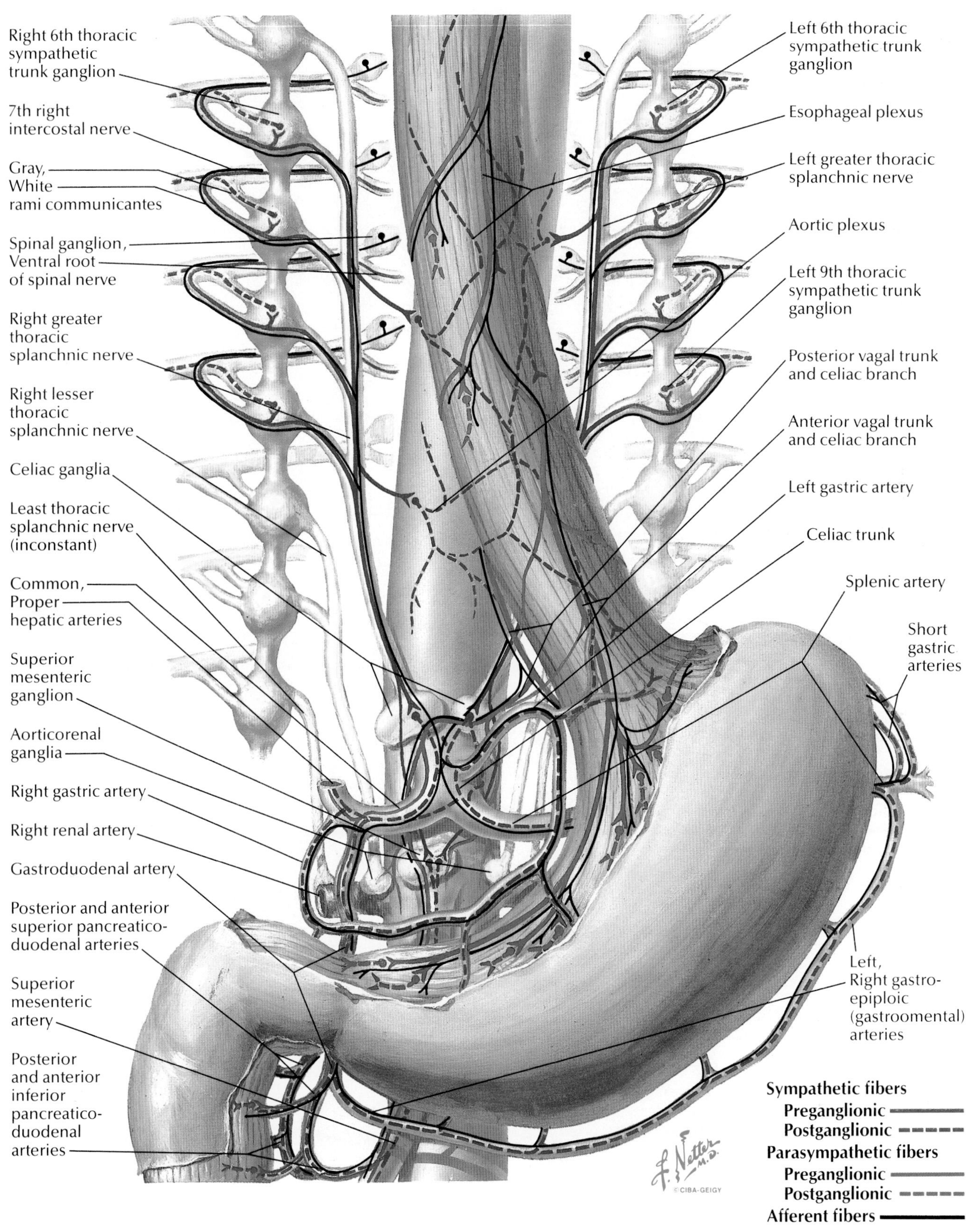

Right 6th thoracic sympathetic trunk ganglion

7th right intercostal nerve

Gray, White rami communicantes

Spinal ganglion, Ventral root of spinal nerve

Right greater thoracic splanchnic nerve

Right lesser thoracic splanchnic nerve

Celiac ganglia

Least thoracic splanchnic nerve (inconstant)

Common, Proper hepatic arteries

Superior mesenteric ganglion

Aorticorenal ganglia

Right gastric artery

Right renal artery

Gastroduodenal artery

Posterior and anterior superior pancreatico-duodenal arteries

Superior mesenteric artery

Posterior and anterior inferior pancreatico-duodenal arteries

Left 6th thoracic sympathetic trunk ganglion

Esophageal plexus

Left greater thoracic splanchnic nerve

Aortic plexus

Left 9th thoracic sympathetic trunk ganglion

Posterior vagal trunk and celiac branch

Anterior vagal trunk and celiac branch

Left gastric artery

Celiac trunk

Splenic artery

Short gastric arteries

Left, Right gastro-epiploic (gastroomental) arteries

Sympathetic fibers
Preganglionic ———
Postganglionic – – –
Parasympathetic fibers
Preganglionic ———
Postganglionic – – –
Afferent fibers ———

f. Netter
M.D.
©CIBA-GEIGY

INNERVATION

PLATE 307

Nerves of Small Intestine

SEE ALSO PLATE 152

Recurrent branch of left inferior phrenic
artery and plexus to esophagus

Anterior vagal trunk

Posterior vagal trunk

Hepatic branch of anterior
vagal trunk in lesser omentum

Celiac branches of anterior
and posterior vagal trunks

Inferior phrenic arteries and plexuses

Left gastric artery and plexus

Hepatic plexus

Greater thoracic splanchnic nerves

Right gastric artery and plexus (cut)

Celiac ganglia and plexus

Gastroduodenal artery and plexus

Lesser thoracic splanchnic nerves

Least thoracic splanchnic nerves

Aorticorenal ganglia

Superior mesenteric ganglion

Intermesenteric (aortic) plexus

Inferior pancreaticoduodenal
arteries and plexuses

Superior mesenteric artery and plexus

Middle colic artery and plexus (cut)

Right colic artery and plexus

Ileocolic artery and plexus

Superior mesenteric
artery and plexus

Peritoneum (cut edge)

Mesenteric branches

Mesoappendix contains
appendicular artery and
nerve plexus

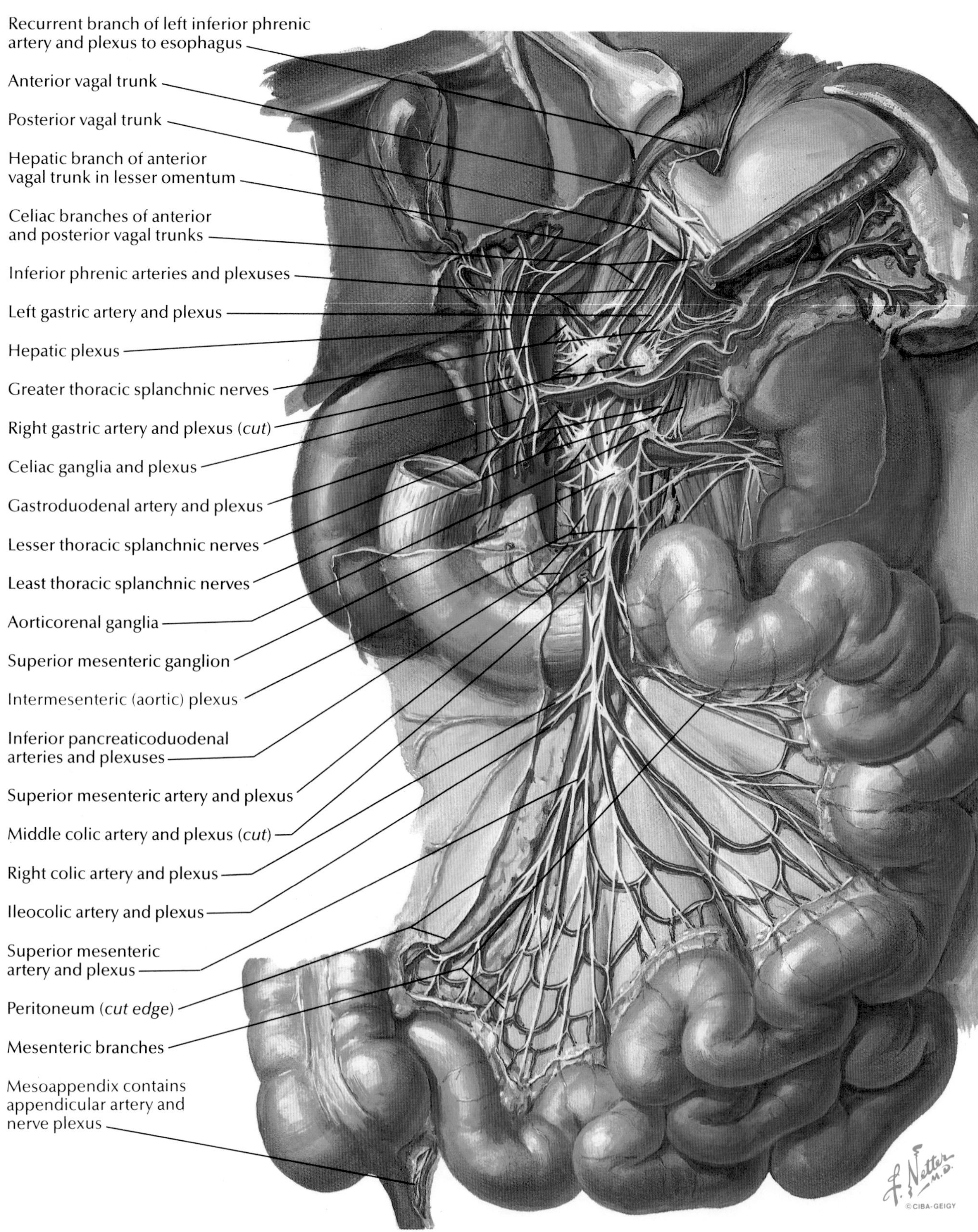

PLATE 308

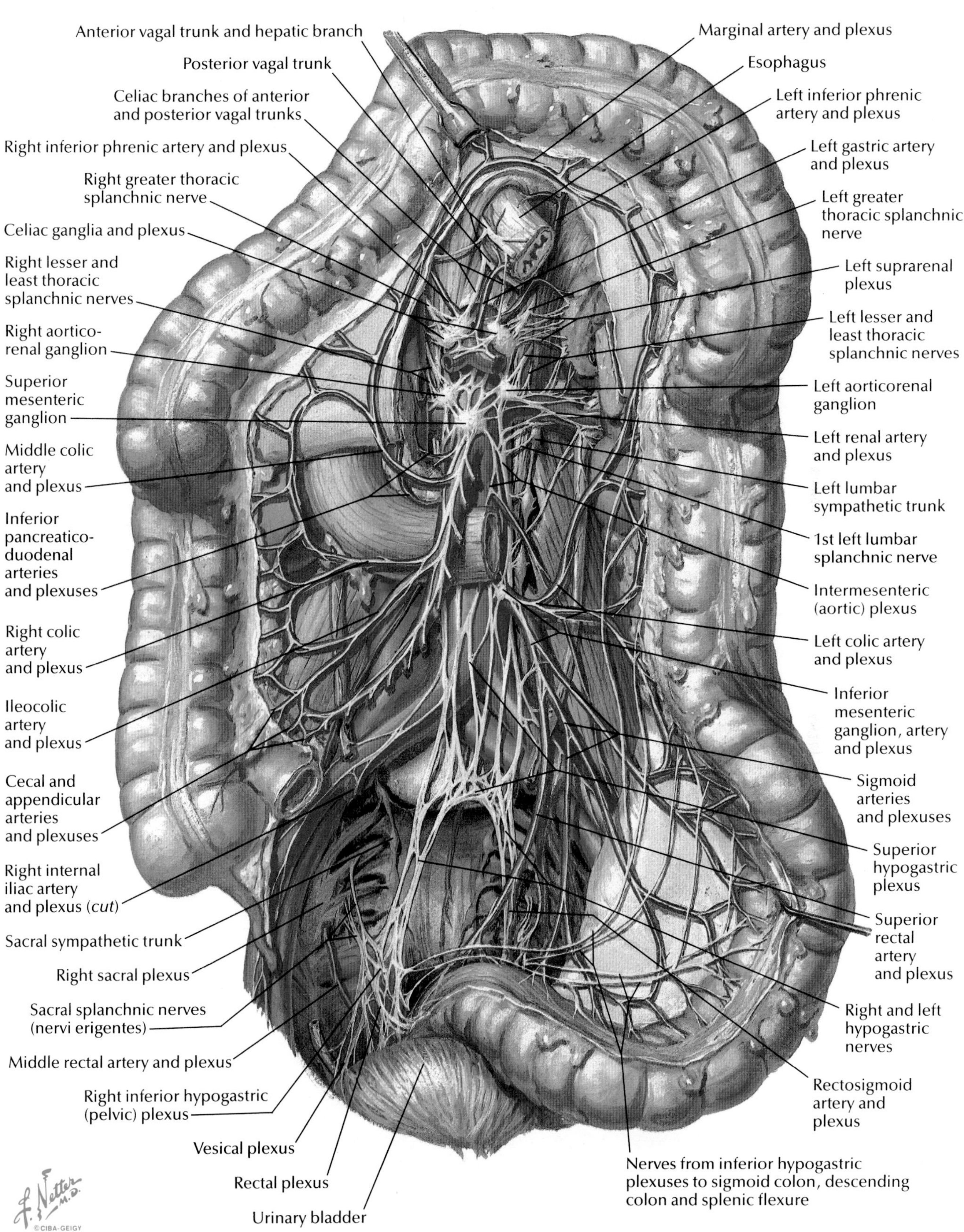

Anterior vagal trunk and hepatic branch

Posterior vagal trunk

Celiac branches of anterior and posterior vagal trunks

Right inferior phrenic artery and plexus

Right greater thoracic splanchnic nerve

Celiac ganglia and plexus

Right lesser and least thoracic splanchnic nerves

Right aortico-renal ganglion

Superior mesenteric ganglion

Middle colic artery and plexus

Inferior pancreatico-duodenal arteries and plexuses

Right colic artery and plexus

Ileocolic artery and plexus

Cecal and appendicular arteries and plexuses

Right internal iliac artery and plexus (*cut*)

Sacral sympathetic trunk

Right sacral plexus

Sacral splanchnic nerves (nervi erigentes)

Middle rectal artery and plexus

Right inferior hypogastric (pelvic) plexus

Vesical plexus

Rectal plexus

Urinary bladder

Marginal artery and plexus

Esophagus

Left inferior phrenic artery and plexus

Left gastric artery and plexus

Left greater thoracic splanchnic nerve

Left suprarenal plexus

Left lesser and least thoracic splanchnic nerves

Left aorticorenal ganglion

Left renal artery and plexus

Left lumbar sympathetic trunk

1st left lumbar splanchnic nerve

Intermesenteric (aortic) plexus

Left colic artery and plexus

Inferior mesenteric ganglion, artery and plexus

Sigmoid arteries and plexuses

Superior hypogastric plexus

Superior rectal artery and plexus

Right and left hypogastric nerves

Rectosigmoid artery and plexus

Nerves from inferior hypogastric plexuses to sigmoid colon, descending colon and splenic flexure

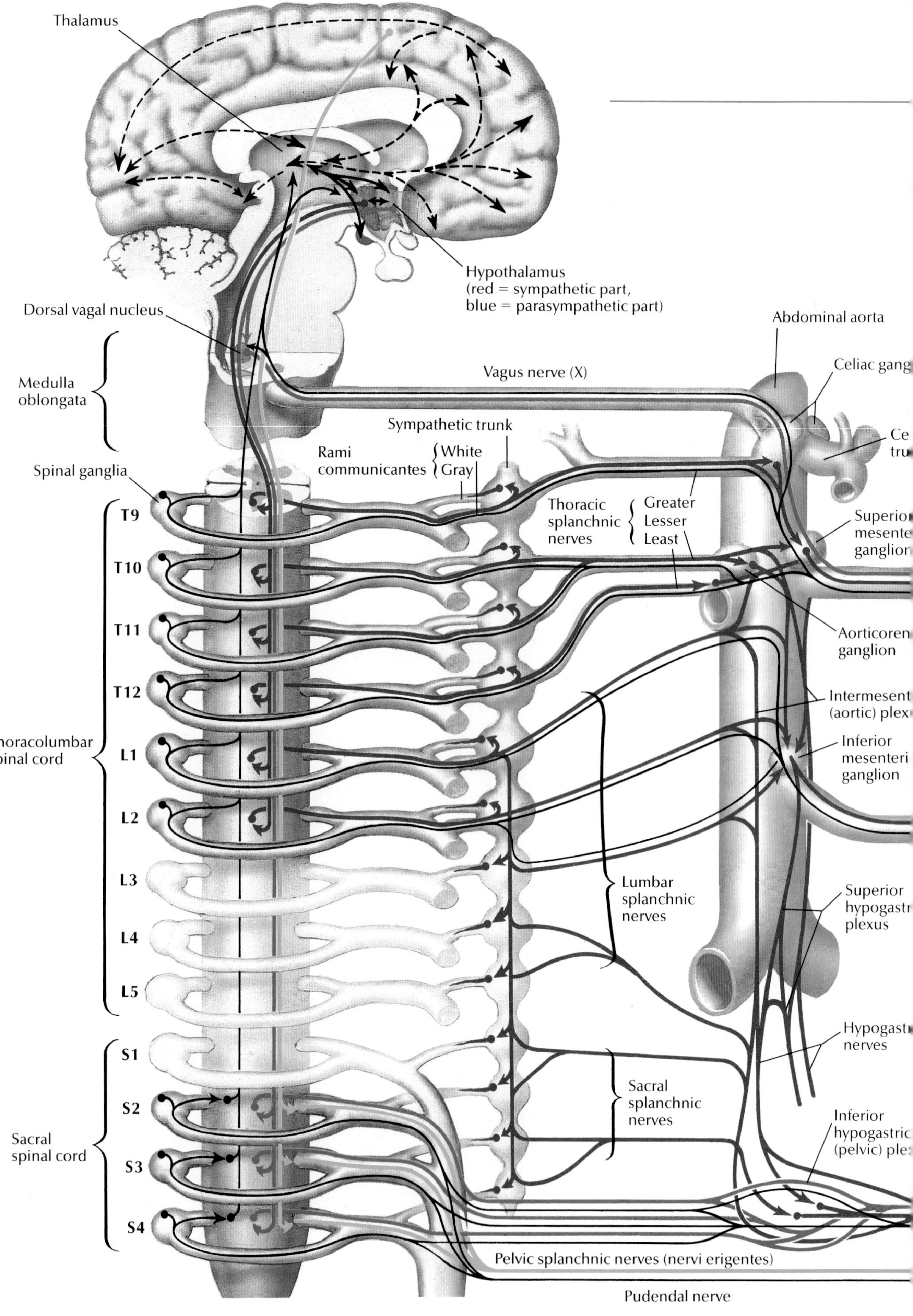

Thalamus

Hypothalamus
(red = sympathetic part,
blue = parasympathetic part)

Dorsal vagal nucleus

Abdominal aorta

Celiac gang

Medulla
oblongata

Vagus nerve (X)

Ce
tru

Sympathetic trunk

Spinal ganglia

Rami
communicantes { White
Gray

Thoracic
splanchnic
nerves { Greater
Lesser
Least

Superior
mesente
ganglior

T9

T10

T11

Aorticoren
ganglion

T12

Intermesent
(aortic) plex

L1

Thoracolumbar
spinal cord

Inferior
mesenteri
ganglion

L2

L3

Lumbar
splanchnic
nerves

Superior
hypogast
plexus

L4

L5

S1

Hypogast
nerves

S2

Sacral
splanchnic
nerves

Sacral
spinal cord

S3

Inferior
hypogastric
(pelvic) ple:

S4

Pelvic splanchnic nerves (nervi erigentes)

Pudendal nerve

PLATE 310

ABDOMEN

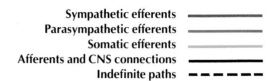

Sympathetic efferents
Parasympathetic efferents
Somatic efferents
Afferents and CNS connections
Indefinite paths

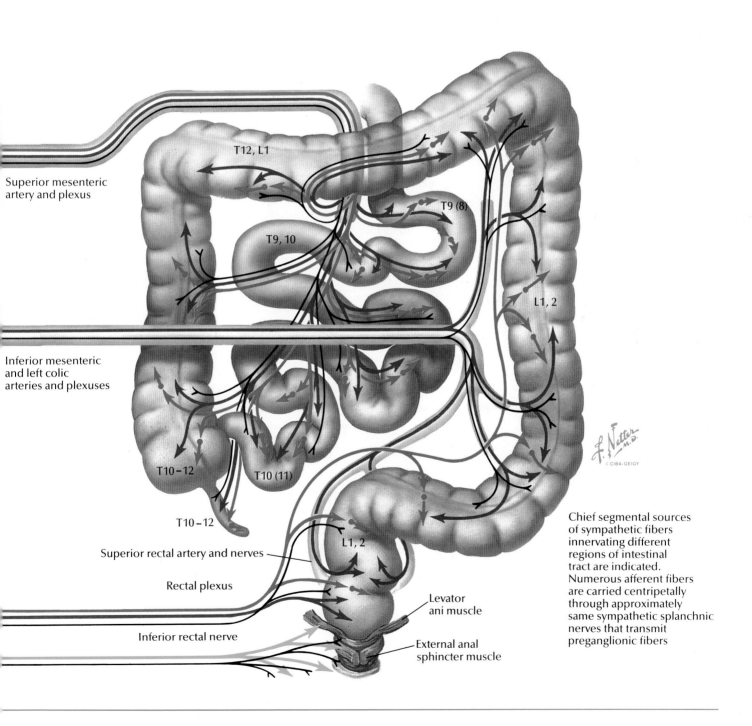

Superior mesenteric
artery and plexus

T12, L1

T9 (8)

T9, 10

L1, 2

Inferior mesenteric
and left colic
arteries and plexuses

T10–12

T10 (11)

T10–12

Superior rectal artery and nerves

L1, 2

Rectal plexus

Inferior rectal nerve

Levator
ani muscle

External anal
sphincter muscle

Chief segmental sources
of sympathetic fibers
innervating different
regions of intestinal
tract are indicated.
Numerous afferent fibers
are carried centripetally
through approximately
same sympathetic splanchnic
nerves that transmit
preganglionic fibers

Autonomic Reflex Pathways: Schema

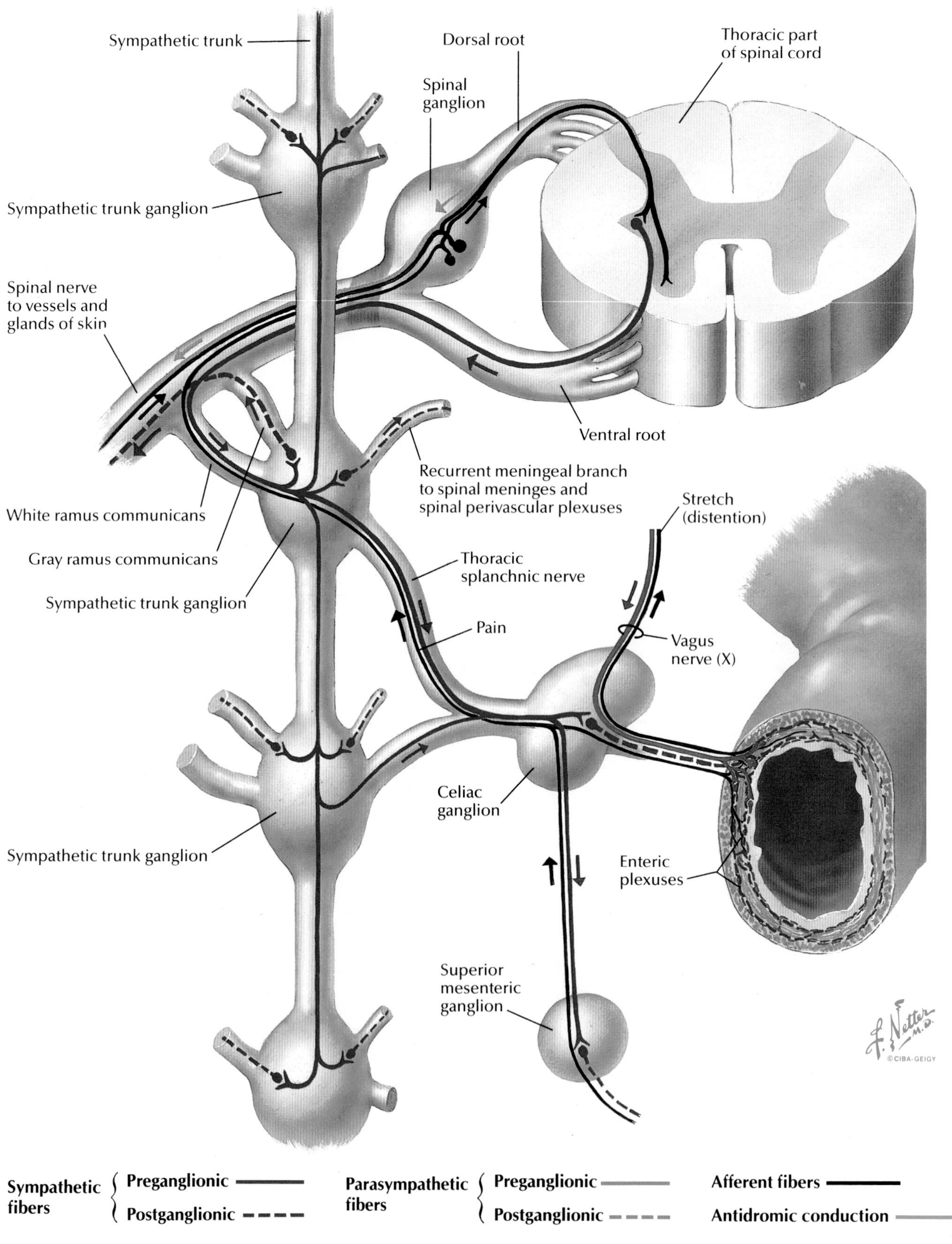

Sympathetic trunk

Dorsal root

Spinal ganglion

Thoracic part of spinal cord

Sympathetic trunk ganglion

Spinal nerve to vessels and glands of skin

Ventral root

White ramus communicans

Recurrent meningeal branch to spinal meninges and spinal perivascular plexuses

Gray ramus communicans

Stretch (distention)

Sympathetic trunk ganglion

Thoracic splanchnic nerve

Pain

Vagus nerve (X)

Celiac ganglion

Enteric plexuses

Sympathetic trunk ganglion

Superior mesenteric ganglion

Sympathetic fibers { Preganglionic ——— / Postganglionic - - - -

Parasympathetic fibers { Preganglionic ——— / Postganglionic - - - -

Afferent fibers ———

Antidromic conduction ———

PLATE 311

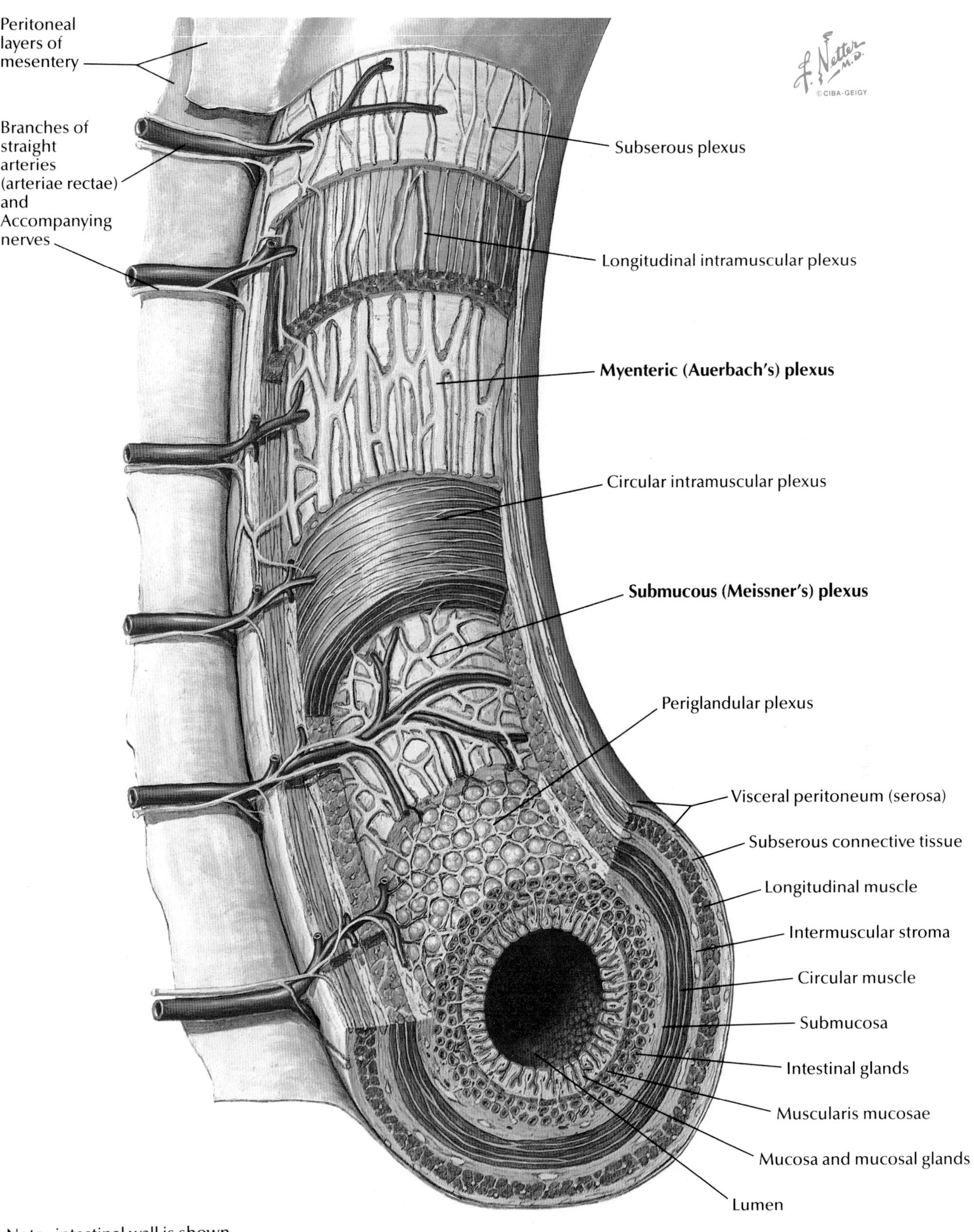

Peritoneal layers of mesentery

Branches of straight arteries (arteriae rectae) and Accompanying nerves

Subserous plexus

Longitudinal intramuscular plexus

Myenteric (Auerbach's) plexus

Circular intramuscular plexus

Submucous (Meissner's) plexus

Periglandular plexus

Visceral peritoneum (serosa)

Subserous connective tissue

Longitudinal muscle

Intermuscular stroma

Circular muscle

Submucosa

Intestinal glands

Muscularis mucosae

Mucosa and mucosal glands

Lumen

Note: intestinal wall is shown much thicker than in actuality

Innervation of Liver and Biliary Tract: Schema

SEE ALSO PLATE 153

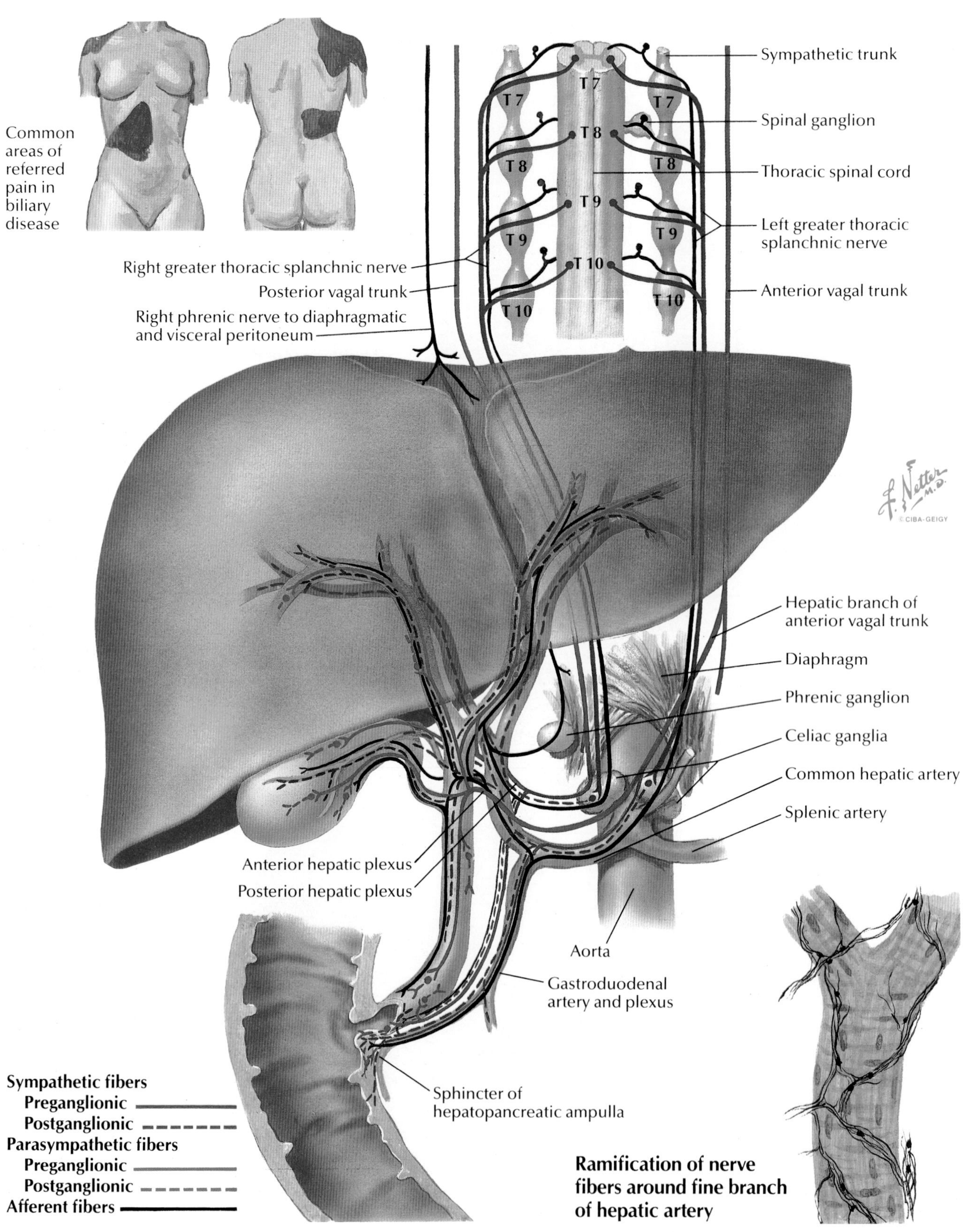

Common areas of referred pain in biliary disease

Sympathetic trunk

Spinal ganglion

Thoracic spinal cord

Left greater thoracic splanchnic nerve

Anterior vagal trunk

T 7 — T 8 — T 9 — T 10

Right greater thoracic splanchnic nerve

Posterior vagal trunk

Right phrenic nerve to diaphragmatic and visceral peritoneum

Hepatic branch of anterior vagal trunk

Diaphragm

Phrenic ganglion

Celiac ganglia

Common hepatic artery

Splenic artery

Anterior hepatic plexus

Posterior hepatic plexus

Aorta

Gastroduodenal artery and plexus

Sphincter of hepatopancreatic ampulla

Sympathetic fibers
  Preganglionic —————
  Postganglionic – – – – –
Parasympathetic fibers
  Preganglionic —————
  Postganglionic – – – – –
Afferent fibers ▬▬▬▬

Ramification of nerve fibers around fine branch of hepatic artery

PLATE 313

ABDOMEN

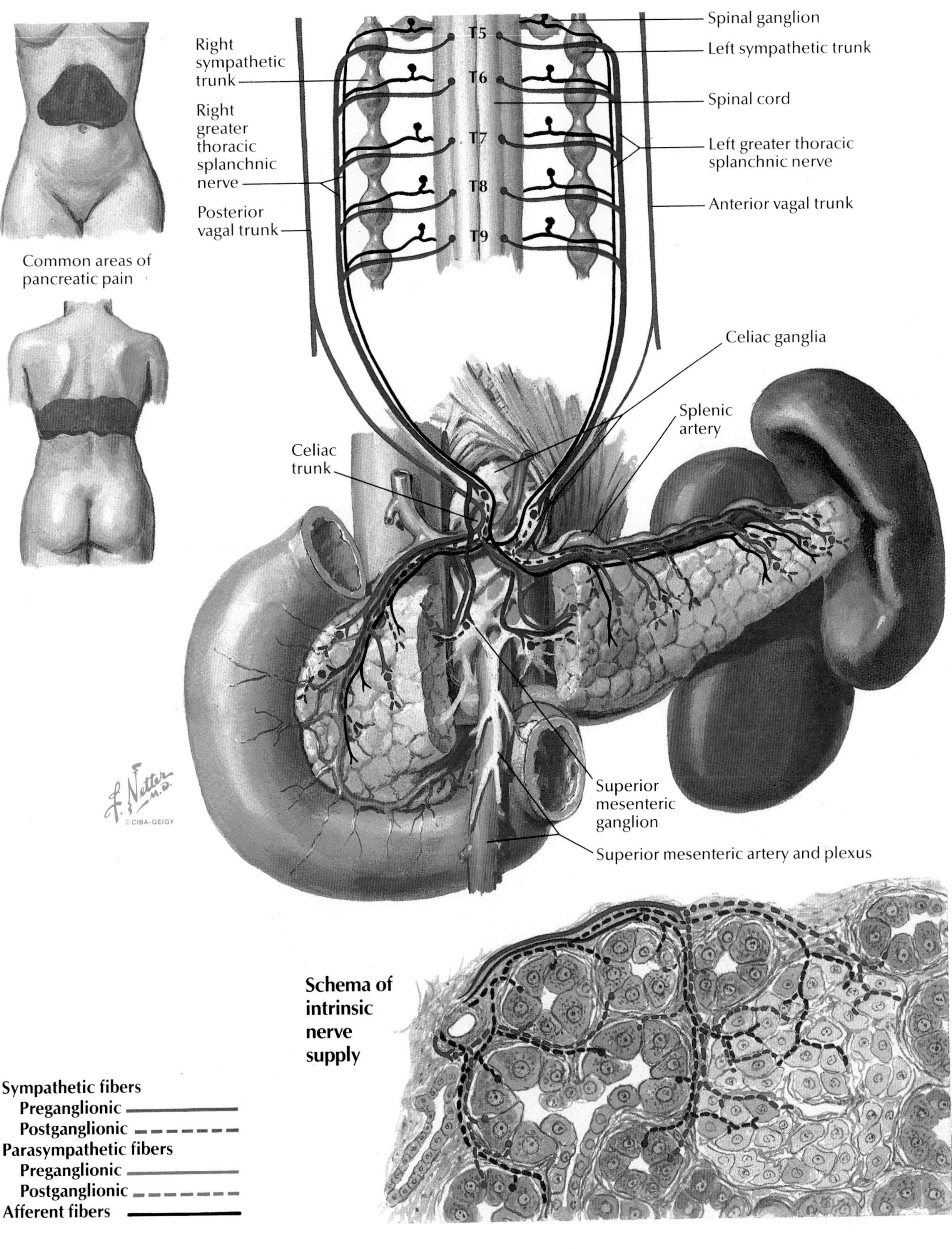

Common areas of pancreatic pain

Right sympathetic trunk

Right greater thoracic splanchnic nerve

Posterior vagal trunk

Spinal ganglion

Left sympathetic trunk

Spinal cord

Left greater thoracic splanchnic nerve

Anterior vagal trunk

T5
T6
T7
T8
T9

Celiac ganglia

Splenic artery

Celiac trunk

Superior mesenteric ganglion

Superior mesenteric artery and plexus

Schema of intrinsic nerve supply

Sympathetic fibers
Preganglionic ———
Postganglionic – – –
Parasympathetic fibers
Preganglionic ———
Postganglionic – – –
Afferent fibers ———

Kidneys In Situ: Anterior Views

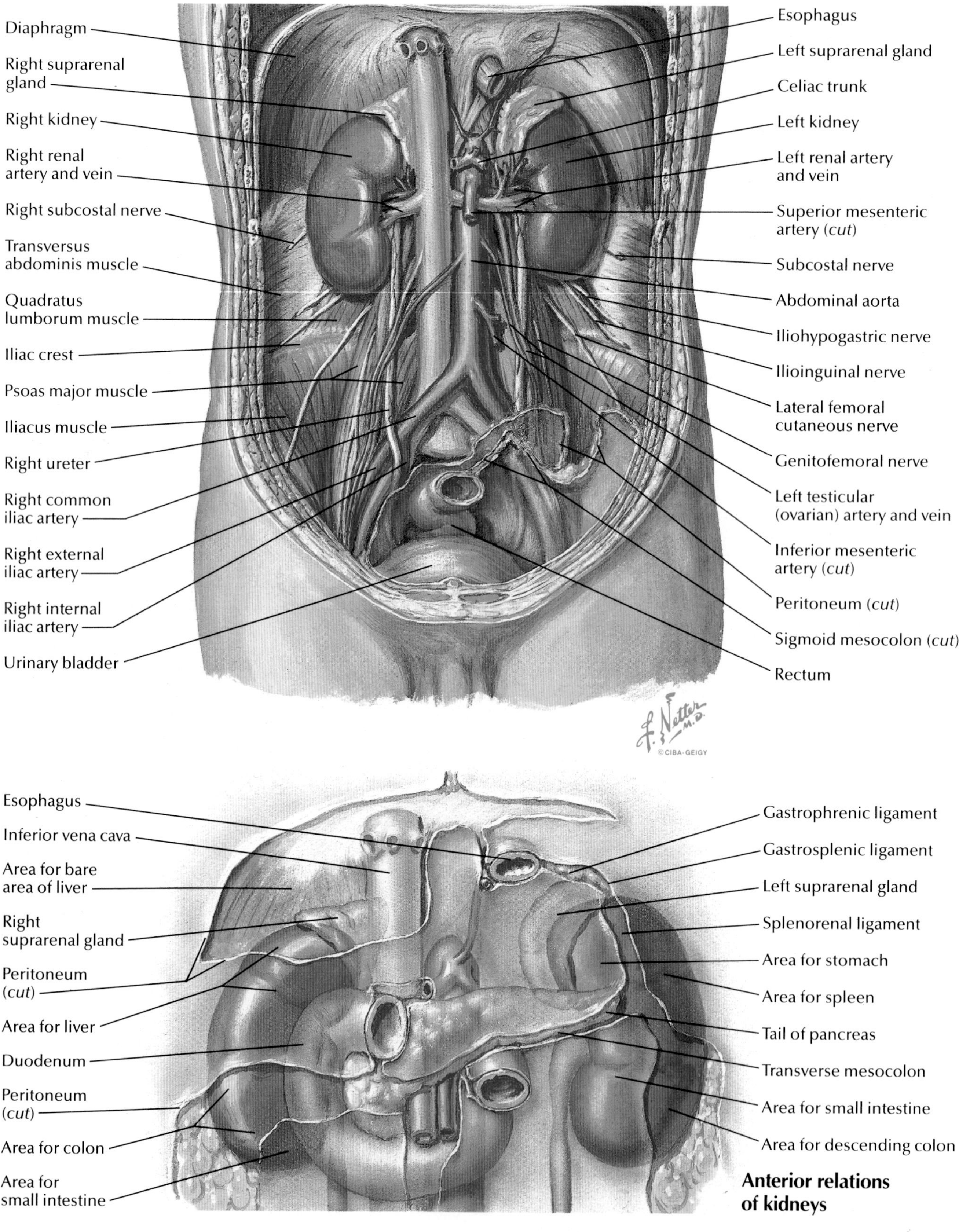

Diaphragm

Right suprarenal gland

Right kidney

Right renal artery and vein

Right subcostal nerve

Transversus abdominis muscle

Quadratus lumborum muscle

Iliac crest

Psoas major muscle

Iliacus muscle

Right ureter

Right common iliac artery

Right external iliac artery

Right internal iliac artery

Urinary bladder

Esophagus

Left suprarenal gland

Celiac trunk

Left kidney

Left renal artery and vein

Superior mesenteric artery (cut)

Subcostal nerve

Abdominal aorta

Iliohypogastric nerve

Ilioinguinal nerve

Lateral femoral cutaneous nerve

Genitofemoral nerve

Left testicular (ovarian) artery and vein

Inferior mesenteric artery (cut)

Peritoneum (cut)

Sigmoid mesocolon (cut)

Rectum

Esophagus

Inferior vena cava

Area for bare area of liver

Right suprarenal gland

Peritoneum (cut)

Area for liver

Duodenum

Peritoneum (cut)

Area for colon

Area for small intestine

Gastrophrenic ligament

Gastrosplenic ligament

Left suprarenal gland

Splenorenal ligament

Area for stomach

Area for spleen

Tail of pancreas

Transverse mesocolon

Area for small intestine

Area for descending colon

Anterior relations of kidneys

PLATE 315

ABDOMEN

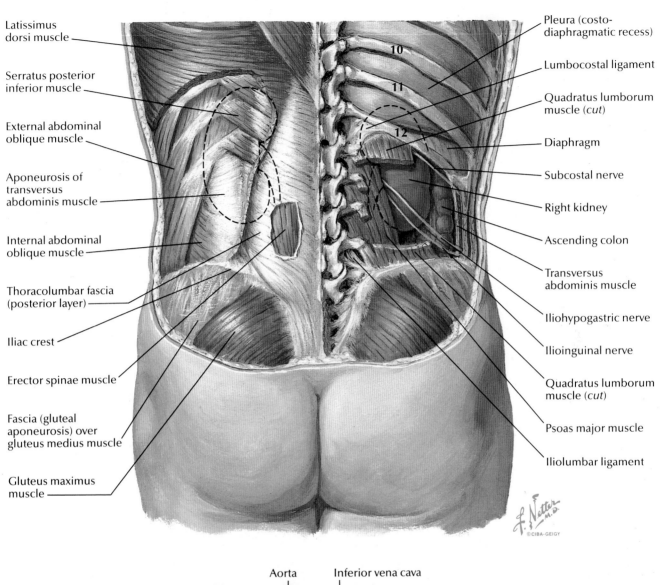

Latissimus dorsi muscle

Serratus posterior inferior muscle

External abdominal oblique muscle

Aponeurosis of transversus abdominis muscle

Internal abdominal oblique muscle

Thoracolumbar fascia (posterior layer)

Iliac crest

Erector spinae muscle

Fascia (gluteal aponeurosis) over gluteus medius muscle

Gluteus maximus muscle

10

11

12

Pleura (costo-diaphragmatic recess)

Lumbocostal ligament

Quadratus lumborum muscle (*cut*)

Diaphragm

Subcostal nerve

Right kidney

Ascending colon

Transversus abdominis muscle

Iliohypogastric nerve

Ilioinguinal nerve

Quadratus lumborum muscle (*cut*)

Psoas major muscle

Iliolumbar ligament

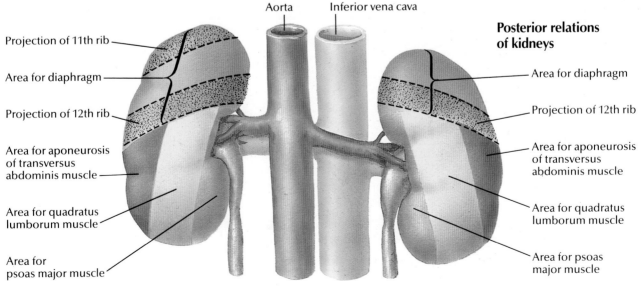

Aorta

Inferior vena cava

Posterior relations of kidneys

Projection of 11th rib

Area for diaphragm

Projection of 12th rib

Area for aponeurosis of transversus abdominis muscle

Area for quadratus lumborum muscle

Area for psoas major muscle

Area for diaphragm

Projection of 12th rib

Area for aponeurosis of transversus abdominis muscle

Area for quadratus lumborum muscle

Area for psoas major muscle

KIDNEYS AND SUPRARENAL GLANDS

PLATE 316

Gross Structure of Kidney

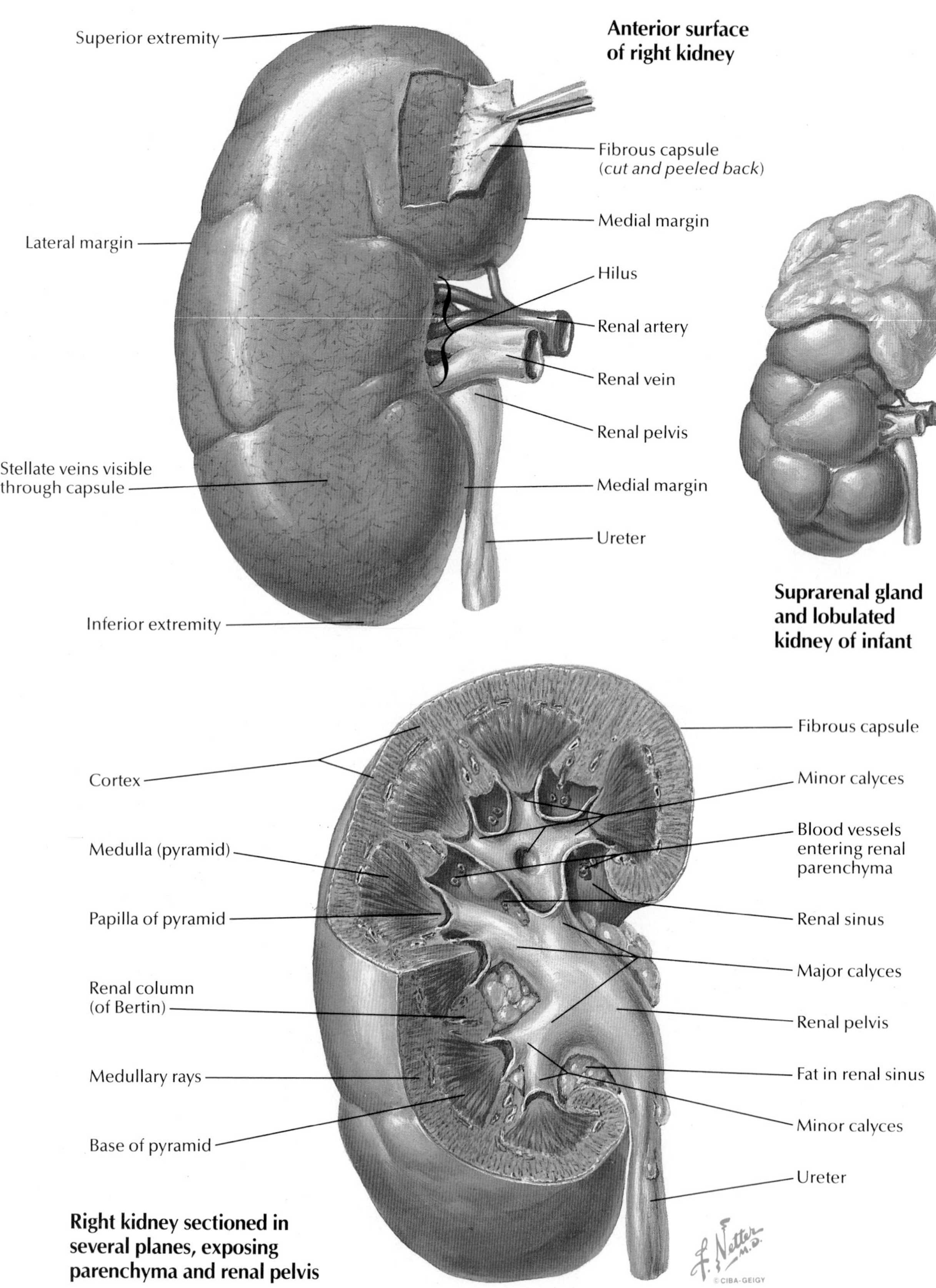

Superior extremity

Anterior surface of right kidney

Fibrous capsule (*cut and peeled back*)

Medial margin

Hilus

Renal artery

Renal vein

Renal pelvis

Lateral margin

Medial margin

Ureter

Stellate veins visible through capsule

Inferior extremity

Suprarenal gland and lobulated kidney of infant

Cortex

Fibrous capsule

Minor calyces

Medulla (pyramid)

Blood vessels entering renal parenchyma

Papilla of pyramid

Renal sinus

Major calyces

Renal column (of Bertin)

Renal pelvis

Medullary rays

Fat in renal sinus

Minor calyces

Base of pyramid

Ureter

Right kidney sectioned in several planes, exposing parenchyma and renal pelvis

PLATE 317

ABDOMEN

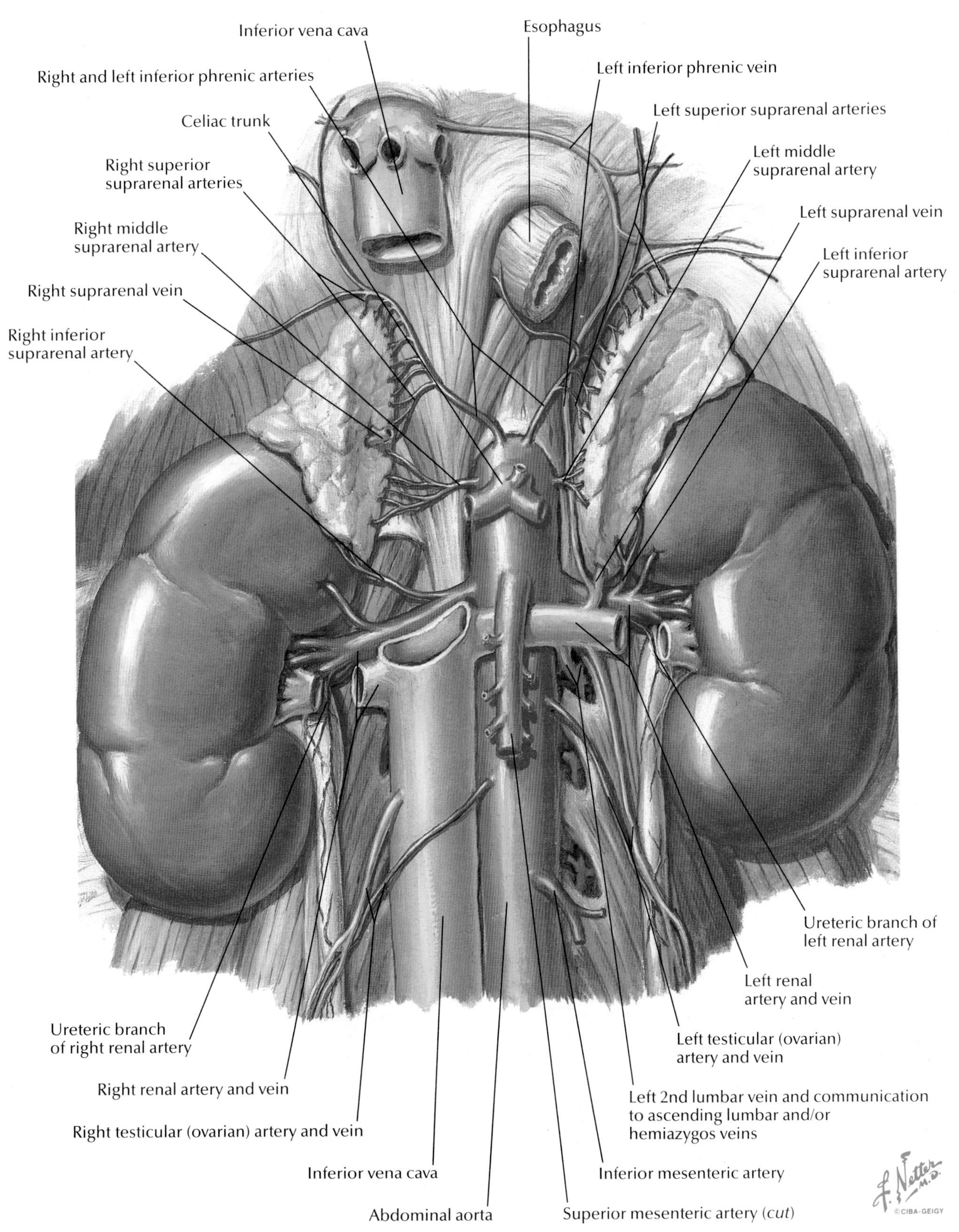

Inferior vena cava

Right and left inferior phrenic arteries

Celiac trunk

Right superior suprarenal arteries

Right middle suprarenal artery

Right suprarenal vein

Right inferior suprarenal artery

Esophagus

Left inferior phrenic vein

Left superior suprarenal arteries

Left middle suprarenal artery

Left suprarenal vein

Left inferior suprarenal artery

Ureteric branch of left renal artery

Left renal artery and vein

Left testicular (ovarian) artery and vein

Left 2nd lumbar vein and communication to ascending lumbar and/or hemiazygos veins

Inferior mesenteric artery

Superior mesenteric artery (cut)

Abdominal aorta

Inferior vena cava

Right testicular (ovarian) artery and vein

Right renal artery and vein

Ureteric branch of right renal artery

Intrarenal Arteries and Kidney Segments

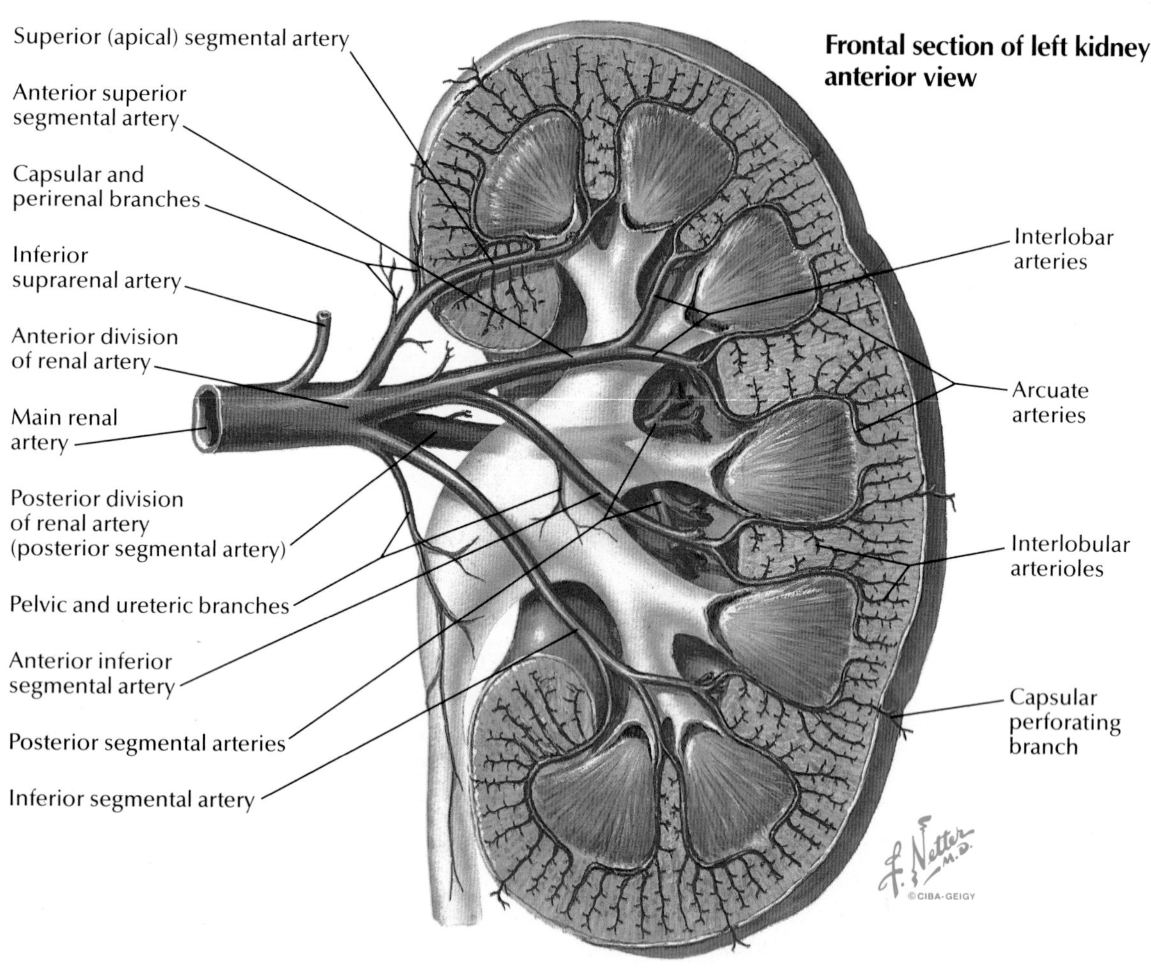

Superior (apical) segmental artery

Anterior superior segmental artery

Capsular and perirenal branches

Inferior suprarenal artery

Anterior division of renal artery

Main renal artery

Posterior division of renal artery (posterior segmental artery)

Pelvic and ureteric branches

Anterior inferior segmental artery

Posterior segmental arteries

Inferior segmental artery

Frontal section of left kidney: anterior view

Interlobar arteries

Arcuate arteries

Interlobular arterioles

Capsular perforating branch

Vascular renal segments

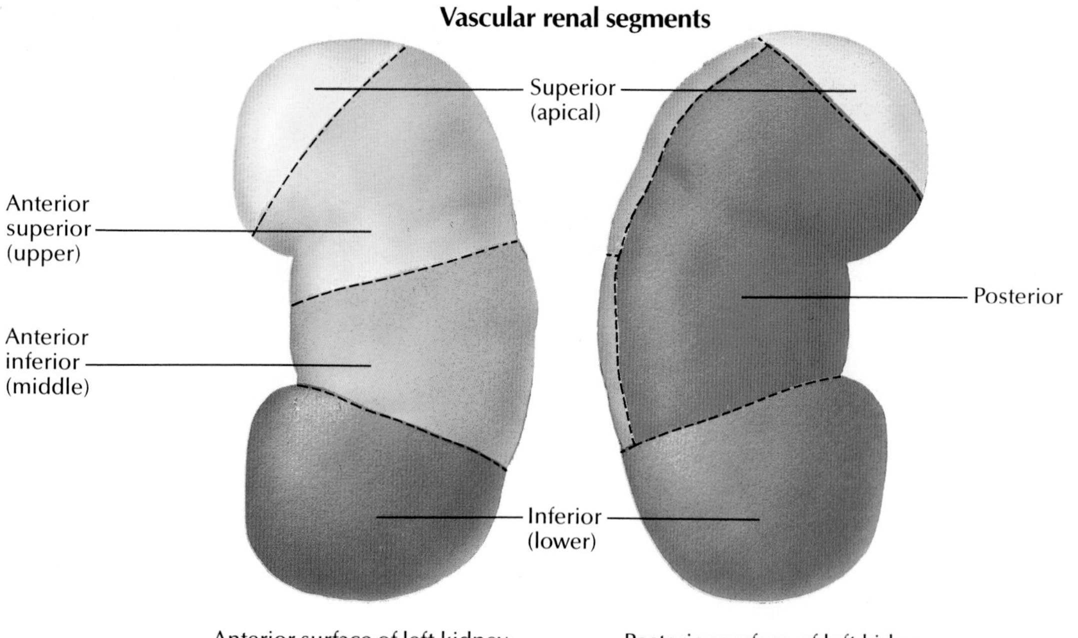

Superior (apical)

Anterior superior (upper)

Anterior inferior (middle)

Posterior

Inferior (lower)

Anterior surface of left kidney

Posterior surface of left kidney

PLATE 319

ABDOMEN

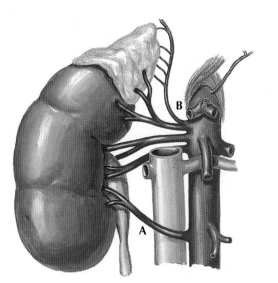

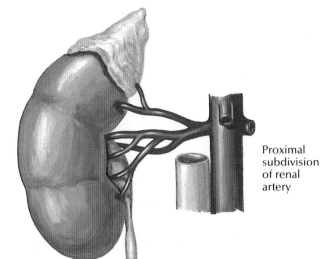

Proximal subdivision of renal artery

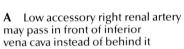

A Low accessory right renal artery may pass in front of inferior vena cava instead of behind it

B Inferior phrenic artery with suprarenal arteries may arise from renal artery

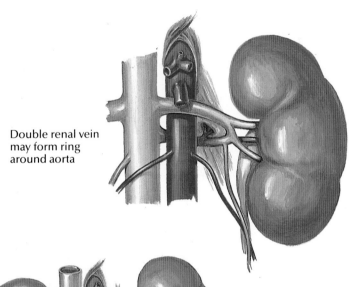

Double renal vein may form ring around aorta

Multiple renal veins

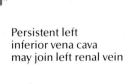

Persistent left inferior vena cava may join left renal vein

Nephron and Collecting Tubule: Schema

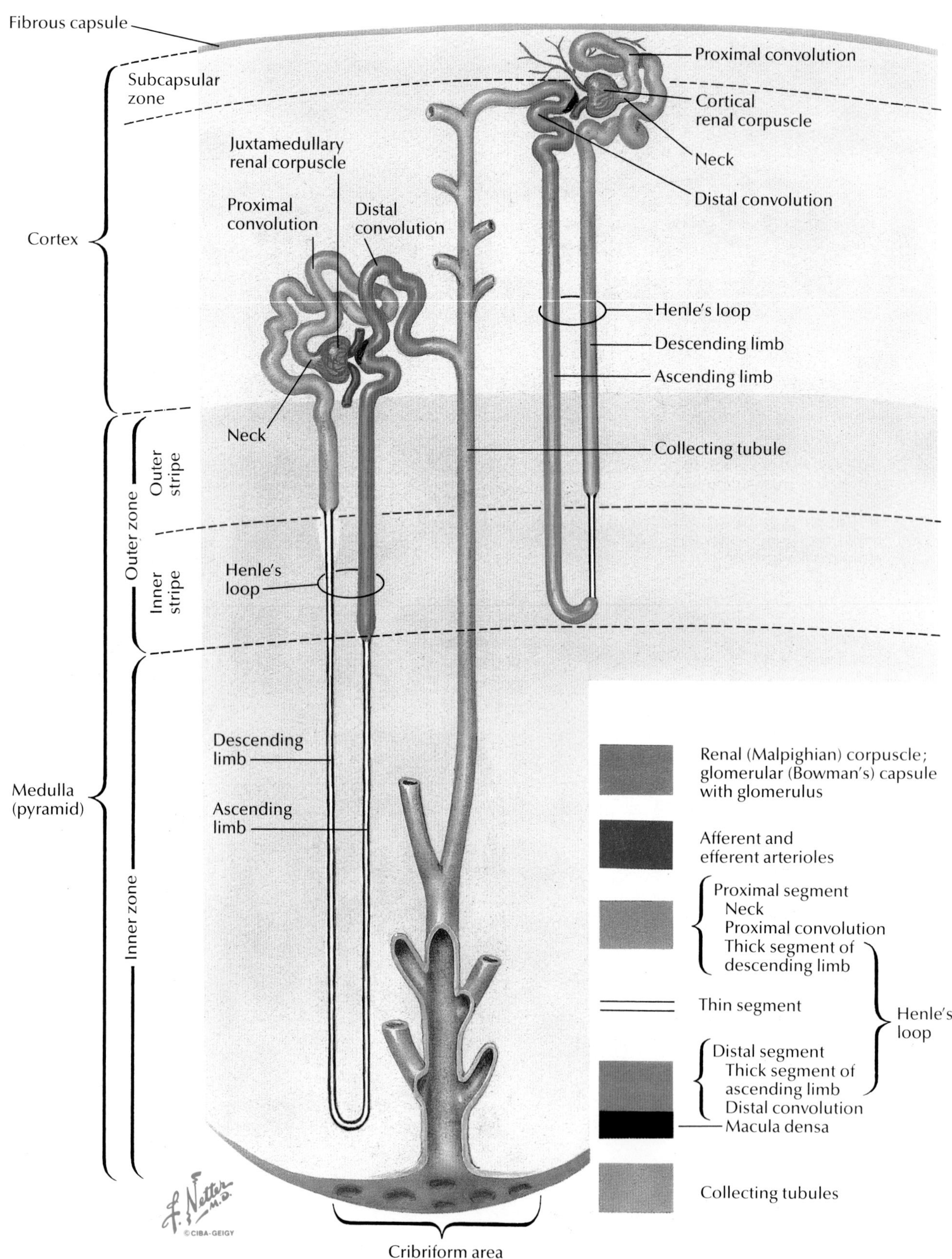

Fibrous capsule

Subcapsular zone

Cortex

Proximal convolution

Cortical renal corpuscle

Neck

Distal convolution

Juxtamedullary renal corpuscle

Proximal convolution

Distal convolution

Henle's loop

Descending limb

Ascending limb

Neck

Collecting tubule

Outer zone

Outer stripe

Inner stripe

Henle's loop

Medulla (pyramid)

Inner zone

Descending limb

Ascending limb

Cribriform area

Renal (Malpighian) corpuscle; glomerular (Bowman's) capsule with glomerulus

Afferent and efferent arterioles

Proximal segment
Neck
Proximal convolution
Thick segment of descending limb

Thin segment

Henle's loop

Distal segment
Thick segment of ascending limb
Distal convolution
Macula densa

Collecting tubules

PLATE 321

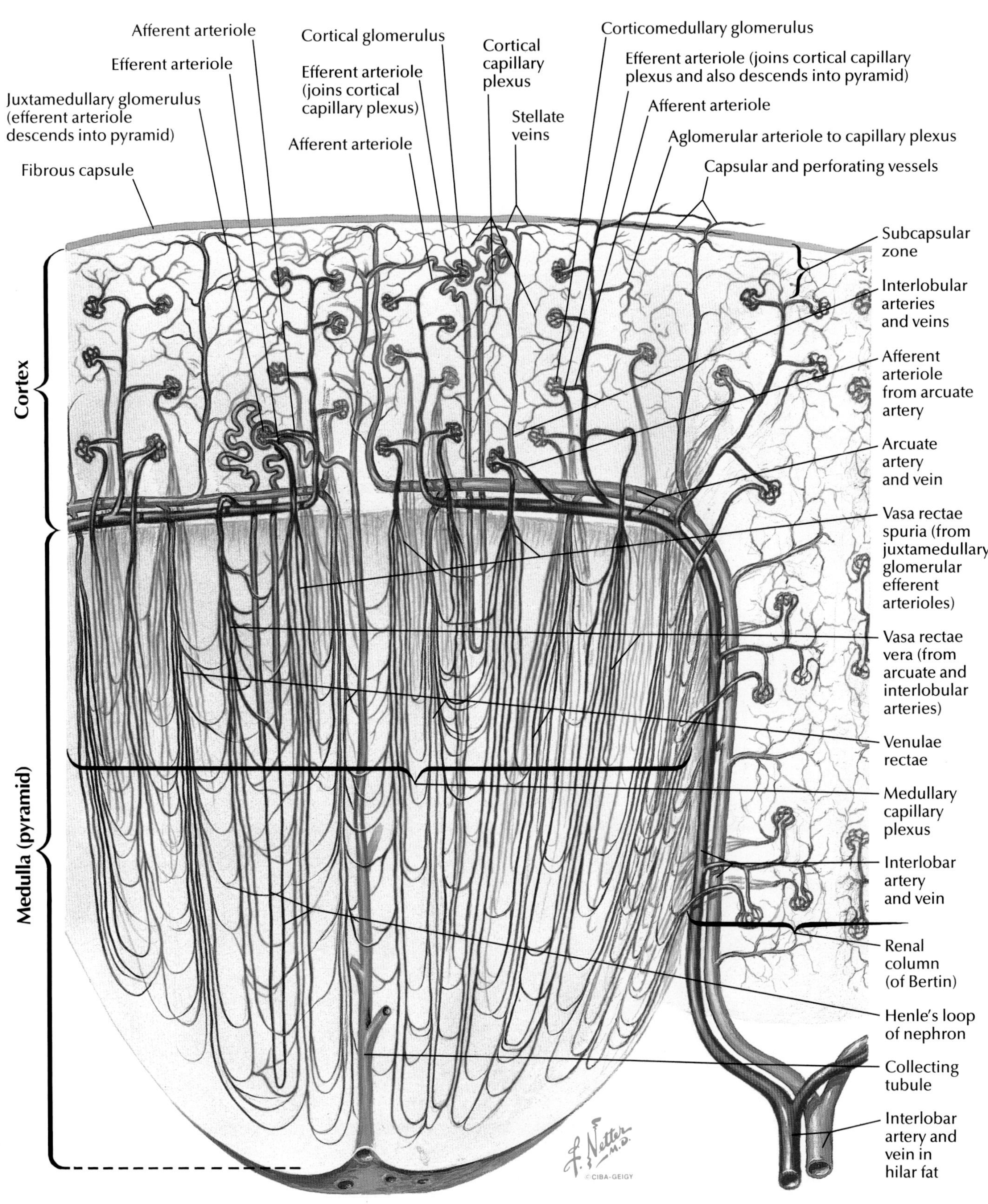

Afferent arteriole

Efferent arteriole

Juxtamedullary glomerulus
(efferent arteriole
descends into pyramid)

Fibrous capsule

Cortical glomerulus

Efferent arteriole
(joins cortical
capillary plexus)

Afferent arteriole

Cortical
capillary
plexus

Stellate
veins

Corticomedullary glomerulus

Efferent arteriole (joins cortical capillary
plexus and also descends into pyramid)

Afferent arteriole

Aglomerular arteriole to capillary plexus

Capsular and perforating vessels

Subcapsular
zone

Interlobular
arteries
and veins

Afferent
arteriole
from arcuate
artery

Arcuate
artery
and vein

Vasa rectae
spuria (from
juxtamedullary
glomerular
efferent
arterioles)

Vasa rectae
vera (from
arcuate and
interlobular
arteries)

Venulae
rectae

Medullary
capillary
plexus

Interlobar
artery
and vein

Renal
column
(of Bertin)

Henle's loop
of nephron

Collecting
tubule

Interlobar
artery and
vein in
hilar fat

Cortex

Medulla (pyramid)

©CIBA-GEIGY

J. Netter
M.D.

Ureters

SEE ALSO PLATES 343, 344, 348

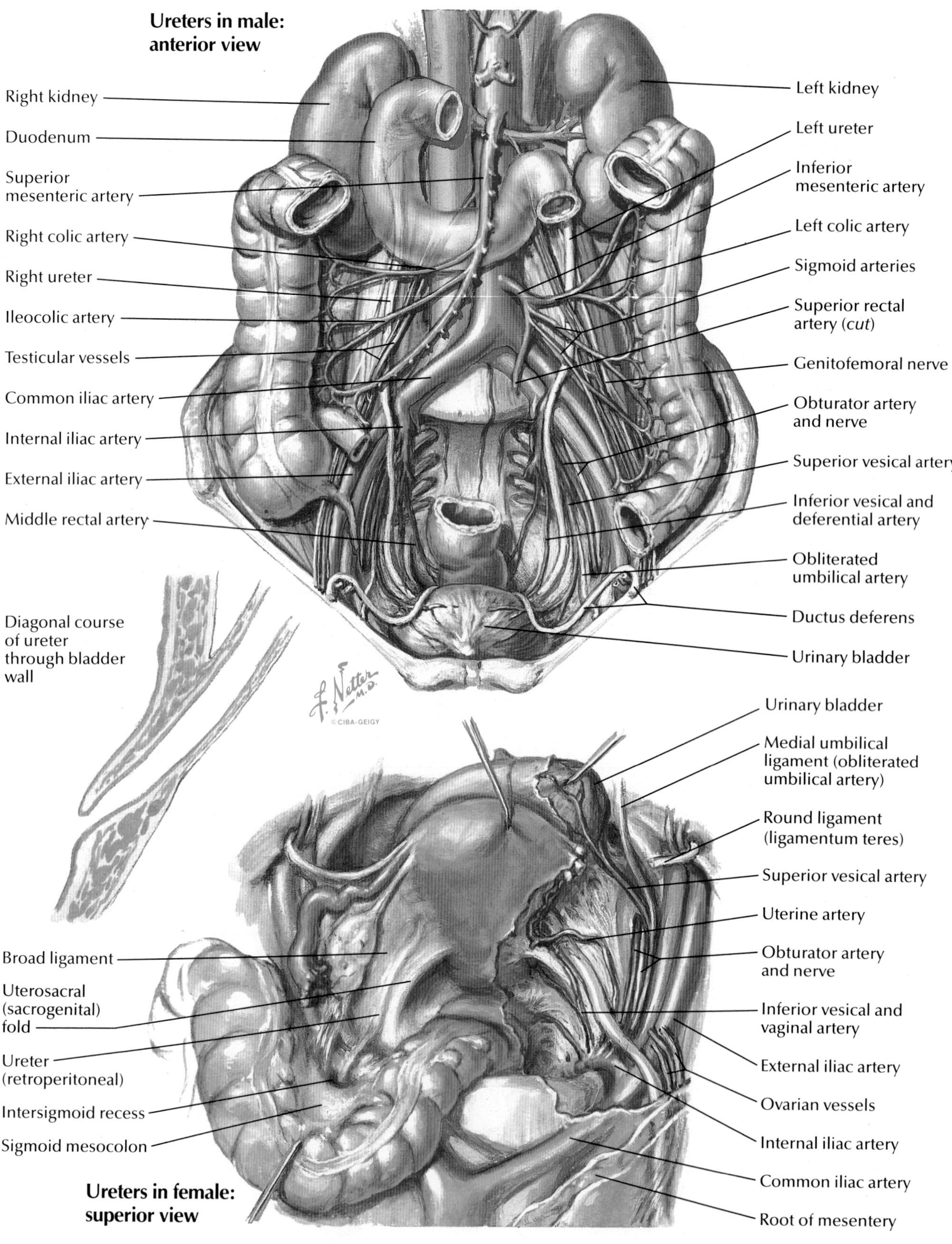

Ureters in male: anterior view

Right kidney

Duodenum

Superior mesenteric artery

Right colic artery

Right ureter

Ileocolic artery

Testicular vessels

Common iliac artery

Internal iliac artery

External iliac artery

Middle rectal artery

Diagonal course of ureter through bladder wall

Left kidney

Left ureter

Inferior mesenteric artery

Left colic artery

Sigmoid arteries

Superior rectal artery (*cut*)

Genitofemoral nerve

Obturator artery and nerve

Superior vesical artery

Inferior vesical and deferential artery

Obliterated umbilical artery

Ductus deferens

Urinary bladder

Urinary bladder

Medial umbilical ligament (obliterated umbilical artery)

Round ligament (ligamentum teres)

Superior vesical artery

Uterine artery

Obturator artery and nerve

Inferior vesical and vaginal artery

External iliac artery

Ovarian vessels

Internal iliac artery

Common iliac artery

Root of mesentery

Broad ligament

Uterosacral (sacrogenital) fold

Ureter (retroperitoneal)

Intersigmoid recess

Sigmoid mesocolon

Ureters in female: superior view

F. Netter M.D.

©CIBA-GEIGY

PLATE 323

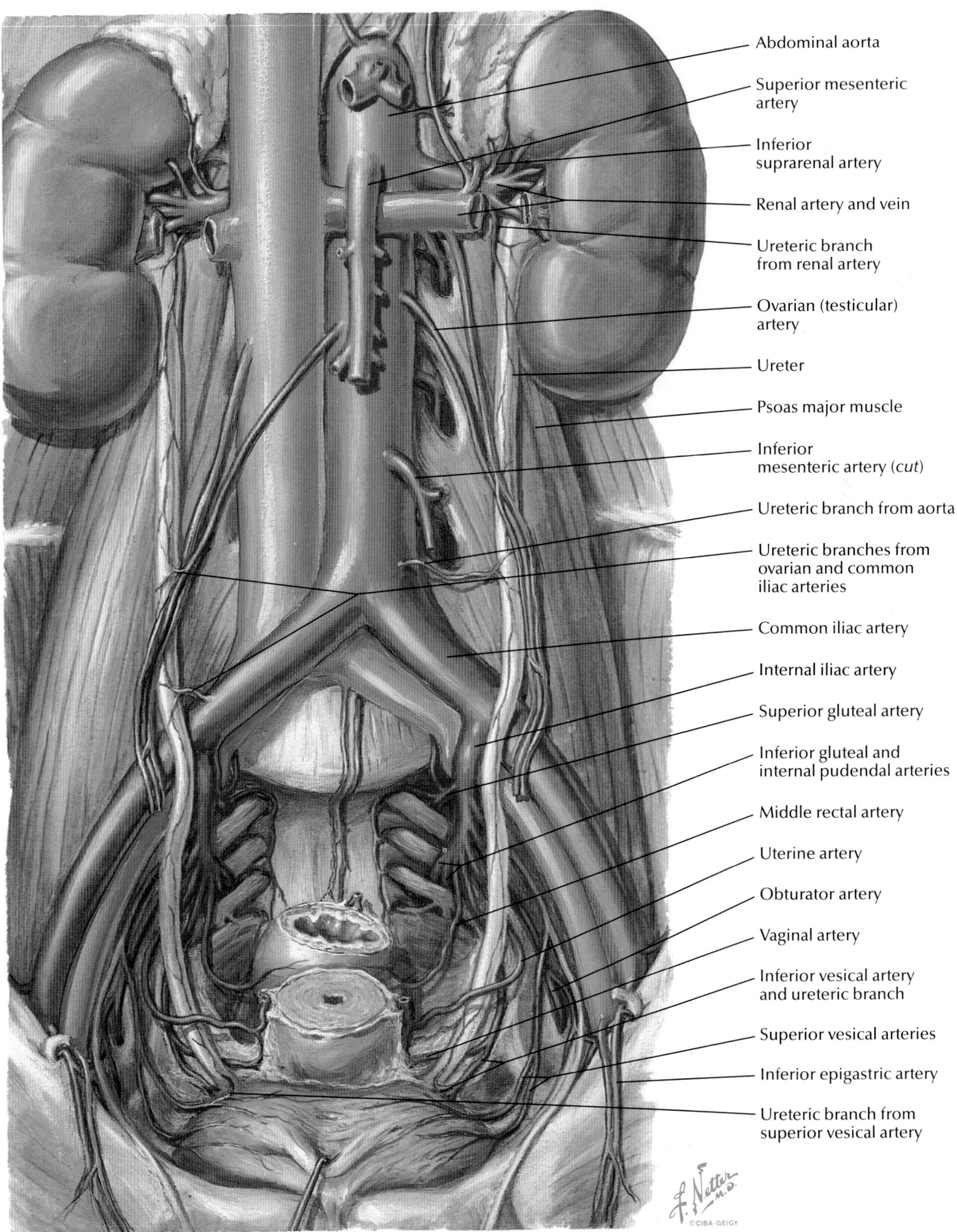

Abdominal aorta

Superior mesenteric artery

Inferior suprarenal artery

Renal artery and vein

Ureteric branch from renal artery

Ovarian (testicular) artery

Ureter

Psoas major muscle

Inferior mesenteric artery (*cut*)

Ureteric branch from aorta

Ureteric branches from ovarian and common iliac arteries

Common iliac artery

Internal iliac artery

Superior gluteal artery

Inferior gluteal and internal pudendal arteries

Middle rectal artery

Uterine artery

Obturator artery

Vaginal artery

Inferior vesical artery and ureteric branch

Superior vesical arteries

Inferior epigastric artery

Ureteric branch from superior vesical artery

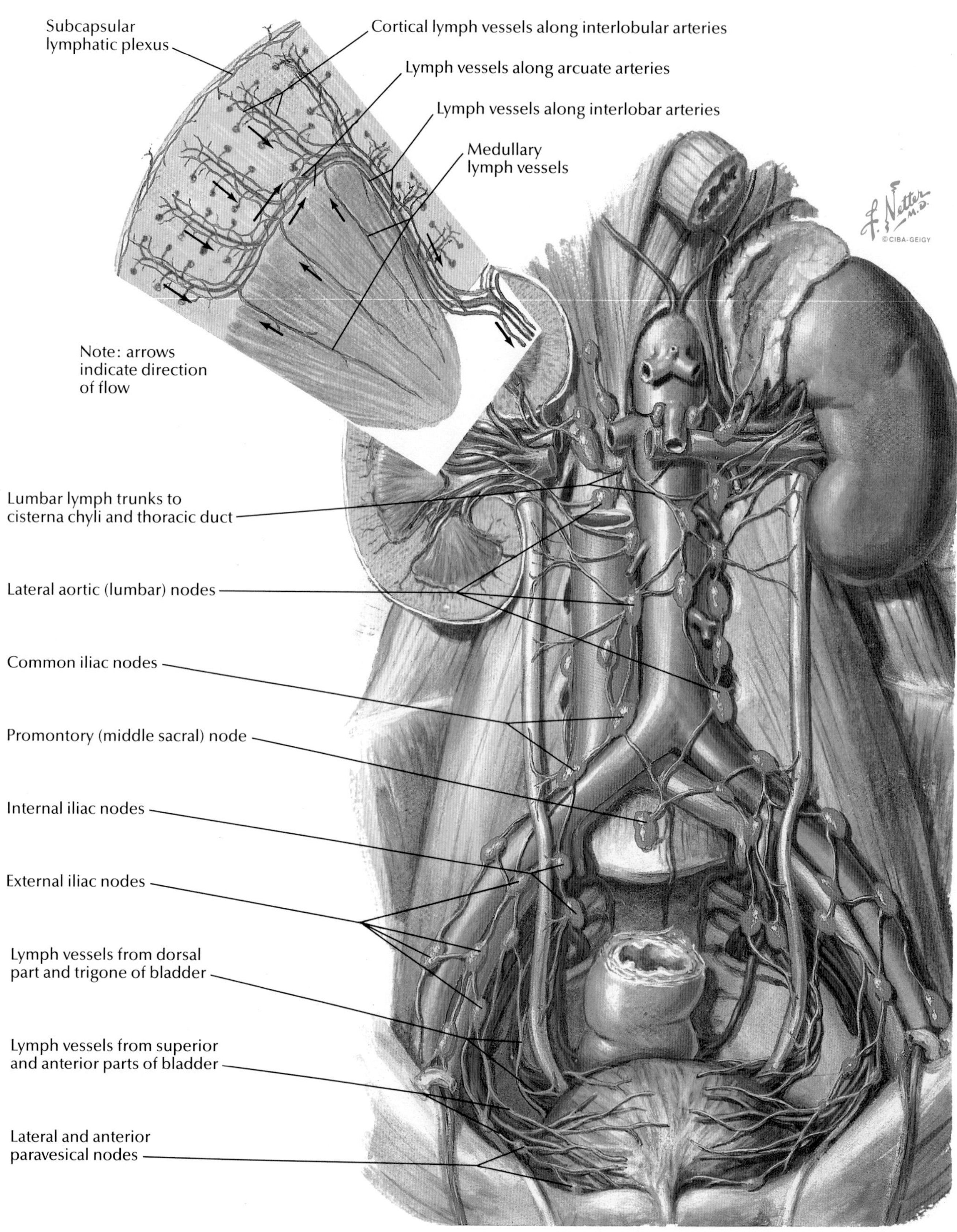

Subcapsular lymphatic plexus

Cortical lymph vessels along interlobular arteries

Lymph vessels along arcuate arteries

Lymph vessels along interlobar arteries

Medullary lymph vessels

Note: arrows indicate direction of flow

Lumbar lymph trunks to cisterna chyli and thoracic duct

Lateral aortic (lumbar) nodes

Common iliac nodes

Promontory (middle sacral) node

Internal iliac nodes

External iliac nodes

Lymph vessels from dorsal part and trigone of bladder

Lymph vessels from superior and anterior parts of bladder

Lateral and anterior paravesical nodes

PLATE 325

ABDOMEN

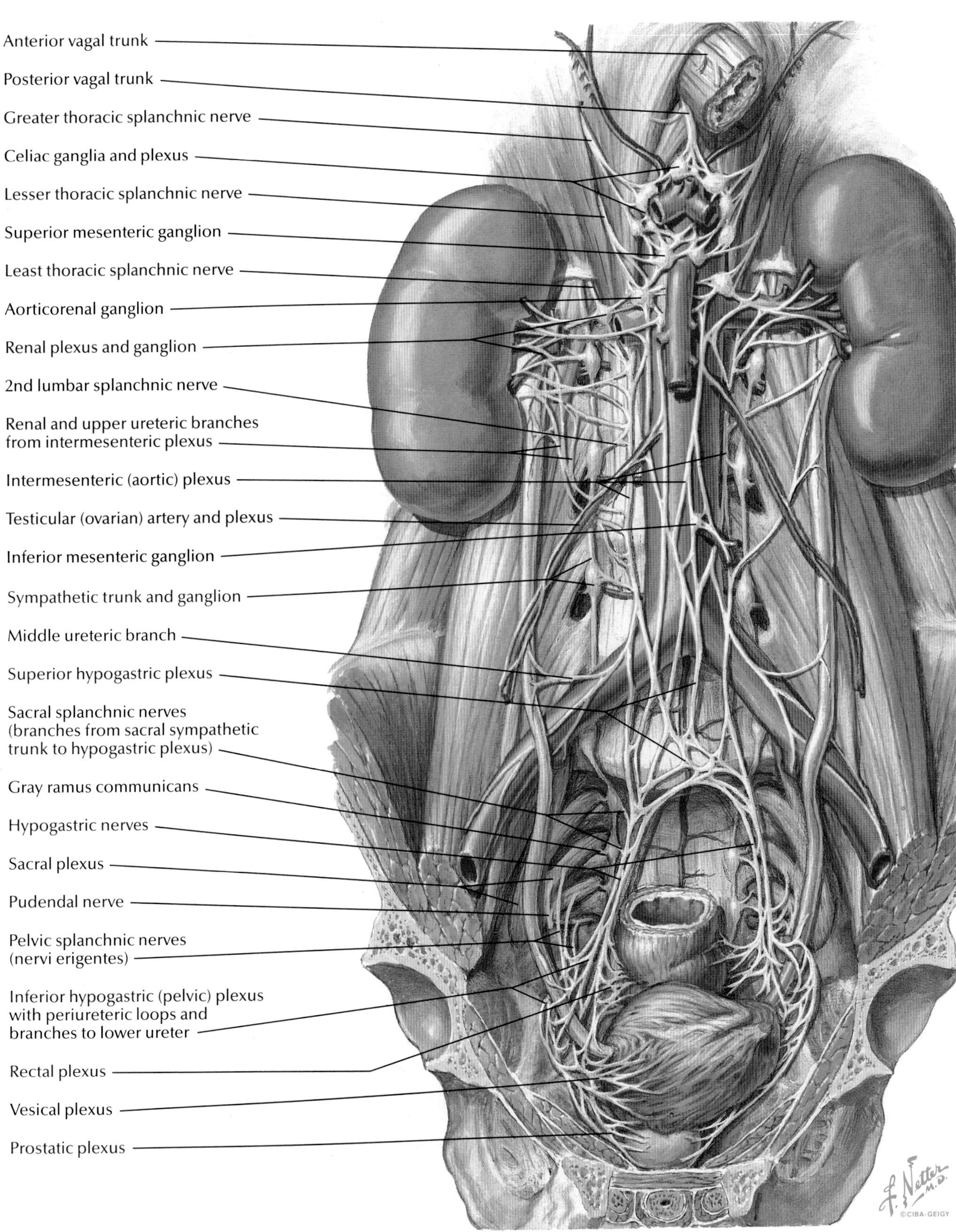

Anterior vagal trunk

Posterior vagal trunk

Greater thoracic splanchnic nerve

Celiac ganglia and plexus

Lesser thoracic splanchnic nerve

Superior mesenteric ganglion

Least thoracic splanchnic nerve

Aorticorenal ganglion

Renal plexus and ganglion

2nd lumbar splanchnic nerve

Renal and upper ureteric branches from intermesenteric plexus

Intermesenteric (aortic) plexus

Testicular (ovarian) artery and plexus

Inferior mesenteric ganglion

Sympathetic trunk and ganglion

Middle ureteric branch

Superior hypogastric plexus

Sacral splanchnic nerves (branches from sacral sympathetic trunk to hypogastric plexus)

Gray ramus communicans

Hypogastric nerves

Sacral plexus

Pudendal nerve

Pelvic splanchnic nerves (nervi erigentes)

Inferior hypogastric (pelvic) plexus with periureteric loops and branches to lower ureter

Rectal plexus

Vesical plexus

Prostatic plexus

Innervation of Kidneys and Upper Ureters: Schema

SEE ALSO PLATES 153, 392

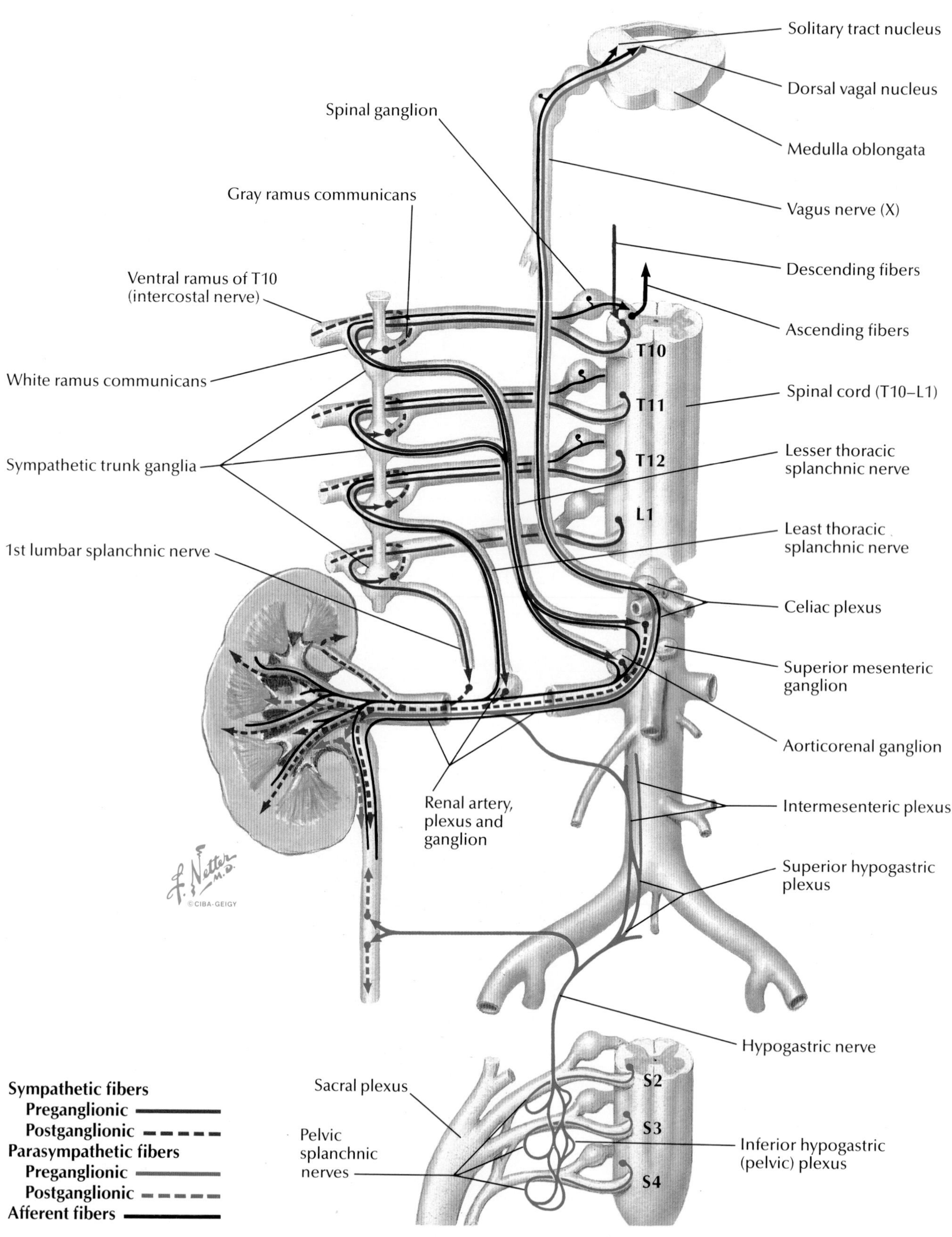

Solitary tract nucleus

Dorsal vagal nucleus

Medulla oblongata

Vagus nerve (X)

Descending fibers

Ascending fibers

Spinal ganglion

Gray ramus communicans

Ventral ramus of T10 (intercostal nerve)

White ramus communicans

Sympathetic trunk ganglia

1st lumbar splanchnic nerve

T10

T11

T12

L1

Spinal cord (T10–L1)

Lesser thoracic splanchnic nerve

Least thoracic splanchnic nerve

Celiac plexus

Superior mesenteric ganglion

Aorticorenal ganglion

Renal artery, plexus and ganglion

Intermesenteric plexus

Superior hypogastric plexus

Hypogastric nerve

Sacral plexus

Pelvic splanchnic nerves

S2

S3

S4

Inferior hypogastric (pelvic) plexus

Sympathetic fibers
Preganglionic ————
Postganglionic – – – –
Parasympathetic fibers
Preganglionic ————
Postganglionic – – – –
Afferent fibers ————

PLATE 327

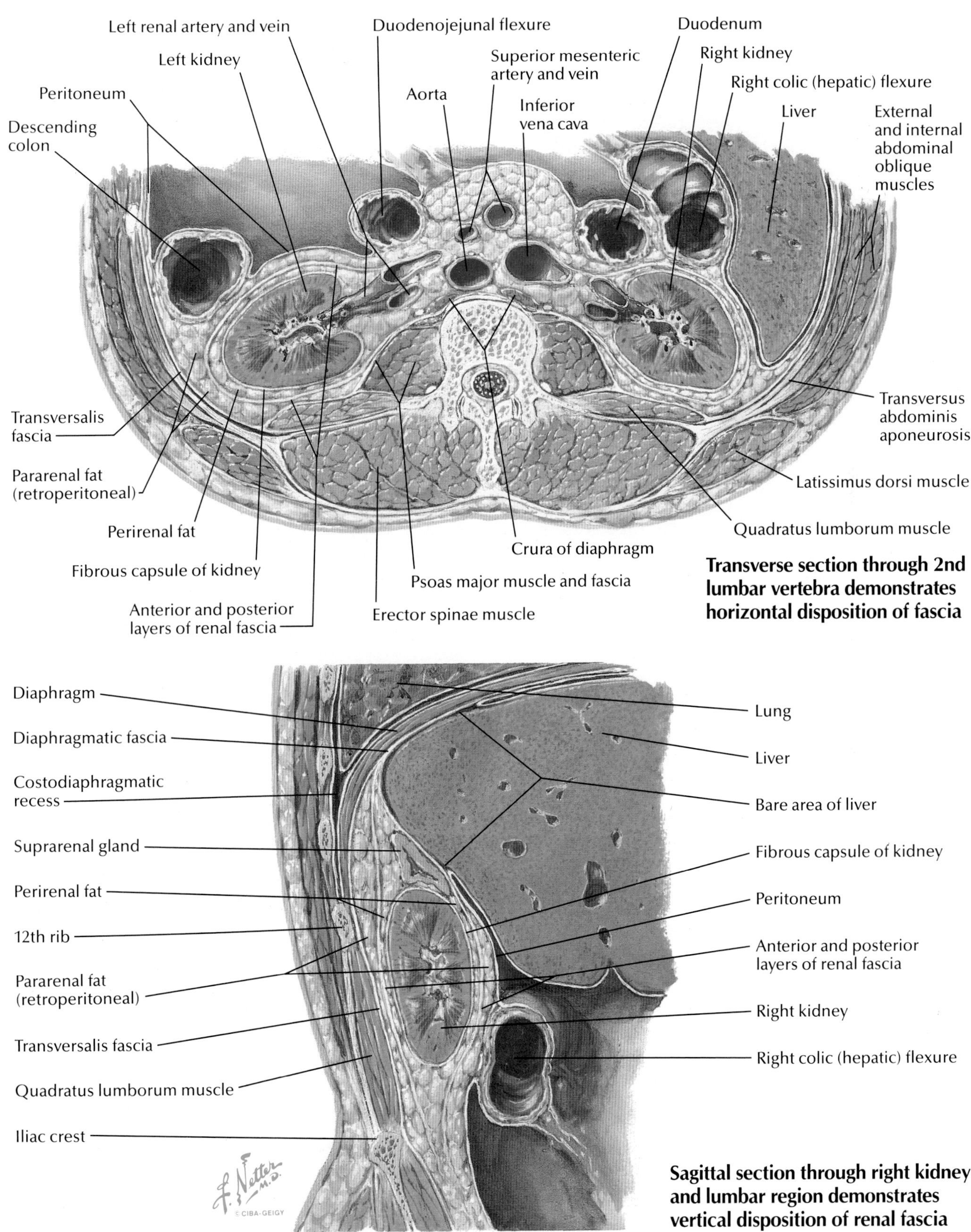

Left renal artery and vein

Left kidney

Peritoneum

Descending colon

Duodenojejunal flexure

Aorta

Superior mesenteric artery and vein

Inferior vena cava

Duodenum

Right kidney

Right colic (hepatic) flexure

Liver

External and internal abdominal oblique muscles

Transversalis fascia

Pararenal fat (retroperitoneal)

Perirenal fat

Fibrous capsule of kidney

Anterior and posterior layers of renal fascia

Erector spinae muscle

Psoas major muscle and fascia

Crura of diaphragm

Quadratus lumborum muscle

Latissimus dorsi muscle

Transversus abdominis aponeurosis

Transverse section through 2nd lumbar vertebra demonstrates horizontal disposition of fascia

Diaphragm

Diaphragmatic fascia

Costodiaphragmatic recess

Suprarenal gland

Perirenal fat

12th rib

Pararenal fat (retroperitoneal)

Transversalis fascia

Quadratus lumborum muscle

Iliac crest

Lung

Liver

Bare area of liver

Fibrous capsule of kidney

Peritoneum

Anterior and posterior layers of renal fascia

Right kidney

Right colic (hepatic) flexure

Sagittal section through right kidney and lumbar region demonstrates vertical disposition of renal fascia

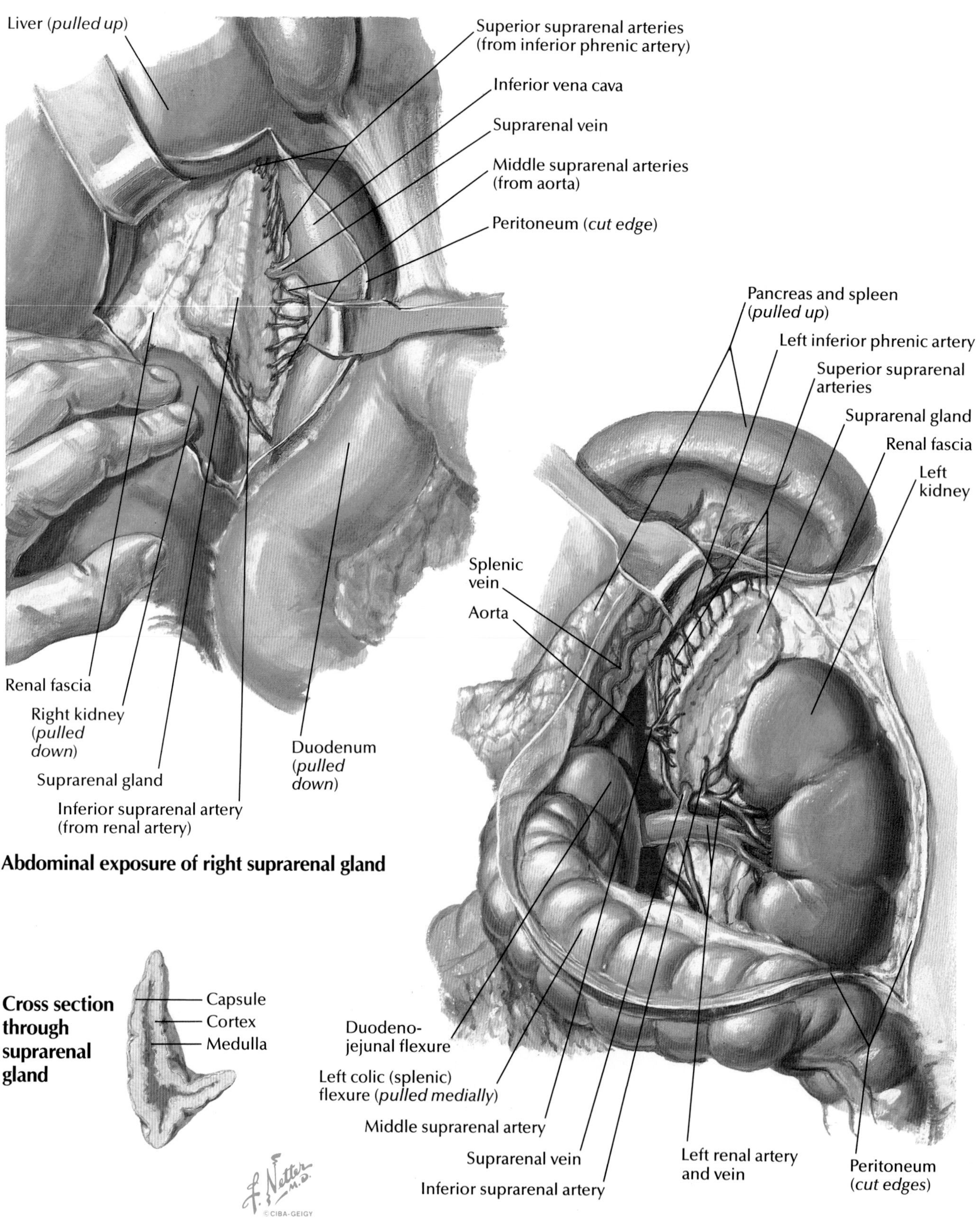

Liver (*pulled up*)

Superior suprarenal arteries (from inferior phrenic artery)

Inferior vena cava

Suprarenal vein

Middle suprarenal arteries (from aorta)

Peritoneum (*cut edge*)

Pancreas and spleen (*pulled up*)

Left inferior phrenic artery

Superior suprarenal arteries

Suprarenal gland

Renal fascia

Left kidney

Splenic vein

Aorta

Renal fascia

Right kidney (*pulled down*)

Suprarenal gland

Inferior suprarenal artery (from renal artery)

Duodenum (*pulled down*)

Abdominal exposure of right suprarenal gland

Cross section through suprarenal gland

Capsule

Cortex

Medulla

Duodeno-jejunal flexure

Left colic (splenic) flexure (*pulled medially*)

Middle suprarenal artery

Suprarenal vein

Inferior suprarenal artery

Left renal artery and vein

Peritoneum (*cut edges*)

Abdominal exposure of left suprarenal gland

PLATE 329

ABDOMEN

Nerves of Suprarenal Glands: Dissection and Schema

SEE ALSO PLATES 152, 153

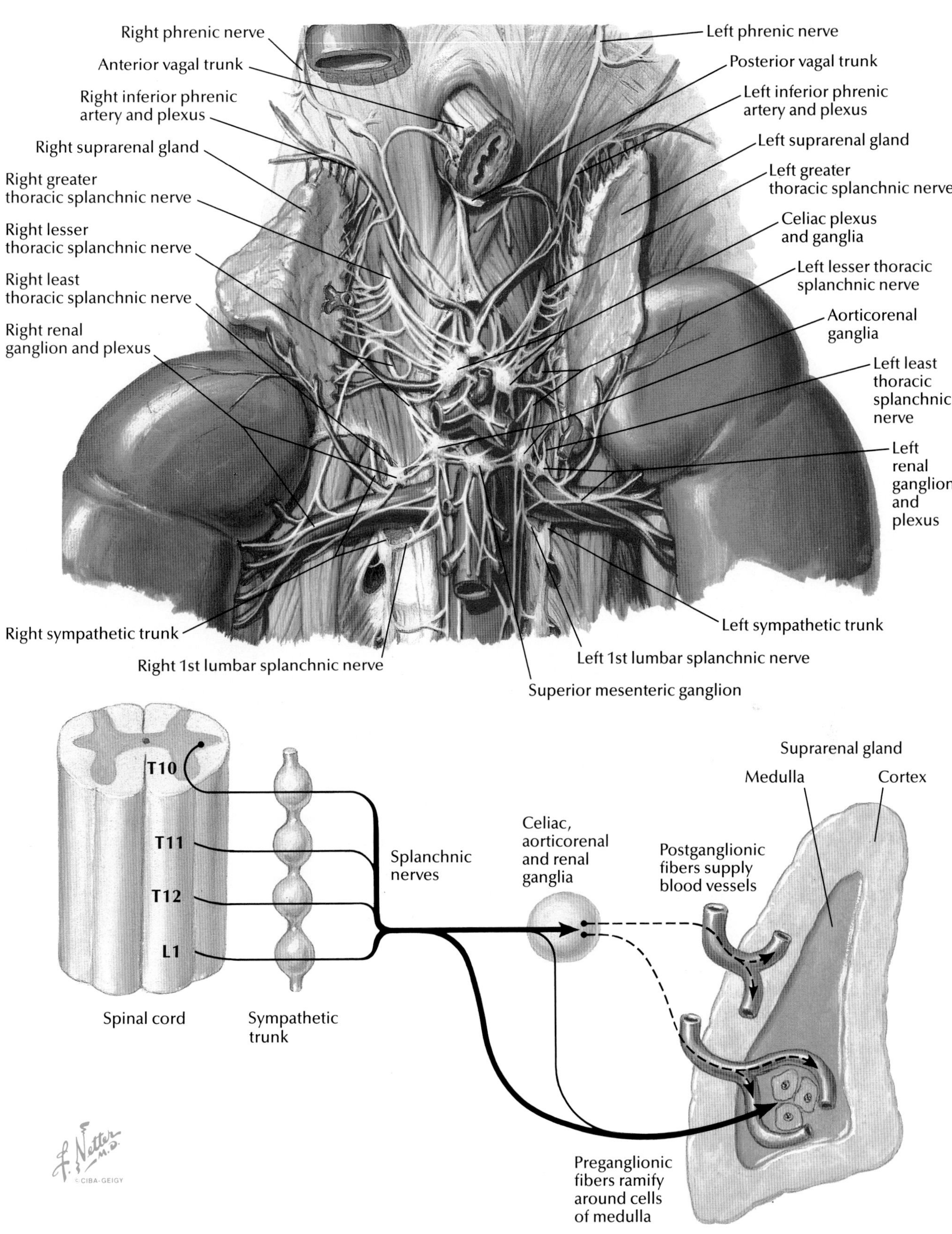

Right phrenic nerve

Anterior vagal trunk

Right inferior phrenic artery and plexus

Right suprarenal gland

Right greater thoracic splanchnic nerve

Right lesser thoracic splanchnic nerve

Right least thoracic splanchnic nerve

Right renal ganglion and plexus

Left phrenic nerve

Posterior vagal trunk

Left inferior phrenic artery and plexus

Left suprarenal gland

Left greater thoracic splanchnic nerve

Celiac plexus and ganglia

Left lesser thoracic splanchnic nerve

Aorticorenal ganglia

Left least thoracic splanchnic nerve

Left renal ganglion and plexus

Right sympathetic trunk

Right 1st lumbar splanchnic nerve

Left 1st lumbar splanchnic nerve

Superior mesenteric ganglion

Left sympathetic trunk

T10

T11

T12

L1

Spinal cord

Sympathetic trunk

Splanchnic nerves

Celiac, aorticorenal and renal ganglia

Postganglionic fibers supply blood vessels

Suprarenal gland

Medulla

Cortex

Preganglionic fibers ramify around cells of medulla

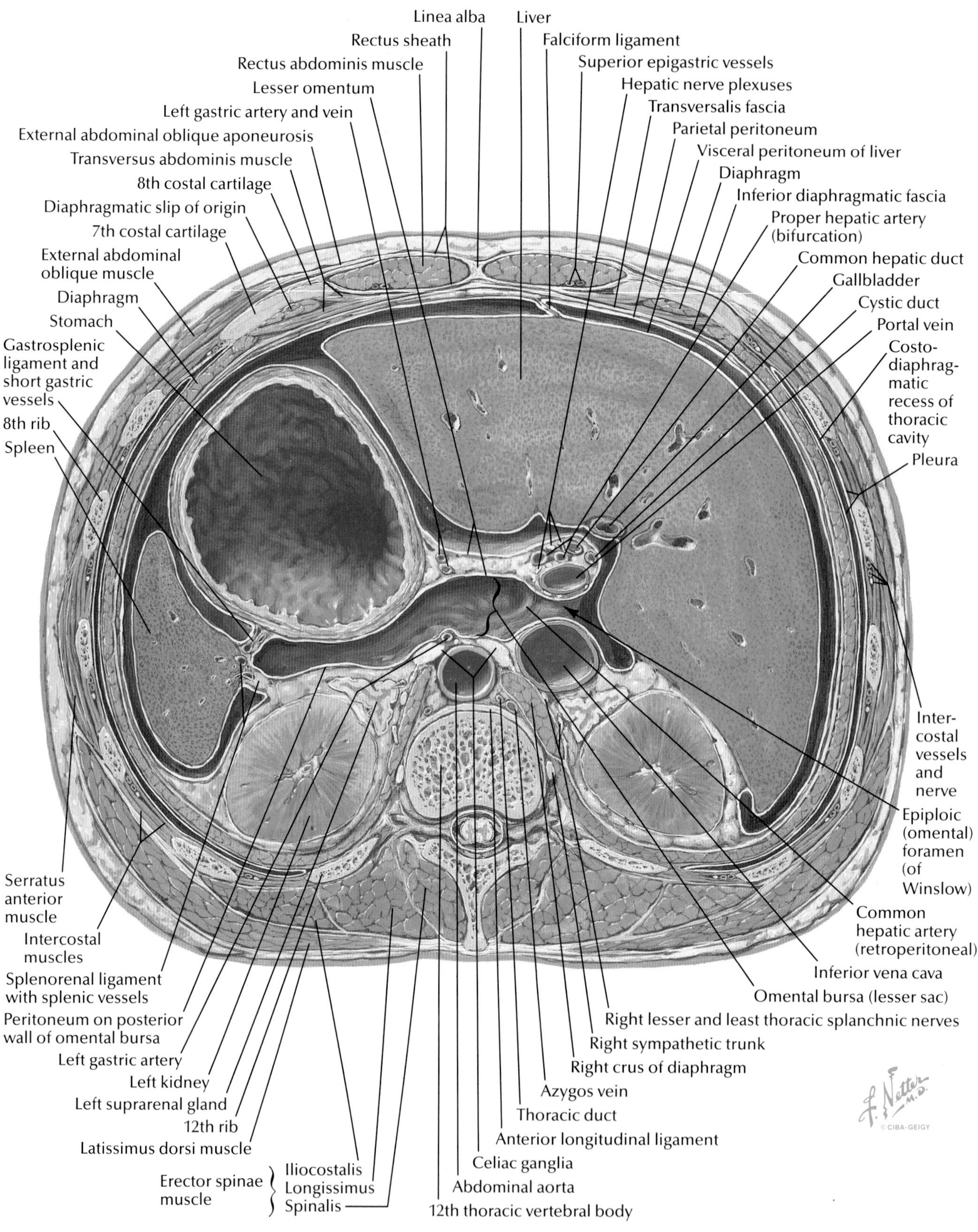

Linea alba
Rectus sheath
Rectus abdominis muscle
Lesser omentum
Left gastric artery and vein
External abdominal oblique aponeurosis
Transversus abdominis muscle
8th costal cartilage
Diaphragmatic slip of origin
7th costal cartilage
External abdominal oblique muscle
Diaphragm
Stomach
Gastrosplenic ligament and short gastric vessels
8th rib
Spleen

Liver
Falciform ligament
Superior epigastric vessels
Hepatic nerve plexuses
Transversalis fascia
Parietal peritoneum
Visceral peritoneum of liver
Diaphragm
Inferior diaphragmatic fascia
Proper hepatic artery (bifurcation)
Common hepatic duct
Gallbladder
Cystic duct
Portal vein
Costo-diaphragmatic recess of thoracic cavity
Pleura

Inter-costal vessels and nerve
Epiploic (omental) foramen (of Winslow)
Common hepatic artery (retroperitoneal)
Inferior vena cava
Omental bursa (lesser sac)
Right lesser and least thoracic splanchnic nerves
Right sympathetic trunk
Right crus of diaphragm
Azygos vein
Thoracic duct
Anterior longitudinal ligament
Celiac ganglia
Abdominal aorta
12th thoracic vertebral body

Serratus anterior muscle
Intercostal muscles
Splenorenal ligament with splenic vessels
Peritoneum on posterior wall of omental bursa
Left gastric artery
Left kidney
Left suprarenal gland
12th rib
Latissimus dorsi muscle
Erector spinae muscle { Iliocostalis Longissimus Spinalis

PLATE 331

ABDOMEN

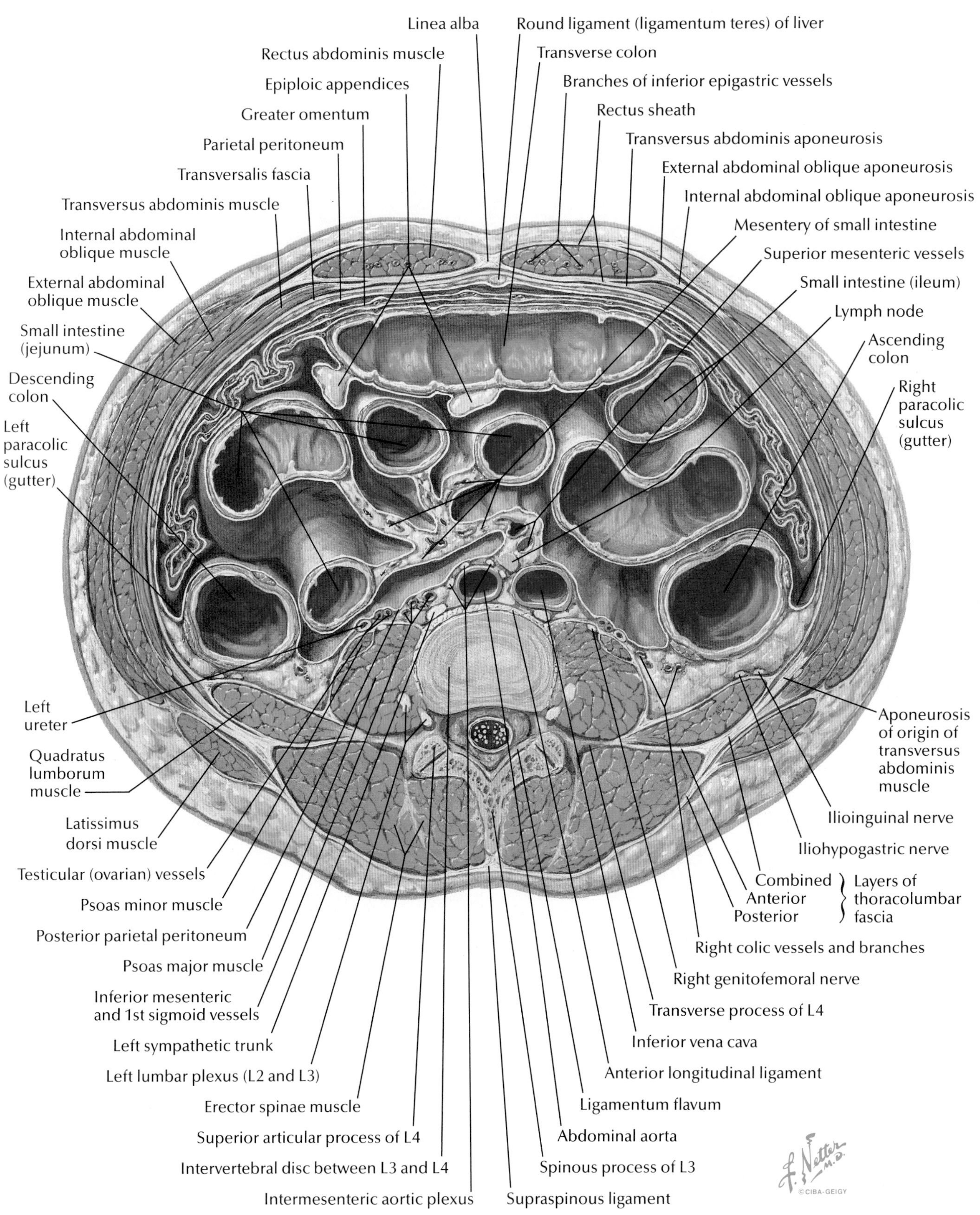

Linea alba

Rectus abdominis muscle

Epiploic appendices

Greater omentum

Parietal peritoneum

Transversalis fascia

Transversus abdominis muscle

Internal abdominal oblique muscle

External abdominal oblique muscle

Small intestine (jejunum)

Descending colon

Left paracolic sulcus (gutter)

Left ureter

Quadratus lumborum muscle

Latissimus dorsi muscle

Testicular (ovarian) vessels

Psoas minor muscle

Posterior parietal peritoneum

Psoas major muscle

Inferior mesenteric and 1st sigmoid vessels

Left sympathetic trunk

Left lumbar plexus (L2 and L3)

Erector spinae muscle

Superior articular process of L4

Intervertebral disc between L3 and L4

Intermesenteric aortic plexus

Round ligament (ligamentum teres) of liver

Transverse colon

Branches of inferior epigastric vessels

Rectus sheath

Transversus abdominis aponeurosis

External abdominal oblique aponeurosis

Internal abdominal oblique aponeurosis

Mesentery of small intestine

Superior mesenteric vessels

Small intestine (ileum)

Lymph node

Ascending colon

Right paracolic sulcus (gutter)

Aponeurosis of origin of transversus abdominis muscle

Ilioinguinal nerve

Iliohypogastric nerve

Combined } Layers of
Anterior } thoracolumbar
Posterior } fascia

Right colic vessels and branches

Right genitofemoral nerve

Transverse process of L4

Inferior vena cava

Anterior longitudinal ligament

Ligamentum flavum

Abdominal aorta

Spinous process of L3

Supraspinous ligament

f. Netter M.D.

©CIBA-GEIGY

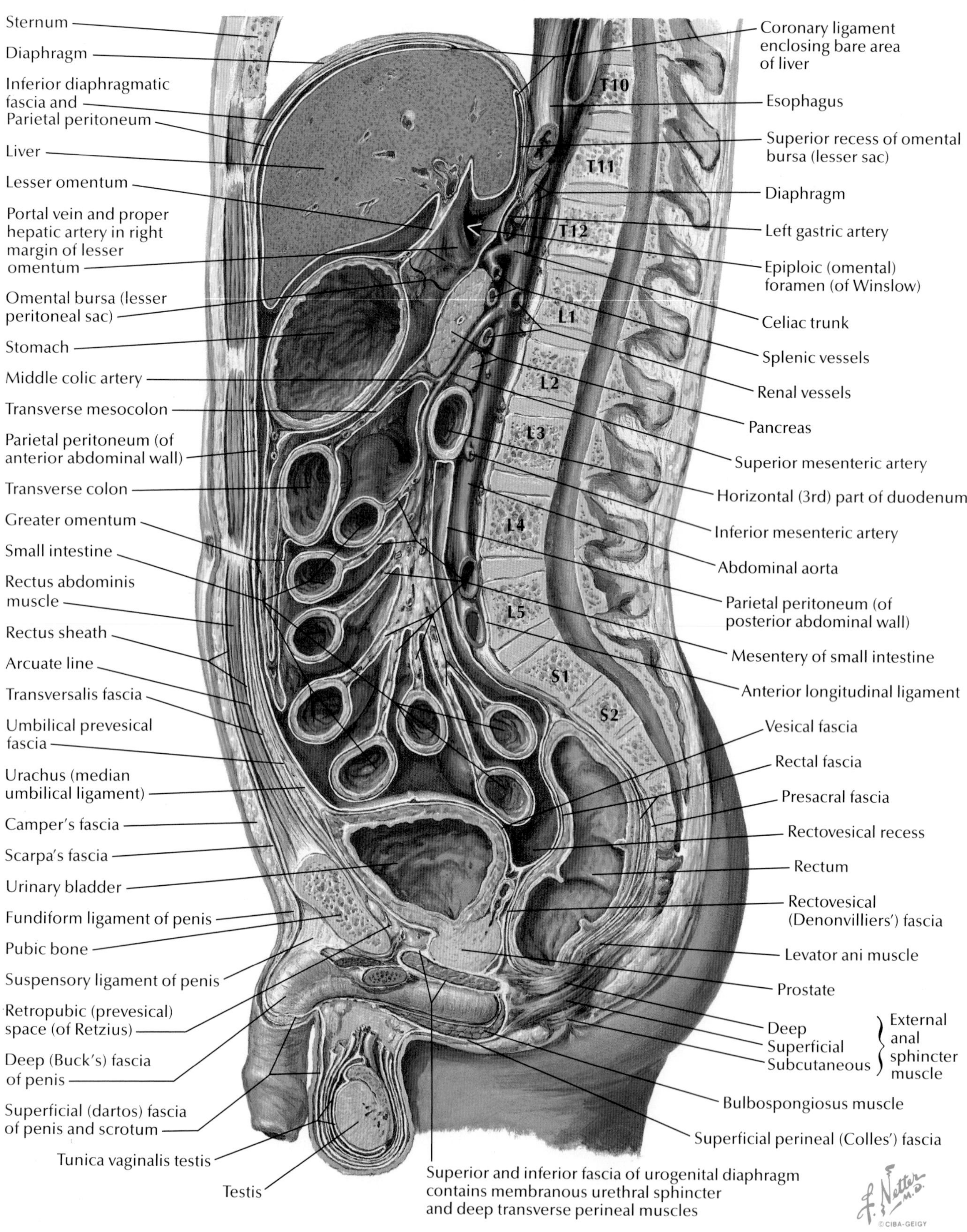

Sternum

Diaphragm

Inferior diaphragmatic fascia and Parietal peritoneum

Liver

Lesser omentum

Portal vein and proper hepatic artery in right margin of lesser omentum

Omental bursa (lesser peritoneal sac)

Stomach

Middle colic artery

Transverse mesocolon

Parietal peritoneum (of anterior abdominal wall)

Transverse colon

Greater omentum

Small intestine

Rectus abdominis muscle

Rectus sheath

Arcuate line

Transversalis fascia

Umbilical prevesical fascia

Urachus (median umbilical ligament)

Camper's fascia

Scarpa's fascia

Urinary bladder

Fundiform ligament of penis

Pubic bone

Suspensory ligament of penis

Retropubic (prevesical) space (of Retzius)

Deep (Buck's) fascia of penis

Superficial (dartos) fascia of penis and scrotum

Tunica vaginalis testis

Testis

Coronary ligament enclosing bare area of liver

Esophagus

Superior recess of omental bursa (lesser sac)

Diaphragm

Left gastric artery

Epiploic (omental) foramen (of Winslow)

Celiac trunk

Splenic vessels

Renal vessels

Pancreas

Superior mesenteric artery

Horizontal (3rd) part of duodenum

Inferior mesenteric artery

Abdominal aorta

Parietal peritoneum (of posterior abdominal wall)

Mesentery of small intestine

Anterior longitudinal ligament

Vesical fascia

Rectal fascia

Presacral fascia

Rectovesical recess

Rectum

Rectovesical (Denonvilliers') fascia

Levator ani muscle

Prostate

Deep
Superficial
Subcutaneous } External anal sphincter muscle

Bulbospongiosus muscle

Superficial perineal (Colles') fascia

T 10

T 11

T 12

L1

L2

L3

L4

L5

S1

S2

Superior and inferior fascia of urogenital diaphragm contains membranous urethral sphincter and deep transverse perineal muscles

PLATE 333

ABDOMEN

Section V

PELVIS AND PERINEUM

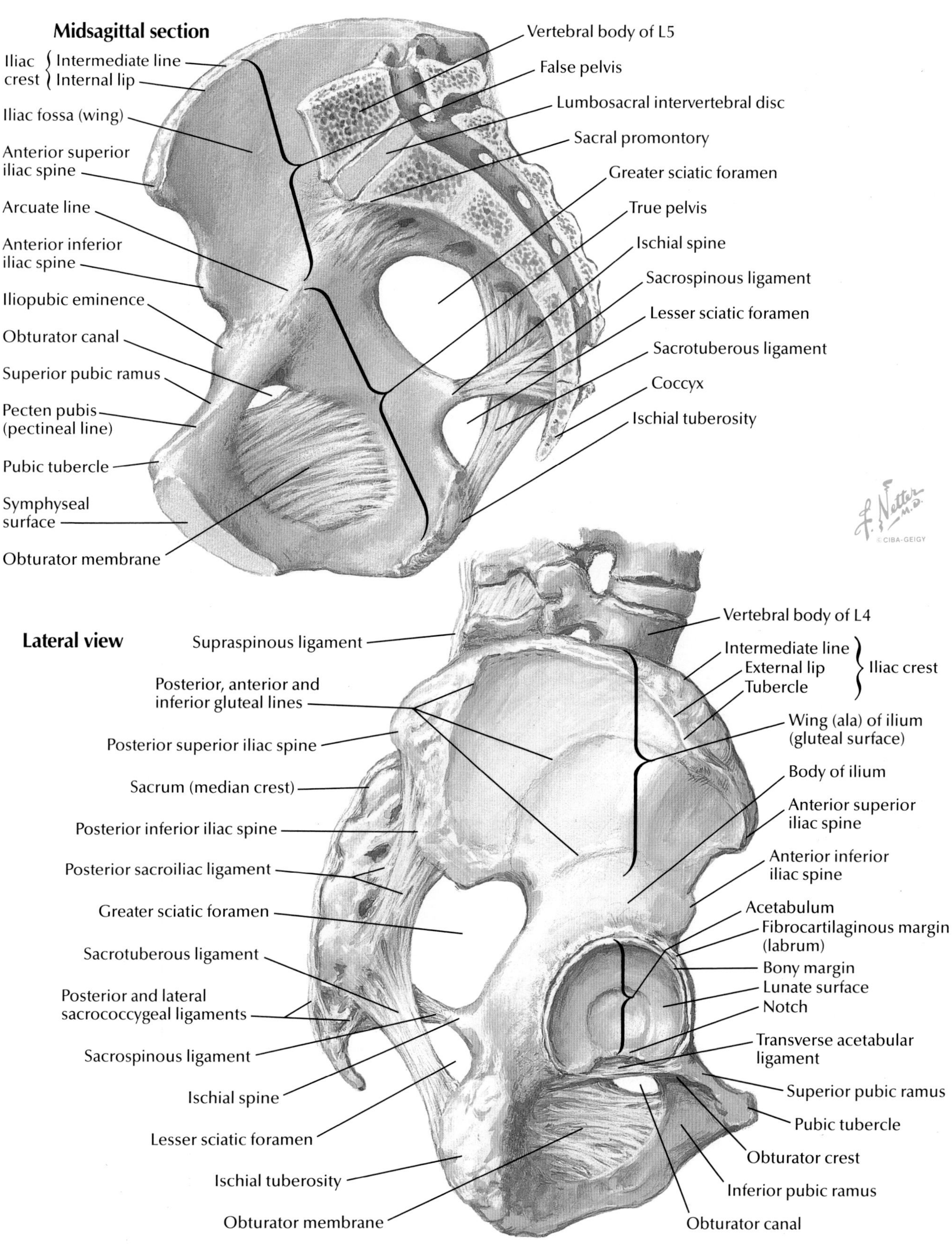

Midsagittal section

Iliac crest { Intermediate line
Iliac crest { Internal lip

Iliac fossa (wing)

Anterior superior iliac spine

Arcuate line

Anterior inferior iliac spine

Iliopubic eminence

Obturator canal

Superior pubic ramus

Pecten pubis (pectineal line)

Pubic tubercle

Symphyseal surface

Obturator membrane

Vertebral body of L5

False pelvis

Lumbosacral intervertebral disc

Sacral promontory

Greater sciatic foramen

True pelvis

Ischial spine

Sacrospinous ligament

Lesser sciatic foramen

Sacrotuberous ligament

Coccyx

Ischial tuberosity

Lateral view

Supraspinous ligament

Posterior, anterior and inferior gluteal lines

Posterior superior iliac spine

Sacrum (median crest)

Posterior inferior iliac spine

Posterior sacroiliac ligament

Greater sciatic foramen

Sacrotuberous ligament

Posterior and lateral sacrococcygeal ligaments

Sacrospinous ligament

Ischial spine

Lesser sciatic foramen

Ischial tuberosity

Obturator membrane

Vertebral body of L4

Intermediate line }
External lip } Iliac crest
Tubercle }

Wing (ala) of ilium (gluteal surface)

Body of ilium

Anterior superior iliac spine

Anterior inferior iliac spine

Acetabulum

Fibrocartilaginous margin (labrum)

Bony margin

Lunate surface

Notch

Transverse acetabular ligament

Superior pubic ramus

Pubic tubercle

Obturator crest

Inferior pubic ramus

Obturator canal

SEE ALSO PLATE 145

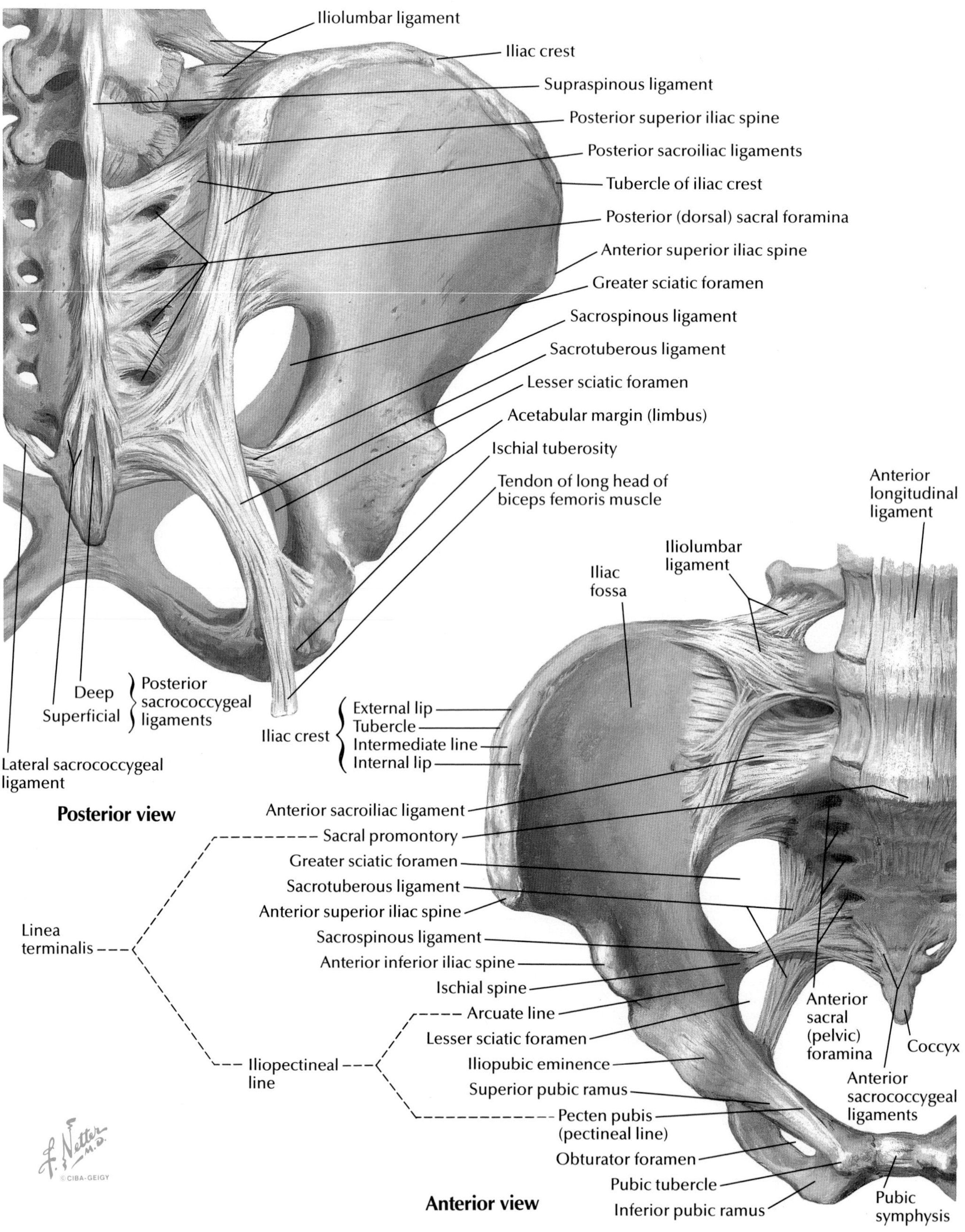

Iliolumbar ligament

Iliac crest

Supraspinous ligament

Posterior superior iliac spine

Posterior sacroiliac ligaments

Tubercle of iliac crest

Posterior (dorsal) sacral foramina

Anterior superior iliac spine

Greater sciatic foramen

Sacrospinous ligament

Sacrotuberous ligament

Lesser sciatic foramen

Acetabular margin (limbus)

Ischial tuberosity

Tendon of long head of biceps femoris muscle

Deep / Superficial } Posterior sacrococcygeal ligaments

Iliac crest {

Lateral sacrococcygeal ligament

Posterior view

Anterior longitudinal ligament

Iliac fossa

Iliolumbar ligament

External lip
Tubercle
Intermediate line
Internal lip

Anterior sacroiliac ligament

Sacral promontory

Greater sciatic foramen

Sacrotuberous ligament

Anterior superior iliac spine

Sacrospinous ligament

Anterior inferior iliac spine

Ischial spine

Arcuate line

Lesser sciatic foramen

Iliopubic eminence

Superior pubic ramus

Pecten pubis (pectineal line)

Obturator foramen

Pubic tubercle

Inferior pubic ramus

Anterior sacral (pelvic) foramina

Coccyx

Anterior sacrococcygeal ligaments

Pubic symphysis

Linea terminalis

Iliopectineal line

Anterior view

PLATE 335   **PELVIS AND PERINEUM**

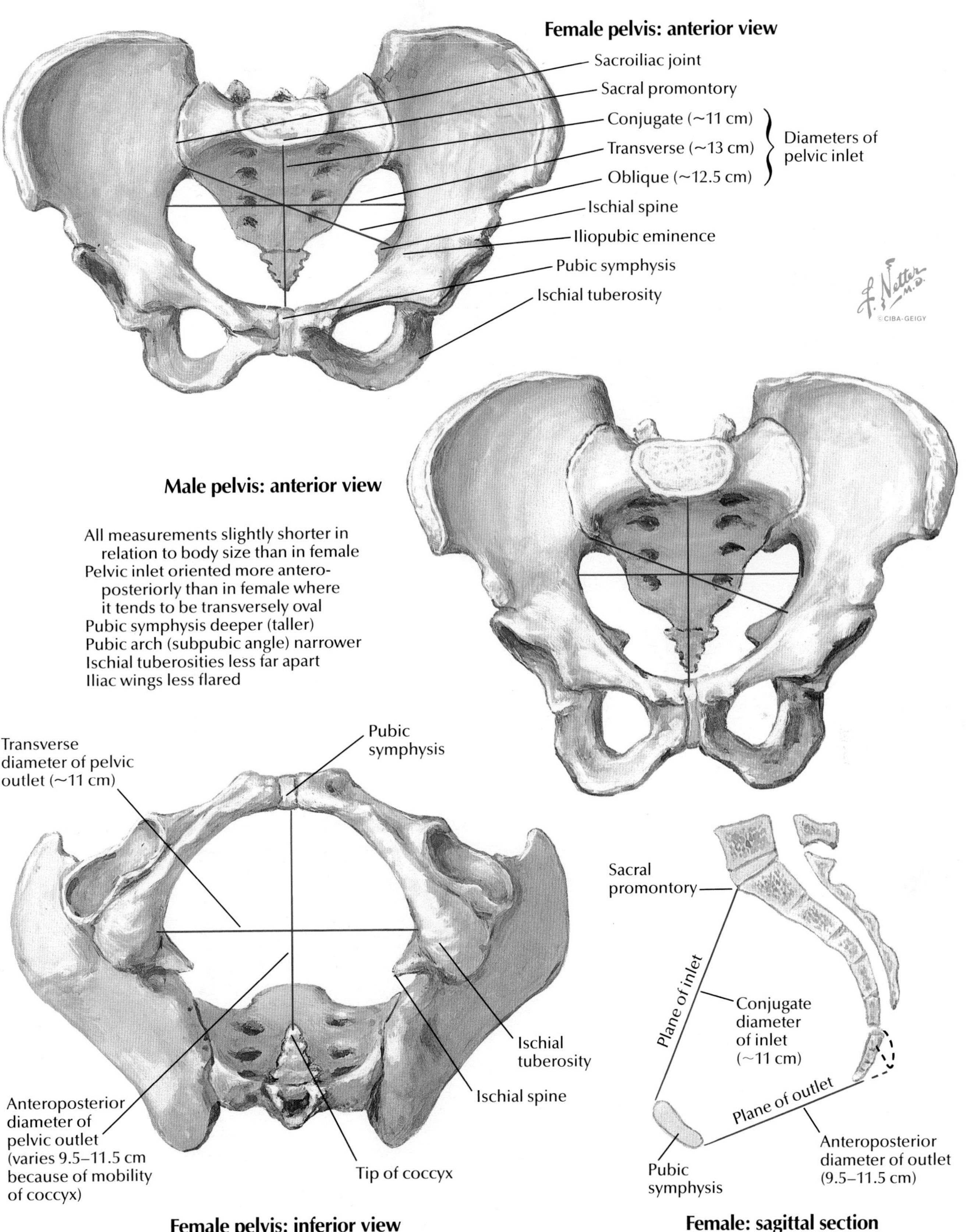

Female pelvis: anterior view

- Sacroiliac joint
- Sacral promontory
- Conjugate (~11 cm) ⎫
- Transverse (~13 cm) ⎬ Diameters of pelvic inlet
- Oblique (~12.5 cm) ⎭
- Ischial spine
- Iliopubic eminence
- Pubic symphysis
- Ischial tuberosity

Male pelvis: anterior view

All measurements slightly shorter in
  relation to body size than in female
Pelvic inlet oriented more antero-
  posteriorly than in female where
  it tends to be transversely oval
Pubic symphysis deeper (taller)
Pubic arch (subpubic angle) narrower
Ischial tuberosities less far apart
Iliac wings less flared

Transverse
diameter of pelvic
outlet (~11 cm)

Pubic
symphysis

Ischial
tuberosity

Ischial spine

Anteroposterior
diameter of
pelvic outlet
(varies 9.5–11.5 cm
because of mobility
of coccyx)

Tip of coccyx

Female pelvis: inferior view

Sacral
promontory

Plane of inlet

Conjugate
diameter
of inlet
(~11 cm)

Plane of outlet

Pubic
symphysis

Anteroposterior
diameter of outlet
(9.5–11.5 cm)

Female: sagittal section

Pelvic Diaphragm: Female

SEE ALSO PLATES 246, 347, 349, 368

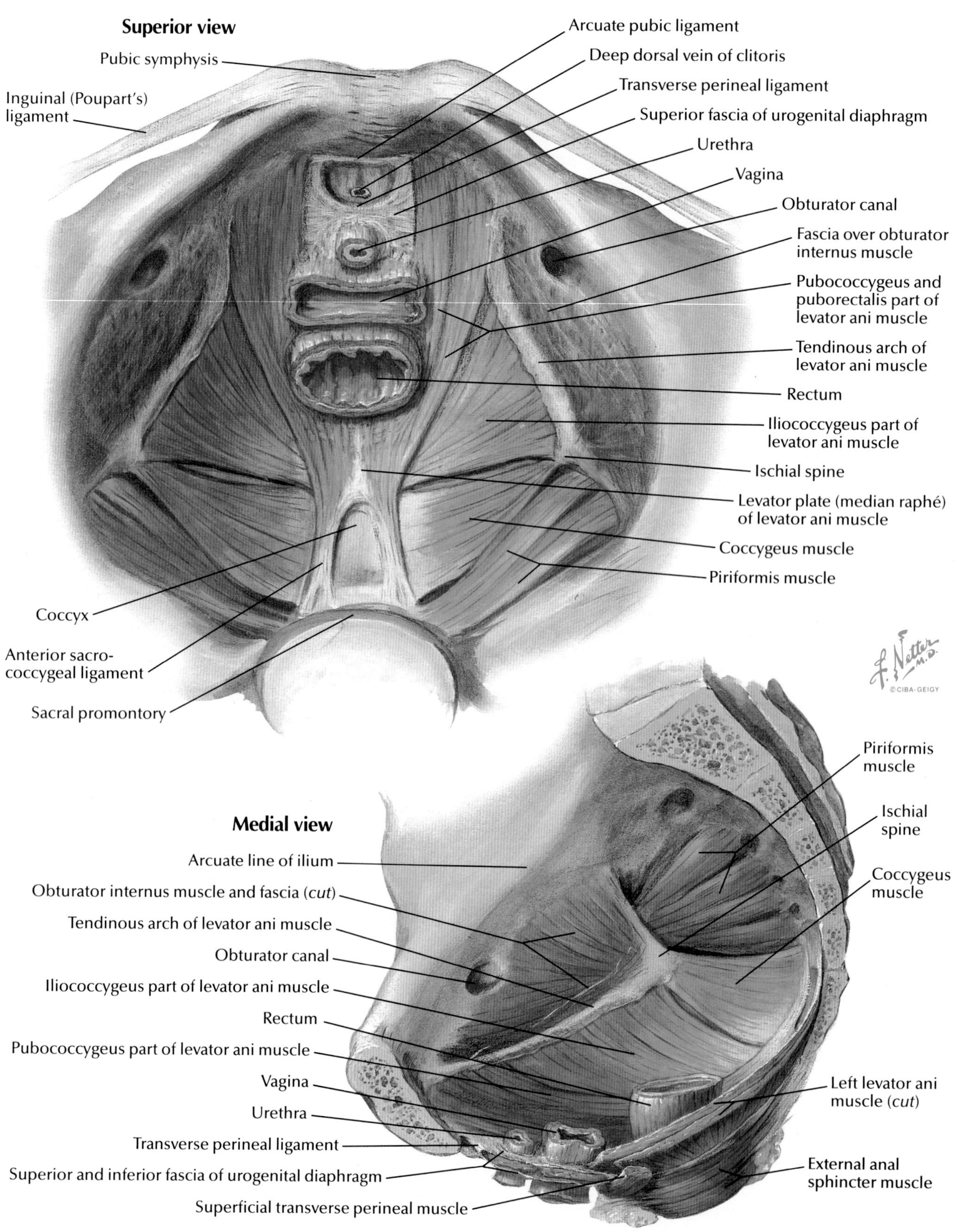

Superior view

Pubic symphysis
Inguinal (Poupart's) ligament
Arcuate pubic ligament
Deep dorsal vein of clitoris
Transverse perineal ligament
Superior fascia of urogenital diaphragm
Urethra
Vagina
Obturator canal
Fascia over obturator internus muscle
Pubococcygeus and puborectalis part of levator ani muscle
Tendinous arch of levator ani muscle
Rectum
Iliococcygeus part of levator ani muscle
Ischial spine
Levator plate (median raphé) of levator ani muscle
Coccygeus muscle
Piriformis muscle
Coccyx
Anterior sacro-coccygeal ligament
Sacral promontory

Medial view

Arcuate line of ilium
Obturator internus muscle and fascia (cut)
Tendinous arch of levator ani muscle
Obturator canal
Iliococcygeus part of levator ani muscle
Rectum
Pubococcygeus part of levator ani muscle
Vagina
Urethra
Transverse perineal ligament
Superior and inferior fascia of urogenital diaphragm
Superficial transverse perineal muscle
Piriformis muscle
Ischial spine
Coccygeus muscle
Left levator ani muscle (cut)
External anal sphincter muscle

PLATE 337

PELVIS AND PERINEUM

FOR UROGENITAL DIAPHRAGM SEE PLATE 356

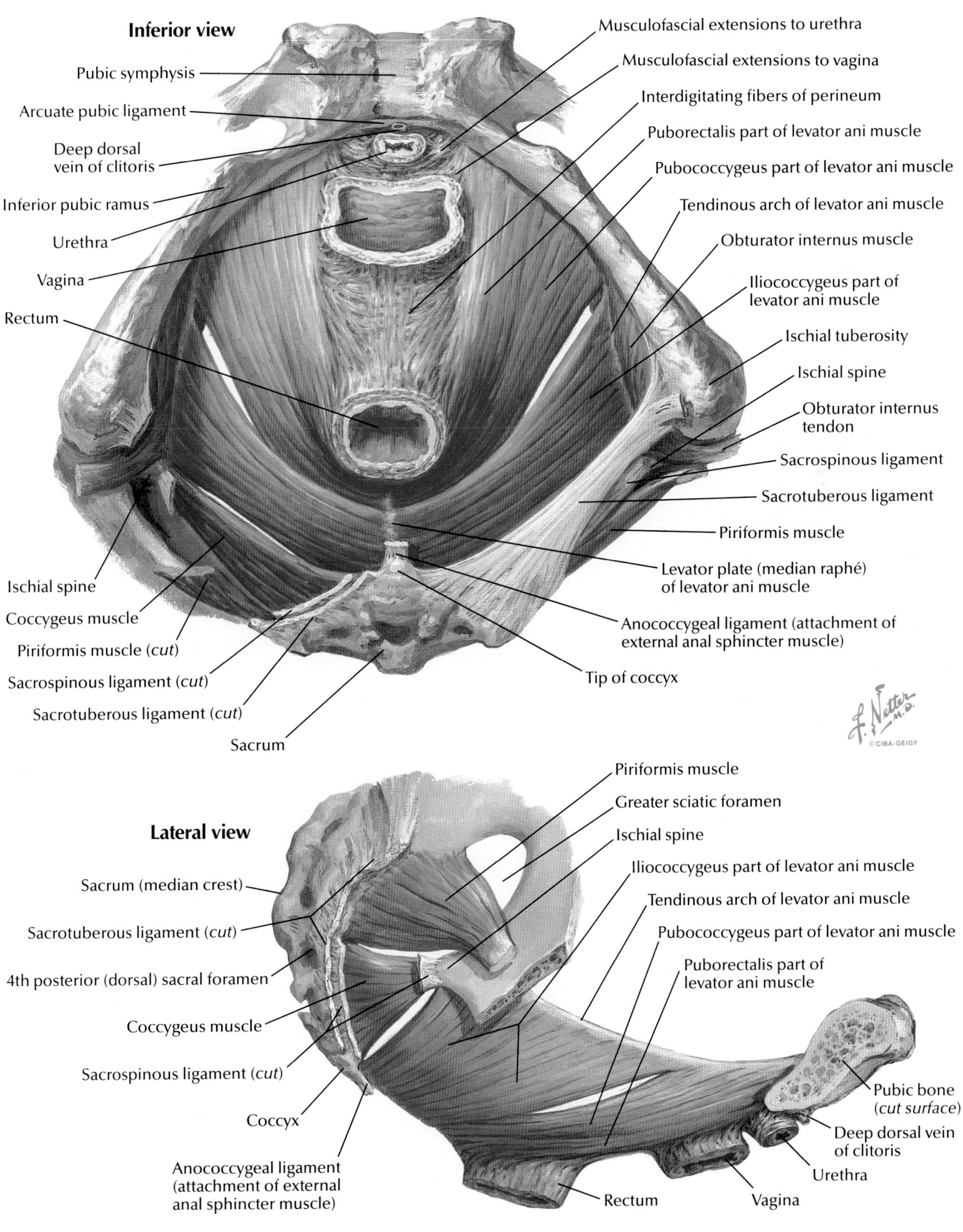

Inferior view

Pubic symphysis

Arcuate pubic ligament

Deep dorsal vein of clitoris

Inferior pubic ramus

Urethra

Vagina

Rectum

Ischial spine

Coccygeus muscle

Piriformis muscle (*cut*)

Sacrospinous ligament (*cut*)

Sacrotuberous ligament (*cut*)

Sacrum

Musculofascial extensions to urethra

Musculofascial extensions to vagina

Interdigitating fibers of perineum

Puborectalis part of levator ani muscle

Pubococcygeus part of levator ani muscle

Tendinous arch of levator ani muscle

Obturator internus muscle

Iliococcygeus part of levator ani muscle

Ischial tuberosity

Ischial spine

Obturator internus tendon

Sacrospinous ligament

Sacrotuberous ligament

Piriformis muscle

Levator plate (median raphé) of levator ani muscle

Anococcygeal ligament (attachment of external anal sphincter muscle)

Tip of coccyx

Lateral view

Sacrum (median crest)

Sacrotuberous ligament (*cut*)

4th posterior (dorsal) sacral foramen

Coccygeus muscle

Sacrospinous ligament (*cut*)

Coccyx

Anococcygeal ligament (attachment of external anal sphincter muscle)

Piriformis muscle

Greater sciatic foramen

Ischial spine

Iliococcygeus part of levator ani muscle

Tendinous arch of levator ani muscle

Pubococcygeus part of levator ani muscle

Puborectalis part of levator ani muscle

Pubic bone (*cut surface*)

Deep dorsal vein of clitoris

Urethra

Vagina

Rectum

Pelvic Diaphragm: Male

SEE ALSO PLATES 246, 347, 368

Superior view (*viscera removed*)

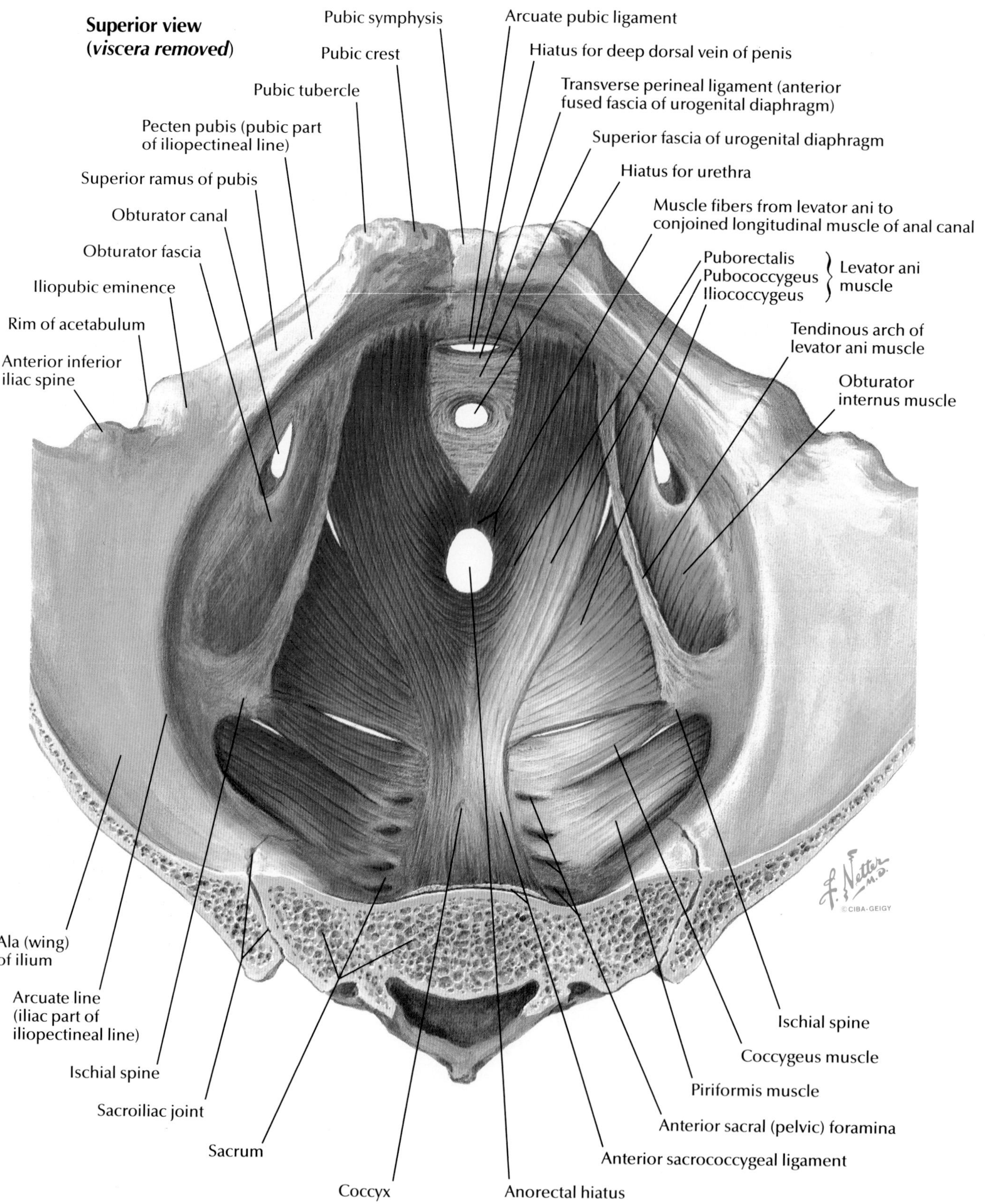

Pubic symphysis

Pubic crest

Pubic tubercle

Pecten pubis (pubic part of iliopectineal line)

Superior ramus of pubis

Obturator canal

Obturator fascia

Iliopubic eminence

Rim of acetabulum

Anterior inferior iliac spine

Arcuate pubic ligament

Hiatus for deep dorsal vein of penis

Transverse perineal ligament (anterior fused fascia of urogenital diaphragm)

Superior fascia of urogenital diaphragm

Hiatus for urethra

Muscle fibers from levator ani to conjoined longitudinal muscle of anal canal

Puborectalis

Pubococcygeus

Iliococcygeus

} Levator ani muscle

Tendinous arch of levator ani muscle

Obturator internus muscle

Ala (wing) of ilium

Arcuate line (iliac part of iliopectineal line)

Ischial spine

Sacroiliac joint

Sacrum

Coccyx

Anorectal hiatus

Anterior sacrococcygeal ligament

Anterior sacral (pelvic) foramina

Piriformis muscle

Coccygeus muscle

Ischial spine

PLATE 339

PELVIS AND PERINEUM

Inferior view

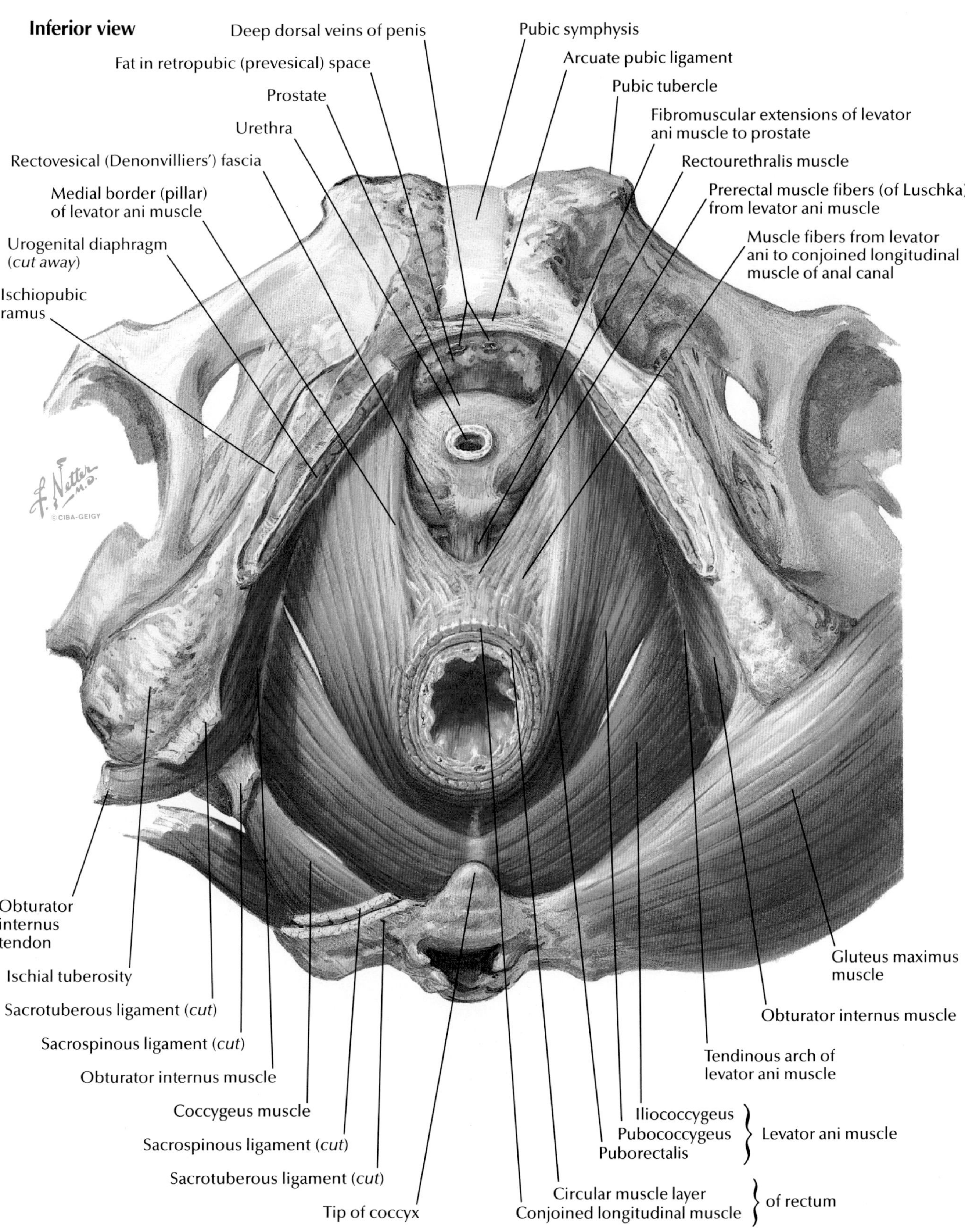

Deep dorsal veins of penis

Fat in retropubic (prevesical) space

Prostate

Urethra

Rectovesical (Denonvilliers') fascia

Medial border (pillar) of levator ani muscle

Urogenital diaphragm (*cut away*)

Ischiopubic ramus

Pubic symphysis

Arcuate pubic ligament

Pubic tubercle

Fibromuscular extensions of levator ani muscle to prostate

Rectourethralis muscle

Prerectal muscle fibers (of Luschka) from levator ani muscle

Muscle fibers from levator ani to conjoined longitudinal muscle of anal canal

Obturator internus tendon

Ischial tuberosity

Sacrotuberous ligament (*cut*)

Sacrospinous ligament (*cut*)

Obturator internus muscle

Coccygeus muscle

Sacrospinous ligament (*cut*)

Sacrotuberous ligament (*cut*)

Tip of coccyx

Gluteus maximus muscle

Obturator internus muscle

Tendinous arch of levator ani muscle

Iliococcygeus ⎫
Pubococcygeus ⎬ Levator ani muscle
Puborectalis ⎭

Circular muscle layer ⎫
Conjoined longitudinal muscle ⎬ of rectum

Pelvic Viscera and Perineum: Female

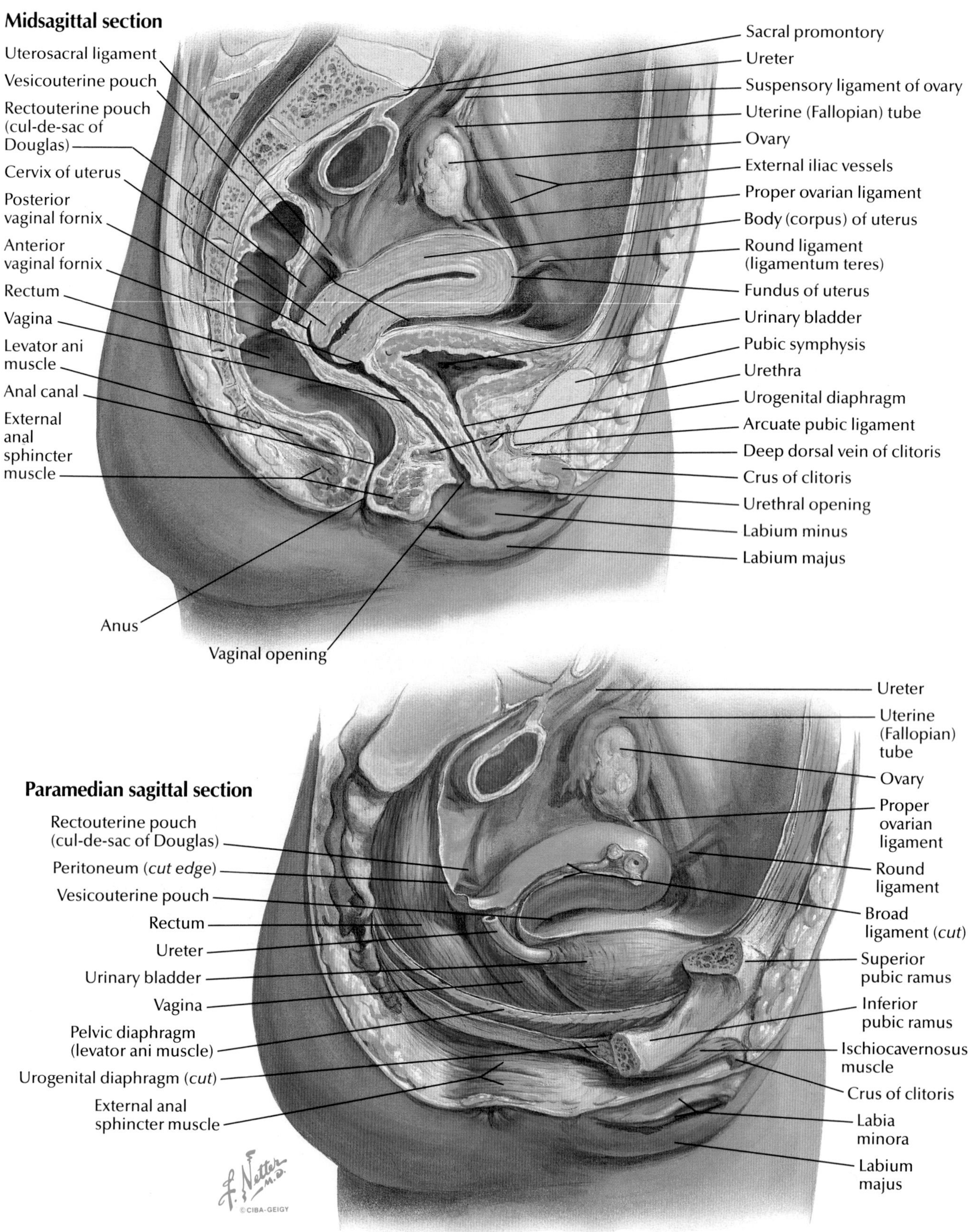

Midsagittal section

Uterosacral ligament
Vesicouterine pouch
Rectouterine pouch (cul-de-sac of Douglas)
Cervix of uterus
Posterior vaginal fornix
Anterior vaginal fornix
Rectum
Vagina
Levator ani muscle
Anal canal
External anal sphincter muscle
Anus
Vaginal opening

Sacral promontory
Ureter
Suspensory ligament of ovary
Uterine (Fallopian) tube
Ovary
External iliac vessels
Proper ovarian ligament
Body (corpus) of uterus
Round ligament (ligamentum teres)
Fundus of uterus
Urinary bladder
Pubic symphysis
Urethra
Urogenital diaphragm
Arcuate pubic ligament
Deep dorsal vein of clitoris
Crus of clitoris
Urethral opening
Labium minus
Labium majus

Paramedian sagittal section

Rectouterine pouch (cul-de-sac of Douglas)
Peritoneum (cut edge)
Vesicouterine pouch
Rectum
Ureter
Urinary bladder
Vagina
Pelvic diaphragm (levator ani muscle)
Urogenital diaphragm (cut)
External anal sphincter muscle

Ureter
Uterine (Fallopian) tube
Ovary
Proper ovarian ligament
Round ligament
Broad ligament (cut)
Superior pubic ramus
Inferior pubic ramus
Ischiocavernosus muscle
Crus of clitoris
Labia minora
Labium majus

PLATE 341

PELVIS AND PERINEUM

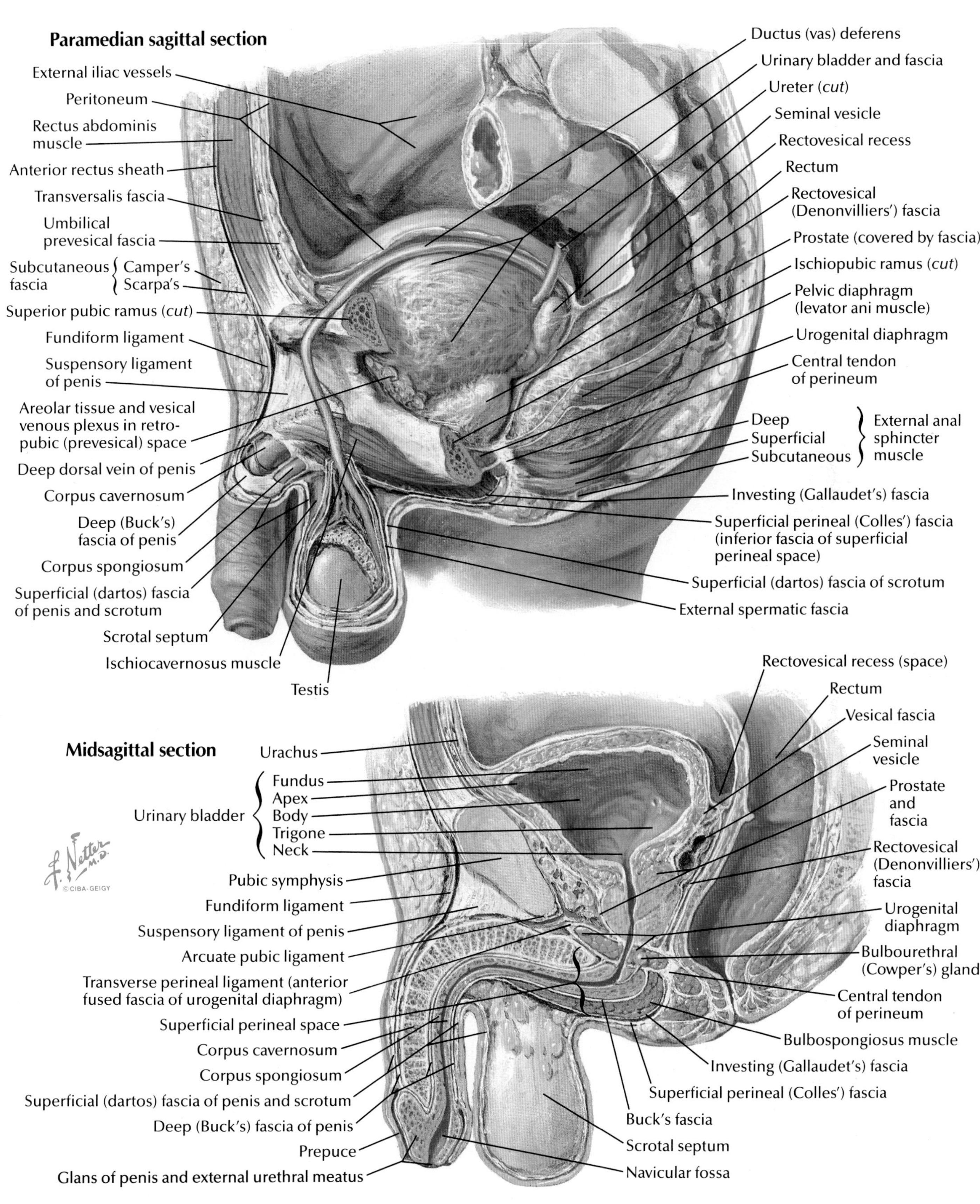

Paramedian sagittal section

External iliac vessels
Peritoneum
Rectus abdominis muscle
Anterior rectus sheath
Transversalis fascia
Umbilical prevesical fascia
Subcutaneous { Camper's fascia { Scarpa's
Superior pubic ramus (cut)
Fundiform ligament
Suspensory ligament of penis
Areolar tissue and vesical venous plexus in retro-pubic (prevesical) space
Deep dorsal vein of penis
Corpus cavernosum
Deep (Buck's) fascia of penis
Corpus spongiosum
Superficial (dartos) fascia of penis and scrotum
Scrotal septum
Ischiocavernosus muscle
Testis

Ductus (vas) deferens
Urinary bladder and fascia
Ureter (cut)
Seminal vesicle
Rectovesical recess
Rectum
Rectovesical (Denonvilliers') fascia
Prostate (covered by fascia)
Ischiopubic ramus (cut)
Pelvic diaphragm (levator ani muscle)
Urogenital diaphragm
Central tendon of perineum
Deep } External anal
Superficial } sphincter
Subcutaneous } muscle
Investing (Gallaudet's) fascia
Superficial perineal (Colles') fascia (inferior fascia of superficial perineal space)
Superficial (dartos) fascia of scrotum
External spermatic fascia

Midsagittal section

Urachus
Urinary bladder { Fundus { Apex { Body { Trigone { Neck
Pubic symphysis
Fundiform ligament
Suspensory ligament of penis
Arcuate pubic ligament
Transverse perineal ligament (anterior fused fascia of urogenital diaphragm)
Superficial perineal space
Corpus cavernosum
Corpus spongiosum
Superficial (dartos) fascia of penis and scrotum
Deep (Buck's) fascia of penis
Prepuce
Glans of penis and external urethral meatus

Rectovesical recess (space)
Rectum
Vesical fascia
Seminal vesicle
Prostate and fascia
Rectovesical (Denonvilliers') fascia
Urogenital diaphragm
Bulbourethral (Cowper's) gland
Central tendon of perineum
Bulbospongiosus muscle
Investing (Gallaudet's) fascia
Superficial perineal (Colles') fascia
Buck's fascia
Scrotal septum
Navicular fossa

f. Netter m.d.
©CIBA-GEIGY

Pelvic Contents: Female

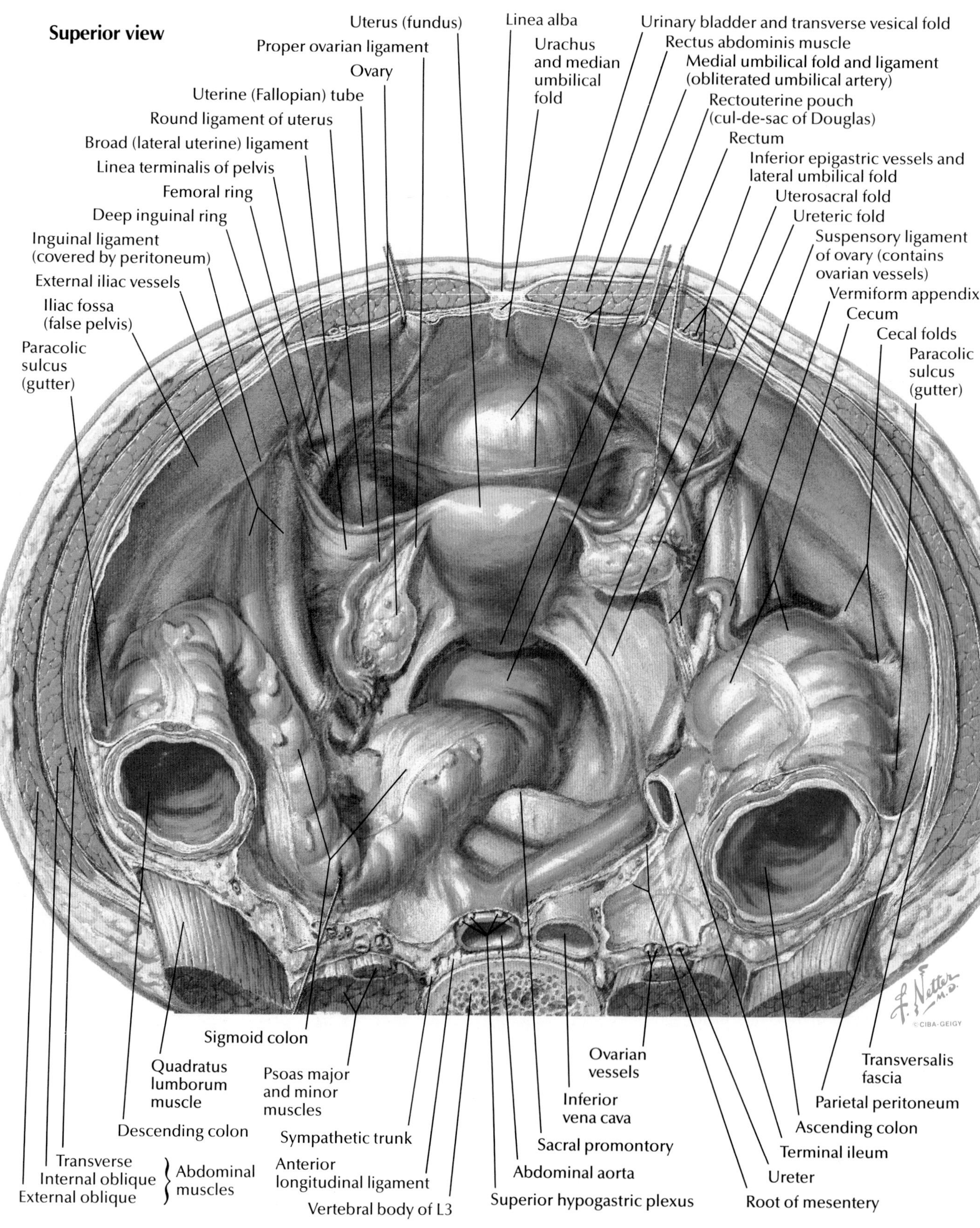

Superior view

Uterus (fundus)

Proper ovarian ligament

Ovary

Uterine (Fallopian) tube

Round ligament of uterus

Broad (lateral uterine) ligament

Linea terminalis of pelvis

Femoral ring

Deep inguinal ring

Inguinal ligament (covered by peritoneum)

External iliac vessels

Iliac fossa (false pelvis)

Paracolic sulcus (gutter)

Linea alba

Urachus and median umbilical fold

Urinary bladder and transverse vesical fold

Rectus abdominis muscle

Medial umbilical fold and ligament (obliterated umbilical artery)

Rectouterine pouch (cul-de-sac of Douglas)

Rectum

Inferior epigastric vessels and lateral umbilical fold

Uterosacral fold

Ureteric fold

Suspensory ligament of ovary (contains ovarian vessels)

Vermiform appendix

Cecum

Cecal folds

Paracolic sulcus (gutter)

Sigmoid colon

Quadratus lumborum muscle

Psoas major and minor muscles

Descending colon

Transverse
Internal oblique } Abdominal muscles
External oblique

Anterior longitudinal ligament

Sympathetic trunk

Vertebral body of L3

Ovarian vessels

Inferior vena cava

Sacral promontory

Abdominal aorta

Superior hypogastric plexus

Transversalis fascia

Parietal peritoneum

Ascending colon

Terminal ileum

Ureter

Root of mesentery

F. Netter M.D.

©CIBA-GEIGY

PLATE 343   **PELVIS AND PERINEUM**

Superior view

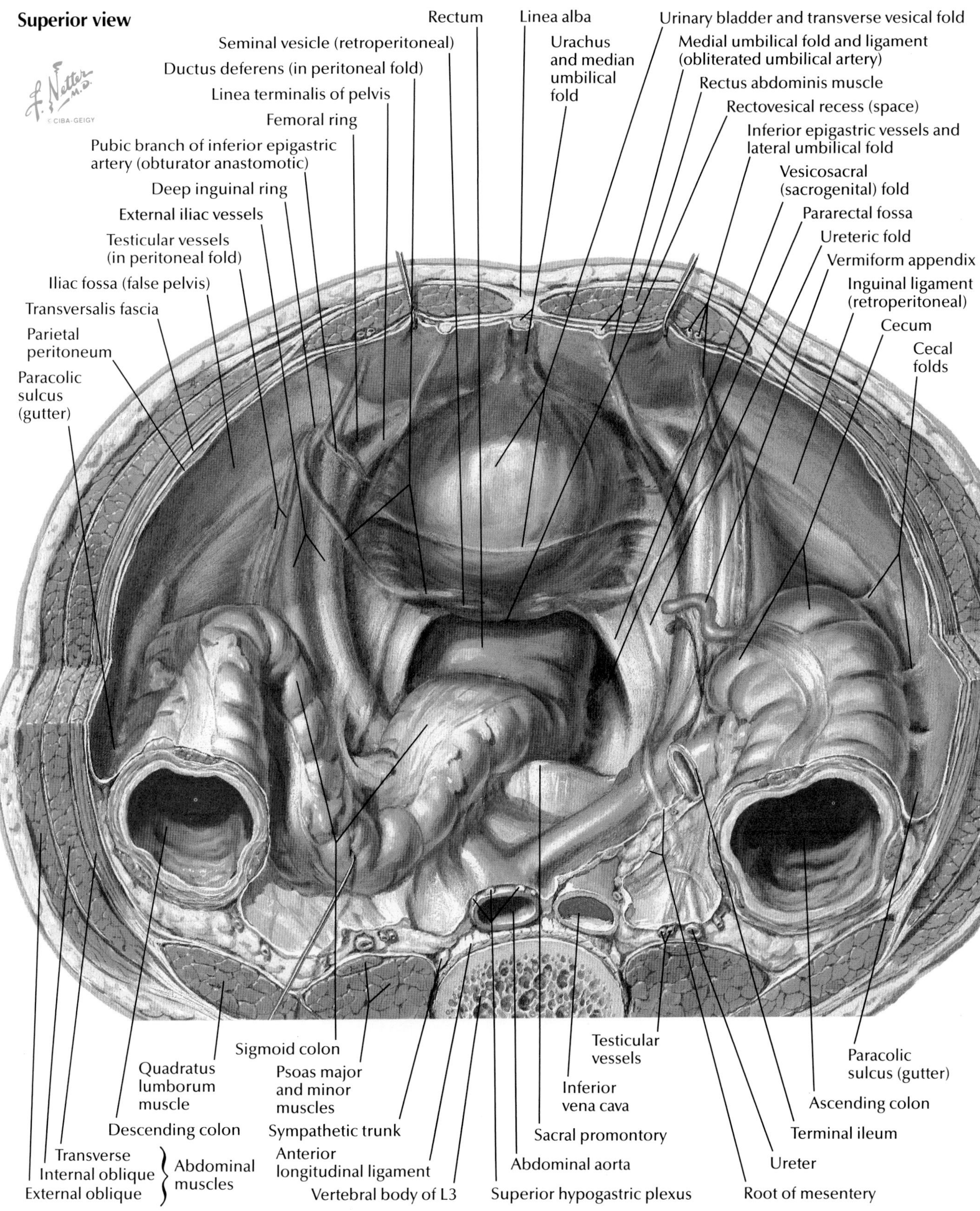

Rectum

Linea alba

Urinary bladder and transverse vesical fold

Seminal vesicle (retroperitoneal)

Urachus and median umbilical fold

Medial umbilical fold and ligament (obliterated umbilical artery)

Ductus deferens (in peritoneal fold)

Linea terminalis of pelvis

Rectus abdominis muscle

Femoral ring

Rectovesical recess (space)

Pubic branch of inferior epigastric artery (obturator anastomotic)

Inferior epigastric vessels and lateral umbilical fold

Deep inguinal ring

Vesicosacral (sacrogenital) fold

External iliac vessels

Pararectal fossa

Testicular vessels (in peritoneal fold)

Ureteric fold

Iliac fossa (false pelvis)

Vermiform appendix

Transversalis fascia

Inguinal ligament (retroperitoneal)

Parietal peritoneum

Cecum

Paracolic sulcus (gutter)

Cecal folds

Quadratus lumborum muscle

Sigmoid colon

Psoas major and minor muscles

Testicular vessels

Paracolic sulcus (gutter)

Descending colon

Sympathetic trunk

Inferior vena cava

Ascending colon

Transverse Internal oblique External oblique } Abdominal muscles

Anterior longitudinal ligament

Sacral promontory

Terminal ileum

Vertebral body of L3

Abdominal aorta

Ureter

Superior hypogastric plexus

Root of mesentery

Endopelvic Fascia and Spaces

Female: superior view

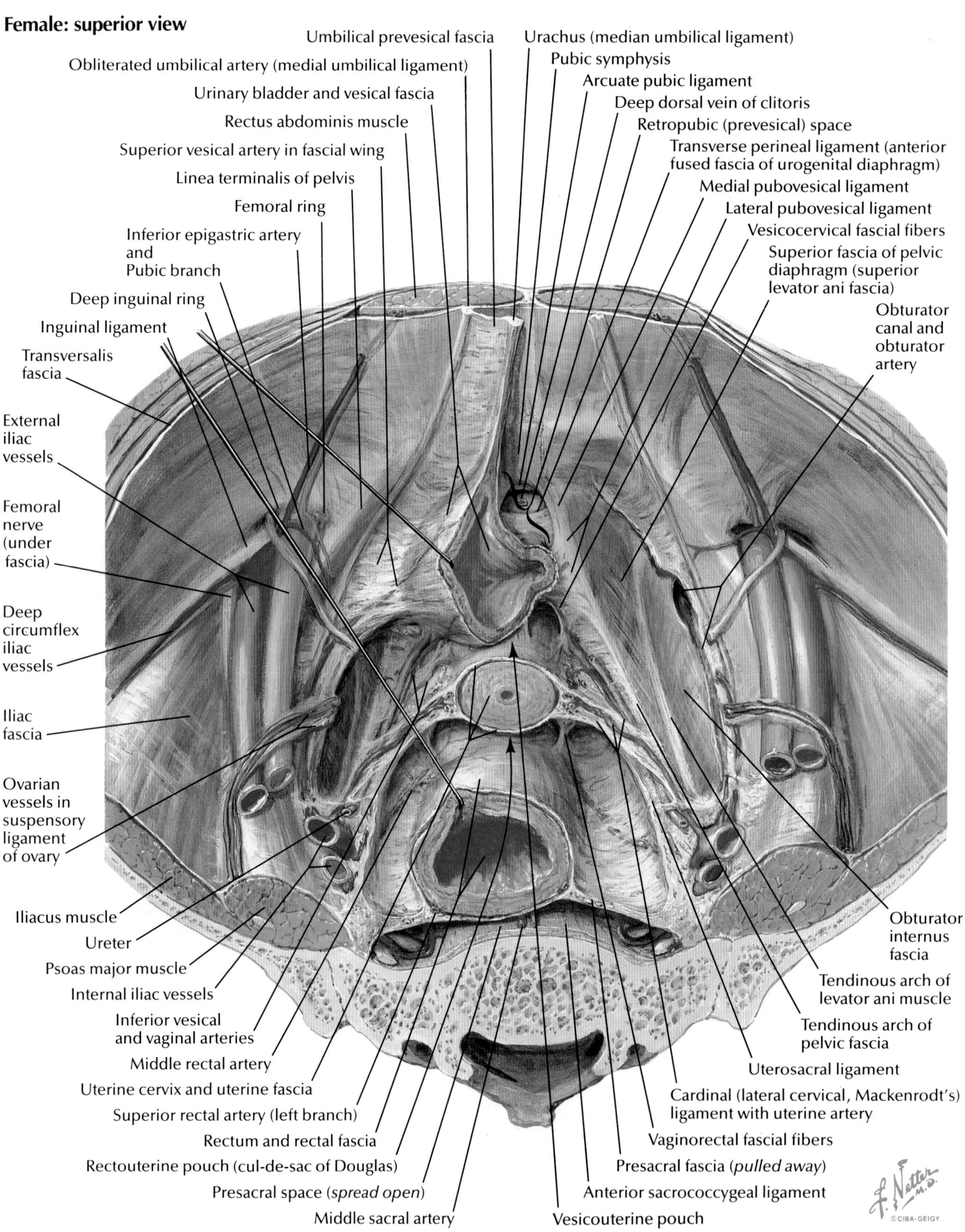

Umbilical prevesical fascia

Obliterated umbilical artery (medial umbilical ligament)

Urinary bladder and vesical fascia

Rectus abdominis muscle

Superior vesical artery in fascial wing

Linea terminalis of pelvis

Femoral ring

Inferior epigastric artery and Pubic branch

Deep inguinal ring

Inguinal ligament

Transversalis fascia

External iliac vessels

Femoral nerve (under fascia)

Deep circumflex iliac vessels

Iliac fascia

Ovarian vessels in suspensory ligament of ovary

Iliacus muscle

Ureter

Psoas major muscle

Internal iliac vessels

Inferior vesical and vaginal arteries

Middle rectal artery

Uterine cervix and uterine fascia

Superior rectal artery (left branch)

Rectum and rectal fascia

Rectouterine pouch (cul-de-sac of Douglas)

Presacral space (*spread open*)

Middle sacral artery

Urachus (median umbilical ligament)

Pubic symphysis

Arcuate pubic ligament

Deep dorsal vein of clitoris

Retropubic (prevesical) space

Transverse perineal ligament (anterior fused fascia of urogenital diaphragm)

Medial pubovesical ligament

Lateral pubovesical ligament

Vesicocervical fascial fibers

Superior fascia of pelvic diaphragm (superior levator ani fascia)

Obturator canal and obturator artery

Obturator internus fascia

Tendinous arch of levator ani muscle

Tendinous arch of pelvic fascia

Uterosacral ligament

Cardinal (lateral cervical, Mackenrodt's) ligament with uterine artery

Vaginorectal fascial fibers

Presacral fascia (*pulled away*)

Anterior sacrococcygeal ligament

Vesicouterine pouch

PLATE 345

PELVIS AND PERINEUM

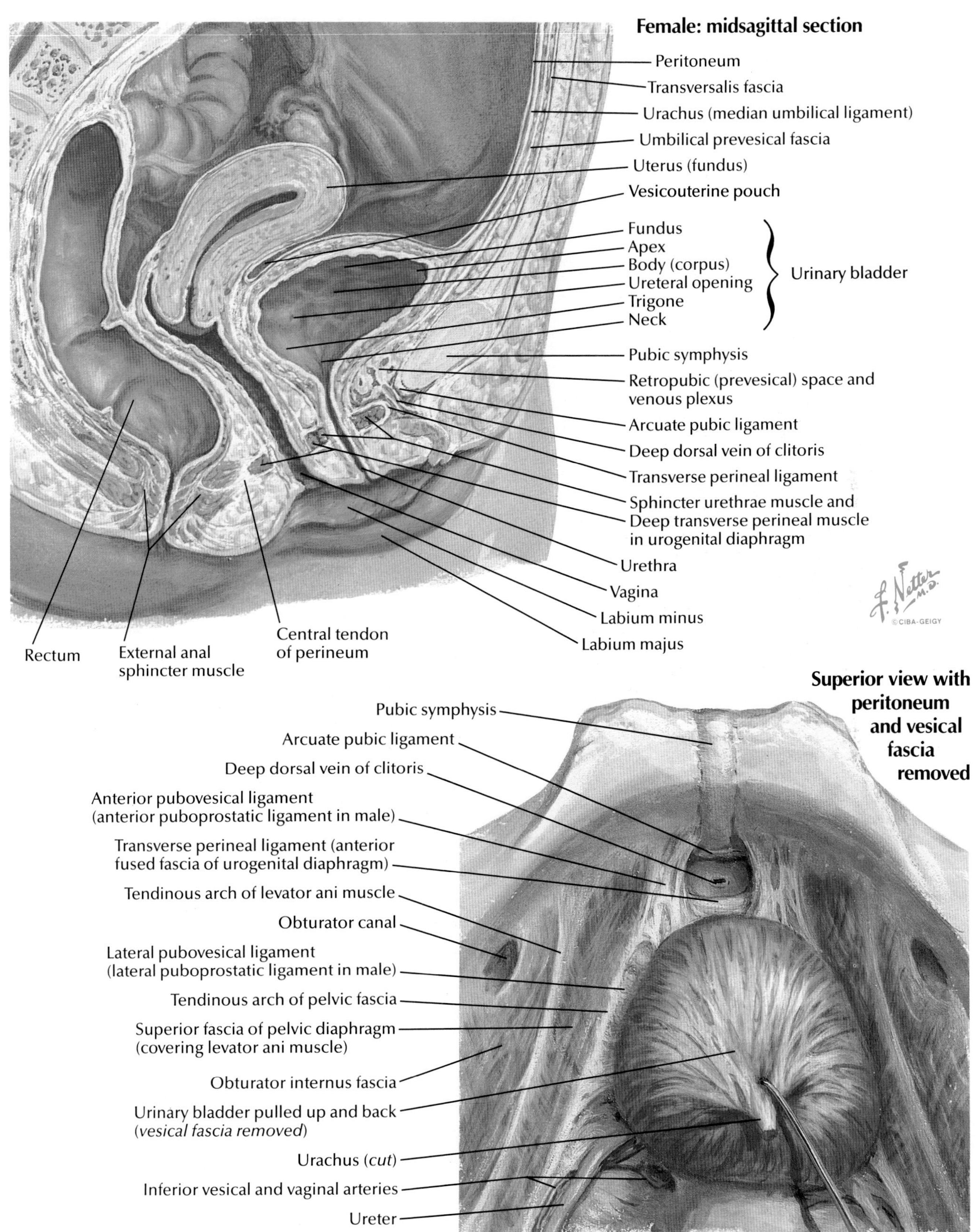

Female: midsagittal section

Peritoneum
Transversalis fascia
Urachus (median umbilical ligament)
Umbilical prevesical fascia
Uterus (fundus)
Vesicouterine pouch
Fundus
Apex
Body (corpus)
Ureteral opening
Trigone
Neck
} Urinary bladder
Pubic symphysis
Retropubic (prevesical) space and venous plexus
Arcuate pubic ligament
Deep dorsal vein of clitoris
Transverse perineal ligament
Sphincter urethrae muscle and
Deep transverse perineal muscle in urogenital diaphragm
Urethra
Vagina
Labium minus
Labium majus

Rectum
External anal sphincter muscle
Central tendon of perineum

Superior view with peritoneum and vesical fascia removed

Pubic symphysis
Arcuate pubic ligament
Deep dorsal vein of clitoris
Anterior pubovesical ligament (anterior puboprostatic ligament in male)
Transverse perineal ligament (anterior fused fascia of urogenital diaphragm)
Tendinous arch of levator ani muscle
Obturator canal
Lateral pubovesical ligament (lateral puboprostatic ligament in male)
Tendinous arch of pelvic fascia
Superior fascia of pelvic diaphragm (covering levator ani muscle)
Obturator internus fascia
Urinary bladder pulled up and back (vesical fascia removed)
Urachus (cut)
Inferior vesical and vaginal arteries
Ureter

Urinary Bladder: Female and Male

SEE ALSO PLATES 325, 341, 342, 346, 375, 377, 378, 392

Female: frontal section

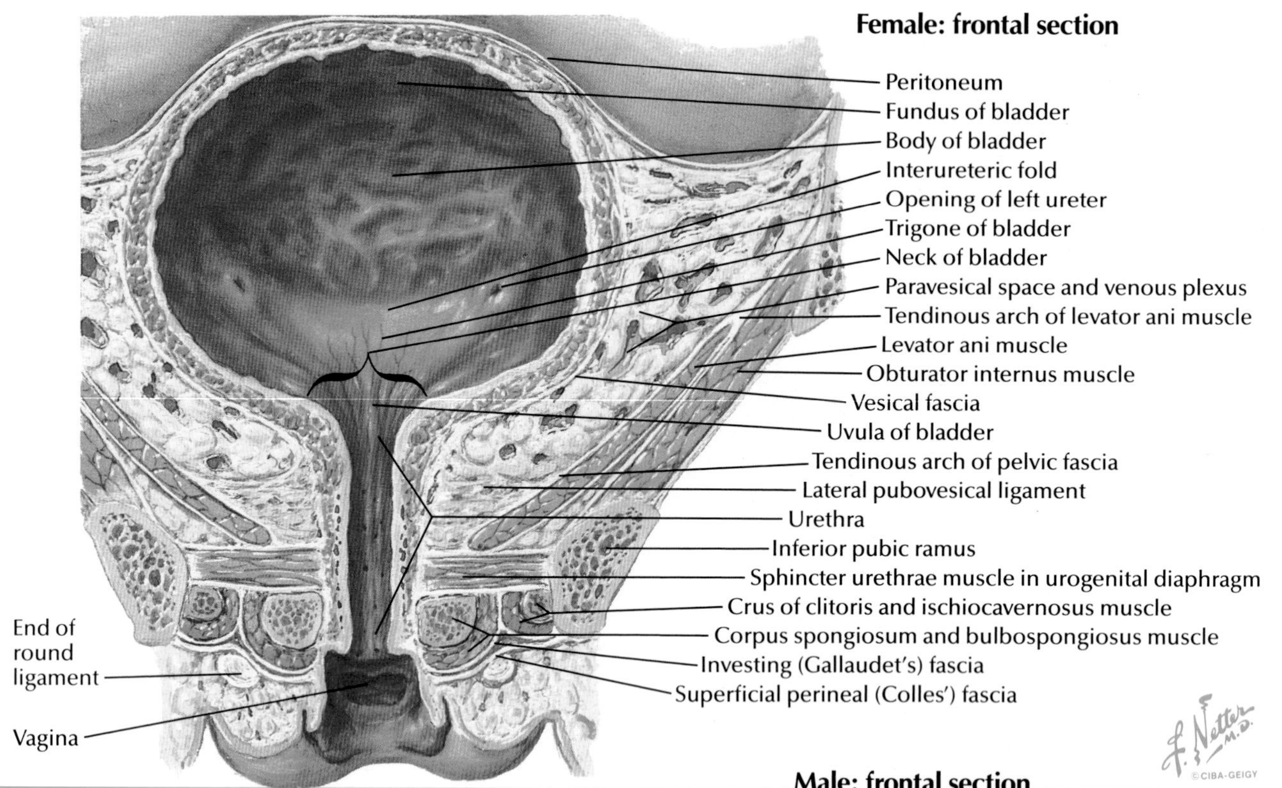

Peritoneum
Fundus of bladder
Body of bladder
Interureteric fold
Opening of left ureter
Trigone of bladder
Neck of bladder
Paravesical space and venous plexus
Tendinous arch of levator ani muscle
Levator ani muscle
Obturator internus muscle
Vesical fascia
Uvula of bladder
Tendinous arch of pelvic fascia
Lateral pubovesical ligament
Urethra
Inferior pubic ramus
Sphincter urethrae muscle in urogenital diaphragm
Crus of clitoris and ischiocavernosus muscle
Corpus spongiosum and bulbospongiosus muscle
Investing (Gallaudet's) fascia
Superficial perineal (Colles') fascia

End of round ligament

Vagina

Male: frontal section

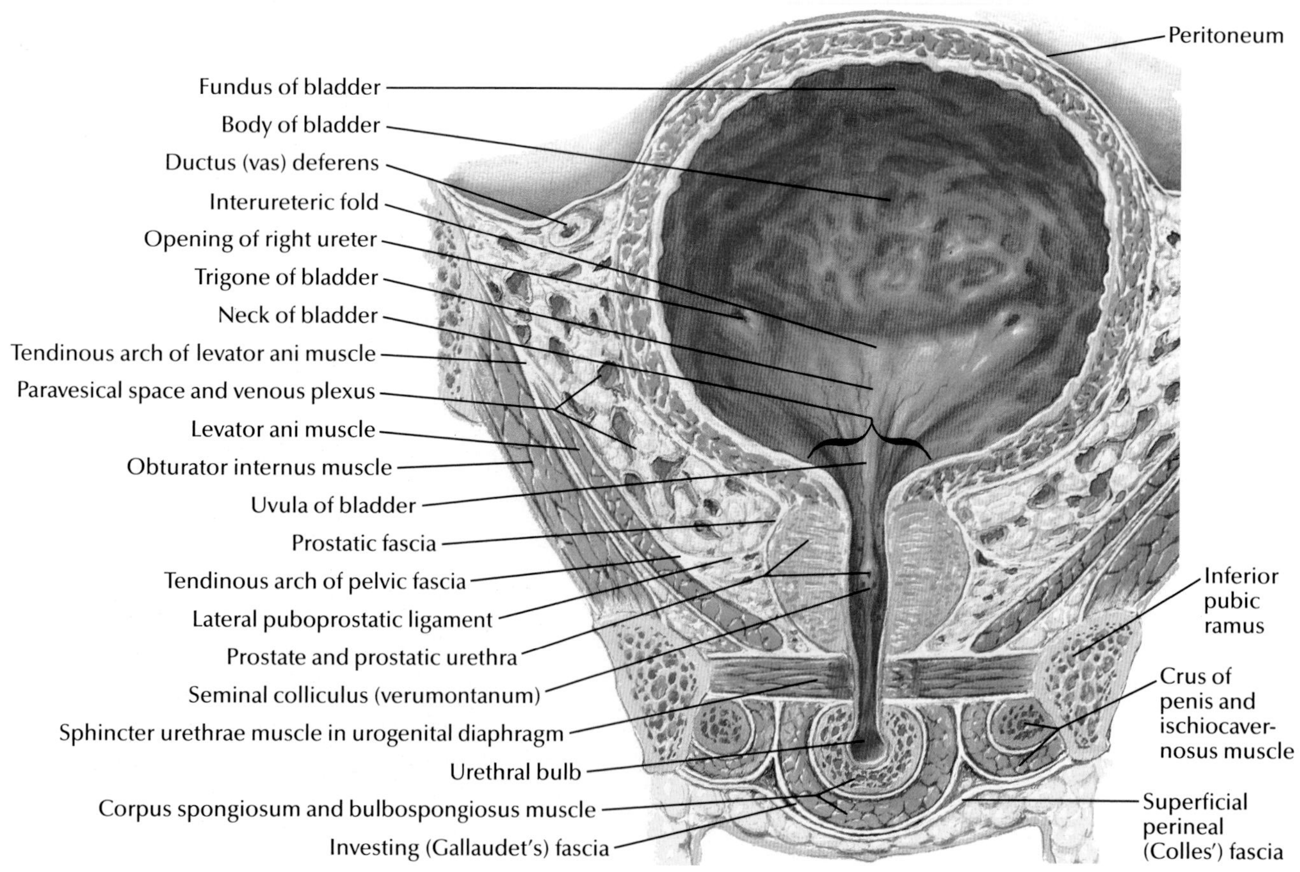

Peritoneum

Fundus of bladder
Body of bladder
Ductus (vas) deferens
Interureteric fold
Opening of right ureter
Trigone of bladder
Neck of bladder
Tendinous arch of levator ani muscle
Paravesical space and venous plexus
Levator ani muscle
Obturator internus muscle
Uvula of bladder
Prostatic fascia
Tendinous arch of pelvic fascia
Lateral puboprostatic ligament
Prostate and prostatic urethra
Seminal colliculus (verumontanum)
Sphincter urethrae muscle in urogenital diaphragm
Urethral bulb
Corpus spongiosum and bulbospongiosus muscle
Investing (Gallaudet's) fascia

Inferior pubic ramus

Crus of penis and ischiocavernosus muscle

Superficial perineal (Colles') fascia

PLATE 347

PELVIS AND PERINEUM

Superior view with peritoneum intact

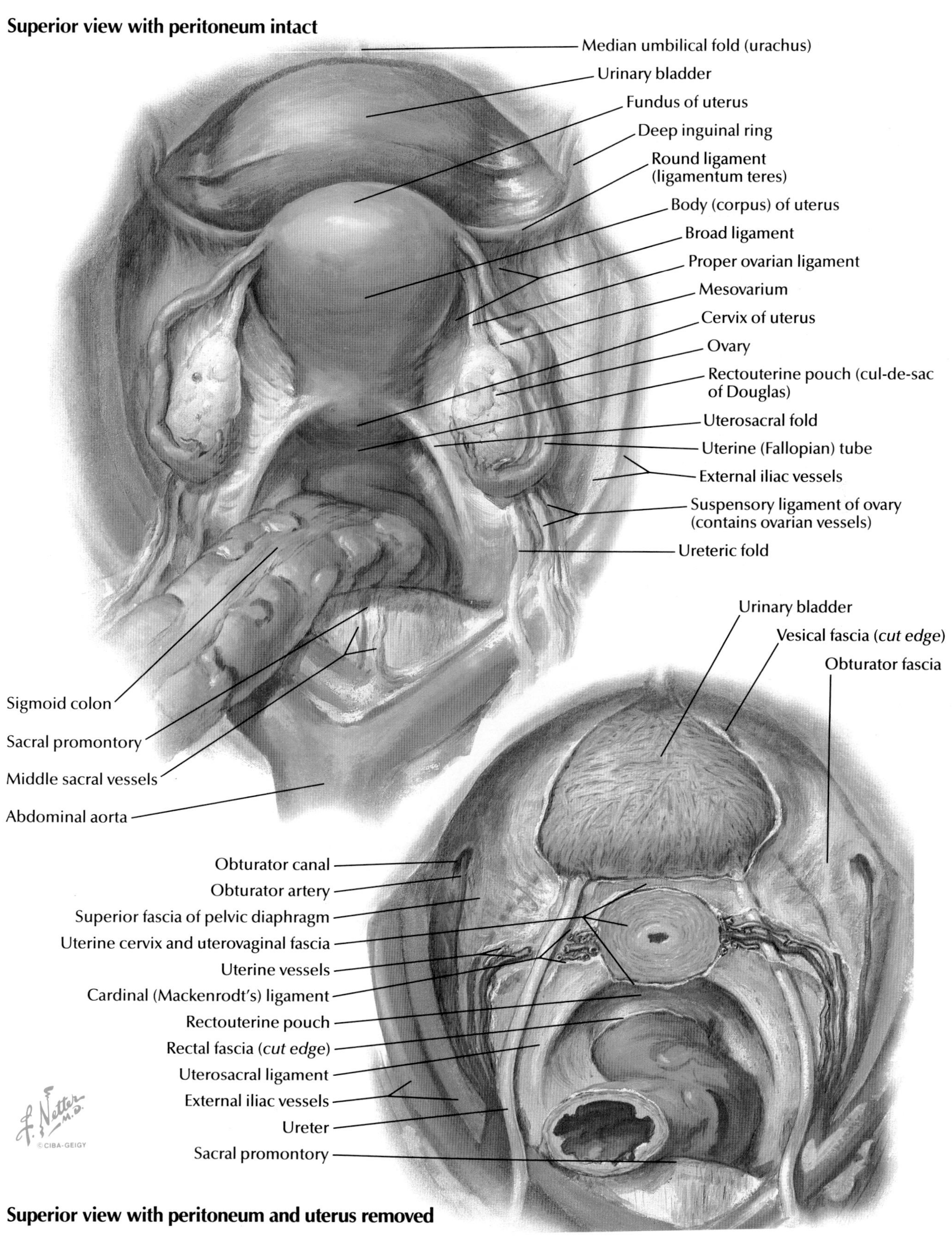

Median umbilical fold (urachus)

Urinary bladder

Fundus of uterus

Deep inguinal ring

Round ligament (ligamentum teres)

Body (corpus) of uterus

Broad ligament

Proper ovarian ligament

Mesovarium

Cervix of uterus

Ovary

Rectouterine pouch (cul-de-sac of Douglas)

Uterosacral fold

Uterine (Fallopian) tube

External iliac vessels

Suspensory ligament of ovary (contains ovarian vessels)

Ureteric fold

Sigmoid colon

Sacral promontory

Middle sacral vessels

Abdominal aorta

Urinary bladder

Vesical fascia (*cut edge*)

Obturator fascia

Obturator canal

Obturator artery

Superior fascia of pelvic diaphragm

Uterine cervix and uterovaginal fascia

Uterine vessels

Cardinal (Mackenrodt's) ligament

Rectouterine pouch

Rectal fascia (*cut edge*)

Uterosacral ligament

External iliac vessels

Ureter

Sacral promontory

Superior view with peritoneum and uterus removed

Uterus, Vagina and Supporting Structures

SEE ALSO PLATES 375, 377, 379, 381, 387, 389, 390

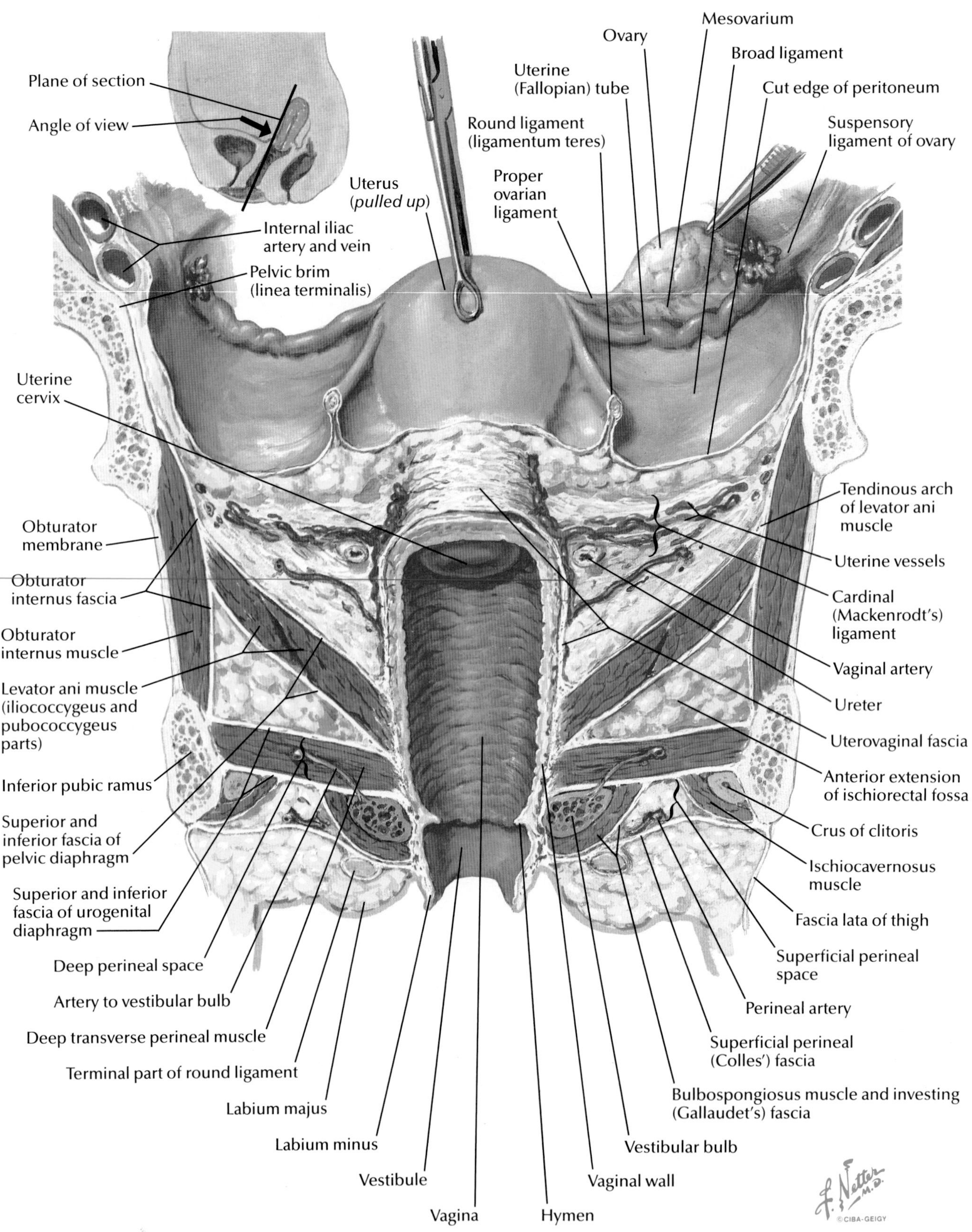

Plane of section

Angle of view

Internal iliac artery and vein

Pelvic brim (linea terminalis)

Uterus (*pulled up*)

Round ligament (ligamentum teres)

Proper ovarian ligament

Uterine (Fallopian) tube

Ovary

Mesovarium

Broad ligament

Cut edge of peritoneum

Suspensory ligament of ovary

Uterine cervix

Obturator membrane

Obturator internus fascia

Obturator internus muscle

Levator ani muscle (iliococcygeus and pubococcygeus parts)

Inferior pubic ramus

Superior and inferior fascia of pelvic diaphragm

Superior and inferior fascia of urogenital diaphragm

Deep perineal space

Artery to vestibular bulb

Deep transverse perineal muscle

Terminal part of round ligament

Labium majus

Labium minus

Vestibule

Vagina

Hymen

Vaginal wall

Vestibular bulb

Bulbospongiosus muscle and investing (Gallaudet's) fascia

Superficial perineal (Colles') fascia

Perineal artery

Superficial perineal space

Fascia lata of thigh

Ischiocavernosus muscle

Crus of clitoris

Anterior extension of ischiorectal fossa

Uterovaginal fascia

Ureter

Vaginal artery

Cardinal (Mackenrodt's) ligament

Uterine vessels

Tendinous arch of levator ani muscle

PLATE 349

PELVIS AND PERINEUM

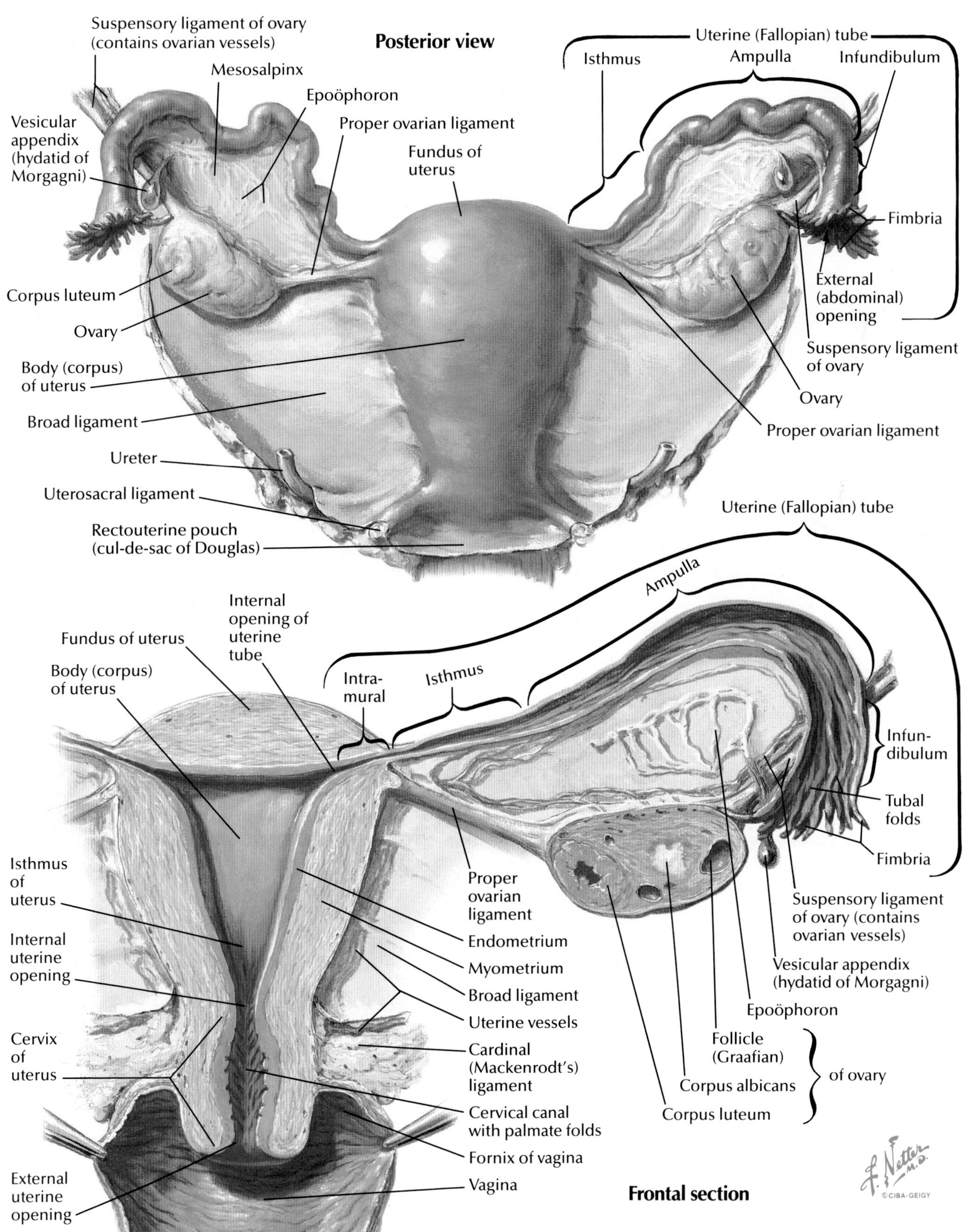

Posterior view

Suspensory ligament of ovary (contains ovarian vessels)

Mesosalpinx

Epoöphoron

Proper ovarian ligament

Fundus of uterus

Uterine (Fallopian) tube

Isthmus

Ampulla

Infundibulum

Vesicular appendix (hydatid of Morgagni)

Fimbria

Corpus luteum

Ovary

External (abdominal) opening

Body (corpus) of uterus

Suspensory ligament of ovary

Broad ligament

Ovary

Ureter

Proper ovarian ligament

Uterosacral ligament

Rectouterine pouch (cul-de-sac of Douglas)

Uterine (Fallopian) tube

Internal opening of uterine tube

Ampulla

Fundus of uterus

Body (corpus) of uterus

Intra-mural

Isthmus

Infundibulum

Tubal folds

Isthmus of uterus

Fimbria

Internal uterine opening

Proper ovarian ligament

Suspensory ligament of ovary (contains ovarian vessels)

Endometrium

Myometrium

Vesicular appendix (hydatid of Morgagni)

Cervix of uterus

Broad ligament

Uterine vessels

Epoöphoron

Cardinal (Mackenrodt's) ligament

Follicle (Graafian)

Cervical canal with palmate folds

Corpus albicans

of ovary

Fornix of vagina

Corpus luteum

External uterine opening

Vagina

Frontal section

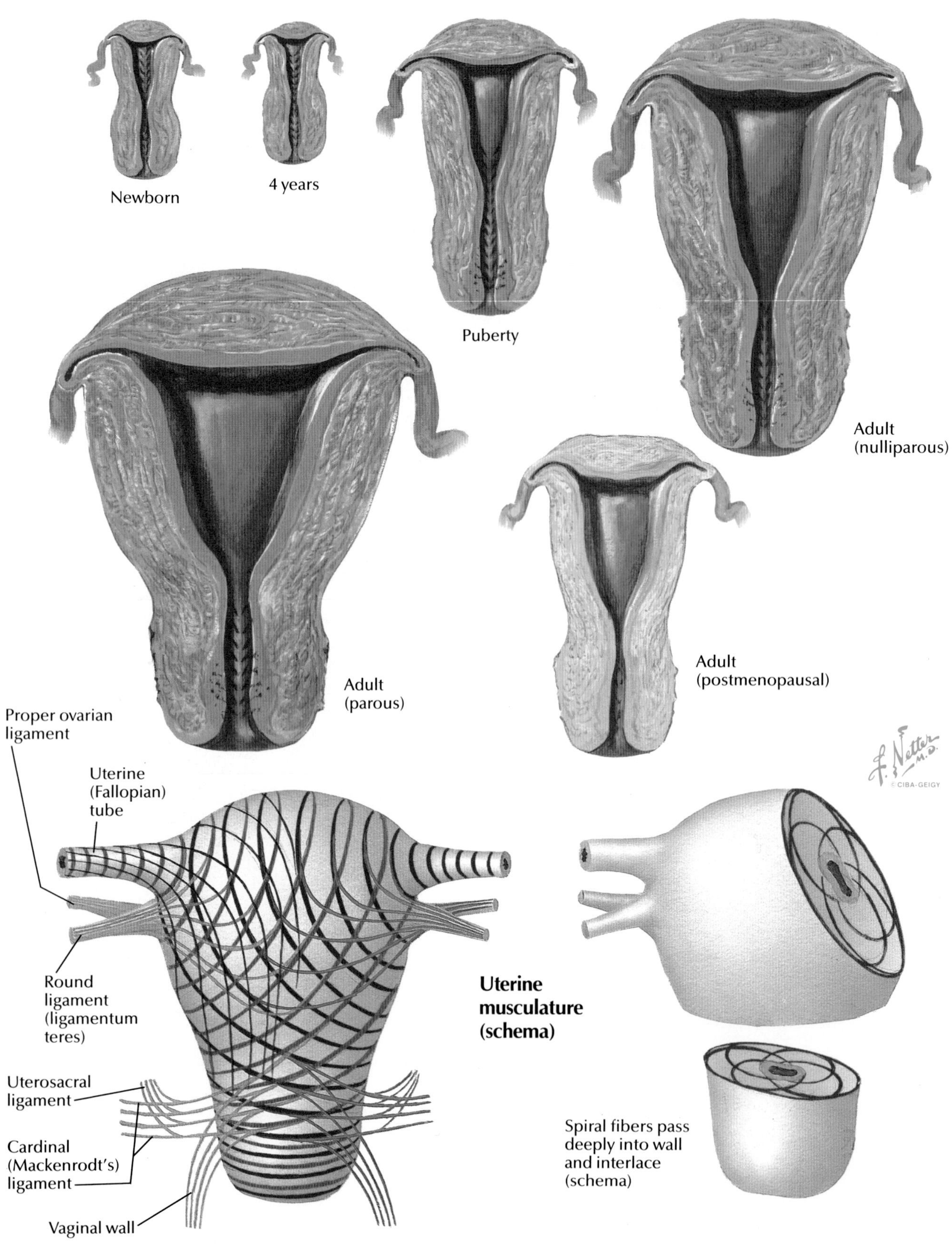

Newborn

4 years

Puberty

Adult
(nulliparous)

Adult
(parous)

Adult
(postmenopausal)

Proper ovarian
ligament

Uterine
(Fallopian)
tube

Round
ligament
(ligamentum
teres)

Uterosacral
ligament

Cardinal
(Mackenrodt's)
ligament

Vaginal wall

**Uterine
musculature
(schema)**

Spiral fibers pass
deeply into wall
and interlace
(schema)

PLATE 351

PELVIS AND PERINEUM

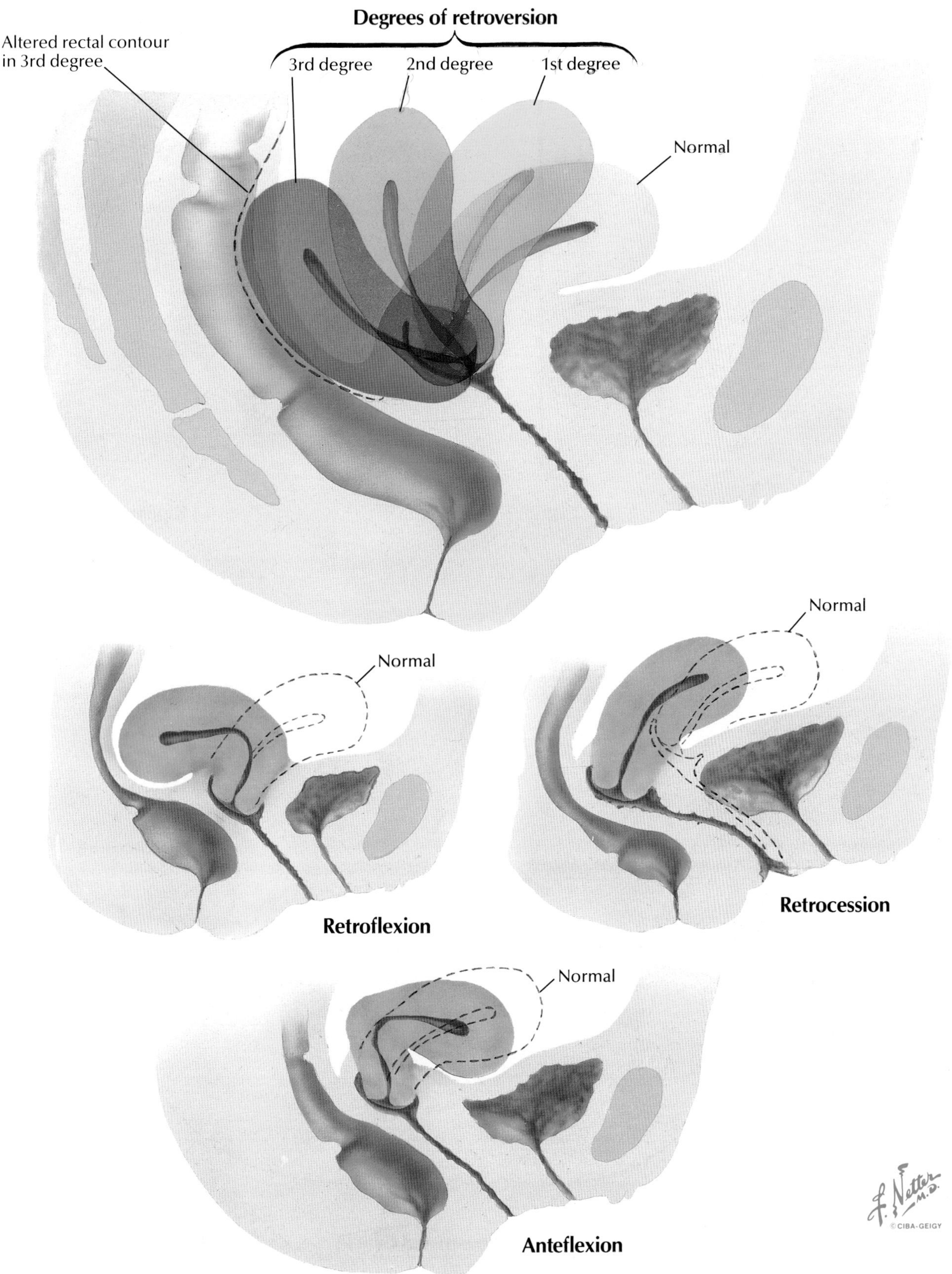

Degrees of retroversion

3rd degree   2nd degree   1st degree

Altered rectal contour
in 3rd degree

Normal

Normal

Retroflexion

Normal

Retrocession

Normal

Anteflexion

Ovary, Ova and Follicles

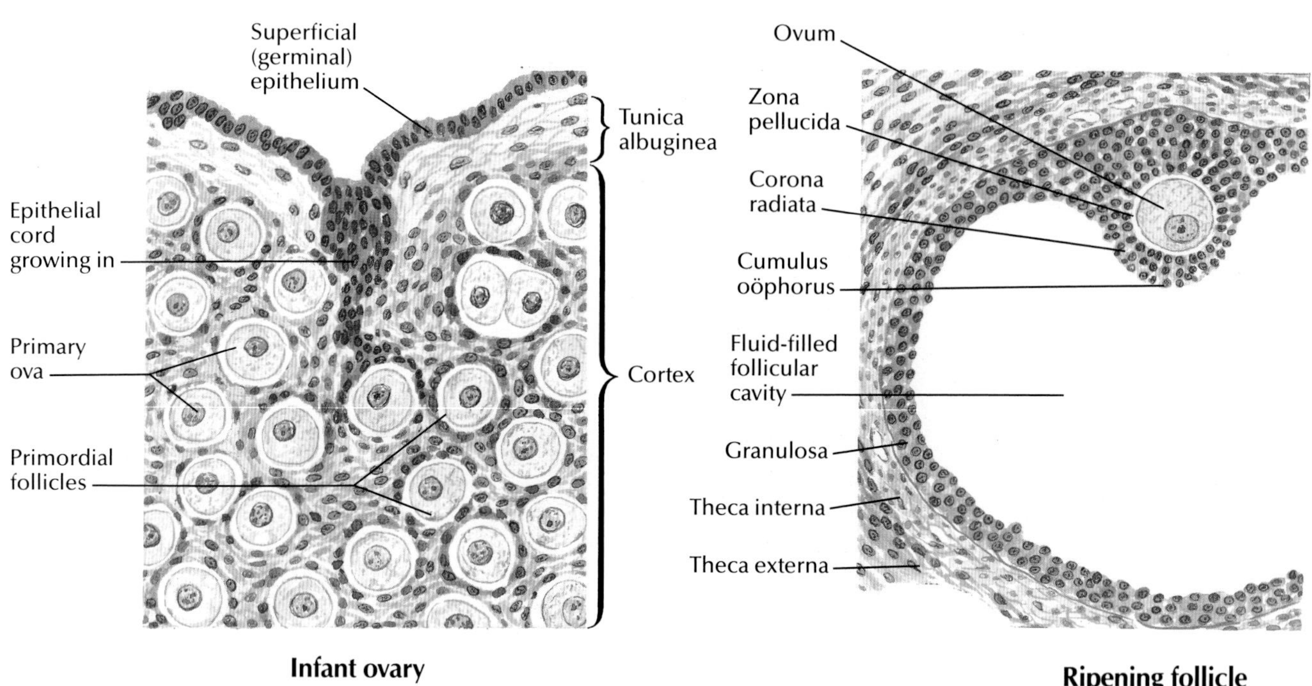

Superficial (germinal) epithelium

Tunica albuginea

Epithelial cord growing in

Primary ova

Primordial follicles

Cortex

Infant ovary

Ovum

Zona pellucida

Corona radiata

Cumulus oöphorus

Fluid-filled follicular cavity

Granulosa

Theca interna

Theca externa

Ripening follicle

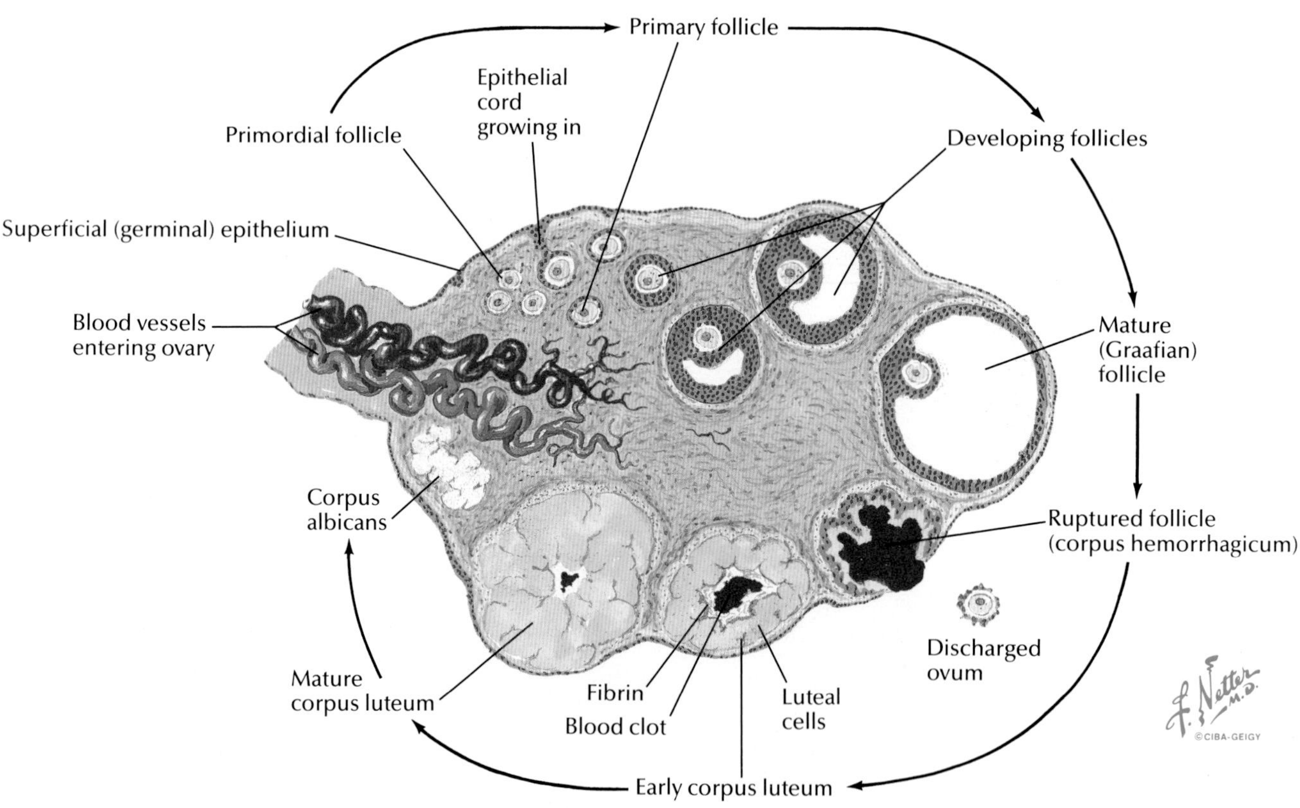

Primary follicle

Epithelial cord growing in

Primordial follicle

Developing follicles

Superficial (germinal) epithelium

Blood vessels entering ovary

Mature (Graafian) follicle

Corpus albicans

Ruptured follicle (corpus hemorrhagicum)

Discharged ovum

Mature corpus luteum

Fibrin

Blood clot

Luteal cells

Early corpus luteum

Stages of ovum and follicle

PLATE 353

PELVIS AND PERINEUM

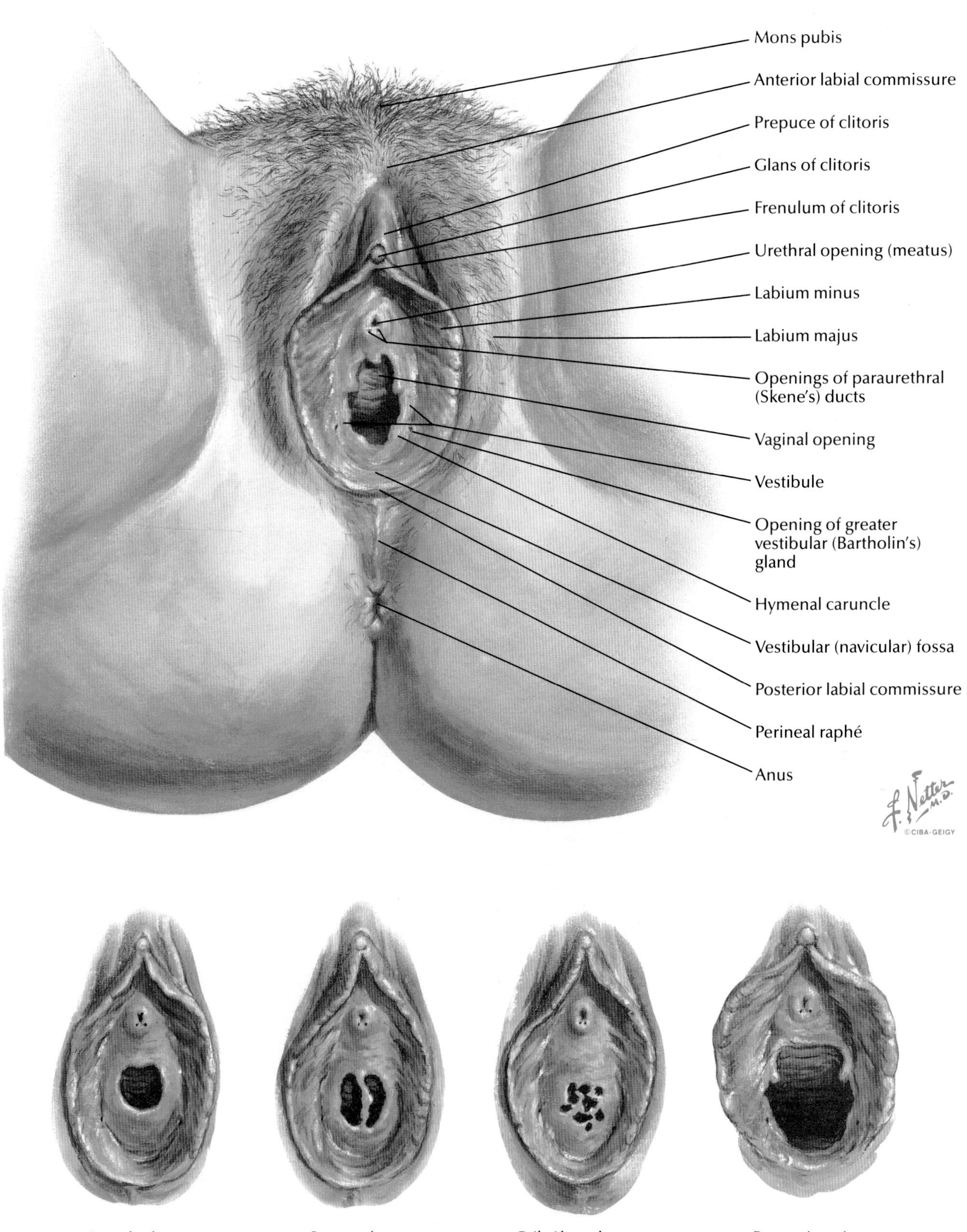

Mons pubis

Anterior labial commissure

Prepuce of clitoris

Glans of clitoris

Frenulum of clitoris

Urethral opening (meatus)

Labium minus

Labium majus

Openings of paraurethral (Skene's) ducts

Vaginal opening

Vestibule

Opening of greater vestibular (Bartholin's) gland

Hymenal caruncle

Vestibular (navicular) fossa

Posterior labial commissure

Perineal raphé

Anus

Annular hymen   Septate hymen   Cribriform hymen   Parous introitus

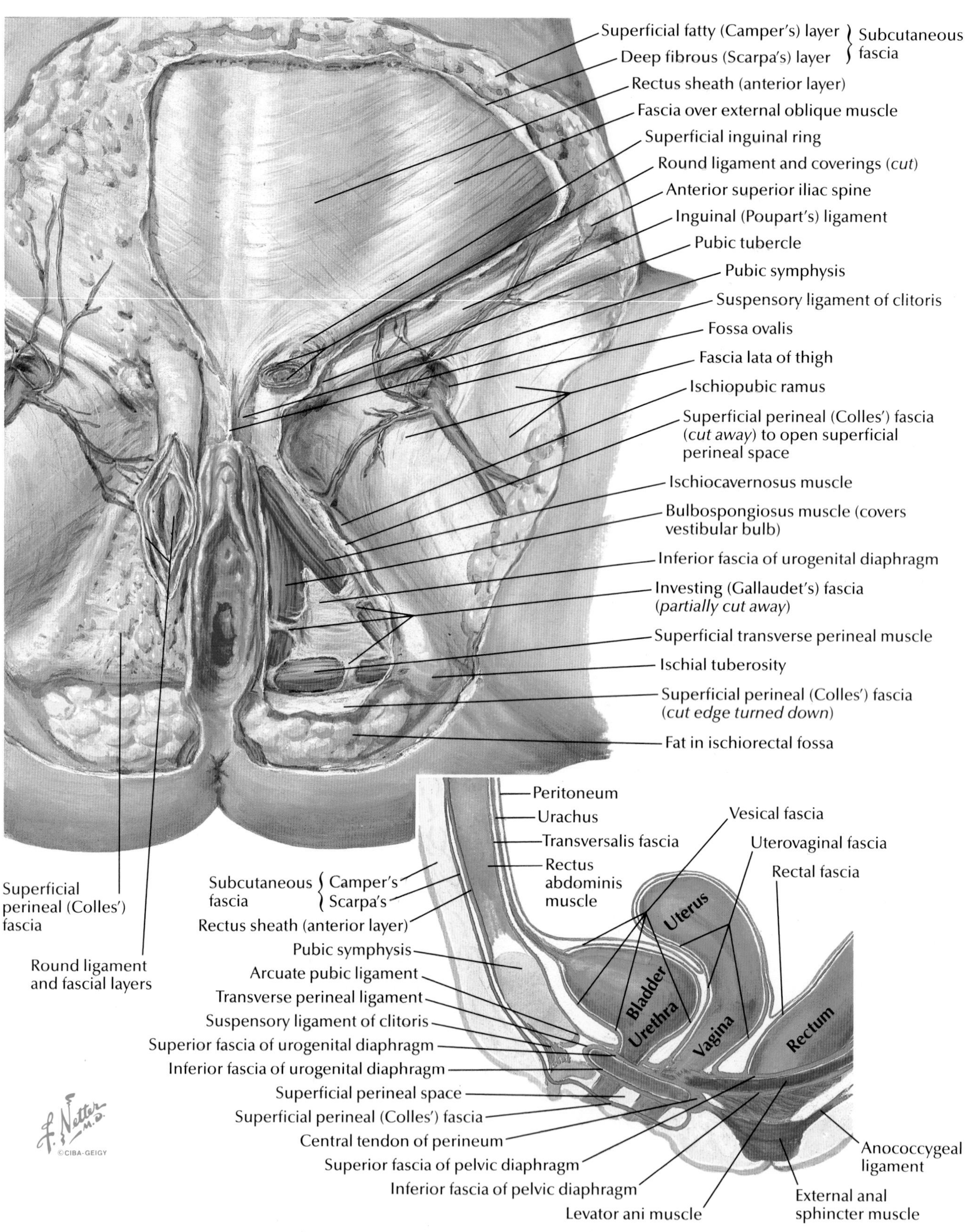

Superficial fatty (Camper's) layer ⎱ Subcutaneous
Deep fibrous (Scarpa's) layer ⎰ fascia
Rectus sheath (anterior layer)
Fascia over external oblique muscle
Superficial inguinal ring
Round ligament and coverings (cut)
Anterior superior iliac spine
Inguinal (Poupart's) ligament
Pubic tubercle
Pubic symphysis
Suspensory ligament of clitoris
Fossa ovalis
Fascia lata of thigh
Ischiopubic ramus
Superficial perineal (Colles') fascia
(cut away) to open superficial
perineal space
Ischiocavernosus muscle
Bulbospongiosus muscle (covers
vestibular bulb)
Inferior fascia of urogenital diaphragm
Investing (Gallaudet's) fascia
(partially cut away)
Superficial transverse perineal muscle
Ischial tuberosity
Superficial perineal (Colles') fascia
(cut edge turned down)
Fat in ischiorectal fossa

Superficial
perineal (Colles')
fascia

Round ligament
and fascial layers

Subcutaneous ⎱ Camper's
fascia ⎰ Scarpa's
Rectus sheath (anterior layer)
Pubic symphysis
Arcuate pubic ligament
Transverse perineal ligament
Suspensory ligament of clitoris
Superior fascia of urogenital diaphragm
Inferior fascia of urogenital diaphragm
Superficial perineal space
Superficial perineal (Colles') fascia
Central tendon of perineum
Superior fascia of pelvic diaphragm
Inferior fascia of pelvic diaphragm
Levator ani muscle

Peritoneum
Urachus
Transversalis fascia
Rectus
abdominis
muscle

Vesical fascia
Uterovaginal fascia
Rectal fascia

Uterus
Bladder
Urethra
Vagina
Rectum

Anococcygeal
ligament

External anal
sphincter muscle

PLATE 355

PELVIS AND PERINEUM

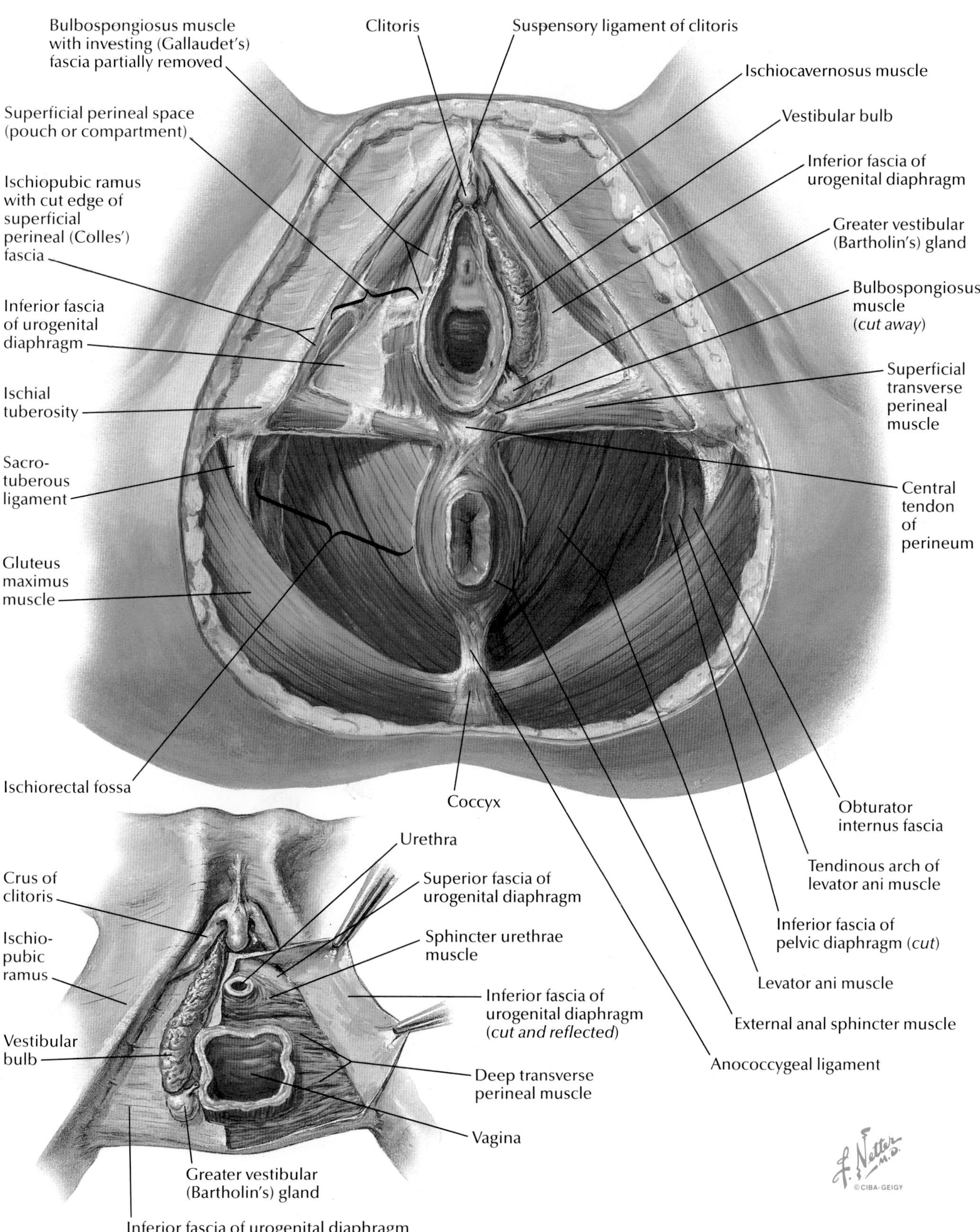

Bulbospongiosus muscle with investing (Gallaudet's) fascia partially removed

Superficial perineal space (pouch or compartment)

Ischiopubic ramus with cut edge of superficial perineal (Colles') fascia

Inferior fascia of urogenital diaphragm

Ischial tuberosity

Sacro-tuberous ligament

Gluteus maximus muscle

Ischiorectal fossa

Clitoris

Suspensory ligament of clitoris

Ischiocavernosus muscle

Vestibular bulb

Inferior fascia of urogenital diaphragm

Greater vestibular (Bartholin's) gland

Bulbospongiosus muscle (*cut away*)

Superficial transverse perineal muscle

Central tendon of perineum

Obturator internus fascia

Tendinous arch of levator ani muscle

Inferior fascia of pelvic diaphragm (*cut*)

Levator ani muscle

External anal sphincter muscle

Anococcygeal ligament

Coccyx

Crus of clitoris

Ischio-pubic ramus

Vestibular bulb

Urethra

Superior fascia of urogenital diaphragm

Sphincter urethrae muscle

Inferior fascia of urogenital diaphragm (*cut and reflected*)

Deep transverse perineal muscle

Vagina

Greater vestibular (Bartholin's) gland

Inferior fascia of urogenital diaphragm

Urethra: Female

SEE ALSO PLATES 341, 346

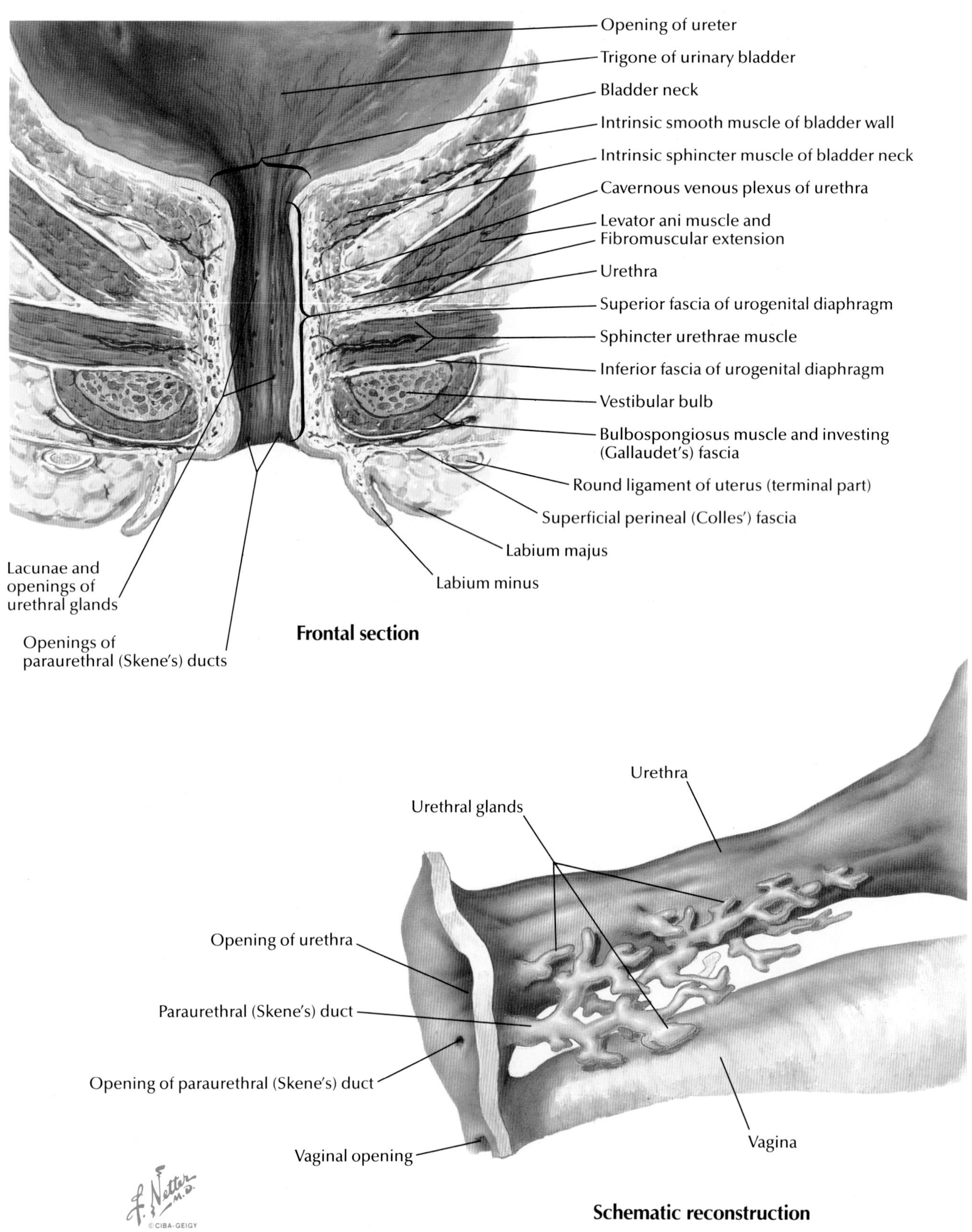

Opening of ureter

Trigone of urinary bladder

Bladder neck

Intrinsic smooth muscle of bladder wall

Intrinsic sphincter muscle of bladder neck

Cavernous venous plexus of urethra

Levator ani muscle and
Fibromuscular extension

Urethra

Superior fascia of urogenital diaphragm

Sphincter urethrae muscle

Inferior fascia of urogenital diaphragm

Vestibular bulb

Bulbospongiosus muscle and investing
(Gallaudet's) fascia

Round ligament of uterus (terminal part)

Superficial perineal (Colles') fascia

Labium majus

Labium minus

Lacunae and openings of urethral glands

Openings of paraurethral (Skene's) ducts

Frontal section

Urethra

Urethral glands

Opening of urethra

Paraurethral (Skene's) duct

Opening of paraurethral (Skene's) duct

Vaginal opening

Vagina

Schematic reconstruction

PLATE 357

PELVIS AND PERINEUM

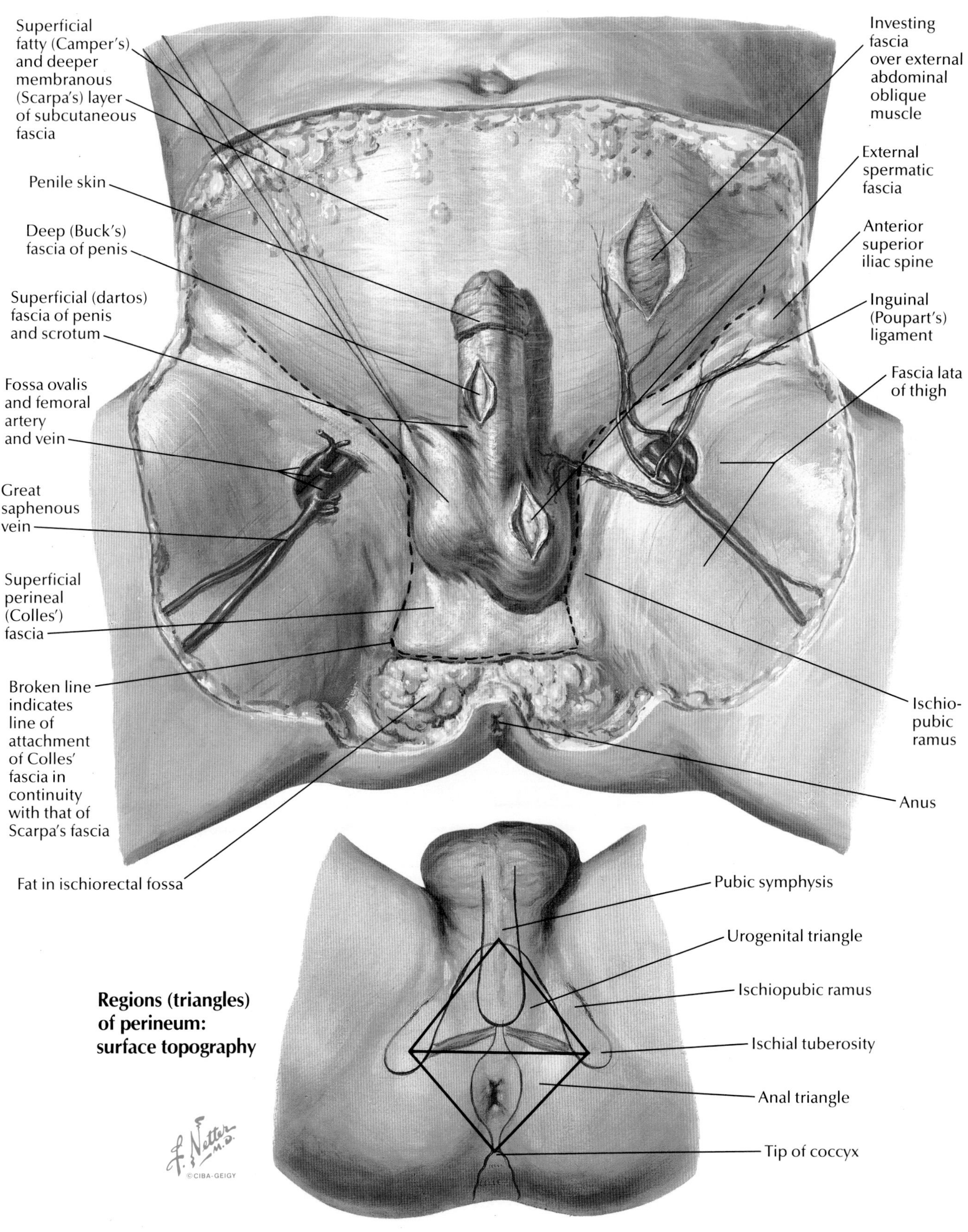

Superficial fatty (Camper's) and deeper membranous (Scarpa's) layer of subcutaneous fascia

Penile skin

Deep (Buck's) fascia of penis

Superficial (dartos) fascia of penis and scrotum

Fossa ovalis and femoral artery and vein

Great saphenous vein

Superficial perineal (Colles') fascia

Broken line indicates line of attachment of Colles' fascia in continuity with that of Scarpa's fascia

Fat in ischiorectal fossa

Investing fascia over external abdominal oblique muscle

External spermatic fascia

Anterior superior iliac spine

Inguinal (Poupart's) ligament

Fascia lata of thigh

Ischio-pubic ramus

Anus

Regions (triangles) of perineum: surface topography

Pubic symphysis

Urogenital triangle

Ischiopubic ramus

Ischial tuberosity

Anal triangle

Tip of coccyx

MALE STRUCTURES

PLATE 358

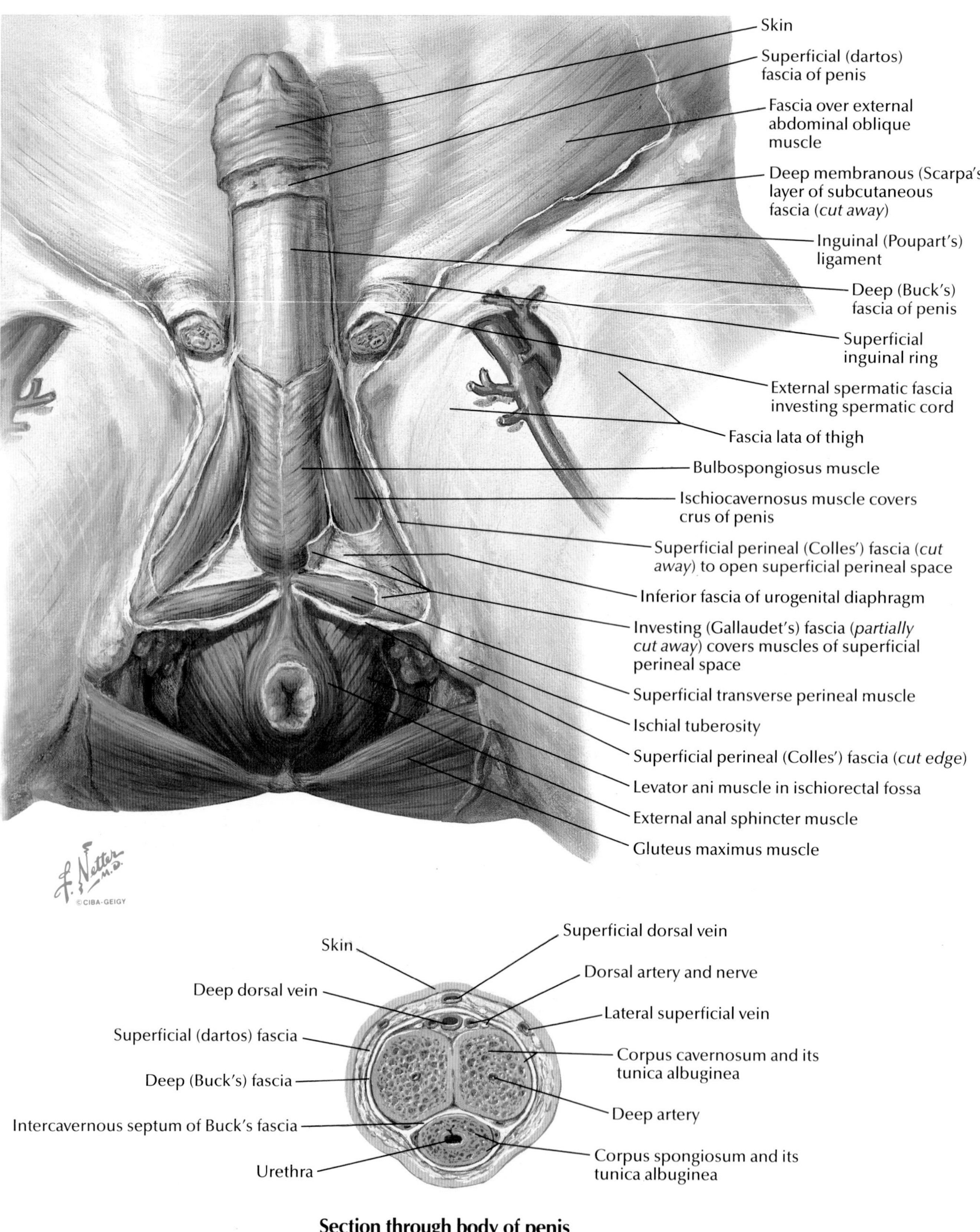

Skin

Superficial (dartos) fascia of penis

Fascia over external abdominal oblique muscle

Deep membranous (Scarpa's) layer of subcutaneous fascia (*cut away*)

Inguinal (Poupart's) ligament

Deep (Buck's) fascia of penis

Superficial inguinal ring

External spermatic fascia investing spermatic cord

Fascia lata of thigh

Bulbospongiosus muscle

Ischiocavernosus muscle covers crus of penis

Superficial perineal (Colles') fascia (*cut away*) to open superficial perineal space

Inferior fascia of urogenital diaphragm

Investing (Gallaudet's) fascia (*partially cut away*) covers muscles of superficial perineal space

Superficial transverse perineal muscle

Ischial tuberosity

Superficial perineal (Colles') fascia (*cut edge*)

Levator ani muscle in ischiorectal fossa

External anal sphincter muscle

Gluteus maximus muscle

Superficial dorsal vein

Skin

Deep dorsal vein

Dorsal artery and nerve

Superficial (dartos) fascia

Lateral superficial vein

Deep (Buck's) fascia

Corpus cavernosum and its tunica albuginea

Intercavernous septum of Buck's fascia

Deep artery

Urethra

Corpus spongiosum and its tunica albuginea

Section through body of penis

PLATE 359

PELVIS AND PERINEUM

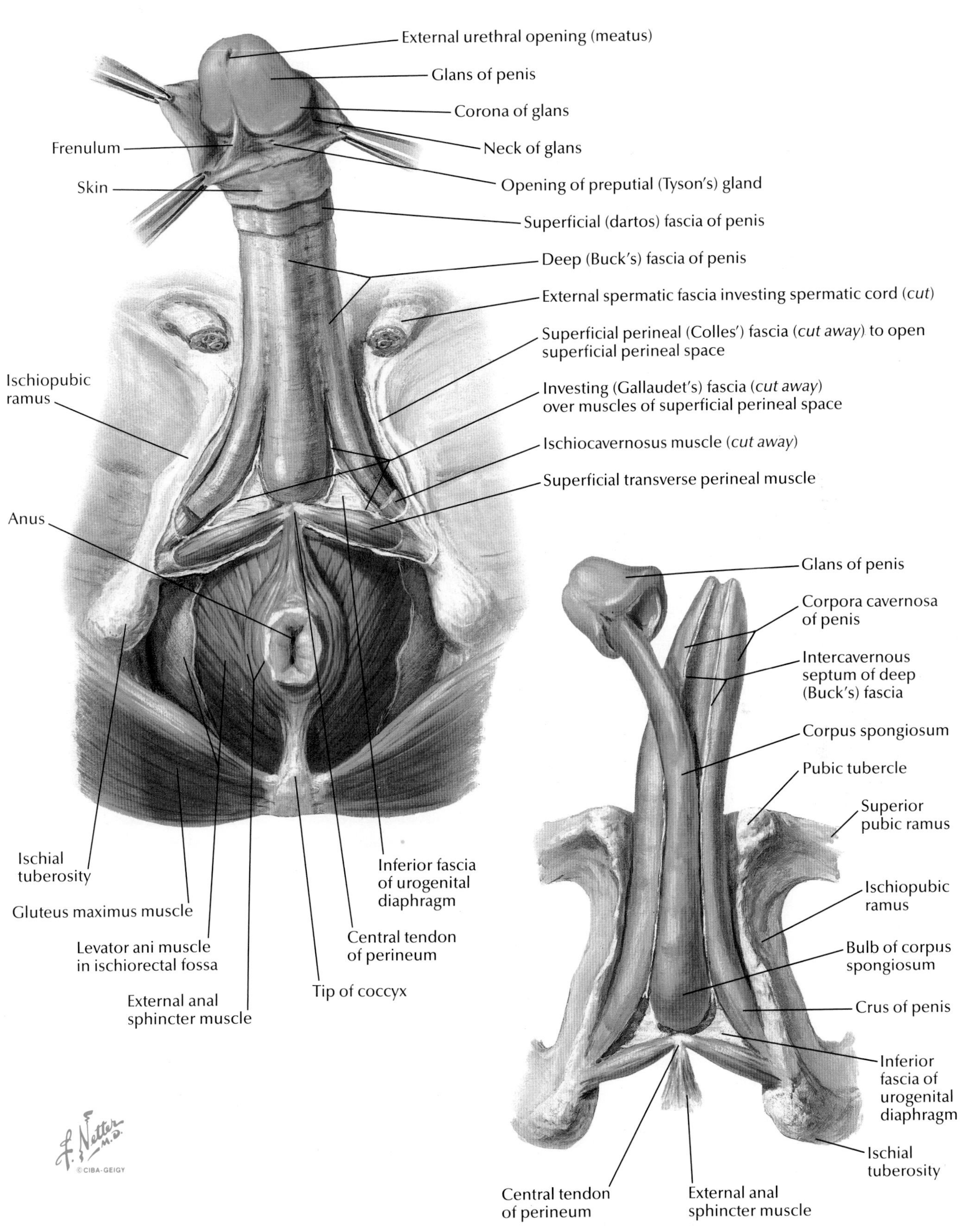

External urethral opening (meatus)

Glans of penis

Corona of glans

Neck of glans

Frenulum

Opening of preputial (Tyson's) gland

Skin

Superficial (dartos) fascia of penis

Deep (Buck's) fascia of penis

External spermatic fascia investing spermatic cord (*cut*)

Superficial perineal (Colles') fascia (*cut away*) to open superficial perineal space

Investing (Gallaudet's) fascia (*cut away*) over muscles of superficial perineal space

Ischiopubic ramus

Ischiocavernosus muscle (*cut away*)

Superficial transverse perineal muscle

Anus

Glans of penis

Corpora cavernosa of penis

Intercavernous septum of deep (Buck's) fascia

Corpus spongiosum

Pubic tubercle

Superior pubic ramus

Ischiopubic ramus

Ischial tuberosity

Gluteus maximus muscle

Levator ani muscle in ischiorectal fossa

External anal sphincter muscle

Tip of coccyx

Central tendon of perineum

Inferior fascia of urogenital diaphragm

Bulb of corpus spongiosum

Crus of penis

Inferior fascia of urogenital diaphragm

Ischial tuberosity

Central tendon of perineum

External anal sphincter muscle

Urogenital Diaphragm: Male

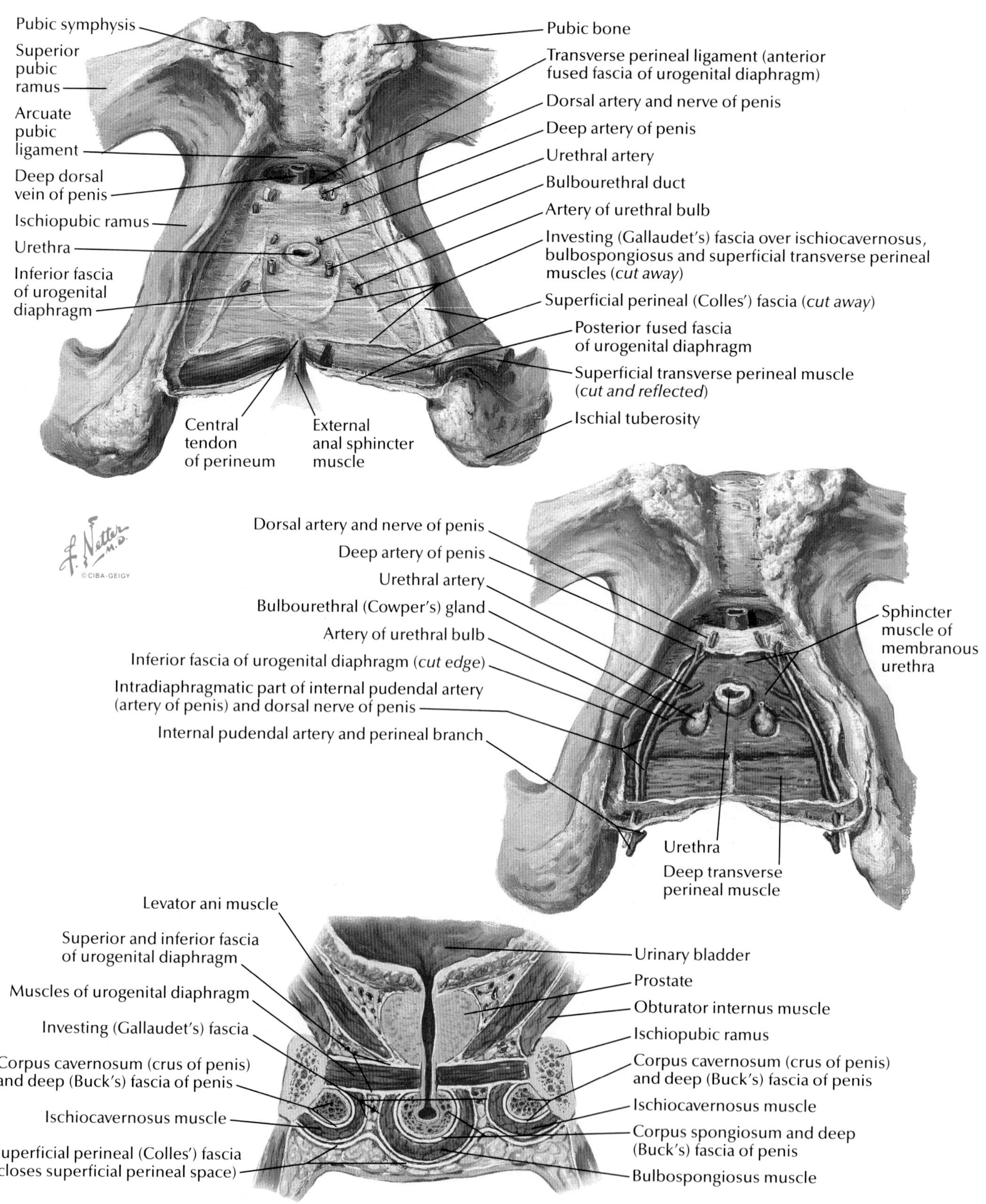

Pubic symphysis

Superior pubic ramus

Arcuate pubic ligament

Deep dorsal vein of penis

Ischiopubic ramus

Urethra

Inferior fascia of urogenital diaphragm

Central tendon of perineum

External anal sphincter muscle

Pubic bone

Transverse perineal ligament (anterior fused fascia of urogenital diaphragm)

Dorsal artery and nerve of penis

Deep artery of penis

Urethral artery

Bulbourethral duct

Artery of urethral bulb

Investing (Gallaudet's) fascia over ischiocavernosus, bulbospongiosus and superficial transverse perineal muscles (cut away)

Superficial perineal (Colles') fascia (cut away)

Posterior fused fascia of urogenital diaphragm

Superficial transverse perineal muscle (cut and reflected)

Ischial tuberosity

Dorsal artery and nerve of penis

Deep artery of penis

Urethral artery

Bulbourethral (Cowper's) gland

Artery of urethral bulb

Inferior fascia of urogenital diaphragm (cut edge)

Intradiaphragmatic part of internal pudendal artery (artery of penis) and dorsal nerve of penis

Internal pudendal artery and perineal branch

Sphincter muscle of membranous urethra

Urethra

Deep transverse perineal muscle

Levator ani muscle

Superior and inferior fascia of urogenital diaphragm

Muscles of urogenital diaphragm

Investing (Gallaudet's) fascia

Corpus cavernosum (crus of penis) and deep (Buck's) fascia of penis

Ischiocavernosus muscle

Superficial perineal (Colles') fascia (closes superficial perineal space)

Urinary bladder

Prostate

Obturator internus muscle

Ischiopubic ramus

Corpus cavernosum (crus of penis) and deep (Buck's) fascia of penis

Ischiocavernosus muscle

Corpus spongiosum and deep (Buck's) fascia of penis

Bulbospongiosus muscle

Frontal section through perineum and urethral bulb: schema

PLATE 361

PELVIS AND PERINEUM

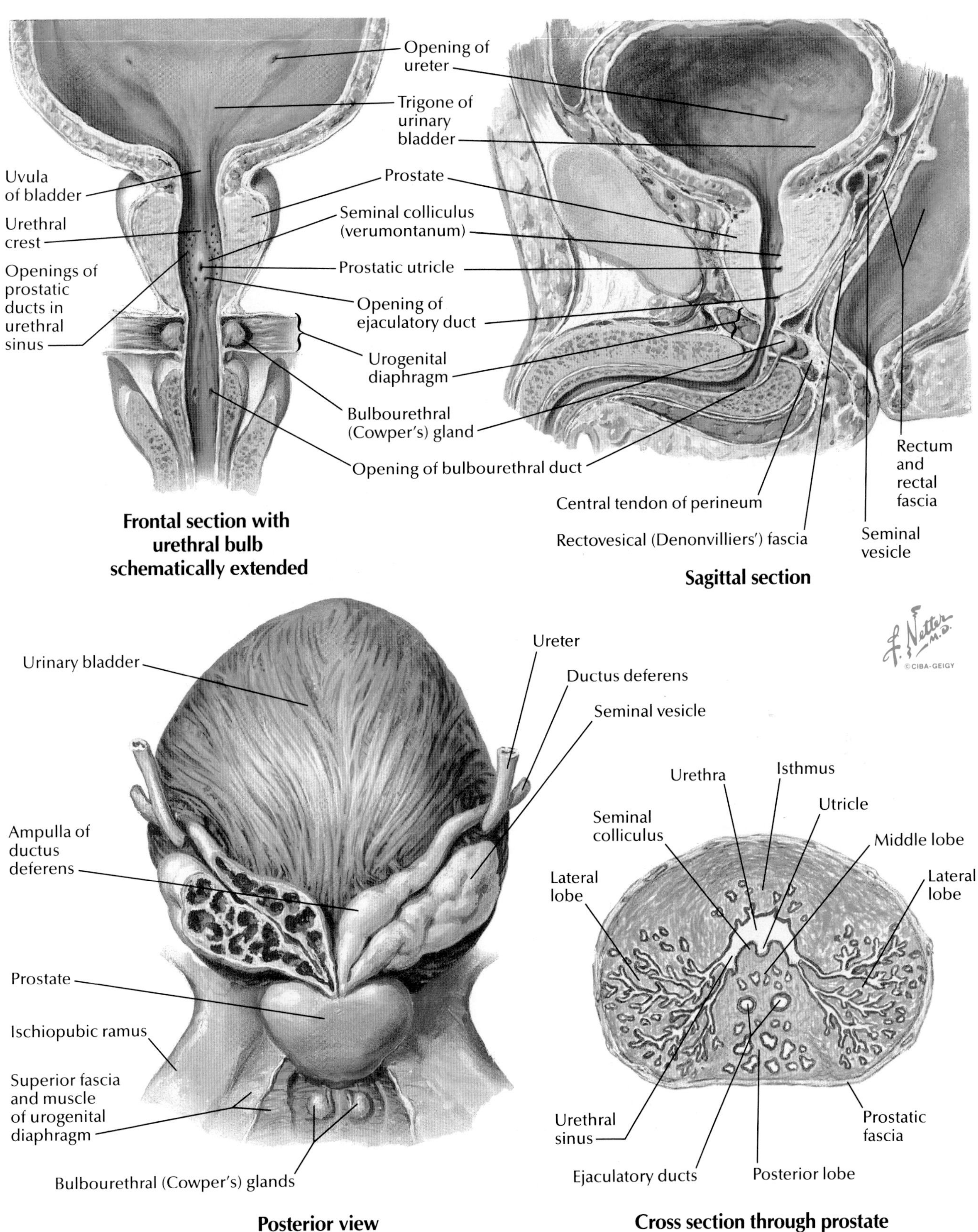

Opening of ureter

Trigone of urinary bladder

Uvula of bladder

Urethral crest

Openings of prostatic ducts in urethral sinus

Prostate

Seminal colliculus (verumontanum)

Prostatic utricle

Opening of ejaculatory duct

Urogenital diaphragm

Bulbourethral (Cowper's) gland

Opening of bulbourethral duct

Rectum and rectal fascia

Central tendon of perineum

Rectovesical (Denonvilliers') fascia

Seminal vesicle

Frontal section with urethral bulb schematically extended

Sagittal section

Urinary bladder

Ureter

Ductus deferens

Seminal vesicle

Ampulla of ductus deferens

Prostate

Ischiopubic ramus

Superior fascia and muscle of urogenital diaphragm

Bulbourethral (Cowper's) glands

Posterior view

Urethra

Isthmus

Utricle

Seminal colliculus

Middle lobe

Lateral lobe

Lateral lobe

Urethral sinus

Ejaculatory ducts

Posterior lobe

Prostatic fascia

Cross section through prostate

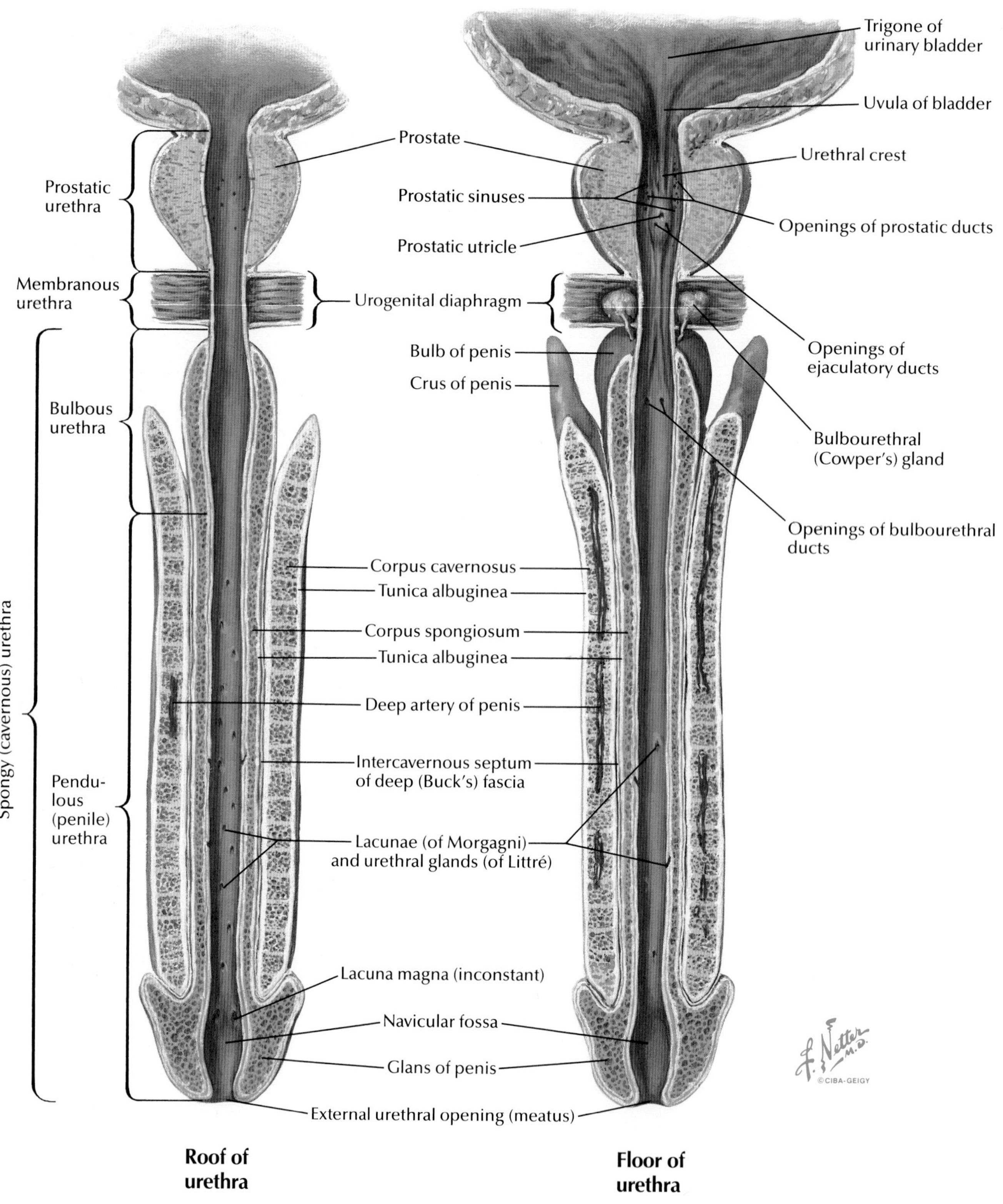

Prostatic urethra

Membranous urethra

Bulbous urethra

Spongy (cavernous) urethra

Pendu-lous (penile) urethra

Prostate

Prostatic sinuses

Prostatic utricle

Urogenital diaphragm

Bulb of penis

Crus of penis

Corpus cavernosus

Tunica albuginea

Corpus spongiosum

Tunica albuginea

Deep artery of penis

Intercavernous septum of deep (Buck's) fascia

Lacunae (of Morgagni) and urethral glands (of Littré)

Lacuna magna (inconstant)

Navicular fossa

Glans of penis

External urethral opening (meatus)

Trigone of urinary bladder

Uvula of bladder

Urethral crest

Openings of prostatic ducts

Openings of ejaculatory ducts

Bulbourethral (Cowper's) gland

Openings of bulbourethral ducts

Roof of urethra

Floor of urethra

PLATE 363

PELVIS AND PERINEUM

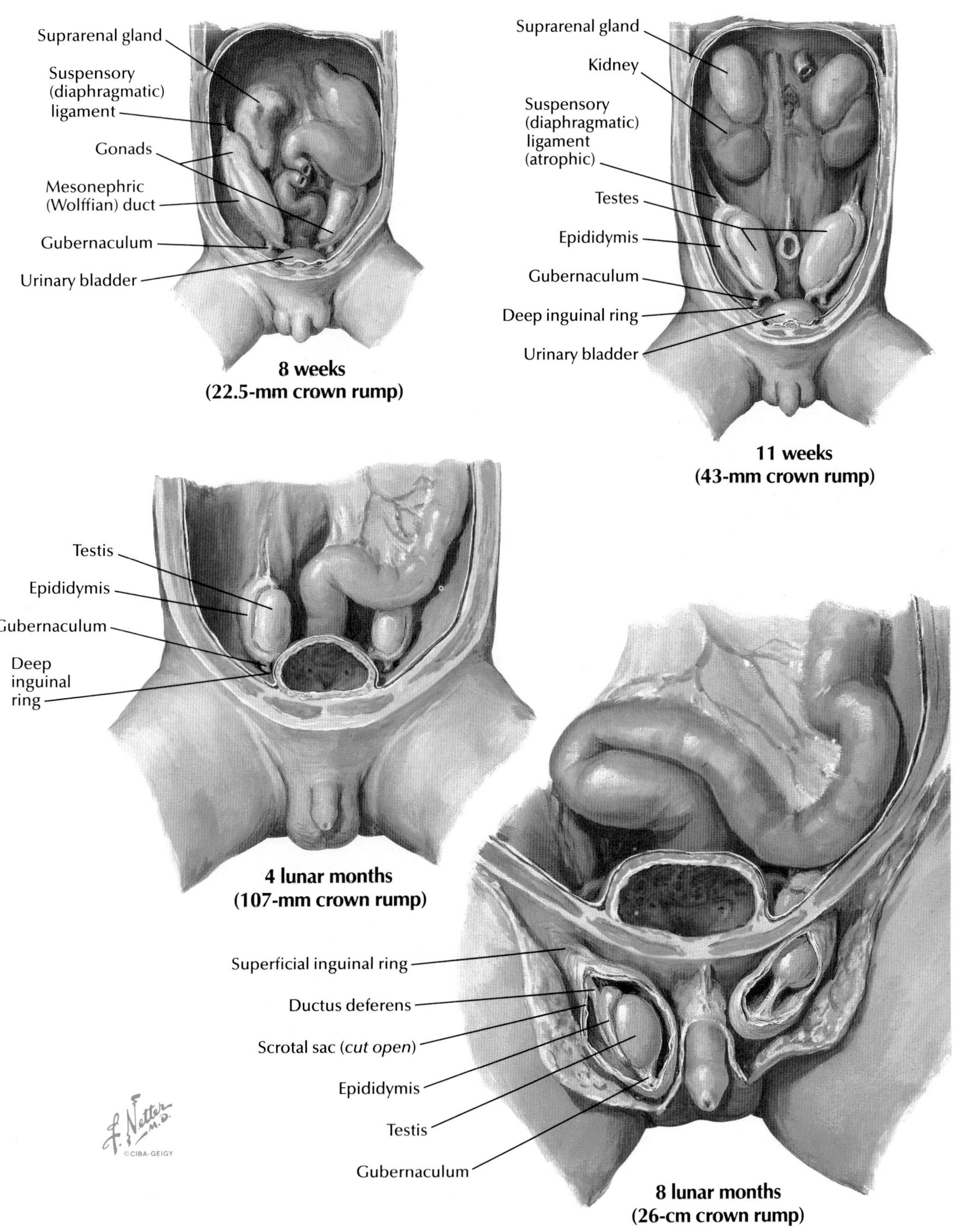

Suprarenal gland
Suspensory (diaphragmatic) ligament
Gonads
Mesonephric (Wolffian) duct
Gubernaculum
Urinary bladder

8 weeks (22.5-mm crown rump)

Suprarenal gland
Kidney
Suspensory (diaphragmatic) ligament (atrophic)
Testes
Epididymis
Gubernaculum
Deep inguinal ring
Urinary bladder

11 weeks (43-mm crown rump)

Testis
Epididymis
Gubernaculum
Deep inguinal ring

4 lunar months (107-mm crown rump)

Superficial inguinal ring
Ductus deferens
Scrotal sac (*cut open*)
Epididymis
Testis
Gubernaculum

8 lunar months (26-cm crown rump)

Scrotum and Contents

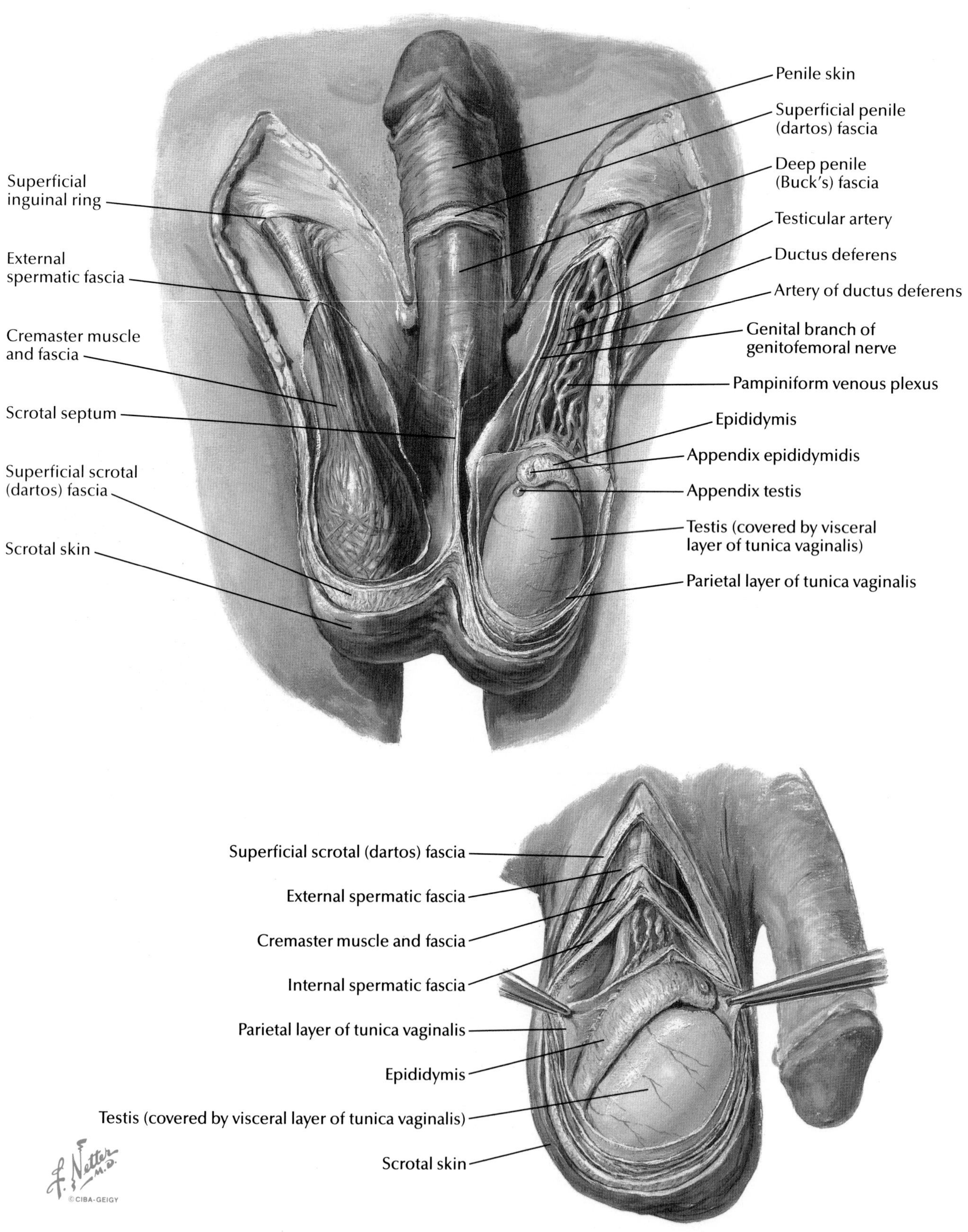

Superficial inguinal ring

External spermatic fascia

Cremaster muscle and fascia

Scrotal septum

Superficial scrotal (dartos) fascia

Scrotal skin

Penile skin

Superficial penile (dartos) fascia

Deep penile (Buck's) fascia

Testicular artery

Ductus deferens

Artery of ductus deferens

Genital branch of genitofemoral nerve

Pampiniform venous plexus

Epididymis

Appendix epididymidis

Appendix testis

Testis (covered by visceral layer of tunica vaginalis)

Parietal layer of tunica vaginalis

Superficial scrotal (dartos) fascia

External spermatic fascia

Cremaster muscle and fascia

Internal spermatic fascia

Parietal layer of tunica vaginalis

Epididymis

Testis (covered by visceral layer of tunica vaginalis)

Scrotal skin

PLATE 365

PELVIS AND PERINEUM

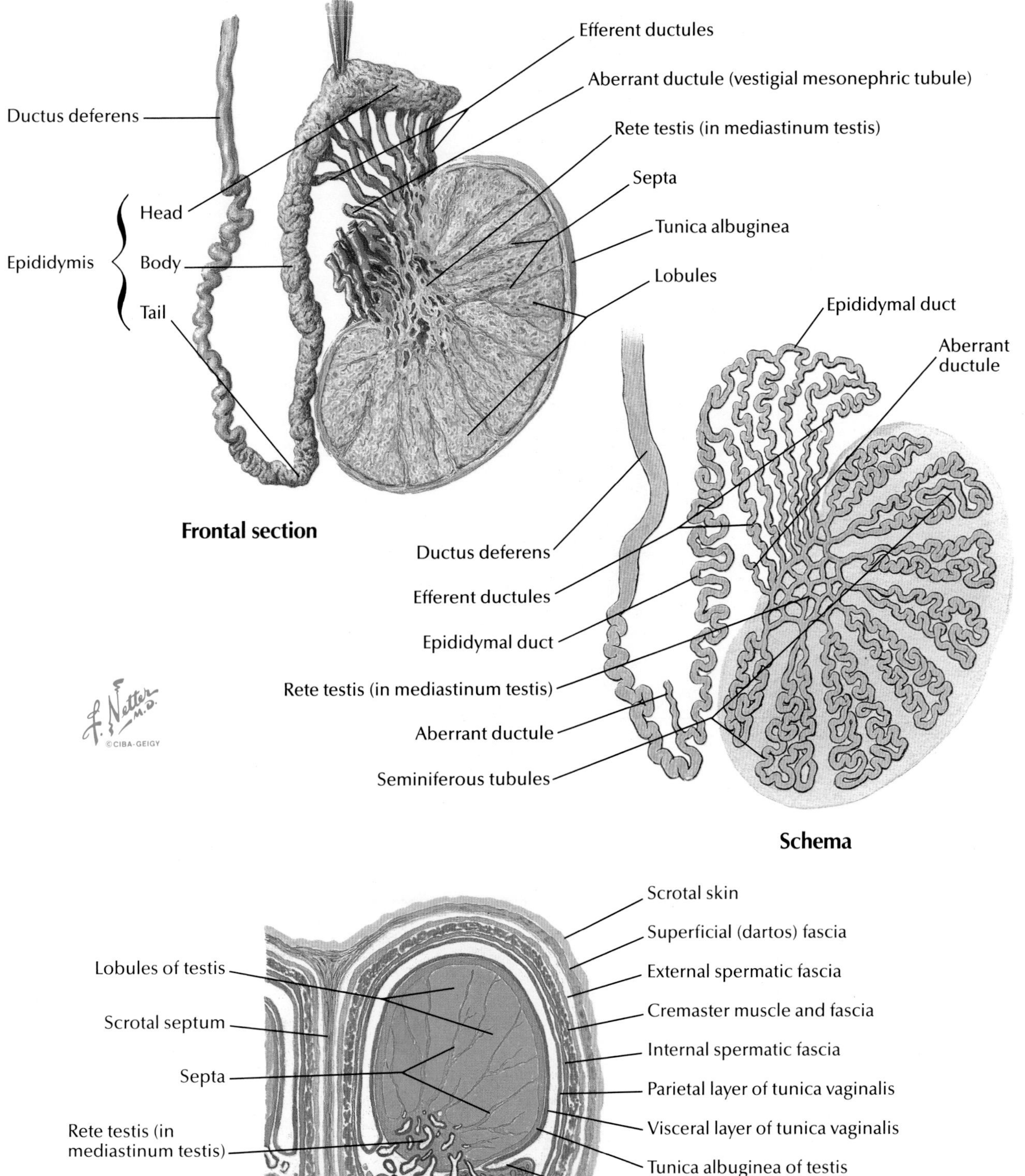

Frontal section

Ductus deferens

Epididymis
- Head
- Body
- Tail

Efferent ductules

Aberrant ductule (vestigial mesonephric tubule)

Rete testis (in mediastinum testis)

Septa

Tunica albuginea

Lobules

Epididymal duct

Aberrant ductule

Ductus deferens

Efferent ductules

Epididymal duct

Rete testis (in mediastinum testis)

Aberrant ductule

Seminiferous tubules

Schema

Lobules of testis

Scrotal septum

Septa

Rete testis (in mediastinum testis)

Ductus deferens

Scrotal skin

Superficial (dartos) fascia

External spermatic fascia

Cremaster muscle and fascia

Internal spermatic fascia

Parietal layer of tunica vaginalis

Visceral layer of tunica vaginalis

Tunica albuginea of testis

Sinus of epididymis

Epididymis

Cross section through scrotum and testis

Rectum In Situ: Female and Male

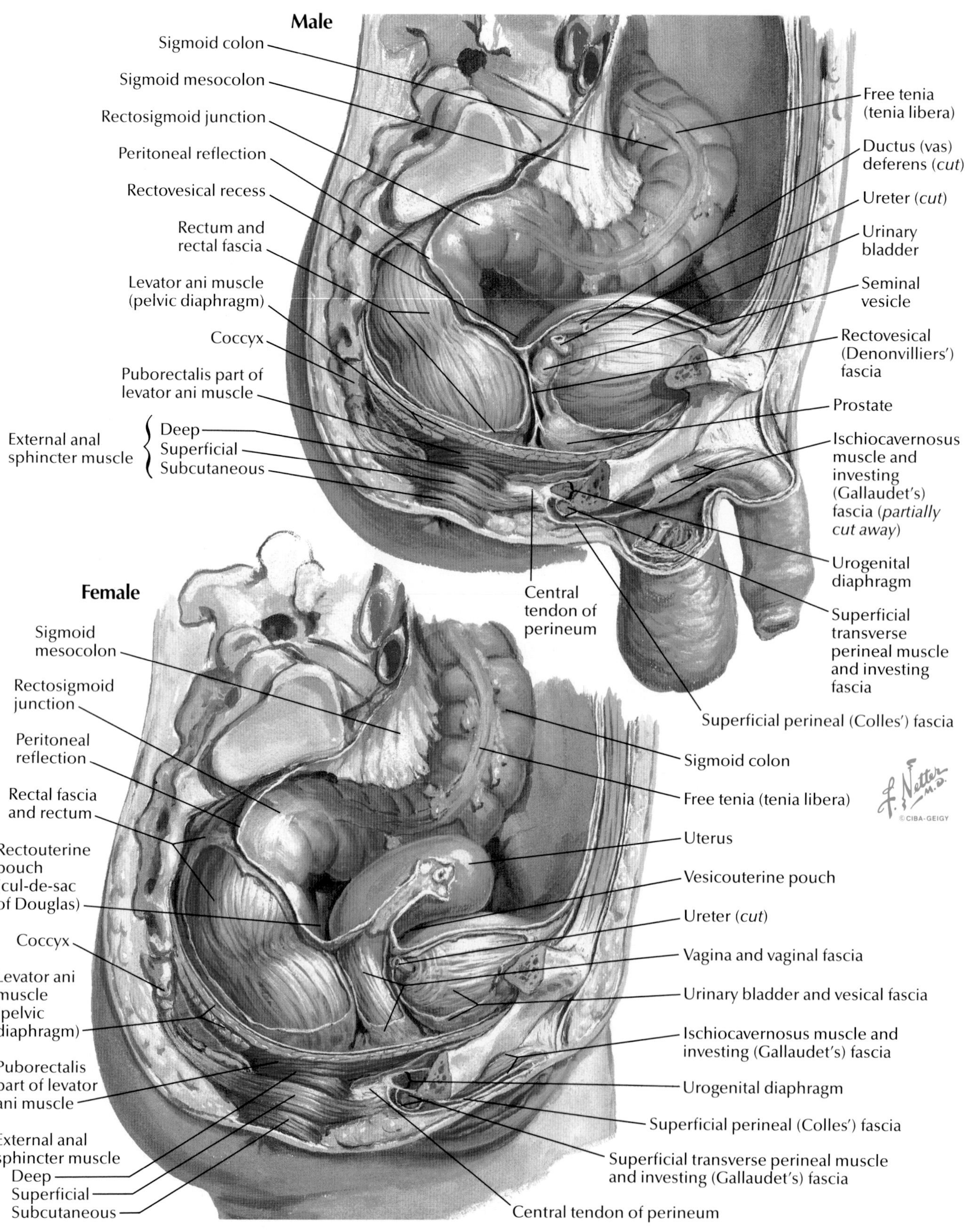

Male

Sigmoid colon

Sigmoid mesocolon

Rectosigmoid junction

Peritoneal reflection

Rectovesical recess

Rectum and rectal fascia

Levator ani muscle (pelvic diaphragm)

Coccyx

Puborectalis part of levator ani muscle

External anal sphincter muscle
{
Deep
Superficial
Subcutaneous
}

Free tenia (tenia libera)

Ductus (vas) deferens (*cut*)

Ureter (*cut*)

Urinary bladder

Seminal vesicle

Rectovesical (Denonvilliers') fascia

Prostate

Ischiocavernosus muscle and investing (Gallaudet's) fascia (*partially cut away*)

Urogenital diaphragm

Superficial transverse perineal muscle and investing fascia

Central tendon of perineum

Superficial perineal (Colles') fascia

Female

Sigmoid mesocolon

Rectosigmoid junction

Peritoneal reflection

Rectal fascia and rectum

Rectouterine pouch (cul-de-sac of Douglas)

Coccyx

Levator ani muscle (pelvic diaphragm)

Puborectalis part of levator ani muscle

External anal sphincter muscle
Deep
Superficial
Subcutaneous

Sigmoid colon

Free tenia (tenia libera)

Uterus

Vesicouterine pouch

Ureter (*cut*)

Vagina and vaginal fascia

Urinary bladder and vesical fascia

Ischiocavernosus muscle and investing (Gallaudet's) fascia

Urogenital diaphragm

Superficial perineal (Colles') fascia

Superficial transverse perineal muscle and investing (Gallaudet's) fascia

Central tendon of perineum

PLATE 367

PELVIS AND PERINEUM

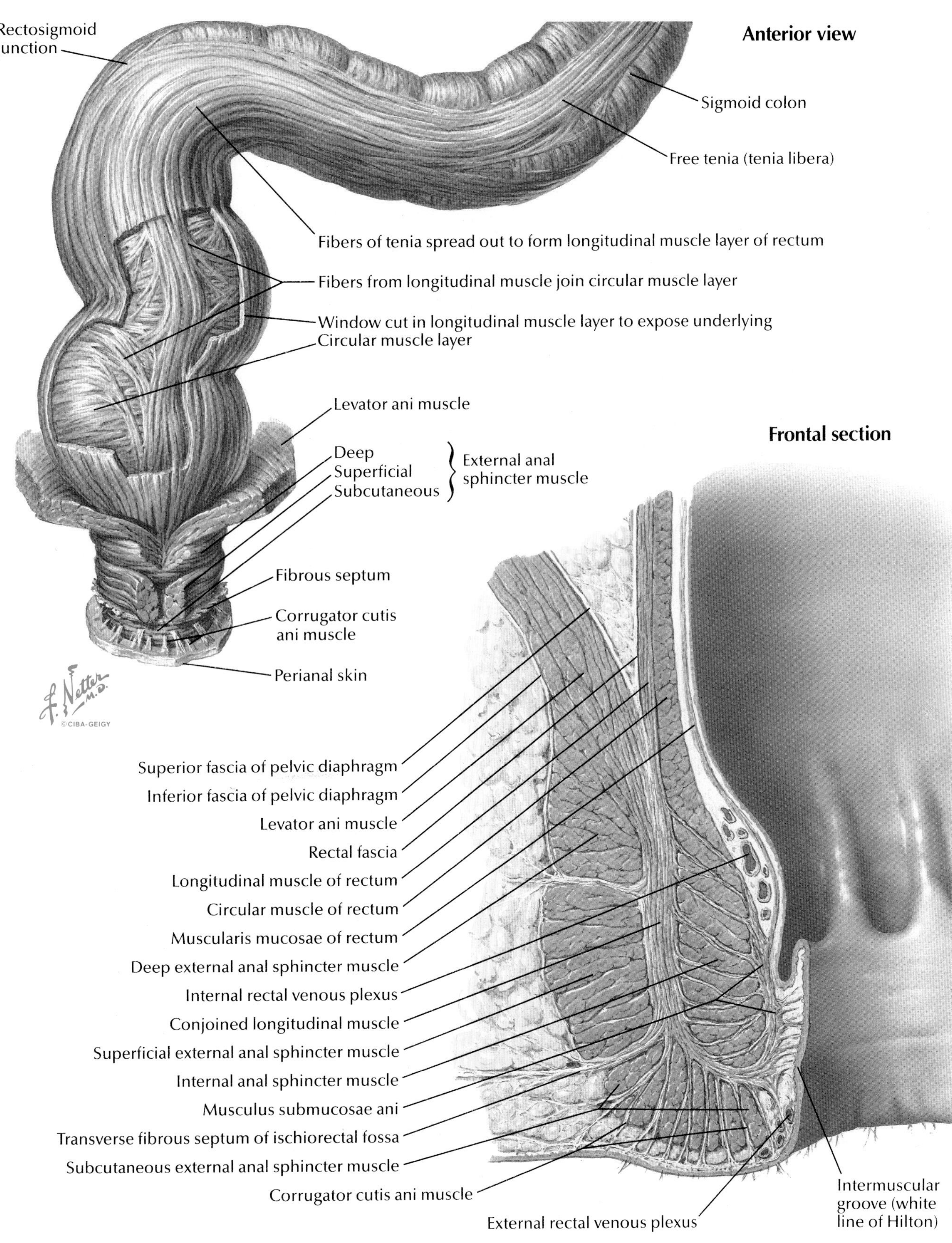

Anterior view

Rectosigmoid junction

Sigmoid colon

Free tenia (tenia libera)

Fibers of tenia spread out to form longitudinal muscle layer of rectum

Fibers from longitudinal muscle join circular muscle layer

Window cut in longitudinal muscle layer to expose underlying Circular muscle layer

Levator ani muscle

Deep
Superficial
Subcutaneous } External anal sphincter muscle

Fibrous septum

Corrugator cutis ani muscle

Perianal skin

Frontal section

Superior fascia of pelvic diaphragm
Inferior fascia of pelvic diaphragm
Levator ani muscle
Rectal fascia
Longitudinal muscle of rectum
Circular muscle of rectum
Muscularis mucosae of rectum
Deep external anal sphincter muscle
Internal rectal venous plexus
Conjoined longitudinal muscle
Superficial external anal sphincter muscle
Internal anal sphincter muscle
Musculus submucosae ani
Transverse fibrous septum of ischiorectal fossa
Subcutaneous external anal sphincter muscle
Corrugator cutis ani muscle

External rectal venous plexus

Intermuscular groove (white line of Hilton)

f. Netter
©CIBA-GEIGY

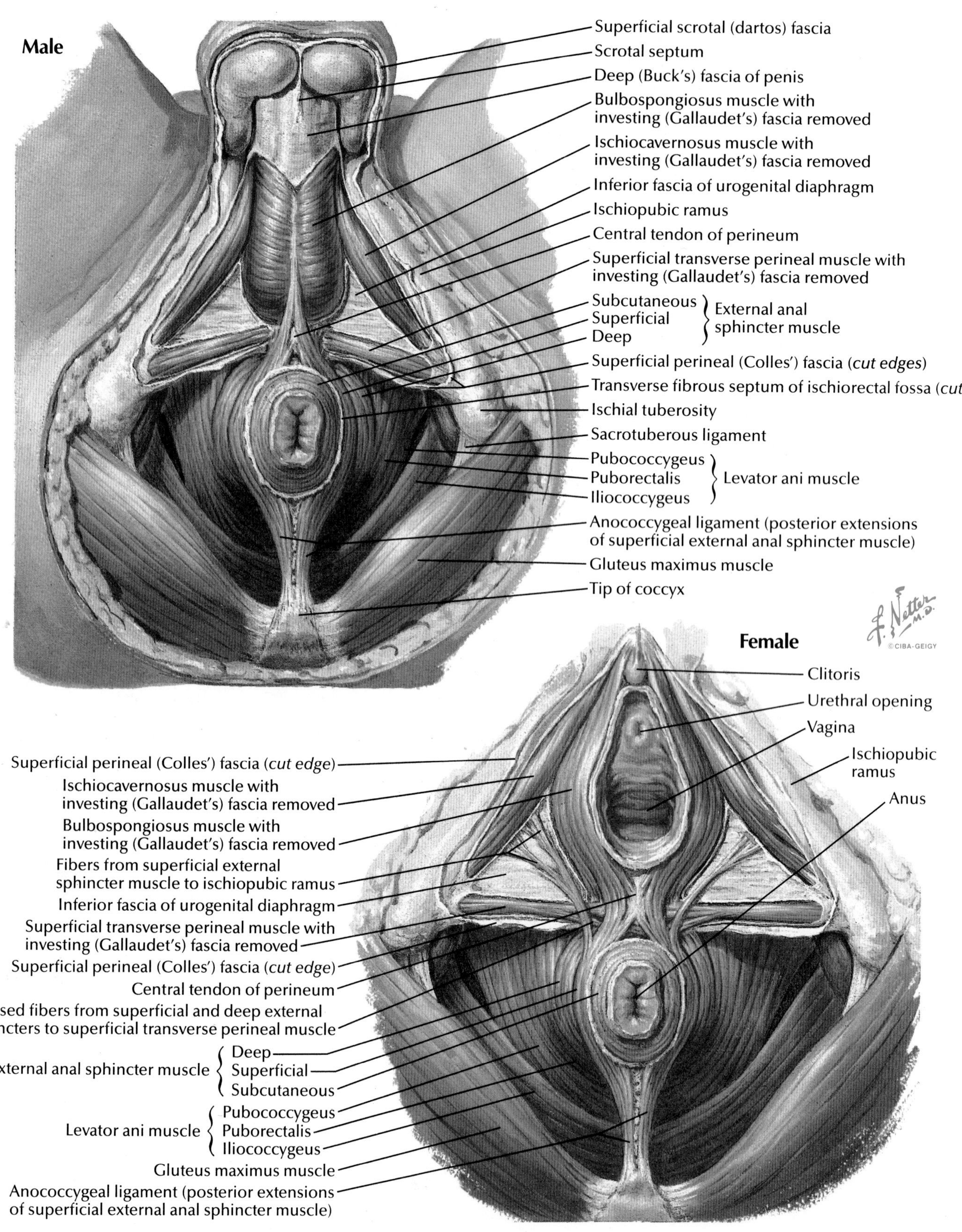

Male

Superficial scrotal (dartos) fascia

Scrotal septum

Deep (Buck's) fascia of penis

Bulbospongiosus muscle with investing (Gallaudet's) fascia removed

Ischiocavernosus muscle with investing (Gallaudet's) fascia removed

Inferior fascia of urogenital diaphragm

Ischiopubic ramus

Central tendon of perineum

Superficial transverse perineal muscle with investing (Gallaudet's) fascia removed

Subcutaneous
Superficial
Deep } External anal sphincter muscle

Superficial perineal (Colles') fascia (*cut edges*)

Transverse fibrous septum of ischiorectal fossa (*cut*)

Ischial tuberosity

Sacrotuberous ligament

Pubococcygeus
Puborectalis } Levator ani muscle
Iliococcygeus

Anococcygeal ligament (posterior extensions of superficial external anal sphincter muscle)

Gluteus maximus muscle

Tip of coccyx

Female

Clitoris

Urethral opening

Vagina

Ischiopubic ramus

Anus

Superficial perineal (Colles') fascia (*cut edge*)

Ischiocavernosus muscle with investing (Gallaudet's) fascia removed

Bulbospongiosus muscle with investing (Gallaudet's) fascia removed

Fibers from superficial external sphincter muscle to ischiopubic ramus

Inferior fascia of urogenital diaphragm

Superficial transverse perineal muscle with investing (Gallaudet's) fascia removed

Superficial perineal (Colles') fascia (*cut edge*)

Central tendon of perineum

Crossed fibers from superficial and deep external sphincters to superficial transverse perineal muscle

External anal sphincter muscle { Deep
Superficial
Subcutaneous

Levator ani muscle { Pubococcygeus
Puborectalis
Iliococcygeus

Gluteus maximus muscle

Anococcygeal ligament (posterior extensions of superficial external anal sphincter muscle)

PLATE 371

PELVIS AND PERINEUM

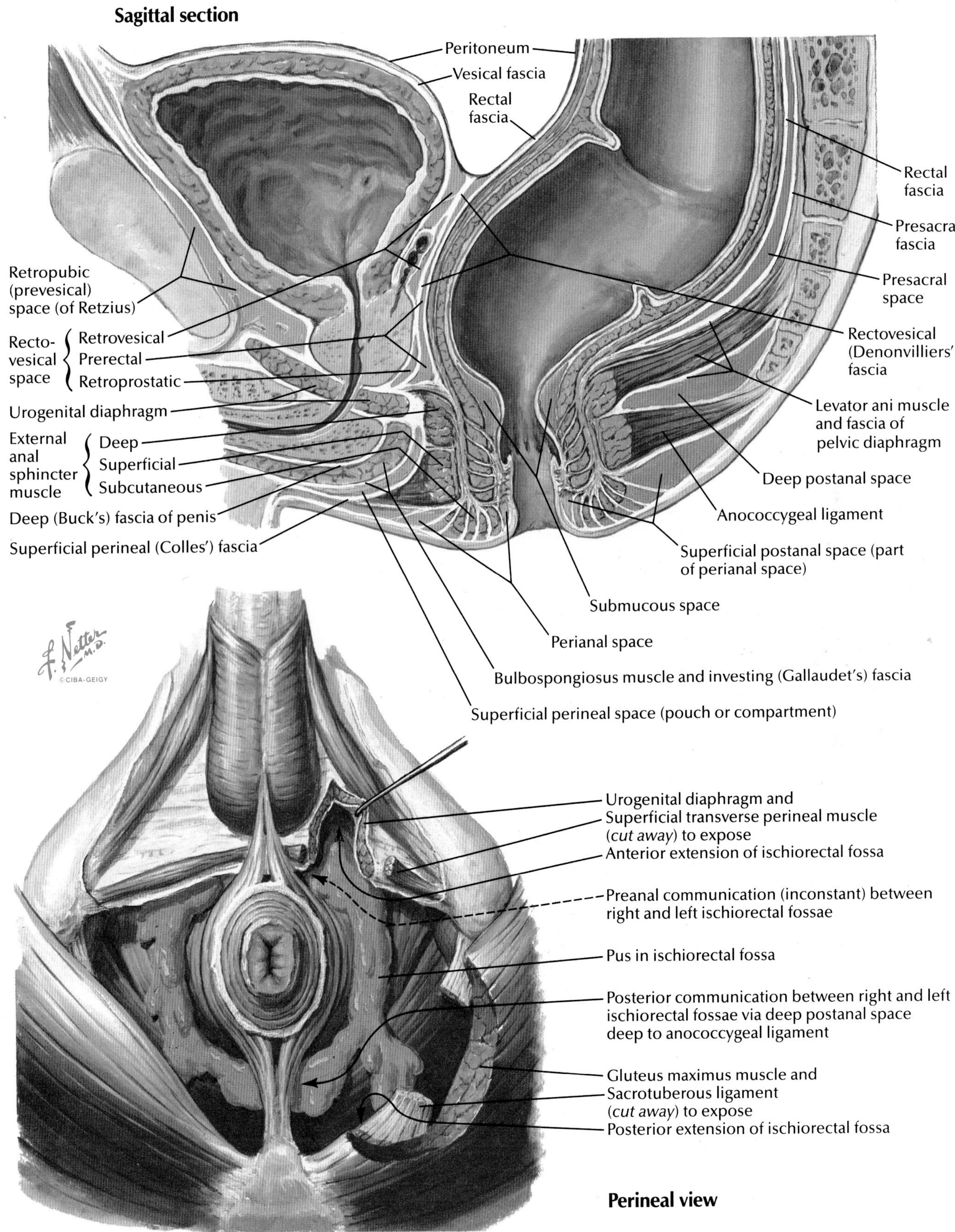

Sagittal section

Peritoneum

Vesical fascia

Rectal fascia

Rectal fascia

Presacral fascia

Presacral space

Rectovesical (Denonvilliers') fascia

Levator ani muscle and fascia of pelvic diaphragm

Deep postanal space

Anococcygeal ligament

Superficial postanal space (part of perianal space)

Submucous space

Perianal space

Bulbospongiosus muscle and investing (Gallaudet's) fascia

Superficial perineal space (pouch or compartment)

Retropubic (prevesical) space (of Retzius)

Recto-vesical space { Retrovesical / Prerectal / Retroprostatic

Urogenital diaphragm

External anal sphincter muscle { Deep / Superficial / Subcutaneous

Deep (Buck's) fascia of penis

Superficial perineal (Colles') fascia

Urogenital diaphragm and Superficial transverse perineal muscle (*cut away*) to expose Anterior extension of ischiorectal fossa

Preanal communication (inconstant) between right and left ischiorectal fossae

Pus in ischiorectal fossa

Posterior communication between right and left ischiorectal fossae via deep postanal space deep to anococcygeal ligament

Gluteus maximus muscle and Sacrotuberous ligament (*cut away*) to expose Posterior extension of ischiorectal fossa

Perineal view

RECTUM

PLATE 372

Arteries of Rectum and Anal Canal

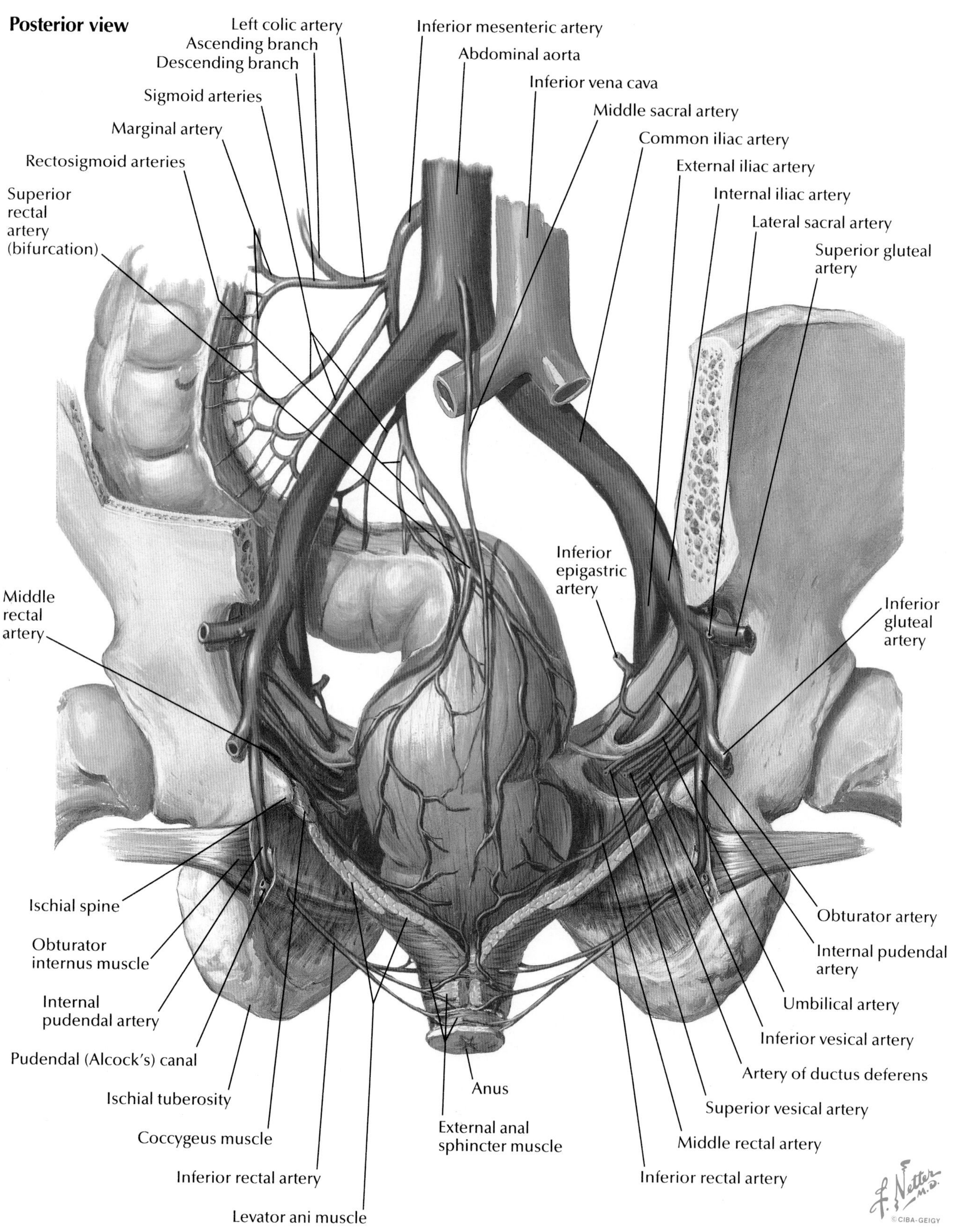

Left colic artery
Ascending branch
Descending branch
Sigmoid arteries
Marginal artery
Rectosigmoid arteries
Superior rectal artery (bifurcation)
Inferior mesenteric artery
Abdominal aorta
Inferior vena cava
Middle sacral artery
Common iliac artery
External iliac artery
Internal iliac artery
Lateral sacral artery
Superior gluteal artery
Middle rectal artery
Inferior epigastric artery
Inferior gluteal artery
Ischial spine
Obturator internus muscle
Internal pudendal artery
Pudendal (Alcock's) canal
Ischial tuberosity
Coccygeus muscle
Inferior rectal artery
Levator ani muscle
Anus
External anal sphincter muscle
Obturator artery
Internal pudendal artery
Umbilical artery
Inferior vesical artery
Artery of ductus deferens
Superior vesical artery
Middle rectal artery
Inferior rectal artery

PLATE 373

PELVIS AND PERINEUM

Anterior view

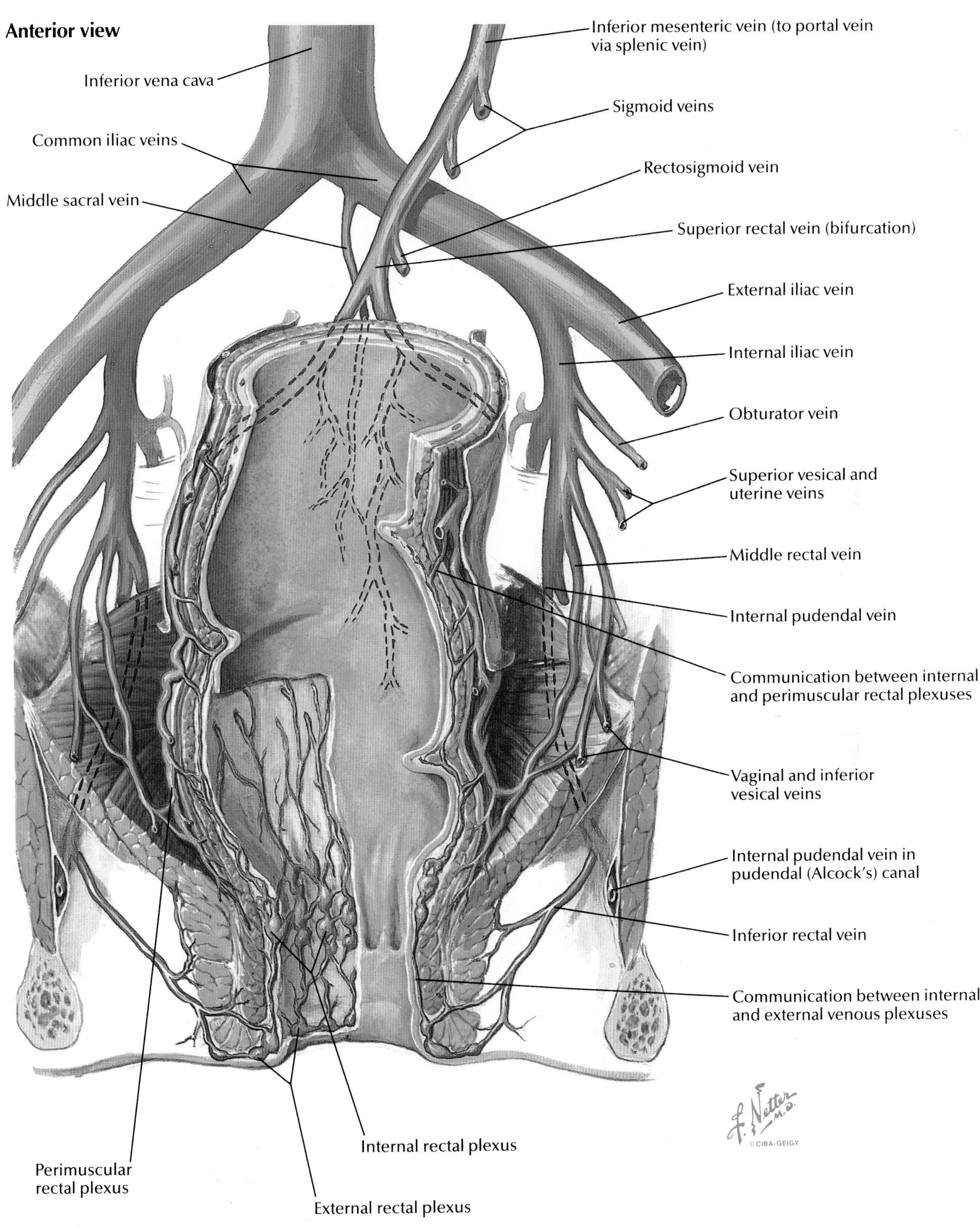

Inferior vena cava

Common iliac veins

Middle sacral vein

Inferior mesenteric vein (to portal vein via splenic vein)

Sigmoid veins

Rectosigmoid vein

Superior rectal vein (bifurcation)

External iliac vein

Internal iliac vein

Obturator vein

Superior vesical and uterine veins

Middle rectal vein

Internal pudendal vein

Communication between internal and perimuscular rectal plexuses

Vaginal and inferior vesical veins

Internal pudendal vein in pudendal (Alcock's) canal

Inferior rectal vein

Communication between internal and external venous plexuses

Internal rectal plexus

Perimuscular rectal plexus

External rectal plexus

Arteries and Veins of Pelvic Organs: Female

Anterior view

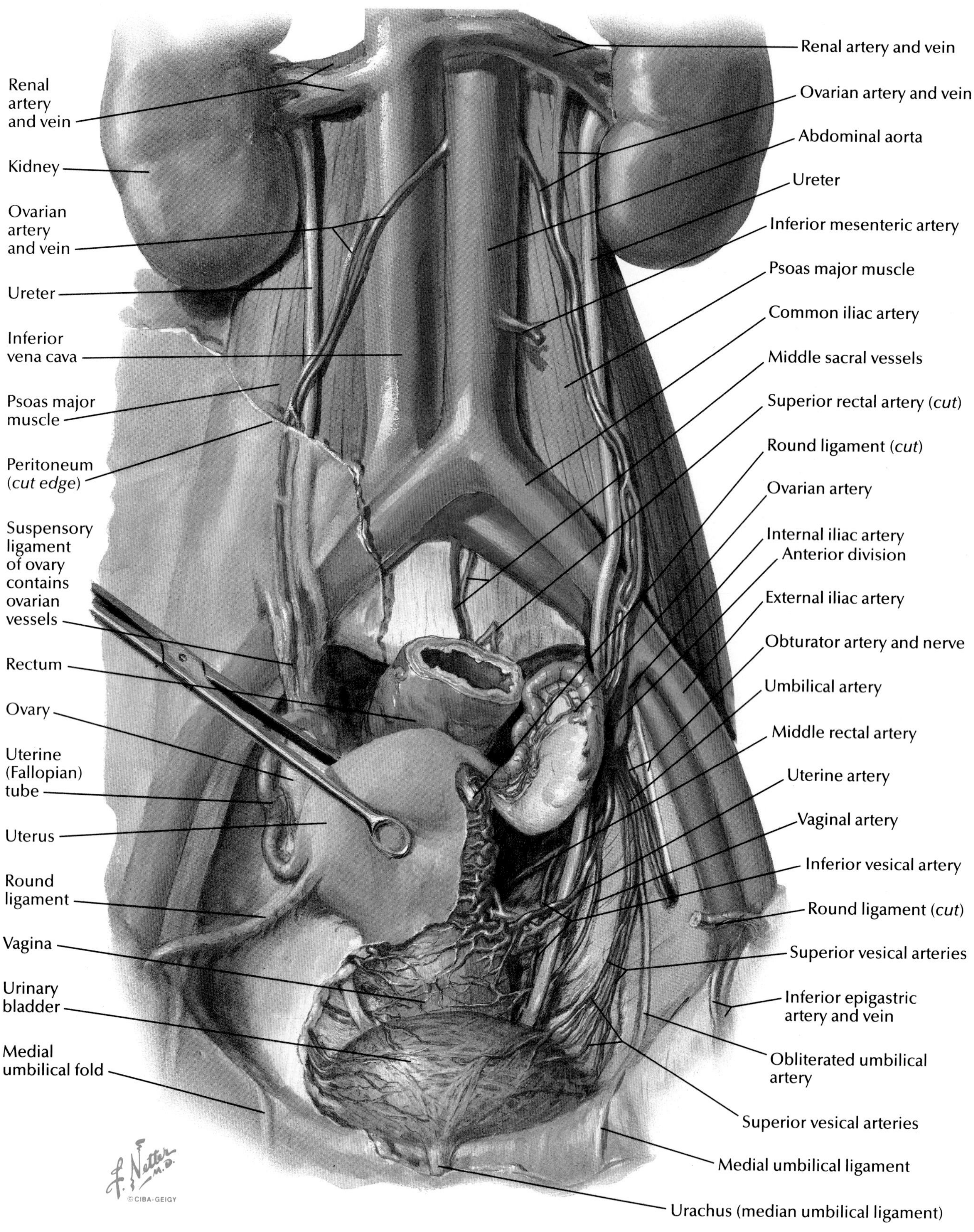

Renal artery and vein

Kidney

Ovarian artery and vein

Ureter

Inferior vena cava

Psoas major muscle

Peritoneum (*cut edge*)

Suspensory ligament of ovary contains ovarian vessels

Rectum

Ovary

Uterine (Fallopian) tube

Uterus

Round ligament

Vagina

Urinary bladder

Medial umbilical fold

Renal artery and vein

Ovarian artery and vein

Abdominal aorta

Ureter

Inferior mesenteric artery

Psoas major muscle

Common iliac artery

Middle sacral vessels

Superior rectal artery (*cut*)

Round ligament (*cut*)

Ovarian artery

Internal iliac artery Anterior division

External iliac artery

Obturator artery and nerve

Umbilical artery

Middle rectal artery

Uterine artery

Vaginal artery

Inferior vesical artery

Round ligament (*cut*)

Superior vesical arteries

Inferior epigastric artery and vein

Obliterated umbilical artery

Superior vesical arteries

Medial umbilical ligament

Urachus (median umbilical ligament)

PLATE 375

PELVIS AND PERINEUM

Anterior view

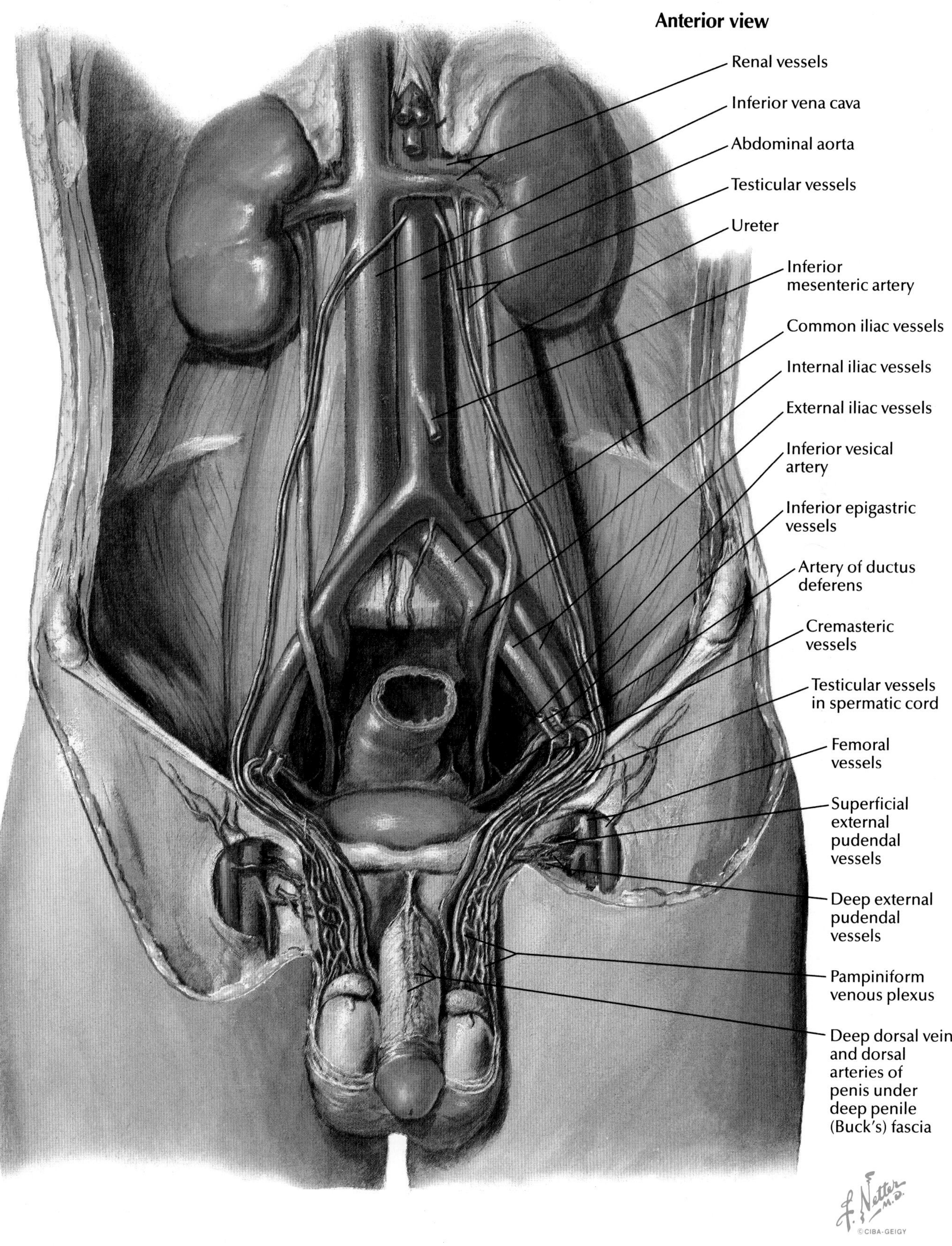

Renal vessels

Inferior vena cava

Abdominal aorta

Testicular vessels

Ureter

Inferior mesenteric artery

Common iliac vessels

Internal iliac vessels

External iliac vessels

Inferior vesical artery

Inferior epigastric vessels

Artery of ductus deferens

Cremasteric vessels

Testicular vessels in spermatic cord

Femoral vessels

Superficial external pudendal vessels

Deep external pudendal vessels

Pampiniform venous plexus

Deep dorsal vein and dorsal arteries of penis under deep penile (Buck's) fascia

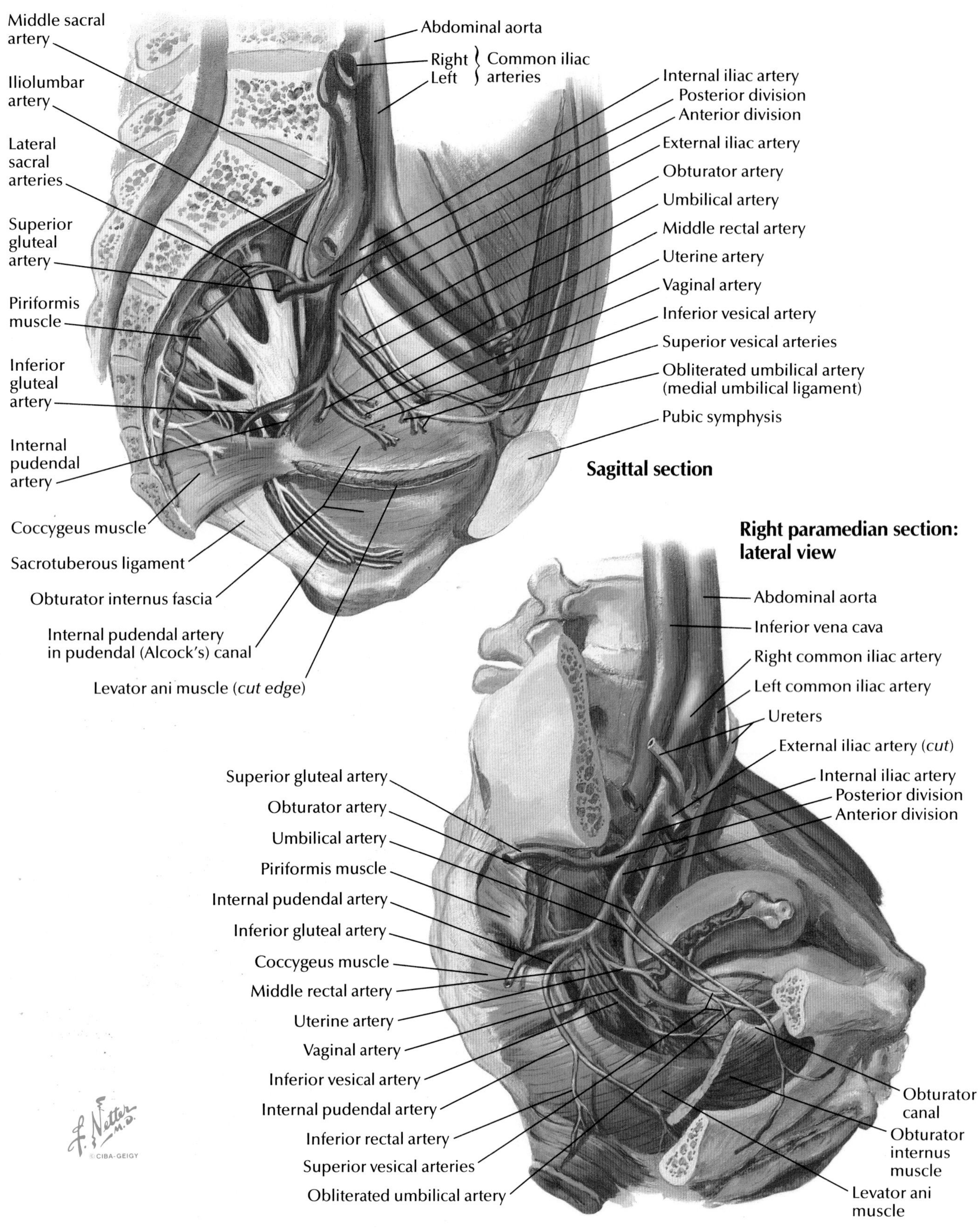

Middle sacral artery

Iliolumbar artery

Lateral sacral arteries

Superior gluteal artery

Piriformis muscle

Inferior gluteal artery

Internal pudendal artery

Coccygeus muscle

Sacrotuberous ligament

Obturator internus fascia

Internal pudendal artery in pudendal (Alcock's) canal

Levator ani muscle (*cut edge*)

Abdominal aorta

Right } Common iliac
Left } arteries

Internal iliac artery
Posterior division
Anterior division

External iliac artery

Obturator artery

Umbilical artery

Middle rectal artery

Uterine artery

Vaginal artery

Inferior vesical artery

Superior vesical arteries

Obliterated umbilical artery (medial umbilical ligament)

Pubic symphysis

Sagittal section

Right paramedian section: lateral view

Abdominal aorta

Inferior vena cava

Right common iliac artery

Left common iliac artery

Ureters

External iliac artery (*cut*)

Internal iliac artery
Posterior division
Anterior division

Superior gluteal artery

Obturator artery

Umbilical artery

Piriformis muscle

Internal pudendal artery

Inferior gluteal artery

Coccygeus muscle

Middle rectal artery

Uterine artery

Vaginal artery

Inferior vesical artery

Internal pudendal artery

Inferior rectal artery

Superior vesical arteries

Obliterated umbilical artery

Obturator canal

Obturator internus muscle

Levator ani muscle

PLATE 377

PELVIS AND PERINEUM

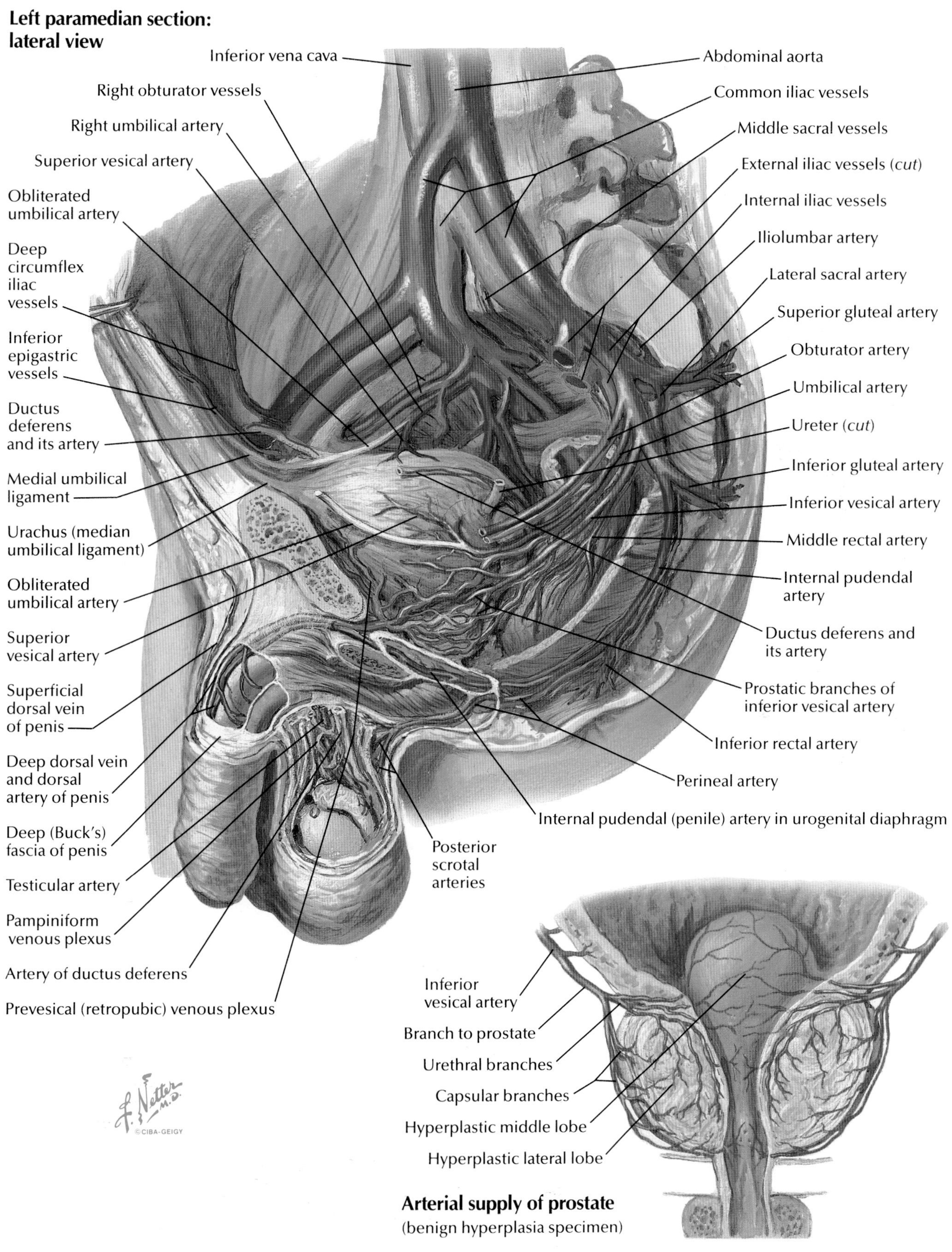

Left paramedian section: lateral view

Inferior vena cava

Right obturator vessels

Right umbilical artery

Superior vesical artery

Obliterated umbilical artery

Deep circumflex iliac vessels

Inferior epigastric vessels

Ductus deferens and its artery

Medial umbilical ligament

Urachus (median umbilical ligament)

Obliterated umbilical artery

Superior vesical artery

Superficial dorsal vein of penis

Deep dorsal vein and dorsal artery of penis

Deep (Buck's) fascia of penis

Testicular artery

Pampiniform venous plexus

Artery of ductus deferens

Prevesical (retropubic) venous plexus

Abdominal aorta

Common iliac vessels

Middle sacral vessels

External iliac vessels *(cut)*

Internal iliac vessels

Iliolumbar artery

Lateral sacral artery

Superior gluteal artery

Obturator artery

Umbilical artery

Ureter *(cut)*

Inferior gluteal artery

Inferior vesical artery

Middle rectal artery

Internal pudendal artery

Ductus deferens and its artery

Prostatic branches of inferior vesical artery

Inferior rectal artery

Perineal artery

Internal pudendal (penile) artery in urogenital diaphragm

Posterior scrotal arteries

Inferior vesical artery

Branch to prostate

Urethral branches

Capsular branches

Hyperplastic middle lobe

Hyperplastic lateral lobe

Arterial supply of prostate
(benign hyperplasia specimen)

Arteries and Veins of Perineum and Uterus

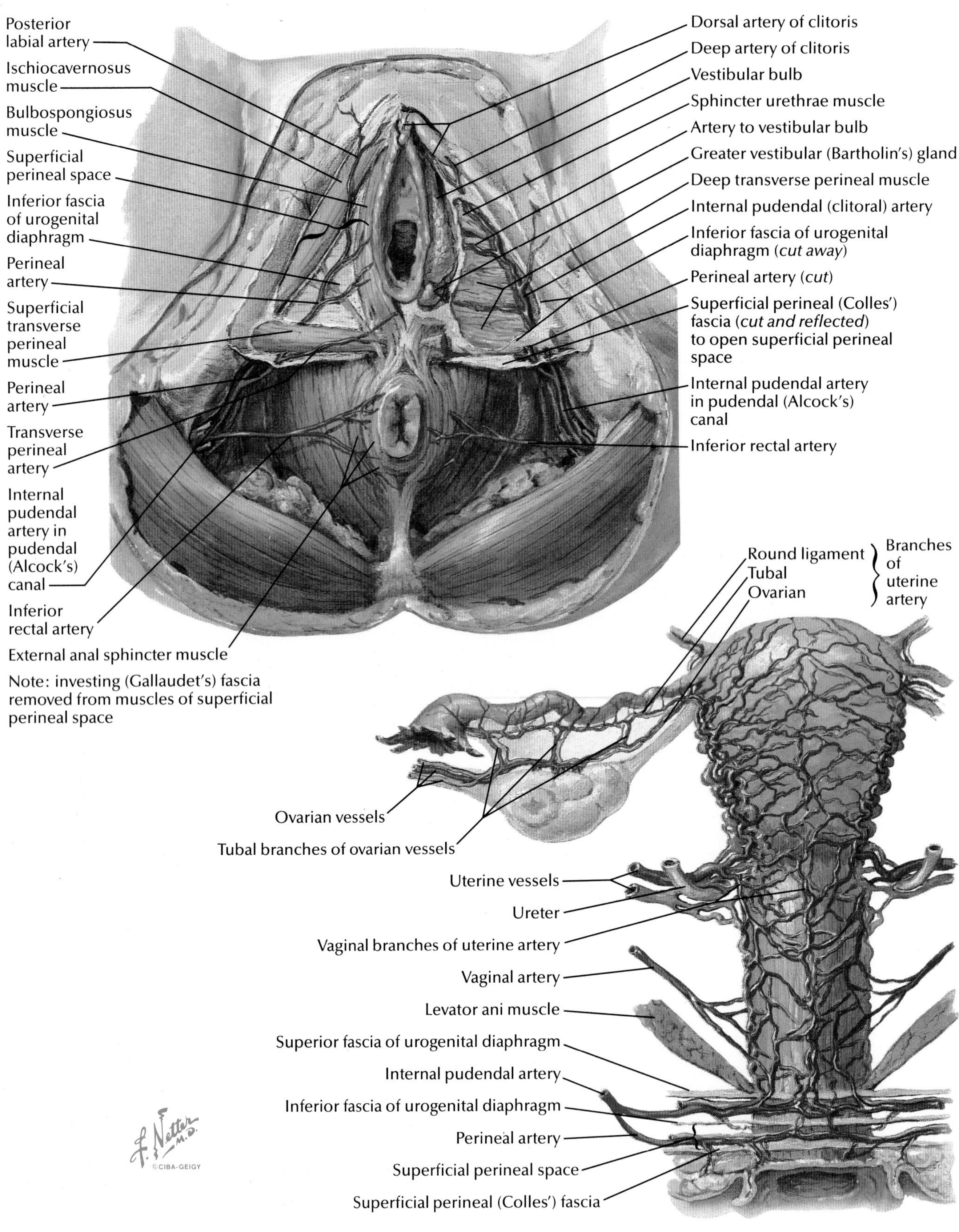

Posterior labial artery

Ischiocavernosus muscle

Bulbospongiosus muscle

Superficial perineal space

Inferior fascia of urogenital diaphragm

Perineal artery

Superficial transverse perineal muscle

Perineal artery

Transverse perineal artery

Internal pudendal artery in pudendal (Alcock's) canal

Inferior rectal artery

External anal sphincter muscle

Note: investing (Gallaudet's) fascia removed from muscles of superficial perineal space

Dorsal artery of clitoris

Deep artery of clitoris

Vestibular bulb

Sphincter urethrae muscle

Artery to vestibular bulb

Greater vestibular (Bartholin's) gland

Deep transverse perineal muscle

Internal pudendal (clitoral) artery

Inferior fascia of urogenital diaphragm (cut away)

Perineal artery (cut)

Superficial perineal (Colles') fascia (cut and reflected) to open superficial perineal space

Internal pudendal artery in pudendal (Alcock's) canal

Inferior rectal artery

Round ligament
Tubal
Ovarian
} Branches of uterine artery

Ovarian vessels

Tubal branches of ovarian vessels

Uterine vessels

Ureter

Vaginal branches of uterine artery

Vaginal artery

Levator ani muscle

Superior fascia of urogenital diaphragm

Internal pudendal artery

Inferior fascia of urogenital diaphragm

Perineal artery

Superficial perineal space

Superficial perineal (Colles') fascia

PLATE 379

PELVIS AND PERINEUM

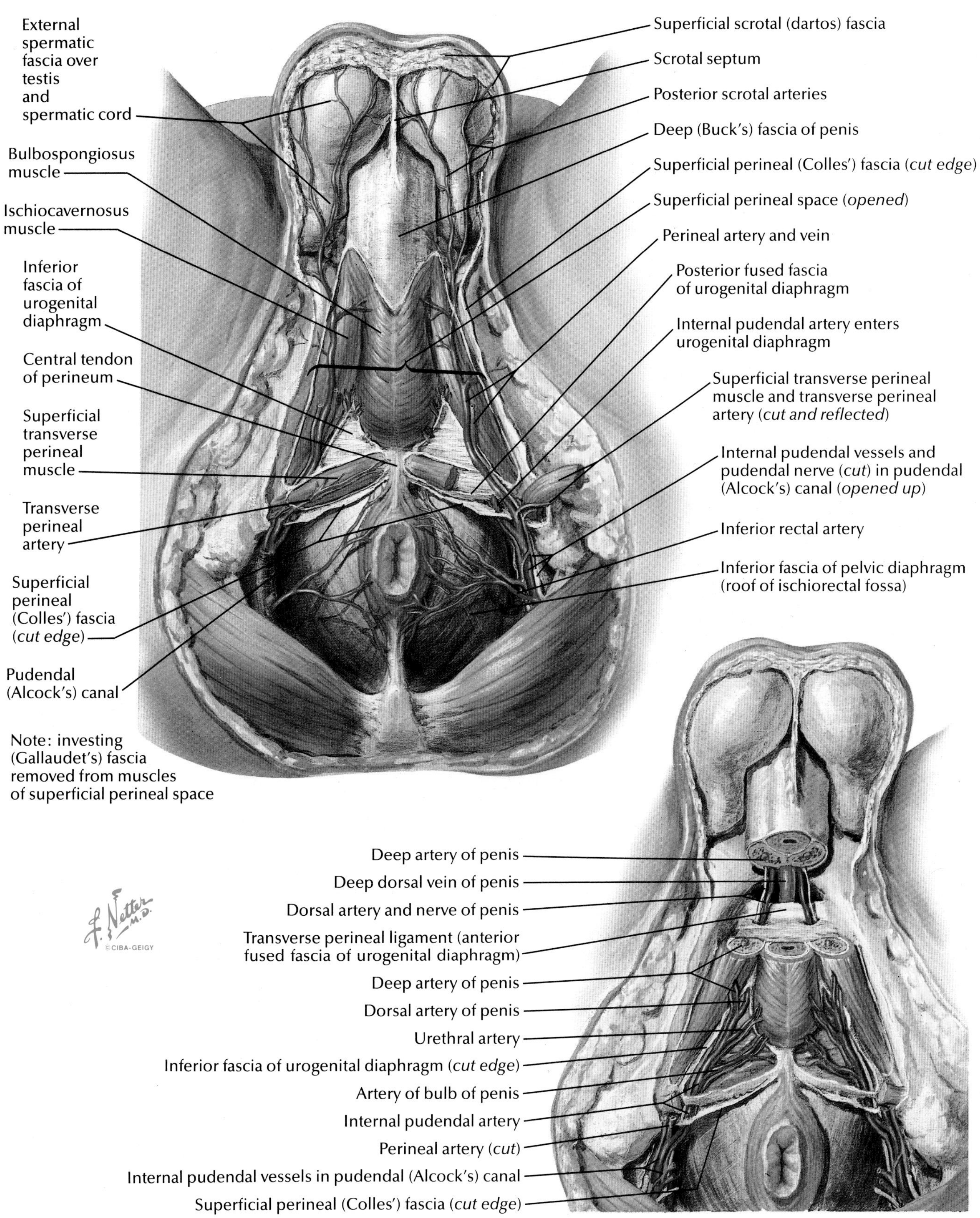

External spermatic fascia over testis and spermatic cord

Bulbospongiosus muscle

Ischiocavernosus muscle

Inferior fascia of urogenital diaphragm

Central tendon of perineum

Superficial transverse perineal muscle

Transverse perineal artery

Superficial perineal (Colles') fascia (cut edge)

Pudendal (Alcock's) canal

Note: investing (Gallaudet's) fascia removed from muscles of superficial perineal space

Superficial scrotal (dartos) fascia

Scrotal septum

Posterior scrotal arteries

Deep (Buck's) fascia of penis

Superficial perineal (Colles') fascia (cut edge)

Superficial perineal space (opened)

Perineal artery and vein

Posterior fused fascia of urogenital diaphragm

Internal pudendal artery enters urogenital diaphragm

Superficial transverse perineal muscle and transverse perineal artery (cut and reflected)

Internal pudendal vessels and pudendal nerve (cut) in pudendal (Alcock's) canal (opened up)

Inferior rectal artery

Inferior fascia of pelvic diaphragm (roof of ischiorectal fossa)

Deep artery of penis

Deep dorsal vein of penis

Dorsal artery and nerve of penis

Transverse perineal ligament (anterior fused fascia of urogenital diaphragm)

Deep artery of penis

Dorsal artery of penis

Urethral artery

Inferior fascia of urogenital diaphragm (cut edge)

Artery of bulb of penis

Internal pudendal artery

Perineal artery (cut)

Internal pudendal vessels in pudendal (Alcock's) canal

Superficial perineal (Colles') fascia (cut edge)

Lymph Vessels and Nodes of Pelvis and Genitalia: Female

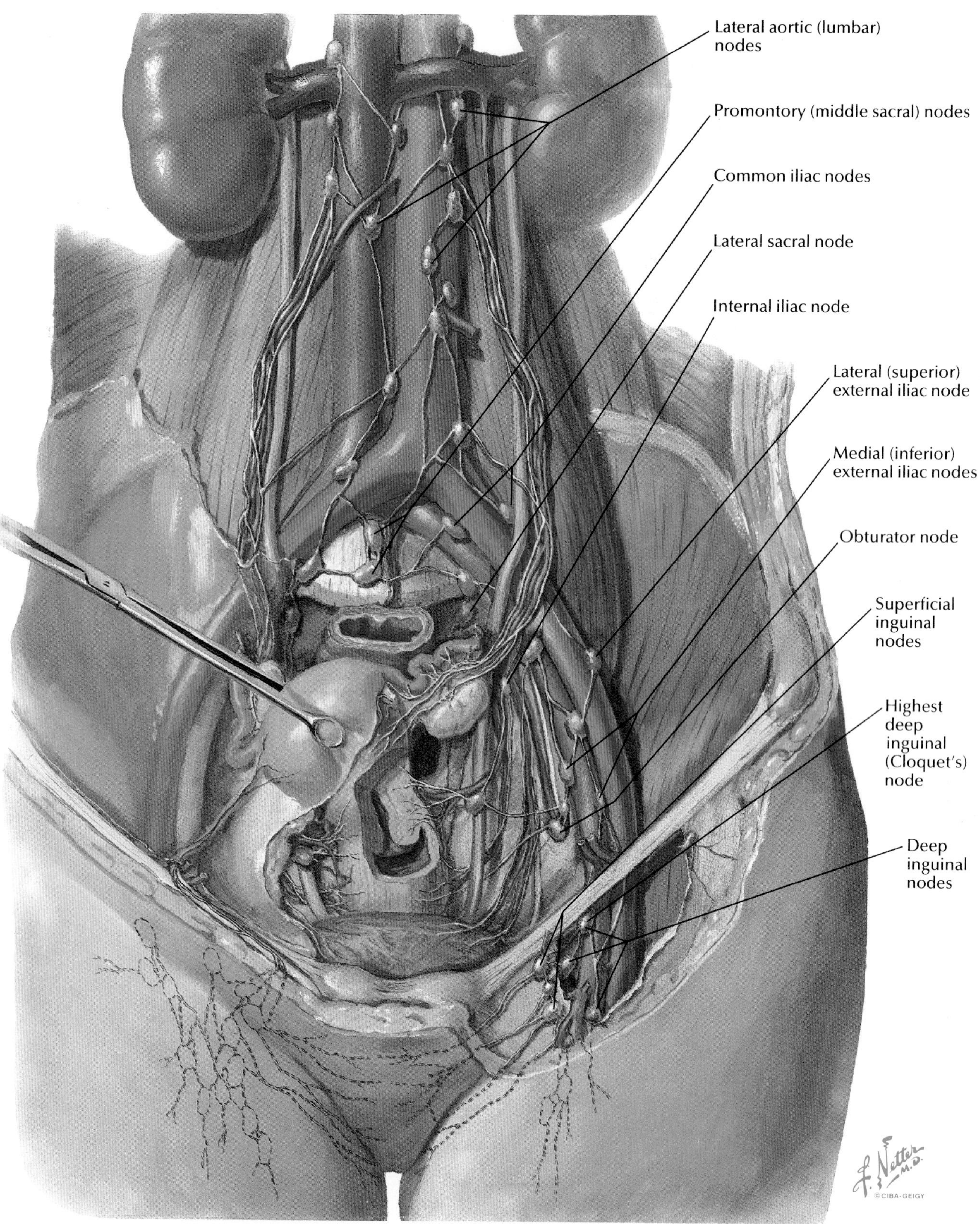

Lateral aortic (lumbar) nodes

Promontory (middle sacral) nodes

Common iliac nodes

Lateral sacral node

Internal iliac node

Lateral (superior) external iliac node

Medial (inferior) external iliac nodes

Obturator node

Superficial inguinal nodes

Highest deep inguinal (Cloquet's) node

Deep inguinal nodes

PLATE 381

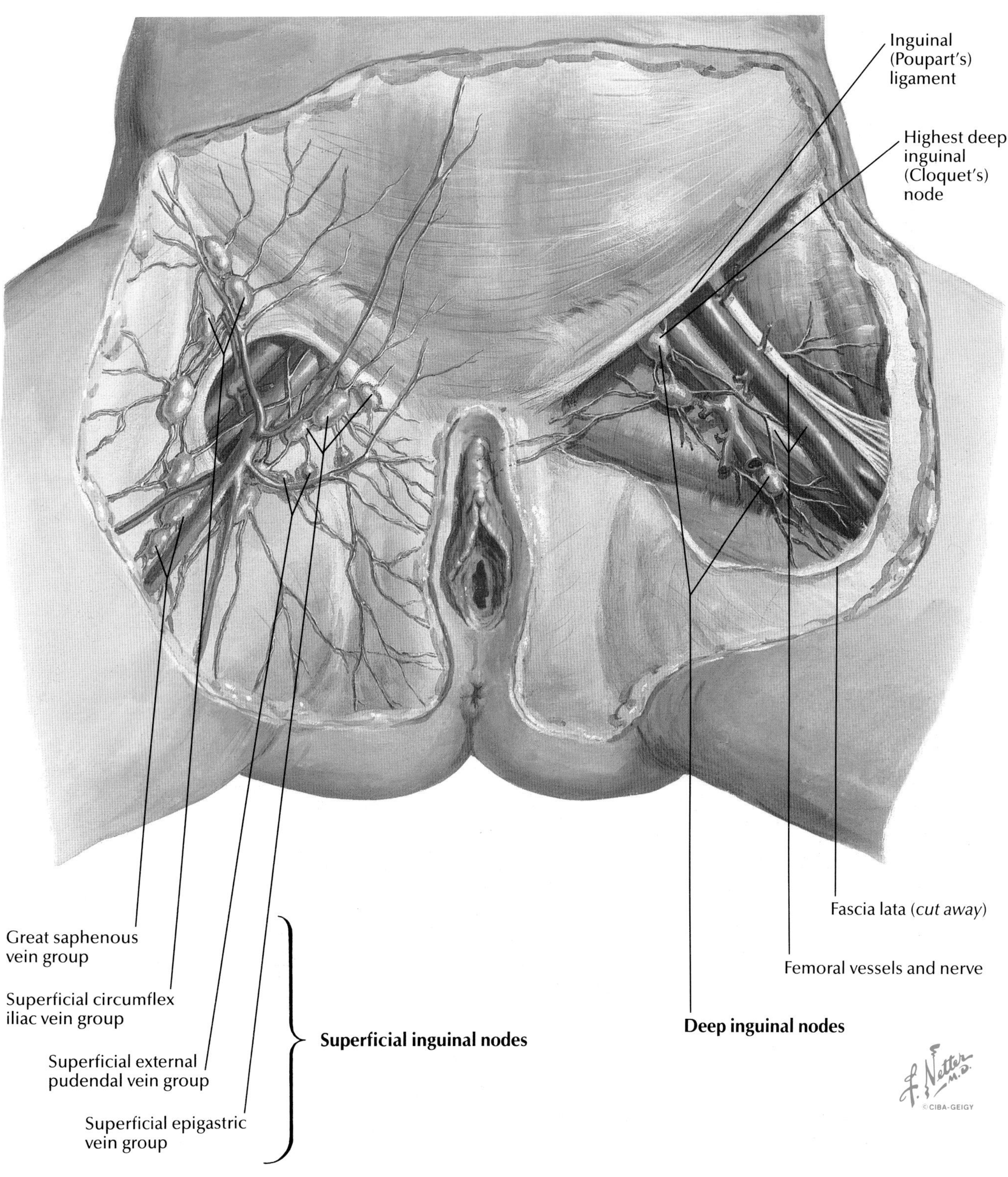

Inguinal
(Poupart's)
ligament

Highest deep
inguinal
(Cloquet's)
node

Great saphenous
vein group

Superficial circumflex
iliac vein group

Superficial external
pudendal vein group

Superficial epigastric
vein group

Superficial inguinal nodes

Fascia lata (*cut away*)

Femoral vessels and nerve

Deep inguinal nodes

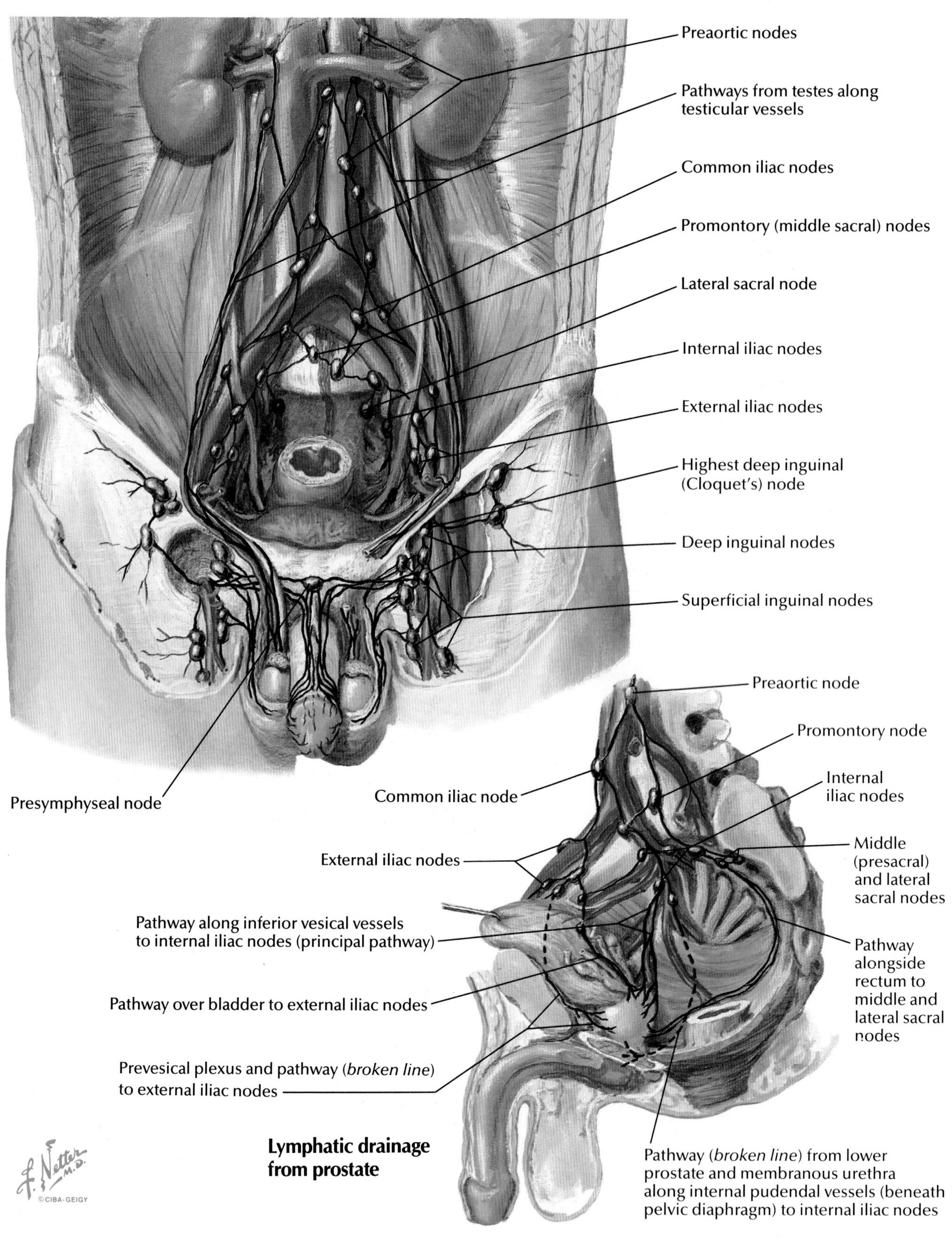

Preaortic nodes

Pathways from testes along testicular vessels

Common iliac nodes

Promontory (middle sacral) nodes

Lateral sacral node

Internal iliac nodes

External iliac nodes

Highest deep inguinal (Cloquet's) node

Deep inguinal nodes

Superficial inguinal nodes

Preaortic node

Promontory node

Internal iliac nodes

Middle (presacral) and lateral sacral nodes

Pathway alongside rectum to middle and lateral sacral nodes

Common iliac node

External iliac nodes

Pathway along inferior vesical vessels to internal iliac nodes (principal pathway)

Pathway over bladder to external iliac nodes

Prevesical plexus and pathway (*broken line*) to external iliac nodes

Presymphyseal node

Lymphatic drainage from prostate

Pathway (*broken line*) from lower prostate and membranous urethra along internal pudendal vessels (beneath pelvic diaphragm) to internal iliac nodes

PLATE 383

PELVIS AND PERINEUM

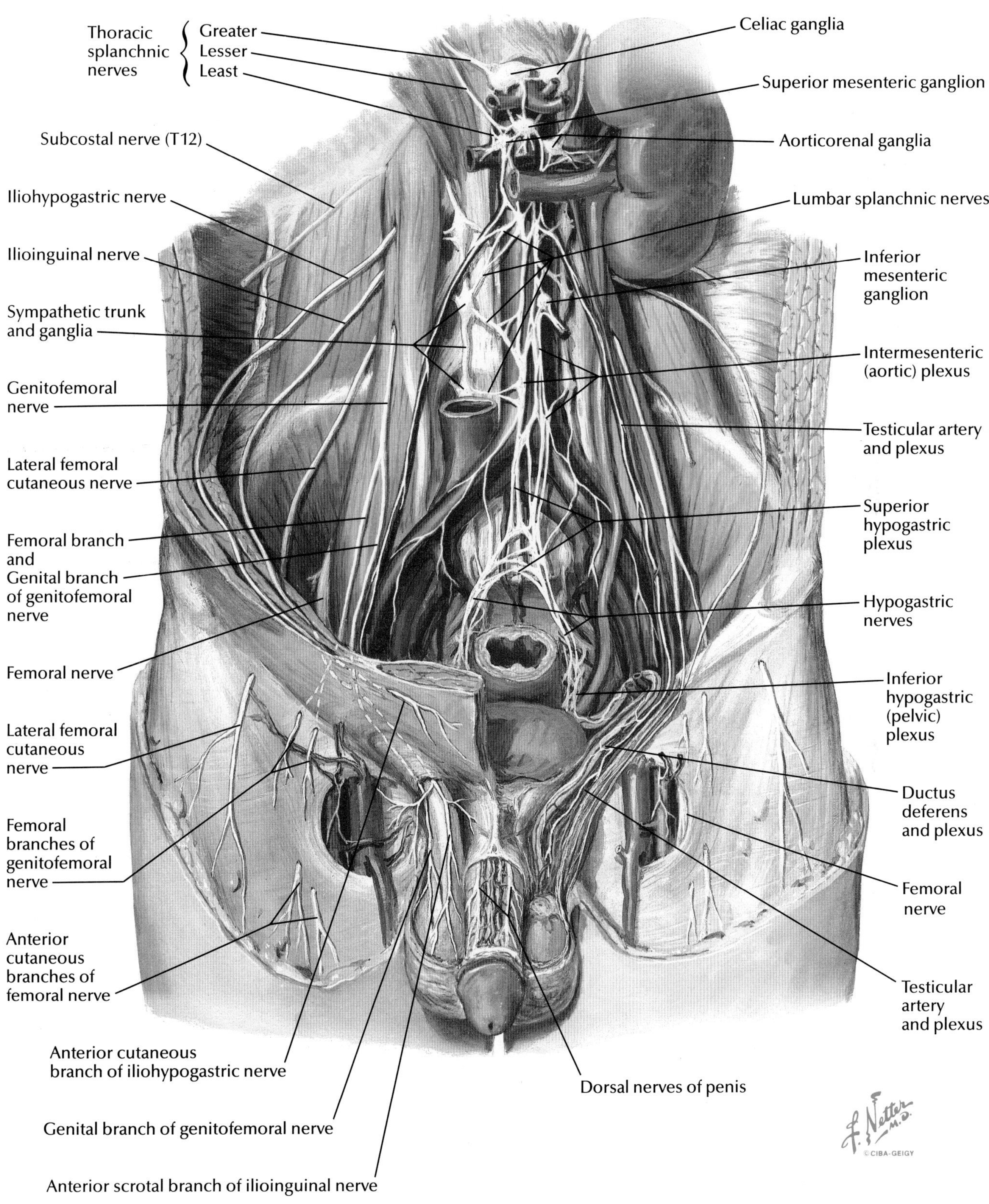

Thoracic splanchnic nerves
— Greater
— Lesser
— Least

Subcostal nerve (T12)

Iliohypogastric nerve

Ilioinguinal nerve

Sympathetic trunk and ganglia

Genitofemoral nerve

Lateral femoral cutaneous nerve

Femoral branch and Genital branch of genitofemoral nerve

Femoral nerve

Lateral femoral cutaneous nerve

Femoral branches of genitofemoral nerve

Anterior cutaneous branches of femoral nerve

Anterior cutaneous branch of iliohypogastric nerve

Genital branch of genitofemoral nerve

Anterior scrotal branch of ilioinguinal nerve

Celiac ganglia

Superior mesenteric ganglion

Aorticorenal ganglia

Lumbar splanchnic nerves

Inferior mesenteric ganglion

Intermesenteric (aortic) plexus

Testicular artery and plexus

Superior hypogastric plexus

Hypogastric nerves

Inferior hypogastric (pelvic) plexus

Ductus deferens and plexus

Femoral nerve

Testicular artery and plexus

Dorsal nerves of penis

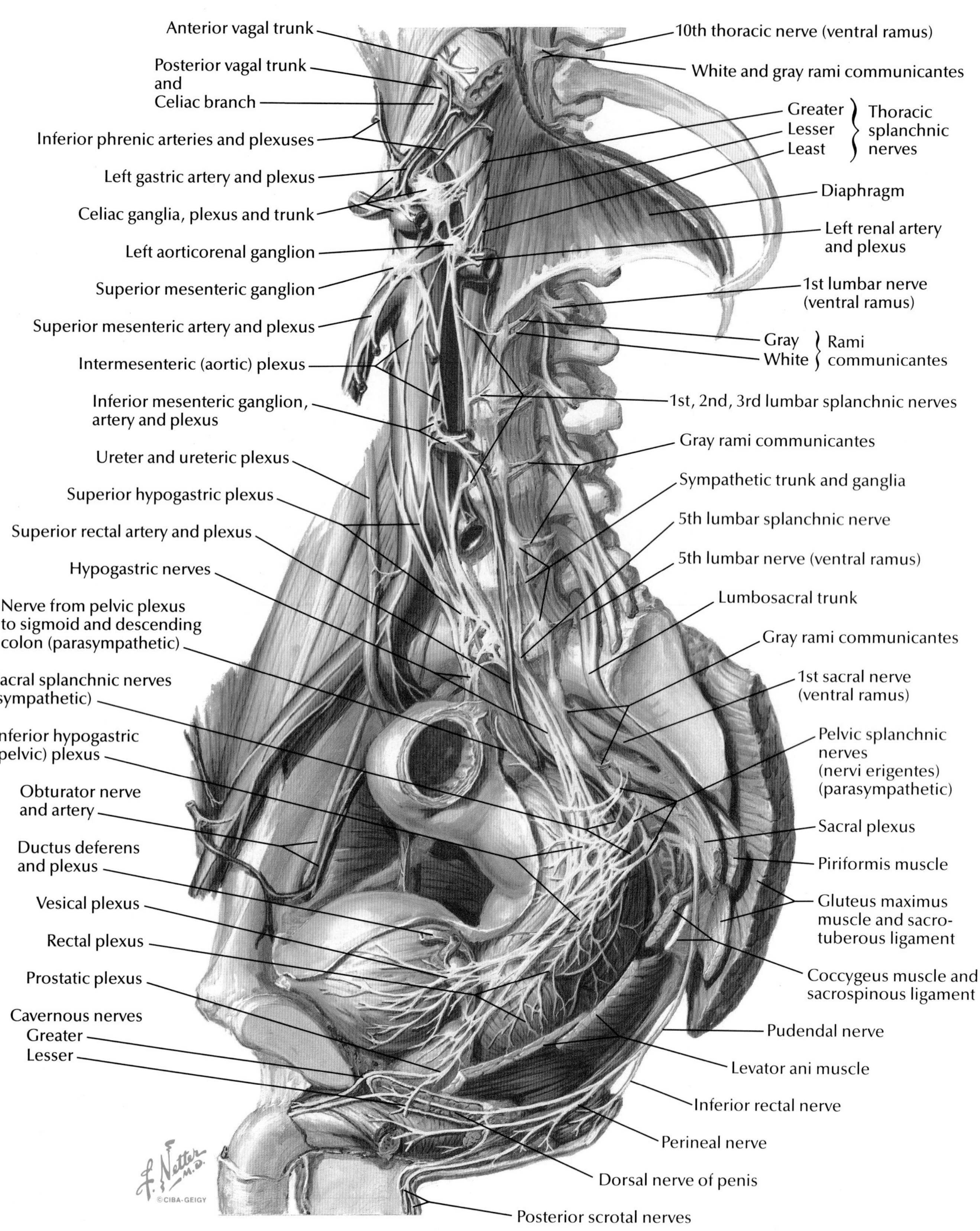

Anterior vagal trunk

Posterior vagal trunk and Celiac branch

Inferior phrenic arteries and plexuses

Left gastric artery and plexus

Celiac ganglia, plexus and trunk

Left aorticorenal ganglion

Superior mesenteric ganglion

Superior mesenteric artery and plexus

Intermesenteric (aortic) plexus

Inferior mesenteric ganglion, artery and plexus

Ureter and ureteric plexus

Superior hypogastric plexus

Superior rectal artery and plexus

Hypogastric nerves

Nerve from pelvic plexus to sigmoid and descending colon (parasympathetic)

Sacral splanchnic nerves (sympathetic)

Inferior hypogastric (pelvic) plexus

Obturator nerve and artery

Ductus deferens and plexus

Vesical plexus

Rectal plexus

Prostatic plexus

Cavernous nerves Greater Lesser

10th thoracic nerve (ventral ramus)

White and gray rami communicantes

Greater / Thoracic
Lesser } splanchnic
Least / nerves

Diaphragm

Left renal artery and plexus

1st lumbar nerve (ventral ramus)

Gray } Rami
White } communicantes

1st, 2nd, 3rd lumbar splanchnic nerves

Gray rami communicantes

Sympathetic trunk and ganglia

5th lumbar splanchnic nerve

5th lumbar nerve (ventral ramus)

Lumbosacral trunk

Gray rami communicantes

1st sacral nerve (ventral ramus)

Pelvic splanchnic nerves (nervi erigentes) (parasympathetic)

Sacral plexus

Piriformis muscle

Gluteus maximus muscle and sacro-tuberous ligament

Coccygeus muscle and sacrospinous ligament

Pudendal nerve

Levator ani muscle

Inferior rectal nerve

Perineal nerve

Dorsal nerve of penis

Posterior scrotal nerves

PLATE 385

PELVIS AND PERINEUM

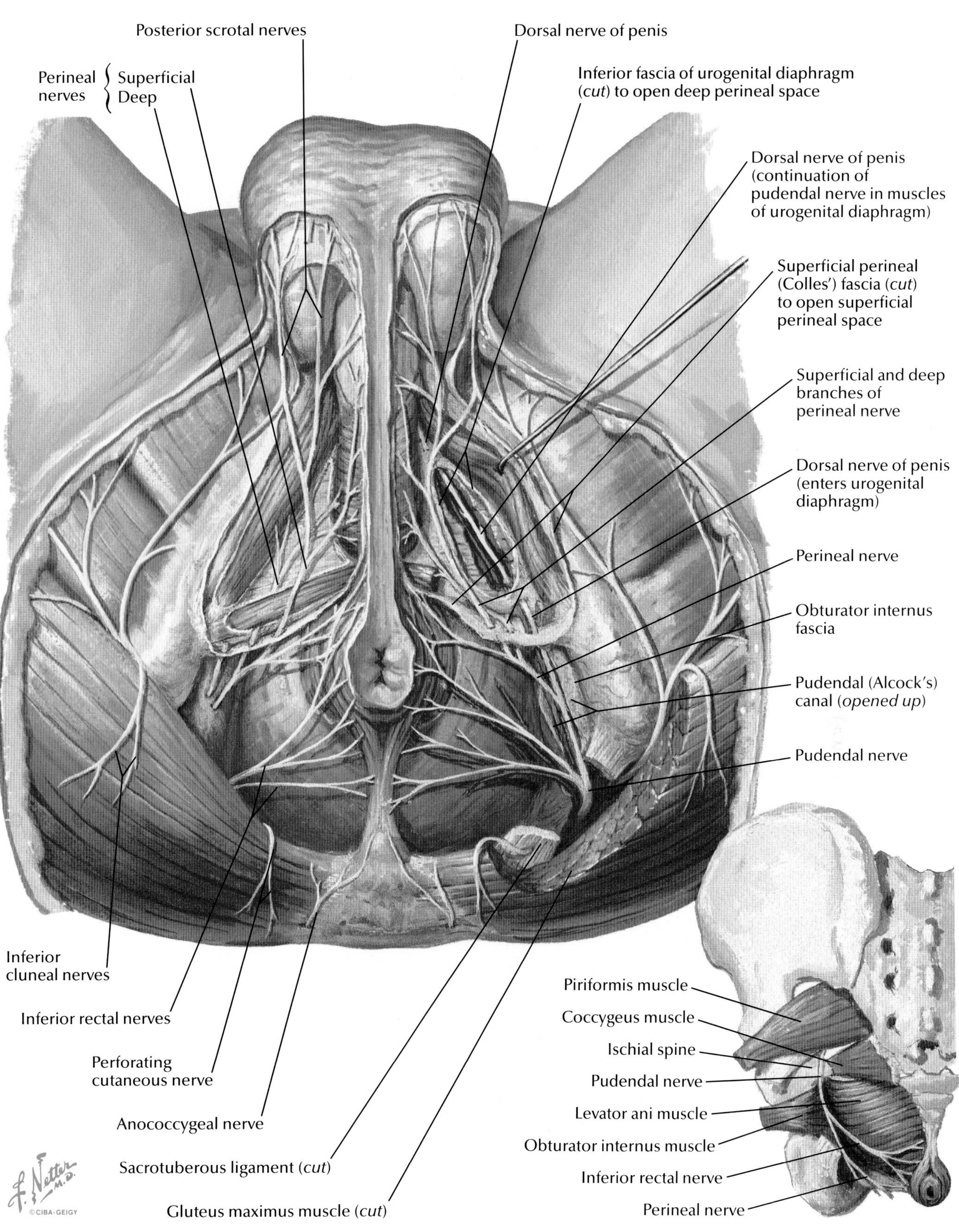

Posterior scrotal nerves

Dorsal nerve of penis

Perineal nerves { Superficial / Deep

Inferior fascia of urogenital diaphragm (*cut*) to open deep perineal space

Dorsal nerve of penis (continuation of pudendal nerve in muscles of urogenital diaphragm)

Superficial perineal (Colles') fascia (*cut*) to open superficial perineal space

Superficial and deep branches of perineal nerve

Dorsal nerve of penis (enters urogenital diaphragm)

Perineal nerve

Obturator internus fascia

Pudendal (Alcock's) canal (*opened up*)

Pudendal nerve

Inferior cluneal nerves

Inferior rectal nerves

Perforating cutaneous nerve

Anococcygeal nerve

Sacrotuberous ligament (*cut*)

Gluteus maximus muscle (*cut*)

Piriformis muscle

Coccygeus muscle

Ischial spine

Pudendal nerve

Levator ani muscle

Obturator internus muscle

Inferior rectal nerve

Perineal nerve

SEE ALSO PLATES 152, 304

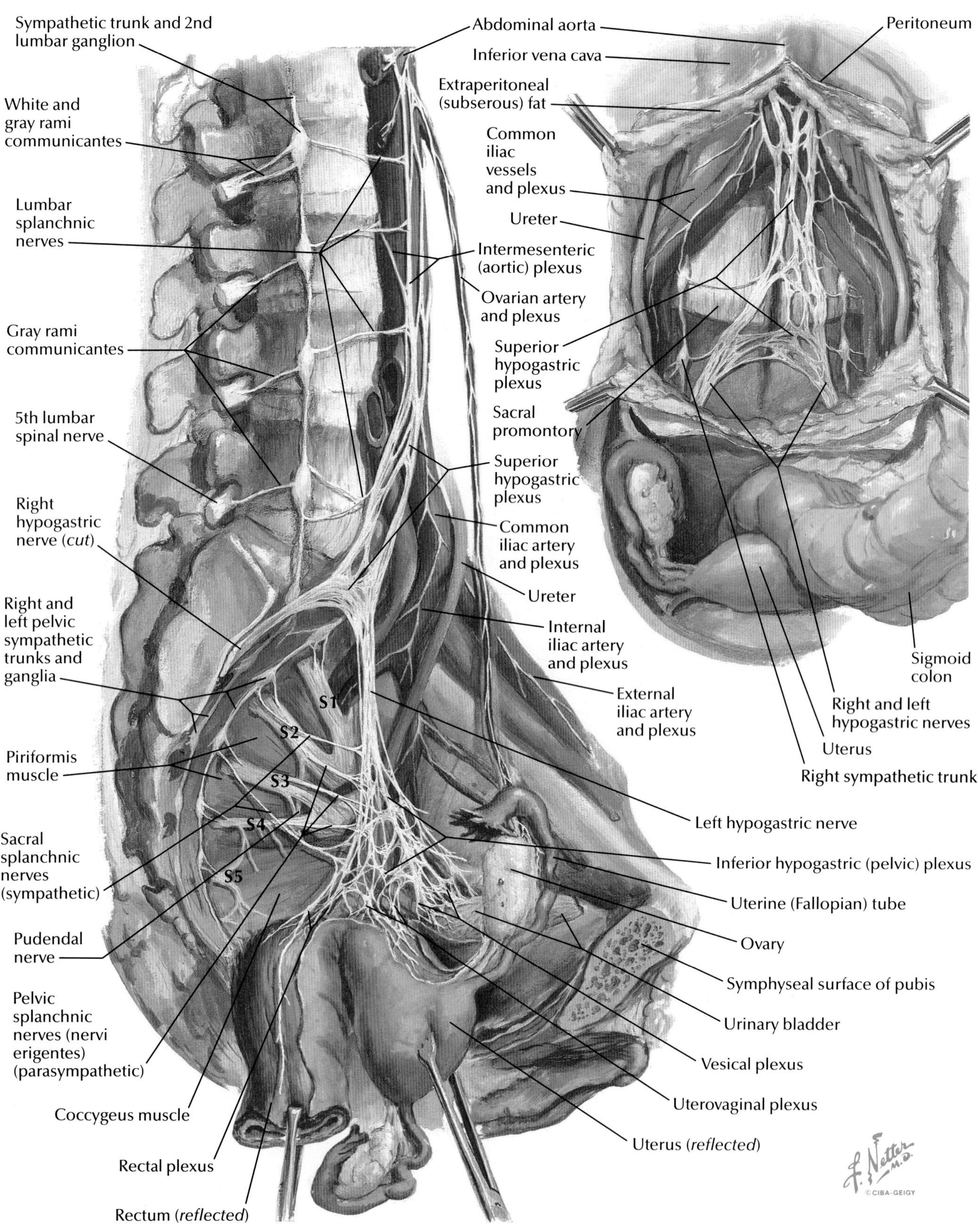

Sympathetic trunk and 2nd lumbar ganglion

White and gray rami communicantes

Lumbar splanchnic nerves

Gray rami communicantes

5th lumbar spinal nerve

Right hypogastric nerve (cut)

Right and left pelvic sympathetic trunks and ganglia

Piriformis muscle

Sacral splanchnic nerves (sympathetic)

Pudendal nerve

Pelvic splanchnic nerves (nervi erigentes) (parasympathetic)

Coccygeus muscle

Rectal plexus

Rectum (reflected)

S1
S2
S3
S4
S5

Abdominal aorta

Inferior vena cava

Extraperitoneal (subserous) fat

Common iliac vessels and plexus

Ureter

Intermesenteric (aortic) plexus

Ovarian artery and plexus

Superior hypogastric plexus

Sacral promontory

Superior hypogastric plexus

Common iliac artery and plexus

Ureter

Internal iliac artery and plexus

External iliac artery and plexus

Peritoneum

Sigmoid colon

Right and left hypogastric nerves

Uterus

Right sympathetic trunk

Left hypogastric nerve

Inferior hypogastric (pelvic) plexus

Uterine (Fallopian) tube

Ovary

Symphyseal surface of pubis

Urinary bladder

Vesical plexus

Uterovaginal plexus

Uterus (reflected)

PLATE 387

PELVIS AND PERINEUM

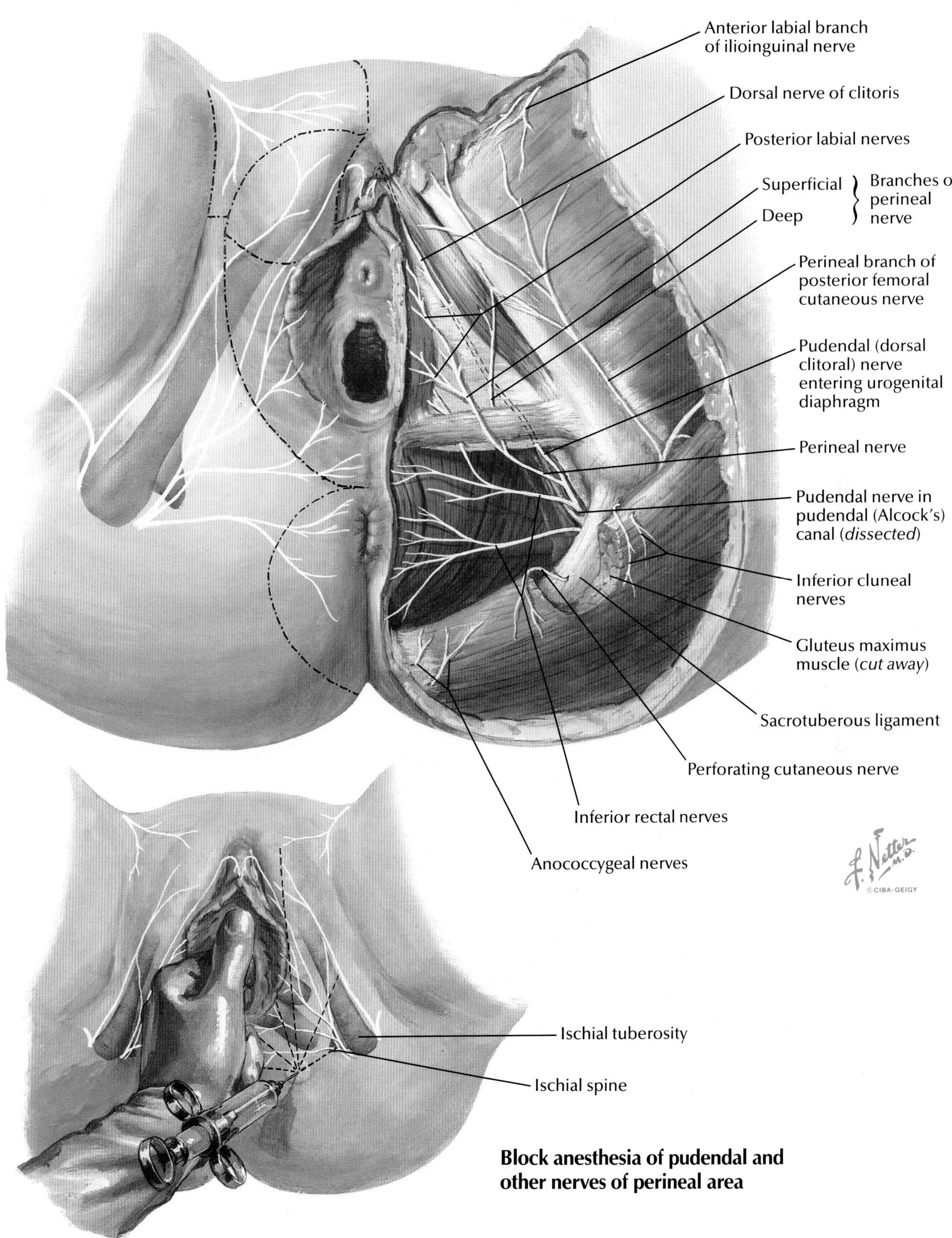

Anterior labial branch
of ilioinguinal nerve

Dorsal nerve of clitoris

Posterior labial nerves

Superficial ⎫ Branches of
⎬ perineal
Deep ⎭ nerve

Perineal branch of
posterior femoral
cutaneous nerve

Pudendal (dorsal
clitoral) nerve
entering urogenital
diaphragm

Perineal nerve

Pudendal nerve in
pudendal (Alcock's)
canal (*dissected*)

Inferior cluneal
nerves

Gluteus maximus
muscle (*cut away*)

Sacrotuberous ligament

Perforating cutaneous nerve

Inferior rectal nerves

Anococcygeal nerves

Ischial tuberosity

Ischial spine

**Block anesthesia of pudendal and
other nerves of perineal area**

SEE ALSO PLATE 152

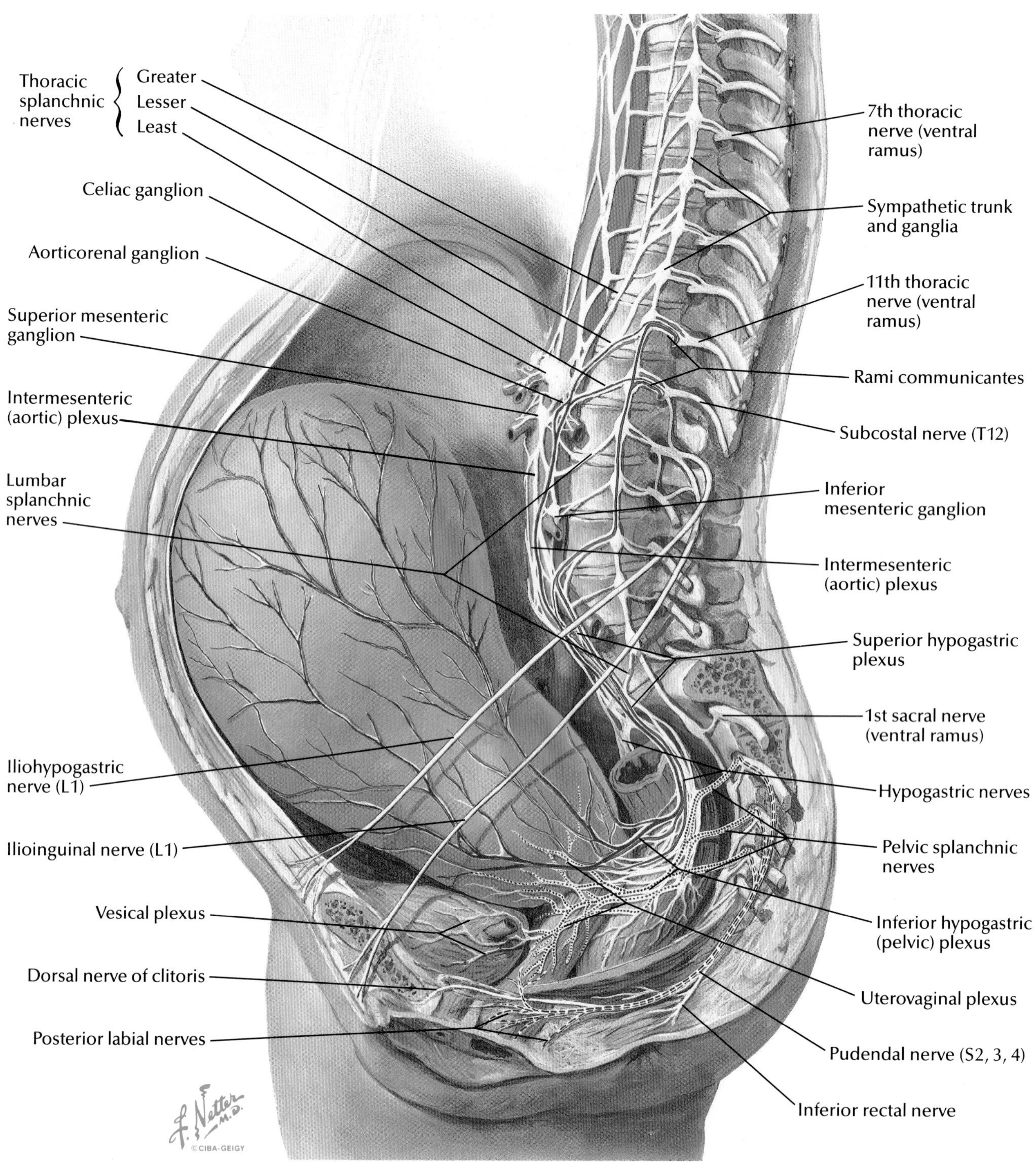

Thoracic splanchnic nerves { Greater / Lesser / Least

Celiac ganglion

Aorticorenal ganglion

Superior mesenteric ganglion

Intermesenteric (aortic) plexus

Lumbar splanchnic nerves

Iliohypogastric nerve (L1)

Ilioinguinal nerve (L1)

Vesical plexus

Dorsal nerve of clitoris

Posterior labial nerves

7th thoracic nerve (ventral ramus)

Sympathetic trunk and ganglia

11th thoracic nerve (ventral ramus)

Rami communicantes

Subcostal nerve (T12)

Inferior mesenteric ganglion

Intermesenteric (aortic) plexus

Superior hypogastric plexus

1st sacral nerve (ventral ramus)

Hypogastric nerves

Pelvic splanchnic nerves

Inferior hypogastric (pelvic) plexus

Uterovaginal plexus

Pudendal nerve (S2, 3, 4)

Inferior rectal nerve

——— Sensory fibers from uterine body and fundus accompany sympathetic fibers via pelvic plexus to T11, 12 (L1?)

——— Motor fibers to uterine body and fundus (sympathetic)

••••••• Sensory fibers from cervix and upper vagina accompany pelvic splanchnic nerves (parasympathetic) to S2, 3, 4

••••••• Motor fibers to lower uterine segment, cervix and upper vagina (parasympathetic)

– – – – – Sensory fibers from lower vagina and perineum accompany somatic fibers via pudendal nerve to S2, 3, 4

– – – – – Motor fibers to lower vagina and perineum via pudendal nerve (somatic)

PLATE 389   **PELVIS AND PERINEUM**

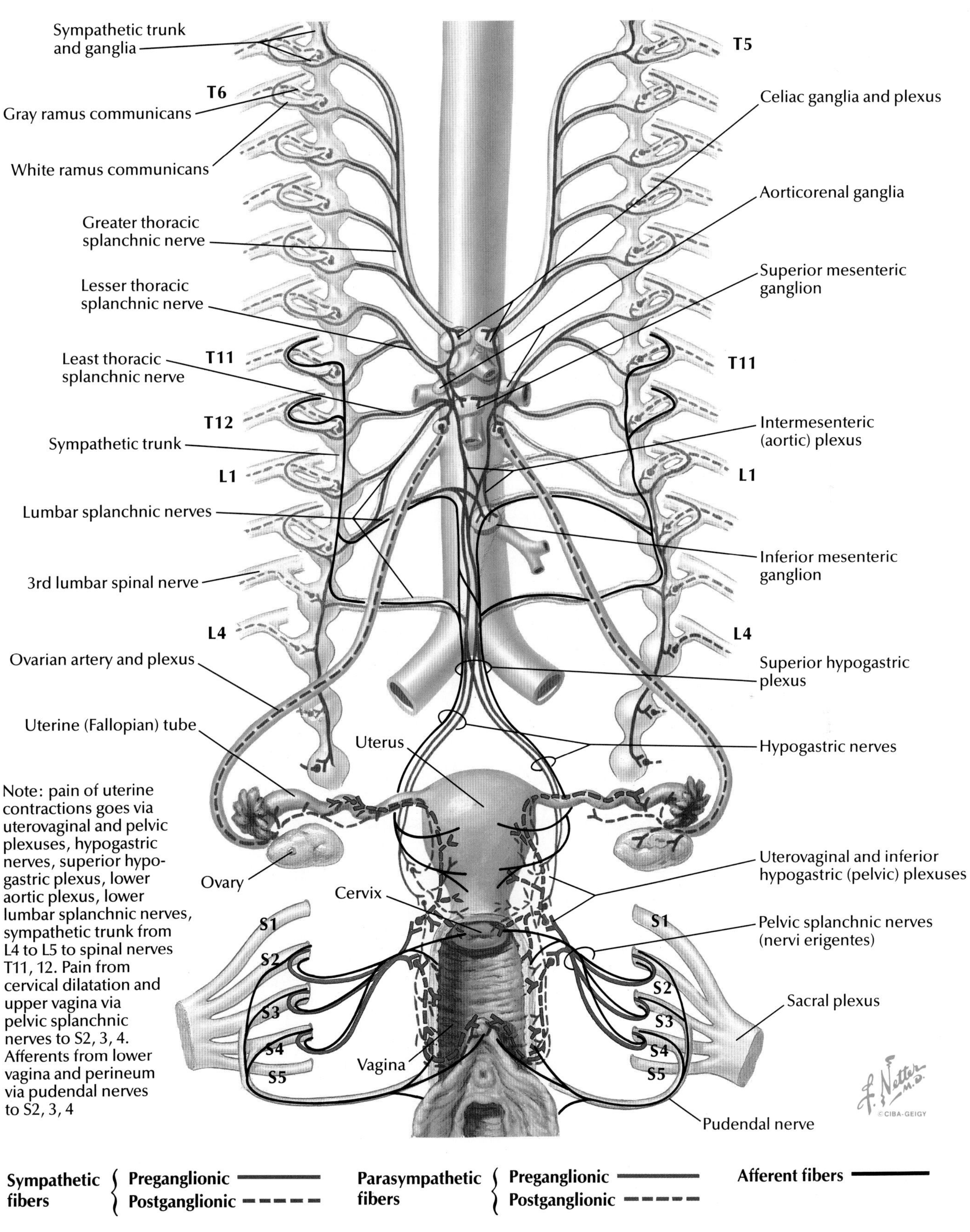

Sympathetic trunk and ganglia

T6

Gray ramus communicans

White ramus communicans

Greater thoracic splanchnic nerve

Lesser thoracic splanchnic nerve

Least thoracic splanchnic nerve — T11

T12

Sympathetic trunk

L1

Lumbar splanchnic nerves

3rd lumbar spinal nerve

L4

Ovarian artery and plexus

Uterine (Fallopian) tube

Note: pain of uterine contractions goes via uterovaginal and pelvic plexuses, hypogastric nerves, superior hypogastric plexus, lower aortic plexus, lower lumbar splanchnic nerves, sympathetic trunk from L4 to L5 to spinal nerves T11, 12. Pain from cervical dilatation and upper vagina via pelvic splanchnic nerves to S2, 3, 4. Afferents from lower vagina and perineum via pudendal nerves to S2, 3, 4

Ovary

Cervix

Vagina

S1
S2
S3
S4
S5

T5

Celiac ganglia and plexus

Aorticorenal ganglia

Superior mesenteric ganglion

T11

Intermesenteric (aortic) plexus

L1

Inferior mesenteric ganglion

L4

Superior hypogastric plexus

Uterus

Hypogastric nerves

Uterovaginal and inferior hypogastric (pelvic) plexuses

Pelvic splanchnic nerves (nervi erigentes)

S1
S2
S3
S4
S5

Sacral plexus

Pudendal nerve

Sympathetic fibers	Preganglionic ————	Parasympathetic fibers	Preganglionic ————	Afferent fibers ————
	Postganglionic - - - - -		Postganglionic - - - - -	

Innervation of Male Reproductive Organs: Schema

SEE ALSO PLATE 153

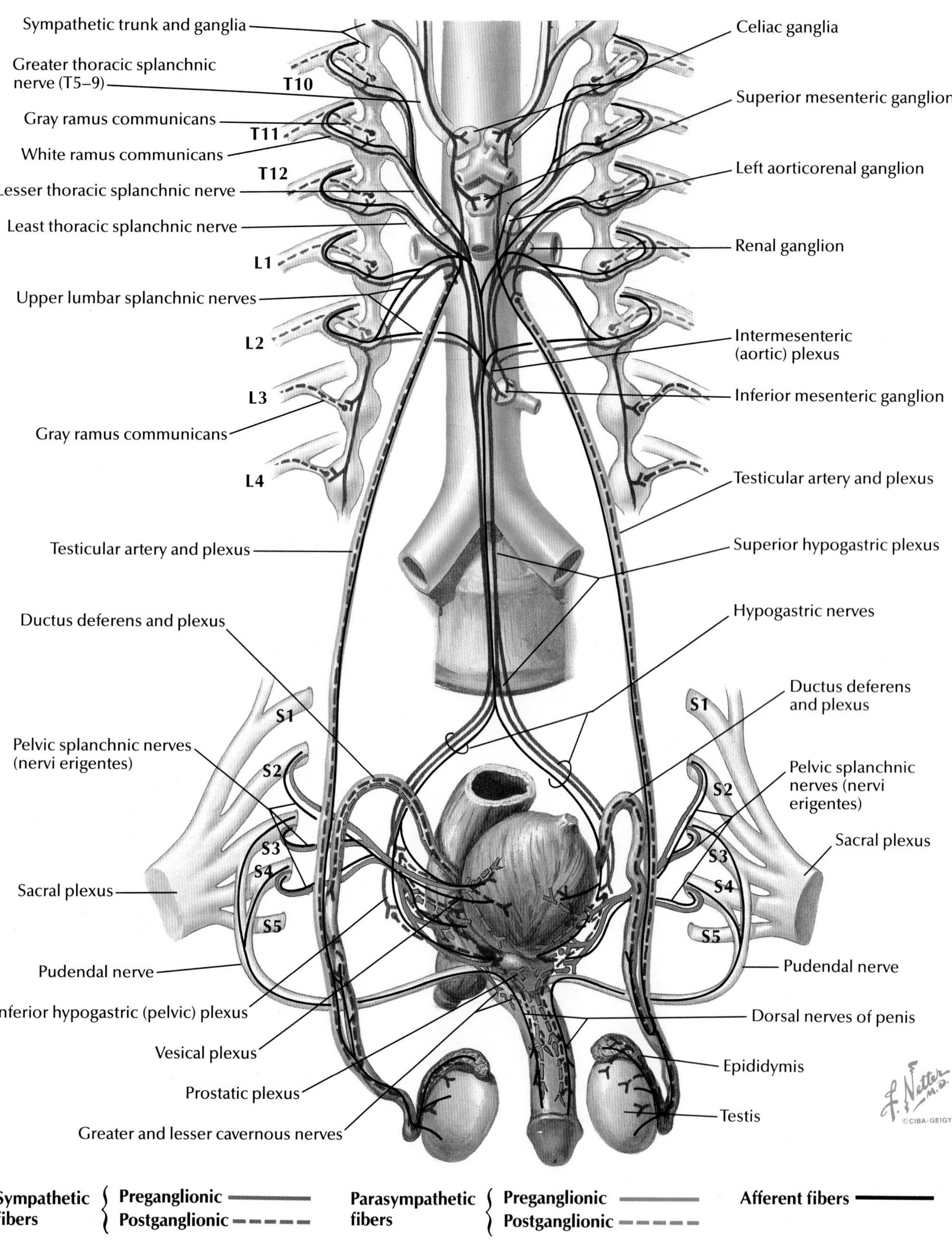

Sympathetic trunk and ganglia

Greater thoracic splanchnic nerve (T5–9)

Gray ramus communicans

White ramus communicans

Lesser thoracic splanchnic nerve

Least thoracic splanchnic nerve

Upper lumbar splanchnic nerves

Gray ramus communicans

Testicular artery and plexus

Ductus deferens and plexus

Pelvic splanchnic nerves (nervi erigentes)

Sacral plexus

Pudendal nerve

Inferior hypogastric (pelvic) plexus

Vesical plexus

Prostatic plexus

Greater and lesser cavernous nerves

T10

T11

T12

L1

L2

L3

L4

S1

S2

S3

S4

S5

Celiac ganglia

Superior mesenteric ganglion

Left aorticorenal ganglion

Renal ganglion

Intermesenteric (aortic) plexus

Inferior mesenteric ganglion

Testicular artery and plexus

Superior hypogastric plexus

Hypogastric nerves

Ductus deferens and plexus

Pelvic splanchnic nerves (nervi erigentes)

Sacral plexus

Pudendal nerve

Dorsal nerves of penis

Epididymis

Testis

S1

S2

S3

S4

S5

Sympathetic fibers	{ Preganglionic ——— Postganglionic - - - - -	Parasympathetic fibers	{ Preganglionic ——— Postganglionic - - - - -	Afferent fibers ———

PLATE 391

PELVIS AND PERINEUM

Innervation of Urinary Bladder and Lower Ureter: Schema

SEE ALSO PLATE 153

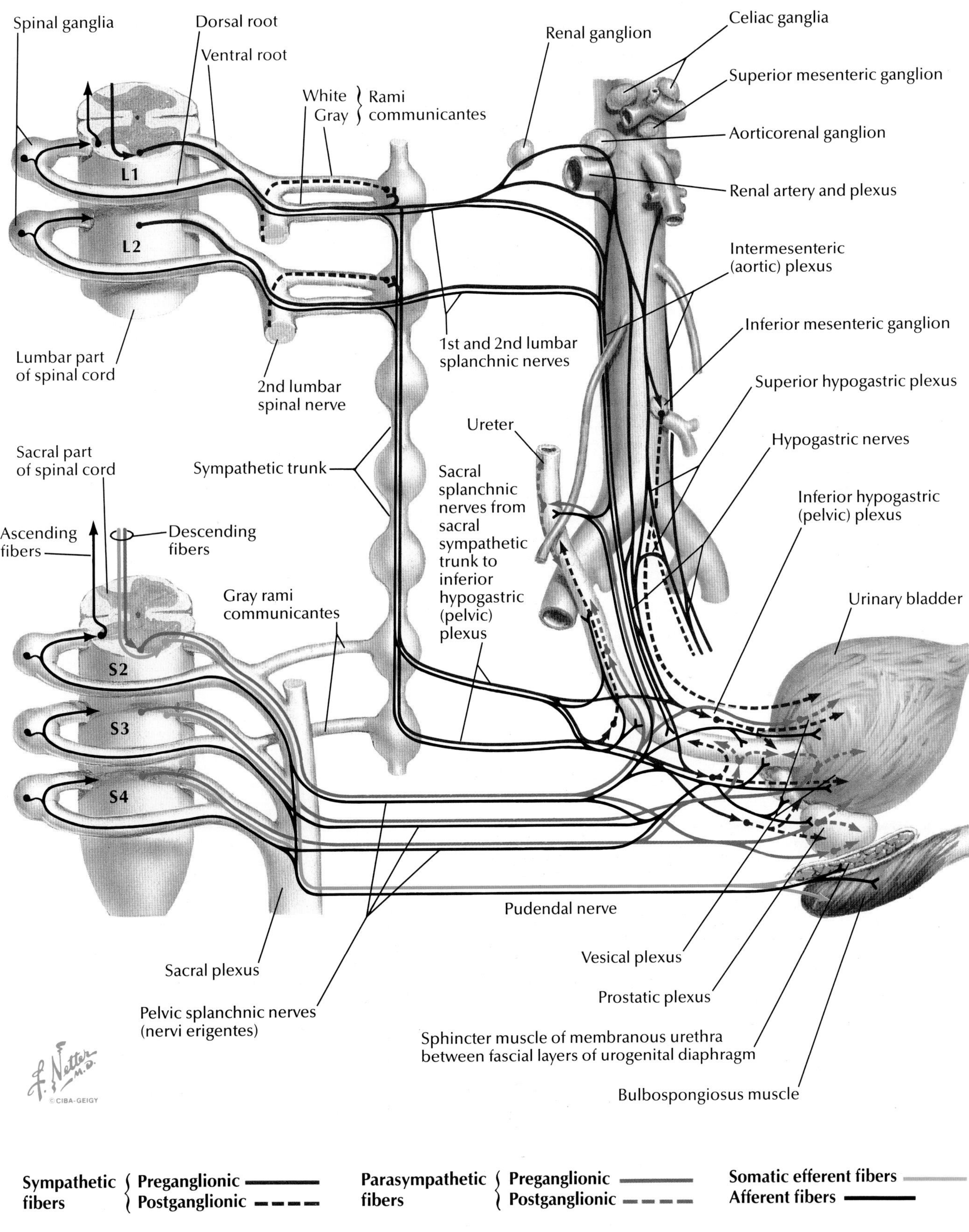

Spinal ganglia

Dorsal root

Ventral root

Renal ganglion

Celiac ganglia

Superior mesenteric ganglion

White } Rami
Gray } communicantes

Aorticorenal ganglion

Renal artery and plexus

L1

L2

Intermesenteric (aortic) plexus

1st and 2nd lumbar splanchnic nerves

Inferior mesenteric ganglion

Lumbar part of spinal cord

2nd lumbar spinal nerve

Superior hypogastric plexus

Sacral part of spinal cord

Sympathetic trunk

Ureter

Hypogastric nerves

Ascending fibers

Descending fibers

Sacral splanchnic nerves from sacral sympathetic trunk to inferior hypogastric (pelvic) plexus

Inferior hypogastric (pelvic) plexus

Gray rami communicantes

Urinary bladder

S2

S3

S4

Pudendal nerve

Sacral plexus

Vesical plexus

Prostatic plexus

Pelvic splanchnic nerves (nervi erigentes)

Sphincter muscle of membranous urethra between fascial layers of urogenital diaphragm

Bulbospongiosus muscle

| Sympathetic fibers | { Preganglionic ———— Postganglionic ━ ━ ━ ━ | Parasympathetic fibers | { Preganglionic ———— Postganglionic ━ ━ ━ ━ | Somatic efferent fibers ———— Afferent fibers ━━━━ |

Homologues of External Genitalia

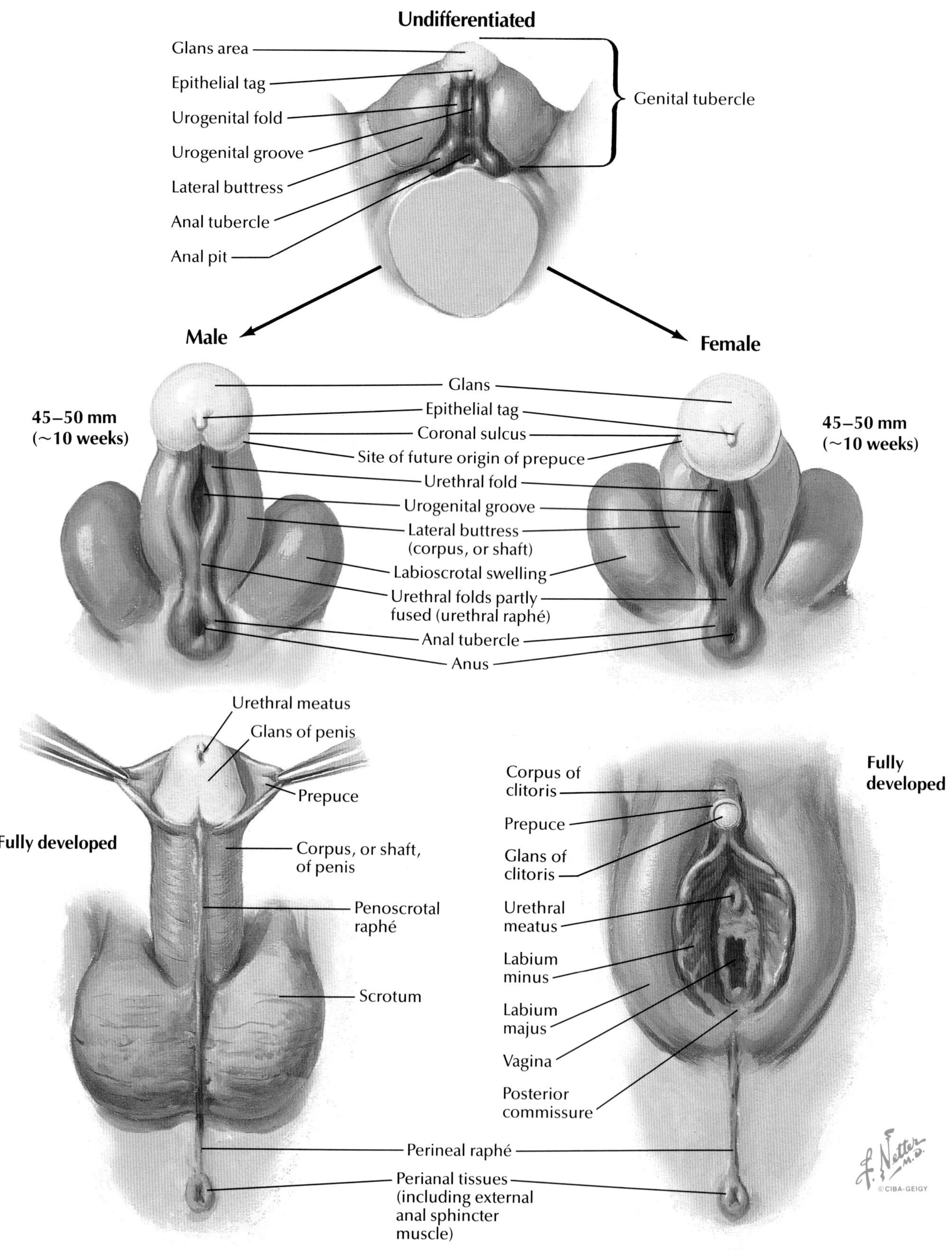

Undifferentiated

Glans area

Epithelial tag

Urogenital fold

Urogenital groove

Lateral buttress

Anal tubercle

Anal pit

Genital tubercle

Male

Female

45–50 mm
(~10 weeks)

45–50 mm
(~10 weeks)

Glans

Epithelial tag

Coronal sulcus

Site of future origin of prepuce

Urethral fold

Urogenital groove

Lateral buttress
(corpus, or shaft)

Labioscrotal swelling

Urethral folds partly
fused (urethral raphé)

Anal tubercle

Anus

Urethral meatus

Glans of penis

Prepuce

Fully developed

Corpus, or shaft,
of penis

Penoscrotal
raphé

Scrotum

Perineal raphé

Perianal tissues
(including external
anal sphincter
muscle)

**Fully
developed**

Corpus of
clitoris

Prepuce

Glans of
clitoris

Urethral
meatus

Labium
minus

Labium
majus

Vagina

Posterior
commissure

PLATE 393

PELVIS AND PERINEUM

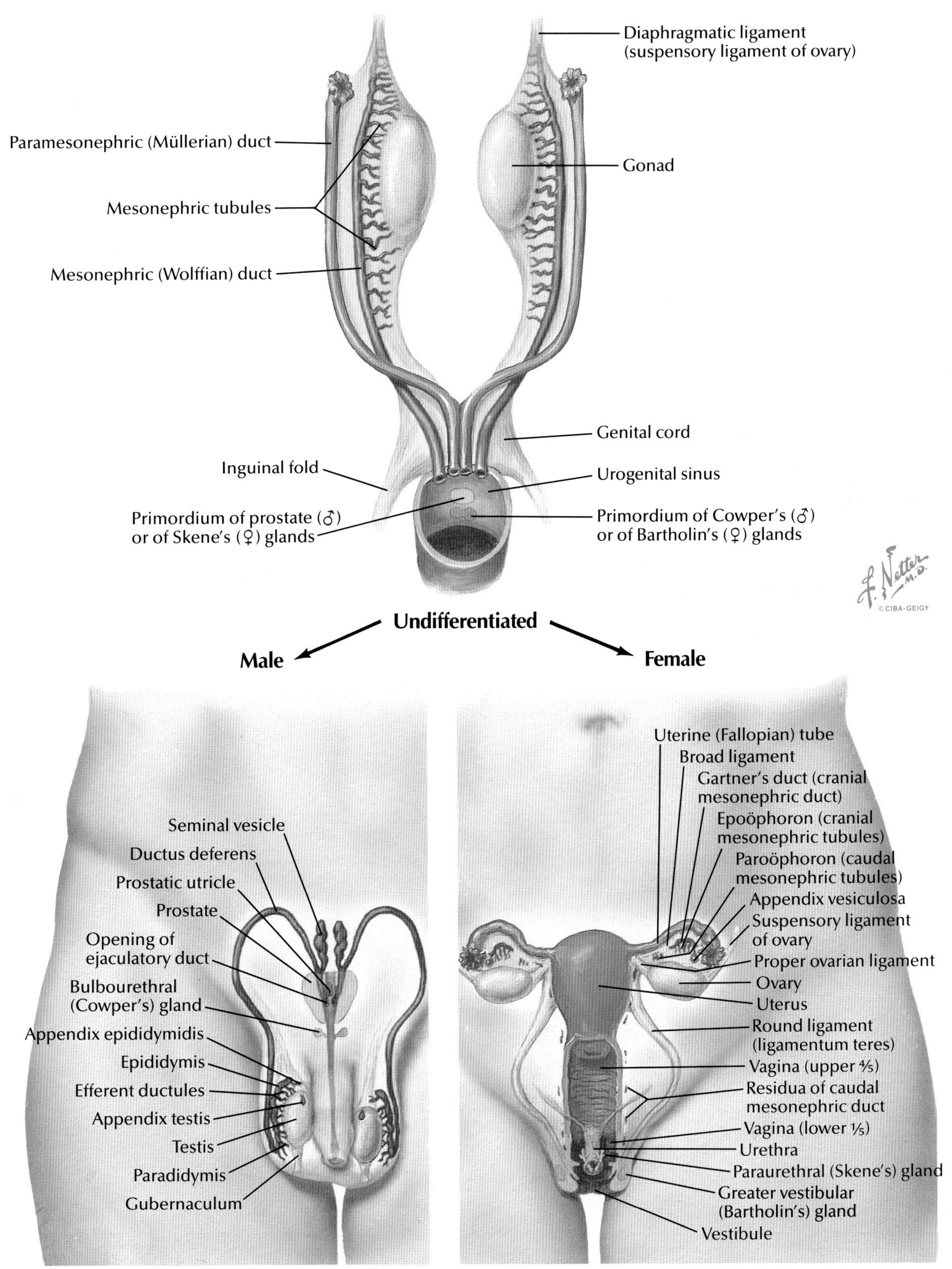

Diaphragmatic ligament
(suspensory ligament of ovary)

Paramesonephric (Müllerian) duct

Mesonephric tubules

Mesonephric (Wolffian) duct

Gonad

Inguinal fold

Primordium of prostate (♂)
or of Skene's (♀) glands

Genital cord

Urogenital sinus

Primordium of Cowper's (♂)
or of Bartholin's (♀) glands

Undifferentiated

Male

Female

Seminal vesicle
Ductus deferens
Prostatic utricle
Prostate
Opening of
ejaculatory duct
Bulbourethral
(Cowper's) gland
Appendix epididymidis
Epididymis
Efferent ductules
Appendix testis
Testis
Paradidymis
Gubernaculum

Uterine (Fallopian) tube
Broad ligament
Gartner's duct (cranial
mesonephric duct)
Epoöphoron (cranial
mesonephric tubules)
Paroöphoron (caudal
mesonephric tubules)
Appendix vesiculosa
Suspensory ligament
of ovary
Proper ovarian ligament
Ovary
Uterus
Round ligament
(ligamentum teres)
Vagina (upper ⅘)
Residua of caudal
mesonephric duct
Vagina (lower ⅕)
Urethra
Paraurethral (Skene's) gland
Greater vestibular
(Bartholin's) gland
Vestibule

Section VI

UPPER LIMB

Right clavicle

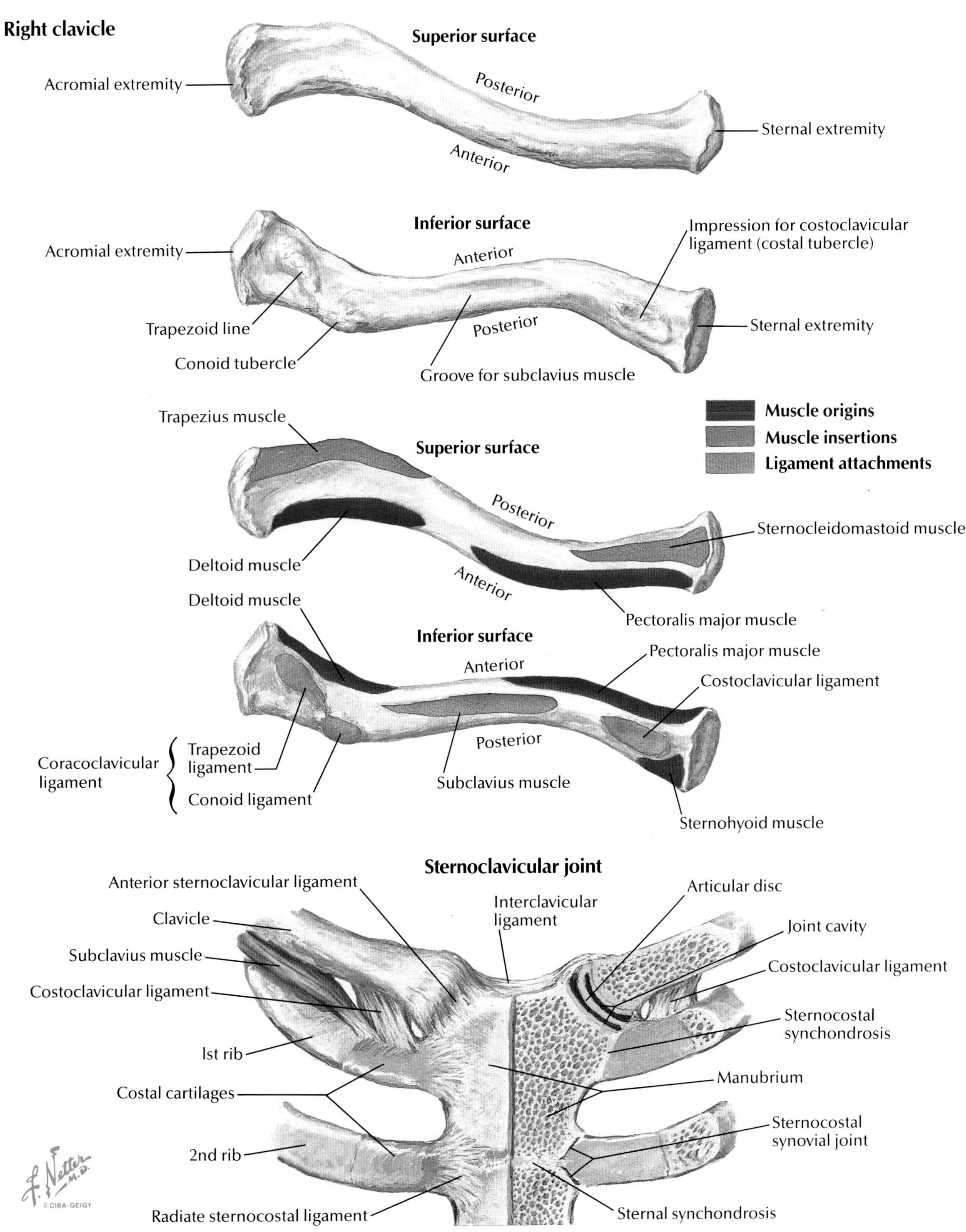

Superior surface

Acromial extremity

Posterior

Anterior

Sternal extremity

Inferior surface

Acromial extremity

Anterior

Posterior

Impression for costoclavicular ligament (costal tubercle)

Trapezoid line

Conoid tubercle

Groove for subclavius muscle

Sternal extremity

Muscle origins
Muscle insertions
Ligament attachments

Trapezius muscle

Superior surface

Posterior

Sternocleidomastoid muscle

Deltoid muscle

Anterior

Pectoralis major muscle

Deltoid muscle

Inferior surface

Anterior

Pectoralis major muscle

Costoclavicular ligament

Coracoclavicular ligament

Trapezoid ligament

Conoid ligament

Posterior

Subclavius muscle

Sternohyoid muscle

Sternoclavicular joint

Anterior sternoclavicular ligament

Clavicle

Subclavius muscle

Costoclavicular ligament

1st rib

Costal cartilages

2nd rib

Radiate sternocostal ligament

Interclavicular ligament

Articular disc

Joint cavity

Costoclavicular ligament

Sternocostal synchondrosis

Manubrium

Sternocostal synovial joint

Sternal synchondrosis

SEE ALSO PLATE 170

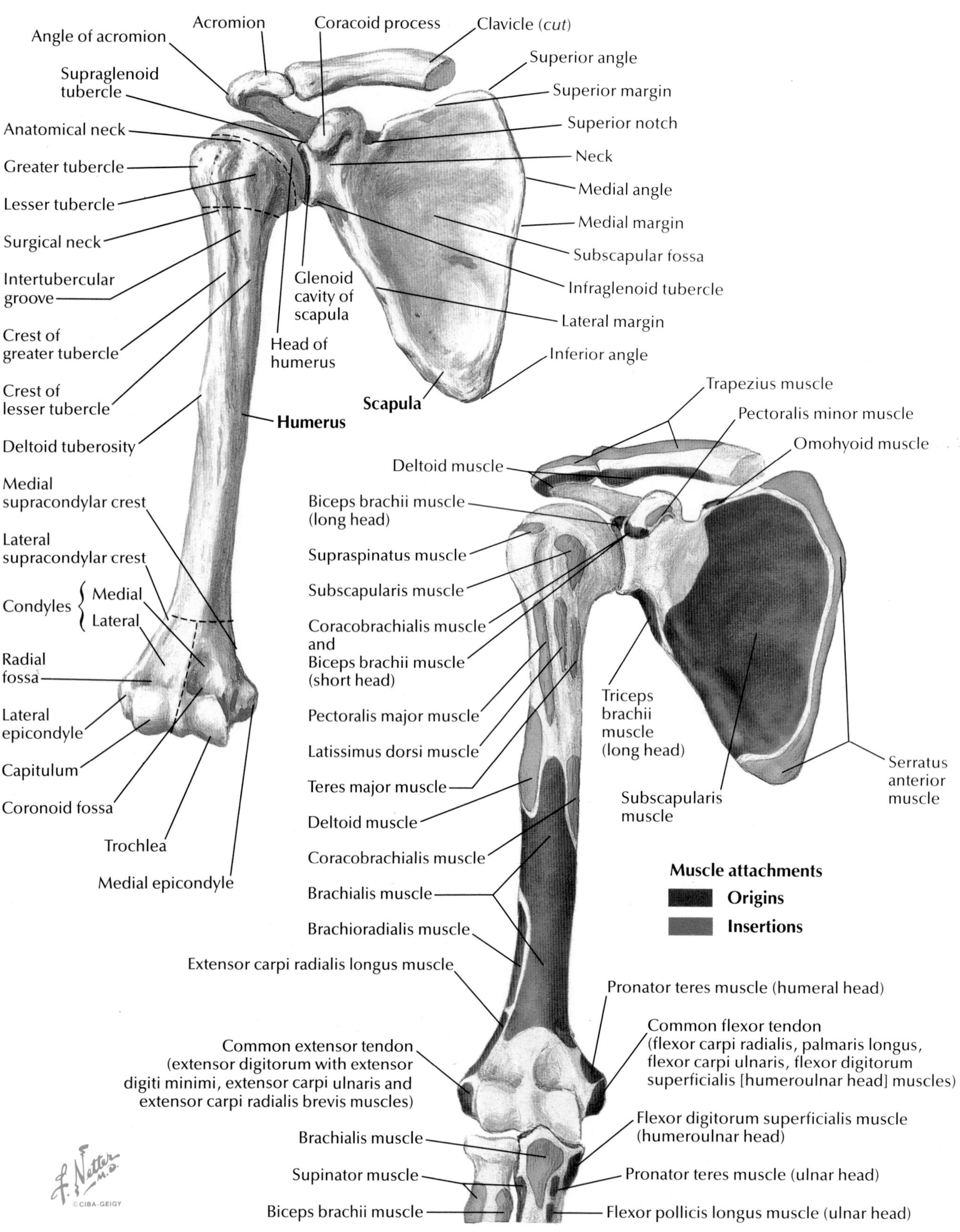

Angle of acromion

Acromion

Coracoid process

Clavicle (*cut*)

Superior angle

Supraglenoid tubercle

Superior margin

Anatomical neck

Superior notch

Greater tubercle

Neck

Lesser tubercle

Medial angle

Surgical neck

Medial margin

Intertubercular groove

Subscapular fossa

Glenoid cavity of scapula

Infraglenoid tubercle

Crest of greater tubercle

Head of humerus

Lateral margin

Crest of lesser tubercle

Inferior angle

Scapula

Deltoid tuberosity

Humerus

Medial supracondylar crest

Lateral supracondylar crest

Condyles { Medial / Lateral }

Radial fossa

Lateral epicondyle

Capitulum

Coronoid fossa

Trochlea

Medial epicondyle

Trapezius muscle

Pectoralis minor muscle

Omohyoid muscle

Deltoid muscle

Biceps brachii muscle (long head)

Supraspinatus muscle

Subscapularis muscle

Coracobrachialis muscle and Biceps brachii muscle (short head)

Pectoralis major muscle

Latissimus dorsi muscle

Teres major muscle

Deltoid muscle

Coracobrachialis muscle

Brachialis muscle

Brachioradialis muscle

Extensor carpi radialis longus muscle

Triceps brachii muscle (long head)

Subscapularis muscle

Serratus anterior muscle

Muscle attachments

■ **Origins**

■ **Insertions**

Pronator teres muscle (humeral head)

Common flexor tendon (flexor carpi radialis, palmaris longus, flexor carpi ulnaris, flexor digitorum superficialis [humeroulnar head] muscles)

Common extensor tendon (extensor digitorum with extensor digiti minimi, extensor carpi ulnaris and extensor carpi radialis brevis muscles)

Brachialis muscle

Supinator muscle

Biceps brachii muscle

Flexor digitorum superficialis muscle (humeroulnar head)

Pronator teres muscle (ulnar head)

Flexor pollicis longus muscle (ulnar head)

PLATE 396

UPPER LIMB

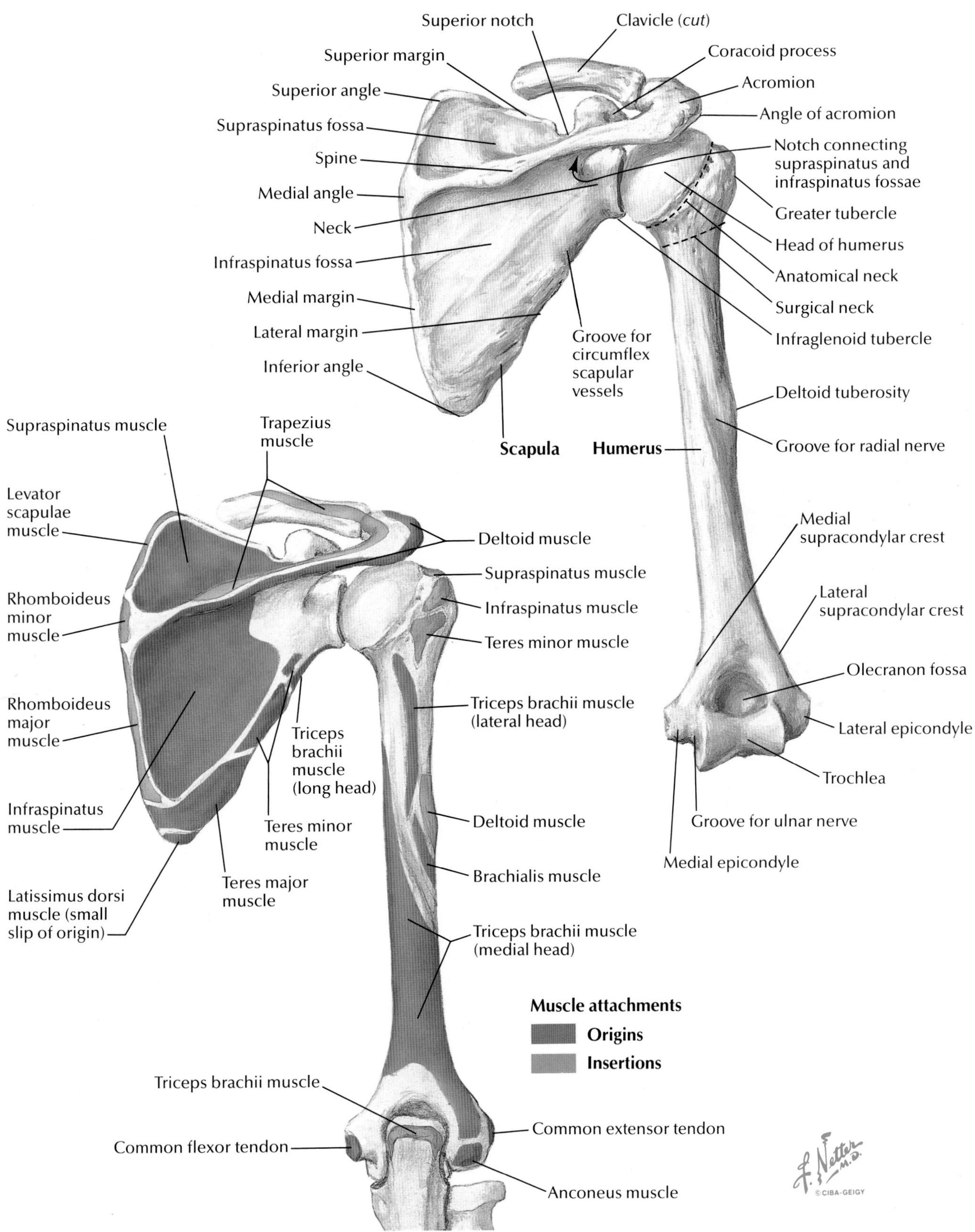

Superior notch

Clavicle (cut)

Superior margin

Coracoid process

Superior angle

Acromion

Supraspinatus fossa

Angle of acromion

Spine

Notch connecting supraspinatus and infraspinatus fossae

Medial angle

Greater tubercle

Neck

Head of humerus

Infraspinatus fossa

Anatomical neck

Medial margin

Surgical neck

Lateral margin

Infraglenoid tubercle

Inferior angle

Groove for circumflex scapular vessels

Scapula

Humerus

Deltoid tuberosity

Groove for radial nerve

Supraspinatus muscle

Trapezius muscle

Levator scapulae muscle

Deltoid muscle

Medial supracondylar crest

Rhomboideus minor muscle

Supraspinatus muscle

Lateral supracondylar crest

Infraspinatus muscle

Olecranon fossa

Teres minor muscle

Rhomboideus major muscle

Triceps brachii muscle (lateral head)

Lateral epicondyle

Triceps brachii muscle (long head)

Trochlea

Infraspinatus muscle

Teres minor muscle

Deltoid muscle

Groove for ulnar nerve

Latissimus dorsi muscle (small slip of origin)

Teres major muscle

Medial epicondyle

Brachialis muscle

Triceps brachii muscle (medial head)

Muscle attachments
- Origins
- Insertions

Triceps brachii muscle

Common flexor tendon

Common extensor tendon

Anconeus muscle

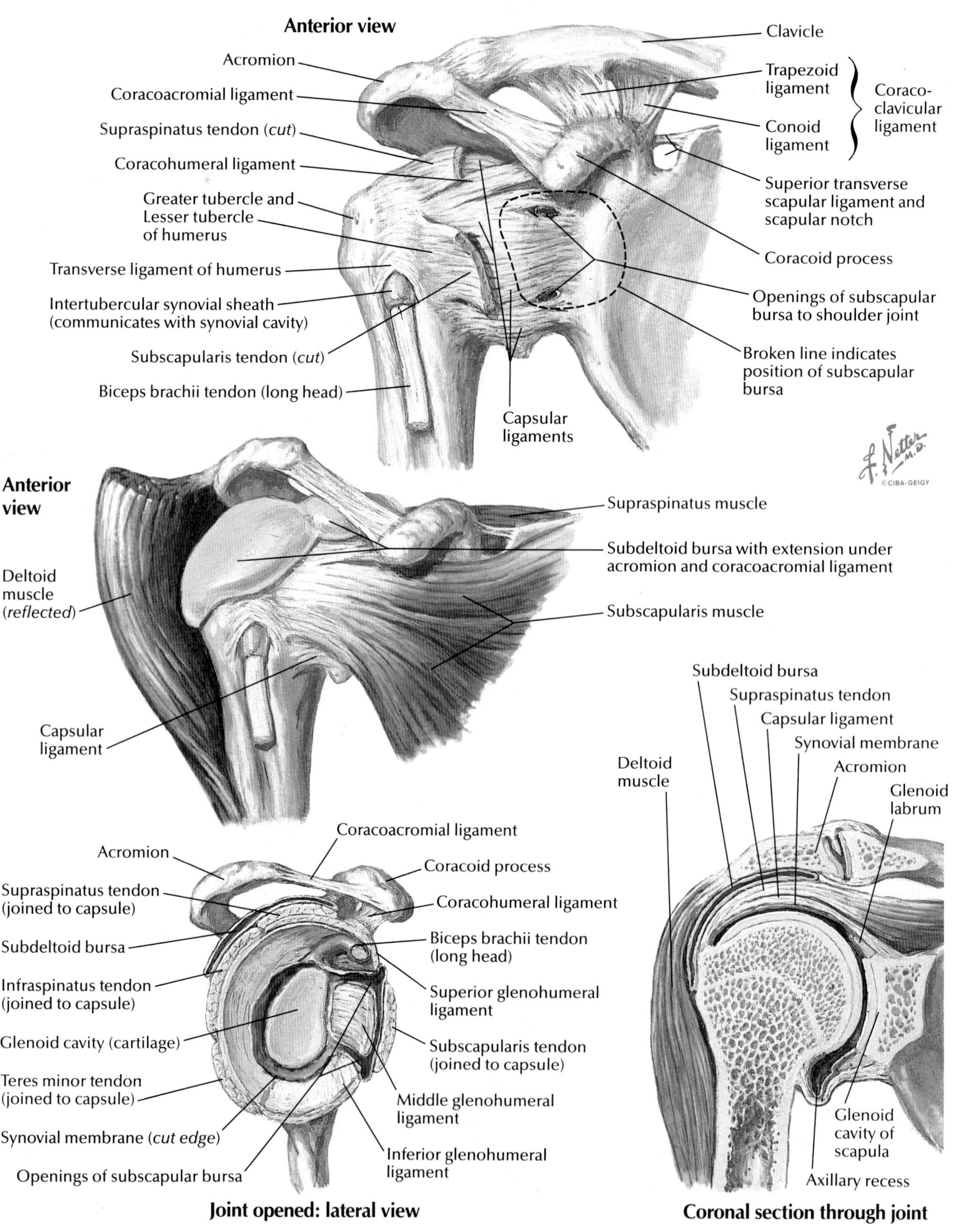

Anterior view

Clavicle

Acromion

Trapezoid ligament

Coracoacromial ligament

Conoid ligament

Coraco-clavicular ligament

Supraspinatus tendon (*cut*)

Coracohumeral ligament

Superior transverse scapular ligament and scapular notch

Greater tubercle and Lesser tubercle of humerus

Coracoid process

Transverse ligament of humerus

Openings of subscapular bursa to shoulder joint

Intertubercular synovial sheath (communicates with synovial cavity)

Broken line indicates position of subscapular bursa

Subscapularis tendon (*cut*)

Biceps brachii tendon (long head)

Capsular ligaments

Anterior view

Supraspinatus muscle

Subdeltoid bursa with extension under acromion and coracoacromial ligament

Deltoid muscle (*reflected*)

Subscapularis muscle

Capsular ligament

Subdeltoid bursa

Supraspinatus tendon

Capsular ligament

Synovial membrane

Acromion

Deltoid muscle

Glenoid labrum

Coracoacromial ligament

Acromion

Coracoid process

Supraspinatus tendon (joined to capsule)

Coracohumeral ligament

Subdeltoid bursa

Biceps brachii tendon (long head)

Infraspinatus tendon (joined to capsule)

Superior glenohumeral ligament

Glenoid cavity (cartilage)

Subscapularis tendon (joined to capsule)

Teres minor tendon (joined to capsule)

Middle glenohumeral ligament

Glenoid cavity of scapula

Synovial membrane (*cut edge*)

Inferior glenohumeral ligament

Openings of subscapular bursa

Axillary recess

Joint opened: lateral view

Coronal section through joint

PLATE 398

UPPER LIMB

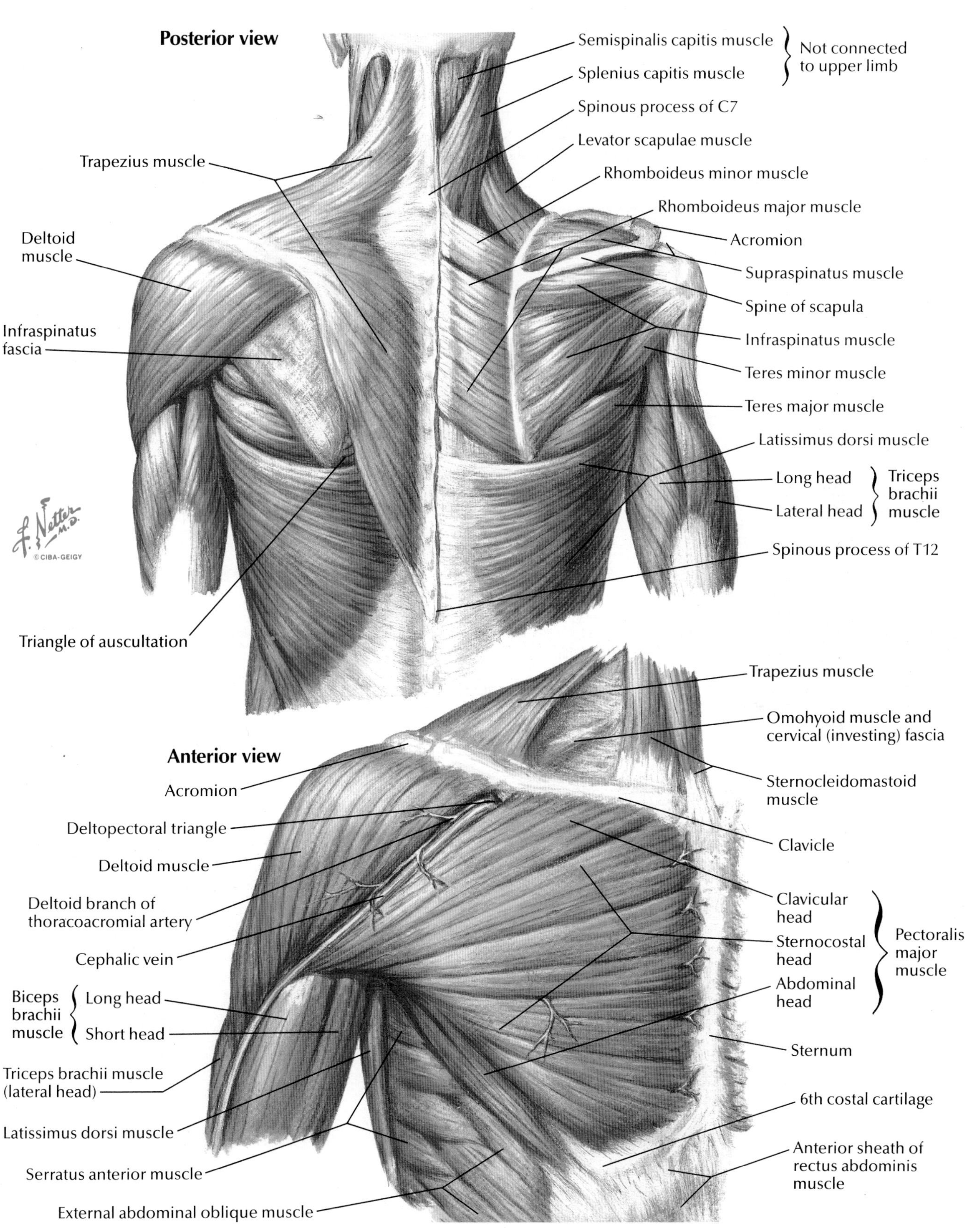

Posterior view

Trapezius muscle

Deltoid muscle

Infraspinatus fascia

Triangle of auscultation

Semispinalis capitis muscle ⎫
Splenius capitis muscle ⎭ Not connected to upper limb

Spinous process of C7

Levator scapulae muscle

Rhomboideus minor muscle

Rhomboideus major muscle

Acromion

Supraspinatus muscle

Spine of scapula

Infraspinatus muscle

Teres minor muscle

Teres major muscle

Latissimus dorsi muscle

Long head ⎫ Triceps
Lateral head ⎭ brachii muscle

Spinous process of T12

Anterior view

Acromion

Deltopectoral triangle

Deltoid muscle

Deltoid branch of thoracoacromial artery

Cephalic vein

Biceps brachii muscle { Long head / Short head

Triceps brachii muscle (lateral head)

Latissimus dorsi muscle

Serratus anterior muscle

External abdominal oblique muscle

Trapezius muscle

Omohyoid muscle and cervical (investing) fascia

Sternocleidomastoid muscle

Clavicle

Clavicular head ⎫
Sternocostal head ⎬ Pectoralis major muscle
Abdominal head ⎭

Sternum

6th costal cartilage

Anterior sheath of rectus abdominis muscle

Muscles of Rotator Cuff

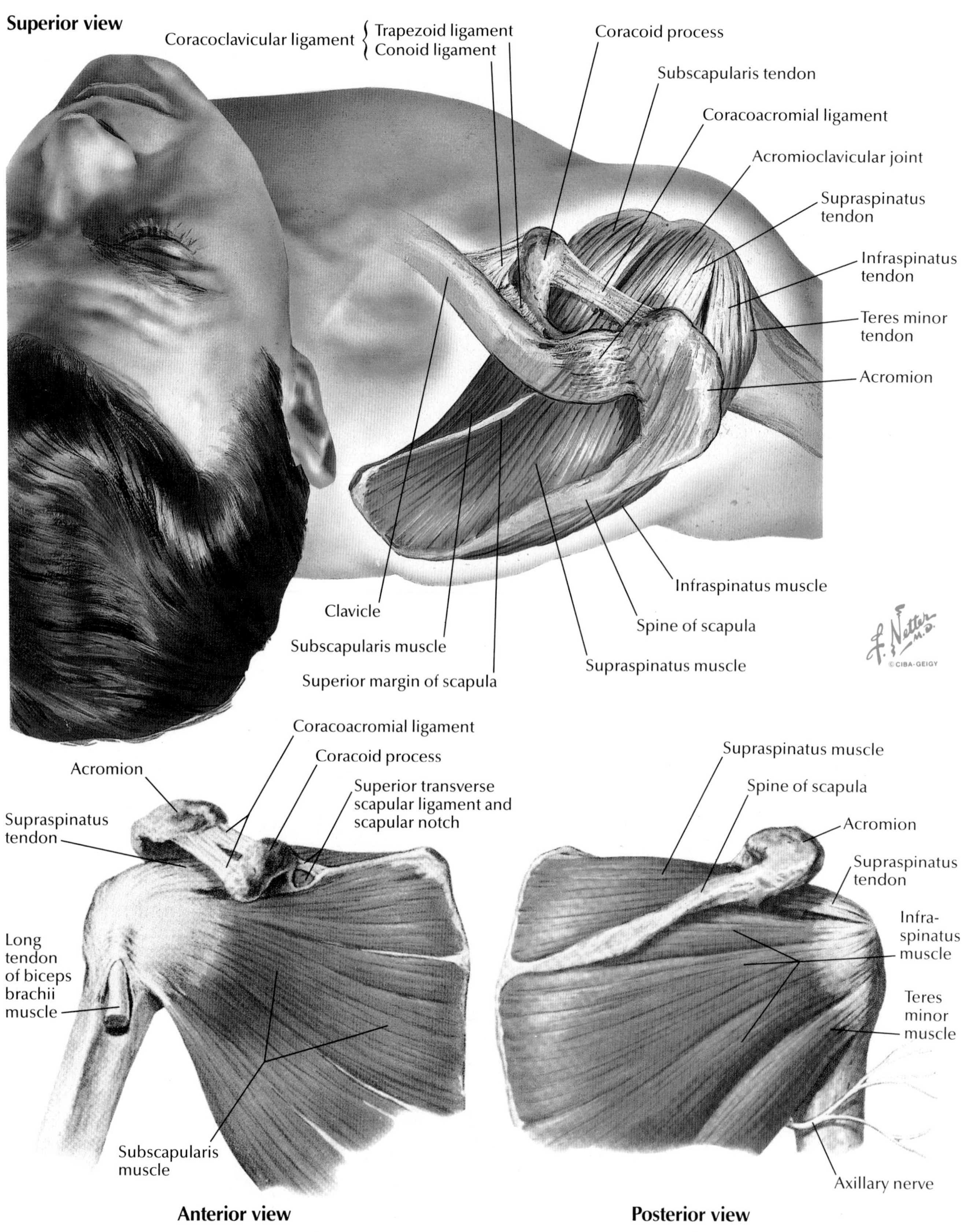

Superior view

Coracoclavicular ligament { Trapezoid ligament / Conoid ligament

Coracoid process

Subscapularis tendon

Coracoacromial ligament

Acromioclavicular joint

Supraspinatus tendon

Infraspinatus tendon

Teres minor tendon

Acromion

Infraspinatus muscle

Spine of scapula

Supraspinatus muscle

Clavicle

Subscapularis muscle

Superior margin of scapula

Coracoacromial ligament

Coracoid process

Superior transverse scapular ligament and scapular notch

Acromion

Supraspinatus tendon

Long tendon of biceps brachii muscle

Subscapularis muscle

Anterior view

Supraspinatus muscle

Spine of scapula

Acromion

Supraspinatus tendon

Infra-spinatus muscle

Teres minor muscle

Axillary nerve

Posterior view

PLATE 400

UPPER LIMB

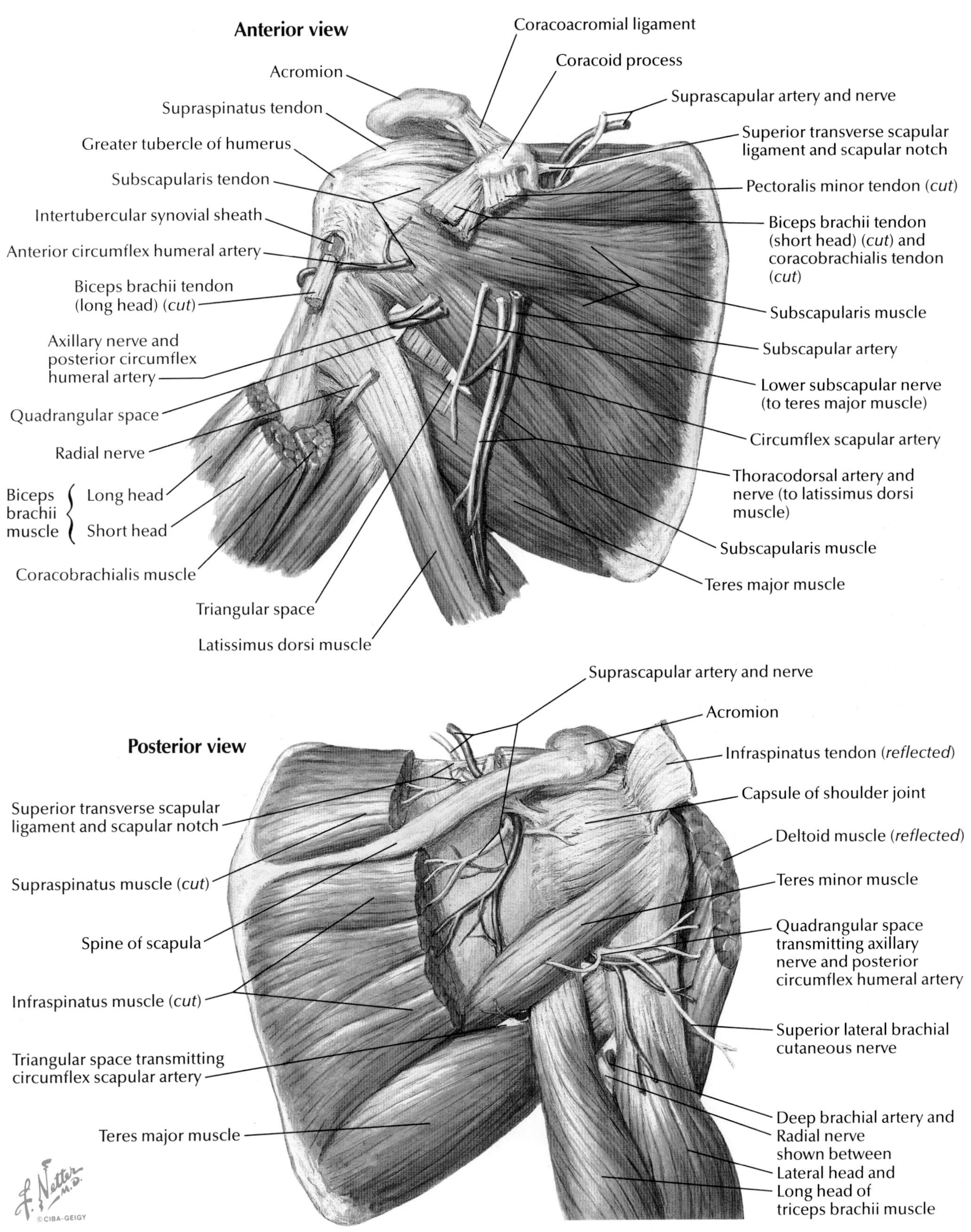

Anterior view

Coracoacromial ligament

Coracoid process

Acromion

Supraspinatus tendon

Greater tubercle of humerus

Subscapularis tendon

Intertubercular synovial sheath

Anterior circumflex humeral artery

Biceps brachii tendon (long head) (*cut*)

Axillary nerve and posterior circumflex humeral artery

Quadrangular space

Radial nerve

Biceps brachii muscle { Long head / Short head }

Coracobrachialis muscle

Triangular space

Latissimus dorsi muscle

Suprascapular artery and nerve

Superior transverse scapular ligament and scapular notch

Pectoralis minor tendon (*cut*)

Biceps brachii tendon (short head) (*cut*) and coracobrachialis tendon (*cut*)

Subscapularis muscle

Subscapular artery

Lower subscapular nerve (to teres major muscle)

Circumflex scapular artery

Thoracodorsal artery and nerve (to latissimus dorsi muscle)

Subscapularis muscle

Teres major muscle

Posterior view

Suprascapular artery and nerve

Acromion

Infraspinatus tendon (*reflected*)

Capsule of shoulder joint

Deltoid muscle (*reflected*)

Teres minor muscle

Quadrangular space transmitting axillary nerve and posterior circumflex humeral artery

Superior lateral brachial cutaneous nerve

Deep brachial artery and Radial nerve shown between Lateral head and Long head of triceps brachii muscle

Superior transverse scapular ligament and scapular notch

Supraspinatus muscle (*cut*)

Spine of scapula

Infraspinatus muscle (*cut*)

Triangular space transmitting circumflex scapular artery

Teres major muscle

Axillary Artery and Anastomoses Around Scapula

SEE ALSO PLATES 28, 409

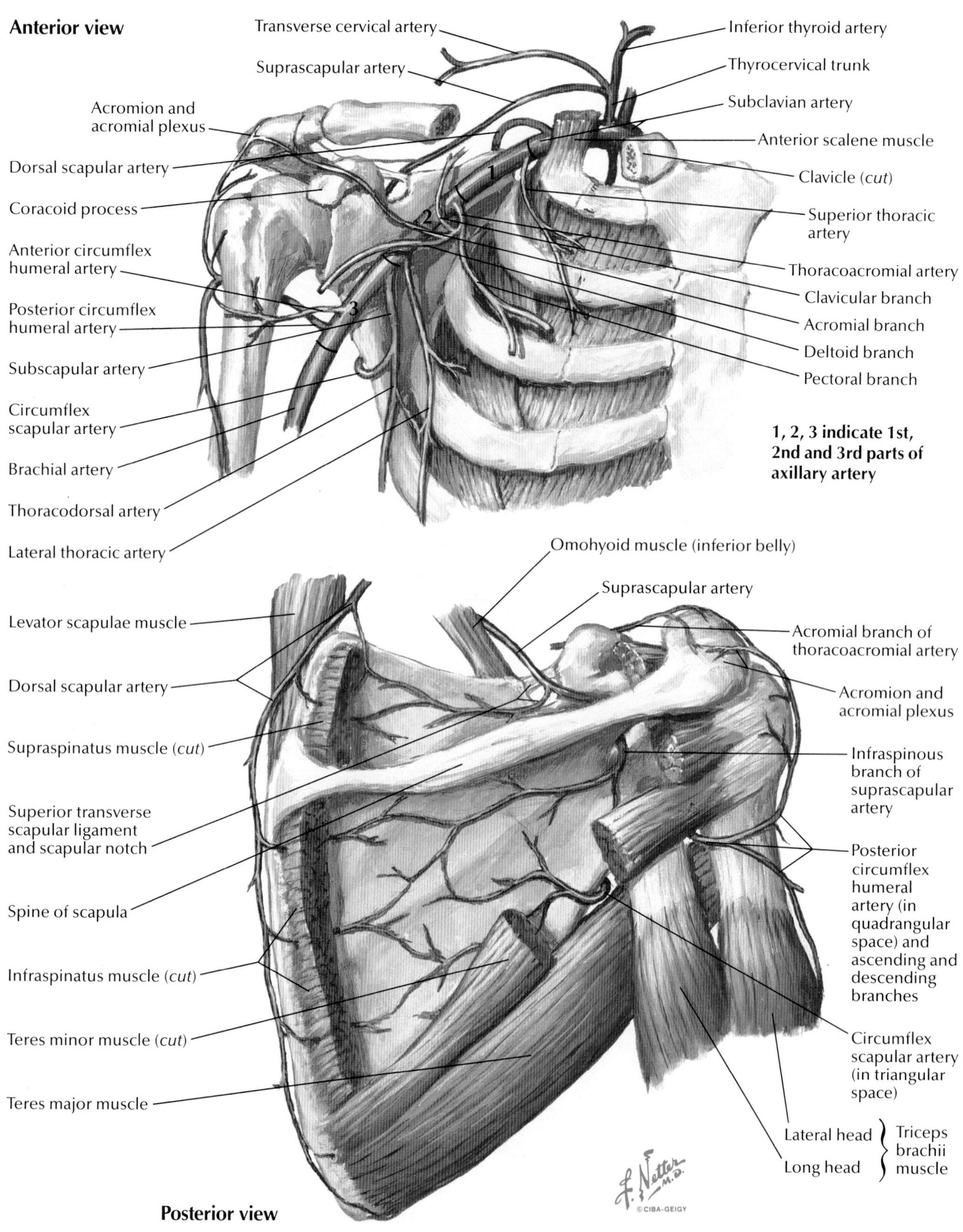

Anterior view

Transverse cervical artery

Suprascapular artery

Acromion and acromial plexus

Dorsal scapular artery

Coracoid process

Anterior circumflex humeral artery

Posterior circumflex humeral artery

Subscapular artery

Circumflex scapular artery

Brachial artery

Thoracodorsal artery

Lateral thoracic artery

Inferior thyroid artery

Thyrocervical trunk

Subclavian artery

Anterior scalene muscle

Clavicle (cut)

Superior thoracic artery

Thoracoacromial artery

Clavicular branch

Acromial branch

Deltoid branch

Pectoral branch

1, 2, 3 indicate 1st, 2nd and 3rd parts of axillary artery

Omohyoid muscle (inferior belly)

Suprascapular artery

Levator scapulae muscle

Dorsal scapular artery

Supraspinatus muscle (cut)

Superior transverse scapular ligament and scapular notch

Spine of scapula

Infraspinatus muscle (cut)

Teres minor muscle (cut)

Teres major muscle

Acromial branch of thoracoacromial artery

Acromion and acromial plexus

Infraspinous branch of suprascapular artery

Posterior circumflex humeral artery (in quadrangular space) and ascending and descending branches

Circumflex scapular artery (in triangular space)

Lateral head ⎫ Triceps
Long head ⎬ brachii
⎭ muscle

Posterior view

PLATE 402

UPPER LIMB

Pectoral, Clavipectoral and Axillary Fasciae

SEE ALSO PLATE 174

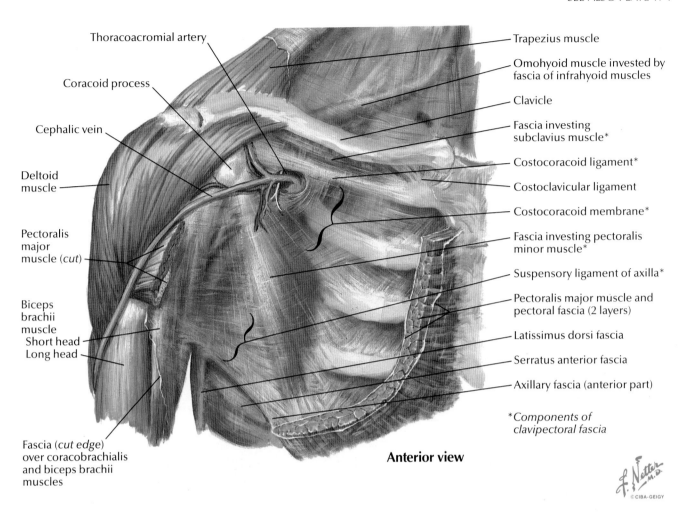

Thoracoacromial artery

Coracoid process

Cephalic vein

Deltoid muscle

Pectoralis major muscle (*cut*)

Biceps brachii muscle
Short head
Long head

Fascia (*cut edge*) over coracobrachialis and biceps brachii muscles

Trapezius muscle

Omohyoid muscle invested by fascia of infrahyoid muscles

Clavicle

Fascia investing subclavius muscle*

Costocoracoid ligament*

Costoclavicular ligament

Costocoracoid membrane*

Fascia investing pectoralis minor muscle*

Suspensory ligament of axilla*

Pectoralis major muscle and pectoral fascia (2 layers)

Latissimus dorsi fascia

Serratus anterior fascia

Axillary fascia (anterior part)

*Components of clavipectoral fascia

Anterior view

Oblique parasagittal section of axilla

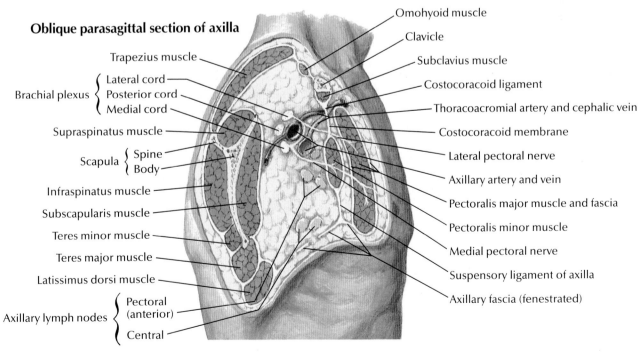

Trapezius muscle

Brachial plexus
Lateral cord
Posterior cord
Medial cord

Supraspinatus muscle

Scapula
Spine
Body

Infraspinatus muscle

Subscapularis muscle

Teres minor muscle

Teres major muscle

Latissimus dorsi muscle

Axillary lymph nodes
Pectoral (anterior)
Central

Omohyoid muscle

Clavicle

Subclavius muscle

Costocoracoid ligament

Thoracoacromial artery and cephalic vein

Costocoracoid membrane

Lateral pectoral nerve

Axillary artery and vein

Pectoralis major muscle and fascia

Pectoralis minor muscle

Medial pectoral nerve

Suspensory ligament of axilla

Axillary fascia (fenestrated)

Axilla (Dissection): Anterior View

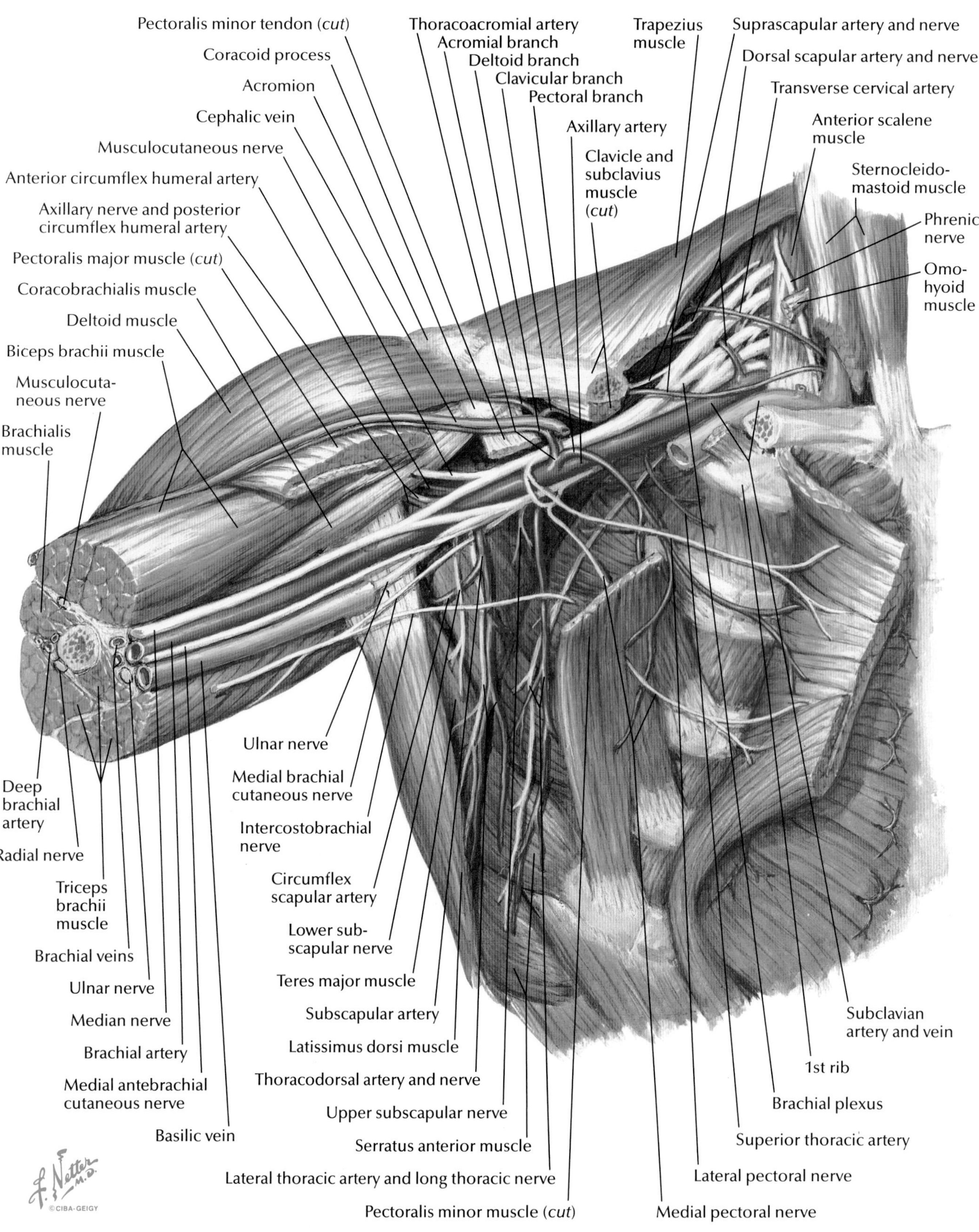

Pectoralis minor tendon (cut)

Coracoid process

Acromion

Cephalic vein

Musculocutaneous nerve

Anterior circumflex humeral artery

Axillary nerve and posterior circumflex humeral artery

Pectoralis major muscle (cut)

Coracobrachialis muscle

Deltoid muscle

Biceps brachii muscle

Musculocuta-neous nerve

Brachialis muscle

Thoracoacromial artery
Acromial branch
Deltoid branch
Clavicular branch
Pectoral branch

Axillary artery

Clavicle and subclavius muscle (cut)

Trapezius muscle

Suprascapular artery and nerve

Dorsal scapular artery and nerve

Transverse cervical artery

Anterior scalene muscle

Sternocleido-mastoid muscle

Phrenic nerve

Omo-hyoid muscle

Deep brachial artery

Radial nerve

Triceps brachii muscle

Brachial veins

Ulnar nerve

Median nerve

Brachial artery

Medial antebrachial cutaneous nerve

Basilic vein

Ulnar nerve

Medial brachial cutaneous nerve

Intercostobrachial nerve

Circumflex scapular artery

Lower sub-scapular nerve

Teres major muscle

Subscapular artery

Latissimus dorsi muscle

Thoracodorsal artery and nerve

Upper subscapular nerve

Serratus anterior muscle

Lateral thoracic artery and long thoracic nerve

Pectoralis minor muscle (cut)

Subclavian artery and vein

1st rib

Brachial plexus

Superior thoracic artery

Lateral pectoral nerve

Medial pectoral nerve

PLATE 404

UPPER LIMB

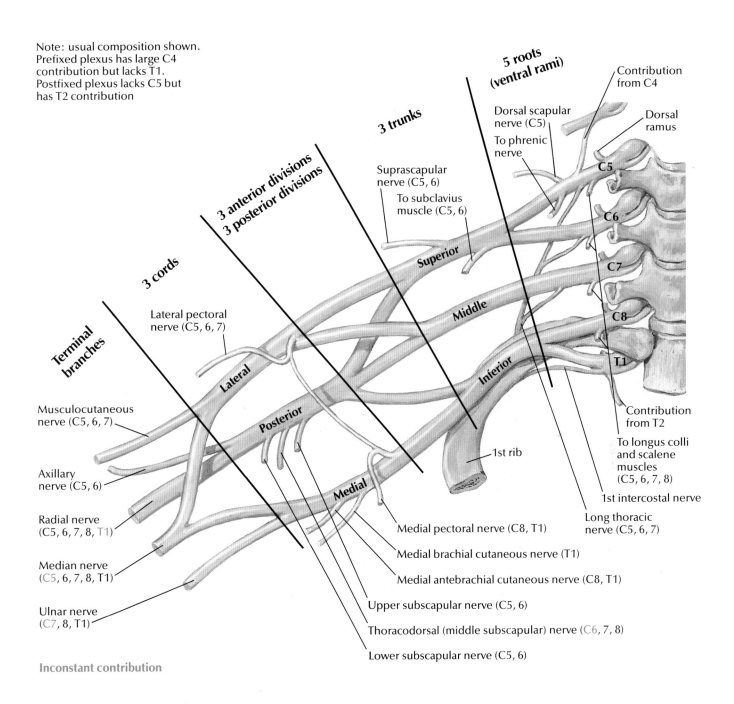

Note: usual composition shown.
Prefixed plexus has large C4
contribution but lacks T1.
Postfixed plexus lacks C5 but
has T2 contribution

5 roots (ventral rami)

Contribution from C4

Dorsal scapular nerve (C5)

Dorsal ramus

To phrenic nerve

3 trunks

C5

Suprascapular nerve (C5, 6)

C6

To subclavius muscle (C5, 6)

C7

3 anterior divisions
3 posterior divisions

Superior

C8

Middle

3 cords

T1

Lateral pectoral nerve (C5, 6, 7)

Lateral

Inferior

Contribution from T2

Terminal branches

Posterior

To longus colli and scalene muscles (C5, 6, 7, 8)

Musculocutaneous nerve (C5, 6, 7)

1st rib

1st intercostal nerve

Axillary nerve (C5, 6)

Medial

Long thoracic nerve (C5, 6, 7)

Radial nerve (C5, 6, 7, 8, T1)

Medial pectoral nerve (C8, T1)

Median nerve (C5, 6, 7, 8, T1)

Medial brachial cutaneous nerve (T1)

Medial antebrachial cutaneous nerve (C8, T1)

Ulnar nerve (C7, 8, T1)

Upper subscapular nerve (C5, 6)

Thoracodorsal (middle subscapular) nerve (C6, 7, 8)

Lower subscapular nerve (C5, 6)

Inconstant contribution

Muscles of Arm: Anterior Views

SEE ALSO PLATE 447

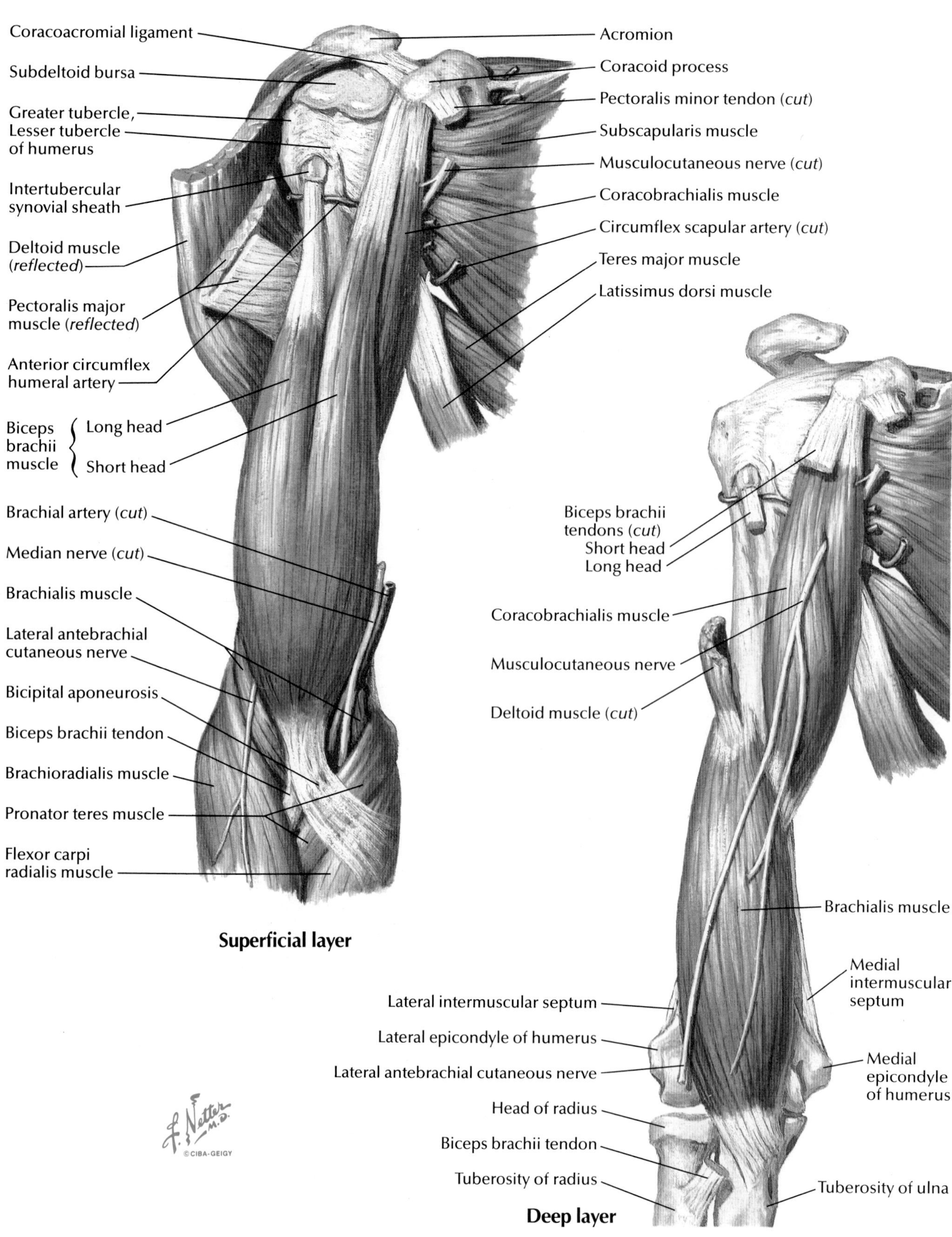

Coracoacromial ligament

Subdeltoid bursa

Greater tubercle,
Lesser tubercle
of humerus

Intertubercular
synovial sheath

Deltoid muscle
(reflected)

Pectoralis major
muscle (reflected)

Anterior circumflex
humeral artery

Biceps
brachii
muscle { Long head

Short head

Brachial artery (cut)

Median nerve (cut)

Brachialis muscle

Lateral antebrachial
cutaneous nerve

Bicipital aponeurosis

Biceps brachii tendon

Brachioradialis muscle

Pronator teres muscle

Flexor carpi
radialis muscle

Acromion

Coracoid process

Pectoralis minor tendon (cut)

Subscapularis muscle

Musculocutaneous nerve (cut)

Coracobrachialis muscle

Circumflex scapular artery (cut)

Teres major muscle

Latissimus dorsi muscle

Superficial layer

Biceps brachii
tendons (cut)
Short head
Long head

Coracobrachialis muscle

Musculocutaneous nerve

Deltoid muscle (cut)

Lateral intermuscular septum

Lateral epicondyle of humerus

Lateral antebrachial cutaneous nerve

Head of radius

Biceps brachii tendon

Tuberosity of radius

Brachialis muscle

Medial
intermuscular
septum

Medial
epicondyle
of humerus

Tuberosity of ulna

Deep layer

PLATE 406

UPPER LIMB

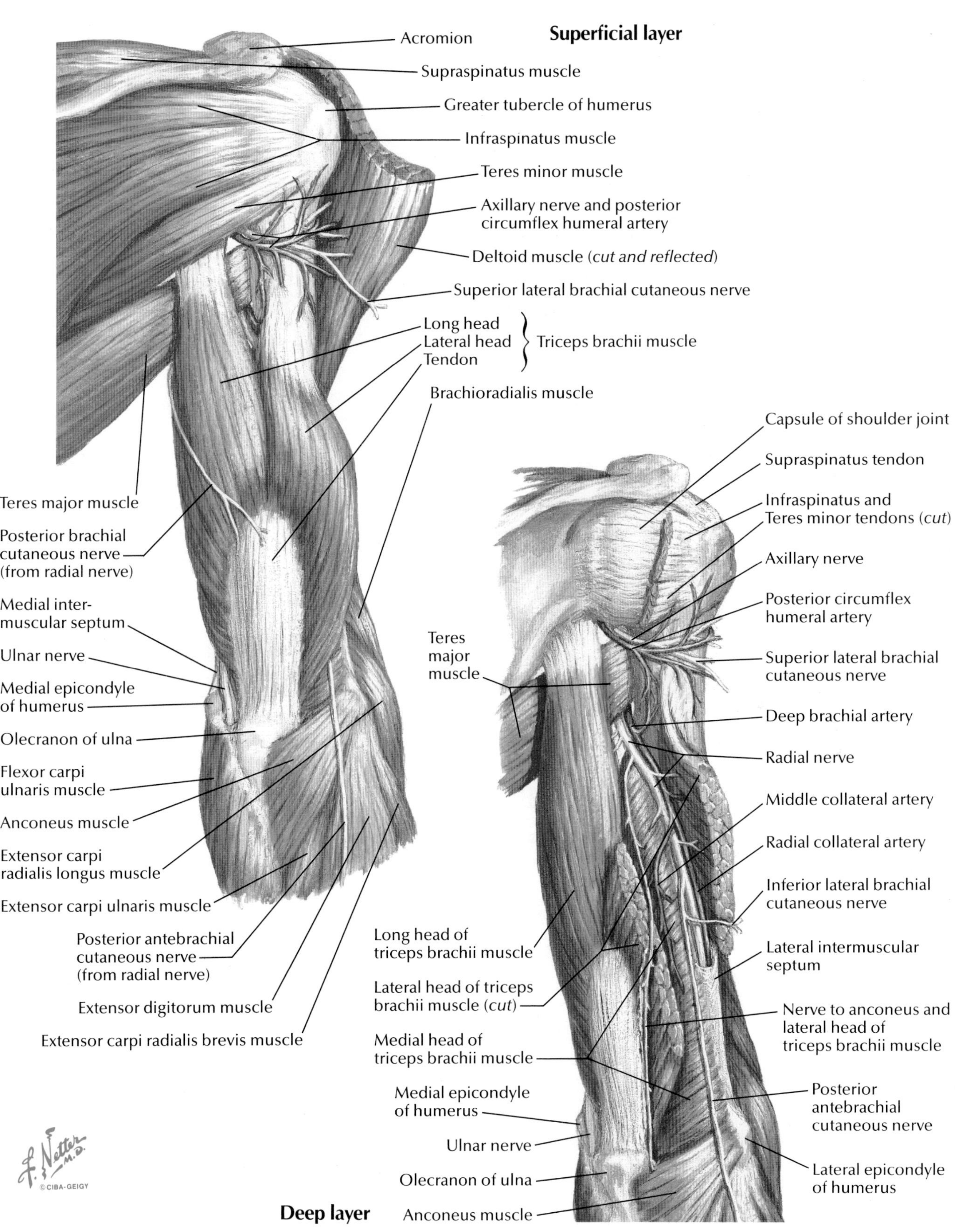

Superficial layer

Acromion

Suprasinatus muscle

Greater tubercle of humerus

Infraspinatus muscle

Teres minor muscle

Axillary nerve and posterior circumflex humeral artery

Deltoid muscle (*cut and reflected*)

Superior lateral brachial cutaneous nerve

Long head
Lateral head } Triceps brachii muscle
Tendon

Brachioradialis muscle

Capsule of shoulder joint

Supraspinatus tendon

Infraspinatus and Teres minor tendons (*cut*)

Axillary nerve

Posterior circumflex humeral artery

Superior lateral brachial cutaneous nerve

Deep brachial artery

Radial nerve

Middle collateral artery

Radial collateral artery

Inferior lateral brachial cutaneous nerve

Lateral intermuscular septum

Nerve to anconeus and lateral head of triceps brachii muscle

Posterior antebrachial cutaneous nerve

Lateral epicondyle of humerus

Teres major muscle

Posterior brachial cutaneous nerve (from radial nerve)

Medial inter-muscular septum

Ulnar nerve

Medial epicondyle of humerus

Olecranon of ulna

Flexor carpi ulnaris muscle

Anconeus muscle

Extensor carpi radialis longus muscle

Extensor carpi ulnaris muscle

Posterior antebrachial cutaneous nerve (from radial nerve)

Extensor digitorum muscle

Extensor carpi radialis brevis muscle

Teres major muscle

Long head of triceps brachii muscle

Lateral head of triceps brachii muscle (*cut*)

Medial head of triceps brachii muscle

Medial epicondyle of humerus

Ulnar nerve

Olecranon of ulna

Deep layer   Anconeus muscle

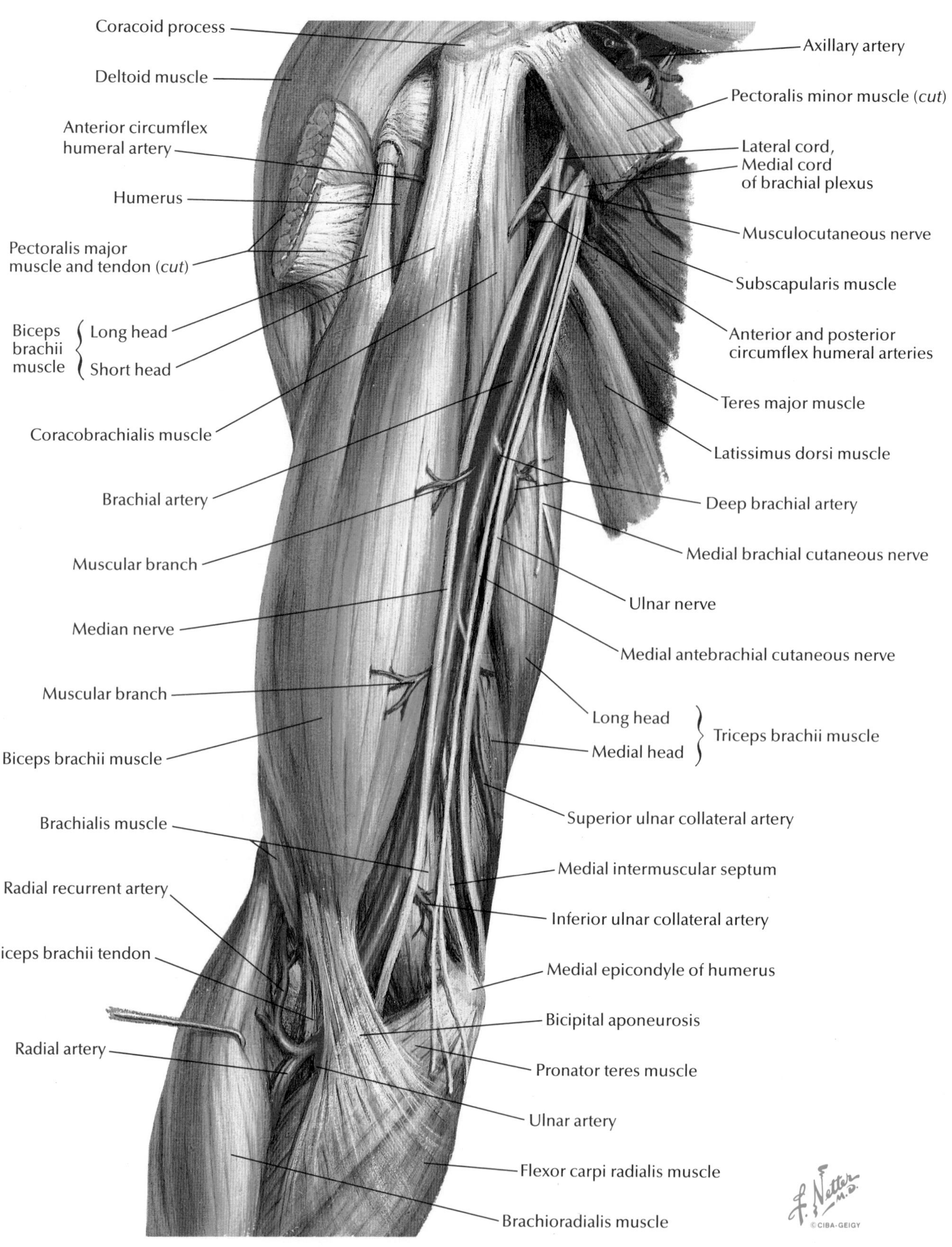

Coracoid process

Deltoid muscle

Anterior circumflex humeral artery

Humerus

Pectoralis major muscle and tendon (*cut*)

Biceps brachii muscle { Long head / Short head

Coracobrachialis muscle

Brachial artery

Muscular branch

Median nerve

Muscular branch

Biceps brachii muscle

Brachialis muscle

Radial recurrent artery

Biceps brachii tendon

Radial artery

Axillary artery

Pectoralis minor muscle (*cut*)

Lateral cord, Medial cord of brachial plexus

Musculocutaneous nerve

Subscapularis muscle

Anterior and posterior circumflex humeral arteries

Teres major muscle

Latissimus dorsi muscle

Deep brachial artery

Medial brachial cutaneous nerve

Ulnar nerve

Medial antebrachial cutaneous nerve

Long head / Medial head } Triceps brachii muscle

Superior ulnar collateral artery

Medial intermuscular septum

Inferior ulnar collateral artery

Medial epicondyle of humerus

Bicipital aponeurosis

Pronator teres muscle

Ulnar artery

Flexor carpi radialis muscle

Brachioradialis muscle

PLATE 408

UPPER LIMB

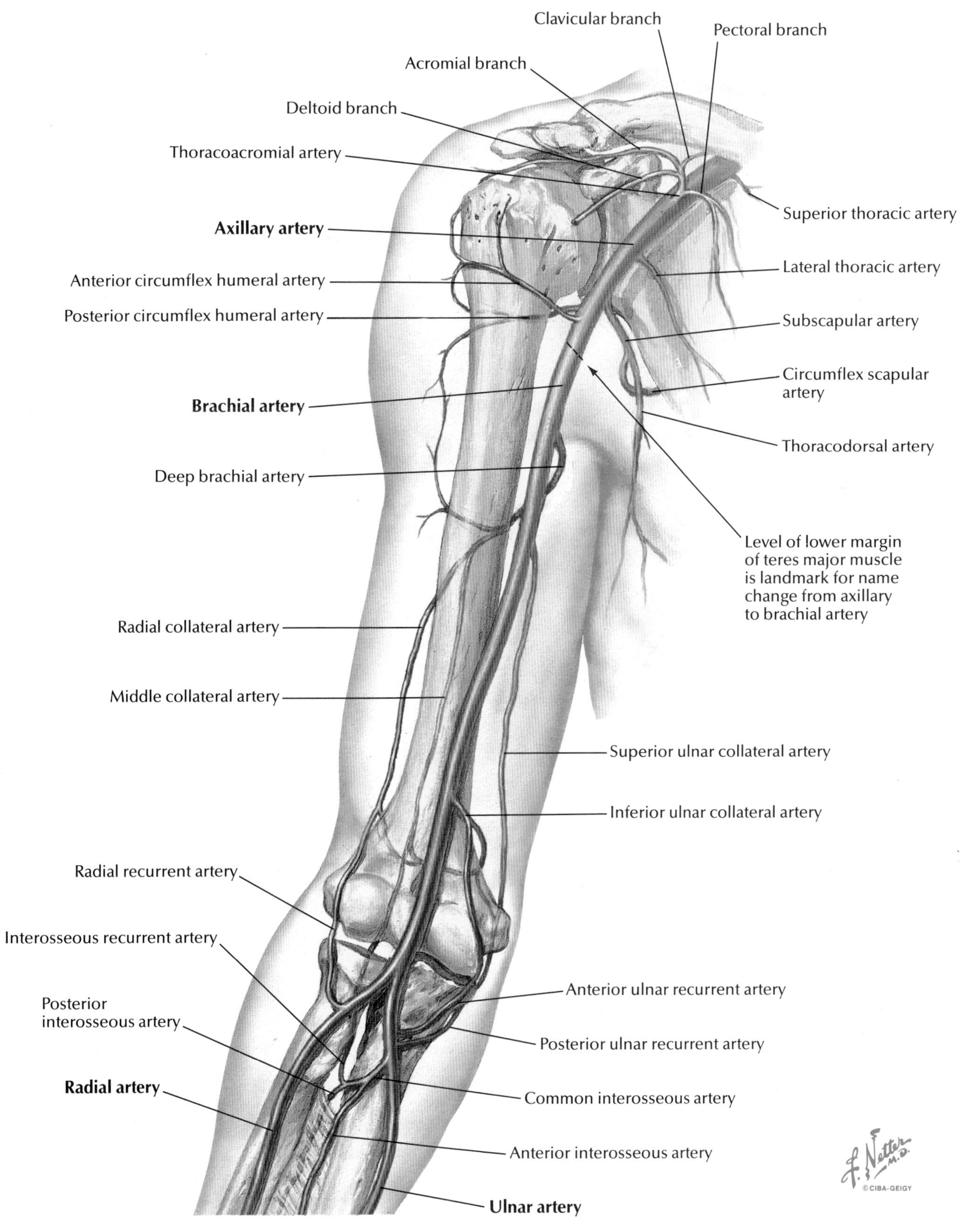

Clavicular branch

Pectoral branch

Acromial branch

Deltoid branch

Thoracoacromial artery

Axillary artery

Anterior circumflex humeral artery

Posterior circumflex humeral artery

Brachial artery

Deep brachial artery

Radial collateral artery

Middle collateral artery

Radial recurrent artery

Interosseous recurrent artery

Posterior interosseous artery

Radial artery

Superior thoracic artery

Lateral thoracic artery

Subscapular artery

Circumflex scapular artery

Thoracodorsal artery

Level of lower margin of teres major muscle is landmark for name change from axillary to brachial artery

Superior ulnar collateral artery

Inferior ulnar collateral artery

Anterior ulnar recurrent artery

Posterior ulnar recurrent artery

Common interosseous artery

Anterior interosseous artery

Ulnar artery

Arm: Serial Cross Sections

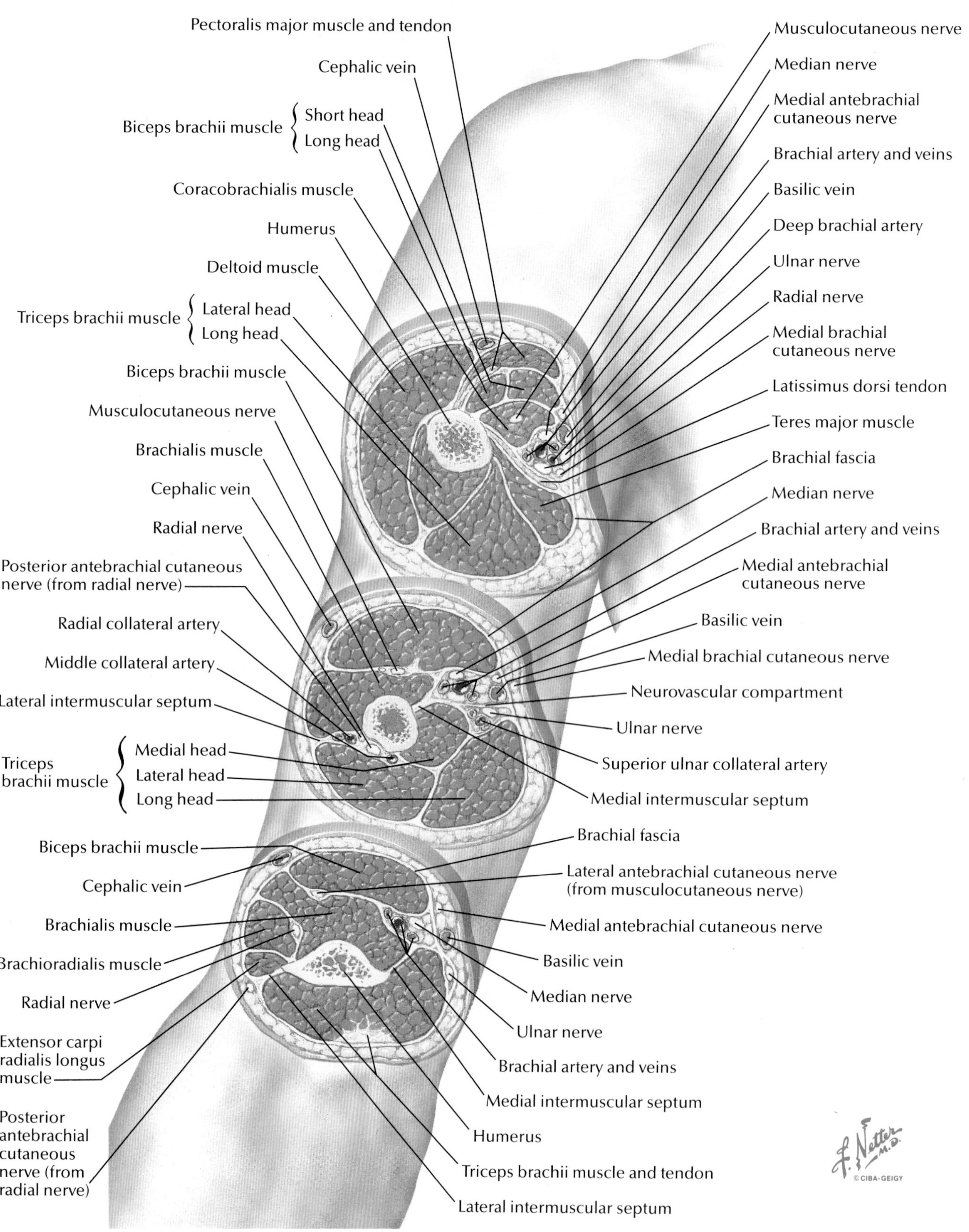

Pectoralis major muscle and tendon

Cephalic vein

Biceps brachii muscle { Short head / Long head

Coracobrachialis muscle

Humerus

Deltoid muscle

Triceps brachii muscle { Lateral head / Long head

Biceps brachii muscle

Musculocutaneous nerve

Brachialis muscle

Cephalic vein

Radial nerve

Posterior antebrachial cutaneous nerve (from radial nerve)

Radial collateral artery

Middle collateral artery

Lateral intermuscular septum

Triceps brachii muscle { Medial head / Lateral head / Long head

Biceps brachii muscle

Cephalic vein

Brachialis muscle

Brachioradialis muscle

Radial nerve

Extensor carpi radialis longus muscle

Posterior antebrachial cutaneous nerve (from radial nerve)

Musculocutaneous nerve

Median nerve

Medial antebrachial cutaneous nerve

Brachial artery and veins

Basilic vein

Deep brachial artery

Ulnar nerve

Radial nerve

Medial brachial cutaneous nerve

Latissimus dorsi tendon

Teres major muscle

Brachial fascia

Median nerve

Brachial artery and veins

Medial antebrachial cutaneous nerve

Basilic vein

Medial brachial cutaneous nerve

Neurovascular compartment

Ulnar nerve

Superior ulnar collateral artery

Medial intermuscular septum

Brachial fascia

Lateral antebrachial cutaneous nerve (from musculocutaneous nerve)

Medial antebrachial cutaneous nerve

Basilic vein

Median nerve

Ulnar nerve

Brachial artery and veins

Medial intermuscular septum

Humerus

Triceps brachii muscle and tendon

Lateral intermuscular septum

PLATE 410

UPPER LIMB

Right elbow

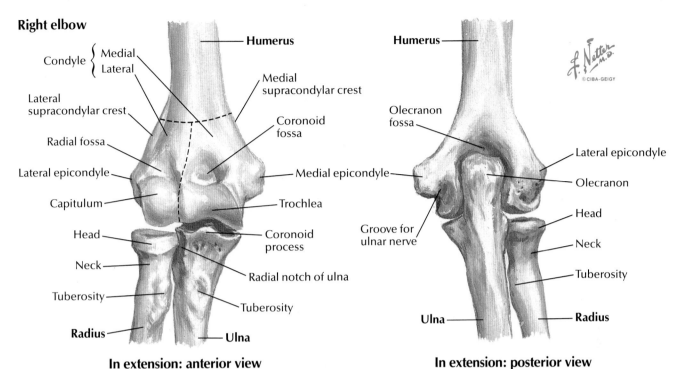

Condyle { Medial
Lateral }

Lateral supracondylar crest

Radial fossa

Lateral epicondyle

Capitulum

Head

Neck

Tuberosity

Radius

Humerus

Medial supracondylar crest

Coronoid fossa

Medial epicondyle

Trochlea

Coronoid process

Radial notch of ulna

Tuberosity

Ulna

In extension: anterior view

Humerus

Olecranon fossa

Lateral epicondyle

Olecranon

Head

Neck

Tuberosity

Groove for ulnar nerve

Ulna

Radius

In extension: posterior view

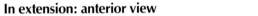

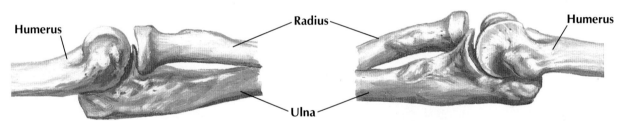

Humerus

Radius

Humerus

Ulna

In extension: lateral view

In extension: medial view

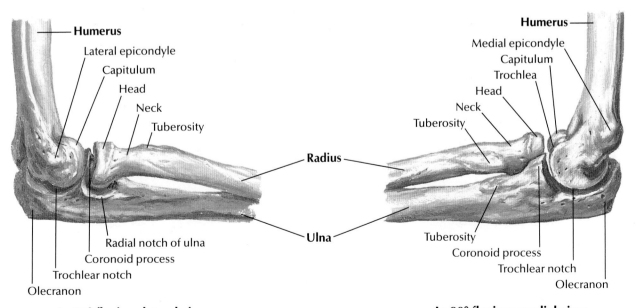

Humerus

Lateral epicondyle

Capitulum

Head

Neck

Tuberosity

Radius

Radial notch of ulna

Coronoid process

Trochlear notch

Olecranon

In 90° flexion: lateral view

Humerus

Medial epicondyle

Capitulum

Trochlea

Head

Neck

Tuberosity

Radius

Ulna

Tuberosity

Coronoid process

Trochlear notch

Olecranon

In 90° flexion: medial view

Ligaments of Elbow

Right elbow

Anterior view

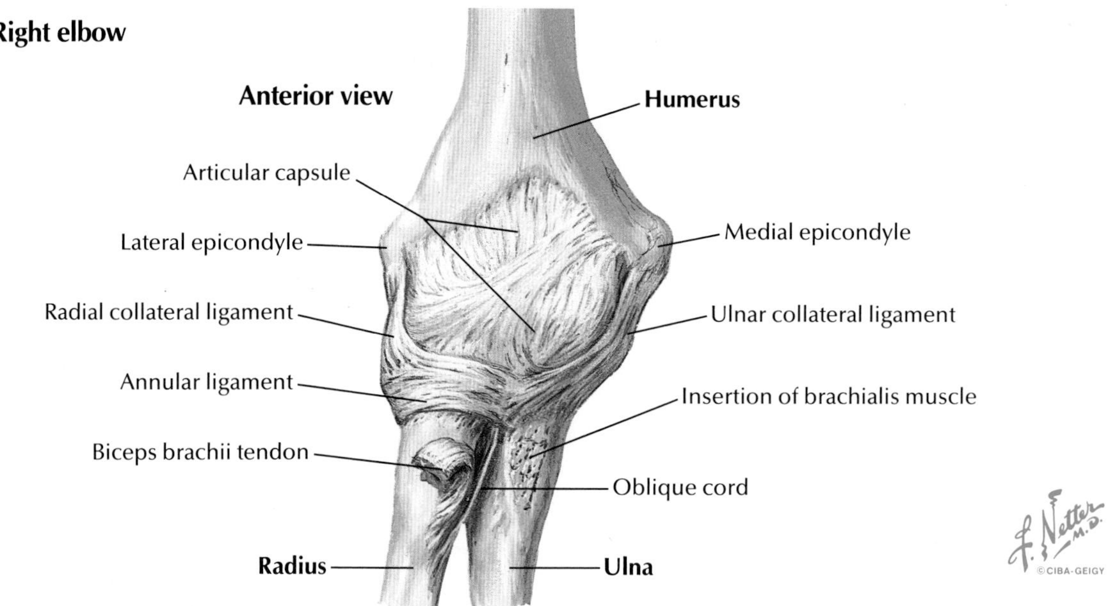

Humerus

Articular capsule

Lateral epicondyle

Medial epicondyle

Radial collateral ligament

Ulnar collateral ligament

Annular ligament

Insertion of brachialis muscle

Biceps brachii tendon

Oblique cord

Radius

Ulna

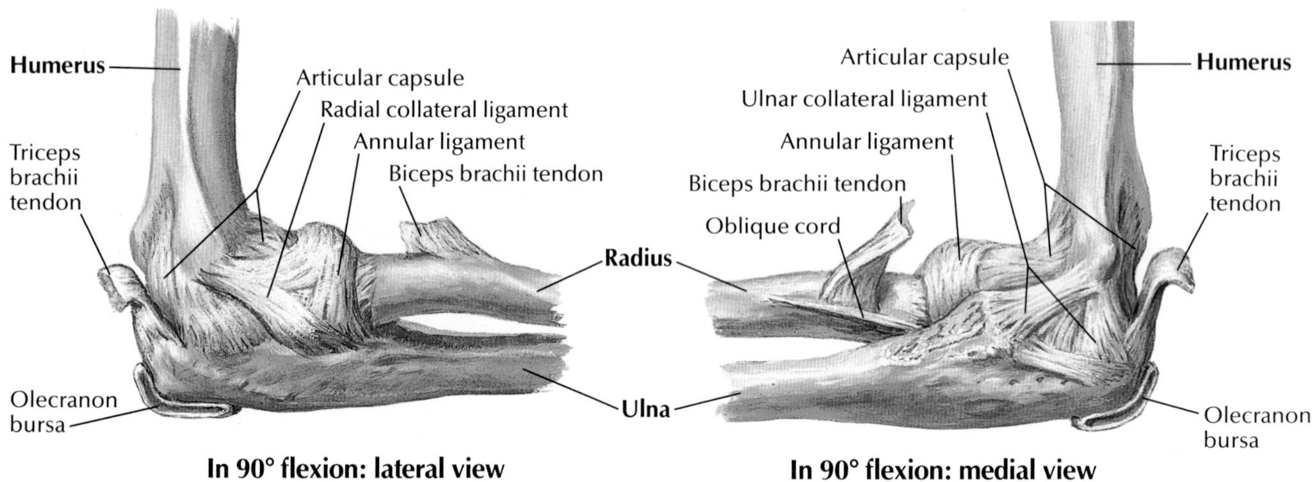

Humerus

Triceps brachii tendon

Articular capsule

Radial collateral ligament

Annular ligament

Biceps brachii tendon

Radius

Olecranon bursa

Ulna

In 90° flexion: lateral view

Articular capsule

Humerus

Ulnar collateral ligament

Annular ligament

Biceps brachii tendon

Oblique cord

Triceps brachii tendon

Olecranon bursa

In 90° flexion: medial view

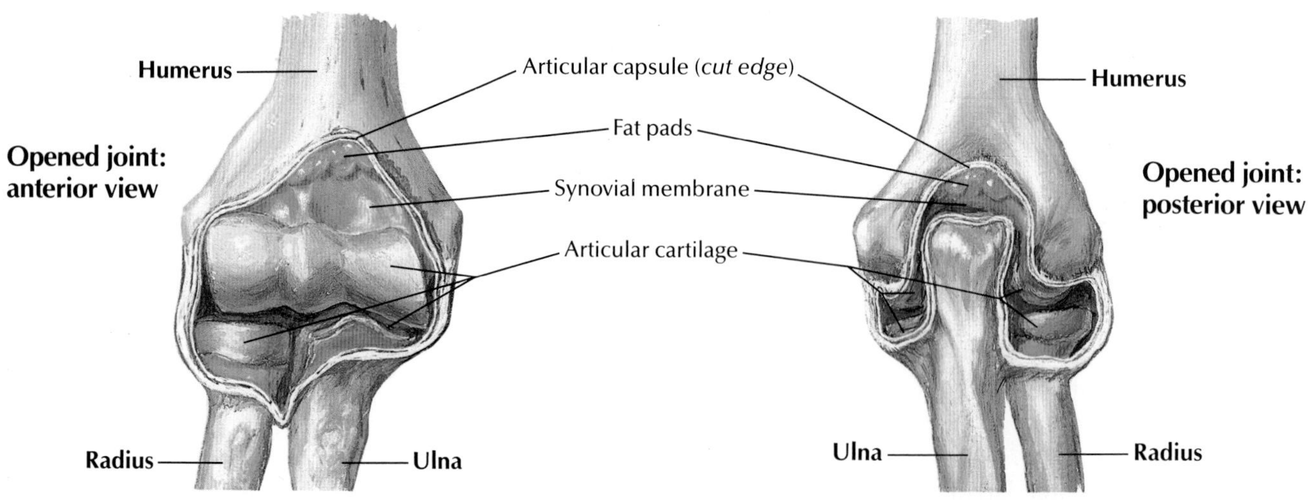

Humerus

Opened joint: anterior view

Articular capsule (*cut edge*)

Fat pads

Synovial membrane

Articular cartilage

Radius

Ulna

Humerus

Opened joint: posterior view

Ulna

Radius

PLATE 412

UPPER LIMB

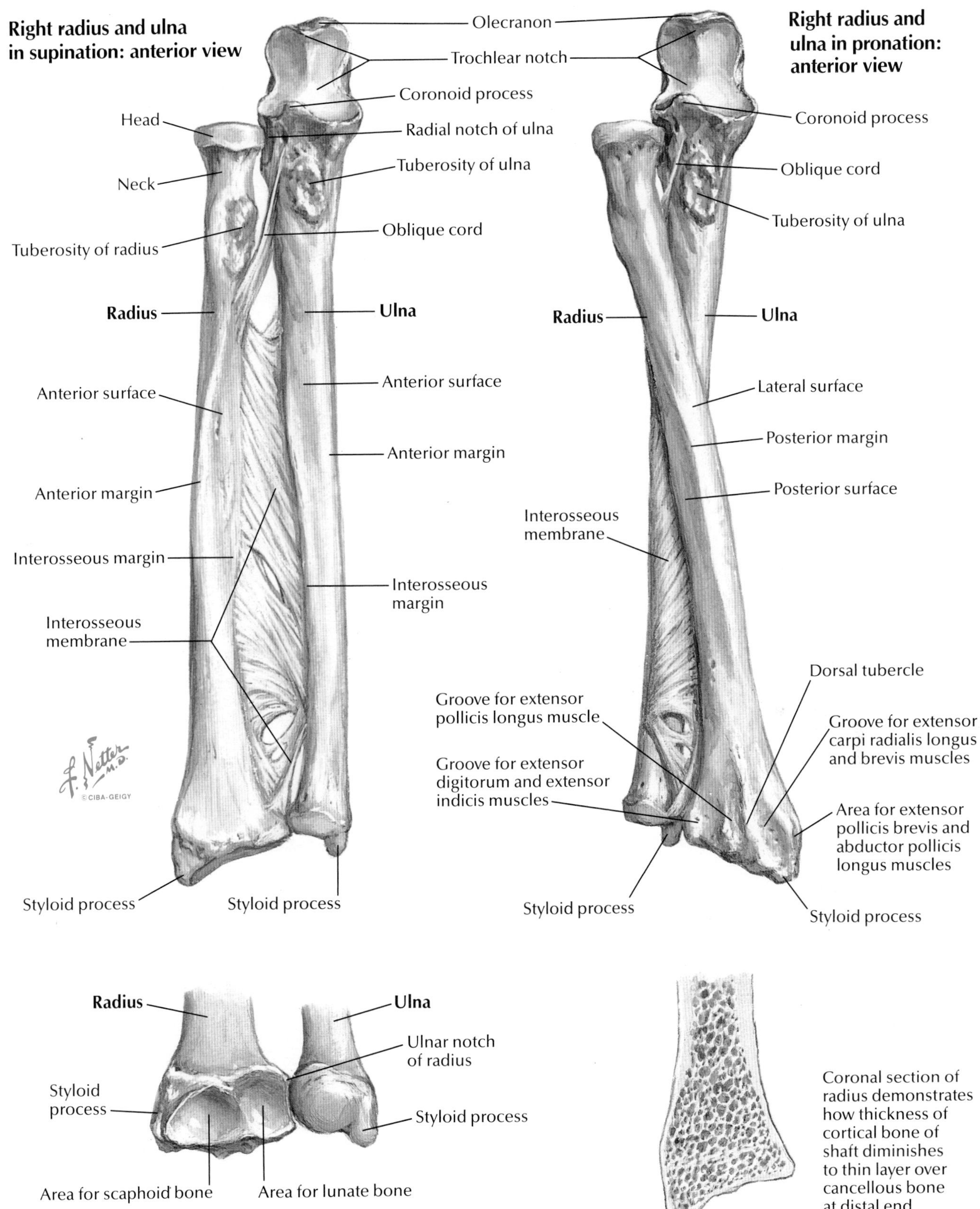

Right radius and ulna in supination: anterior view

Olecranon

Trochlear notch

Coronoid process

Head

Radial notch of ulna

Neck

Tuberosity of ulna

Tuberosity of radius

Oblique cord

Radius

Ulna

Anterior surface

Anterior surface

Anterior margin

Anterior margin

Interosseous margin

Interosseous margin

Interosseous membrane

Interosseous margin

Right radius and ulna in pronation: anterior view

Coronoid process

Oblique cord

Tuberosity of ulna

Radius

Ulna

Lateral surface

Posterior margin

Posterior surface

Interosseous membrane

Dorsal tubercle

Groove for extensor pollicis longus muscle

Groove for extensor digitorum and extensor indicis muscles

Groove for extensor carpi radialis longus and brevis muscles

Area for extensor pollicis brevis and abductor pollicis longus muscles

Styloid process

Styloid process

Styloid process

Styloid process

Radius

Ulna

Styloid process

Ulnar notch of radius

Styloid process

Area for scaphoid bone

Area for lunate bone

Carpal articular surface

Coronal section of radius demonstrates how thickness of cortical bone of shaft diminishes to thin layer over cancellous bone at distal end

Right forearm: anterior view

Supination

Pronation

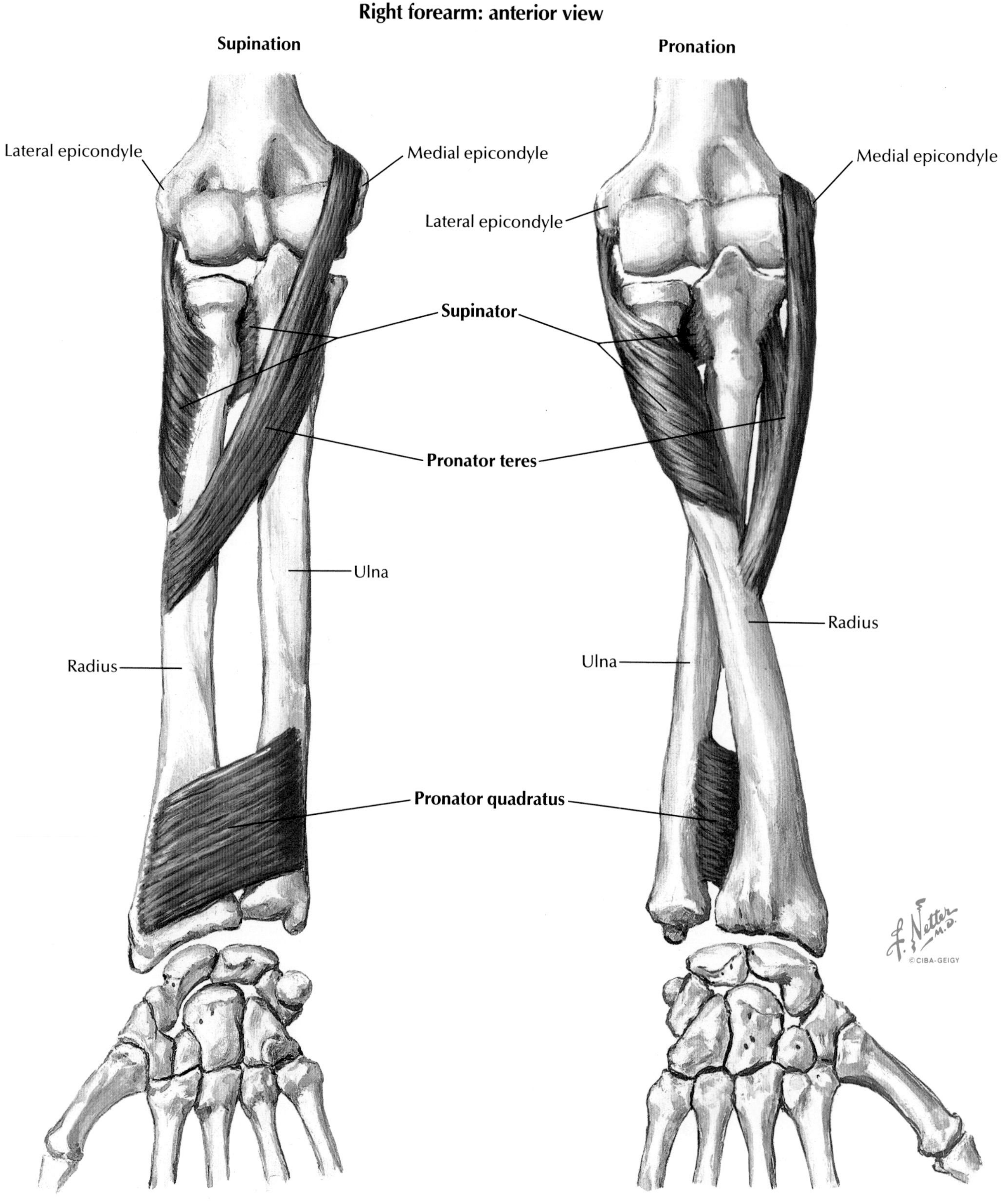

Lateral epicondyle

Medial epicondyle

Medial epicondyle

Lateral epicondyle

Supinator

Pronator teres

Ulna

Radius

Radius

Ulna

Pronator quadratus

PLATE 414

UPPER LIMB

Individual Muscles of Forearm: Extensors of Wrist and Digits

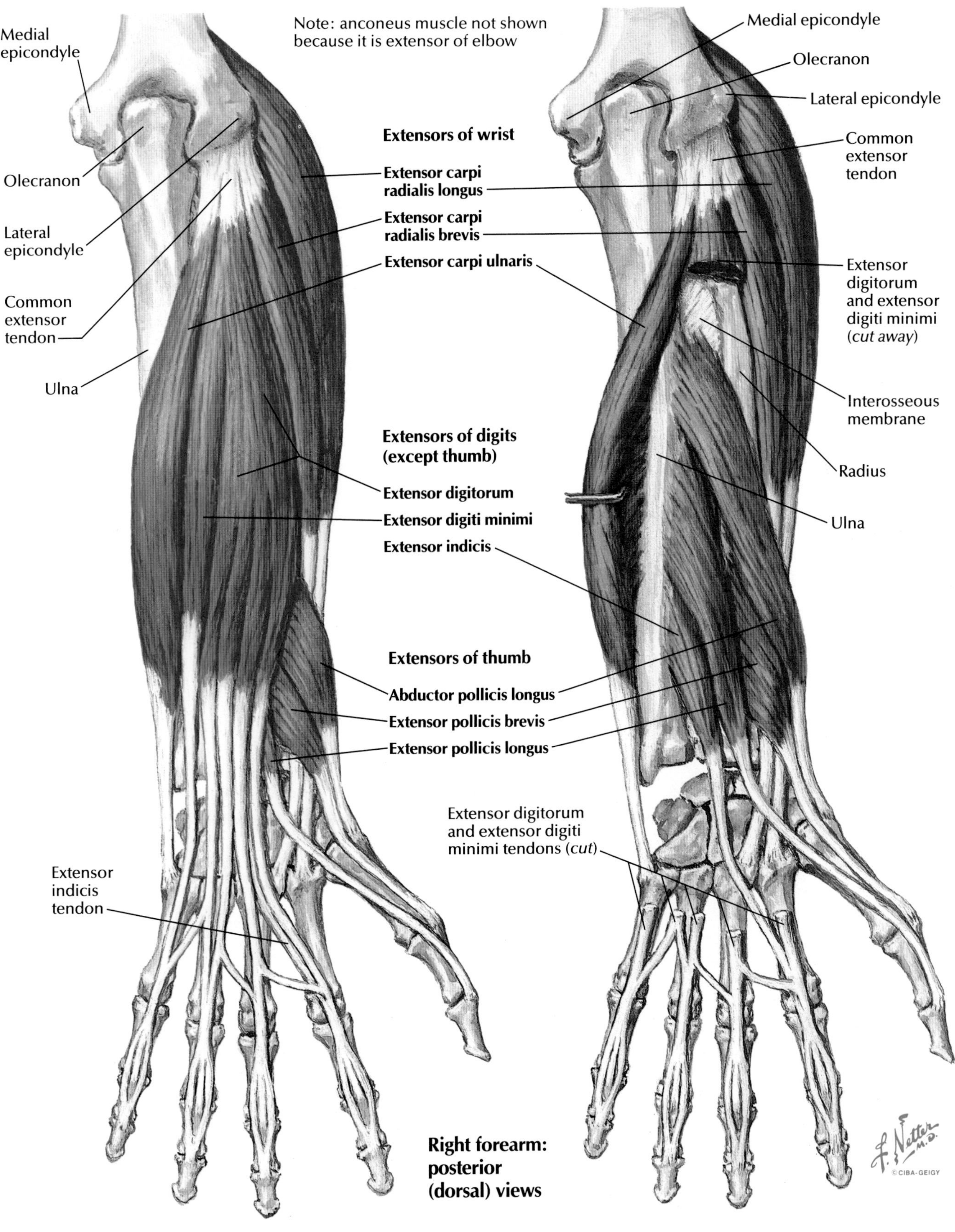

Medial epicondyle

Olecranon

Lateral epicondyle

Common extensor tendon

Ulna

Note: anconeus muscle not shown because it is extensor of elbow

Extensors of wrist

Extensor carpi radialis longus

Extensor carpi radialis brevis

Extensor carpi ulnaris

Extensors of digits (except thumb)

Extensor digitorum

Extensor digiti minimi

Extensor indicis

Extensors of thumb

Abductor pollicis longus

Extensor pollicis brevis

Extensor pollicis longus

Extensor digitorum and extensor digiti minimi tendons (*cut*)

Extensor indicis tendon

Medial epicondyle

Olecranon

Lateral epicondyle

Common extensor tendon

Extensor digitorum and extensor digiti minimi (*cut away*)

Interosseous membrane

Radius

Ulna

Right forearm: posterior (dorsal) views

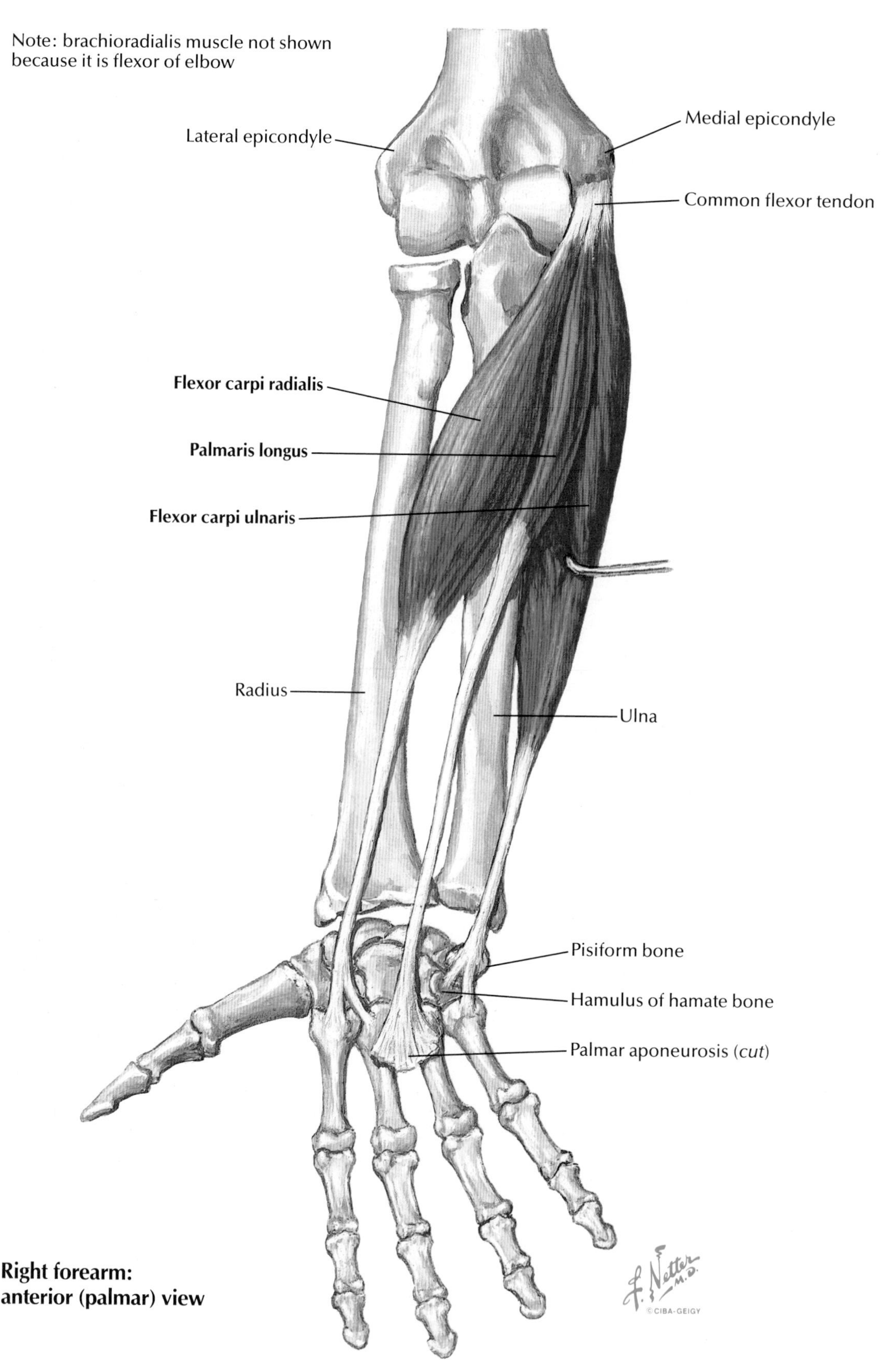

Note: brachioradialis muscle not shown
because it is flexor of elbow

Lateral epicondyle

Medial epicondyle

Common flexor tendon

Flexor carpi radialis

Palmaris longus

Flexor carpi ulnaris

Radius

Ulna

Pisiform bone

Hamulus of hamate bone

Palmar aponeurosis *(cut)*

**Right forearm:
anterior (palmar) view**

PLATE 416

UPPER LIMB

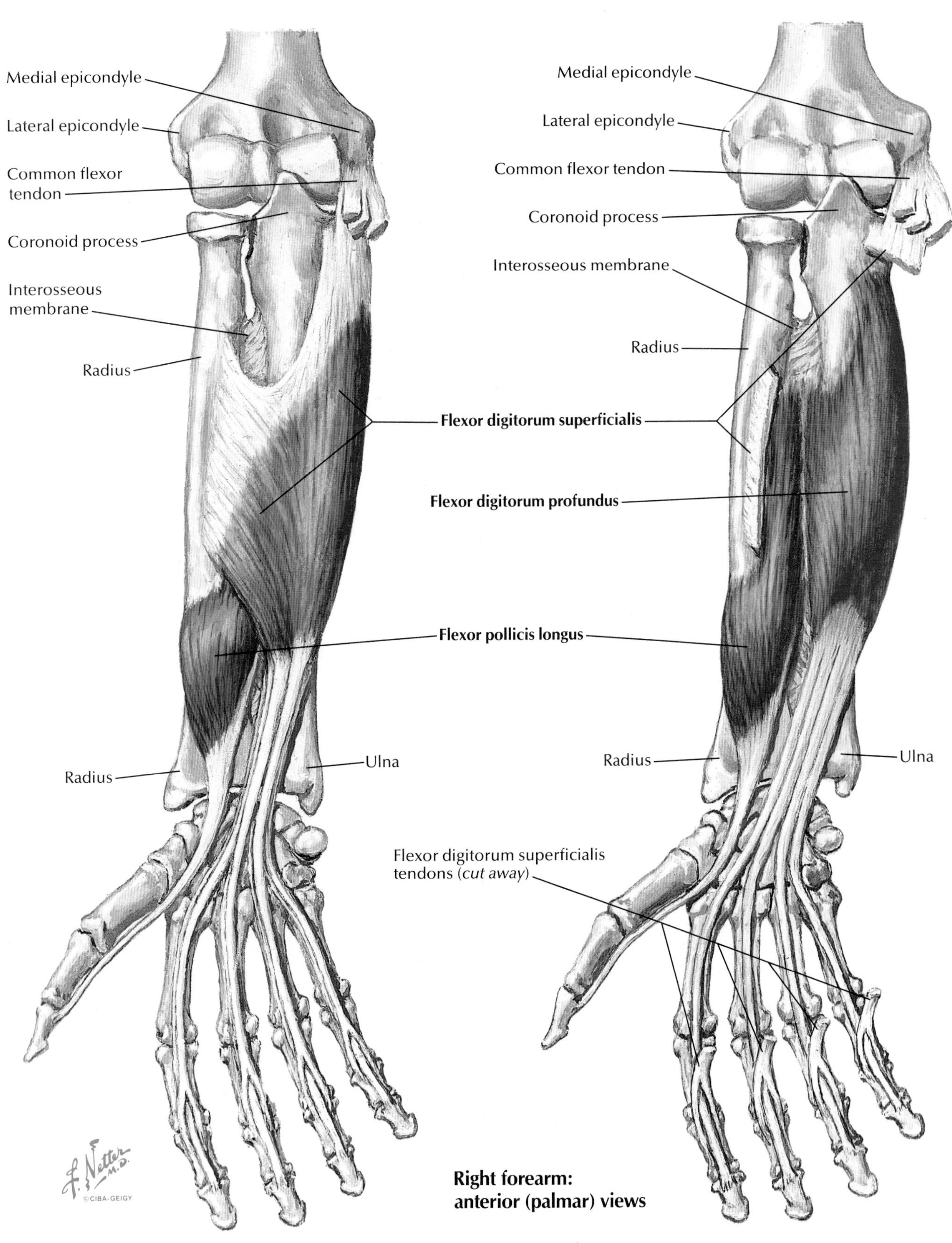

Medial epicondyle

Lateral epicondyle

Common flexor tendon

Coronoid process

Interosseous membrane

Radius

Flexor digitorum superficialis

Flexor digitorum profundus

Flexor pollicis longus

Radius

Ulna

Flexor digitorum superficialis tendons (*cut away*)

Medial epicondyle

Lateral epicondyle

Common flexor tendon

Coronoid process

Interosseous membrane

Radius

Radius

Ulna

Right forearm: anterior (palmar) views

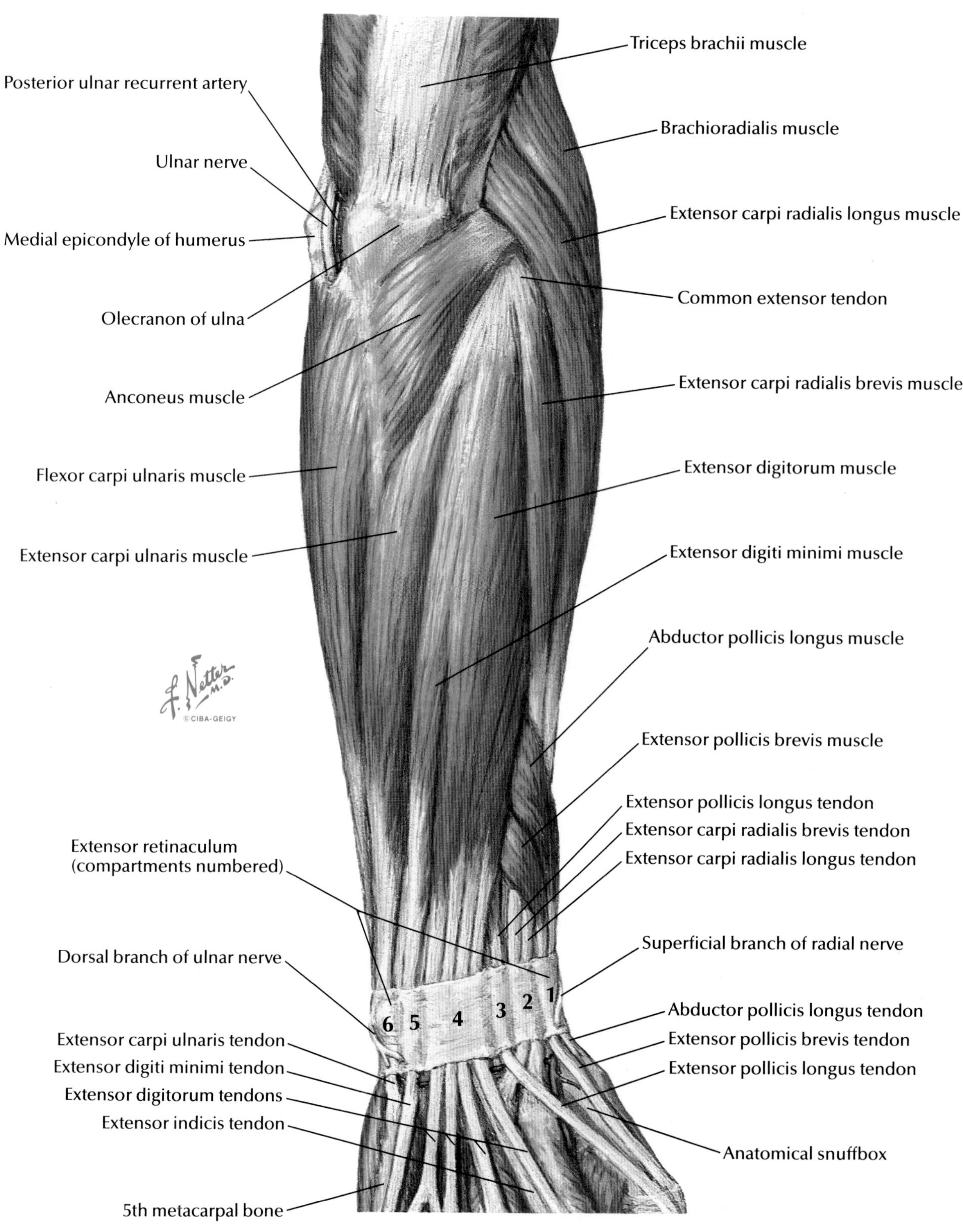

Triceps brachii muscle

Posterior ulnar recurrent artery

Brachioradialis muscle

Ulnar nerve

Extensor carpi radialis longus muscle

Medial epicondyle of humerus

Common extensor tendon

Olecranon of ulna

Extensor carpi radialis brevis muscle

Anconeus muscle

Extensor digitorum muscle

Flexor carpi ulnaris muscle

Extensor digiti minimi muscle

Extensor carpi ulnaris muscle

Abductor pollicis longus muscle

Extensor pollicis brevis muscle

Extensor pollicis longus tendon
Extensor carpi radialis brevis tendon
Extensor carpi radialis longus tendon

Extensor retinaculum
(compartments numbered)

Superficial branch of radial nerve

Dorsal branch of ulnar nerve

Abductor pollicis longus tendon
Extensor pollicis brevis tendon

Extensor carpi ulnaris tendon
Extensor digiti minimi tendon
Extensor digitorum tendons
Extensor indicis tendon

Extensor pollicis longus tendon

Anatomical snuffbox

5th metacarpal bone

6 5 4 3 2 1

PLATE 418

UPPER LIMB

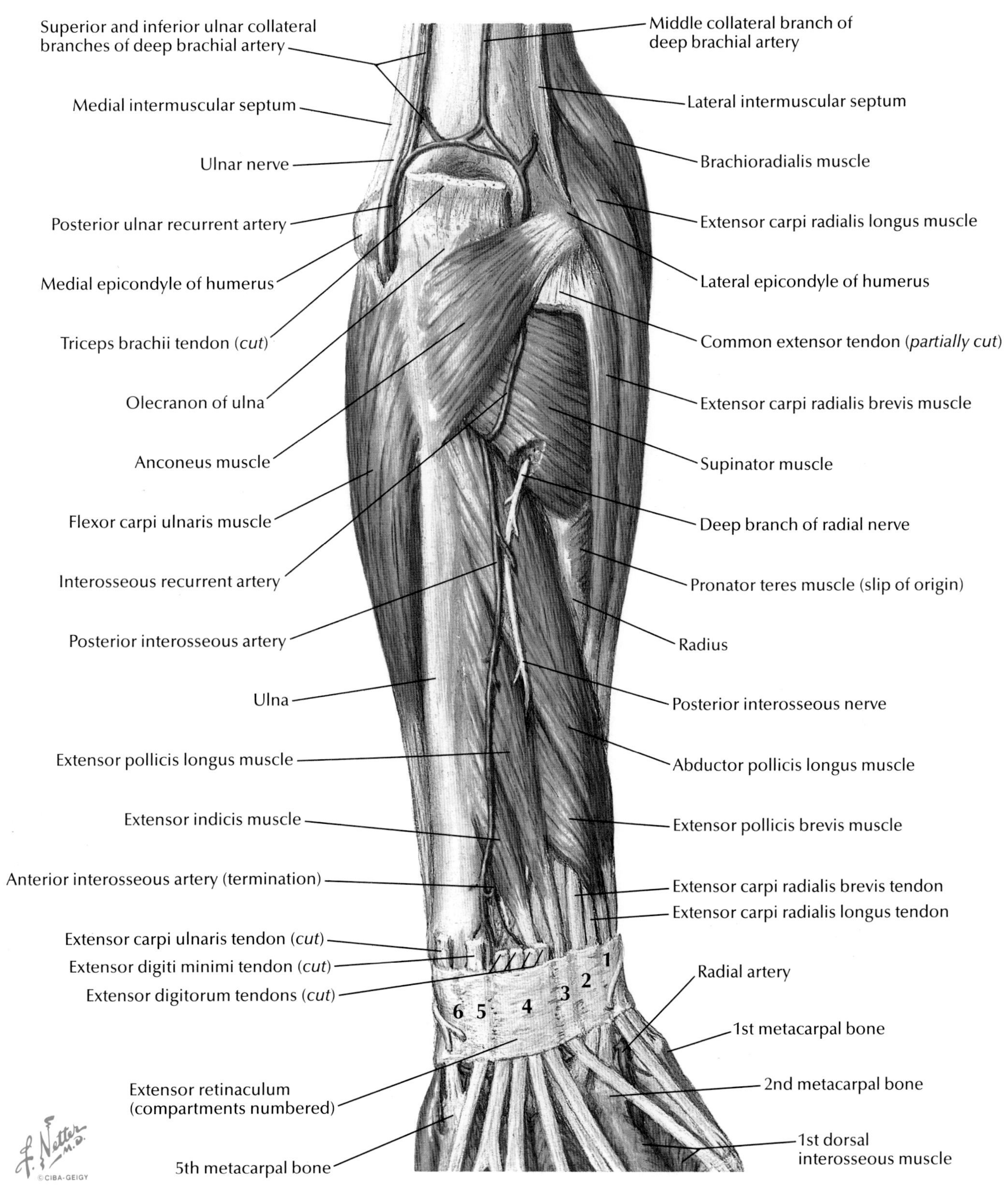

Superior and inferior ulnar collateral branches of deep brachial artery

Medial intermuscular septum

Ulnar nerve

Posterior ulnar recurrent artery

Medial epicondyle of humerus

Triceps brachii tendon (*cut*)

Olecranon of ulna

Anconeus muscle

Flexor carpi ulnaris muscle

Interosseous recurrent artery

Posterior interosseous artery

Ulna

Extensor pollicis longus muscle

Extensor indicis muscle

Anterior interosseous artery (termination)

Extensor carpi ulnaris tendon (*cut*)

Extensor digiti minimi tendon (*cut*)

Extensor digitorum tendons (*cut*)

Extensor retinaculum (compartments numbered)

5th metacarpal bone

Middle collateral branch of deep brachial artery

Lateral intermuscular septum

Brachioradialis muscle

Extensor carpi radialis longus muscle

Lateral epicondyle of humerus

Common extensor tendon (*partially cut*)

Extensor carpi radialis brevis muscle

Supinator muscle

Deep branch of radial nerve

Pronator teres muscle (slip of origin)

Radius

Posterior interosseous nerve

Abductor pollicis longus muscle

Extensor pollicis brevis muscle

Extensor carpi radialis brevis tendon

Extensor carpi radialis longus tendon

Radial artery

1st metacarpal bone

2nd metacarpal bone

1st dorsal interosseous muscle

SEE ALSO PLATES 448, 449

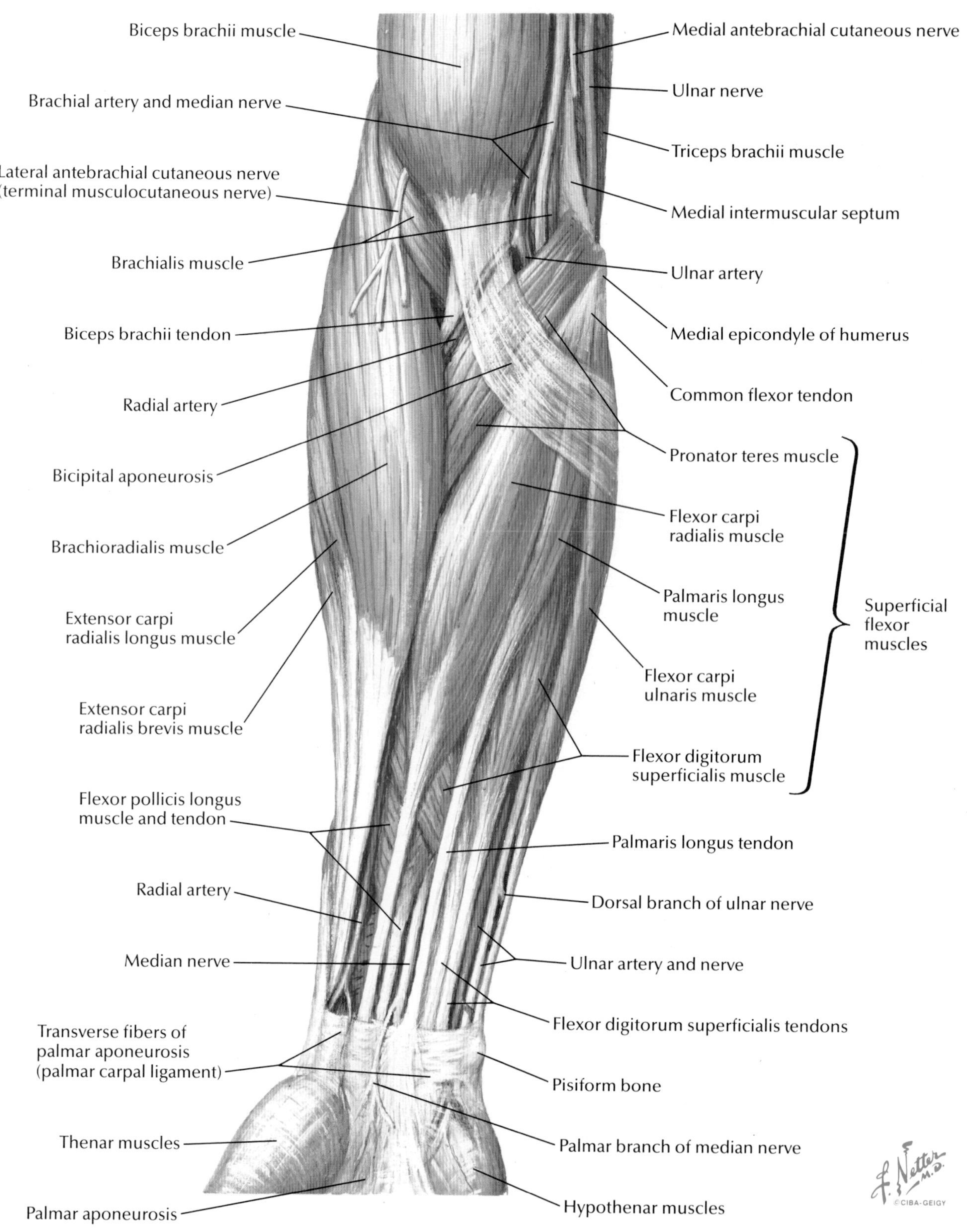

Biceps brachii muscle

Brachial artery and median nerve

Lateral antebrachial cutaneous nerve (terminal musculocutaneous nerve)

Brachialis muscle

Biceps brachii tendon

Radial artery

Bicipital aponeurosis

Brachioradialis muscle

Extensor carpi radialis longus muscle

Extensor carpi radialis brevis muscle

Flexor pollicis longus muscle and tendon

Radial artery

Median nerve

Transverse fibers of palmar aponeurosis (palmar carpal ligament)

Thenar muscles

Palmar aponeurosis

Medial antebrachial cutaneous nerve

Ulnar nerve

Triceps brachii muscle

Medial intermuscular septum

Ulnar artery

Medial epicondyle of humerus

Common flexor tendon

Pronator teres muscle

Flexor carpi radialis muscle

Palmaris longus muscle

Flexor carpi ulnaris muscle

Flexor digitorum superficialis muscle

Superficial flexor muscles

Palmaris longus tendon

Dorsal branch of ulnar nerve

Ulnar artery and nerve

Flexor digitorum superficialis tendons

Pisiform bone

Palmar branch of median nerve

Hypothenar muscles

PLATE 420

UPPER LIMB

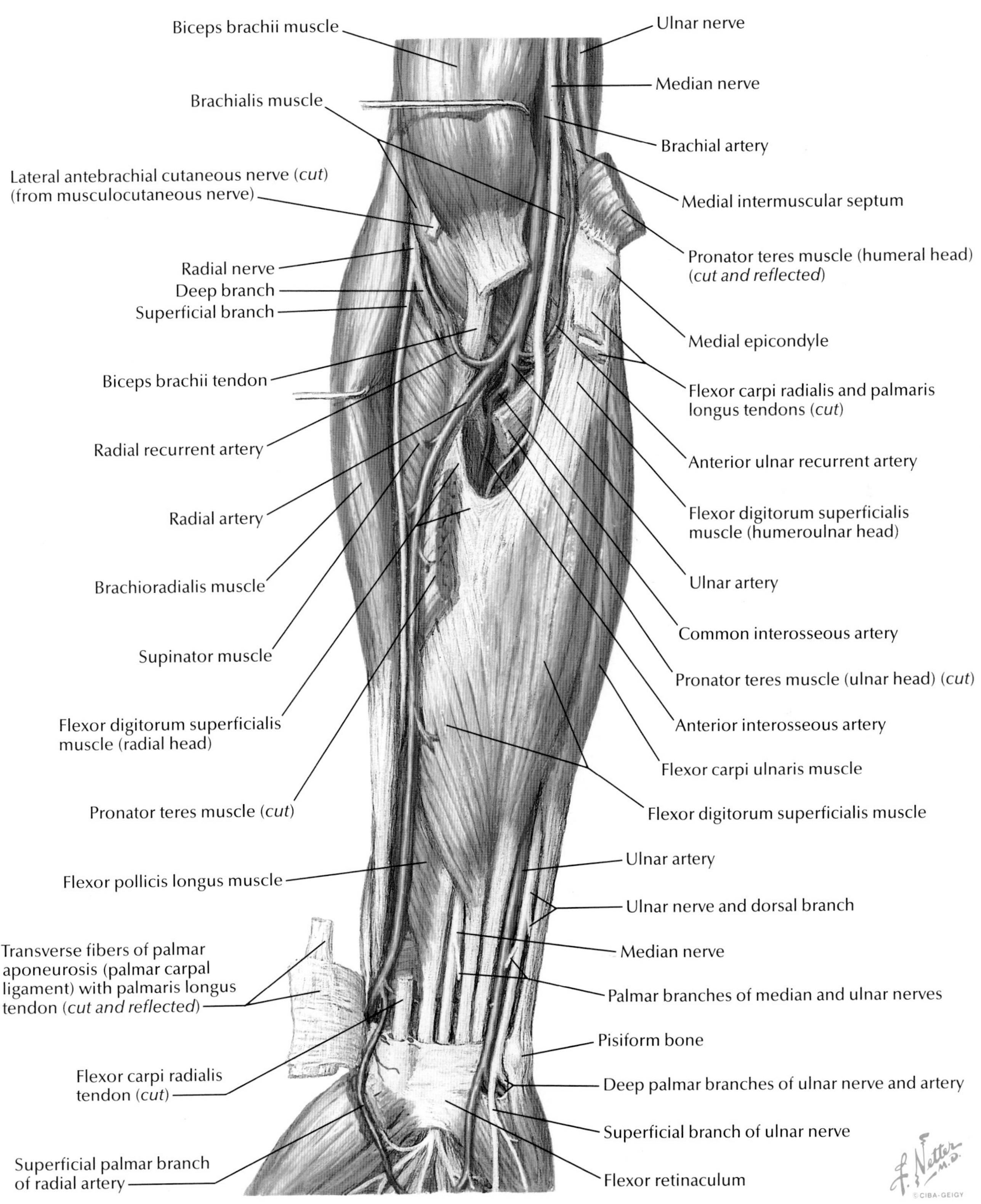

Biceps brachii muscle

Brachialis muscle

Lateral antebrachial cutaneous nerve (*cut*)
(from musculocutaneous nerve)

Radial nerve
Deep branch
Superficial branch

Biceps brachii tendon

Radial recurrent artery

Radial artery

Brachioradialis muscle

Supinator muscle

Flexor digitorum superficialis
muscle (radial head)

Pronator teres muscle (*cut*)

Flexor pollicis longus muscle

Transverse fibers of palmar
aponeurosis (palmar carpal
ligament) with palmaris longus
tendon (*cut and reflected*)

Flexor carpi radialis
tendon (*cut*)

Superficial palmar branch
of radial artery

Ulnar nerve

Median nerve

Brachial artery

Medial intermuscular septum

Pronator teres muscle (humeral head)
(*cut and reflected*)

Medial epicondyle

Flexor carpi radialis and palmaris
longus tendons (*cut*)

Anterior ulnar recurrent artery

Flexor digitorum superficialis
muscle (humeroulnar head)

Ulnar artery

Common interosseous artery

Pronator teres muscle (ulnar head) (*cut*)

Anterior interosseous artery

Flexor carpi ulnaris muscle

Flexor digitorum superficialis muscle

Ulnar artery

Ulnar nerve and dorsal branch

Median nerve

Palmar branches of median and ulnar nerves

Pisiform bone

Deep palmar branches of ulnar nerve and artery

Superficial branch of ulnar nerve

Flexor retinaculum

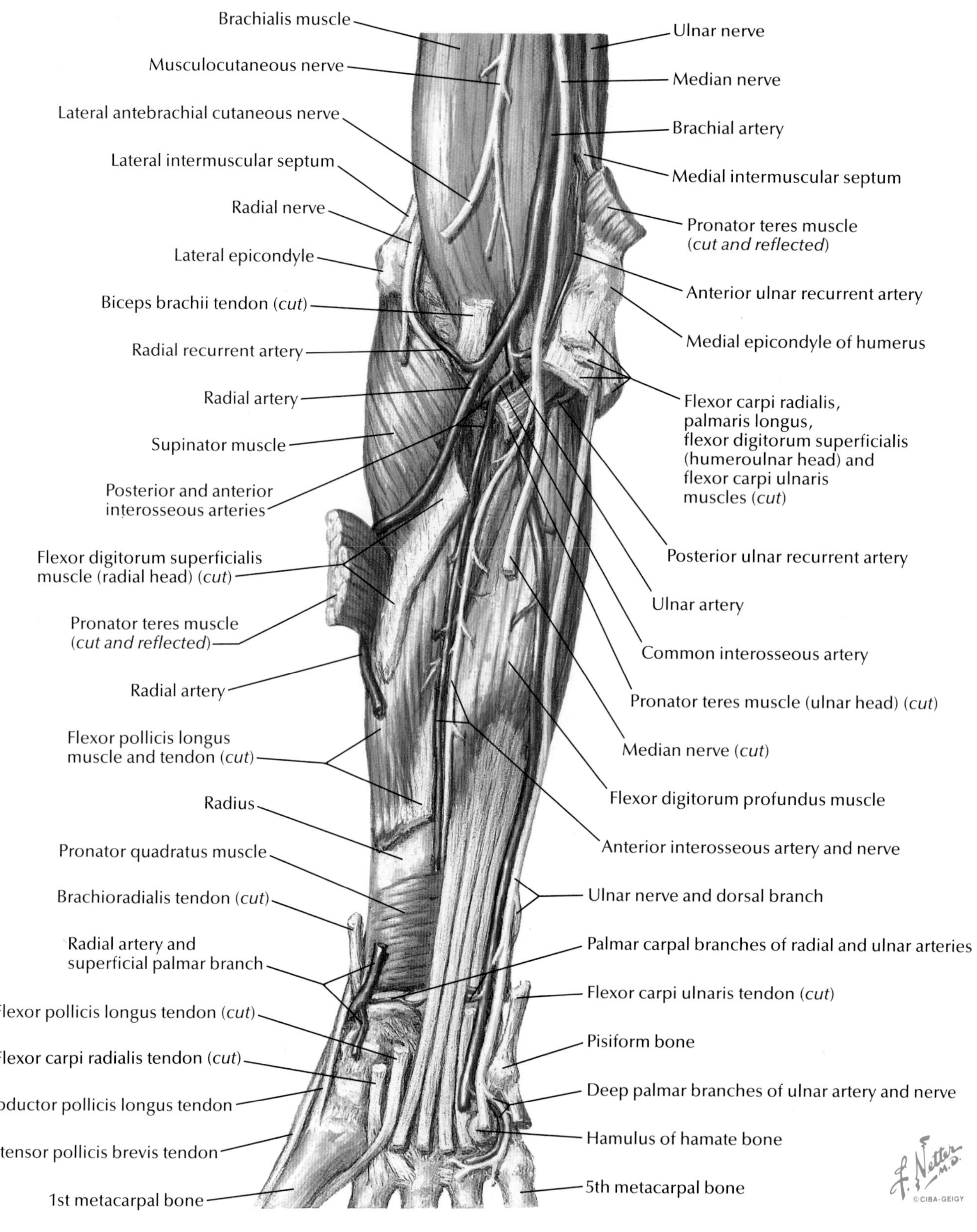

Brachialis muscle

Musculocutaneous nerve

Lateral antebrachial cutaneous nerve

Lateral intermuscular septum

Radial nerve

Lateral epicondyle

Biceps brachii tendon (*cut*)

Radial recurrent artery

Radial artery

Supinator muscle

Posterior and anterior interosseous arteries

Flexor digitorum superficialis muscle (radial head) (*cut*)

Pronator teres muscle (*cut and reflected*)

Radial artery

Flexor pollicis longus muscle and tendon (*cut*)

Radius

Pronator quadratus muscle

Brachioradialis tendon (*cut*)

Radial artery and superficial palmar branch

Flexor pollicis longus tendon (*cut*)

Flexor carpi radialis tendon (*cut*)

Abductor pollicis longus tendon

Extensor pollicis brevis tendon

1st metacarpal bone

Ulnar nerve

Median nerve

Brachial artery

Medial intermuscular septum

Pronator teres muscle (*cut and reflected*)

Anterior ulnar recurrent artery

Medial epicondyle of humerus

Flexor carpi radialis, palmaris longus, flexor digitorum superficialis (humeroulnar head) and flexor carpi ulnaris muscles (*cut*)

Posterior ulnar recurrent artery

Ulnar artery

Common interosseous artery

Pronator teres muscle (ulnar head) (*cut*)

Median nerve (*cut*)

Flexor digitorum profundus muscle

Anterior interosseous artery and nerve

Ulnar nerve and dorsal branch

Palmar carpal branches of radial and ulnar arteries

Flexor carpi ulnaris tendon (*cut*)

Pisiform bone

Deep palmar branches of ulnar artery and nerve

Hamulus of hamate bone

5th metacarpal bone

PLATE 422

UPPER LIMB

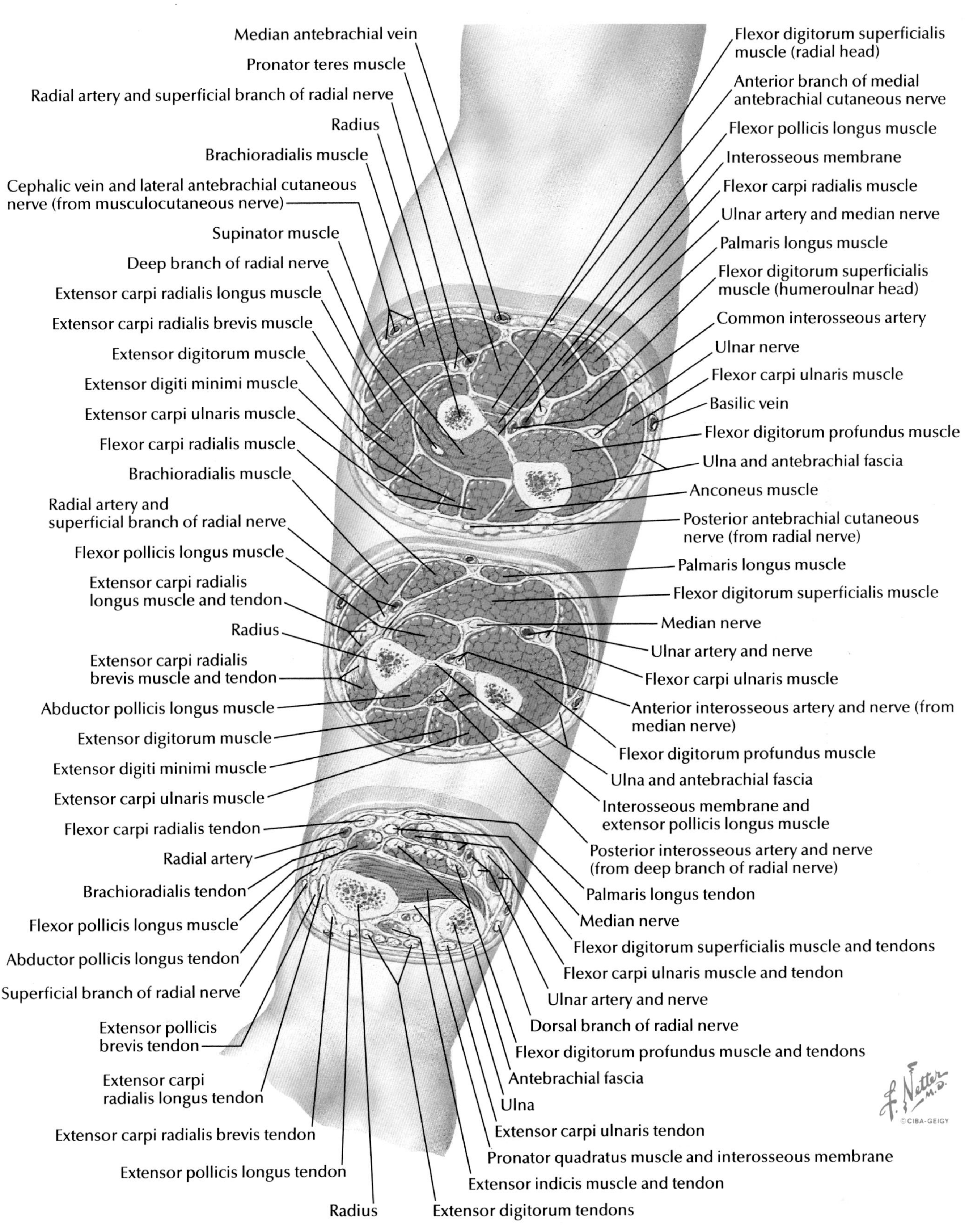

Median antebrachial vein

Pronator teres muscle

Radial artery and superficial branch of radial nerve

Radius

Brachioradialis muscle

Cephalic vein and lateral antebrachial cutaneous nerve (from musculocutaneous nerve)

Supinator muscle

Deep branch of radial nerve

Extensor carpi radialis longus muscle

Extensor carpi radialis brevis muscle

Extensor digitorum muscle

Extensor digiti minimi muscle

Extensor carpi ulnaris muscle

Flexor carpi radialis muscle

Brachioradialis muscle

Radial artery and superficial branch of radial nerve

Flexor pollicis longus muscle

Extensor carpi radialis longus muscle and tendon

Radius

Extensor carpi radialis brevis muscle and tendon

Abductor pollicis longus muscle

Extensor digitorum muscle

Extensor digiti minimi muscle

Extensor carpi ulnaris muscle

Flexor carpi radialis tendon

Radial artery

Brachioradialis tendon

Flexor pollicis longus muscle

Abductor pollicis longus tendon

Superficial branch of radial nerve

Extensor pollicis brevis tendon

Extensor carpi radialis longus tendon

Extensor carpi radialis brevis tendon

Extensor pollicis longus tendon

Radius

Flexor digitorum superficialis muscle (radial head)

Anterior branch of medial antebrachial cutaneous nerve

Flexor pollicis longus muscle

Interosseous membrane

Flexor carpi radialis muscle

Ulnar artery and median nerve

Palmaris longus muscle

Flexor digitorum superficialis muscle (humeroulnar head)

Common interosseous artery

Ulnar nerve

Flexor carpi ulnaris muscle

Basilic vein

Flexor digitorum profundus muscle

Ulna and antebrachial fascia

Anconeus muscle

Posterior antebrachial cutaneous nerve (from radial nerve)

Palmaris longus muscle

Flexor digitorum superficialis muscle

Median nerve

Ulnar artery and nerve

Flexor carpi ulnaris muscle

Anterior interosseous artery and nerve (from median nerve)

Flexor digitorum profundus muscle

Ulna and antebrachial fascia

Interosseous membrane and extensor pollicis longus muscle

Posterior interosseous artery and nerve (from deep branch of radial nerve)

Palmaris longus tendon

Median nerve

Flexor digitorum superficialis muscle and tendons

Flexor carpi ulnaris muscle and tendon

Ulnar artery and nerve

Dorsal branch of radial nerve

Flexor digitorum profundus muscle and tendons

Antebrachial fascia

Ulna

Extensor carpi ulnaris tendon

Pronator quadratus muscle and interosseous membrane

Extensor indicis muscle and tendon

Extensor digitorum tendons

Bony Attachments of Muscles of Forearm: Anterior View

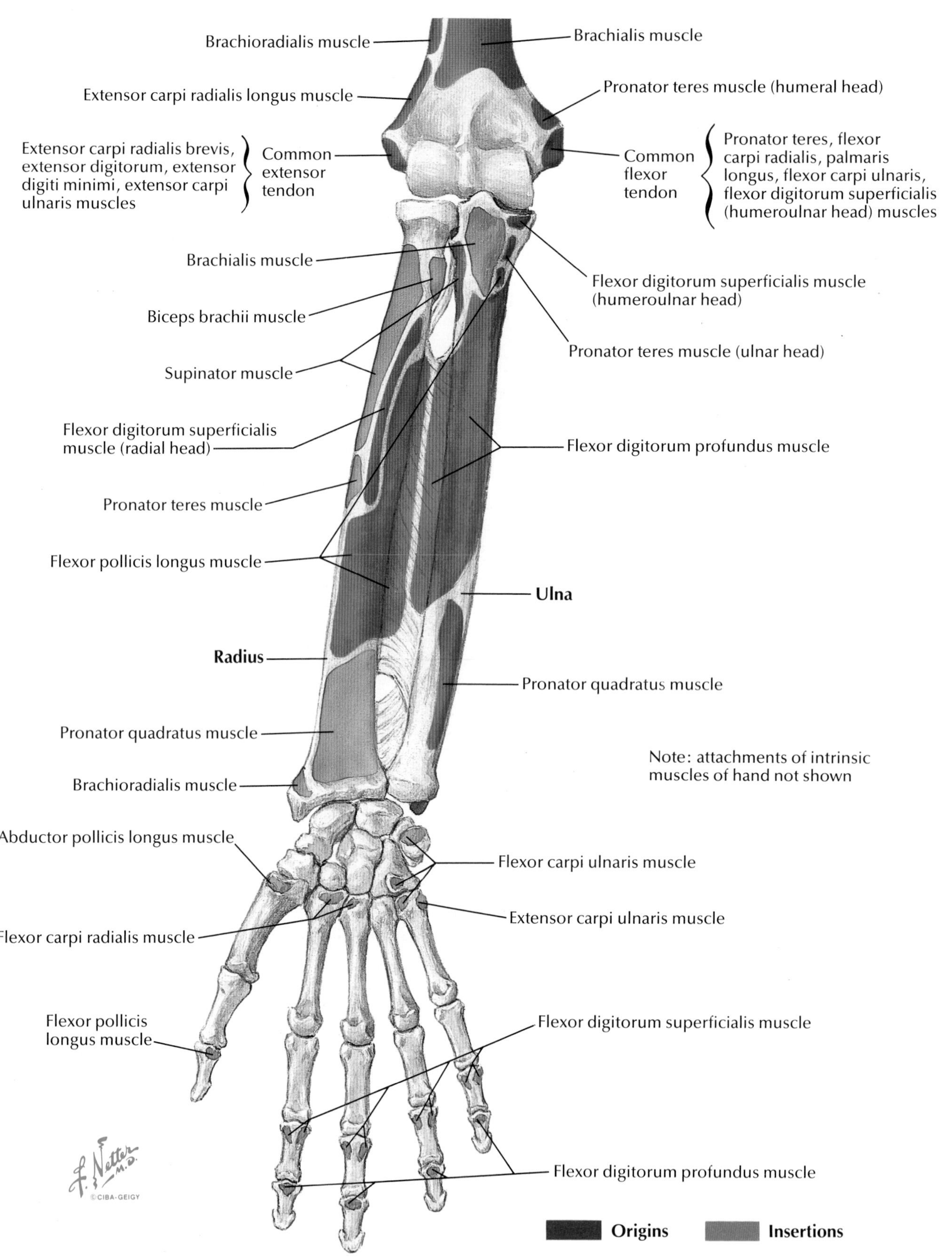

Brachioradialis muscle

Brachialis muscle

Extensor carpi radialis longus muscle

Pronator teres muscle (humeral head)

Extensor carpi radialis brevis, extensor digitorum, extensor digiti minimi, extensor carpi ulnaris muscles } Common extensor tendon

Common flexor tendon { Pronator teres, flexor carpi radialis, palmaris longus, flexor carpi ulnaris, flexor digitorum superficialis (humeroulnar head) muscles

Flexor digitorum superficialis muscle (humeroulnar head)

Brachialis muscle

Biceps brachii muscle

Supinator muscle

Pronator teres muscle (ulnar head)

Flexor digitorum superficialis muscle (radial head)

Flexor digitorum profundus muscle

Pronator teres muscle

Flexor pollicis longus muscle

Ulna

Radius

Pronator quadratus muscle

Pronator quadratus muscle

Note: attachments of intrinsic muscles of hand not shown

Brachioradialis muscle

Abductor pollicis longus muscle

Flexor carpi ulnaris muscle

Extensor carpi ulnaris muscle

Flexor carpi radialis muscle

Flexor pollicis longus muscle

Flexor digitorum superficialis muscle

Flexor digitorum profundus muscle

Origins   Insertions

PLATE 424

UPPER LIMB

Bony Attachments of Muscles of Forearm: Posterior View

Note: attachments of intrinsic muscles of hand not shown

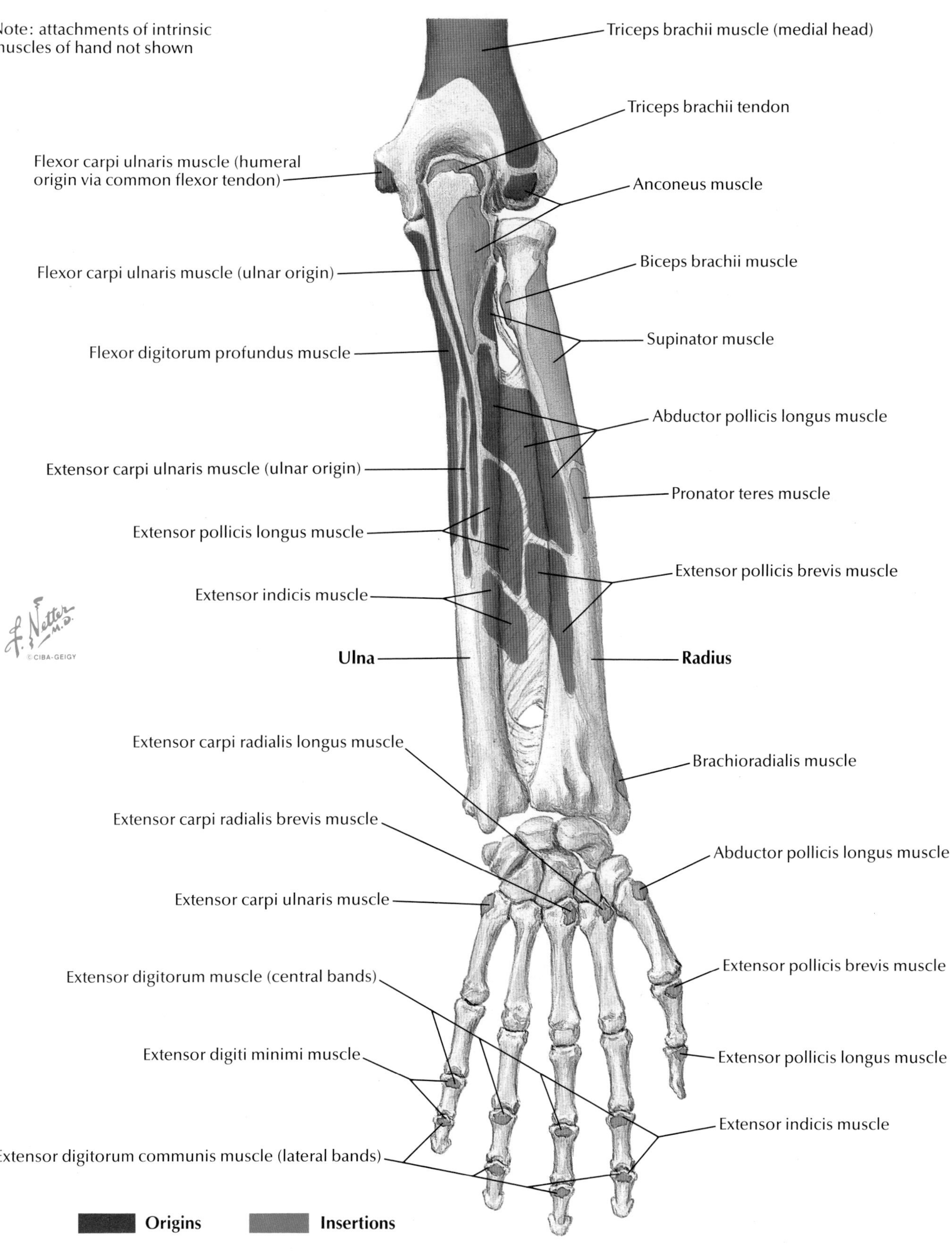

Triceps brachii muscle (medial head)

Triceps brachii tendon

Flexor carpi ulnaris muscle (humeral origin via common flexor tendon)

Anconeus muscle

Flexor carpi ulnaris muscle (ulnar origin)

Biceps brachii muscle

Flexor digitorum profundus muscle

Supinator muscle

Abductor pollicis longus muscle

Extensor carpi ulnaris muscle (ulnar origin)

Pronator teres muscle

Extensor pollicis longus muscle

Extensor pollicis brevis muscle

Extensor indicis muscle

Ulna

Radius

Extensor carpi radialis longus muscle

Brachioradialis muscle

Extensor carpi radialis brevis muscle

Abductor pollicis longus muscle

Extensor carpi ulnaris muscle

Extensor pollicis brevis muscle

Extensor digitorum muscle (central bands)

Extensor pollicis longus muscle

Extensor digiti minimi muscle

Extensor indicis muscle

Extensor digitorum communis muscle (lateral bands)

■ Origins ■ Insertions

Carpal Bones

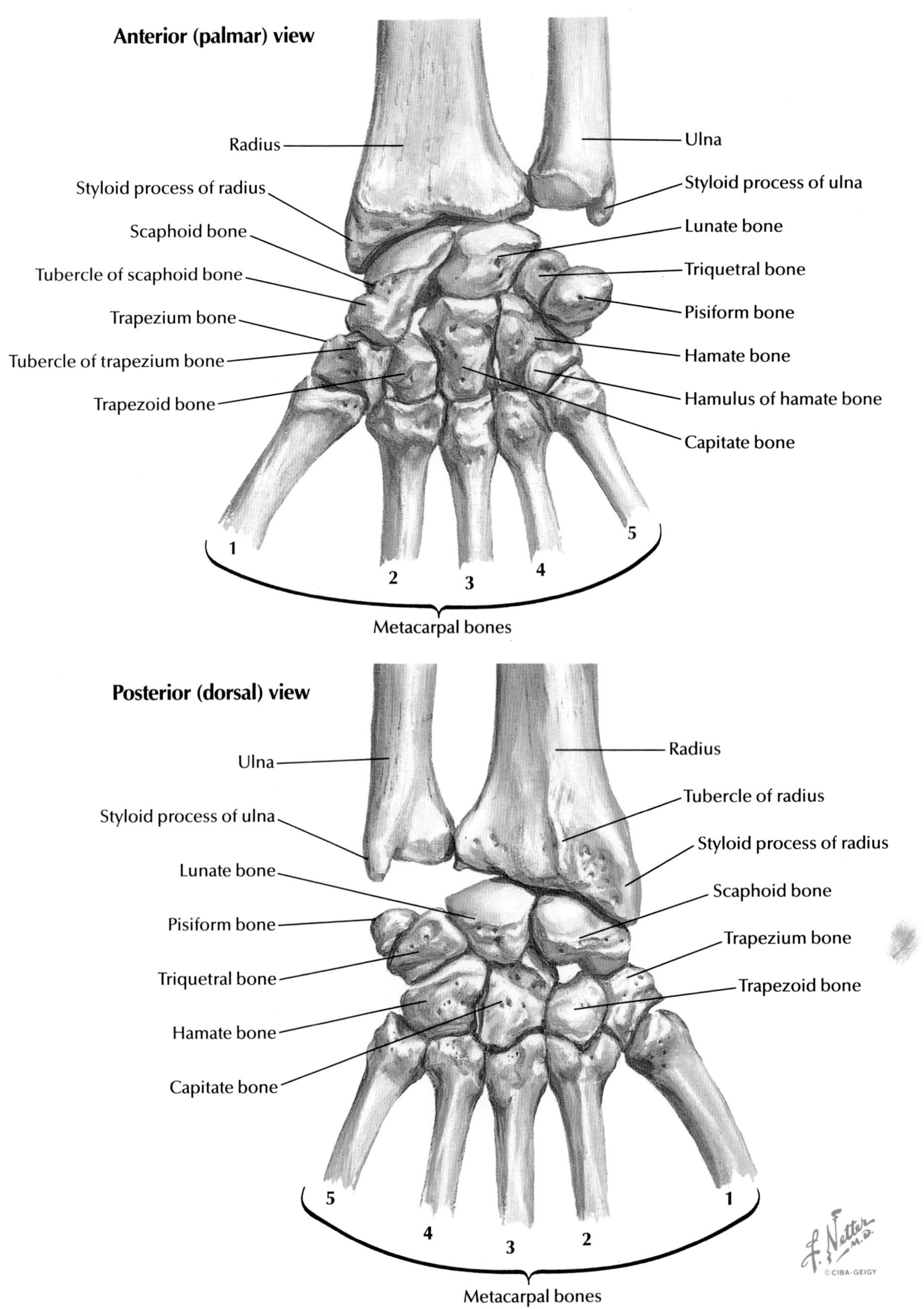

Anterior (palmar) view

Radius

Styloid process of radius

Scaphoid bone

Tubercle of scaphoid bone

Trapezium bone

Tubercle of trapezium bone

Trapezoid bone

Ulna

Styloid process of ulna

Lunate bone

Triquetral bone

Pisiform bone

Hamate bone

Hamulus of hamate bone

Capitate bone

1   2   3   4   5

Metacarpal bones

Posterior (dorsal) view

Ulna

Styloid process of ulna

Lunate bone

Pisiform bone

Triquetral bone

Hamate bone

Capitate bone

Radius

Tubercle of radius

Styloid process of radius

Scaphoid bone

Trapezium bone

Trapezoid bone

5   4   3   2   1

Metacarpal bones

PLATE 426

UPPER LIMB

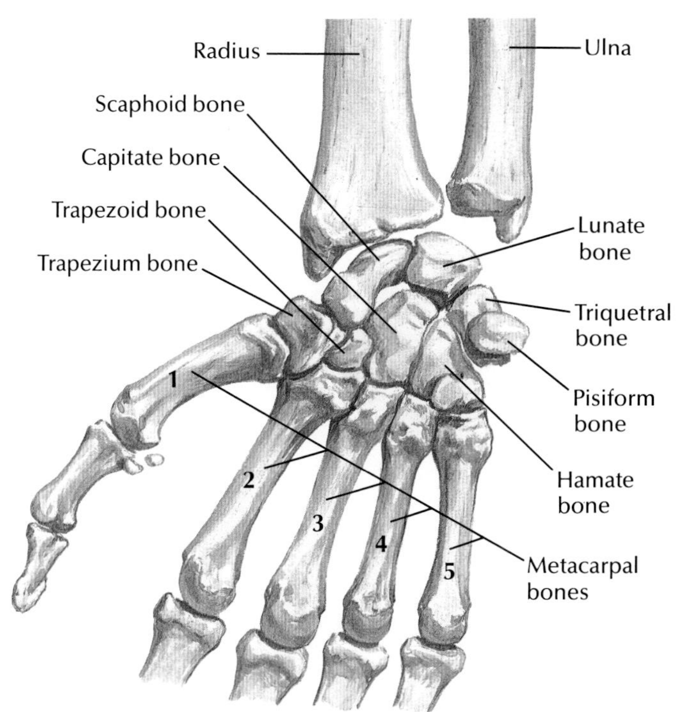

Radius

Ulna

Scaphoid bone

Capitate bone

Trapezoid bone

Trapezium bone

Lunate bone

Triquetral bone

Pisiform bone

Hamate bone

1

2

3

4

5

Metacarpal bones

Position of carpal bones with hand in abduction: anterior (palmar) view

Radius

Ulna

Lunate bone

Triquetral bone

Scaphoid bone

Pisiform bone

Capitate bone

Hamate bone

Trapezoid bone

Trapezium bone

5

4

3

2

1

Metacarpal bones

Position of carpal bones with hand in adduction: anterior (palmar) view

Radius

Radiocarpal articulation

Articular disc

Lunate bone

Intercarpal (midcarpal) articulation

Capitate bone

Carpometacarpal articulation

3rd metacarpal bone

Dorsum

Palm

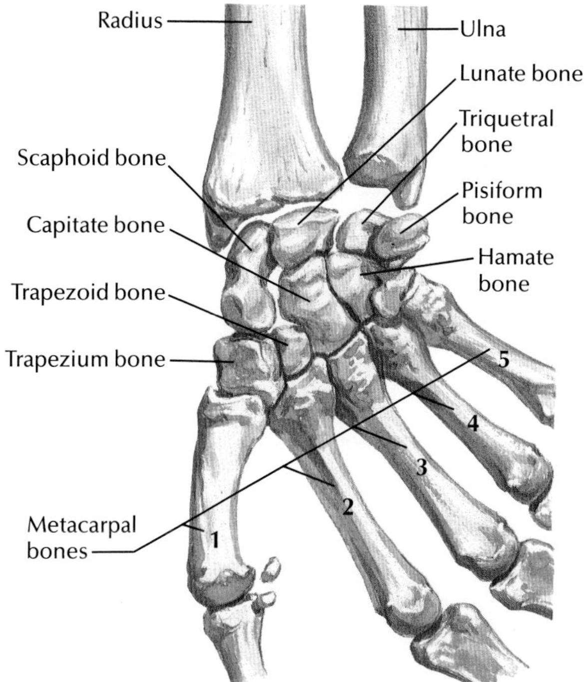

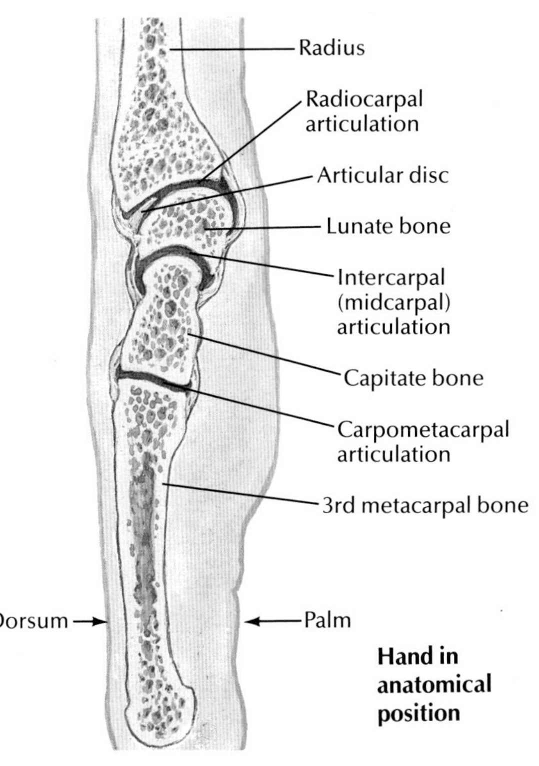

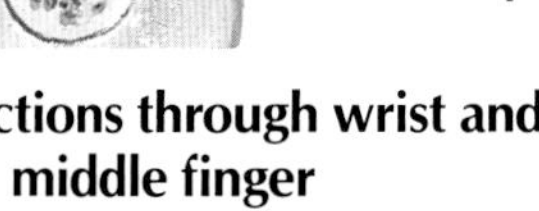

Hand in anatomical position

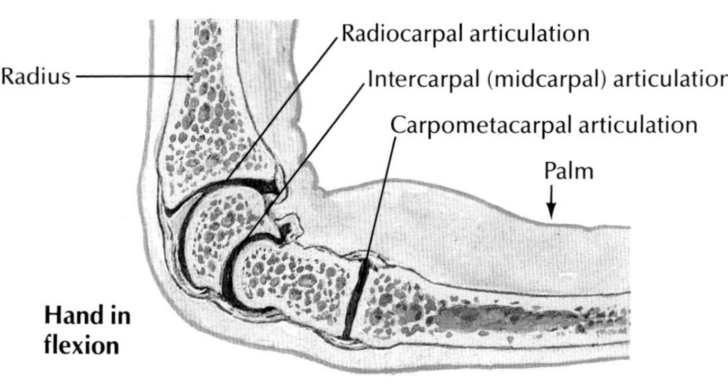

Sagittal sections through wrist and middle finger

Radius

Radiocarpal articulation

Intercarpal (midcarpal) articulation

Carpometacarpal articulation

Palm

Hand in flexion

Radiocarpal articulation

Intercarpal (midcarpal) articulation

Carpometacarpal articulation

Hand in extension

Palm

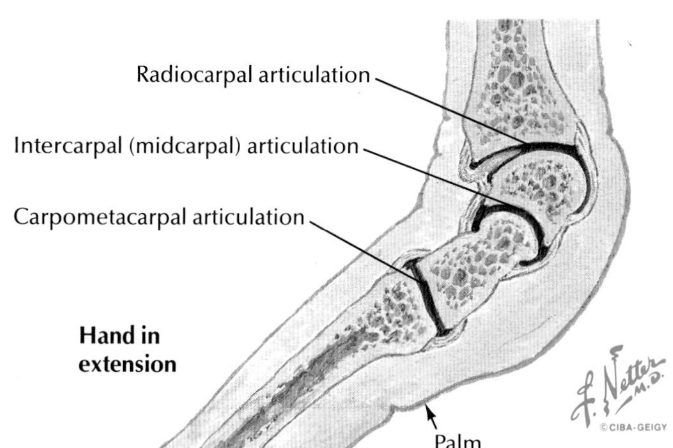

Ligaments of Wrist

Carpal tunnel: palmar view

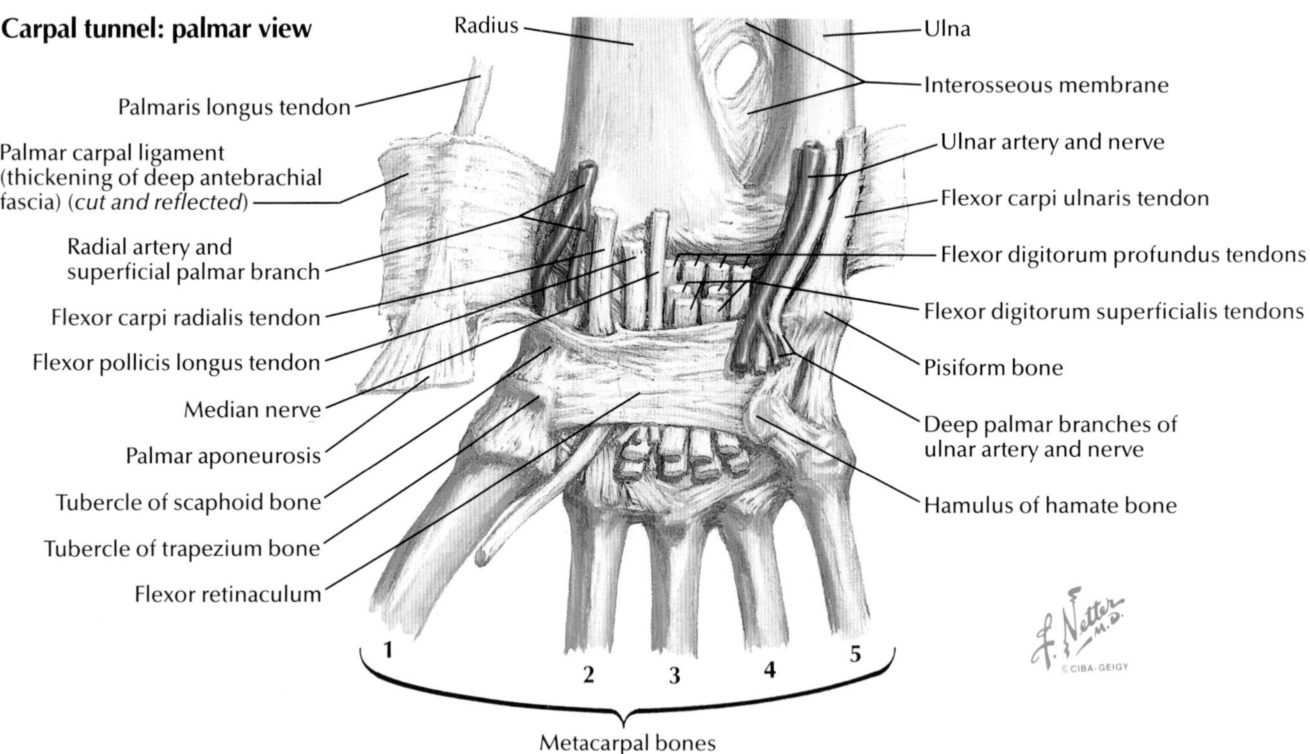

Radius

Ulna

Interosseous membrane

Palmaris longus tendon

Palmar carpal ligament (thickening of deep antebrachial fascia) (cut and reflected)

Ulnar artery and nerve

Flexor carpi ulnaris tendon

Radial artery and superficial palmar branch

Flexor digitorum profundus tendons

Flexor carpi radialis tendon

Flexor digitorum superficialis tendons

Flexor pollicis longus tendon

Pisiform bone

Median nerve

Deep palmar branches of ulnar artery and nerve

Palmar aponeurosis

Tubercle of scaphoid bone

Hamulus of hamate bone

Tubercle of trapezium bone

Flexor retinaculum

1   2   3   4   5

Metacarpal bones

Flexor retinaculum removed: palmar view

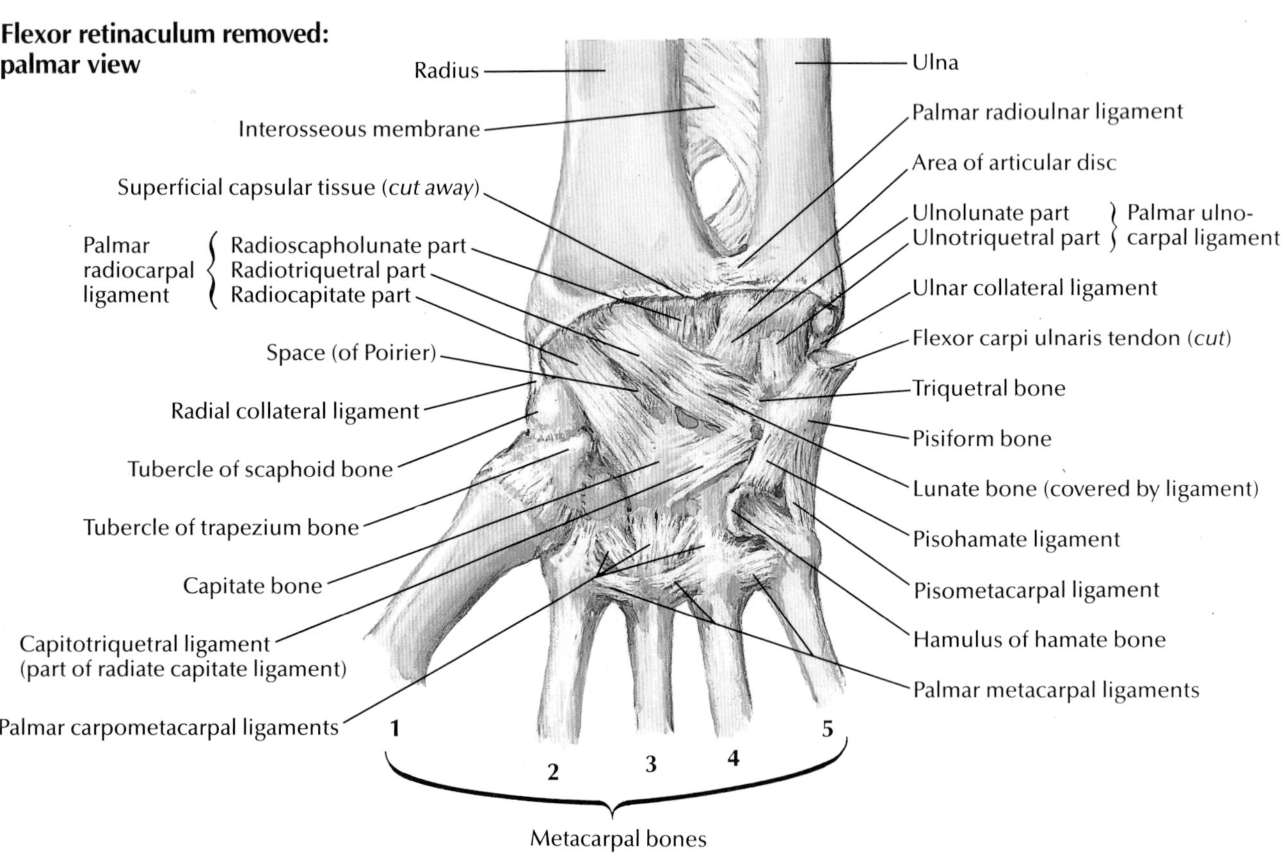

Radius

Ulna

Palmar radioulnar ligament

Interosseous membrane

Area of articular disc

Superficial capsular tissue (cut away)

Ulnolunate part } Palmar ulno-
Ulnotriquetral part } carpal ligament

Palmar radiocarpal ligament { Radioscapholunate part
Radiotriquetral part
Radiocapitate part

Ulnar collateral ligament

Flexor carpi ulnaris tendon (cut)

Space (of Poirier)

Triquetral bone

Radial collateral ligament

Pisiform bone

Tubercle of scaphoid bone

Lunate bone (covered by ligament)

Tubercle of trapezium bone

Pisohamate ligament

Capitate bone

Pisometacarpal ligament

Capitotriquetral ligament (part of radiate capitate ligament)

Hamulus of hamate bone

Palmar metacarpal ligaments

Palmar carpometacarpal ligaments

1   2   3   4   5

Metacarpal bones

PLATE 428

UPPER LIMB

Posterior (dorsal) view

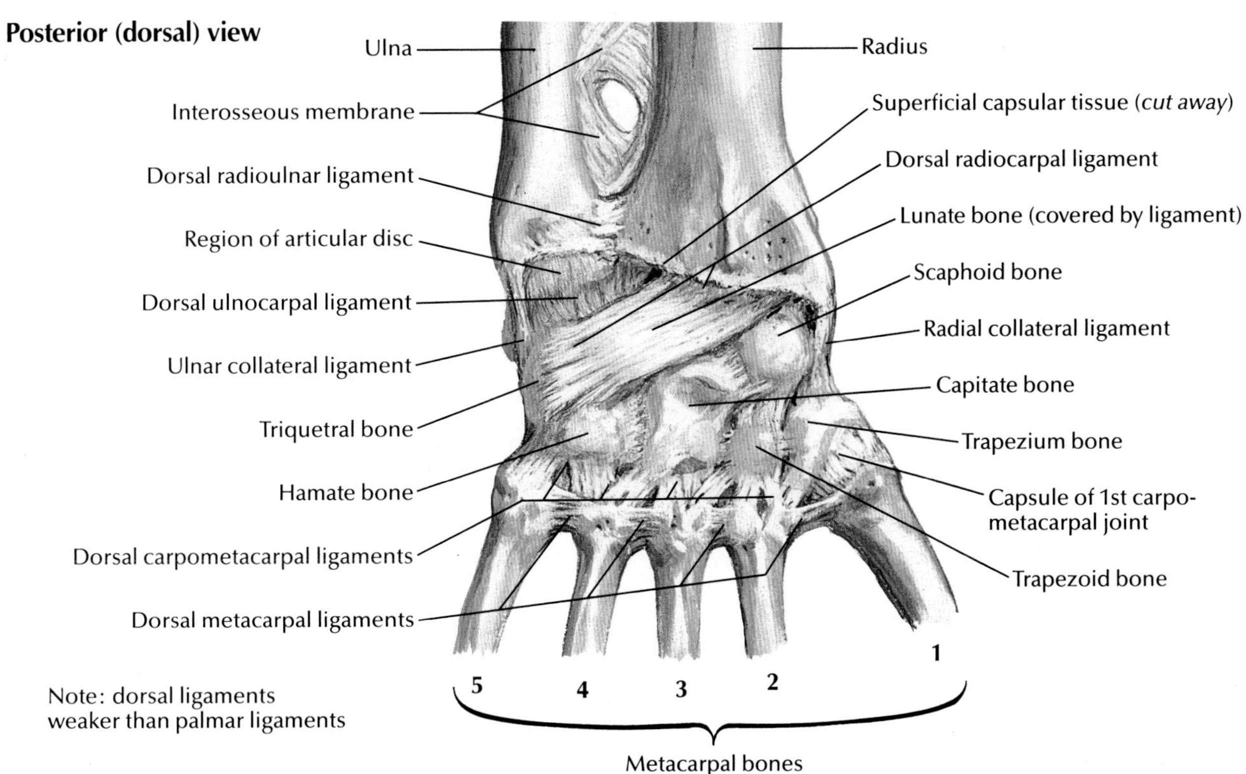

Ulna

Interosseous membrane

Dorsal radioulnar ligament

Region of articular disc

Dorsal ulnocarpal ligament

Ulnar collateral ligament

Triquetral bone

Hamate bone

Dorsal carpometacarpal ligaments

Dorsal metacarpal ligaments

Radius

Superficial capsular tissue (*cut away*)

Dorsal radiocarpal ligament

Lunate bone (covered by ligament)

Scaphoid bone

Radial collateral ligament

Capitate bone

Trapezium bone

Capsule of 1st carpo-metacarpal joint

Trapezoid bone

Note: dorsal ligaments weaker than palmar ligaments

5   4   3   2   1

Metacarpal bones

Coronal section: dorsal view

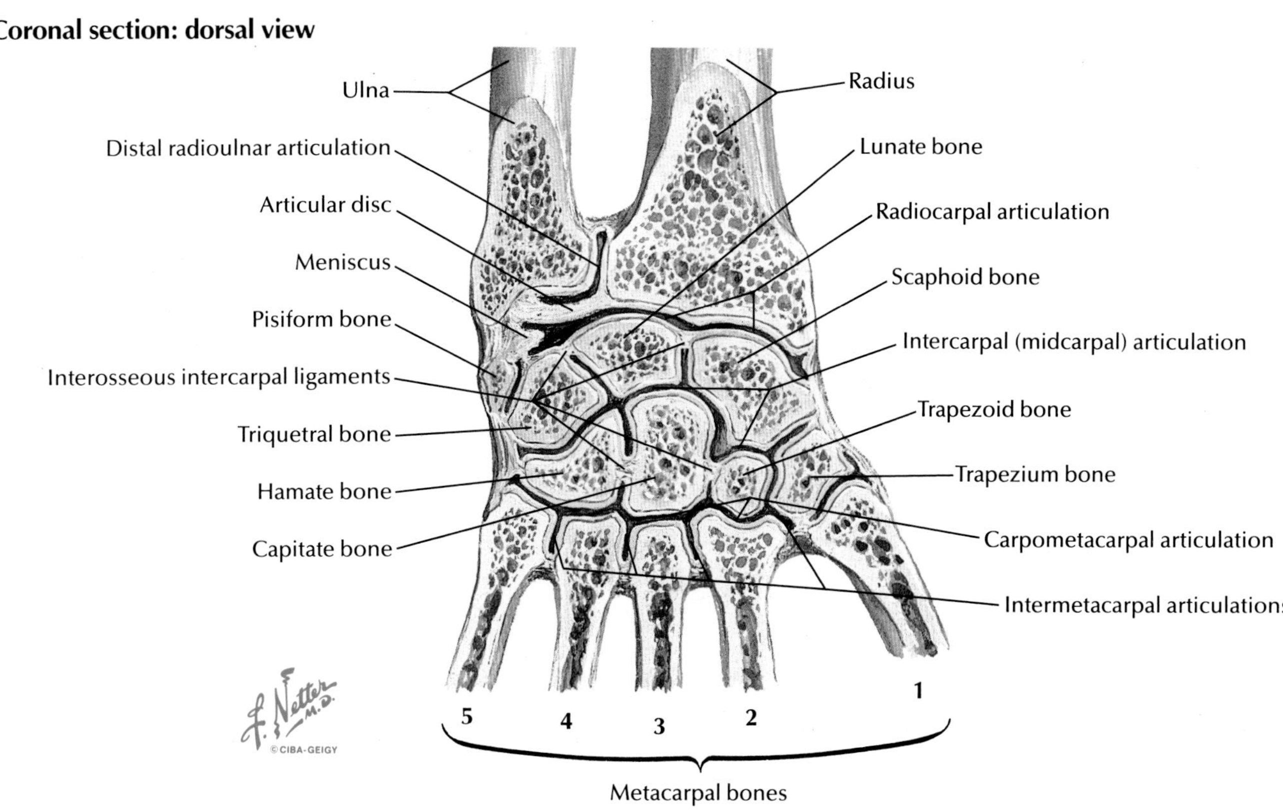

Ulna

Distal radioulnar articulation

Articular disc

Meniscus

Pisiform bone

Interosseous intercarpal ligaments

Triquetral bone

Hamate bone

Capitate bone

Radius

Lunate bone

Radiocarpal articulation

Scaphoid bone

Intercarpal (midcarpal) articulation

Trapezoid bone

Trapezium bone

Carpometacarpal articulation

Intermetacarpal articulations

5   4   3   2   1

Metacarpal bones

WRIST AND HAND

PLATE 429

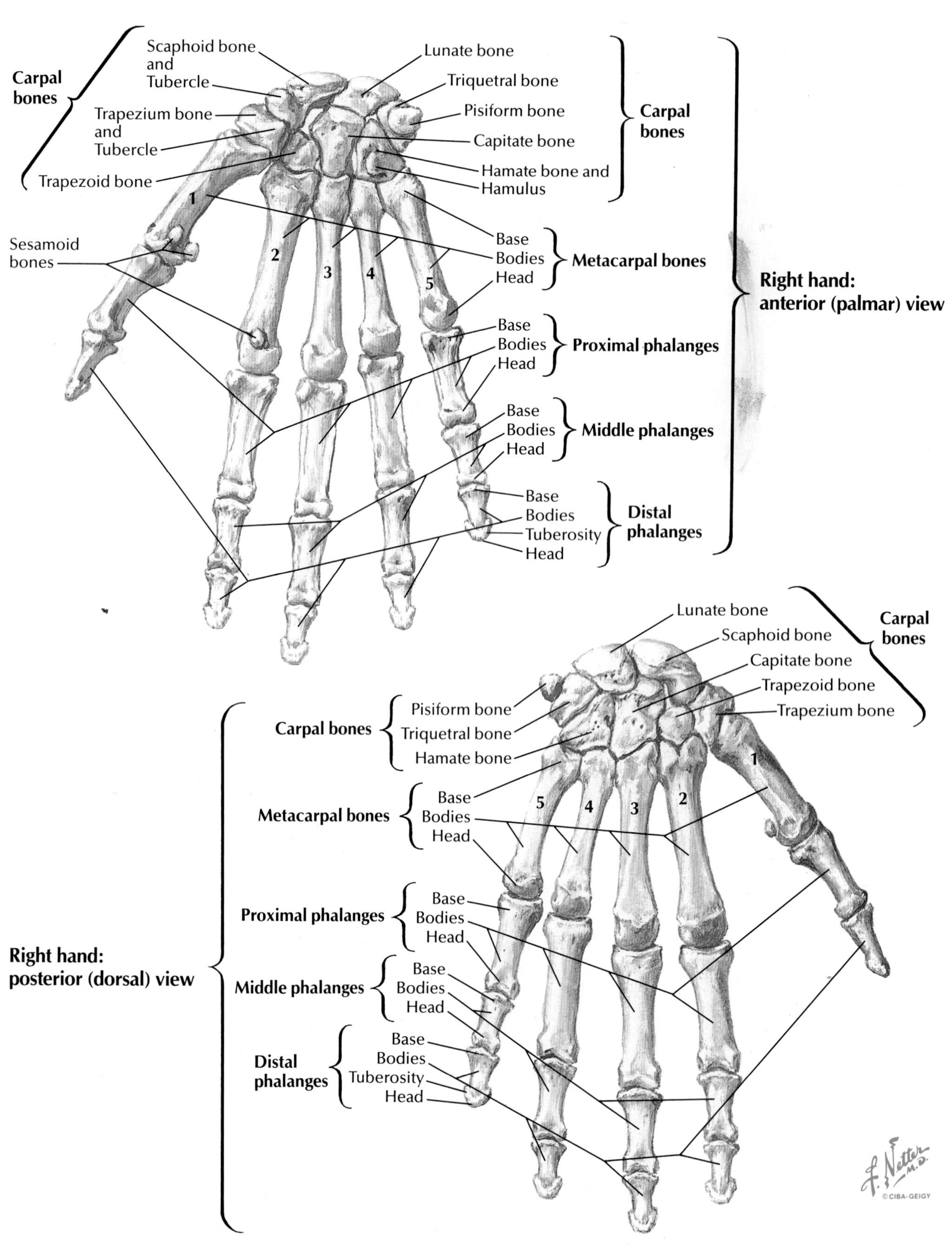

Carpal bones
Scaphoid bone and Tubercle
Trapezium bone and Tubercle
Trapezoid bone

Sesamoid bones

Lunate bone
Triquetral bone
Pisiform bone
Capitate bone
Hamate bone and Hamulus

Carpal bones

1
2
3
4
5

Base
Bodies
Head
} **Metacarpal bones**

Base
Bodies
Head
} **Proximal phalanges**

Base
Bodies
Head
} **Middle phalanges**

Base
Bodies
Tuberosity
Head
} **Distal phalanges**

Right hand: anterior (palmar) view

Lunate bone
Scaphoid bone
Capitate bone
Trapezoid bone
Trapezium bone
Carpal bones

Pisiform bone
Triquetral bone
Hamate bone
Carpal bones

Base
Bodies
Head
Metacarpal bones

5 4 3 2 1

Base
Bodies
Head
Proximal phalanges

Base
Bodies
Head
Middle phalanges

Base
Bodies
Tuberosity
Head
Distal phalanges

Right hand: posterior (dorsal) view

PLATE 430

UPPER LIMB

Metacarpophalangeal and Interphalangeal Ligaments

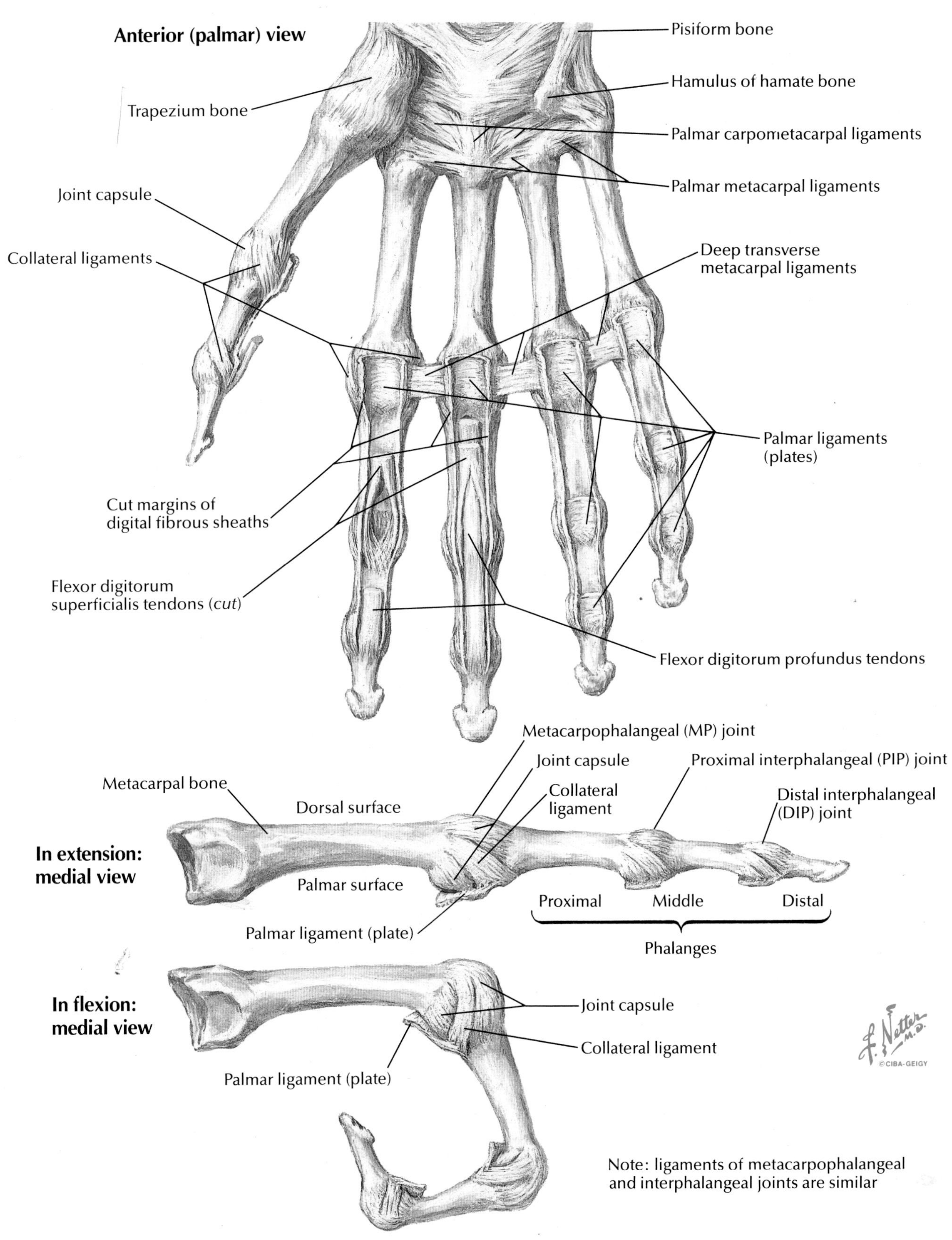

Anterior (palmar) view

Pisiform bone

Hamulus of hamate bone

Palmar carpometacarpal ligaments

Palmar metacarpal ligaments

Trapezium bone

Joint capsule

Collateral ligaments

Deep transverse metacarpal ligaments

Palmar ligaments (plates)

Cut margins of digital fibrous sheaths

Flexor digitorum superficialis tendons (*cut*)

Flexor digitorum profundus tendons

Metacarpophalangeal (MP) joint

Joint capsule

Collateral ligament

Proximal interphalangeal (PIP) joint

Distal interphalangeal (DIP) joint

Metacarpal bone

Dorsal surface

In extension: medial view

Palmar surface

Proximal   Middle   Distal

Phalanges

Palmar ligament (plate)

In flexion: medial view

Joint capsule

Collateral ligament

Palmar ligament (plate)

Note: ligaments of metacarpophalangeal and interphalangeal joints are similar

Wrist and Hand: *Superficial Palmar Dissections*

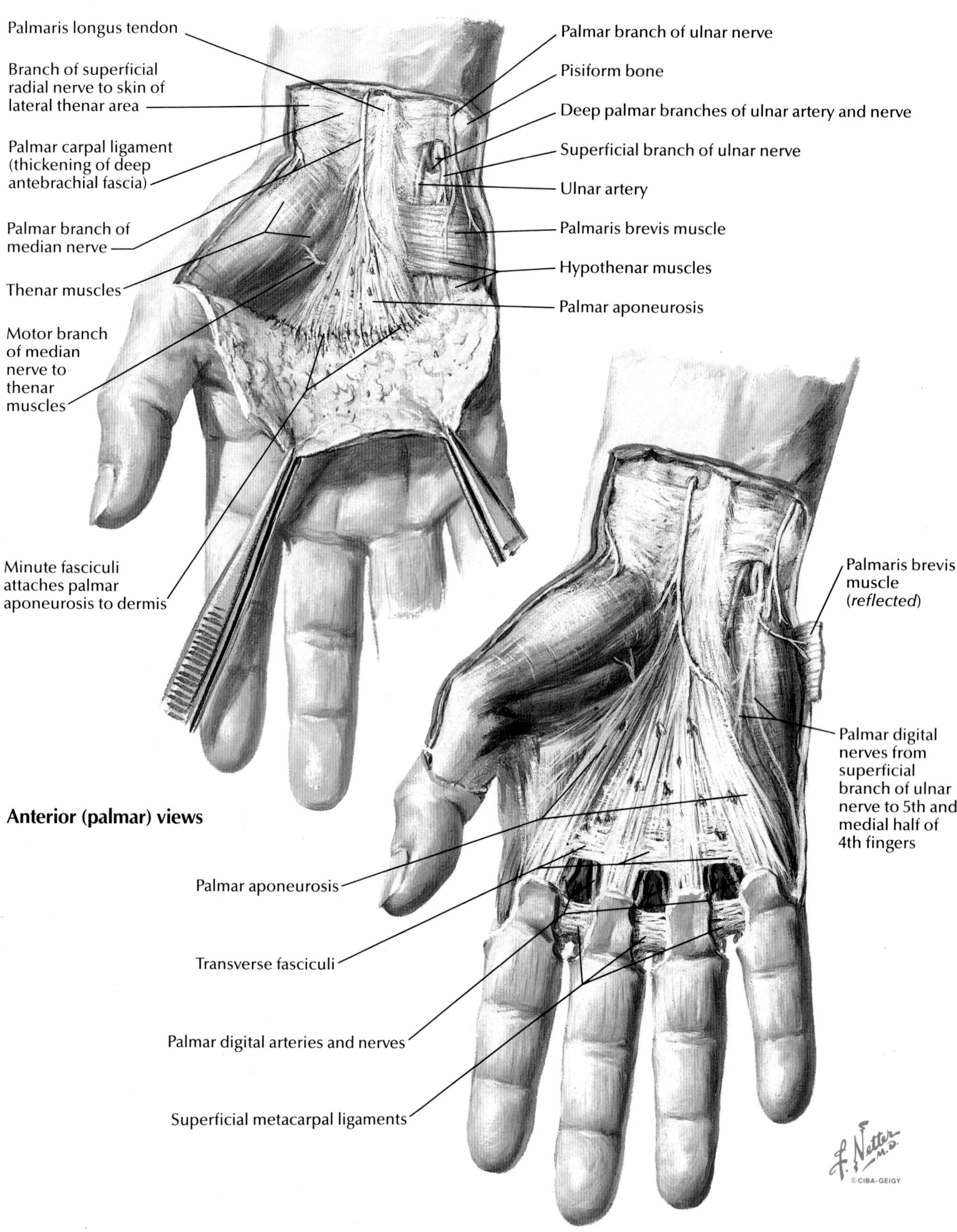

Palmaris longus tendon

Branch of superficial radial nerve to skin of lateral thenar area

Palmar carpal ligament (thickening of deep antebrachial fascia)

Palmar branch of median nerve

Thenar muscles

Motor branch of median nerve to thenar muscles

Minute fasciculi attaches palmar aponeurosis to dermis

Anterior (palmar) views

Palmar branch of ulnar nerve

Pisiform bone

Deep palmar branches of ulnar artery and nerve

Superficial branch of ulnar nerve

Ulnar artery

Palmaris brevis muscle

Hypothenar muscles

Palmar aponeurosis

Palmaris brevis muscle (*reflected*)

Palmar digital nerves from superficial branch of ulnar nerve to 5th and medial half of 4th fingers

Palmar aponeurosis

Transverse fasciculi

Palmar digital arteries and nerves

Superficial metacarpal ligaments

PLATE 432

UPPER LIMB

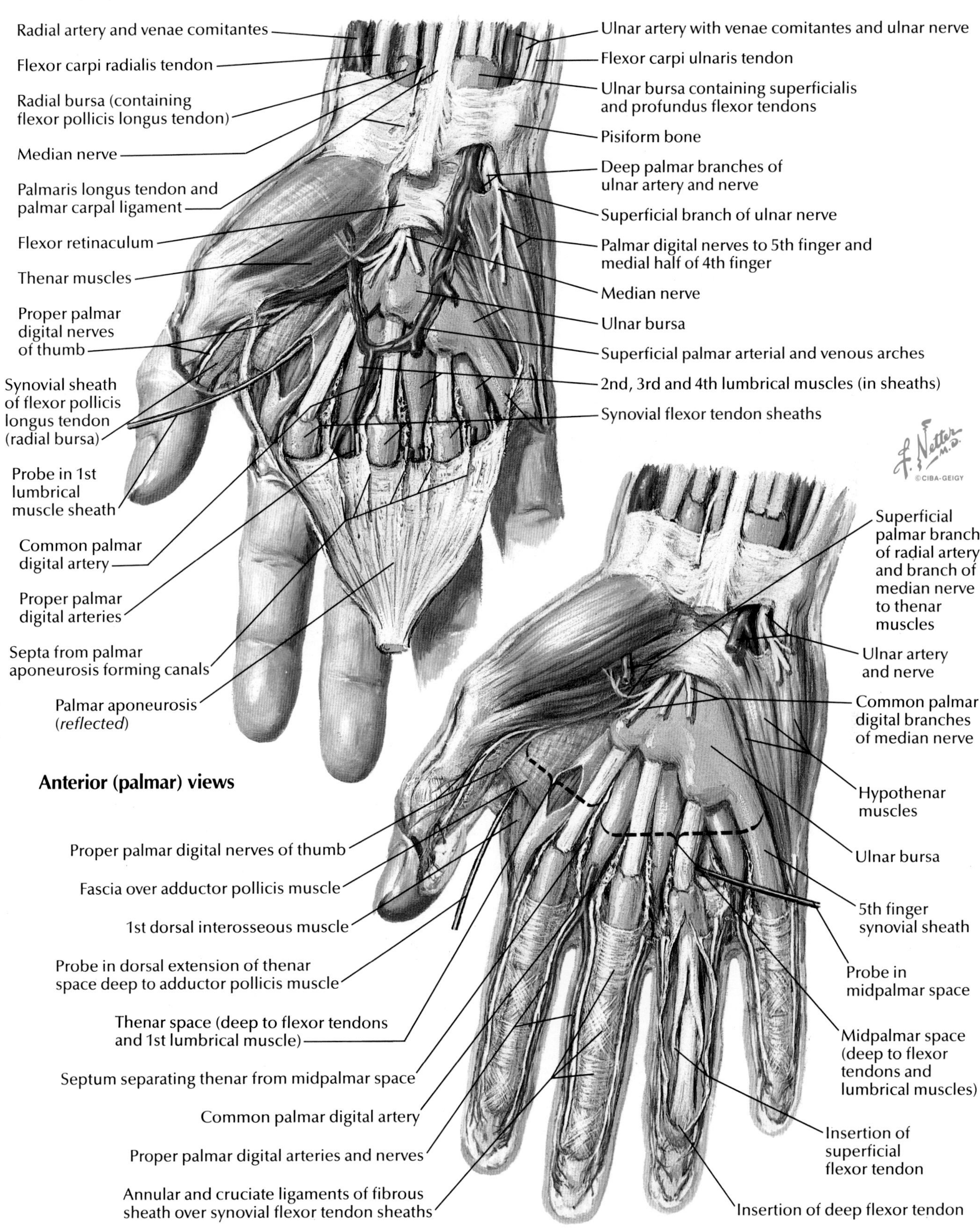

Radial artery and venae comitantes

Flexor carpi radialis tendon

Radial bursa (containing flexor pollicis longus tendon)

Median nerve

Palmaris longus tendon and palmar carpal ligament

Flexor retinaculum

Thenar muscles

Proper palmar digital nerves of thumb

Synovial sheath of flexor pollicis longus tendon (radial bursa)

Probe in 1st lumbrical muscle sheath

Common palmar digital artery

Proper palmar digital arteries

Septa from palmar aponeurosis forming canals

Palmar aponeurosis (*reflected*)

Anterior (palmar) views

Ulnar artery with venae comitantes and ulnar nerve

Flexor carpi ulnaris tendon

Ulnar bursa containing superficialis and profundus flexor tendons

Pisiform bone

Deep palmar branches of ulnar artery and nerve

Superficial branch of ulnar nerve

Palmar digital nerves to 5th finger and medial half of 4th finger

Median nerve

Ulnar bursa

Superficial palmar arterial and venous arches

2nd, 3rd and 4th lumbrical muscles (in sheaths)

Synovial flexor tendon sheaths

Superficial palmar branch of radial artery and branch of median nerve to thenar muscles

Ulnar artery and nerve

Common palmar digital branches of median nerve

Hypothenar muscles

Ulnar bursa

5th finger synovial sheath

Probe in midpalmar space

Midpalmar space (deep to flexor tendons and lumbrical muscles)

Insertion of superficial flexor tendon

Insertion of deep flexor tendon

Proper palmar digital nerves of thumb

Fascia over adductor pollicis muscle

1st dorsal interosseous muscle

Probe in dorsal extension of thenar space deep to adductor pollicis muscle

Thenar space (deep to flexor tendons and 1st lumbrical muscle)

Septum separating thenar from midpalmar space

Common palmar digital artery

Proper palmar digital arteries and nerves

Annular and cruciate ligaments of fibrous sheath over synovial flexor tendon sheaths

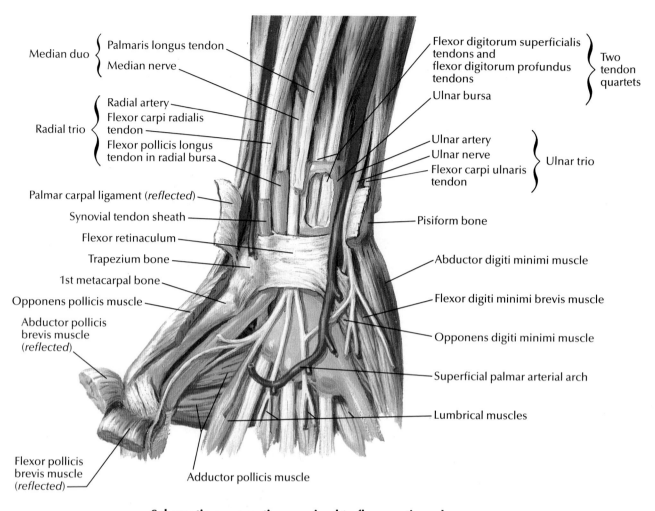

Median duo { Palmaris longus tendon
Median nerve

Radial trio { Radial artery
Flexor carpi radialis tendon
Flexor pollicis longus tendon in radial bursa

Palmar carpal ligament (*reflected*)
Synovial tendon sheath
Flexor retinaculum
Trapezium bone
1st metacarpal bone
Opponens pollicis muscle
Abductor pollicis brevis muscle (*reflected*)
Flexor pollicis brevis muscle (*reflected*)
Adductor pollicis muscle

Flexor digitorum superficialis tendons and flexor digitorum profundus tendons } Two tendon quartets
Ulnar bursa

Ulnar artery
Ulnar nerve
Flexor carpi ulnaris tendon } Ulnar trio

Pisiform bone
Abductor digiti minimi muscle
Flexor digiti minimi brevis muscle
Opponens digiti minimi muscle
Superficial palmar arterial arch
Lumbrical muscles

Schematic cross section proximal to flexor retinaculum

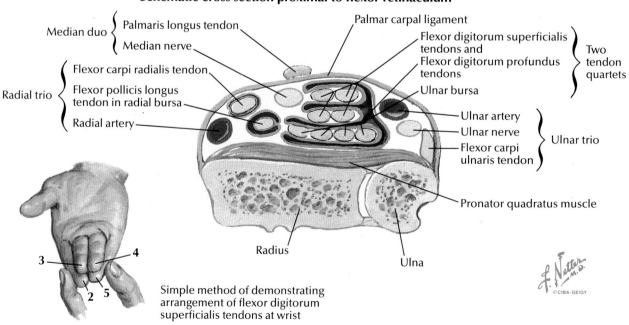

Median duo { Palmaris longus tendon
Median nerve

Radial trio { Flexor carpi radialis tendon
Flexor pollicis longus tendon in radial bursa
Radial artery

Palmar carpal ligament

Flexor digitorum superficialis tendons and Flexor digitorum profundus tendons } Two tendon quartets
Ulnar bursa

Ulnar artery
Ulnar nerve
Flexor carpi ulnaris tendon } Ulnar trio

Pronator quadratus muscle

Radius
Ulna

3 4
2 5

Simple method of demonstrating arrangement of flexor digitorum superficialis tendons at wrist

PLATE 434

UPPER LIMB

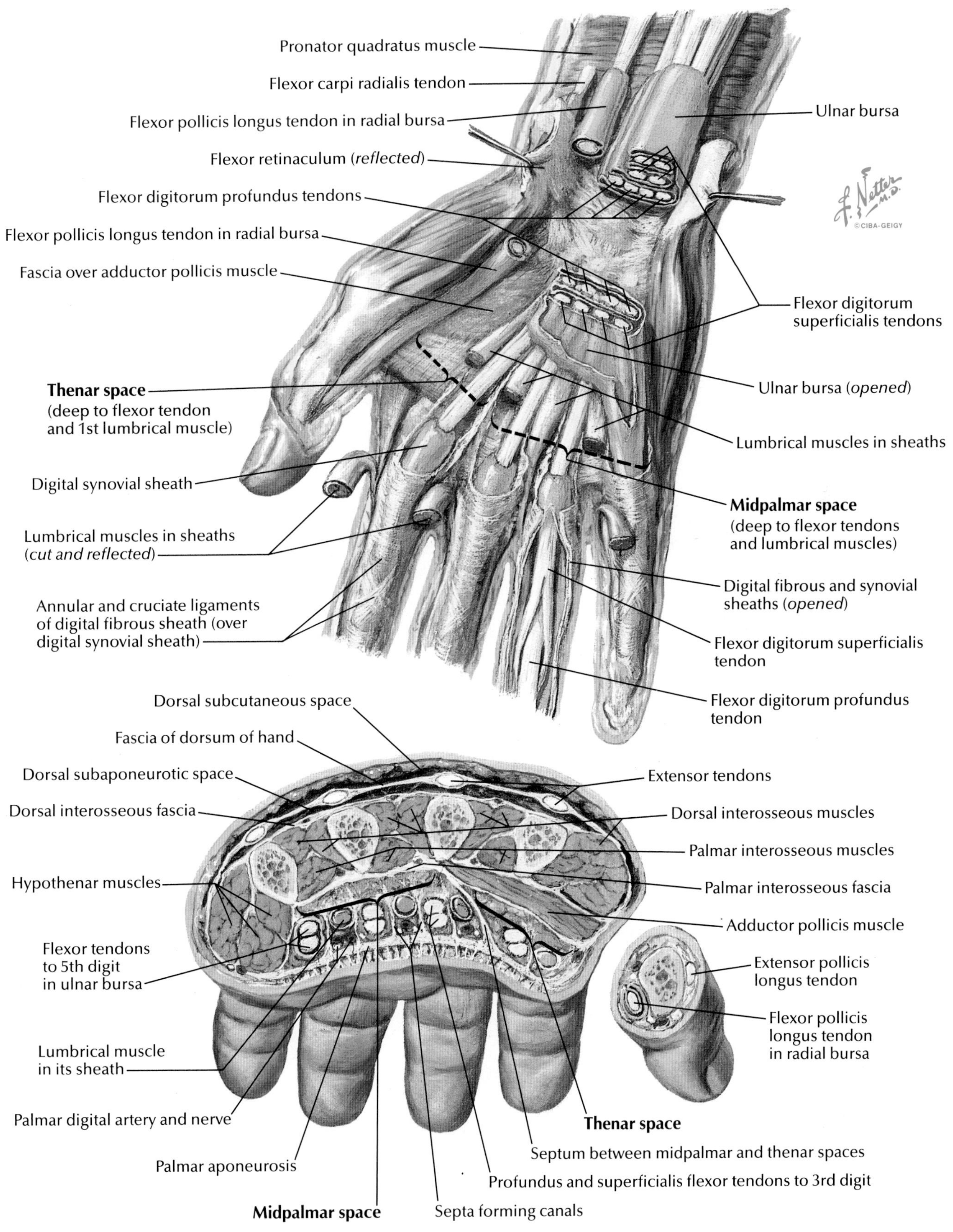

Pronator quadratus muscle

Flexor carpi radialis tendon

Flexor pollicis longus tendon in radial bursa

Flexor retinaculum (*reflected*)

Flexor digitorum profundus tendons

Flexor pollicis longus tendon in radial bursa

Fascia over adductor pollicis muscle

Thenar space
(deep to flexor tendon
and 1st lumbrical muscle)

Digital synovial sheath

Lumbrical muscles in sheaths
(*cut and reflected*)

Annular and cruciate ligaments
of digital fibrous sheath (over
digital synovial sheath)

Ulnar bursa

Flexor digitorum
superficialis tendons

Ulnar bursa (*opened*)

Lumbrical muscles in sheaths

Midpalmar space
(deep to flexor tendons
and lumbrical muscles)

Digital fibrous and synovial
sheaths (*opened*)

Flexor digitorum superficialis
tendon

Flexor digitorum profundus
tendon

Dorsal subcutaneous space

Fascia of dorsum of hand

Dorsal subaponeurotic space

Dorsal interosseous fascia

Hypothenar muscles

Flexor tendons
to 5th digit
in ulnar bursa

Lumbrical muscle
in its sheath

Palmar digital artery and nerve

Palmar aponeurosis

Midpalmar space

Extensor tendons

Dorsal interosseous muscles

Palmar interosseous muscles

Palmar interosseous fascia

Adductor pollicis muscle

Extensor pollicis
longus tendon

Flexor pollicis
longus tendon
in radial bursa

Thenar space

Septum between midpalmar and thenar spaces

Profundus and superficialis flexor tendons to 3rd digit

Septa forming canals

Lumbrical Muscles and Bursae, Spaces and Sheaths: Schema

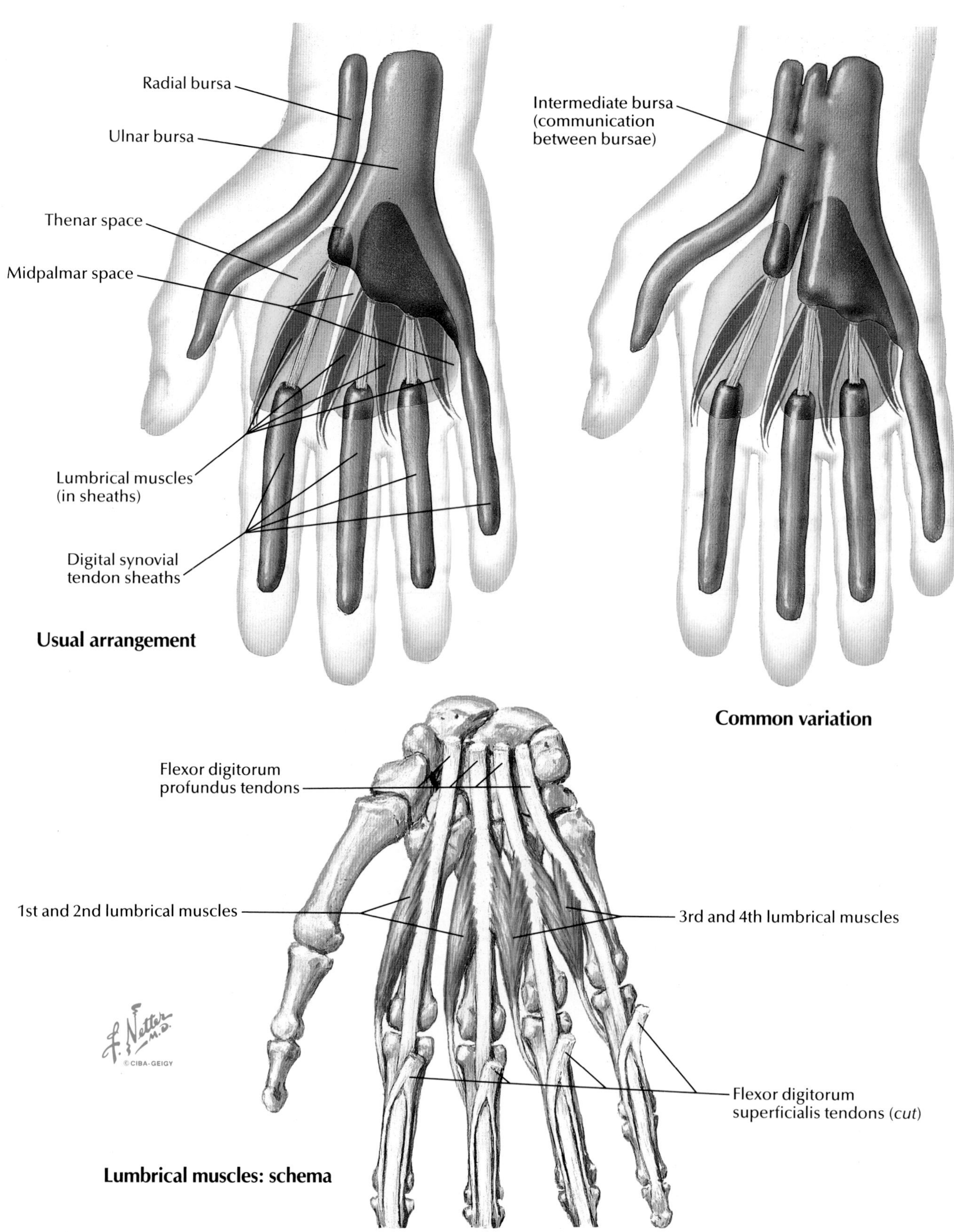

Radial bursa

Ulnar bursa

Thenar space

Midpalmar space

Lumbrical muscles
(in sheaths)

Digital synovial
tendon sheaths

Usual arrangement

Intermediate bursa
(communication
between bursae)

Common variation

Flexor digitorum
profundus tendons

1st and 2nd lumbrical muscles

3rd and 4th lumbrical muscles

Flexor digitorum
superficialis tendons (*cut*)

Lumbrical muscles: schema

PLATE 436

UPPER LIMB

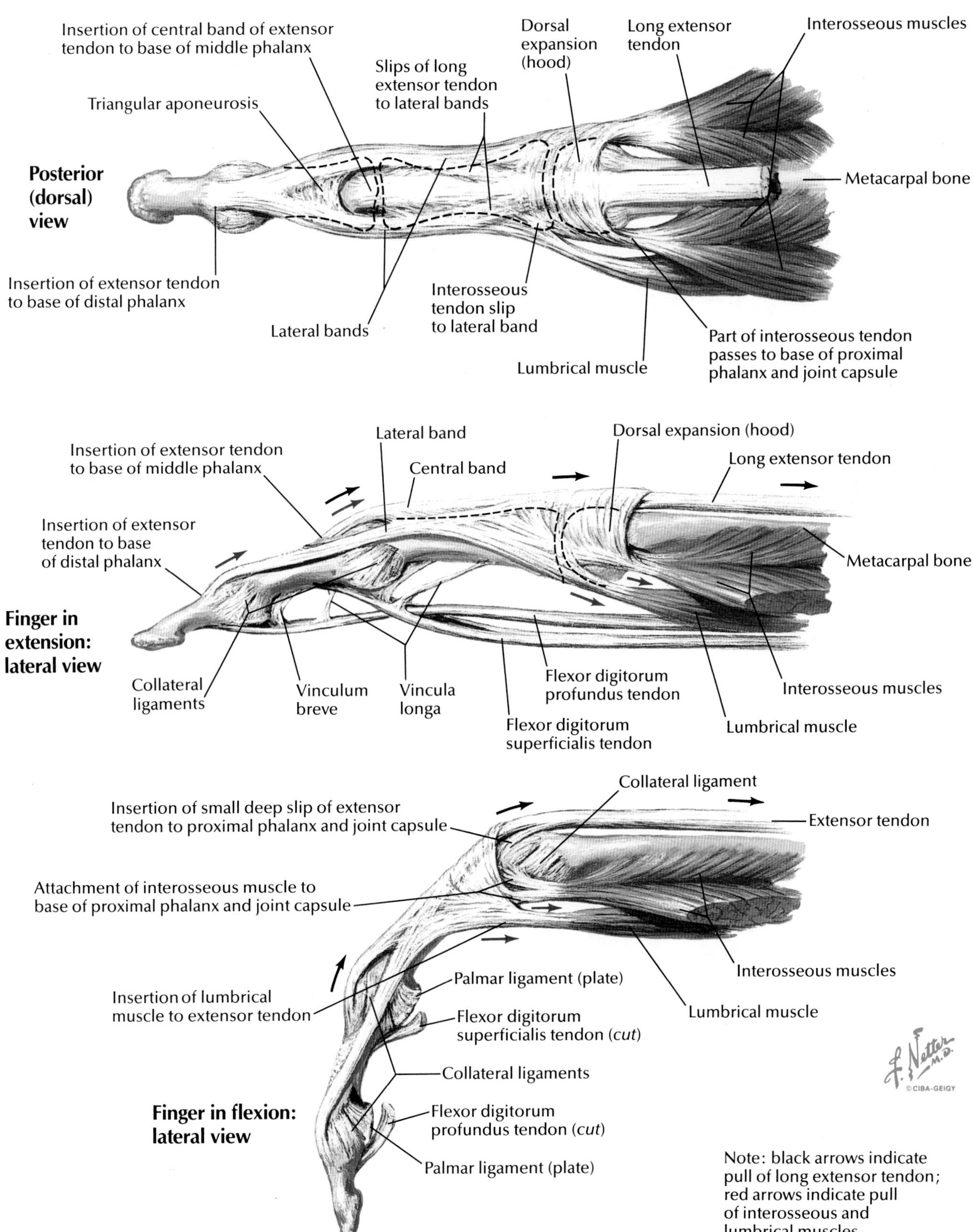

Posterior (dorsal) view

Insertion of central band of extensor tendon to base of middle phalanx

Triangular aponeurosis

Slips of long extensor tendon to lateral bands

Dorsal expansion (hood)

Long extensor tendon

Interosseous muscles

Metacarpal bone

Insertion of extensor tendon to base of distal phalanx

Lateral bands

Interosseous tendon slip to lateral band

Lumbrical muscle

Part of interosseous tendon passes to base of proximal phalanx and joint capsule

Finger in extension: lateral view

Insertion of extensor tendon to base of middle phalanx

Insertion of extensor tendon to base of distal phalanx

Lateral band

Central band

Dorsal expansion (hood)

Long extensor tendon

Metacarpal bone

Collateral ligaments

Vinculum breve

Vincula longa

Flexor digitorum profundus tendon

Flexor digitorum superficialis tendon

Interosseous muscles

Lumbrical muscle

Finger in flexion: lateral view

Insertion of small deep slip of extensor tendon to proximal phalanx and joint capsule

Attachment of interosseous muscle to base of proximal phalanx and joint capsule

Insertion of lumbrical muscle to extensor tendon

Collateral ligament

Extensor tendon

Palmar ligament (plate)

Flexor digitorum superficialis tendon (*cut*)

Collateral ligaments

Flexor digitorum profundus tendon (*cut*)

Palmar ligament (plate)

Interosseous muscles

Lumbrical muscle

Note: black arrows indicate pull of long extensor tendon; red arrows indicate pull of interosseous and lumbrical muscles

Intrinsic Muscles of Hand

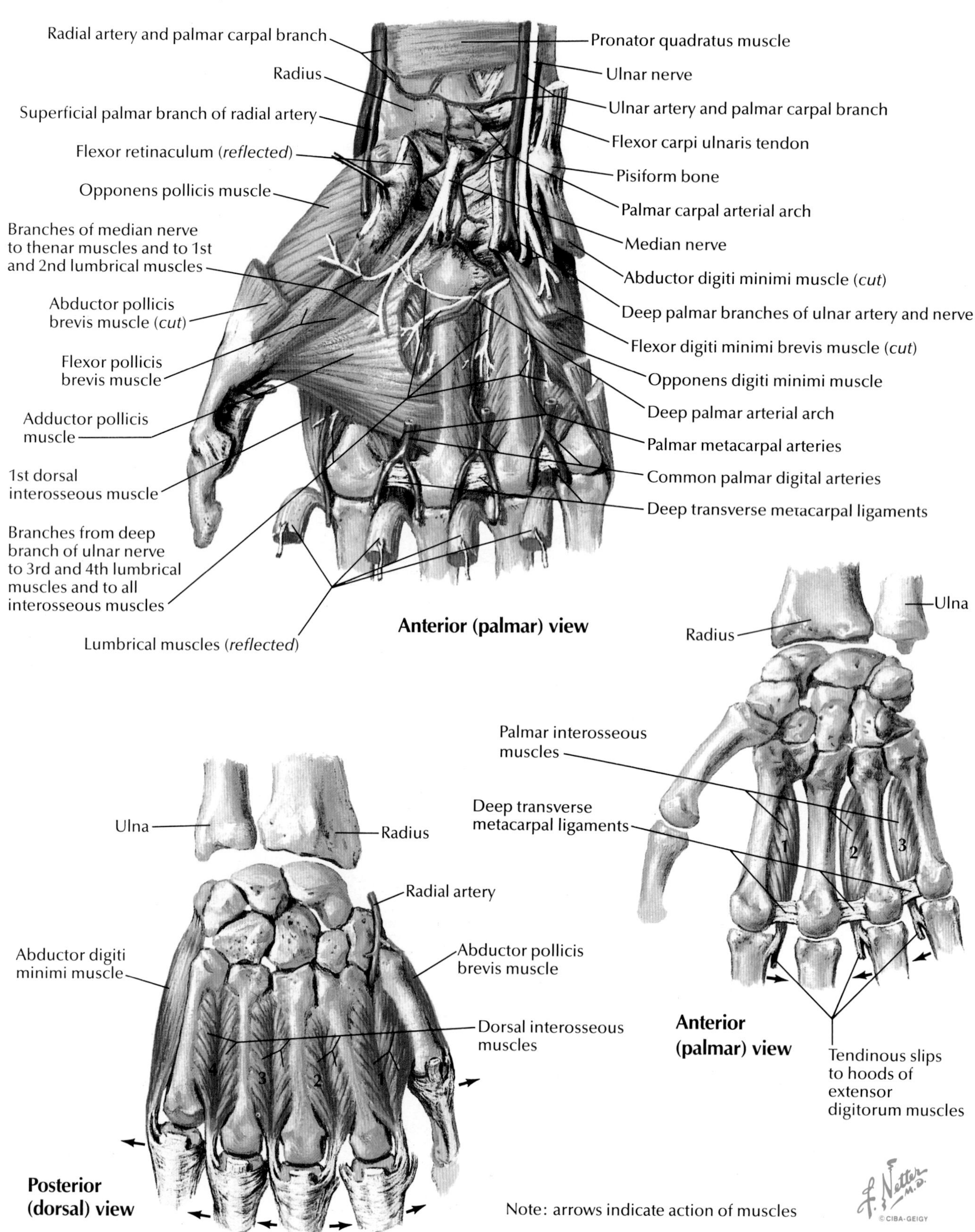

Radial artery and palmar carpal branch

Radius

Superficial palmar branch of radial artery

Flexor retinaculum (*reflected*)

Opponens pollicis muscle

Branches of median nerve to thenar muscles and to 1st and 2nd lumbrical muscles

Abductor pollicis brevis muscle (*cut*)

Flexor pollicis brevis muscle

Adductor pollicis muscle

1st dorsal interosseous muscle

Branches from deep branch of ulnar nerve to 3rd and 4th lumbrical muscles and to all interosseous muscles

Lumbrical muscles (*reflected*)

Pronator quadratus muscle

Ulnar nerve

Ulnar artery and palmar carpal branch

Flexor carpi ulnaris tendon

Pisiform bone

Palmar carpal arterial arch

Median nerve

Abductor digiti minimi muscle (*cut*)

Deep palmar branches of ulnar artery and nerve

Flexor digiti minimi brevis muscle (*cut*)

Opponens digiti minimi muscle

Deep palmar arterial arch

Palmar metacarpal arteries

Common palmar digital arteries

Deep transverse metacarpal ligaments

Anterior (palmar) view

Ulna

Radius

Abductor digiti minimi muscle

Radial artery

Abductor pollicis brevis muscle

Dorsal interosseous muscles

Posterior (dorsal) view

Radius

Ulna

Palmar interosseous muscles

Deep transverse metacarpal ligaments

Anterior (palmar) view

Tendinous slips to hoods of extensor digitorum muscles

Note: arrows indicate action of muscles

PLATE 438

UPPER LIMB

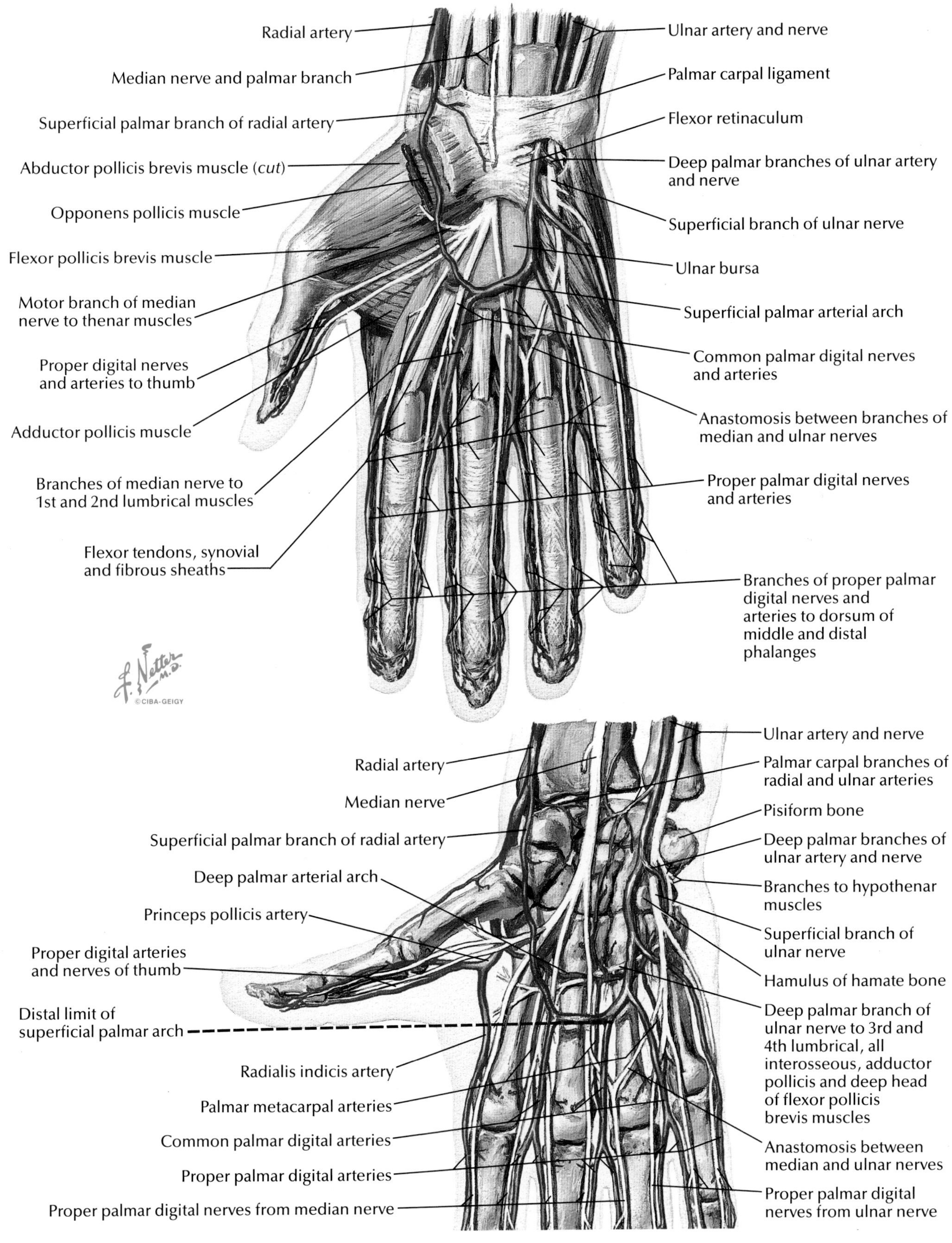

Radial artery

Median nerve and palmar branch

Superficial palmar branch of radial artery

Abductor pollicis brevis muscle (*cut*)

Opponens pollicis muscle

Flexor pollicis brevis muscle

Motor branch of median nerve to thenar muscles

Proper digital nerves and arteries to thumb

Adductor pollicis muscle

Branches of median nerve to 1st and 2nd lumbrical muscles

Flexor tendons, synovial and fibrous sheaths

Ulnar artery and nerve

Palmar carpal ligament

Flexor retinaculum

Deep palmar branches of ulnar artery and nerve

Superficial branch of ulnar nerve

Ulnar bursa

Superficial palmar arterial arch

Common palmar digital nerves and arteries

Anastomosis between branches of median and ulnar nerves

Proper palmar digital nerves and arteries

Branches of proper palmar digital nerves and arteries to dorsum of middle and distal phalanges

Radial artery

Median nerve

Superficial palmar branch of radial artery

Deep palmar arterial arch

Princeps pollicis artery

Proper digital arteries and nerves of thumb

Distal limit of superficial palmar arch

Radialis indicis artery

Palmar metacarpal arteries

Common palmar digital arteries

Proper palmar digital arteries

Proper palmar digital nerves from median nerve

Ulnar artery and nerve

Palmar carpal branches of radial and ulnar arteries

Pisiform bone

Deep palmar branches of ulnar artery and nerve

Branches to hypothenar muscles

Superficial branch of ulnar nerve

Hamulus of hamate bone

Deep palmar branch of ulnar nerve to 3rd and 4th lumbrical, all interosseous, adductor pollicis and deep head of flexor pollicis brevis muscles

Anastomosis between median and ulnar nerves

Proper palmar digital nerves from ulnar nerve

Wrist and Hand: Superficial Radial Dissection

Lateral (radial) view

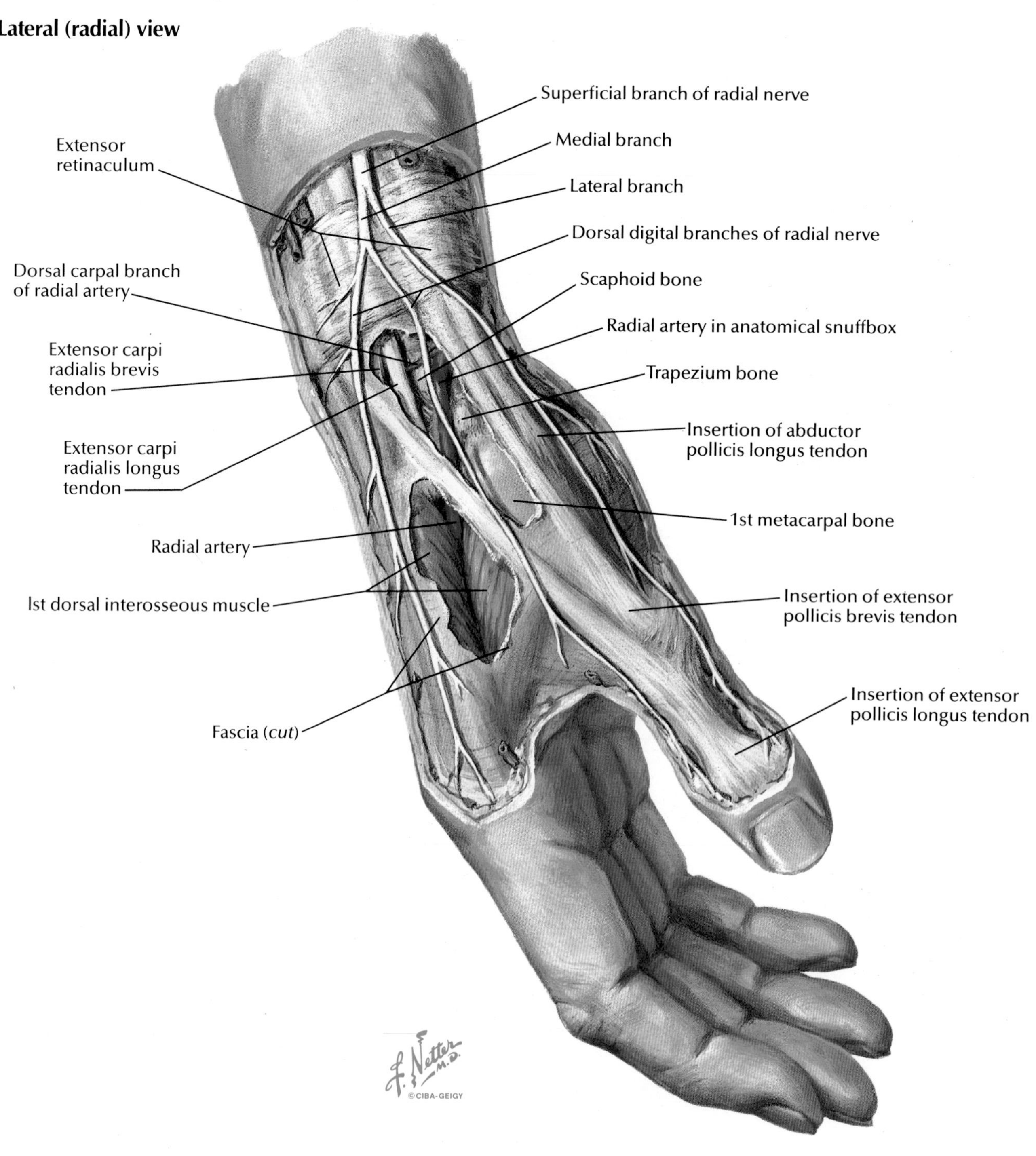

Superficial branch of radial nerve

Medial branch

Lateral branch

Dorsal digital branches of radial nerve

Scaphoid bone

Radial artery in anatomical snuffbox

Trapezium bone

Insertion of abductor pollicis longus tendon

1st metacarpal bone

Insertion of extensor pollicis brevis tendon

Insertion of extensor pollicis longus tendon

Extensor retinaculum

Dorsal carpal branch of radial artery

Extensor carpi radialis brevis tendon

Extensor carpi radialis longus tendon

Radial artery

Ist dorsal interosseous muscle

Fascia (cut)

PLATE 440

UPPER LIMB

Posterior (dorsal) view

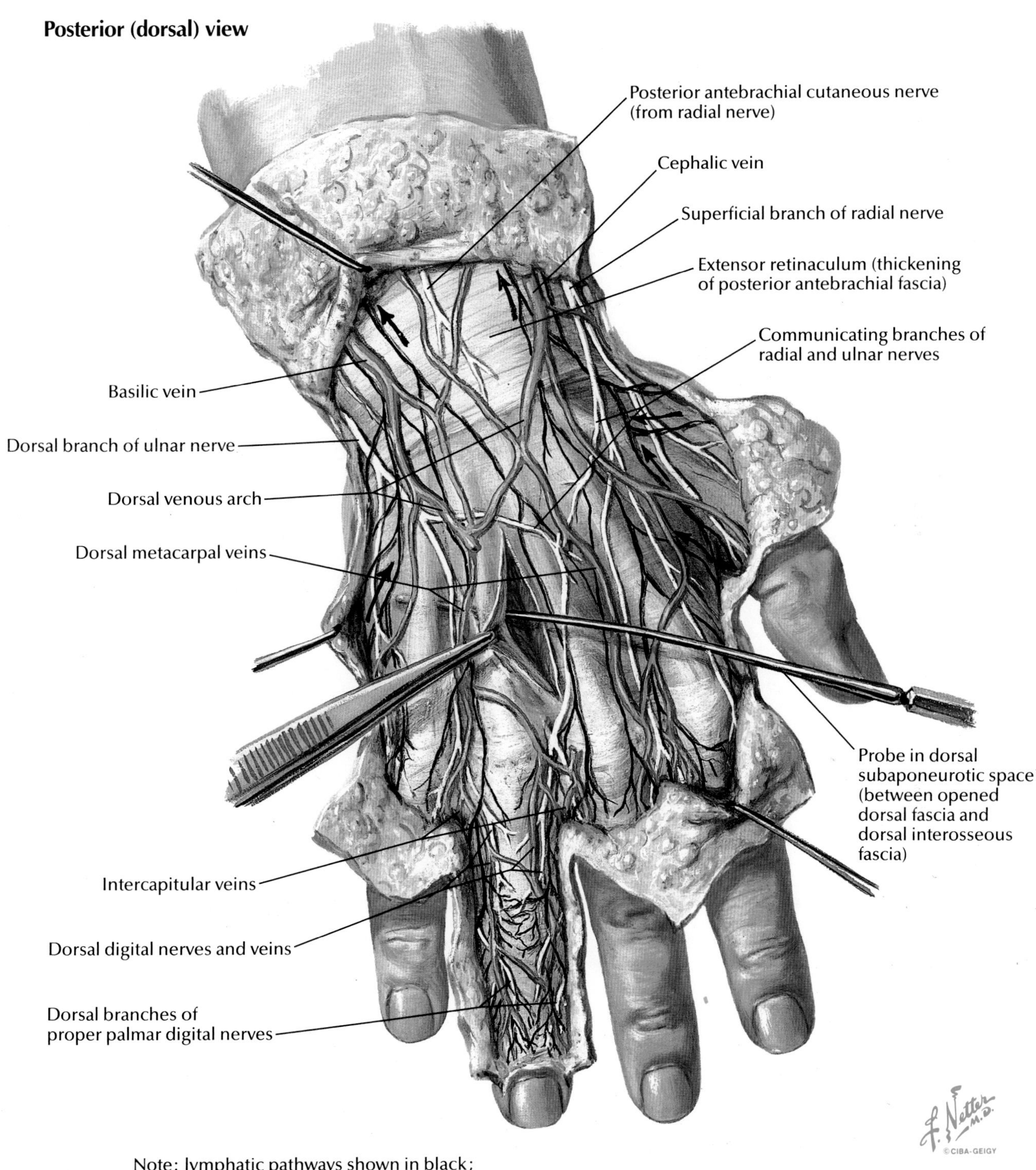

Posterior antebrachial cutaneous nerve (from radial nerve)

Cephalic vein

Superficial branch of radial nerve

Extensor retinaculum (thickening of posterior antebrachial fascia)

Communicating branches of radial and ulnar nerves

Basilic vein

Dorsal branch of ulnar nerve

Dorsal venous arch

Dorsal metacarpal veins

Probe in dorsal subaponeurotic space (between opened dorsal fascia and dorsal interosseous fascia)

Intercapitular veins

Dorsal digital nerves and veins

Dorsal branches of proper palmar digital nerves

Note: lymphatic pathways shown in black; arrows indicate direction of drainage

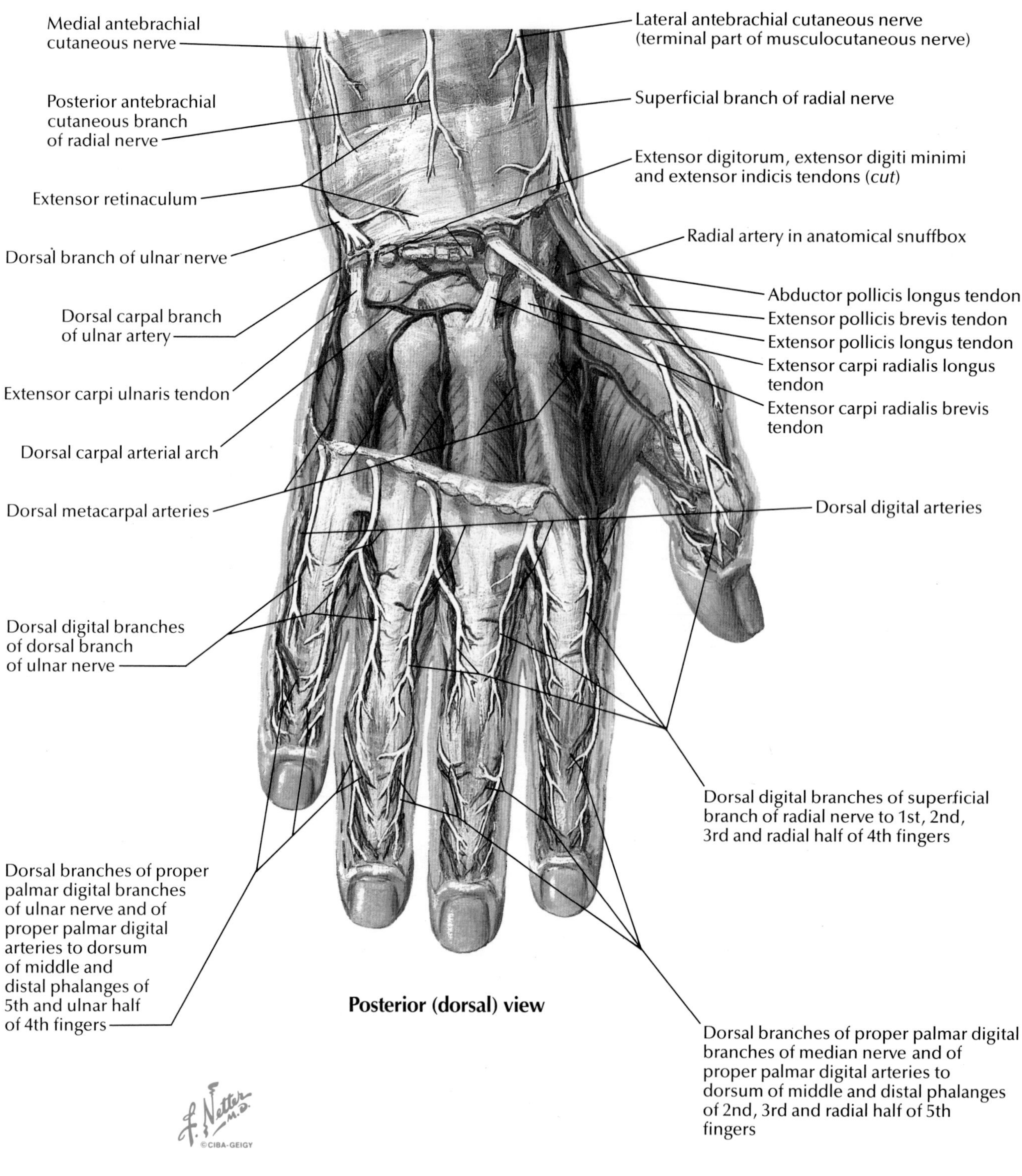

Medial antebrachial cutaneous nerve

Posterior antebrachial cutaneous branch of radial nerve

Extensor retinaculum

Dorsal branch of ulnar nerve

Dorsal carpal branch of ulnar artery

Extensor carpi ulnaris tendon

Dorsal carpal arterial arch

Dorsal metacarpal arteries

Dorsal digital branches of dorsal branch of ulnar nerve

Dorsal branches of proper palmar digital branches of ulnar nerve and of proper palmar digital arteries to dorsum of middle and distal phalanges of 5th and ulnar half of 4th fingers

Lateral antebrachial cutaneous nerve (terminal part of musculocutaneous nerve)

Superficial branch of radial nerve

Extensor digitorum, extensor digiti minimi and extensor indicis tendons (cut)

Radial artery in anatomical snuffbox

Abductor pollicis longus tendon
Extensor pollicis brevis tendon
Extensor pollicis longus tendon
Extensor carpi radialis longus tendon
Extensor carpi radialis brevis tendon

Dorsal digital arteries

Dorsal digital branches of superficial branch of radial nerve to 1st, 2nd, 3rd and radial half of 4th fingers

Posterior (dorsal) view

Dorsal branches of proper palmar digital branches of median nerve and of proper palmar digital arteries to dorsum of middle and distal phalanges of 2nd, 3rd and radial half of 5th fingers

PLATE 442

UPPER LIMB

Posterior (dorsal) view

Extensor carpi ulnaris — **Compartment 6**

Extensor digiti minimi — **Compartment 5**

Extensor digitorum
Extensor indicis } **Compartment 4**

Extensor pollicis longus — **Compartment 3**

Extensor carpi radialis brevis
Extensor carpi radialis longus } **Compartment 2**

Abductor pollicis longus
Extensor pollicis brevis } **Compartment 1**

Extensor retinaculum

Radial artery in anatomical snuffbox

Abductor digiti
minimi muscle

Dorsal interosseous muscles

Intertendinous connections

Transverse fibers of
dorsal expansions (hoods)

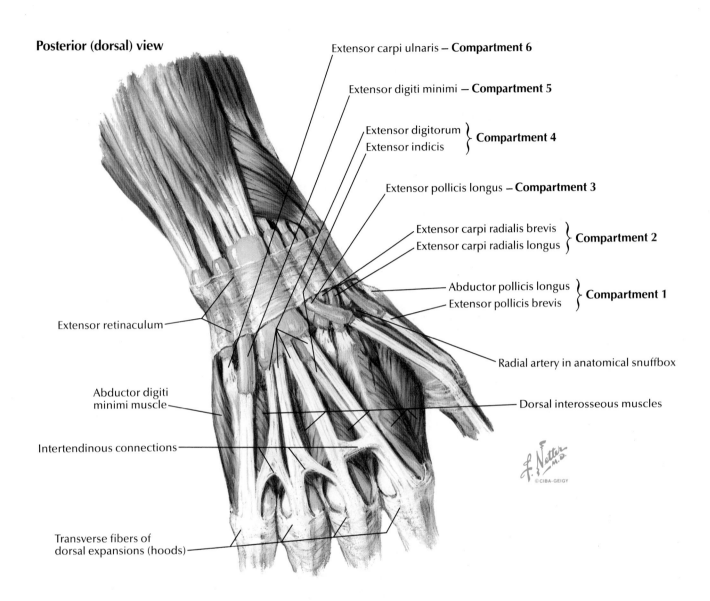

Cross section at proximal wrist

Extensor retinaculum

Extensor pollicis longus — **Compartment 3**

Compartment 4 { Extensor digitorum and
extensor indicis

Extensor carpi
radialis brevis
} **Compartment 2**
Extensor carpi
radialis longus

Compartment 5 { Extensor
digiti minimi

Compartment 6 { Extensor
carpi
ulnaris

Extensor
pollicis brevis
} **Compartment 1**
Abductor
pollicis longus

Ulna

Radius

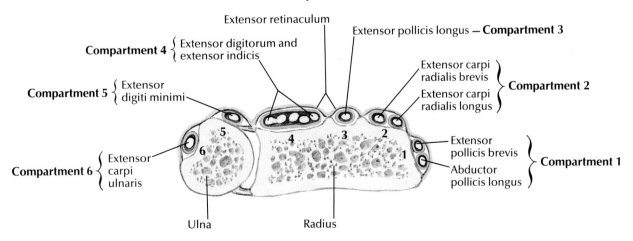

Fingers

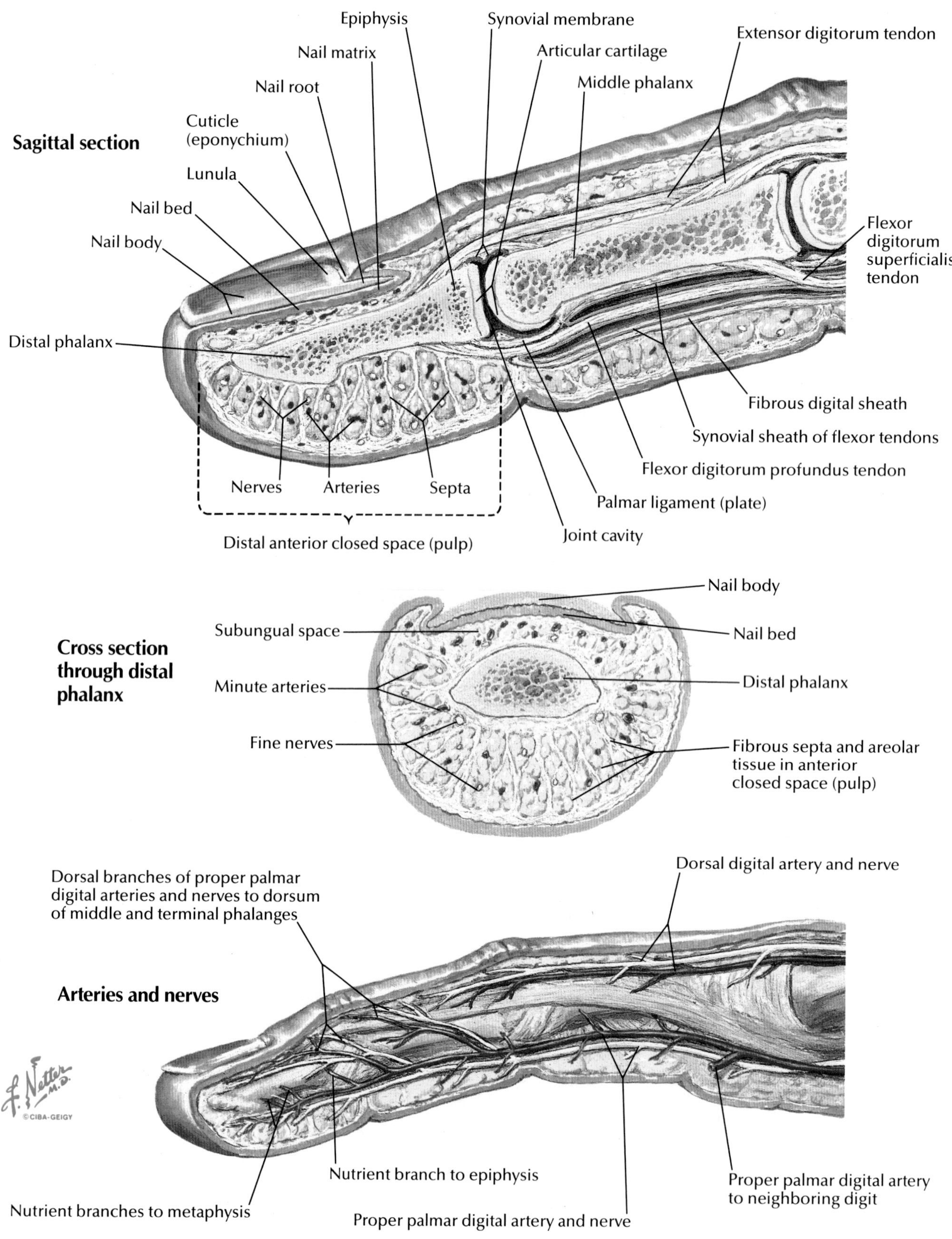

Sagittal section

Epiphysis

Synovial membrane

Nail matrix

Articular cartilage

Extensor digitorum tendon

Nail root

Middle phalanx

Cuticle (eponychium)

Lunula

Nail bed

Nail body

Flexor digitorum superficialis tendon

Distal phalanx

Fibrous digital sheath

Synovial sheath of flexor tendons

Flexor digitorum profundus tendon

Nerves   Arteries   Septa

Palmar ligament (plate)

Joint cavity

Distal anterior closed space (pulp)

Cross section through distal phalanx

Nail body

Subungual space

Nail bed

Minute arteries

Distal phalanx

Fine nerves

Fibrous septa and areolar tissue in anterior closed space (pulp)

Dorsal digital artery and nerve

Dorsal branches of proper palmar digital arteries and nerves to dorsum of middle and terminal phalanges

Arteries and nerves

Nutrient branch to epiphysis

Proper palmar digital artery to neighboring digit

Nutrient branches to metaphysis

Proper palmar digital artery and nerve

PLATE 444

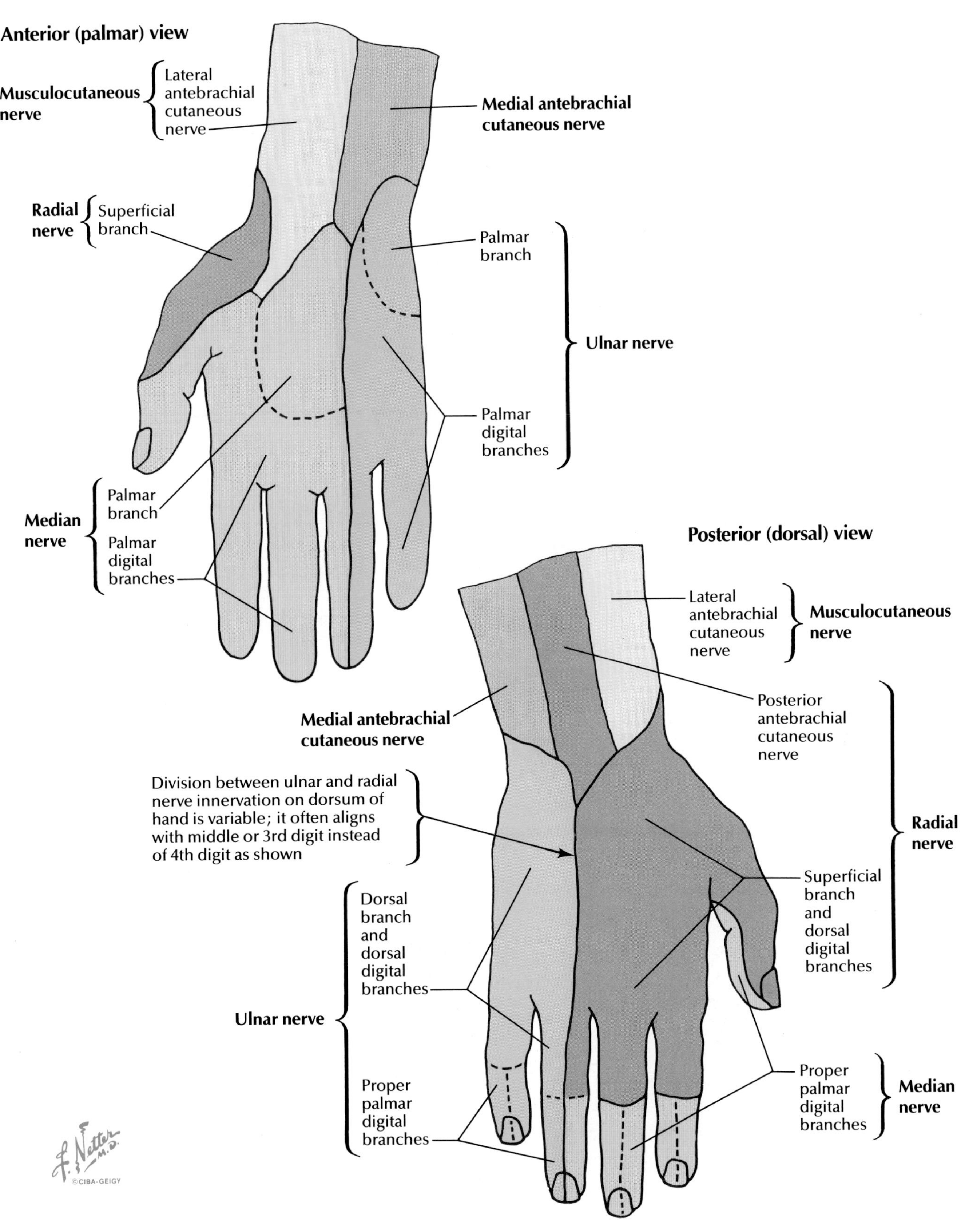

Anterior (palmar) view

Musculocutaneous nerve { Lateral antebrachial cutaneous nerve

Medial antebrachial cutaneous nerve

Radial nerve { Superficial branch

Palmar branch

Ulnar nerve

Palmar digital branches

Median nerve { Palmar branch / Palmar digital branches

Posterior (dorsal) view

Lateral antebrachial cutaneous nerve } **Musculocutaneous nerve**

Posterior antebrachial cutaneous nerve

Medial antebrachial cutaneous nerve

Division between ulnar and radial nerve innervation on dorsum of hand is variable; it often aligns with middle or 3rd digit instead of 4th digit as shown

Radial nerve

Superficial branch and dorsal digital branches

Ulnar nerve { Dorsal branch and dorsal digital branches / Proper palmar digital branches

Proper palmar digital branches } **Median nerve**

Arteries and Nerves of Upper Limb

Anterior view

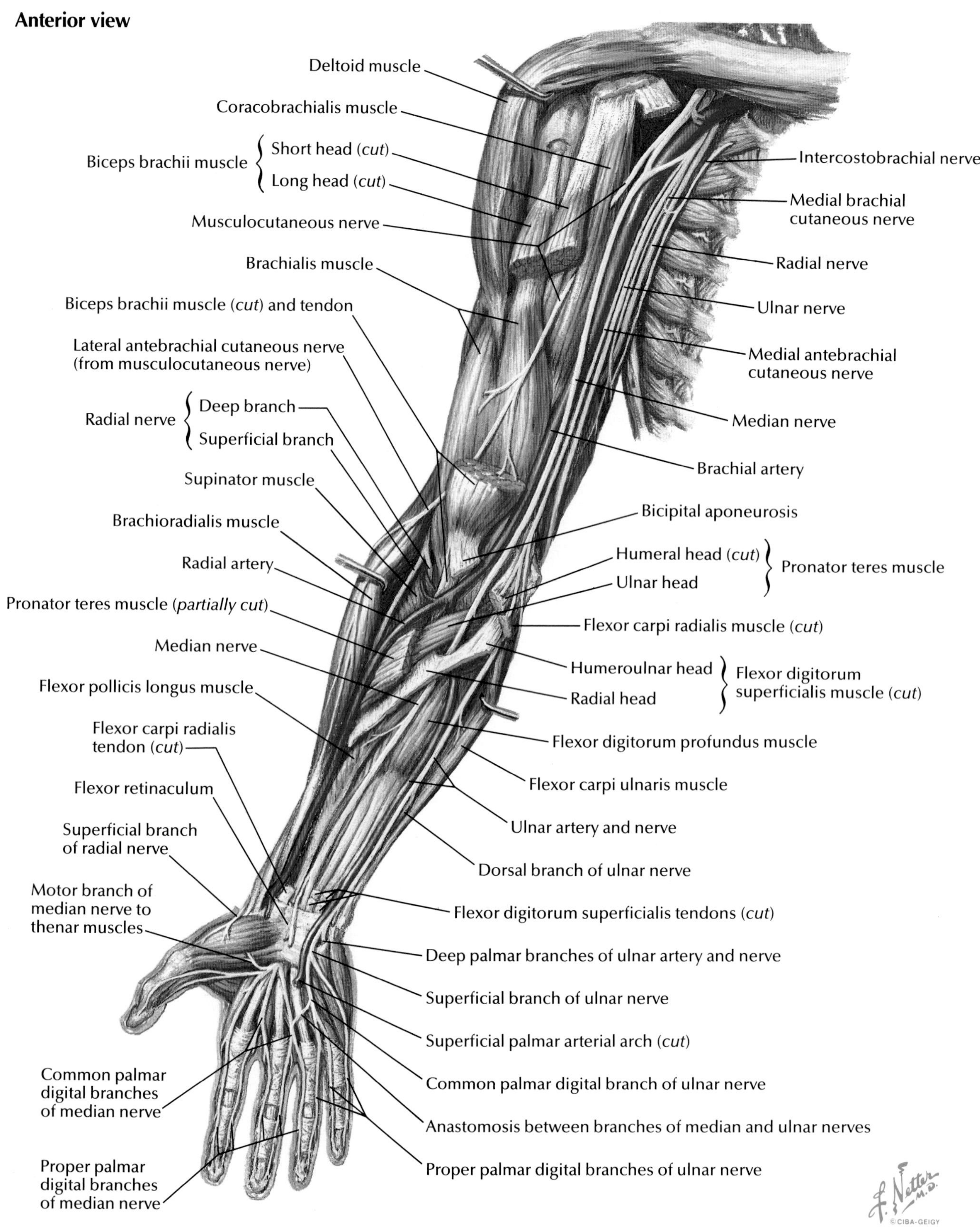

Deltoid muscle

Coracobrachialis muscle

Biceps brachii muscle { Short head (*cut*)
Long head (*cut*)

Musculocutaneous nerve

Brachialis muscle

Biceps brachii muscle (*cut*) and tendon

Lateral antebrachial cutaneous nerve (from musculocutaneous nerve)

Radial nerve { Deep branch
Superficial branch

Supinator muscle

Brachioradialis muscle

Radial artery

Pronator teres muscle (*partially cut*)

Median nerve

Flexor pollicis longus muscle

Flexor carpi radialis tendon (*cut*)

Flexor retinaculum

Superficial branch of radial nerve

Motor branch of median nerve to thenar muscles

Common palmar digital branches of median nerve

Proper palmar digital branches of median nerve

Intercostobrachial nerve

Medial brachial cutaneous nerve

Radial nerve

Ulnar nerve

Medial antebrachial cutaneous nerve

Median nerve

Brachial artery

Bicipital aponeurosis

Humeral head (*cut*) } Pronator teres muscle
Ulnar head

Flexor carpi radialis muscle (*cut*)

Humeroulnar head } Flexor digitorum superficialis muscle (*cut*)
Radial head

Flexor digitorum profundus muscle

Flexor carpi ulnaris muscle

Ulnar artery and nerve

Dorsal branch of ulnar nerve

Flexor digitorum superficialis tendons (*cut*)

Deep palmar branches of ulnar artery and nerve

Superficial branch of ulnar nerve

Superficial palmar arterial arch (*cut*)

Common palmar digital branch of ulnar nerve

Anastomosis between branches of median and ulnar nerves

Proper palmar digital branches of ulnar nerve

f. Netter M.D.
©CIBA-GEIGY

PLATE 446

UPPER LIMB

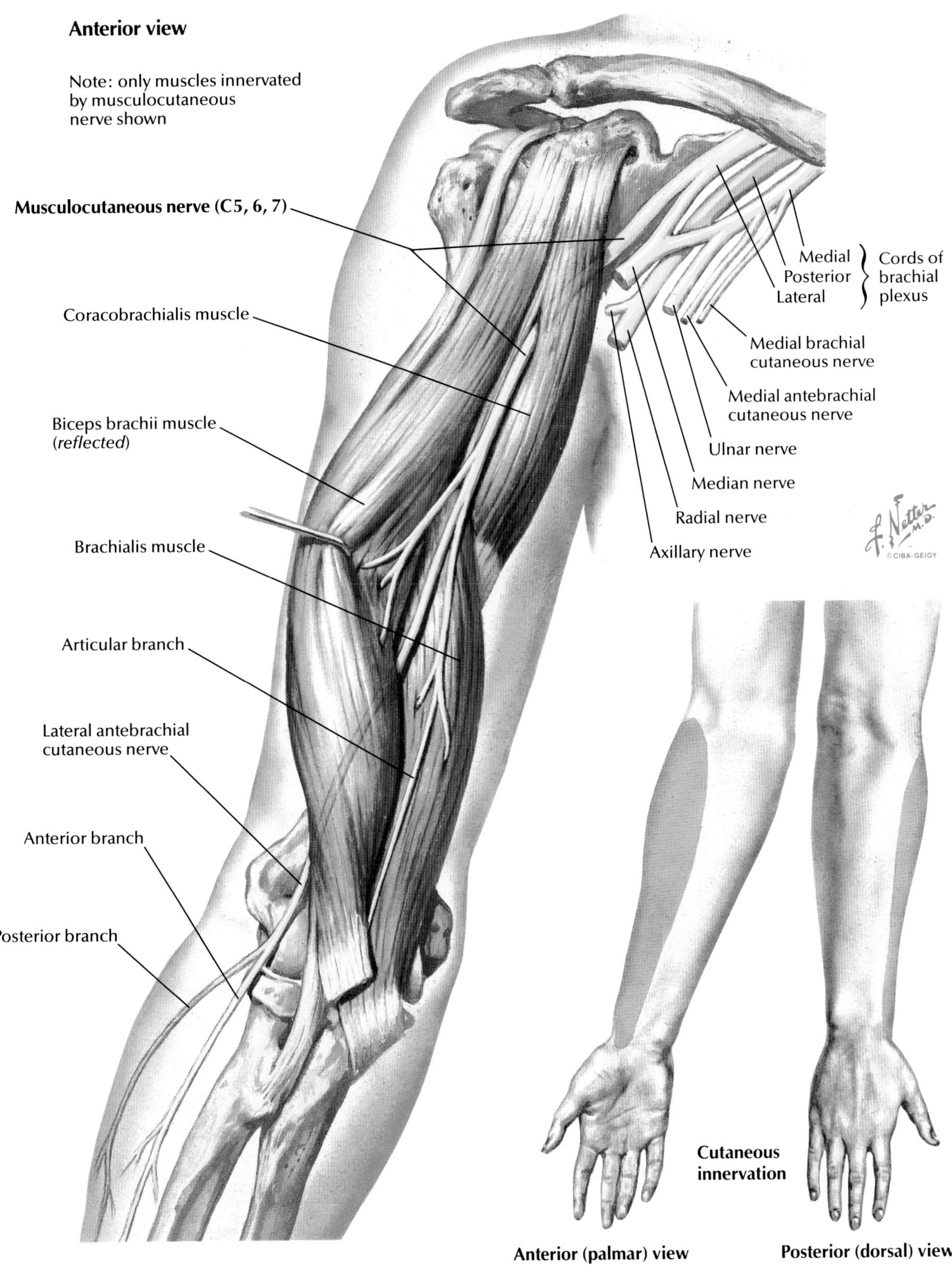

Anterior view

Note: only muscles innervated by musculocutaneous nerve shown

Musculocutaneous nerve (C5, 6, 7)

Coracobrachialis muscle

Biceps brachii muscle (*reflected*)

Brachialis muscle

Articular branch

Lateral antebrachial cutaneous nerve

Anterior branch

Posterior branch

Medial
Posterior } Cords of
Lateral } brachial
plexus

Medial brachial cutaneous nerve

Medial antebrachial cutaneous nerve

Ulnar nerve

Median nerve

Radial nerve

Axillary nerve

Cutaneous innervation

Anterior (palmar) view

Posterior (dorsal) view

Median Nerve

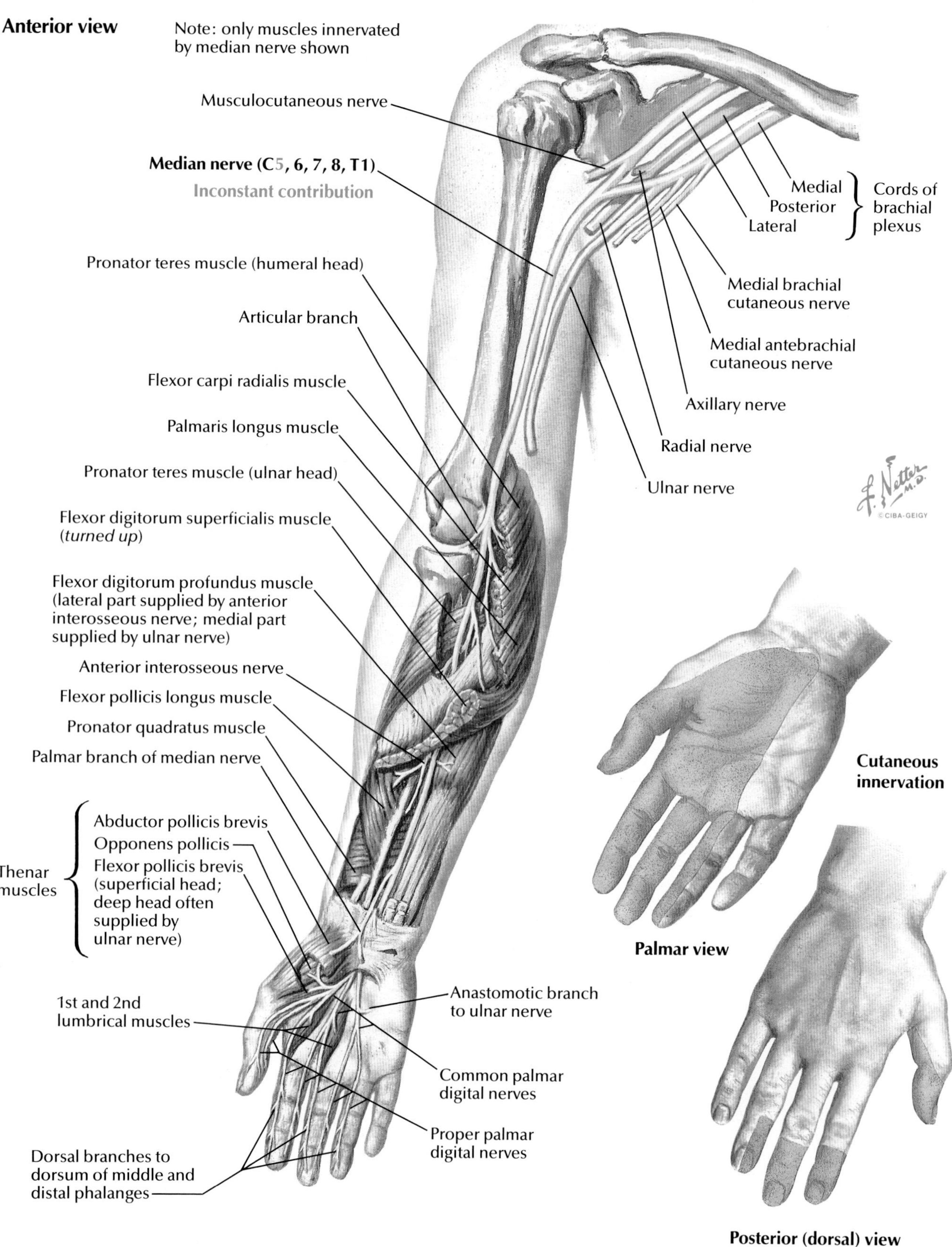

Anterior view

Note: only muscles innervated by median nerve shown

Musculocutaneous nerve

Median nerve (C5, 6, 7, 8, T1)
Inconstant contribution

Pronator teres muscle (humeral head)

Articular branch

Flexor carpi radialis muscle

Palmaris longus muscle

Pronator teres muscle (ulnar head)

Flexor digitorum superficialis muscle (*turned up*)

Flexor digitorum profundus muscle (lateral part supplied by anterior interosseous nerve; medial part supplied by ulnar nerve)

Anterior interosseous nerve

Flexor pollicis longus muscle

Pronator quadratus muscle

Palmar branch of median nerve

Thenar muscles
- Abductor pollicis brevis
- Opponens pollicis
- Flexor pollicis brevis (superficial head; deep head often supplied by ulnar nerve)

1st and 2nd lumbrical muscles

Dorsal branches to dorsum of middle and distal phalanges

Medial
Posterior
Lateral

Cords of brachial plexus

Medial brachial cutaneous nerve

Medial antebrachial cutaneous nerve

Axillary nerve

Radial nerve

Ulnar nerve

Anastomotic branch to ulnar nerve

Common palmar digital nerves

Proper palmar digital nerves

Cutaneous innervation

Palmar view

Posterior (dorsal) view

PLATE 448

UPPER LIMB

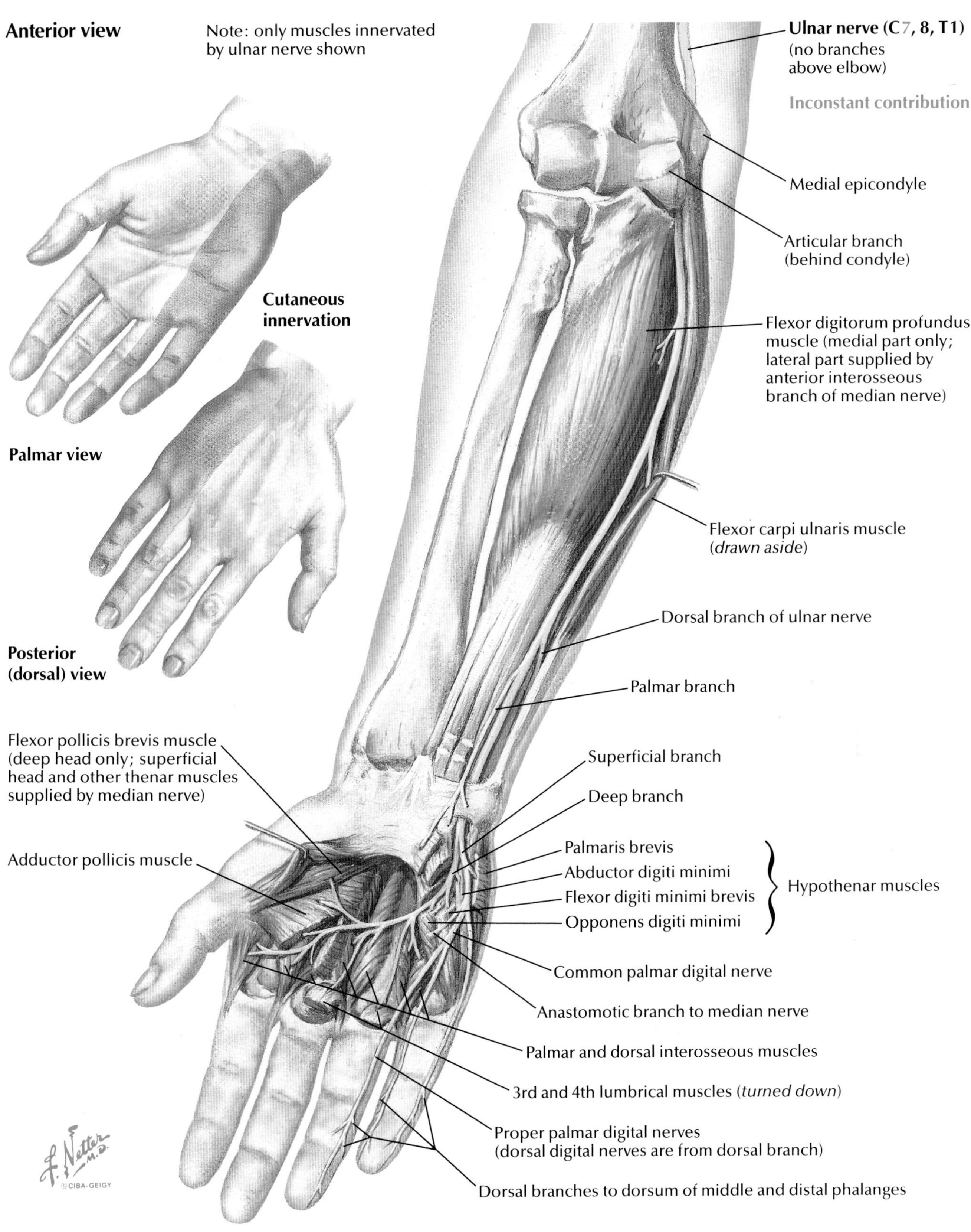

Anterior view

Note: only muscles innervated by ulnar nerve shown

Cutaneous innervation

Palmar view

Posterior (dorsal) view

Ulnar nerve (C7, 8, T1) (no branches above elbow)

Inconstant contribution

Medial epicondyle

Articular branch (behind condyle)

Flexor digitorum profundus muscle (medial part only; lateral part supplied by anterior interosseous branch of median nerve)

Flexor carpi ulnaris muscle (*drawn aside*)

Dorsal branch of ulnar nerve

Palmar branch

Flexor pollicis brevis muscle (deep head only; superficial head and other thenar muscles supplied by median nerve)

Adductor pollicis muscle

Superficial branch

Deep branch

Palmaris brevis
Abductor digiti minimi
Flexor digiti minimi brevis
Opponens digiti minimi
} Hypothenar muscles

Common palmar digital nerve

Anastomotic branch to median nerve

Palmar and dorsal interosseous muscles

3rd and 4th lumbrical muscles (*turned down*)

Proper palmar digital nerves (dorsal digital nerves are from dorsal branch)

Dorsal branches to dorsum of middle and distal phalanges

©CIBA-GEIGY

NEUROVASCULATURE

PLATE 449

Radial Nerve in Arm and Nerves of Posterior Shoulder

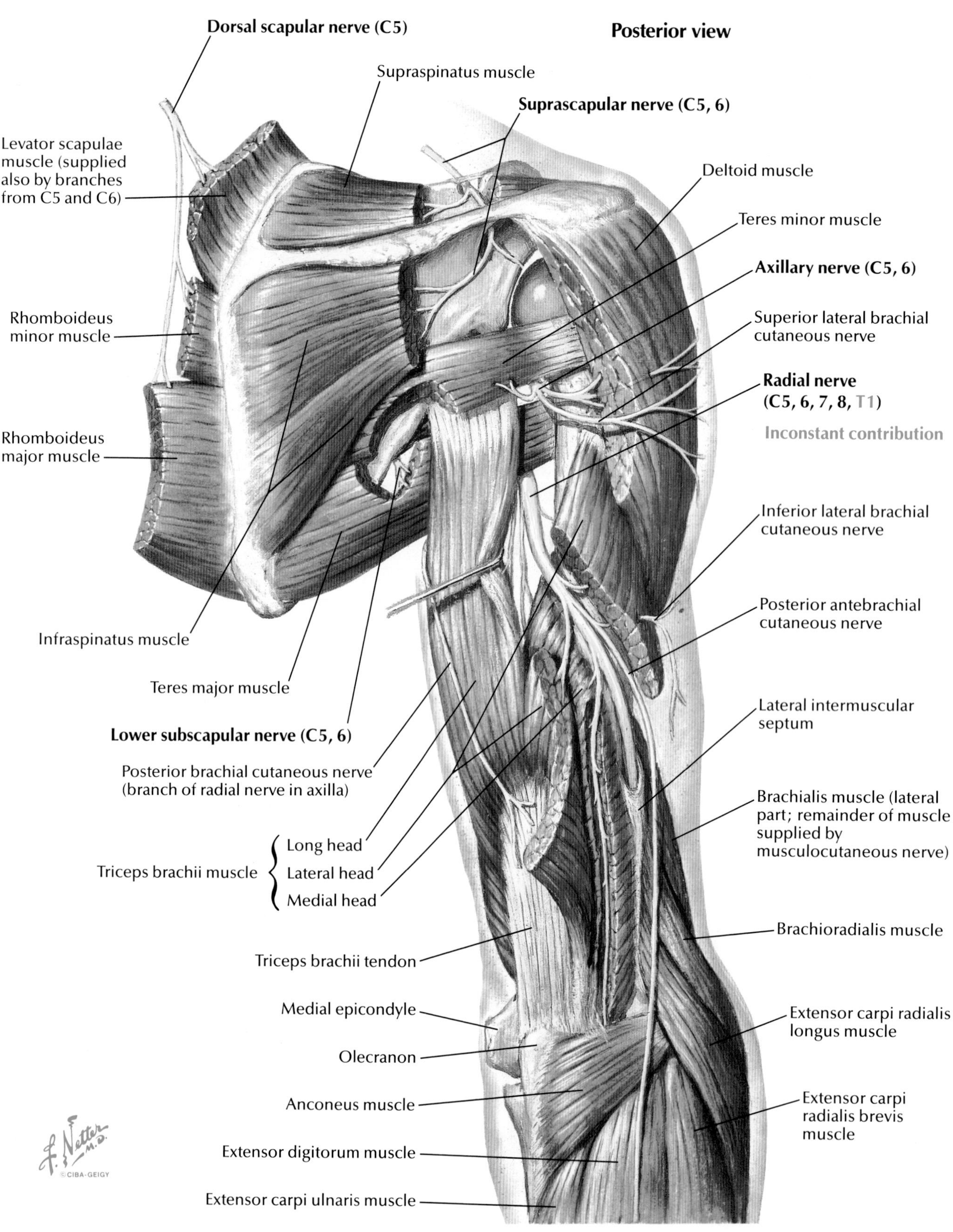

Dorsal scapular nerve (C5)

Posterior view

Supraspinatus muscle

Suprascapular nerve (C5, 6)

Levator scapulae muscle (supplied also by branches from C5 and C6)

Deltoid muscle

Teres minor muscle

Axillary nerve (C5, 6)

Rhomboideus minor muscle

Superior lateral brachial cutaneous nerve

Radial nerve (C5, 6, 7, 8, T1)

Inconstant contribution

Rhomboideus major muscle

Inferior lateral brachial cutaneous nerve

Posterior antebrachial cutaneous nerve

Infraspinatus muscle

Teres major muscle

Lateral intermuscular septum

Lower subscapular nerve (C5, 6)

Posterior brachial cutaneous nerve (branch of radial nerve in axilla)

Brachialis muscle (lateral part; remainder of muscle supplied by musculocutaneous nerve)

Long head
Lateral head
Medial head

Triceps brachii muscle

Brachioradialis muscle

Triceps brachii tendon

Medial epicondyle

Extensor carpi radialis longus muscle

Olecranon

Anconeus muscle

Extensor carpi radialis brevis muscle

Extensor digitorum muscle

Extensor carpi ulnaris muscle

PLATE 450

UPPER LIMB

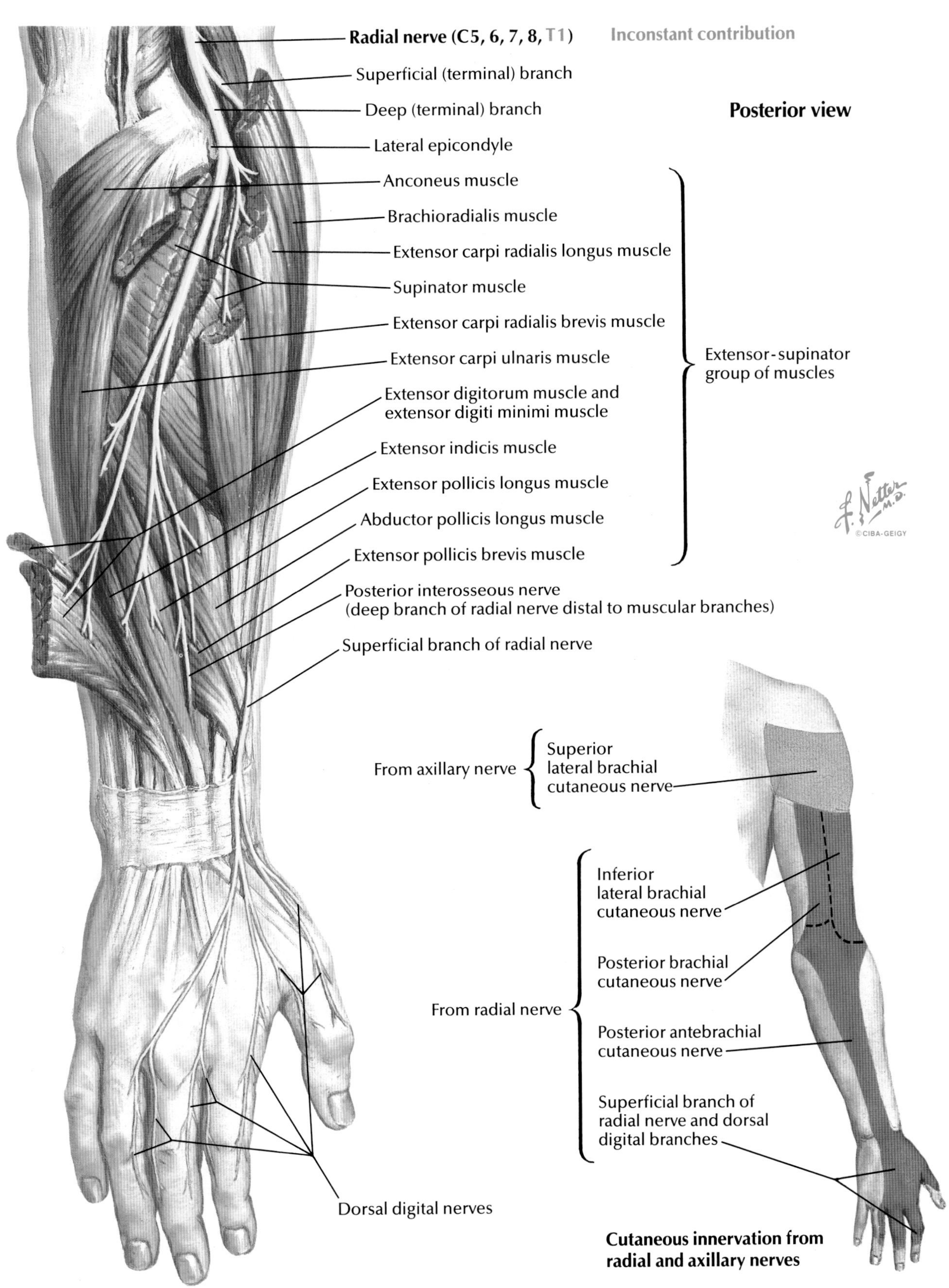

Radial nerve (C5, 6, 7, 8, T1) Inconstant contribution

Superficial (terminal) branch

Deep (terminal) branch

Lateral epicondyle

Posterior view

Anconeus muscle

Brachioradialis muscle

Extensor carpi radialis longus muscle

Supinator muscle

Extensor carpi radialis brevis muscle

Extensor carpi ulnaris muscle

Extensor digitorum muscle and extensor digiti minimi muscle

Extensor indicis muscle

Extensor pollicis longus muscle

Abductor pollicis longus muscle

Extensor pollicis brevis muscle

Extensor-supinator group of muscles

Posterior interosseous nerve (deep branch of radial nerve distal to muscular branches)

Superficial branch of radial nerve

From axillary nerve {
Superior lateral brachial cutaneous nerve

From radial nerve {
Inferior lateral brachial cutaneous nerve

Posterior brachial cutaneous nerve

Posterior antebrachial cutaneous nerve

Superficial branch of radial nerve and dorsal digital branches

Dorsal digital nerves

Cutaneous innervation from radial and axillary nerves

Cutaneous Nerves and Superficial Veins of Shoulder and Arm

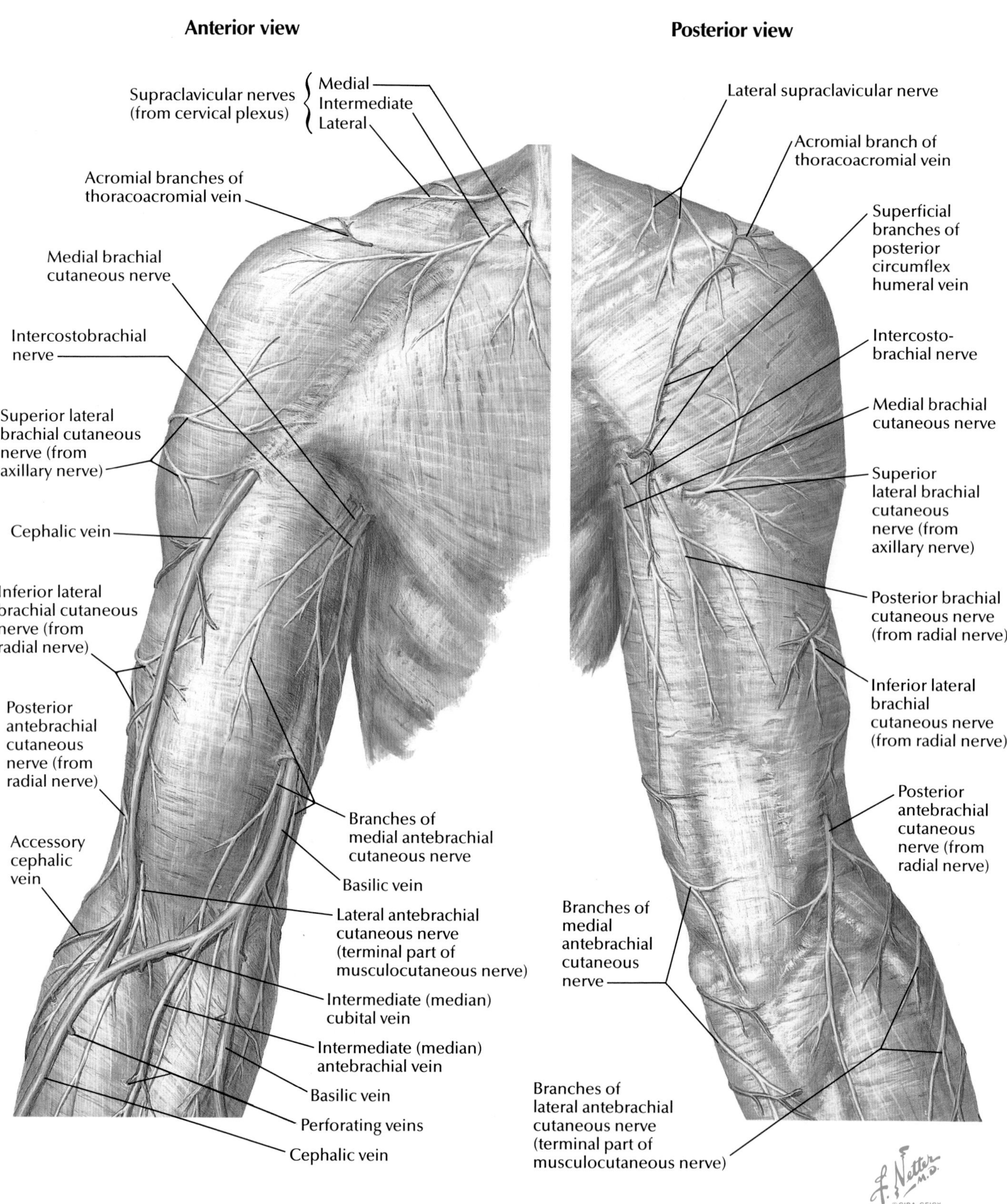

Anterior view

Supraclavicular nerves (from cervical plexus) { Medial, Intermediate, Lateral

Acromial branches of thoracoacromial vein

Medial brachial cutaneous nerve

Intercostobrachial nerve

Superior lateral brachial cutaneous nerve (from axillary nerve)

Cephalic vein

Inferior lateral brachial cutaneous nerve (from radial nerve)

Posterior antebrachial cutaneous nerve (from radial nerve)

Accessory cephalic vein

Branches of medial antebrachial cutaneous nerve

Basilic vein

Lateral antebrachial cutaneous nerve (terminal part of musculocutaneous nerve)

Intermediate (median) cubital vein

Intermediate (median) antebrachial vein

Basilic vein

Perforating veins

Cephalic vein

Posterior view

Lateral supraclavicular nerve

Acromial branch of thoracoacromial vein

Superficial branches of posterior circumflex humeral vein

Intercostobrachial nerve

Medial brachial cutaneous nerve

Superior lateral brachial cutaneous nerve (from axillary nerve)

Posterior brachial cutaneous nerve (from radial nerve)

Inferior lateral brachial cutaneous nerve (from radial nerve)

Posterior antebrachial cutaneous nerve (from radial nerve)

Branches of medial antebrachial cutaneous nerve

Branches of lateral antebrachial cutaneous nerve (terminal part of musculocutaneous nerve)

PLATE 452

Cutaneous Nerves and Superficial Veins of Forearm

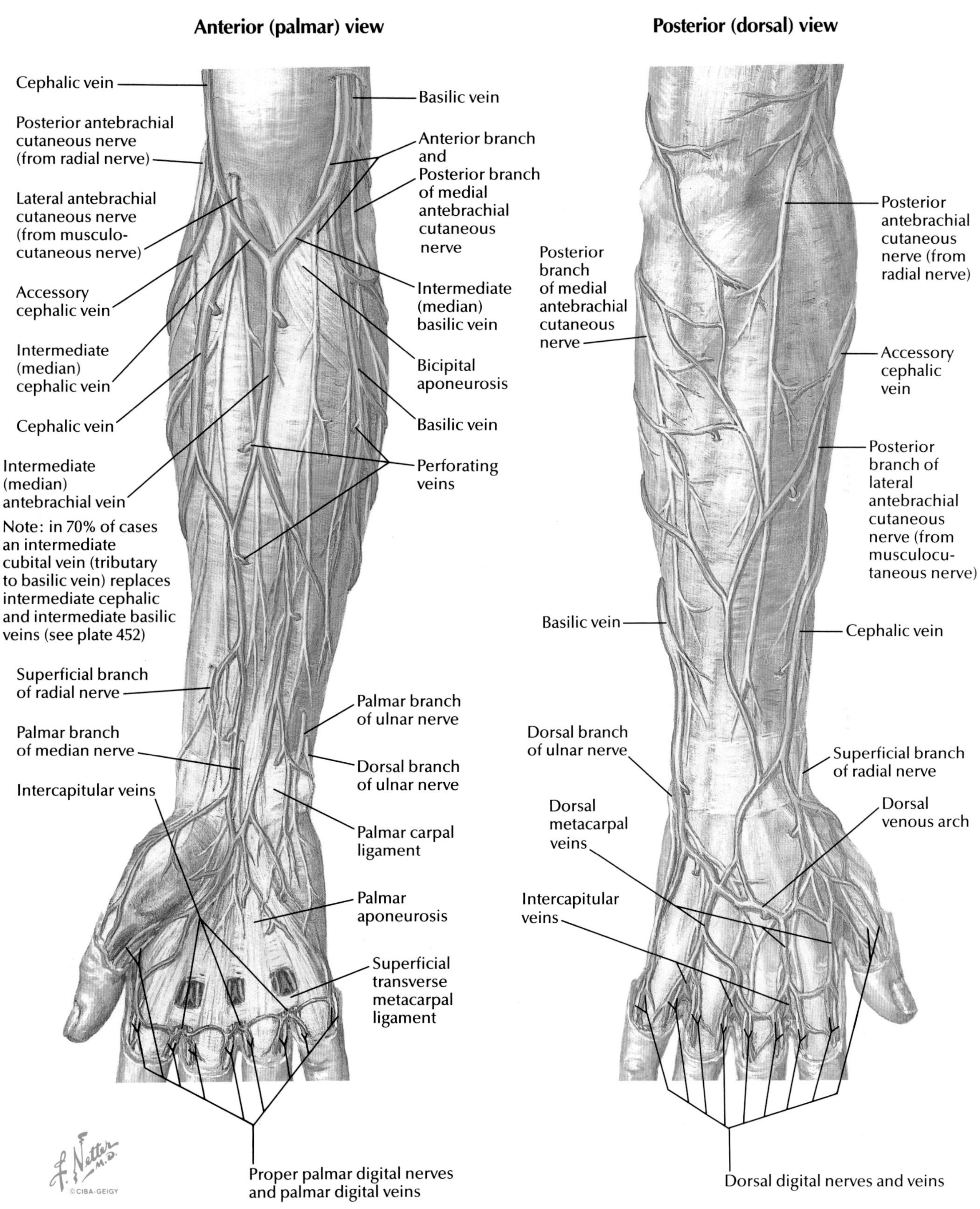

Anterior (palmar) view

Cephalic vein

Posterior antebrachial cutaneous nerve (from radial nerve)

Lateral antebrachial cutaneous nerve (from musculo-cutaneous nerve)

Accessory cephalic vein

Intermediate (median) cephalic vein

Cephalic vein

Intermediate (median) antebrachial vein

Note: in 70% of cases an intermediate cubital vein (tributary to basilic vein) replaces intermediate cephalic and intermediate basilic veins (see plate 452)

Superficial branch of radial nerve

Palmar branch of median nerve

Intercapitular veins

Basilic vein

Anterior branch and Posterior branch of medial antebrachial cutaneous nerve

Intermediate (median) basilic vein

Bicipital aponeurosis

Basilic vein

Perforating veins

Palmar branch of ulnar nerve

Dorsal branch of ulnar nerve

Palmar carpal ligament

Palmar aponeurosis

Superficial transverse metacarpal ligament

Proper palmar digital nerves and palmar digital veins

Posterior (dorsal) view

Posterior branch of medial antebrachial cutaneous nerve

Posterior antebrachial cutaneous nerve (from radial nerve)

Accessory cephalic vein

Posterior branch of lateral antebrachial cutaneous nerve (from musculocutaneous nerve)

Cephalic vein

Basilic vein

Dorsal branch of ulnar nerve

Dorsal metacarpal veins

Intercapitular veins

Superficial branch of radial nerve

Dorsal venous arch

Dorsal digital nerves and veins

NEUROVASCULATURE

PLATE 453

Cutaneous Innervation of Upper Limb

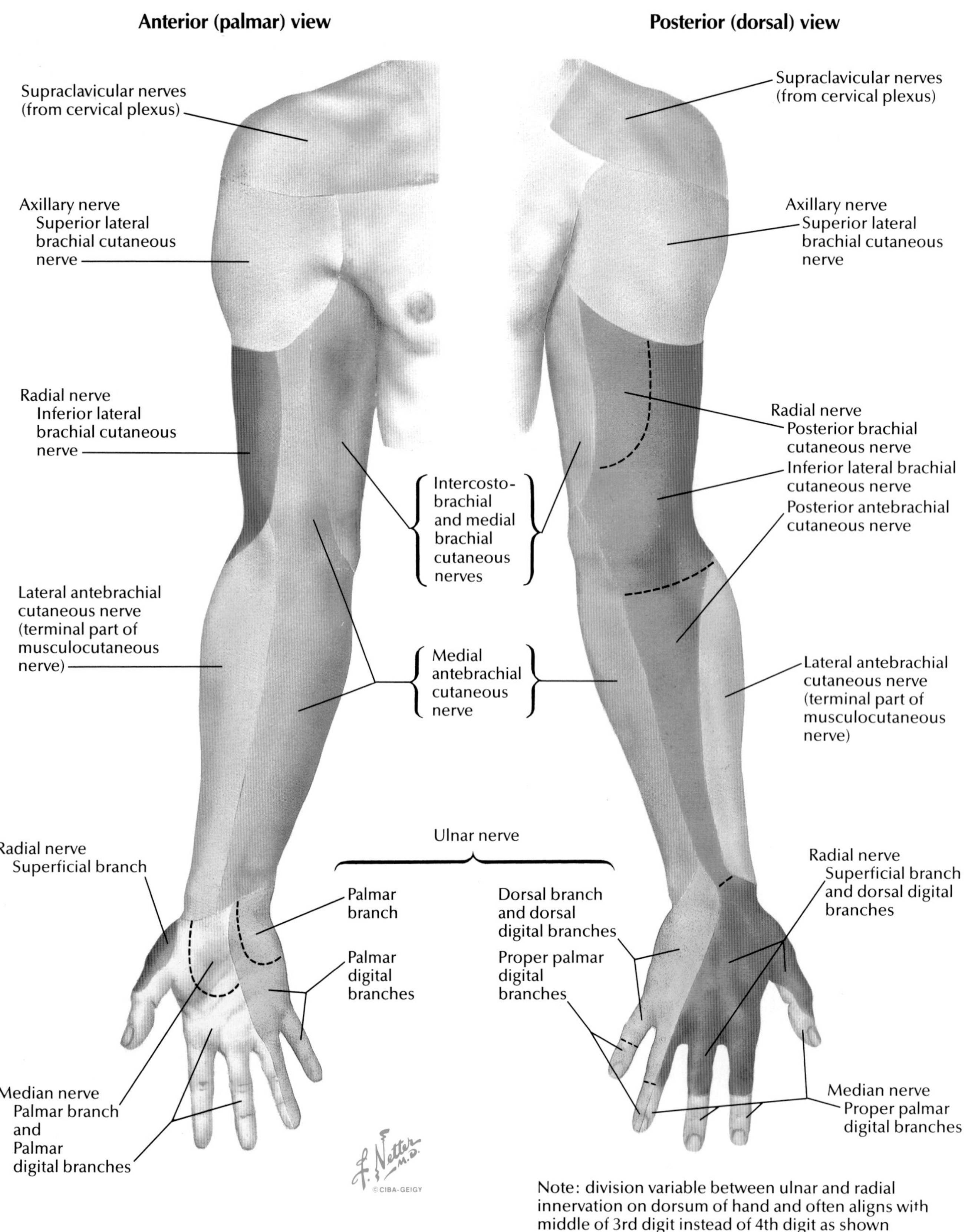

Anterior (palmar) view

Supraclavicular nerves (from cervical plexus)

Axillary nerve
Superior lateral brachial cutaneous nerve

Radial nerve
Inferior lateral brachial cutaneous nerve

Lateral antebrachial cutaneous nerve (terminal part of musculocutaneous nerve)

Intercosto-brachial and medial brachial cutaneous nerves

Medial antebrachial cutaneous nerve

Radial nerve
Superficial branch

Median nerve
Palmar branch and
Palmar digital branches

Posterior (dorsal) view

Supraclavicular nerves (from cervical plexus)

Axillary nerve
Superior lateral brachial cutaneous nerve

Radial nerve
Posterior brachial cutaneous nerve
Inferior lateral brachial cutaneous nerve
Posterior antebrachial cutaneous nerve

Lateral antebrachial cutaneous nerve (terminal part of musculocutaneous nerve)

Radial nerve
Superficial branch and dorsal digital branches

Median nerve
Proper palmar digital branches

Ulnar nerve

Palmar branch

Palmar digital branches

Dorsal branch and dorsal digital branches

Proper palmar digital branches

Note: division variable between ulnar and radial innervation on dorsum of hand and often aligns with middle of 3rd digit instead of 4th digit as shown

PLATE 454

UPPER LIMB

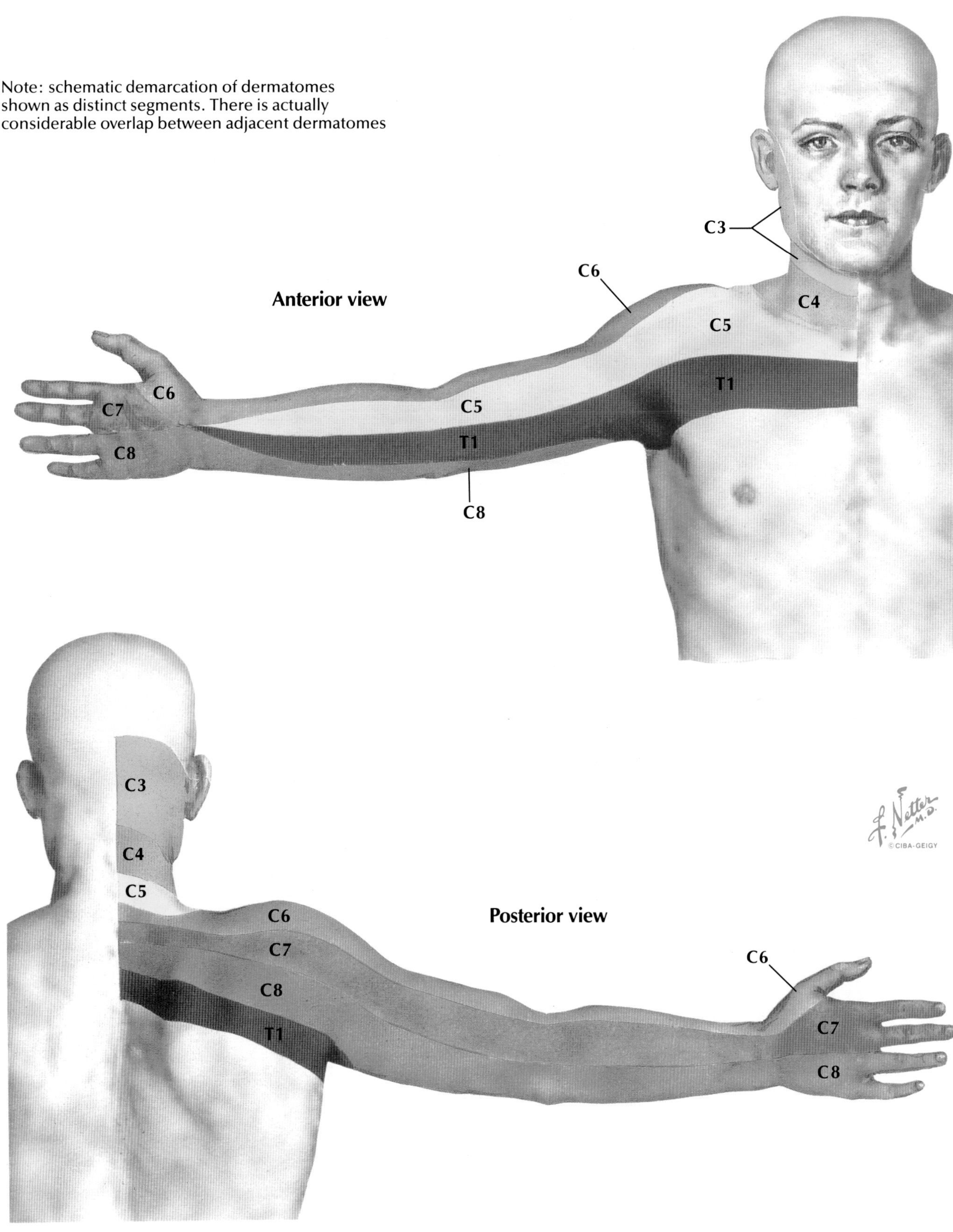

Note: schematic demarcation of dermatomes shown as distinct segments. There is actually considerable overlap between adjacent dermatomes

Anterior view

Posterior view

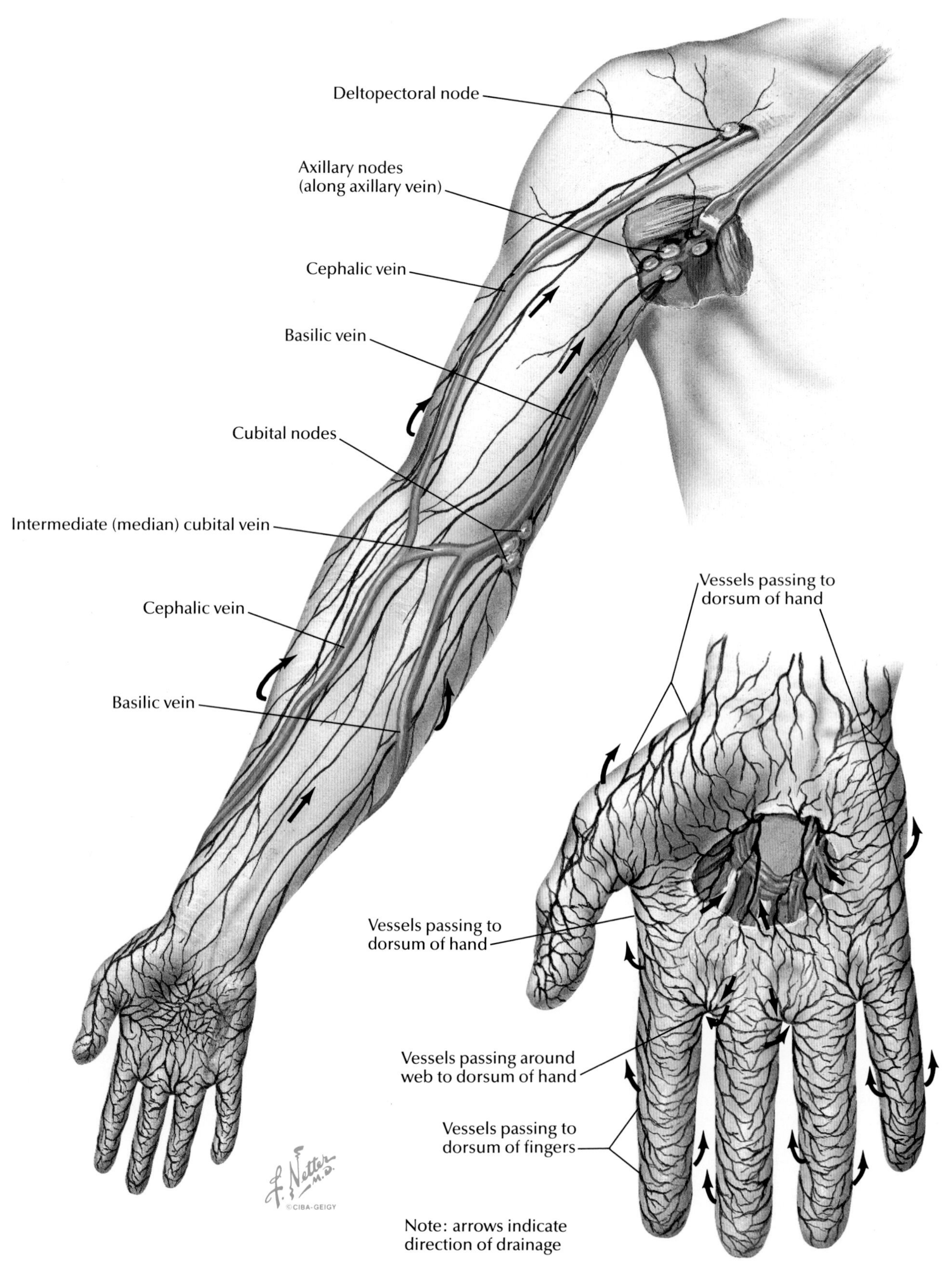

Deltopectoral node

Axillary nodes
(along axillary vein)

Cephalic vein

Basilic vein

Cubital nodes

Intermediate (median) cubital vein

Cephalic vein

Basilic vein

Vessels passing to
dorsum of hand

Vessels passing to
dorsum of hand

Vessels passing around
web to dorsum of hand

Vessels passing to
dorsum of fingers

Note: arrows indicate
direction of drainage

PLATE 456

UPPER LIMB

Section VII

LOWER LIMB

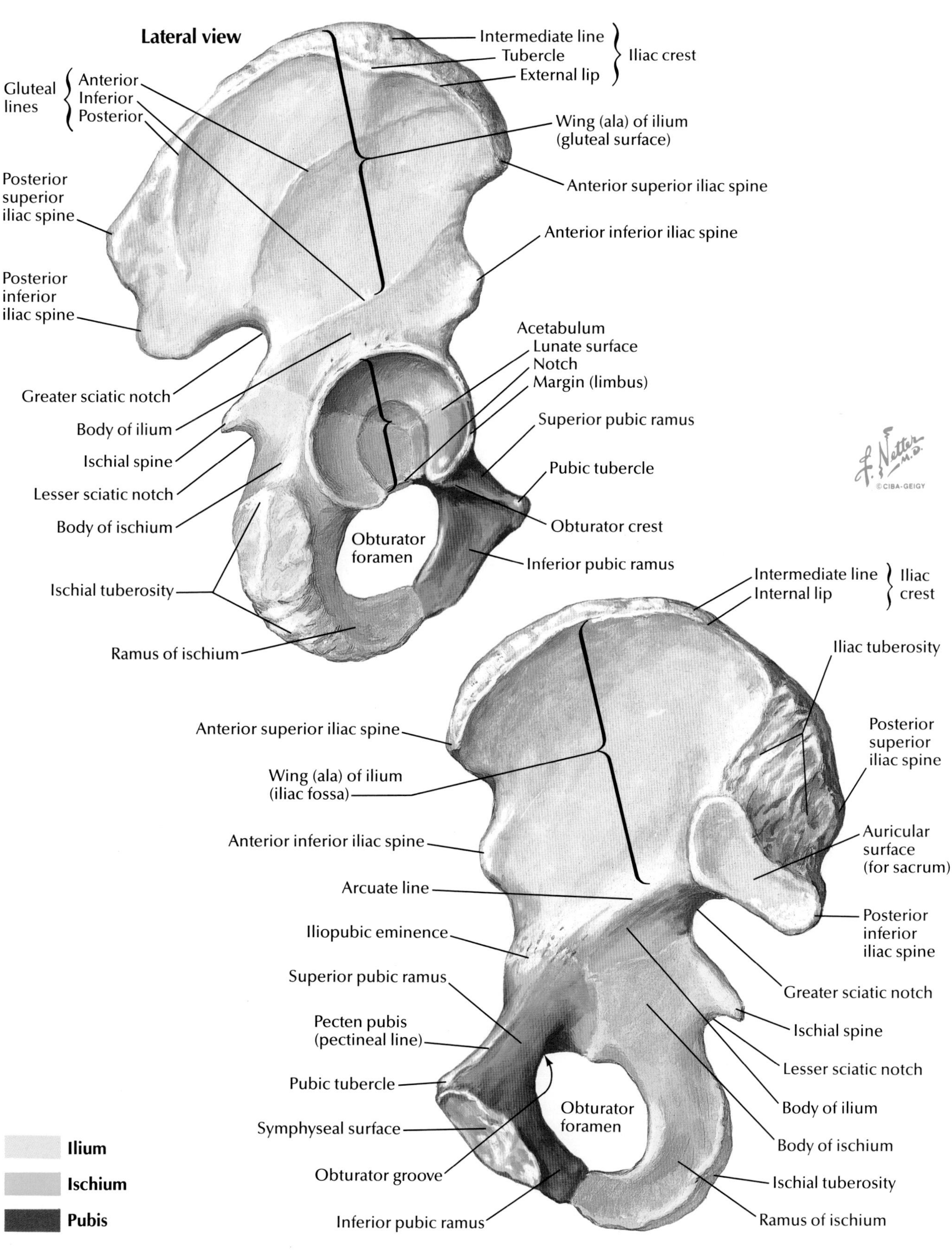

Lateral view

Intermediate line
Tubercle } Iliac crest
External lip

Gluteal lines {
Anterior
Inferior
Posterior

Wing (ala) of ilium (gluteal surface)

Anterior superior iliac spine

Posterior superior iliac spine

Anterior inferior iliac spine

Posterior inferior iliac spine

Acetabulum
Lunate surface
Notch
Margin (limbus)

Greater sciatic notch

Superior pubic ramus

Body of ilium

Ischial spine

Pubic tubercle

Lesser sciatic notch

Body of ischium

Obturator crest

Ischial tuberosity

Obturator foramen

Inferior pubic ramus

Ramus of ischium

Intermediate line
Internal lip } Iliac crest

Iliac tuberosity

Anterior superior iliac spine

Posterior superior iliac spine

Wing (ala) of ilium (iliac fossa)

Anterior inferior iliac spine

Auricular surface (for sacrum)

Arcuate line

Iliopubic eminence

Posterior inferior iliac spine

Superior pubic ramus

Pecten pubis (pectineal line)

Greater sciatic notch

Pubic tubercle

Ischial spine

Symphyseal surface

Lesser sciatic notch

Obturator foramen

Body of ilium

Obturator groove

Body of ischium

Inferior pubic ramus

Ischial tuberosity

Ramus of ischium

Ilium
Ischium
Pubis

Hip Joint

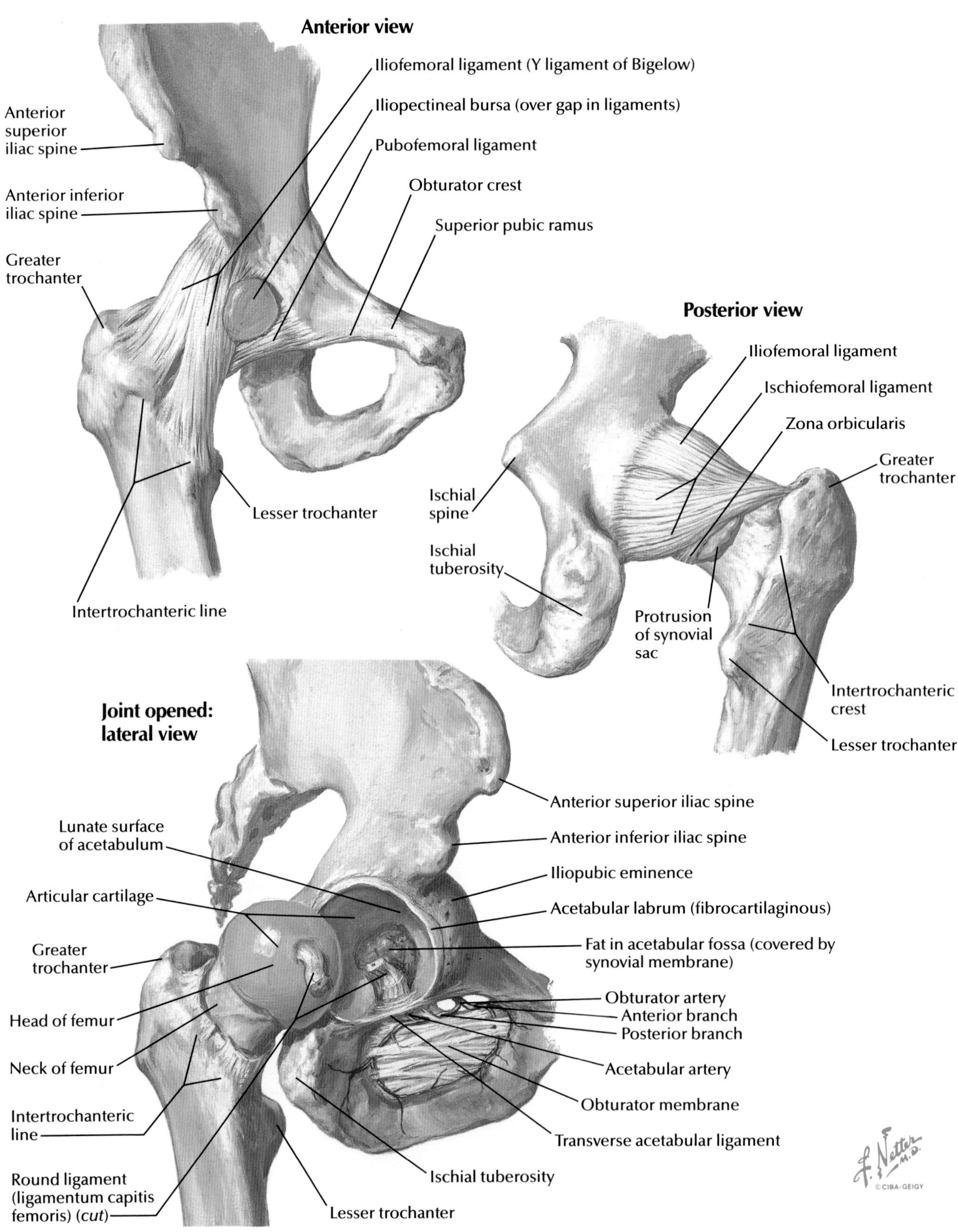

Anterior view

Anterior superior iliac spine

Anterior inferior iliac spine

Greater trochanter

Intertrochanteric line

Iliofemoral ligament (Y ligament of Bigelow)

Iliopectineal bursa (over gap in ligaments)

Pubofemoral ligament

Obturator crest

Superior pubic ramus

Lesser trochanter

Posterior view

Iliofemoral ligament

Ischiofemoral ligament

Zona orbicularis

Greater trochanter

Ischial spine

Ischial tuberosity

Protrusion of synovial sac

Intertrochanteric crest

Lesser trochanter

Joint opened: lateral view

Lunate surface of acetabulum

Articular cartilage

Greater trochanter

Head of femur

Neck of femur

Intertrochanteric line

Round ligament (ligamentum capitis femoris) (*cut*)

Anterior superior iliac spine

Anterior inferior iliac spine

Iliopubic eminence

Acetabular labrum (fibrocartilaginous)

Fat in acetabular fossa (covered by synovial membrane)

Obturator artery

Anterior branch

Posterior branch

Acetabular artery

Obturator membrane

Transverse acetabular ligament

Ischial tuberosity

Lesser trochanter

PLATE 458

LOWER LIMB

Femur

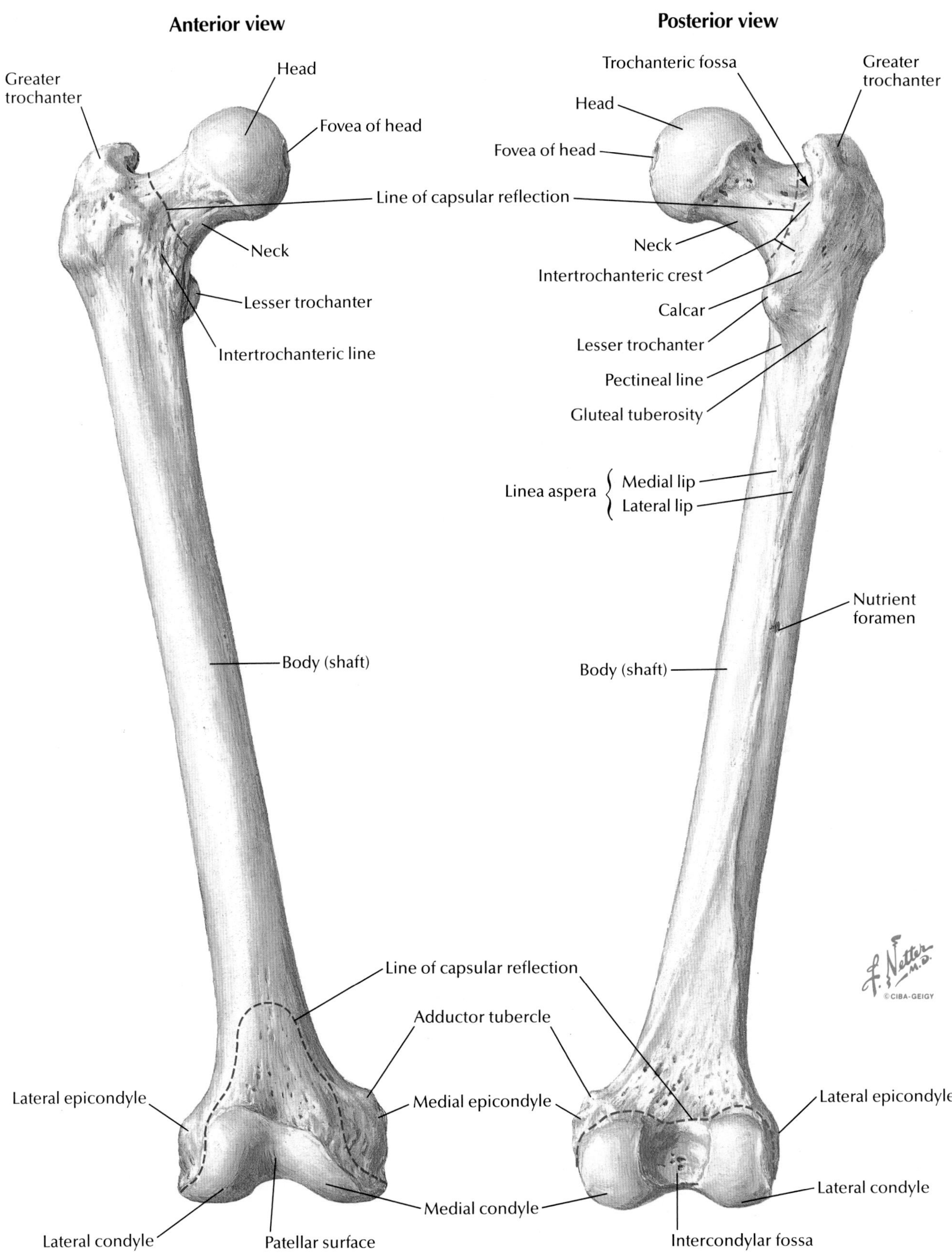

Anterior view

Greater trochanter

Head

Fovea of head

Line of capsular reflection

Neck

Lesser trochanter

Intertrochanteric line

Body (shaft)

Line of capsular reflection

Adductor tubercle

Lateral epicondyle

Medial epicondyle

Lateral condyle

Medial condyle

Patellar surface

Posterior view

Trochanteric fossa

Greater trochanter

Head

Fovea of head

Neck

Intertrochanteric crest

Calcar

Lesser trochanter

Pectineal line

Gluteal tuberosity

Linea aspera { Medial lip / Lateral lip }

Nutrient foramen

Body (shaft)

Lateral epicondyle

Lateral condyle

Intercondylar fossa

Bony Attachments of Muscles of Hip and Thigh: Anterior View

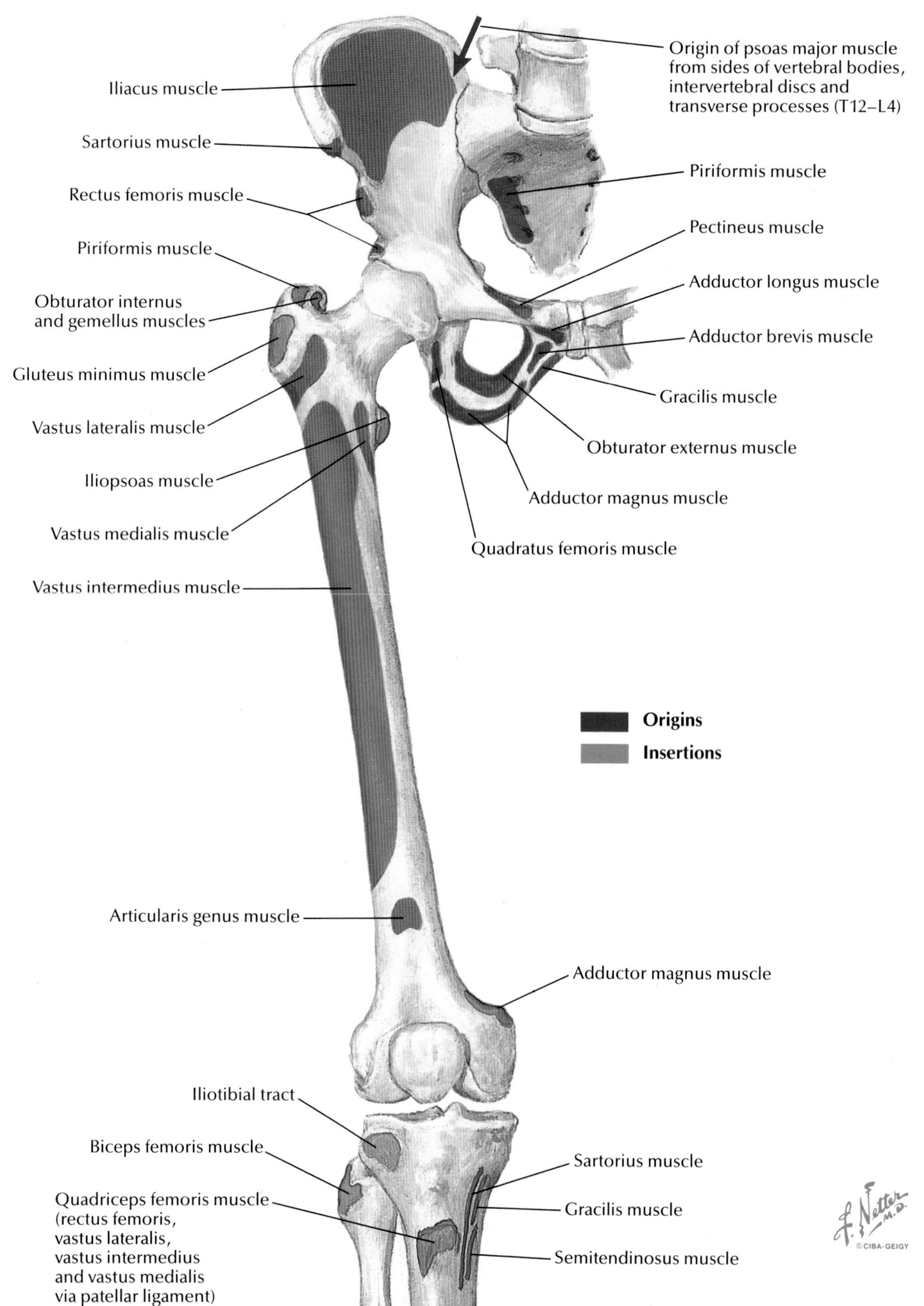

Iliacus muscle

Sartorius muscle

Rectus femoris muscle

Piriformis muscle

Obturator internus and gemellus muscles

Gluteus minimus muscle

Vastus lateralis muscle

Iliopsoas muscle

Vastus medialis muscle

Vastus intermedius muscle

Origin of psoas major muscle from sides of vertebral bodies, intervertebral discs and transverse processes (T12–L4)

Piriformis muscle

Pectineus muscle

Adductor longus muscle

Adductor brevis muscle

Gracilis muscle

Obturator externus muscle

Adductor magnus muscle

Quadratus femoris muscle

Origins

Insertions

Articularis genus muscle

Adductor magnus muscle

Iliotibial tract

Biceps femoris muscle

Quadriceps femoris muscle (rectus femoris, vastus lateralis, vastus intermedius and vastus medialis via patellar ligament)

Sartorius muscle

Gracilis muscle

Semitendinosus muscle

PLATE 460

LOWER LIMB

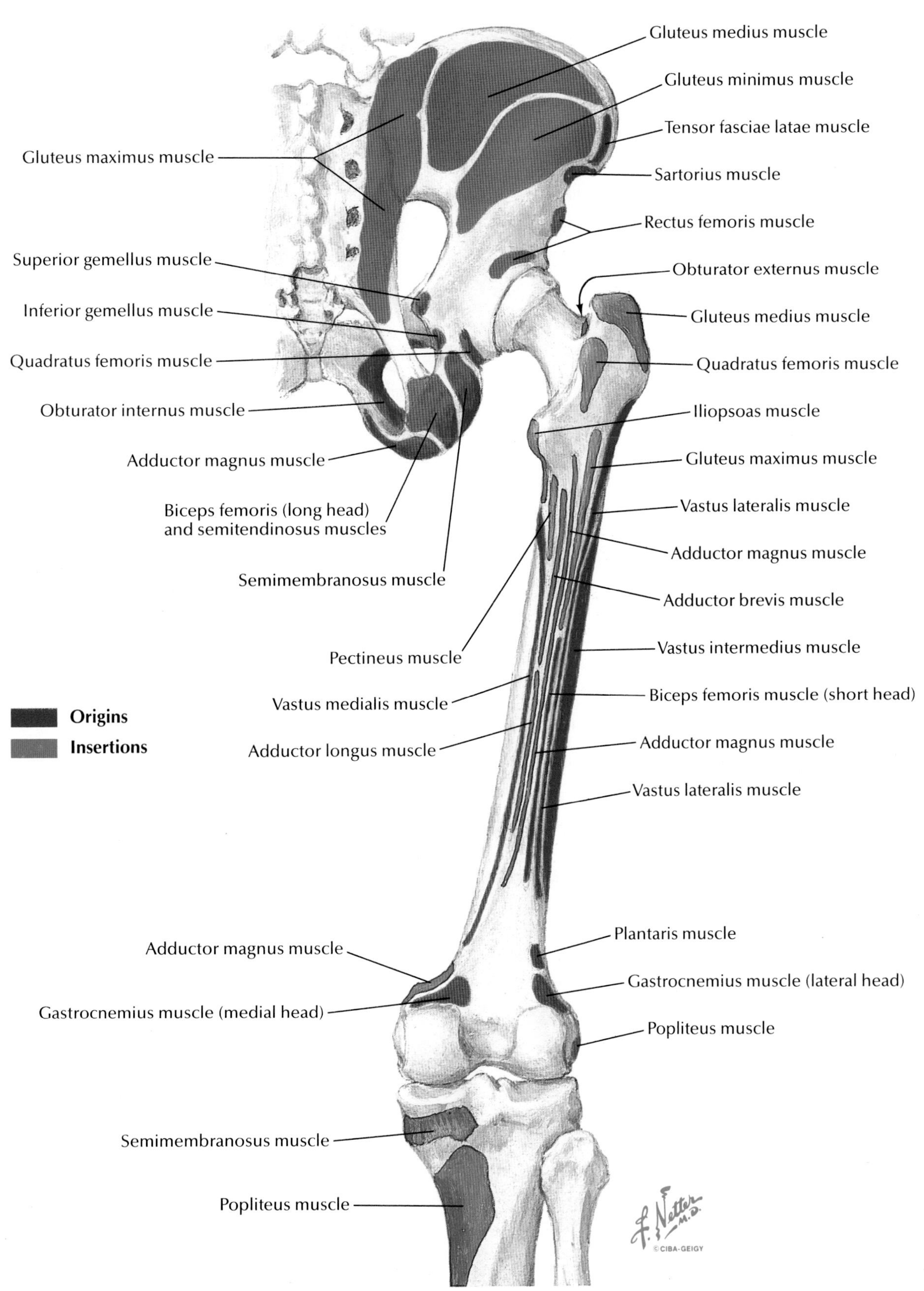

Gluteus medius muscle

Gluteus minimus muscle

Tensor fasciae latae muscle

Sartorius muscle

Rectus femoris muscle

Obturator externus muscle

Gluteus medius muscle

Quadratus femoris muscle

Iliopsoas muscle

Gluteus maximus muscle

Vastus lateralis muscle

Adductor magnus muscle

Adductor brevis muscle

Vastus intermedius muscle

Biceps femoris muscle (short head)

Adductor magnus muscle

Vastus lateralis muscle

Plantaris muscle

Gastrocnemius muscle (lateral head)

Popliteus muscle

Gluteus maximus muscle

Superior gemellus muscle

Inferior gemellus muscle

Quadratus femoris muscle

Obturator internus muscle

Adductor magnus muscle

Biceps femoris (long head)
and semitendinosus muscles

Semimembranosus muscle

Pectineus muscle

Vastus medialis muscle

Adductor longus muscle

Adductor magnus muscle

Gastrocnemius muscle (medial head)

Semimembranosus muscle

Popliteus muscle

Origins
Insertions

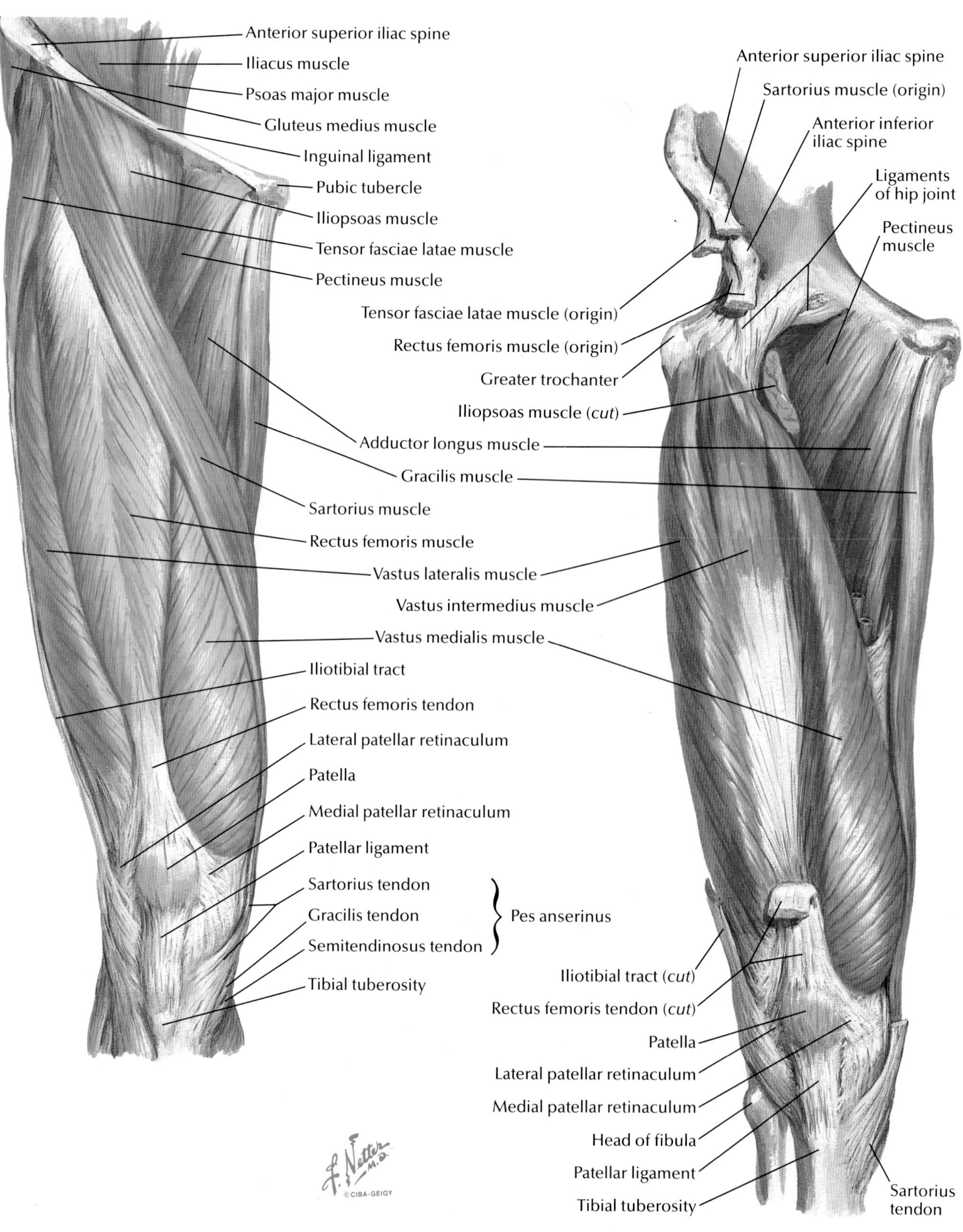

Anterior superior iliac spine
Iliacus muscle
Psoas major muscle
Gluteus medius muscle
Inguinal ligament
Pubic tubercle
Iliopsoas muscle
Tensor fasciae latae muscle
Pectineus muscle
Tensor fasciae latae muscle (origin)
Rectus femoris muscle (origin)
Greater trochanter
Iliopsoas muscle (cut)
Adductor longus muscle
Gracilis muscle
Sartorius muscle
Rectus femoris muscle
Vastus lateralis muscle
Vastus intermedius muscle
Vastus medialis muscle
Iliotibial tract
Rectus femoris tendon
Lateral patellar retinaculum
Patella
Medial patellar retinaculum
Patellar ligament
Sartorius tendon
Gracilis tendon
Semitendinosus tendon
Tibial tuberosity

} Pes anserinus

Anterior superior iliac spine
Sartorius muscle (origin)
Anterior inferior iliac spine
Ligaments of hip joint
Pectineus muscle

Iliotibial tract (cut)
Rectus femoris tendon (cut)
Patella
Lateral patellar retinaculum
Medial patellar retinaculum
Head of fibula
Patellar ligament
Tibial tuberosity
Sartorius tendon

PLATE 462

LOWER LIMB

Deep dissection

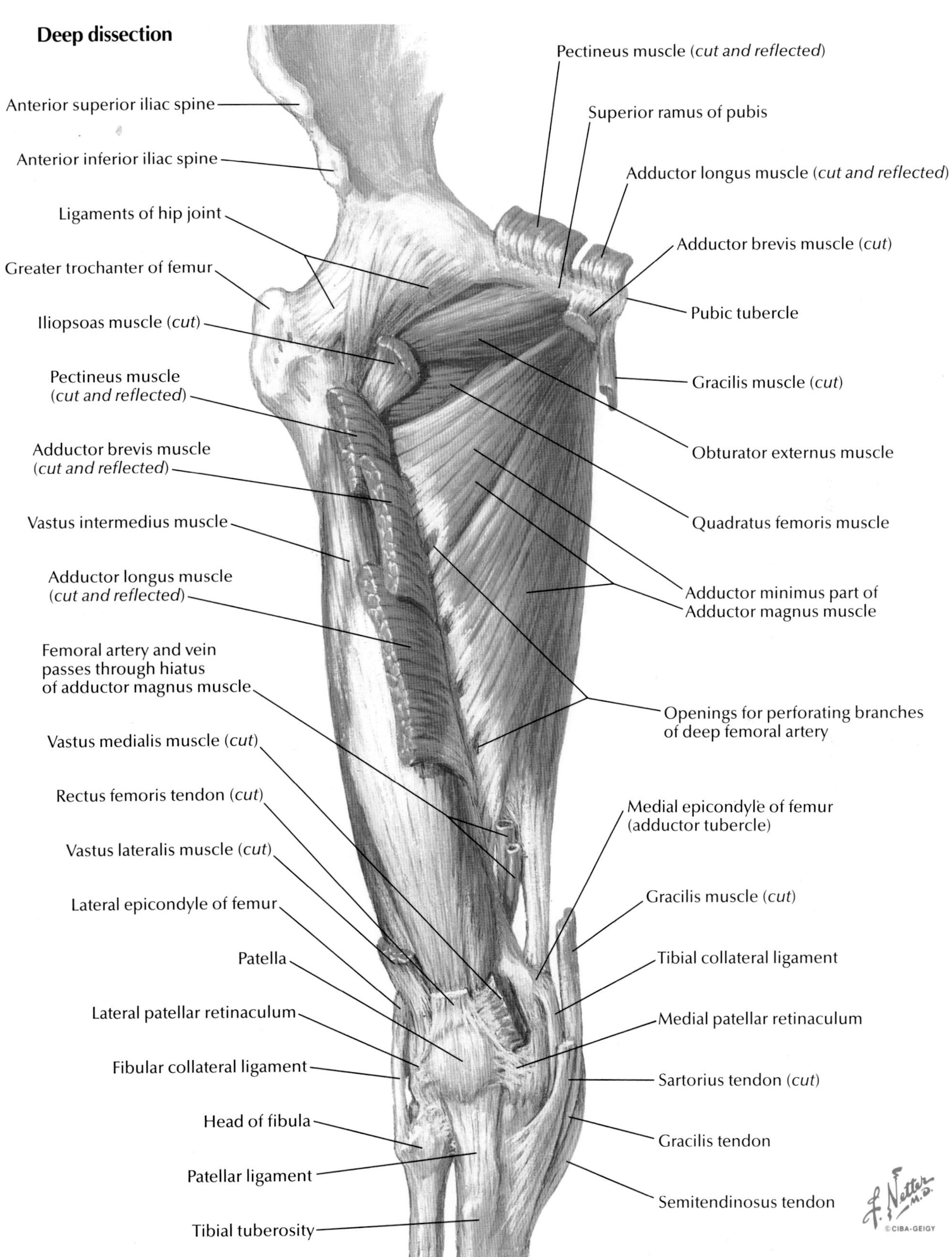

Pectineus muscle (*cut and reflected*)

Superior ramus of pubis

Adductor longus muscle (*cut and reflected*)

Adductor brevis muscle (*cut*)

Pubic tubercle

Gracilis muscle (*cut*)

Obturator externus muscle

Quadratus femoris muscle

Adductor minimus part of Adductor magnus muscle

Openings for perforating branches of deep femoral artery

Medial epicondyle of femur (adductor tubercle)

Gracilis muscle (*cut*)

Tibial collateral ligament

Medial patellar retinaculum

Sartorius tendon (*cut*)

Gracilis tendon

Semitendinosus tendon

Anterior superior iliac spine

Anterior inferior iliac spine

Ligaments of hip joint

Greater trochanter of femur

Iliopsoas muscle (*cut*)

Pectineus muscle (*cut and reflected*)

Adductor brevis muscle (*cut and reflected*)

Vastus intermedius muscle

Adductor longus muscle (*cut and reflected*)

Femoral artery and vein passes through hiatus of adductor magnus muscle

Vastus medialis muscle (*cut*)

Rectus femoris tendon (*cut*)

Vastus lateralis muscle (*cut*)

Lateral epicondyle of femur

Patella

Lateral patellar retinaculum

Fibular collateral ligament

Head of fibula

Patellar ligament

Tibial tuberosity

Muscles of Hip and Thigh: Lateral View

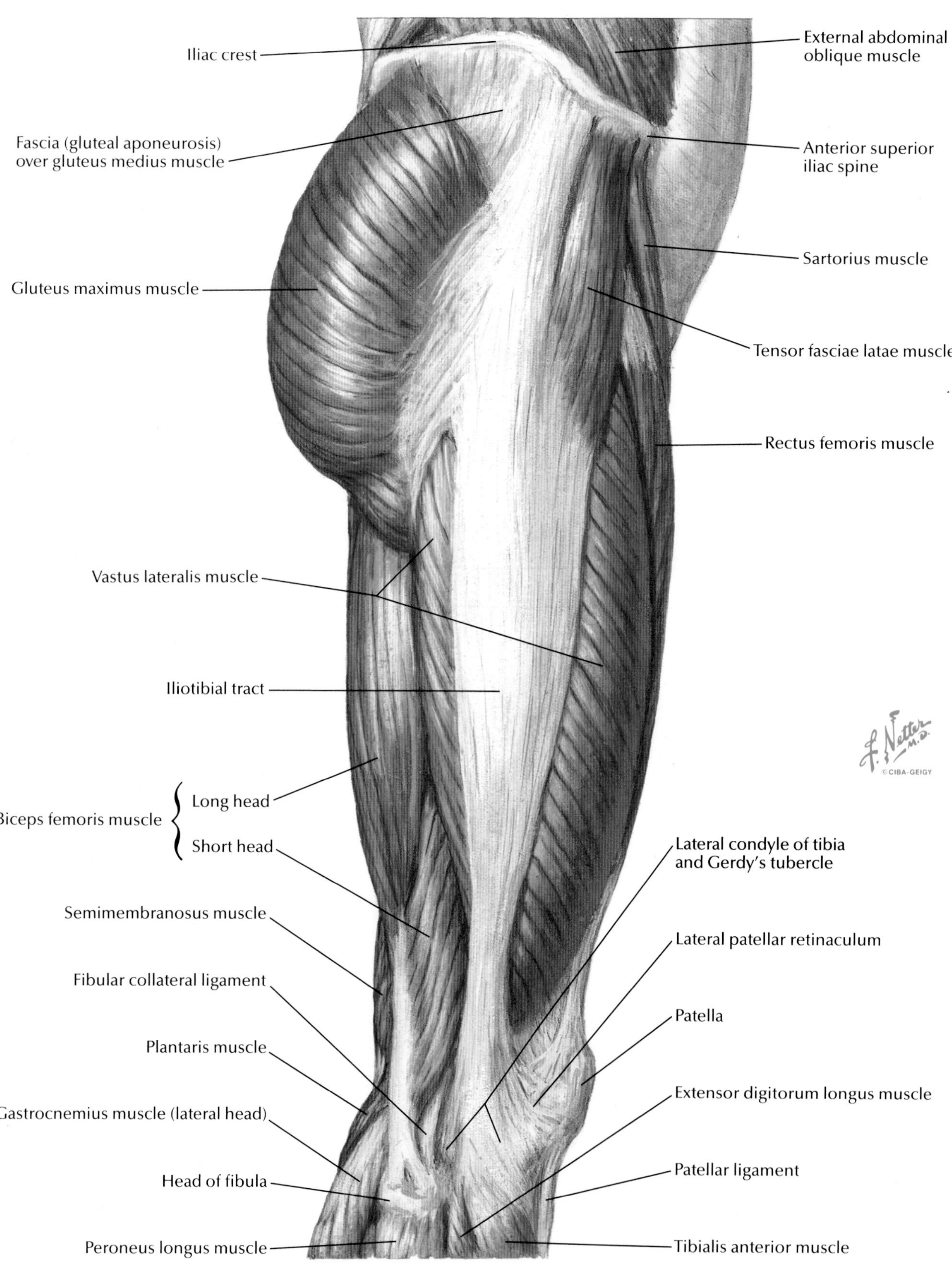

Iliac crest

External abdominal oblique muscle

Fascia (gluteal aponeurosis) over gluteus medius muscle

Anterior superior iliac spine

Gluteus maximus muscle

Sartorius muscle

Tensor fasciae latae muscle

Rectus femoris muscle

Vastus lateralis muscle

Iliotibial tract

Biceps femoris muscle { Long head / Short head

Lateral condyle of tibia and Gerdy's tubercle

Semimembranosus muscle

Lateral patellar retinaculum

Fibular collateral ligament

Patella

Plantaris muscle

Extensor digitorum longus muscle

Gastrocnemius muscle (lateral head)

Head of fibula

Patellar ligament

Peroneus longus muscle

Tibialis anterior muscle

PLATE 464

LOWER LIMB

FOR PIRIFORMIS AND OBTURATOR INTERNUS SEE ALSO PLATES 337, 338; FOR OBTURATOR EXTERNUS SEE PLATE 463

Superficial dissection

Deeper dissection

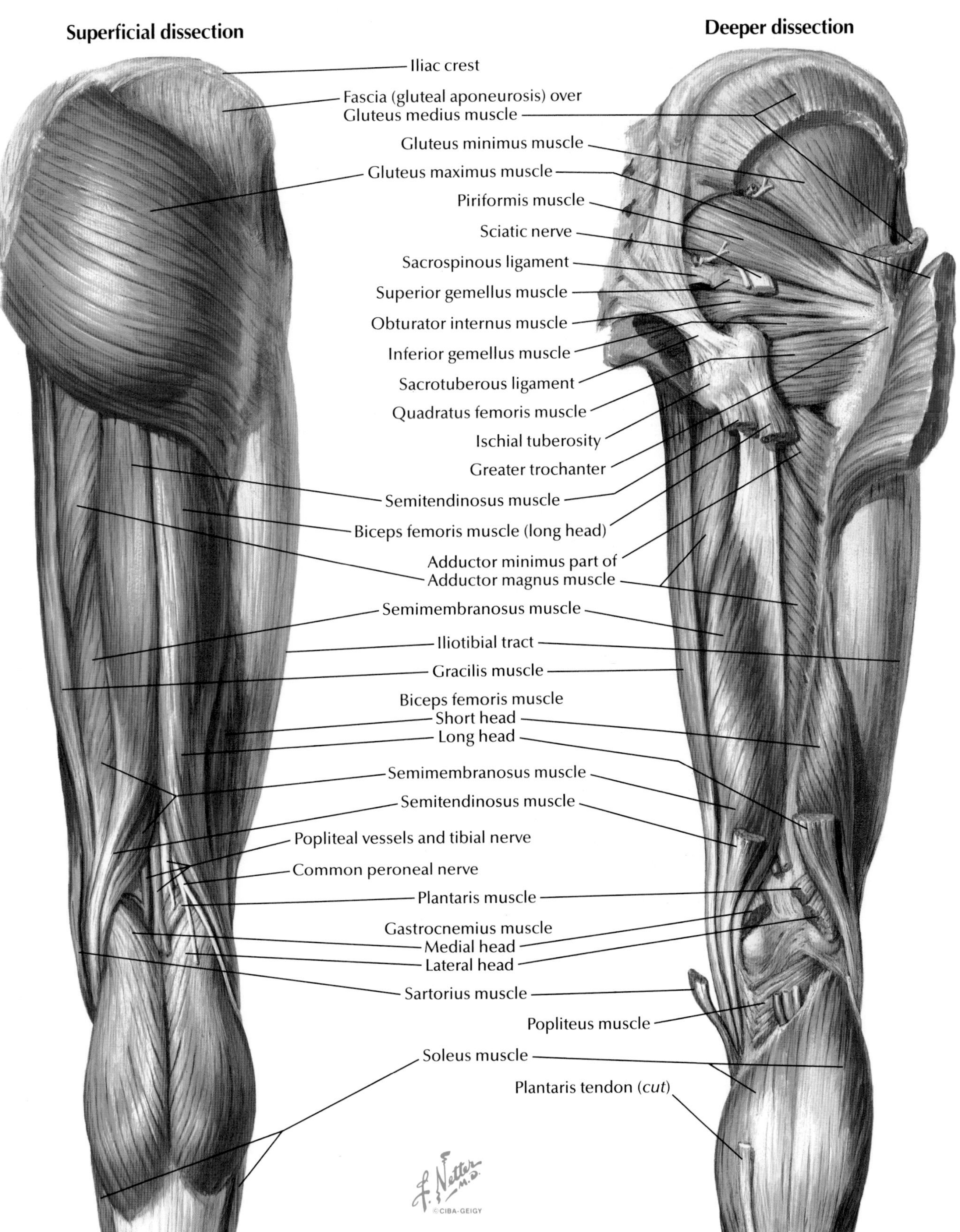

Iliac crest

Fascia (gluteal aponeurosis) over
Gluteus medius muscle

Gluteus minimus muscle

Gluteus maximus muscle

Piriformis muscle

Sciatic nerve

Sacrospinous ligament

Superior gemellus muscle

Obturator internus muscle

Inferior gemellus muscle

Sacrotuberous ligament

Quadratus femoris muscle

Ischial tuberosity

Greater trochanter

Semitendinosus muscle

Biceps femoris muscle (long head)

Adductor minimus part of
Adductor magnus muscle

Semimembranosus muscle

Iliotibial tract

Gracilis muscle

Biceps femoris muscle
Short head
Long head

Semimembranosus muscle

Semitendinosus muscle

Popliteal vessels and tibial nerve

Common peroneal nerve

Plantaris muscle

Gastrocnemius muscle
Medial head
Lateral head

Sartorius muscle

Popliteus muscle

Soleus muscle

Plantaris tendon (*cut*)

Psoas and Iliacus Muscles

SEE ALSO PLATE 246

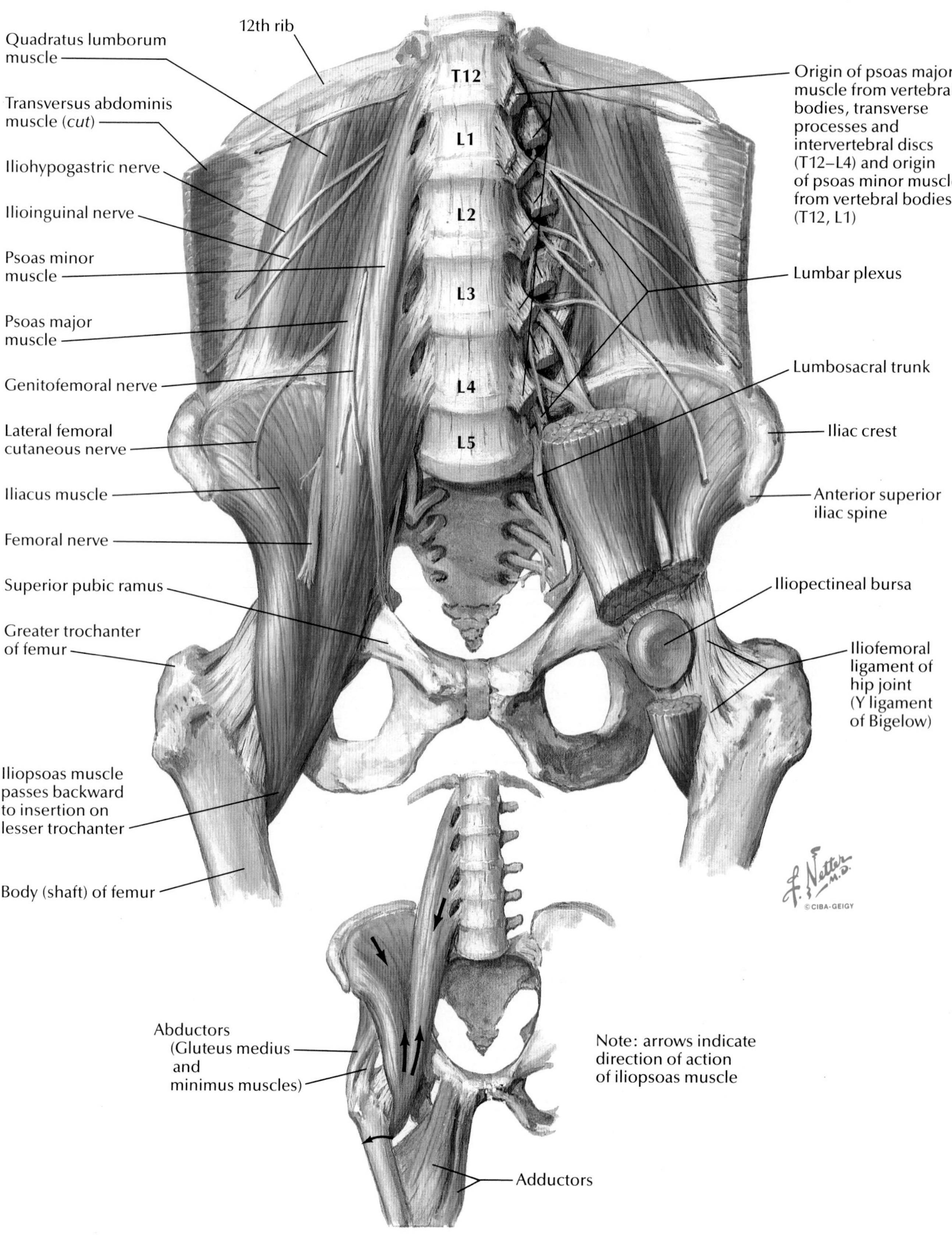

Quadratus lumborum muscle

12th rib

Transversus abdominis muscle (*cut*)

Iliohypogastric nerve

Ilioinguinal nerve

Psoas minor muscle

Psoas major muscle

Genitofemoral nerve

Lateral femoral cutaneous nerve

Iliacus muscle

Femoral nerve

Superior pubic ramus

Greater trochanter of femur

Iliopsoas muscle passes backward to insertion on lesser trochanter

Body (shaft) of femur

T12

L1

L2

L3

L4

L5

Origin of psoas major muscle from vertebral bodies, transverse processes and intervertebral discs (T12–L4) and origin of psoas minor muscle from vertebral bodies (T12, L1)

Lumbar plexus

Lumbosacral trunk

Iliac crest

Anterior superior iliac spine

Iliopectineal bursa

Iliofemoral ligament of hip joint (Y ligament of Bigelow)

Abductors (Gluteus medius and minimus muscles)

Note: arrows indicate direction of action of iliopsoas muscle

Adductors

PLATE 466

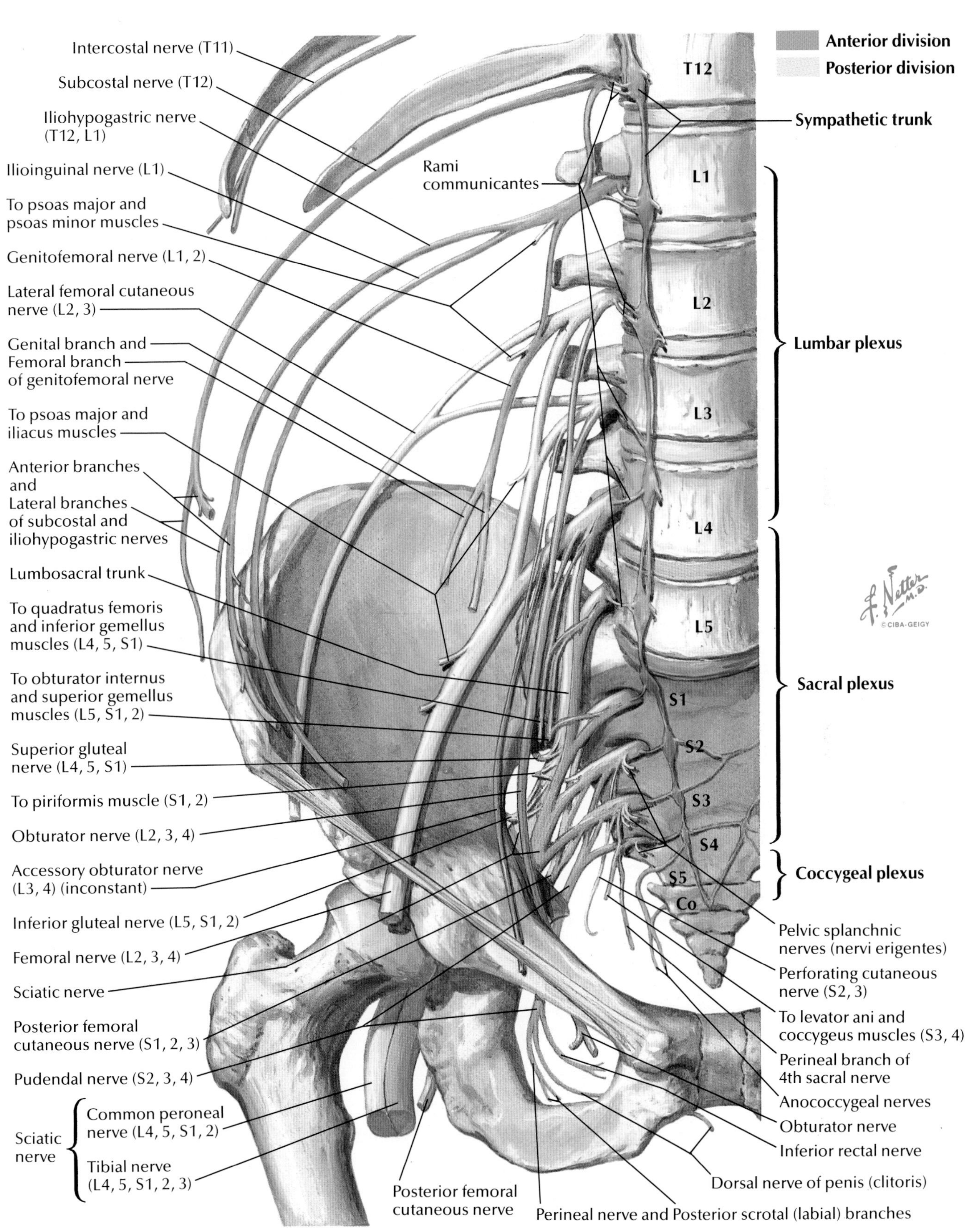

Intercostal nerve (T11)

Subcostal nerve (T12)

Iliohypogastric nerve (T12, L1)

Ilioinguinal nerve (L1)

To psoas major and psoas minor muscles

Genitofemoral nerve (L1, 2)

Lateral femoral cutaneous nerve (L2, 3)

Genital branch and Femoral branch of genitofemoral nerve

To psoas major and iliacus muscles

Anterior branches and Lateral branches of subcostal and iliohypogastric nerves

Lumbosacral trunk

To quadratus femoris and inferior gemellus muscles (L4, 5, S1)

To obturator internus and superior gemellus muscles (L5, S1, 2)

Superior gluteal nerve (L4, 5, S1)

To piriformis muscle (S1, 2)

Obturator nerve (L2, 3, 4)

Accessory obturator nerve (L3, 4) (inconstant)

Inferior gluteal nerve (L5, S1, 2)

Femoral nerve (L2, 3, 4)

Sciatic nerve

Posterior femoral cutaneous nerve (S1, 2, 3)

Pudendal nerve (S2, 3, 4)

Sciatic nerve { Common peroneal nerve (L4, 5, S1, 2)

Tibial nerve (L4, 5, S1, 2, 3)

Rami communicantes

T12

L1

L2

L3

L4

L5

S1

S2

S3

S4

S5

Co

Anterior division

Posterior division

Sympathetic trunk

Lumbar plexus

Sacral plexus

Coccygeal plexus

Pelvic splanchnic nerves (nervi erigentes)

Perforating cutaneous nerve (S2, 3)

To levator ani and coccygeus muscles (S3, 4)

Perineal branch of 4th sacral nerve

Anococcygeal nerves

Obturator nerve

Inferior rectal nerve

Dorsal nerve of penis (clitoris)

Posterior femoral cutaneous nerve

Perineal nerve and Posterior scrotal (labial) branches

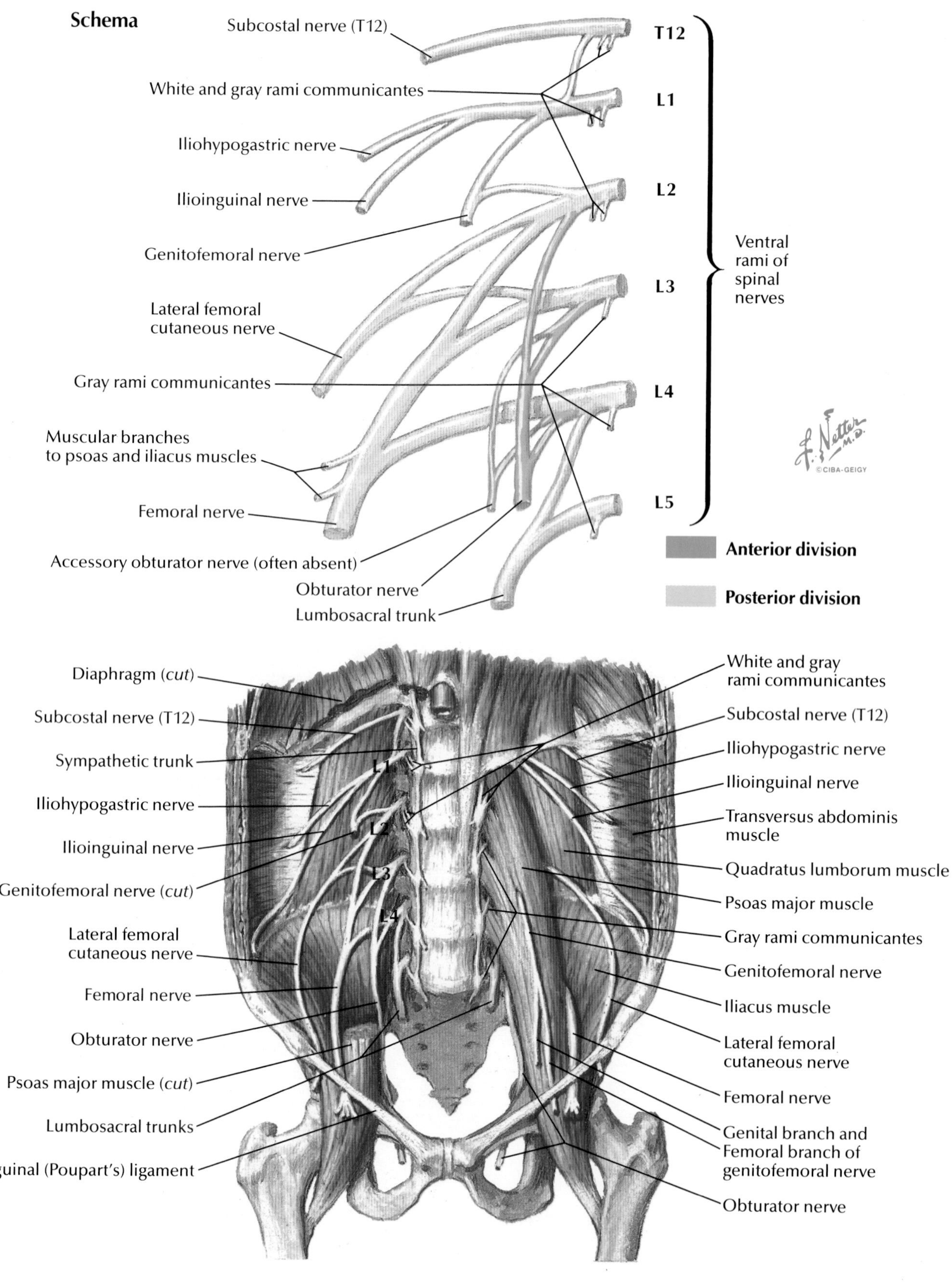

Schema

Subcostal nerve (T12)

White and gray rami communicantes

Iliohypogastric nerve

Ilioinguinal nerve

Genitofemoral nerve

Lateral femoral cutaneous nerve

Gray rami communicantes

Muscular branches to psoas and iliacus muscles

Femoral nerve

Accessory obturator nerve (often absent)

Obturator nerve
Lumbosacral trunk

T12
L1
L2
L3
L4
L5

Ventral rami of spinal nerves

Anterior division

Posterior division

Diaphragm (cut)
Subcostal nerve (T12)
Sympathetic trunk
Iliohypogastric nerve
Ilioinguinal nerve
Genitofemoral nerve (cut)
Lateral femoral cutaneous nerve
Femoral nerve
Obturator nerve
Psoas major muscle (cut)
Lumbosacral trunks
Inguinal (Poupart's) ligament

White and gray rami communicantes
Subcostal nerve (T12)
Iliohypogastric nerve
Ilioinguinal nerve
Transversus abdominis muscle
Quadratus lumborum muscle
Psoas major muscle
Gray rami communicantes
Genitofemoral nerve
Iliacus muscle
Lateral femoral cutaneous nerve
Femoral nerve
Genital branch and Femoral branch of genitofemoral nerve
Obturator nerve

PLATE 468

LOWER LIMB

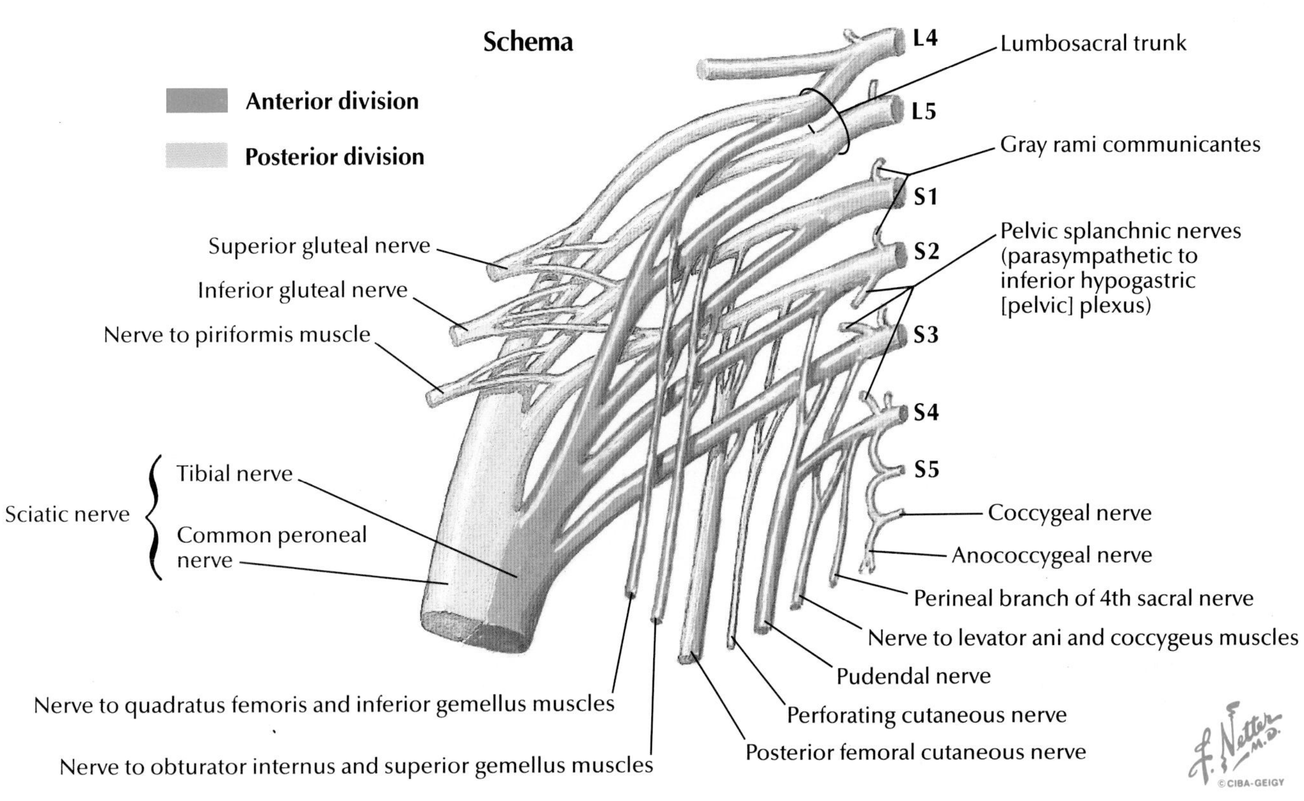

Schema

Anterior division

Posterior division

Superior gluteal nerve

Inferior gluteal nerve

Nerve to piriformis muscle

L4 — Lumbosacral trunk

L5

Gray rami communicantes

S1

S2 — Pelvic splanchnic nerves (parasympathetic to inferior hypogastric [pelvic] plexus)

S3

S4

S5

Sciatic nerve { Tibial nerve

Common peroneal nerve

Coccygeal nerve

Anococcygeal nerve

Perineal branch of 4th sacral nerve

Nerve to levator ani and coccygeus muscles

Pudendal nerve

Nerve to quadratus femoris and inferior gemellus muscles

Perforating cutaneous nerve

Nerve to obturator internus and superior gemellus muscles

Posterior femoral cutaneous nerve

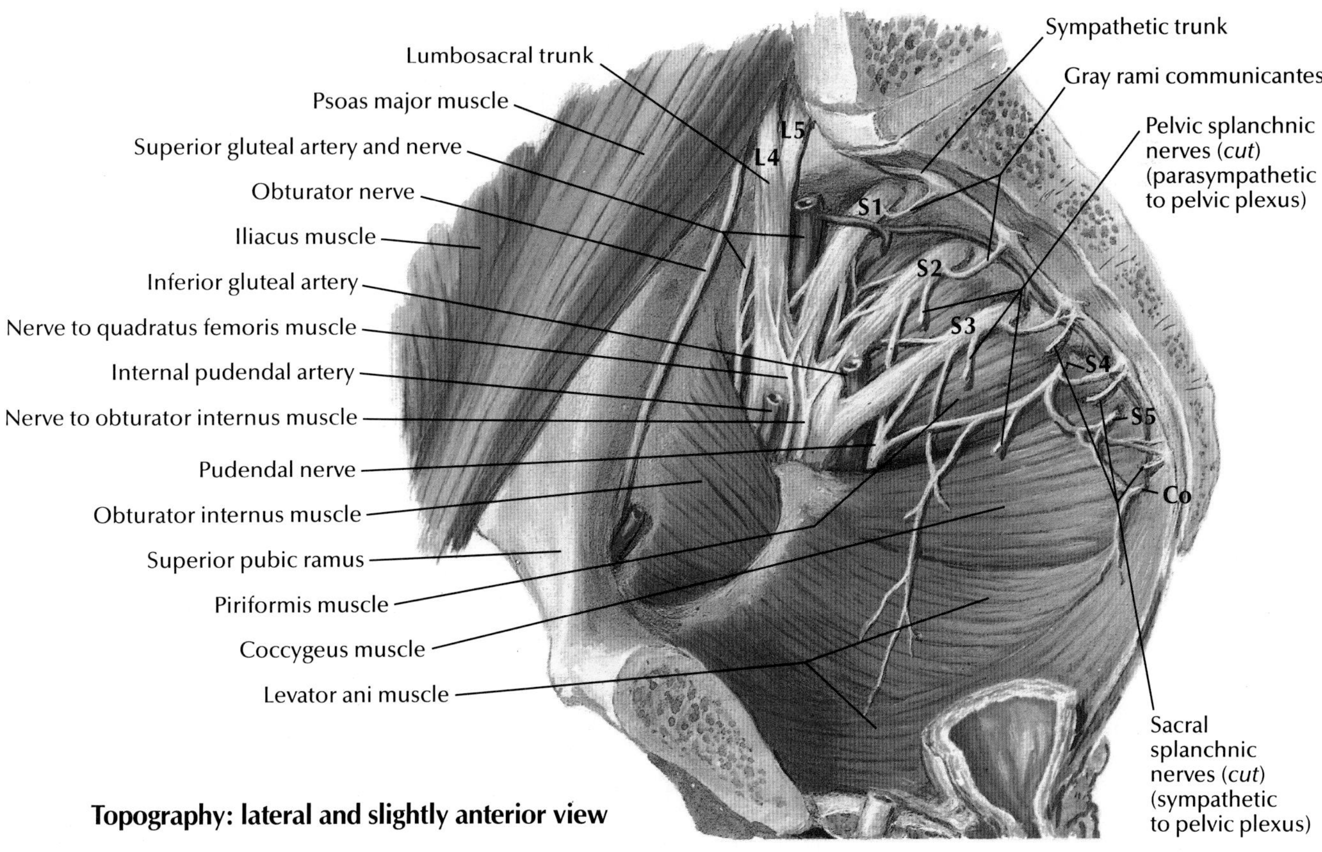

Lumbosacral trunk

Psoas major muscle

Superior gluteal artery and nerve

Obturator nerve

Iliacus muscle

Inferior gluteal artery

Nerve to quadratus femoris muscle

Internal pudendal artery

Nerve to obturator internus muscle

Pudendal nerve

Obturator internus muscle

Superior pubic ramus

Piriformis muscle

Coccygeus muscle

Levator ani muscle

Sympathetic trunk

Gray rami communicantes

Pelvic splanchnic nerves (cut) (parasympathetic to pelvic plexus)

L5

L4

S1

S2

S3

S4

S5

Co

Sacral splanchnic nerves (cut) (sympathetic to pelvic plexus)

Topography: lateral and slightly anterior view

Superficial dissections

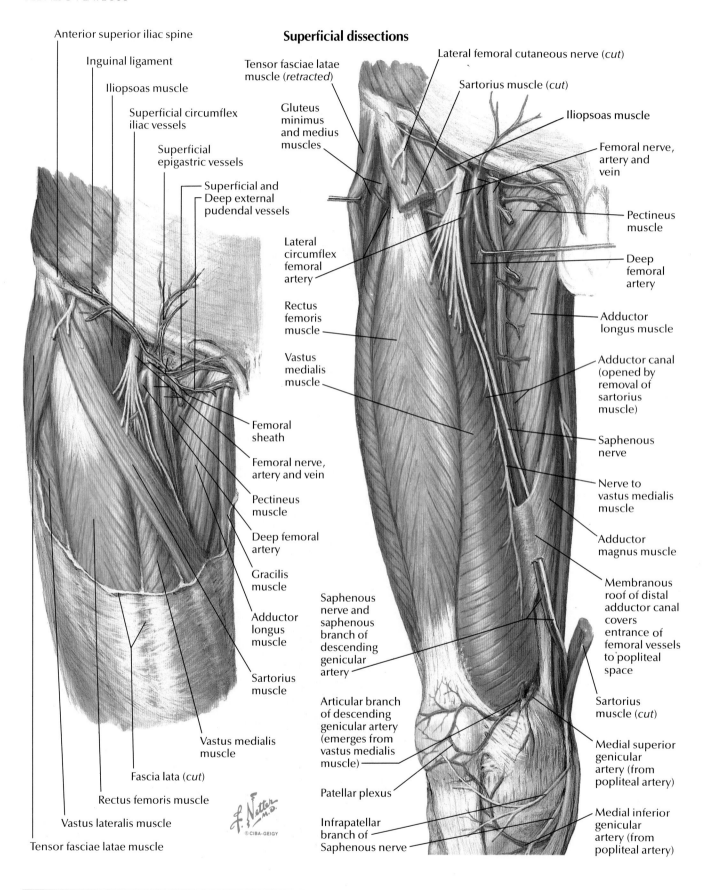

Anterior superior iliac spine

Inguinal ligament

Iliopsoas muscle

Superficial circumflex iliac vessels

Superficial epigastric vessels

Superficial and Deep external pudendal vessels

Tensor fasciae latae muscle (*retracted*)

Gluteus minimus and medius muscles

Lateral circumflex femoral artery

Rectus femoris muscle

Vastus medialis muscle

Femoral sheath

Femoral nerve, artery and vein

Pectineus muscle

Deep femoral artery

Gracilis muscle

Adductor longus muscle

Sartorius muscle

Vastus medialis muscle

Fascia lata (*cut*)

Rectus femoris muscle

Vastus lateralis muscle

Tensor fasciae latae muscle

Lateral femoral cutaneous nerve (*cut*)

Sartorius muscle (*cut*)

Iliopsoas muscle

Femoral nerve, artery and vein

Pectineus muscle

Deep femoral artery

Adductor longus muscle

Adductor canal (opened by removal of sartorius muscle)

Saphenous nerve

Nerve to vastus medialis muscle

Adductor magnus muscle

Membranous roof of distal adductor canal covers entrance of femoral vessels to popliteal space

Sartorius muscle (*cut*)

Medial superior genicular artery (from popliteal artery)

Medial inferior genicular artery (from popliteal artery)

Saphenous nerve and saphenous branch of descending genicular artery

Articular branch of descending genicular artery (emerges from vastus medialis muscle)

Patellar plexus

Infrapatellar branch of Saphenous nerve

PLATE 470

LOWER LIMB

Deep dissection

Deep circumflex iliac artery

Lateral femoral cutaneous nerve

Sartorius muscle (*cut*)

Iliopsoas muscle

Tensor fasciae latae muscle (*retracted*)

Gluteus medius and gluteus minimus muscles

Femoral nerve

Rectus femoris muscle (*cut*)

Ascending, transverse and descending branches of Lateral circumflex femoral artery

Medial circumflex femoral artery

Pectineus muscle (*cut*)

Deep femoral artery

Perforating branches

Adductor longus muscle (*cut*)

Vastus lateralis muscle

Vastus intermedius muscle

Rectus femoris muscle (*cut*)

Saphenous nerve

Membranous roof of adductor canal (*opened*)

Vastus medialis muscle

Quadriceps femoris tendon

Patella and patellar plexus

Medial patellar retinaculum

Patellar ligament

External iliac artery and vein

Inguinal (Poupart's) ligament

Femoral artery and vein (*cut*)

Pectineus muscle (*cut*)

Obturator foramen

Obturator externus muscle

Adductor longus muscle (*cut*)

Anterior division and Posterior division of obturator nerve

Quadratus femoris muscle

Adductor brevis muscle

Branches of posterior division of obturator nerve

Adductor magnus muscle

Gracilis muscle

Cutaneous branch of obturator nerve

Femoral artery and vein (*cut*)

Descending genicular artery
Articular branch
Saphenous branch

Adductor hiatus

Sartorius muscle (*cut*)

Adductor magnus tendon

Medial epicondyle of femur (adductor tubercle)

Medial superior genicular artery (from popliteal artery)

Infrapatellar branch of Saphenous nerve

Medial inferior genicular artery (from popliteal artery)

f. Netter m.d.

©CIBA-GEIGY

HIP AND THIGH

PLATE 471

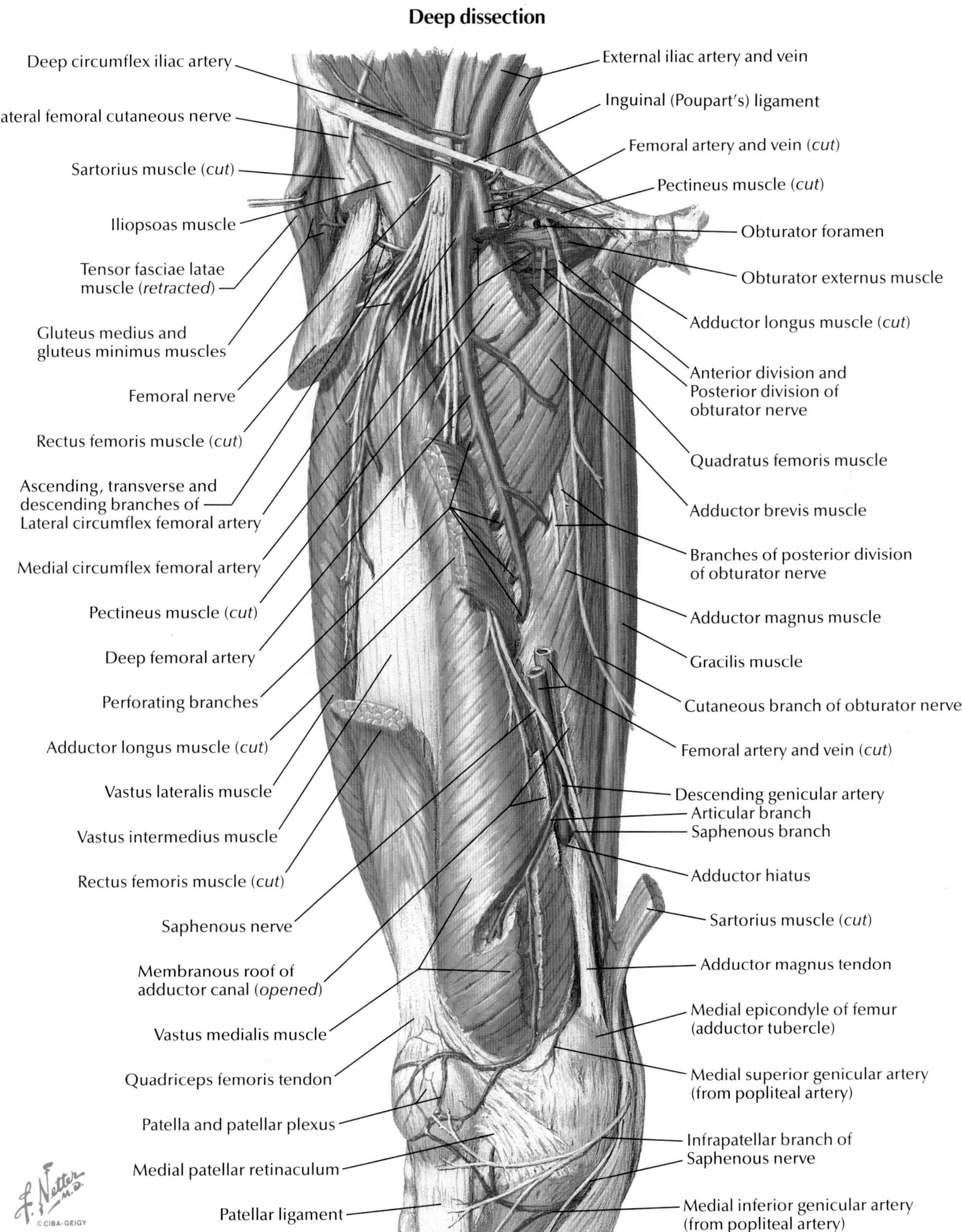

Deep dissection

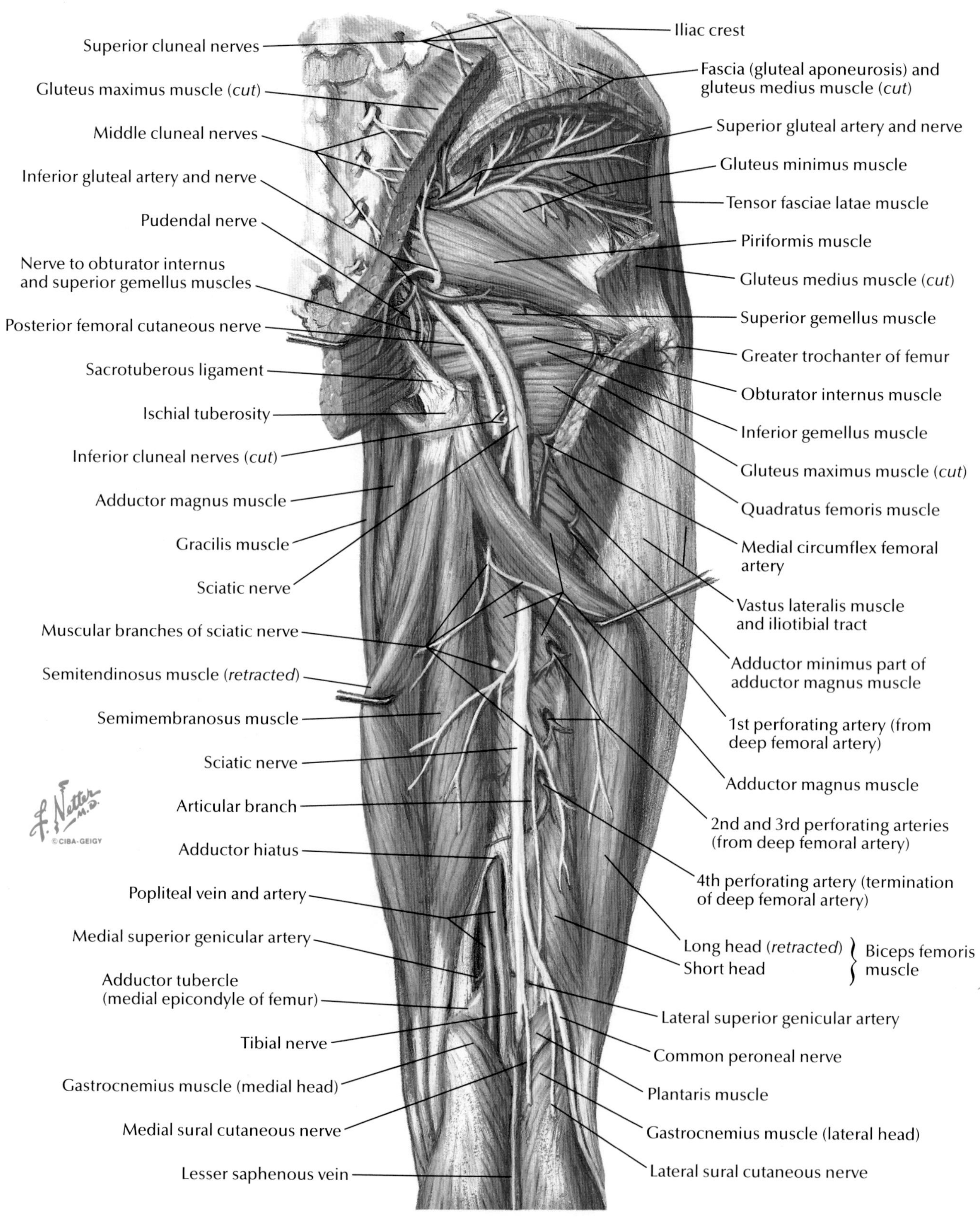

Superior cluneal nerves

Gluteus maximus muscle (*cut*)

Middle cluneal nerves

Inferior gluteal artery and nerve

Pudendal nerve

Nerve to obturator internus and superior gemellus muscles

Posterior femoral cutaneous nerve

Sacrotuberous ligament

Ischial tuberosity

Inferior cluneal nerves (*cut*)

Adductor magnus muscle

Gracilis muscle

Sciatic nerve

Muscular branches of sciatic nerve

Semitendinosus muscle (*retracted*)

Semimembranosus muscle

Sciatic nerve

Articular branch

Adductor hiatus

Popliteal vein and artery

Medial superior genicular artery

Adductor tubercle (medial epicondyle of femur)

Tibial nerve

Gastrocnemius muscle (medial head)

Medial sural cutaneous nerve

Lesser saphenous vein

Iliac crest

Fascia (gluteal aponeurosis) and gluteus medius muscle (*cut*)

Superior gluteal artery and nerve

Gluteus minimus muscle

Tensor fasciae latae muscle

Piriformis muscle

Gluteus medius muscle (*cut*)

Superior gemellus muscle

Greater trochanter of femur

Obturator internus muscle

Inferior gemellus muscle

Gluteus maximus muscle (*cut*)

Quadratus femoris muscle

Medial circumflex femoral artery

Vastus lateralis muscle and iliotibial tract

Adductor minimus part of adductor magnus muscle

1st perforating artery (from deep femoral artery)

Adductor magnus muscle

2nd and 3rd perforating arteries (from deep femoral artery)

4th perforating artery (termination of deep femoral artery)

Long head (*retracted*) } Biceps femoris
Short head } muscle

Lateral superior genicular artery

Common peroneal nerve

Plantaris muscle

Gastrocnemius muscle (lateral head)

Lateral sural cutaneous nerve

PLATE 472

LOWER LIMB

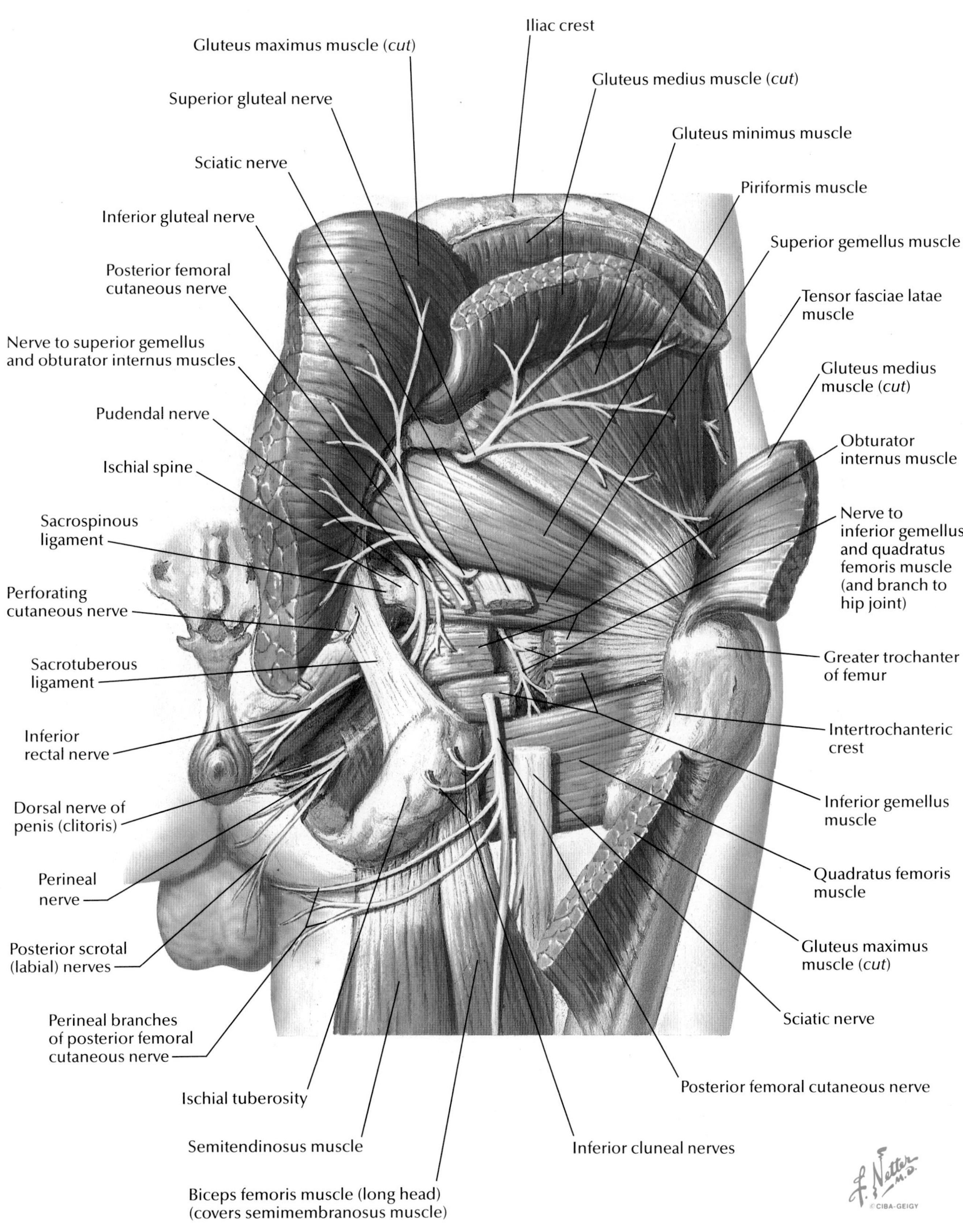

Gluteus maximus muscle (*cut*)

Iliac crest

Superior gluteal nerve

Gluteus medius muscle (*cut*)

Sciatic nerve

Gluteus minimus muscle

Inferior gluteal nerve

Piriformis muscle

Posterior femoral cutaneous nerve

Superior gemellus muscle

Nerve to superior gemellus and obturator internus muscles

Tensor fasciae latae muscle

Gluteus medius muscle (*cut*)

Pudendal nerve

Obturator internus muscle

Ischial spine

Nerve to inferior gemellus and quadratus femoris muscle (and branch to hip joint)

Sacrospinous ligament

Perforating cutaneous nerve

Greater trochanter of femur

Sacrotuberous ligament

Intertrochanteric crest

Inferior rectal nerve

Inferior gemellus muscle

Dorsal nerve of penis (clitoris)

Quadratus femoris muscle

Perineal nerve

Gluteus maximus muscle (*cut*)

Posterior scrotal (labial) nerves

Sciatic nerve

Perineal branches of posterior femoral cutaneous nerve

Posterior femoral cutaneous nerve

Ischial tuberosity

Inferior cluneal nerves

Semitendinosus muscle

Biceps femoris muscle (long head) (covers semimembranosus muscle)

Arteries of Femoral Head and Neck

SEE ALSO PLATE 481

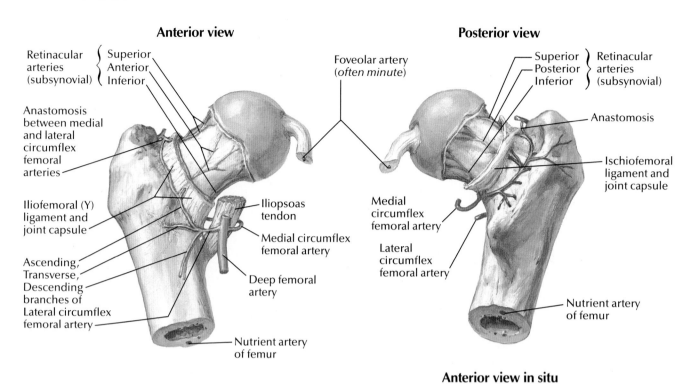

Anterior view

Retinacular arteries (subsynovial) { Superior / Anterior / Inferior

Anastomosis between medial and lateral circumflex femoral arteries

Iliofemoral (Y) ligament and joint capsule

Ascending, Transverse, Descending branches of Lateral circumflex femoral artery

Iliopsoas tendon

Medial circumflex femoral artery

Deep femoral artery

Nutrient artery of femur

Foveolar artery (*often minute*)

Posterior view

Superior / Posterior / Inferior } Retinacular arteries (subsynovial)

Anastomosis

Ischiofemoral ligament and joint capsule

Medial circumflex femoral artery

Lateral circumflex femoral artery

Nutrient artery of femur

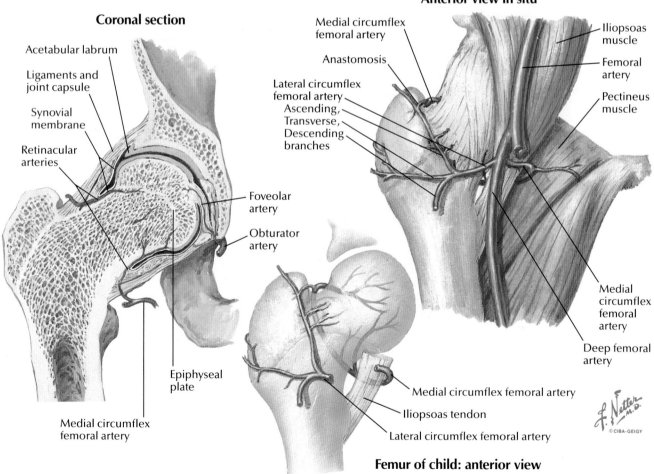

Coronal section

Acetabular labrum

Ligaments and joint capsule

Synovial membrane

Retinacular arteries

Foveolar artery

Obturator artery

Epiphyseal plate

Medial circumflex femoral artery

Anterior view in situ

Medial circumflex femoral artery

Anastomosis

Lateral circumflex femoral artery

Ascending, Transverse, Descending branches

Iliopsoas muscle

Femoral artery

Pectineus muscle

Medial circumflex femoral artery

Deep femoral artery

Medial circumflex femoral artery

Iliopsoas tendon

Lateral circumflex femoral artery

Femur of child: anterior view

PLATE 474

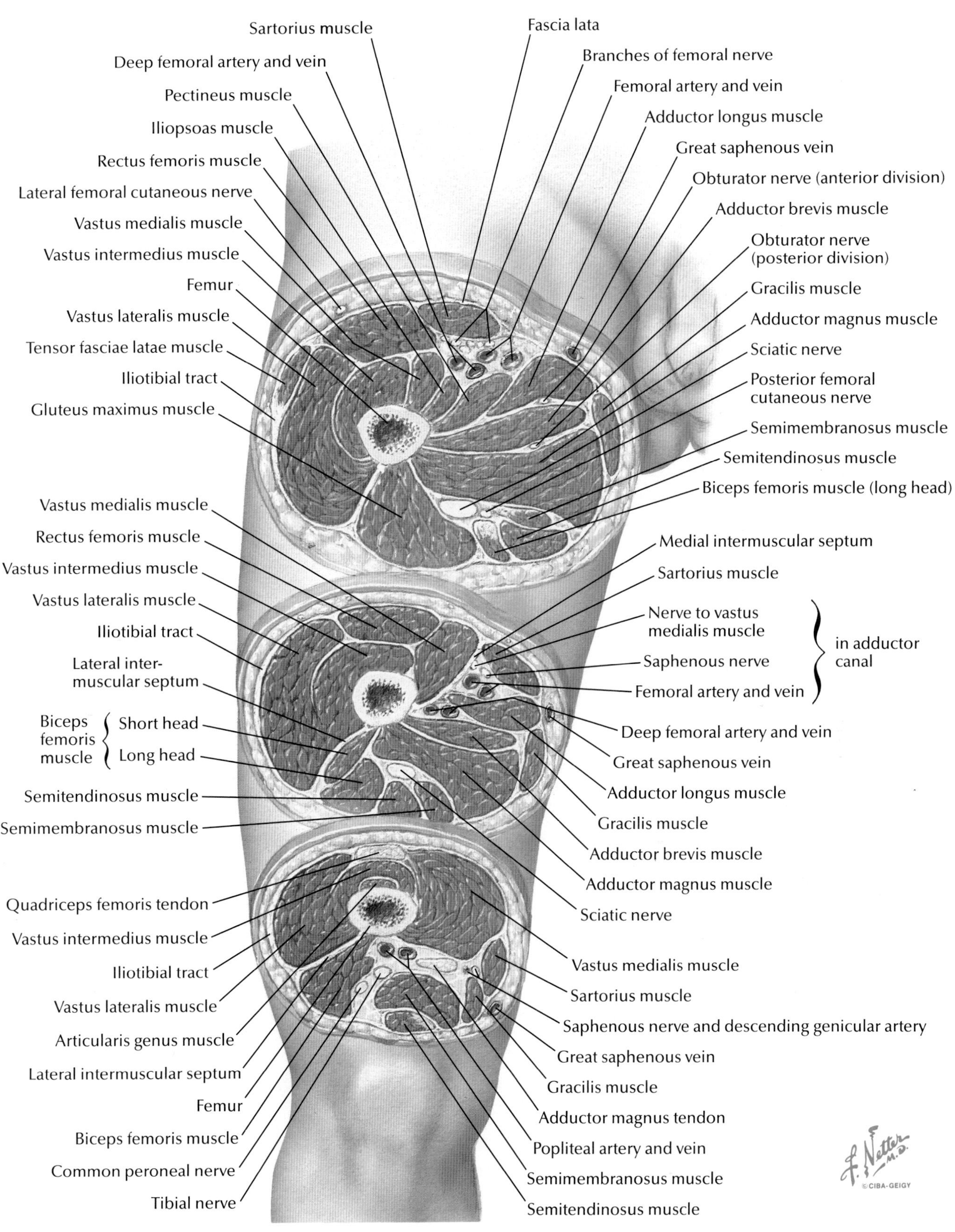

Sartorius muscle

Deep femoral artery and vein

Pectineus muscle

Iliopsoas muscle

Rectus femoris muscle

Lateral femoral cutaneous nerve

Vastus medialis muscle

Vastus intermedius muscle

Femur

Vastus lateralis muscle

Tensor fasciae latae muscle

Iliotibial tract

Gluteus maximus muscle

Vastus medialis muscle

Rectus femoris muscle

Vastus intermedius muscle

Vastus lateralis muscle

Iliotibial tract

Lateral inter-muscular septum

Biceps femoris muscle { Short head / Long head }

Semitendinosus muscle

Semimembranosus muscle

Quadriceps femoris tendon

Vastus intermedius muscle

Iliotibial tract

Vastus lateralis muscle

Articularis genus muscle

Lateral intermuscular septum

Femur

Biceps femoris muscle

Common peroneal nerve

Tibial nerve

Fascia lata

Branches of femoral nerve

Femoral artery and vein

Adductor longus muscle

Great saphenous vein

Obturator nerve (anterior division)

Adductor brevis muscle

Obturator nerve (posterior division)

Gracilis muscle

Adductor magnus muscle

Sciatic nerve

Posterior femoral cutaneous nerve

Semimembranosus muscle

Semitendinosus muscle

Biceps femoris muscle (long head)

Medial intermuscular septum

Sartorius muscle

Nerve to vastus medialis muscle

Saphenous nerve

} in adductor canal

Femoral artery and vein

Deep femoral artery and vein

Great saphenous vein

Adductor longus muscle

Gracilis muscle

Adductor brevis muscle

Adductor magnus muscle

Sciatic nerve

Vastus medialis muscle

Sartorius muscle

Saphenous nerve and descending genicular artery

Great saphenous vein

Gracilis muscle

Adductor magnus tendon

Popliteal artery and vein

Semimembranosus muscle

Semitendinosus muscle

Knee: Lateral and Medial Views

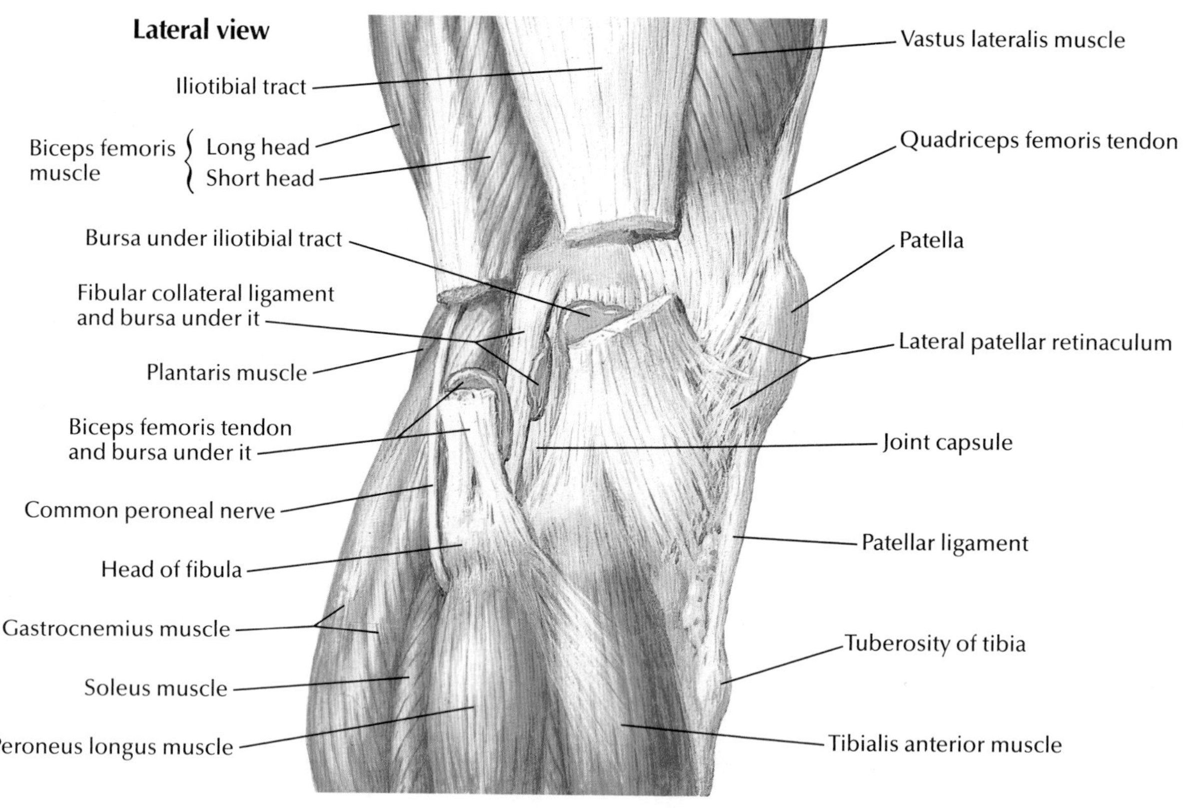

Lateral view

Iliotibial tract

Biceps femoris muscle { Long head / Short head

Bursa under iliotibial tract

Fibular collateral ligament and bursa under it

Plantaris muscle

Biceps femoris tendon and bursa under it

Common peroneal nerve

Head of fibula

Gastrocnemius muscle

Soleus muscle

Peroneus longus muscle

Vastus lateralis muscle

Quadriceps femoris tendon

Patella

Lateral patellar retinaculum

Joint capsule

Patellar ligament

Tuberosity of tibia

Tibialis anterior muscle

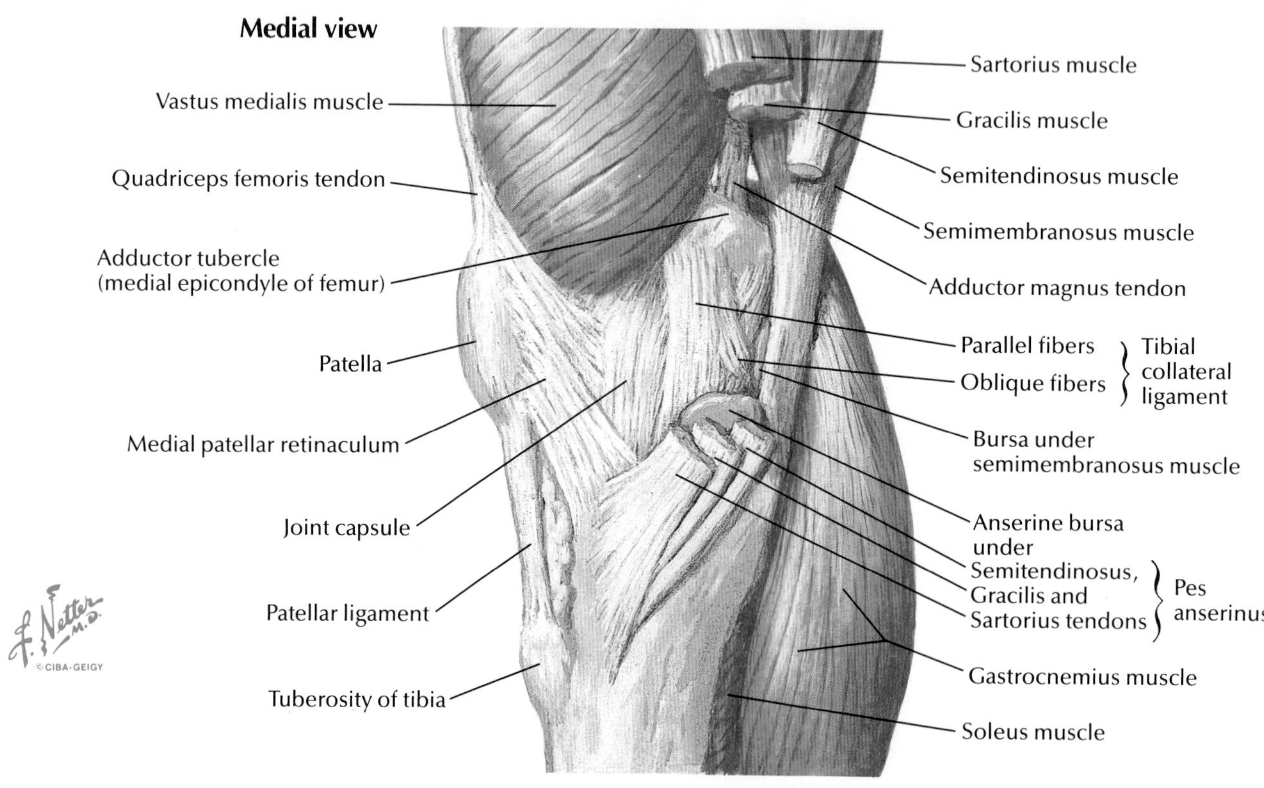

Medial view

Vastus medialis muscle

Quadriceps femoris tendon

Adductor tubercle (medial epicondyle of femur)

Patella

Medial patellar retinaculum

Joint capsule

Patellar ligament

Tuberosity of tibia

Sartorius muscle

Gracilis muscle

Semitendinosus muscle

Semimembranosus muscle

Adductor magnus tendon

Parallel fibers } Tibial collateral ligament

Oblique fibers

Bursa under semimembranosus muscle

Anserine bursa under Semitendinosus, Gracilis and Sartorius tendons } Pes anserinus

Gastrocnemius muscle

Soleus muscle

PLATE 476

LOWER LIMB

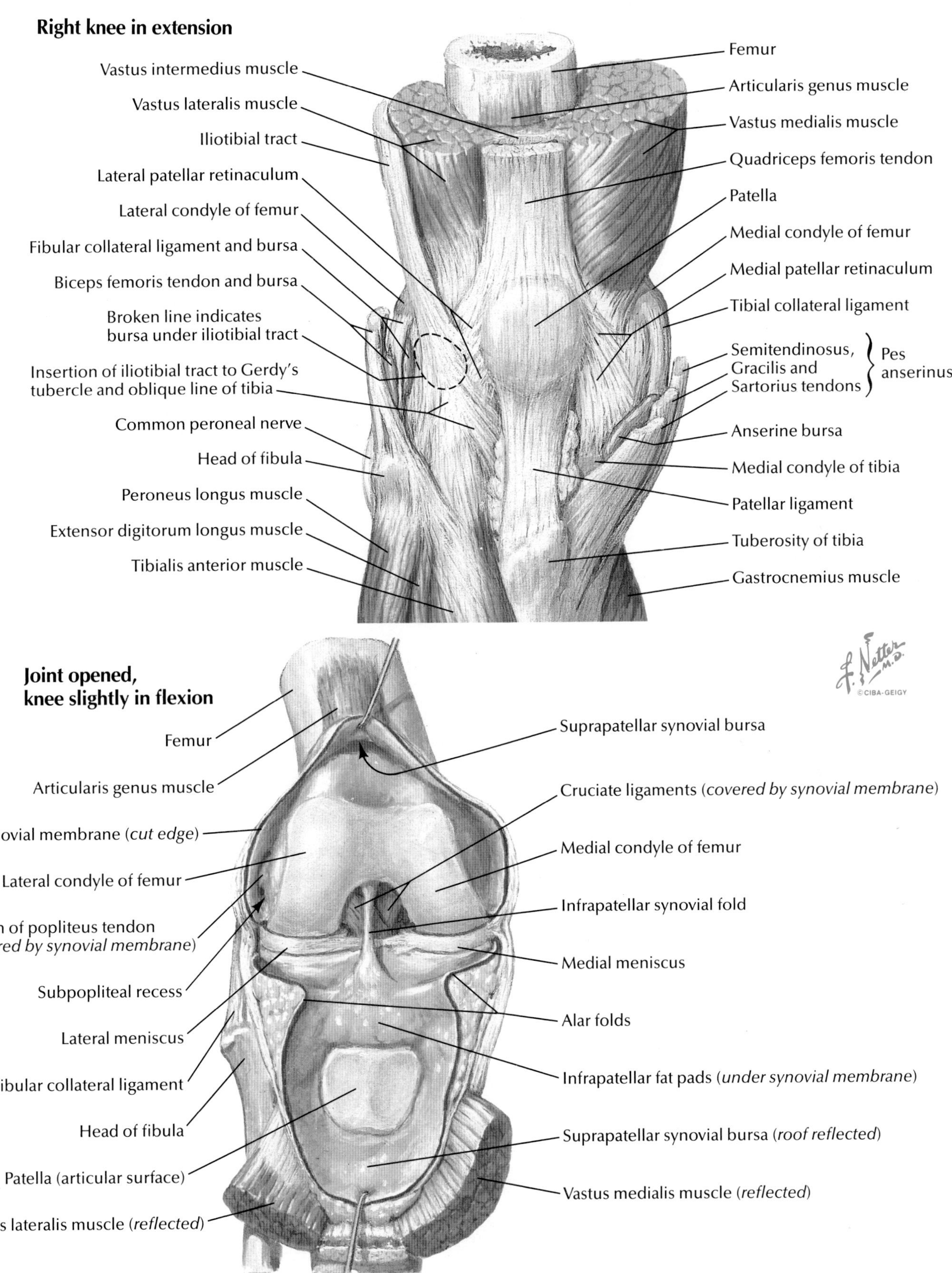

Right knee in extension

Vastus intermedius muscle

Vastus lateralis muscle

Iliotibial tract

Lateral patellar retinaculum

Lateral condyle of femur

Fibular collateral ligament and bursa

Biceps femoris tendon and bursa

Broken line indicates bursa under iliotibial tract

Insertion of iliotibial tract to Gerdy's tubercle and oblique line of tibia

Common peroneal nerve

Head of fibula

Peroneus longus muscle

Extensor digitorum longus muscle

Tibialis anterior muscle

Femur

Articularis genus muscle

Vastus medialis muscle

Quadriceps femoris tendon

Patella

Medial condyle of femur

Medial patellar retinaculum

Tibial collateral ligament

Semitendinosus, Gracilis and Sartorius tendons } Pes anserinus

Anserine bursa

Medial condyle of tibia

Patellar ligament

Tuberosity of tibia

Gastrocnemius muscle

Joint opened, knee slightly in flexion

Femur

Articularis genus muscle

Synovial membrane (*cut edge*)

Lateral condyle of femur

Origin of popliteus tendon (*covered by synovial membrane*)

Subpopliteal recess

Lateral meniscus

Fibular collateral ligament

Head of fibula

Patella (articular surface)

Vastus lateralis muscle (*reflected*)

Suprapatellar synovial bursa

Cruciate ligaments (*covered by synovial membrane*)

Medial condyle of femur

Infrapatellar synovial fold

Medial meniscus

Alar folds

Infrapatellar fat pads (*under synovial membrane*)

Suprapatellar synovial bursa (*roof reflected*)

Vastus medialis muscle (*reflected*)

Inferior view

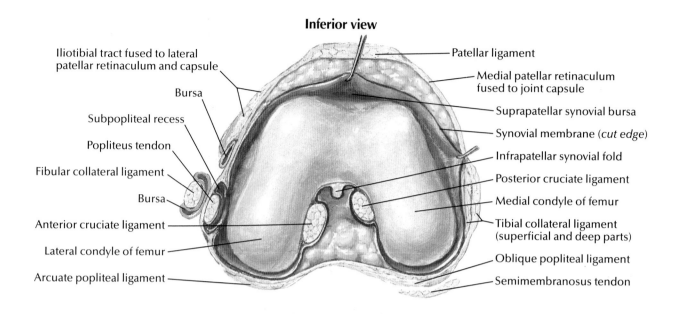

Iliotibial tract fused to lateral patellar retinaculum and capsule

Bursa

Subpopliteal recess

Popliteus tendon

Fibular collateral ligament

Bursa

Anterior cruciate ligament

Lateral condyle of femur

Arcuate popliteal ligament

Patellar ligament

Medial patellar retinaculum fused to joint capsule

Suprapatellar synovial bursa

Synovial membrane (cut edge)

Infrapatellar synovial fold

Posterior cruciate ligament

Medial condyle of femur

Tibial collateral ligament (superficial and deep parts)

Oblique popliteal ligament

Semimembranosus tendon

Superior view

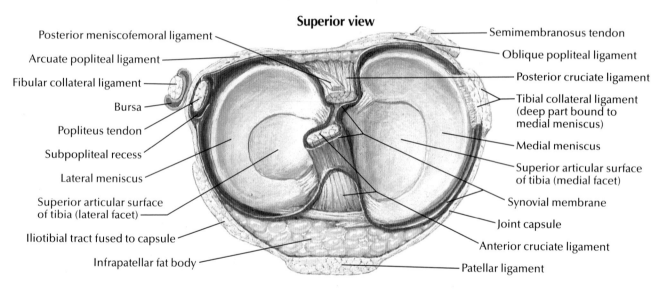

Posterior meniscofemoral ligament

Arcuate popliteal ligament

Fibular collateral ligament

Bursa

Popliteus tendon

Subpopliteal recess

Lateral meniscus

Superior articular surface of tibia (lateral facet)

Iliotibial tract fused to capsule

Infrapatellar fat body

Semimembranosus tendon

Oblique popliteal ligament

Posterior cruciate ligament

Tibial collateral ligament (deep part bound to medial meniscus)

Medial meniscus

Superior articular surface of tibia (medial facet)

Synovial membrane

Joint capsule

Anterior cruciate ligament

Patellar ligament

Superior view: ligaments and cartilage removed

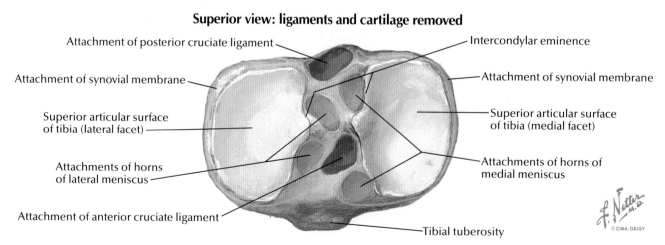

Attachment of posterior cruciate ligament

Attachment of synovial membrane

Superior articular surface of tibia (lateral facet)

Attachments of horns of lateral meniscus

Attachment of anterior cruciate ligament

Intercondylar eminence

Attachment of synovial membrane

Superior articular surface of tibia (medial facet)

Attachments of horns of medial meniscus

Tibial tuberosity

PLATE 478

Knee: Cruciate and Collateral Ligaments

Right knee in flexion: anterior view

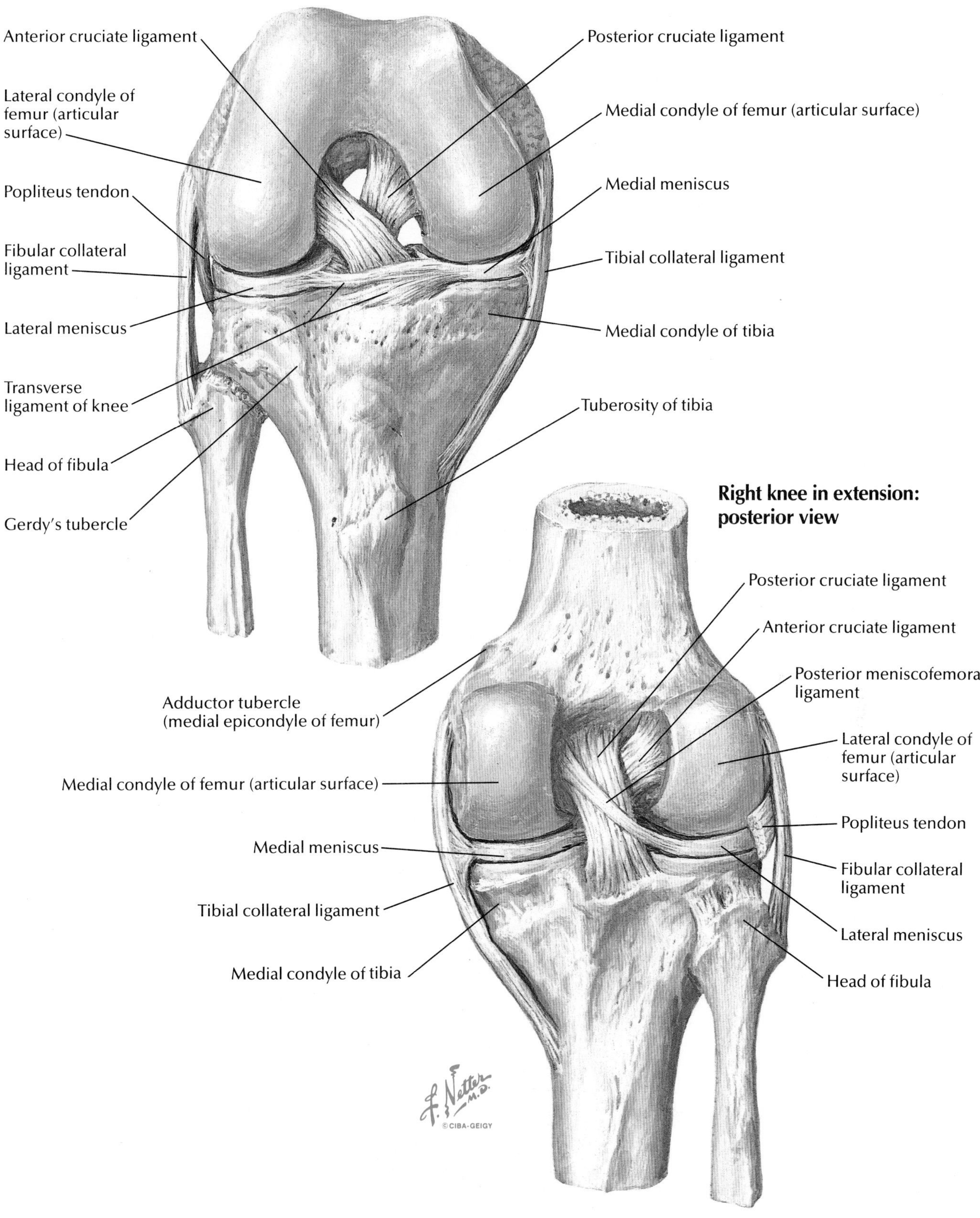

Anterior cruciate ligament

Lateral condyle of femur (articular surface)

Popliteus tendon

Fibular collateral ligament

Lateral meniscus

Transverse ligament of knee

Head of fibula

Gerdy's tubercle

Posterior cruciate ligament

Medial condyle of femur (articular surface)

Medial meniscus

Tibial collateral ligament

Medial condyle of tibia

Tuberosity of tibia

Right knee in extension: posterior view

Posterior cruciate ligament

Anterior cruciate ligament

Posterior meniscofemoral ligament

Lateral condyle of femur (articular surface)

Popliteus tendon

Fibular collateral ligament

Lateral meniscus

Head of fibula

Adductor tubercle (medial epicondyle of femur)

Medial condyle of femur (articular surface)

Medial meniscus

Tibial collateral ligament

Medial condyle of tibia

F. Netter M.D.

©CIBA-GEIGY

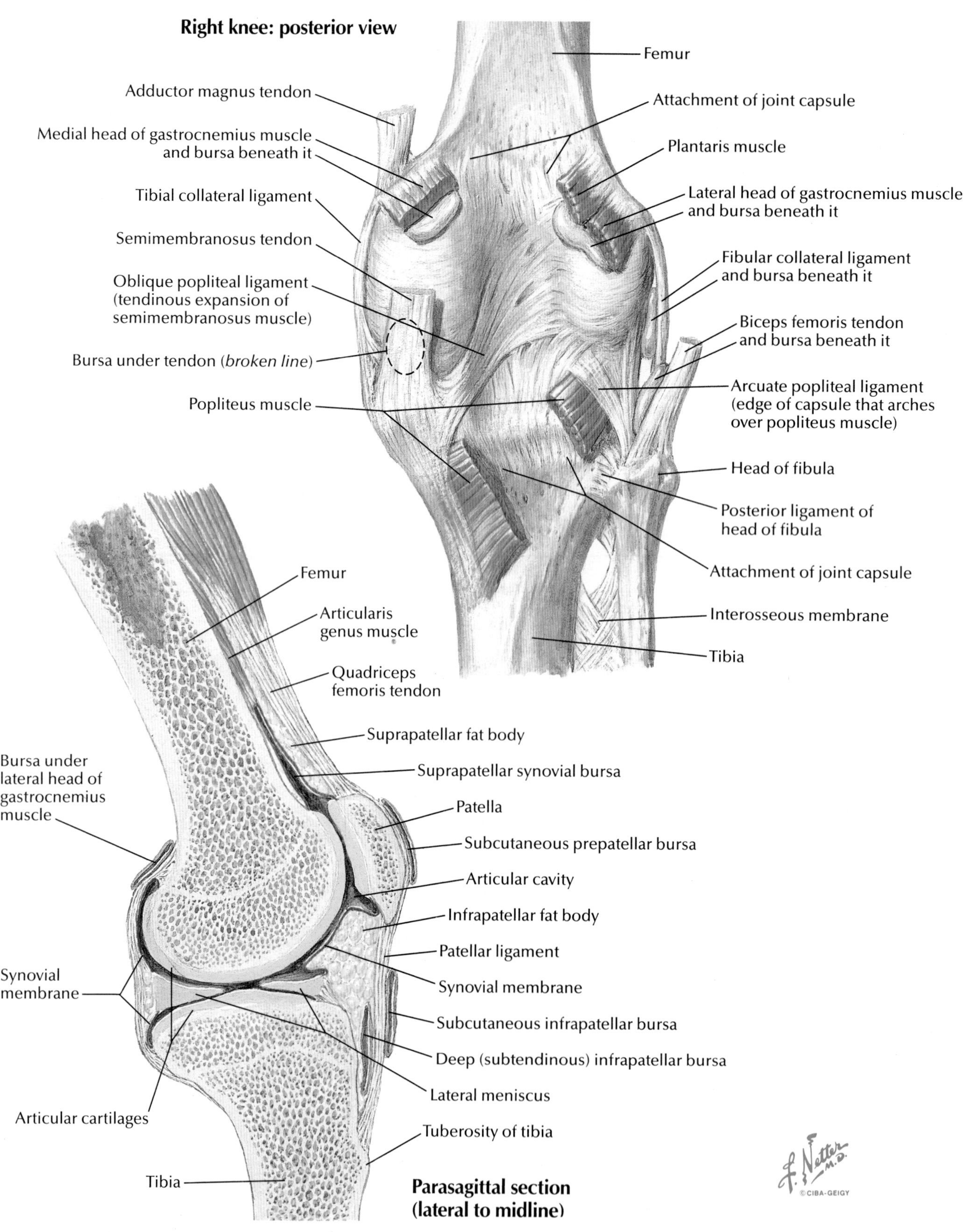

Right knee: posterior view

Adductor magnus tendon

Medial head of gastrocnemius muscle and bursa beneath it

Tibial collateral ligament

Semimembranosus tendon

Oblique popliteal ligament (tendinous expansion of semimembranosus muscle)

Bursa under tendon (*broken line*)

Popliteus muscle

Femur

Attachment of joint capsule

Plantaris muscle

Lateral head of gastrocnemius muscle and bursa beneath it

Fibular collateral ligament and bursa beneath it

Biceps femoris tendon and bursa beneath it

Arcuate popliteal ligament (edge of capsule that arches over popliteus muscle)

Head of fibula

Posterior ligament of head of fibula

Attachment of joint capsule

Interosseous membrane

Tibia

Bursa under lateral head of gastrocnemius muscle

Synovial membrane

Articular cartilages

Tibia

Femur

Articularis genus muscle

Quadriceps femoris tendon

Suprapatellar fat body

Suprapatellar synovial bursa

Patella

Subcutaneous prepatellar bursa

Articular cavity

Infrapatellar fat body

Patellar ligament

Synovial membrane

Subcutaneous infrapatellar bursa

Deep (subtendinous) infrapatellar bursa

Lateral meniscus

Tuberosity of tibia

Parasagittal section (lateral to midline)

PLATE 480

LOWER LIMB

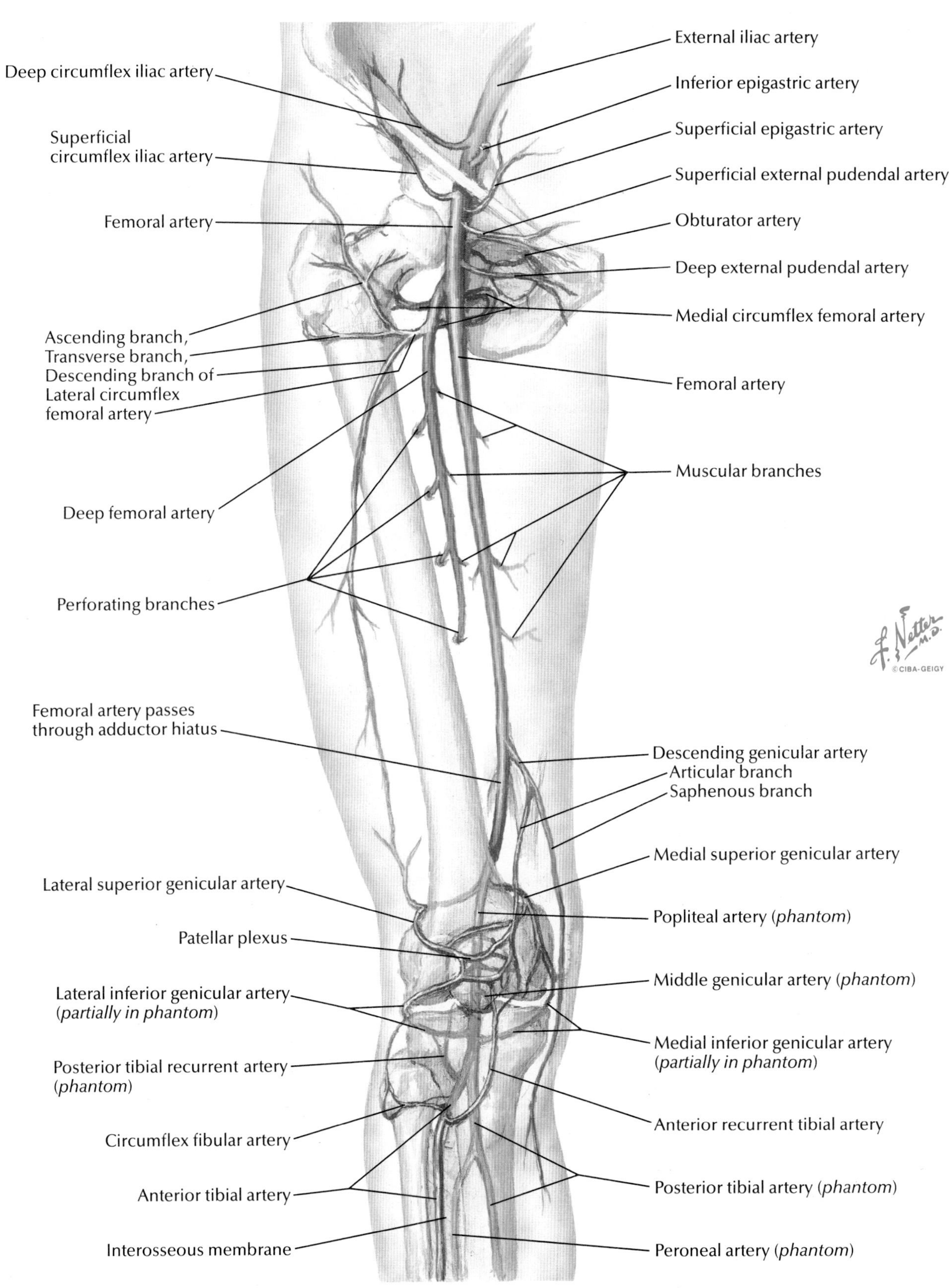

Deep circumflex iliac artery

Superficial circumflex iliac artery

Femoral artery

Ascending branch,
Transverse branch,
Descending branch of
Lateral circumflex
femoral artery

Deep femoral artery

Perforating branches

Femoral artery passes
through adductor hiatus

Lateral superior genicular artery

Patellar plexus

Lateral inferior genicular artery
(*partially in phantom*)

Posterior tibial recurrent artery
(*phantom*)

Circumflex fibular artery

Anterior tibial artery

Interosseous membrane

External iliac artery

Inferior epigastric artery

Superficial epigastric artery

Superficial external pudendal artery

Obturator artery

Deep external pudendal artery

Medial circumflex femoral artery

Femoral artery

Muscular branches

Descending genicular artery
Articular branch
Saphenous branch

Medial superior genicular artery

Popliteal artery (*phantom*)

Middle genicular artery (*phantom*)

Medial inferior genicular artery
(*partially in phantom*)

Anterior recurrent tibial artery

Posterior tibial artery (*phantom*)

Peroneal artery (*phantom*)

Tibia and Fibula

Bones of right leg

Anterior view

Intercondylar eminence
- Lateral intercondylar tubercle
- Medial intercondylar tubercle

Anterior intercondylar area

Lateral condyle

Apex, Head, Neck of fibula

Medial condyle

Gerdy's tubercle (insertion of iliotibial tract)

Oblique line

Tuberosity

Lateral surface

Lateral surface

Anterior border

Anterior border

Interosseous border

Interosseous border

Medial surface

Medial surface

Medial border

Fibula

Tibia

Lateral malleolus

Medial malleolus

Malleolar articular surface

Inferior articular surface

Malleolar articular surface

Posterior view

Intercondylar eminence
- Medial intercondylar tubercle
- Lateral intercondylar tubercle

Posterior intercondylar area

Superior articular surfaces (medial and lateral facets)

Lateral condyle

Apex, Head, Neck of fibula

Groove for insertion of semimembranosus tendon

Soleal line

Nutrient foramen

Interosseous border

Posterior surface

Posterior surface

Medial crest

Medial border

Lateral surface

Tibia

Fibula

Posterior border

Groove for tibialis posterior and flexor digitorum longus tendons

Medial malleolus

Fibular notch

Lateral malleolus

Fossa of lateral malleolus

Malleolar articular surface

Inferior articular surface

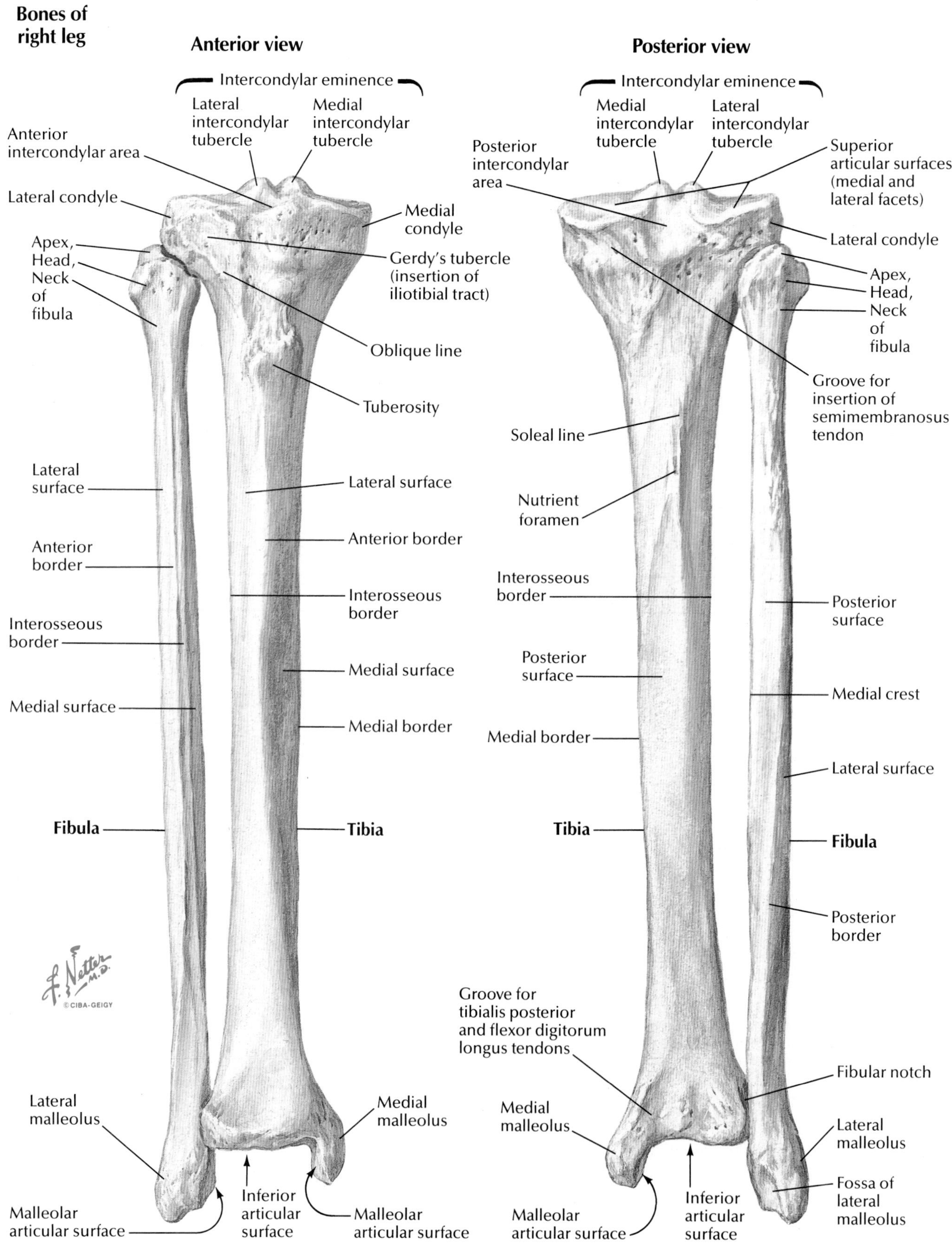

PLATE 482

LOWER LIMB

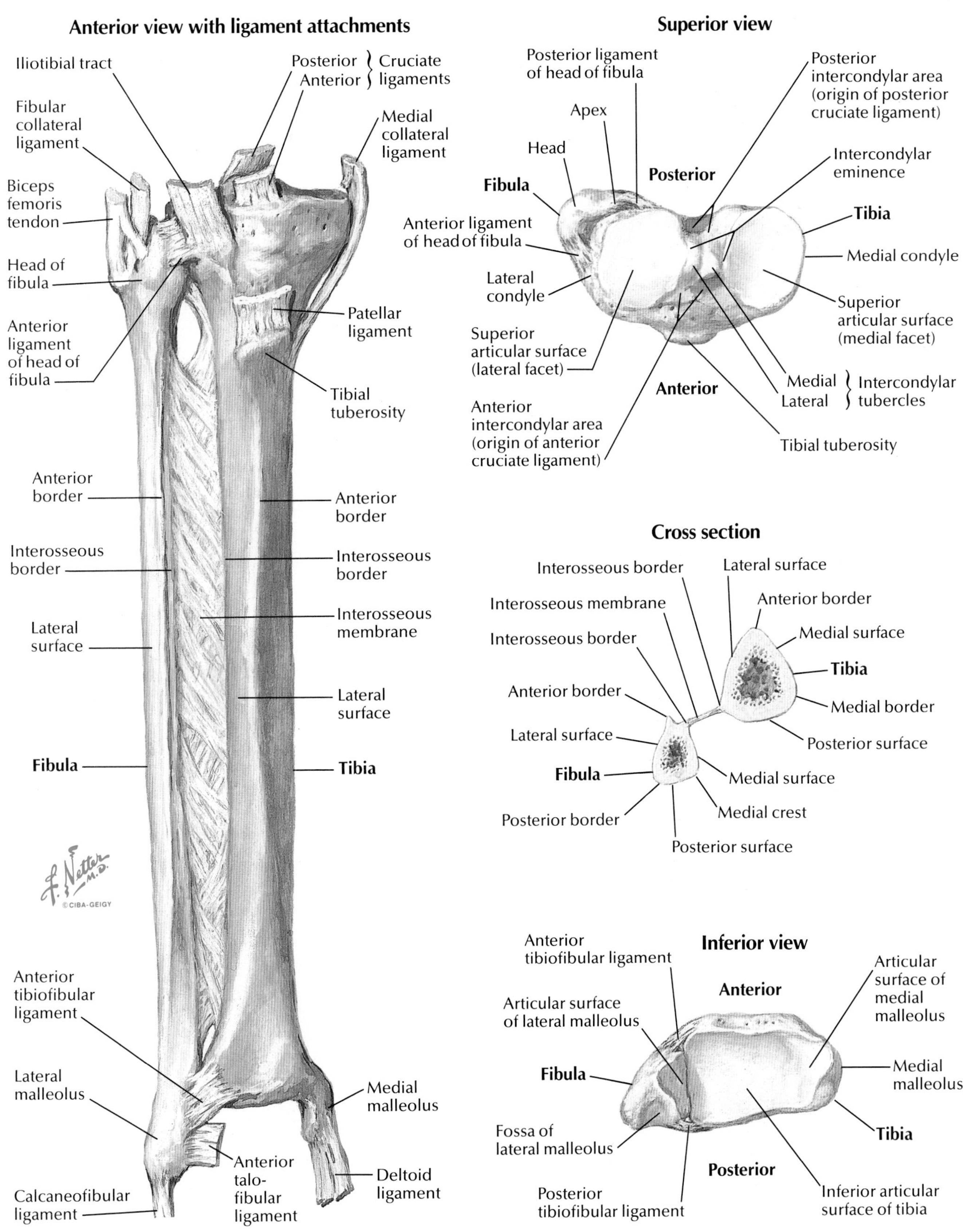

Anterior view with ligament attachments

Iliotibial tract

Fibular collateral ligament

Biceps femoris tendon

Head of fibula

Anterior ligament of head of fibula

Anterior border

Interosseous border

Lateral surface

Fibula

Anterior tibiofibular ligament

Lateral malleolus

Calcaneofibular ligament

Posterior } Cruciate
Anterior } ligaments

Medial collateral ligament

Patellar ligament

Tibial tuberosity

Anterior border

Interosseous border

Interosseous membrane

Lateral surface

Tibia

Anterior talo-fibular ligament

Medial malleolus

Deltoid ligament

Superior view

Posterior ligament of head of fibula

Apex

Head

Fibula

Anterior ligament of head of fibula

Lateral condyle

Superior articular surface (lateral facet)

Anterior intercondylar area (origin of anterior cruciate ligament)

Posterior

Anterior

Posterior intercondylar area (origin of posterior cruciate ligament)

Intercondylar eminence

Tibia

Medial condyle

Superior articular surface (medial facet)

Medial } Intercondylar
Lateral } tubercles

Tibial tuberosity

Cross section

Interosseous border

Interosseous membrane

Interosseous border

Anterior border

Lateral surface

Fibula

Posterior border

Lateral surface

Anterior border

Medial surface

Tibia

Medial border

Posterior surface

Medial surface

Medial crest

Posterior surface

Inferior view

Anterior tibiofibular ligament

Articular surface of lateral malleolus

Fibula

Fossa of lateral malleolus

Posterior tibiofibular ligament

Anterior

Posterior

Articular surface of medial malleolus

Medial malleolus

Tibia

Inferior articular surface of tibia

Bony Attachments of Muscles of Leg

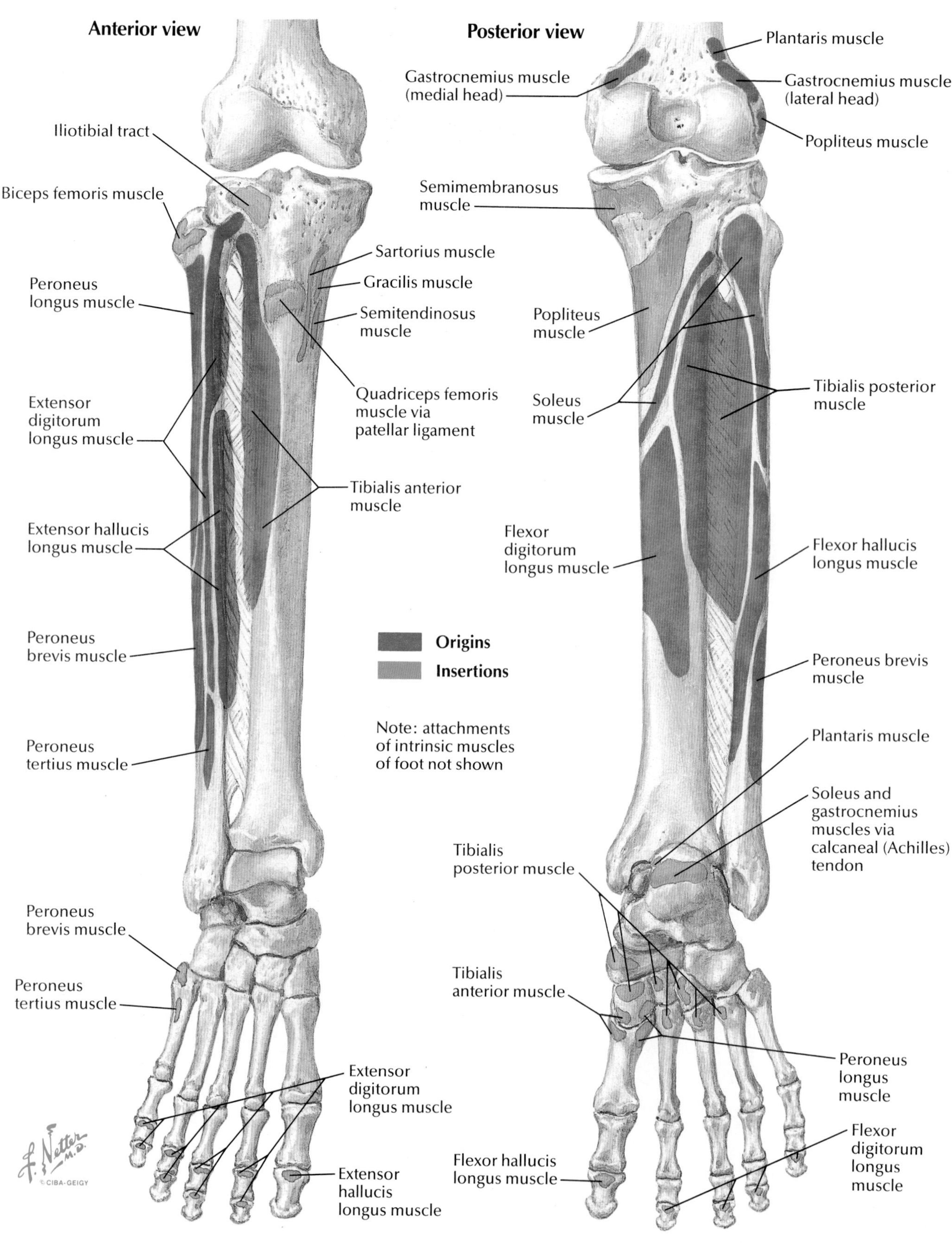

Anterior view

Iliotibial tract

Biceps femoris muscle

Peroneus longus muscle

Extensor digitorum longus muscle

Extensor hallucis longus muscle

Peroneus brevis muscle

Peroneus tertius muscle

Peroneus brevis muscle

Peroneus tertius muscle

Extensor digitorum longus muscle

Extensor hallucis longus muscle

Sartorius muscle

Gracilis muscle

Semitendinosus muscle

Quadriceps femoris muscle via patellar ligament

Tibialis anterior muscle

Posterior view

Gastrocnemius muscle (medial head)

Semimembranosus muscle

Popliteus muscle

Soleus muscle

Flexor digitorum longus muscle

Plantaris muscle

Gastrocnemius muscle (lateral head)

Popliteus muscle

Tibialis posterior muscle

Flexor hallucis longus muscle

Peroneus brevis muscle

Plantaris muscle

Soleus and gastrocnemius muscles via calcaneal (Achilles) tendon

Tibialis posterior muscle

Tibialis anterior muscle

Flexor hallucis longus muscle

Peroneus longus muscle

Flexor digitorum longus muscle

Origins

Insertions

Note: attachments of intrinsic muscles of foot not shown

PLATE 484

LOWER LIMB

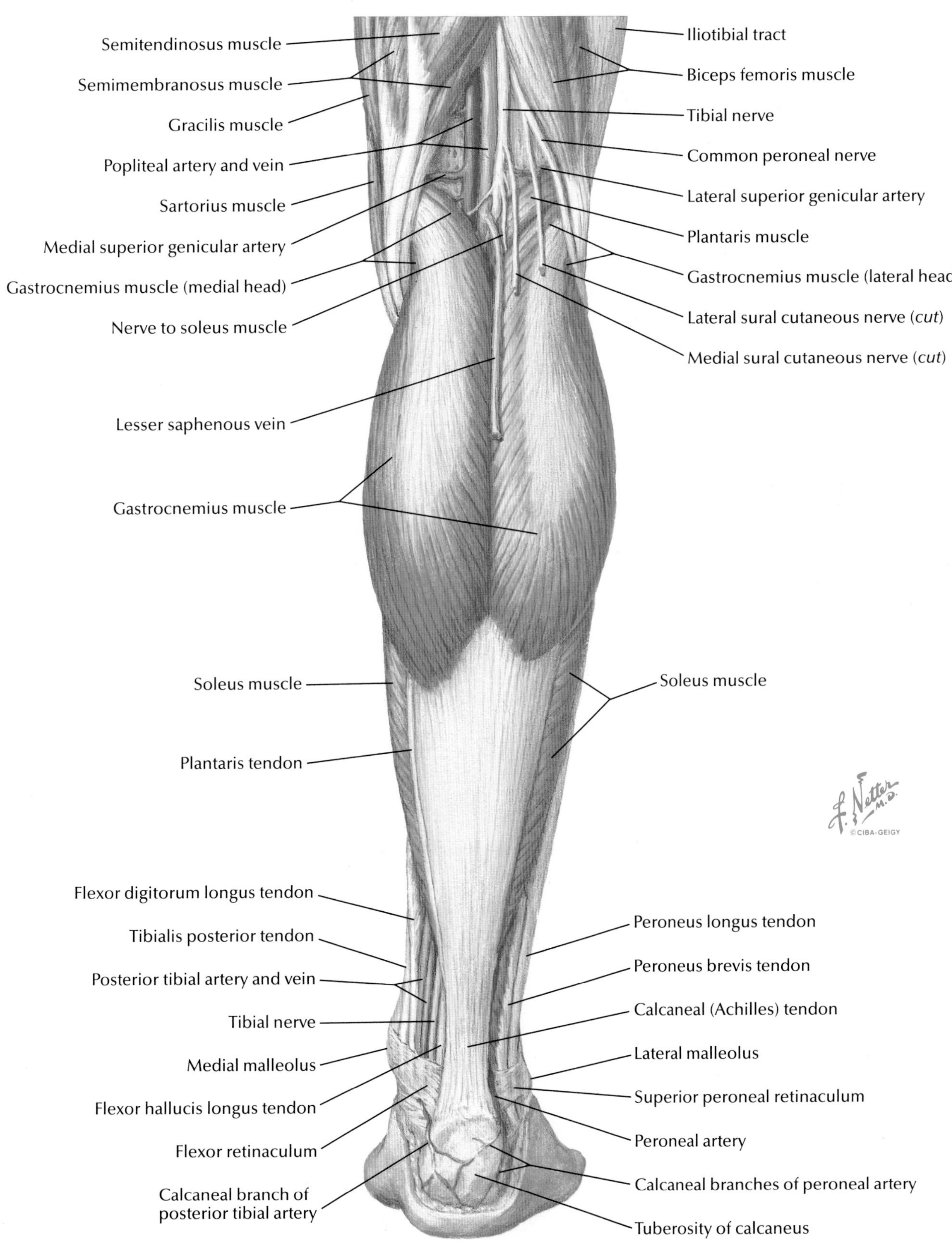

Semitendinosus muscle

Semimembranosus muscle

Gracilis muscle

Popliteal artery and vein

Sartorius muscle

Medial superior genicular artery

Gastrocnemius muscle (medial head)

Nerve to soleus muscle

Lesser saphenous vein

Gastrocnemius muscle

Soleus muscle

Plantaris tendon

Flexor digitorum longus tendon

Tibialis posterior tendon

Posterior tibial artery and vein

Tibial nerve

Medial malleolus

Flexor hallucis longus tendon

Flexor retinaculum

Calcaneal branch of posterior tibial artery

Iliotibial tract

Biceps femoris muscle

Tibial nerve

Common peroneal nerve

Lateral superior genicular artery

Plantaris muscle

Gastrocnemius muscle (lateral head)

Lateral sural cutaneous nerve (*cut*)

Medial sural cutaneous nerve (*cut*)

Soleus muscle

Peroneus longus tendon

Peroneus brevis tendon

Calcaneal (Achilles) tendon

Lateral malleolus

Superior peroneal retinaculum

Peroneal artery

Calcaneal branches of peroneal artery

Tuberosity of calcaneus

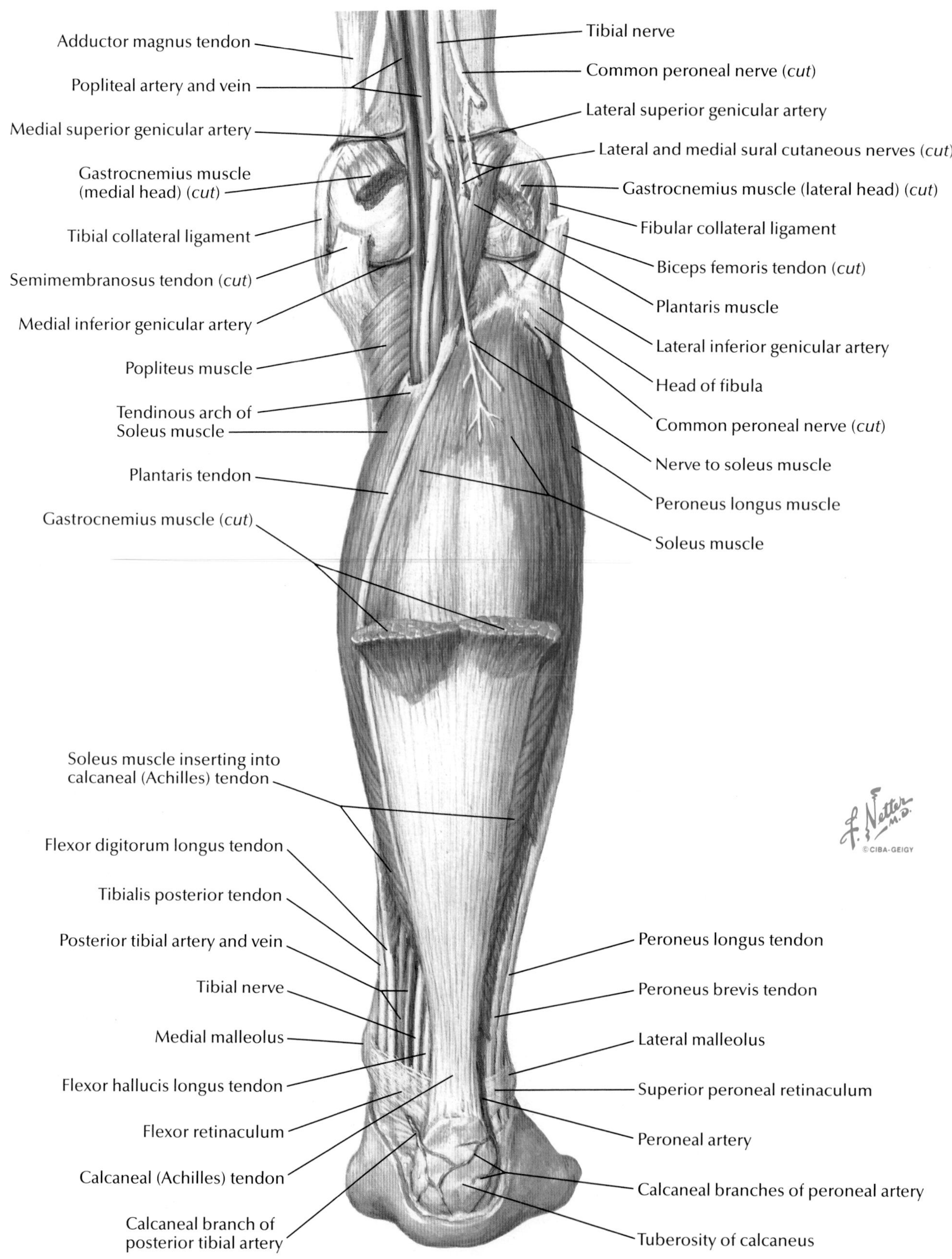

Adductor magnus tendon

Popliteal artery and vein

Medial superior genicular artery

Gastrocnemius muscle (medial head) (cut)

Tibial collateral ligament

Semimembranosus tendon (cut)

Medial inferior genicular artery

Popliteus muscle

Tendinous arch of Soleus muscle

Plantaris tendon

Gastrocnemius muscle (cut)

Soleus muscle inserting into calcaneal (Achilles) tendon

Flexor digitorum longus tendon

Tibialis posterior tendon

Posterior tibial artery and vein

Tibial nerve

Medial malleolus

Flexor hallucis longus tendon

Flexor retinaculum

Calcaneal (Achilles) tendon

Calcaneal branch of posterior tibial artery

Tibial nerve

Common peroneal nerve (cut)

Lateral superior genicular artery

Lateral and medial sural cutaneous nerves (cut)

Gastrocnemius muscle (lateral head) (cut)

Fibular collateral ligament

Biceps femoris tendon (cut)

Plantaris muscle

Lateral inferior genicular artery

Head of fibula

Common peroneal nerve (cut)

Nerve to soleus muscle

Peroneus longus muscle

Soleus muscle

Peroneus longus tendon

Peroneus brevis tendon

Lateral malleolus

Superior peroneal retinaculum

Peroneal artery

Calcaneal branches of peroneal artery

Tuberosity of calcaneus

PLATE 486

LOWER LIMB

SEE ALSO PLATE 509

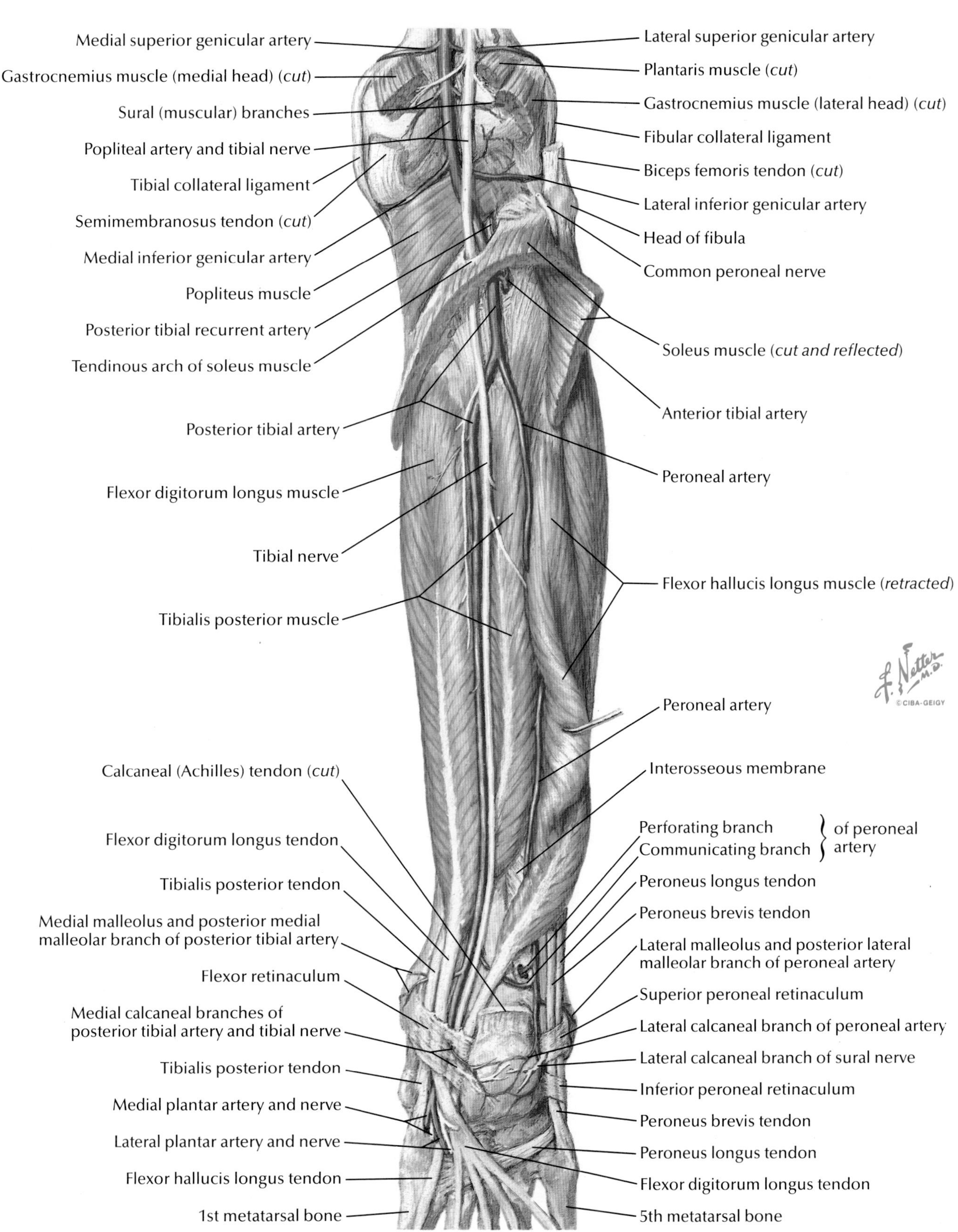

Medial superior genicular artery

Gastrocnemius muscle (medial head) (*cut*)

Sural (muscular) branches

Popliteal artery and tibial nerve

Tibial collateral ligament

Semimembranosus tendon (*cut*)

Medial inferior genicular artery

Popliteus muscle

Posterior tibial recurrent artery

Tendinous arch of soleus muscle

Posterior tibial artery

Flexor digitorum longus muscle

Tibial nerve

Tibialis posterior muscle

Calcaneal (Achilles) tendon (*cut*)

Flexor digitorum longus tendon

Tibialis posterior tendon

Medial malleolus and posterior medial malleolar branch of posterior tibial artery

Flexor retinaculum

Medial calcaneal branches of posterior tibial artery and tibial nerve

Tibialis posterior tendon

Medial plantar artery and nerve

Lateral plantar artery and nerve

Flexor hallucis longus tendon

1st metatarsal bone

Lateral superior genicular artery

Plantaris muscle (*cut*)

Gastrocnemius muscle (lateral head) (*cut*)

Fibular collateral ligament

Biceps femoris tendon (*cut*)

Lateral inferior genicular artery

Head of fibula

Common peroneal nerve

Soleus muscle (*cut and reflected*)

Anterior tibial artery

Peroneal artery

Flexor hallucis longus muscle (*retracted*)

Peroneal artery

Interosseous membrane

Perforating branch } of peroneal
Communicating branch } artery

Peroneus longus tendon

Peroneus brevis tendon

Lateral malleolus and posterior lateral malleolar branch of peroneal artery

Superior peroneal retinaculum

Lateral calcaneal branch of peroneal artery

Lateral calcaneal branch of sural nerve

Inferior peroneal retinaculum

Peroneus brevis tendon

Peroneus longus tendon

Flexor digitorum longus tendon

5th metatarsal bone

f. Netter
M.D.
©CIBA-GEIGY

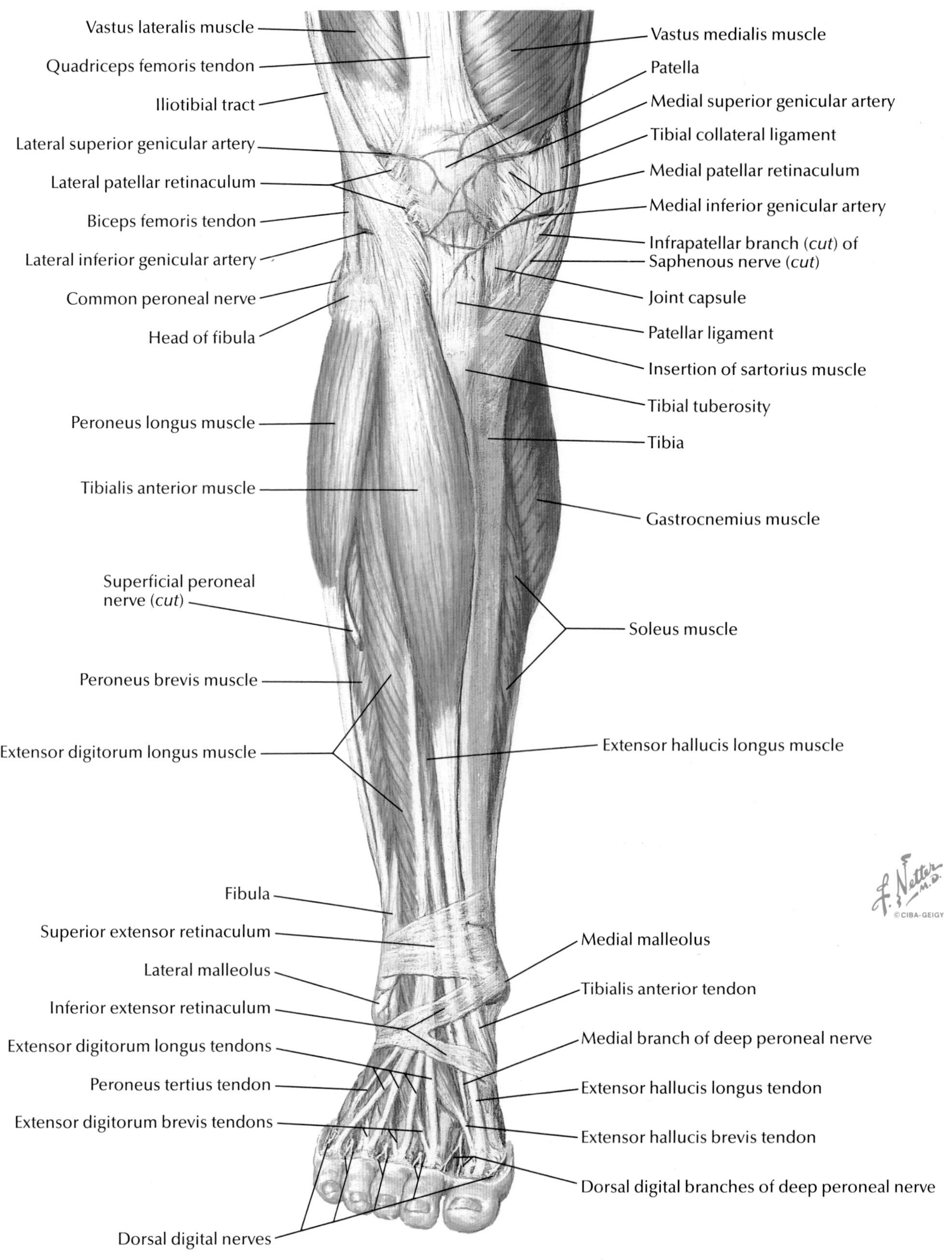

Vastus lateralis muscle

Quadriceps femoris tendon

Iliotibial tract

Lateral superior genicular artery

Lateral patellar retinaculum

Biceps femoris tendon

Lateral inferior genicular artery

Common peroneal nerve

Head of fibula

Peroneus longus muscle

Tibialis anterior muscle

Superficial peroneal nerve (*cut*)

Peroneus brevis muscle

Extensor digitorum longus muscle

Fibula

Superior extensor retinaculum

Lateral malleolus

Inferior extensor retinaculum

Extensor digitorum longus tendons

Peroneus tertius tendon

Extensor digitorum brevis tendons

Dorsal digital nerves

Vastus medialis muscle

Patella

Medial superior genicular artery

Tibial collateral ligament

Medial patellar retinaculum

Medial inferior genicular artery

Infrapatellar branch (*cut*) of Saphenous nerve (*cut*)

Joint capsule

Patellar ligament

Insertion of sartorius muscle

Tibial tuberosity

Tibia

Gastrocnemius muscle

Soleus muscle

Extensor hallucis longus muscle

Medial malleolus

Tibialis anterior tendon

Medial branch of deep peroneal nerve

Extensor hallucis longus tendon

Extensor hallucis brevis tendon

Dorsal digital branches of deep peroneal nerve

PLATE 488

LOWER LIMB

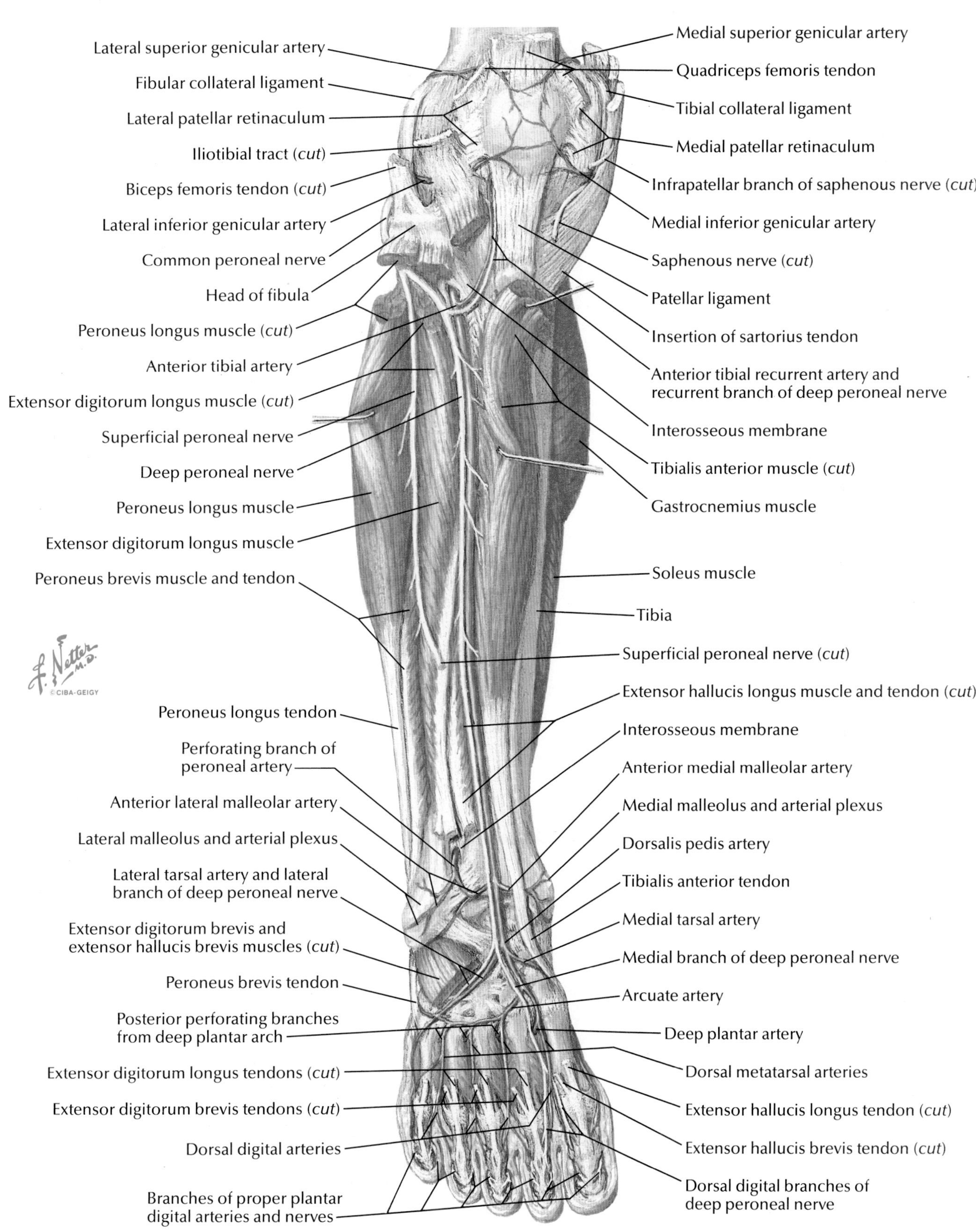

Lateral superior genicular artery

Fibular collateral ligament

Lateral patellar retinaculum

Iliotibial tract (cut)

Biceps femoris tendon (cut)

Lateral inferior genicular artery

Common peroneal nerve

Head of fibula

Peroneus longus muscle (cut)

Anterior tibial artery

Extensor digitorum longus muscle (cut)

Superficial peroneal nerve

Deep peroneal nerve

Peroneus longus muscle

Extensor digitorum longus muscle

Peroneus brevis muscle and tendon

Peroneus longus tendon

Perforating branch of peroneal artery

Anterior lateral malleolar artery

Lateral malleolus and arterial plexus

Lateral tarsal artery and lateral branch of deep peroneal nerve

Extensor digitorum brevis and extensor hallucis brevis muscles (cut)

Peroneus brevis tendon

Posterior perforating branches from deep plantar arch

Extensor digitorum longus tendons (cut)

Extensor digitorum brevis tendons (cut)

Dorsal digital arteries

Branches of proper plantar digital arteries and nerves

Medial superior genicular artery

Quadriceps femoris tendon

Tibial collateral ligament

Medial patellar retinaculum

Infrapatellar branch of saphenous nerve (cut)

Medial inferior genicular artery

Saphenous nerve (cut)

Patellar ligament

Insertion of sartorius tendon

Anterior tibial recurrent artery and recurrent branch of deep peroneal nerve

Interosseous membrane

Tibialis anterior muscle (cut)

Gastrocnemius muscle

Soleus muscle

Tibia

Superficial peroneal nerve (cut)

Extensor hallucis longus muscle and tendon (cut)

Interosseous membrane

Anterior medial malleolar artery

Medial malleolus and arterial plexus

Dorsalis pedis artery

Tibialis anterior tendon

Medial tarsal artery

Medial branch of deep peroneal nerve

Arcuate artery

Deep plantar artery

Dorsal metatarsal arteries

Extensor hallucis longus tendon (cut)

Extensor hallucis brevis tendon (cut)

Dorsal digital branches of deep peroneal nerve

SEE ALSO PLATE 510

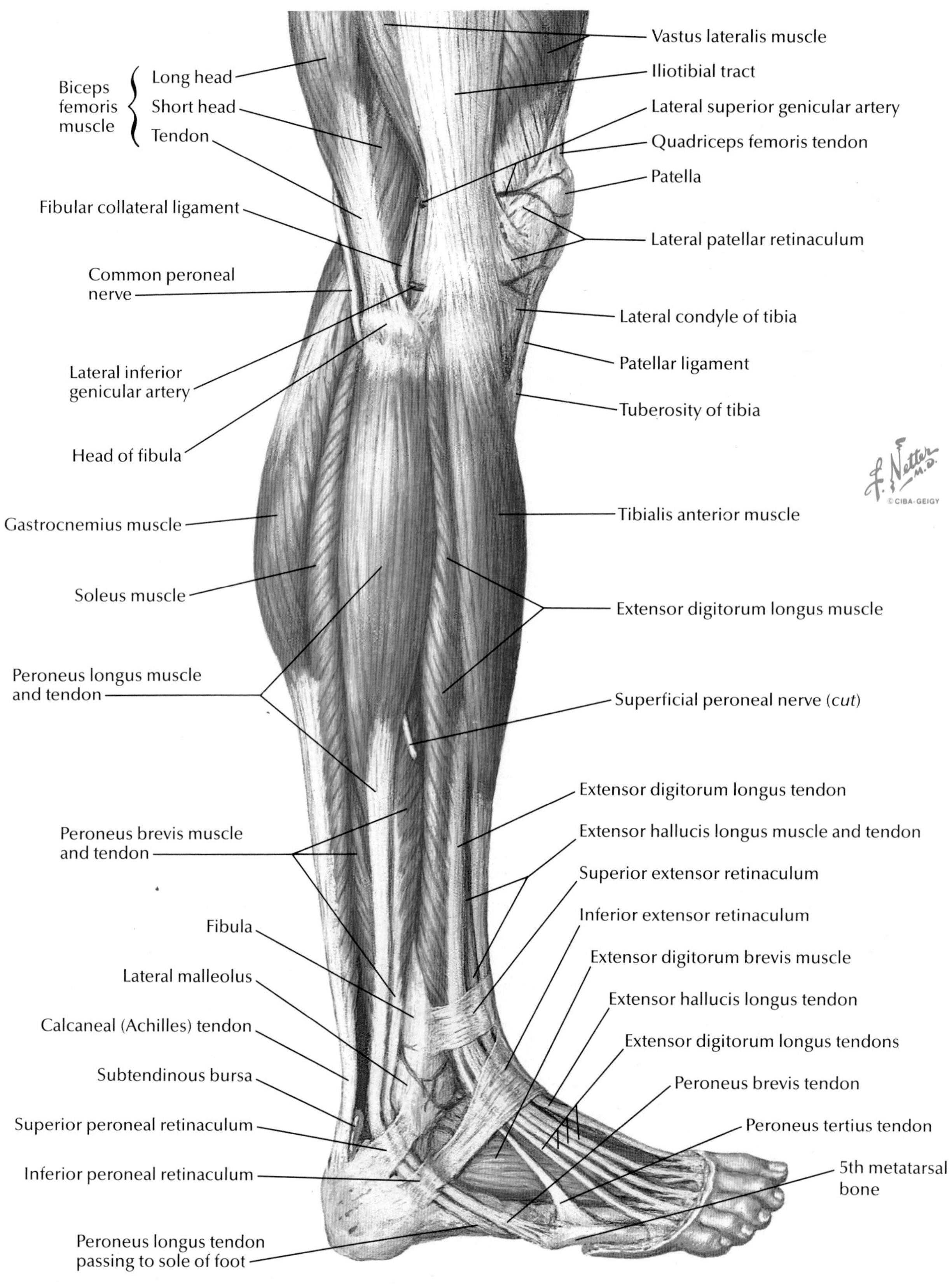

Biceps femoris muscle { Long head / Short head / Tendon

Vastus lateralis muscle

Iliotibial tract

Lateral superior genicular artery

Quadriceps femoris tendon

Patella

Fibular collateral ligament

Lateral patellar retinaculum

Common peroneal nerve

Lateral condyle of tibia

Patellar ligament

Lateral inferior genicular artery

Tuberosity of tibia

Head of fibula

Tibialis anterior muscle

Gastrocnemius muscle

Soleus muscle

Extensor digitorum longus muscle

Peroneus longus muscle and tendon

Superficial peroneal nerve (cut)

Peroneus brevis muscle and tendon

Extensor digitorum longus tendon

Extensor hallucis longus muscle and tendon

Superior extensor retinaculum

Inferior extensor retinaculum

Fibula

Lateral malleolus

Extensor digitorum brevis muscle

Calcaneal (Achilles) tendon

Extensor hallucis longus tendon

Subtendinous bursa

Extensor digitorum longus tendons

Superior peroneal retinaculum

Peroneus brevis tendon

Inferior peroneal retinaculum

Peroneus tertius tendon

5th metatarsal bone

Peroneus longus tendon passing to sole of foot

PLATE 490

LOWER LIMB

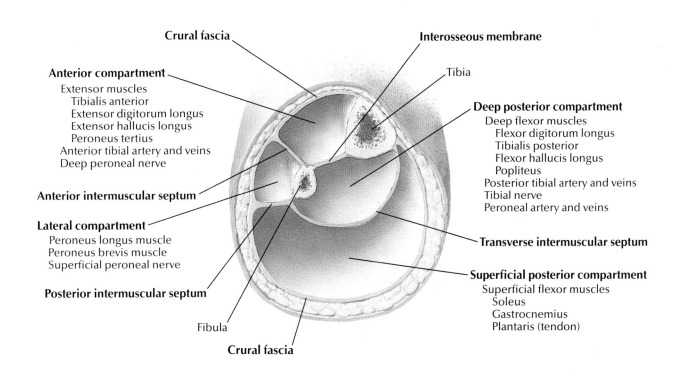

Crural fascia

Interosseous membrane

Tibia

Anterior compartment
Extensor muscles
Tibialis anterior
Extensor digitorum longus
Extensor hallucis longus
Peroneus tertius
Anterior tibial artery and veins
Deep peroneal nerve

Deep posterior compartment
Deep flexor muscles
Flexor digitorum longus
Tibialis posterior
Flexor hallucis longus
Popliteus
Posterior tibial artery and veins
Tibial nerve
Peroneal artery and veins

Anterior intermuscular septum

Transverse intermuscular septum

Lateral compartment
Peroneus longus muscle
Peroneus brevis muscle
Superficial peroneal nerve

Superficial posterior compartment
Superficial flexor muscles
Soleus
Gastrocnemius
Plantaris (tendon)

Posterior intermuscular septum

Fibula

Crural fascia

Cross section just above middle of left leg

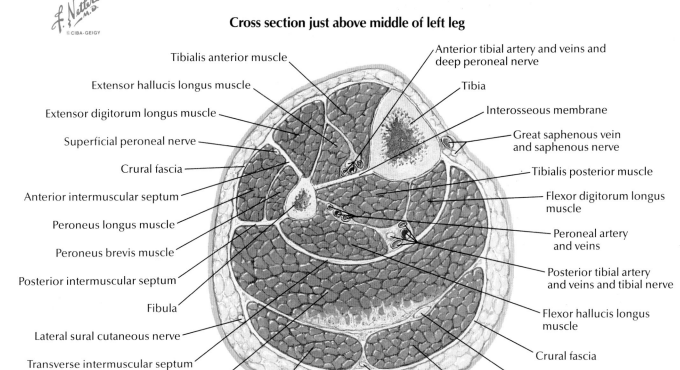

Tibialis anterior muscle

Anterior tibial artery and veins and deep peroneal nerve

Extensor hallucis longus muscle

Tibia

Extensor digitorum longus muscle

Interosseous membrane

Superficial peroneal nerve

Great saphenous vein and saphenous nerve

Crural fascia

Tibialis posterior muscle

Anterior intermuscular septum

Flexor digitorum longus muscle

Peroneus longus muscle

Peroneal artery and veins

Peroneus brevis muscle

Posterior tibial artery and veins and tibial nerve

Posterior intermuscular septum

Fibula

Flexor hallucis longus muscle

Lateral sural cutaneous nerve

Crural fascia

Transverse intermuscular septum

Plantaris tendon

Soleus muscle

Gastrocnemius muscle (medial belly)

Gastrocnemius muscle (lateral belly)

Medial sural cutaneous nerve

Peroneal communicating branch of lateral sural cutaneous nerve

Lesser saphenous vein

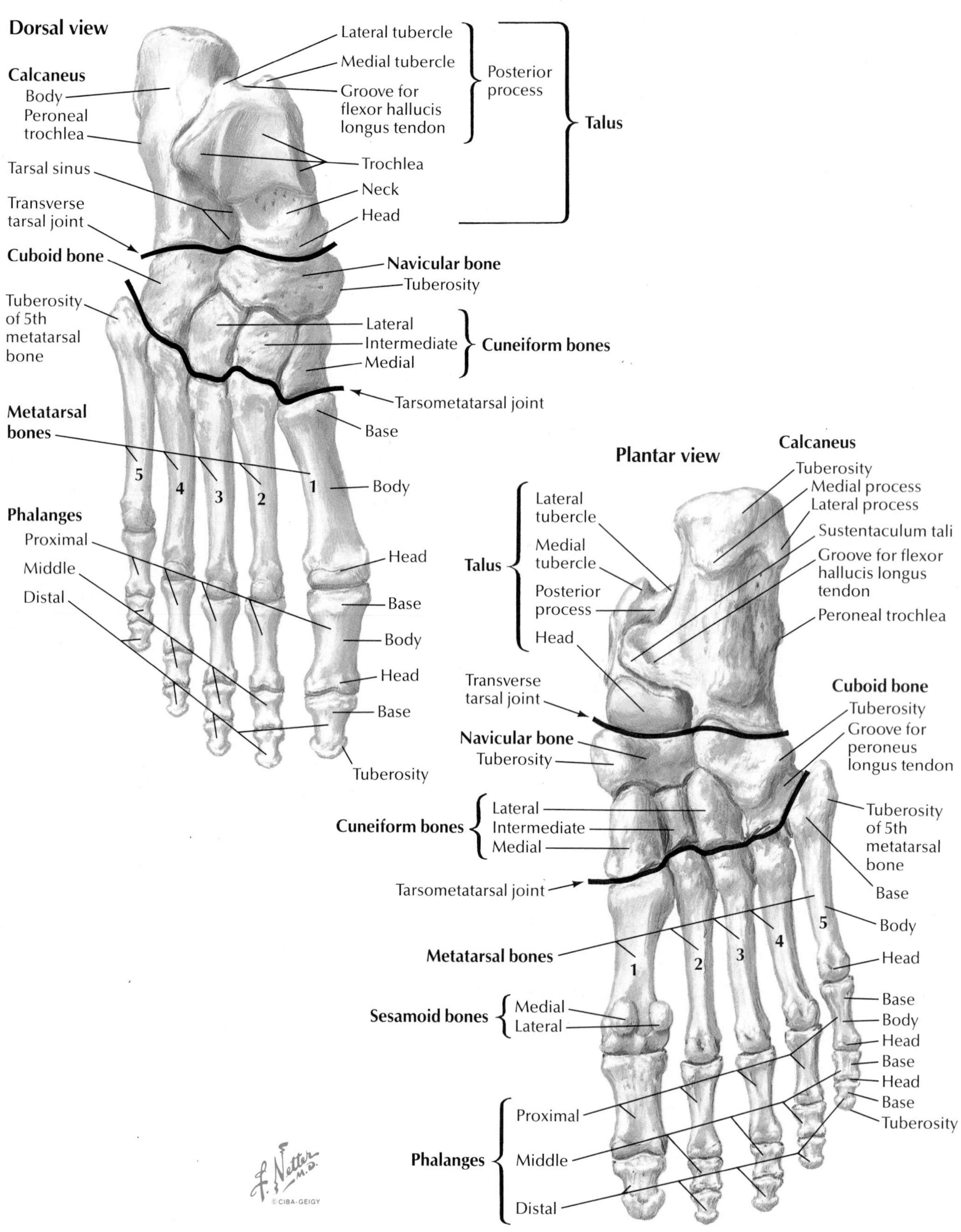

Dorsal view

Calcaneus
Body
Peroneal trochlea

Tarsal sinus

Transverse tarsal joint

Cuboid bone

Tuberosity of 5th metatarsal bone

Metatarsal bones

5 4 3 2 1

Phalanges
Proximal
Middle
Distal

Lateral tubercle
Medial tubercle
Groove for flexor hallucis longus tendon

Posterior process

Trochlea
Neck
Head

Talus

Navicular bone
Tuberosity

Lateral
Intermediate
Medial

Cuneiform bones

Tarsometatarsal joint

Base

Body

Head
Base
Body
Head
Base

Tuberosity

Plantar view

Calcaneus
Tuberosity
Medial process
Lateral process
Sustentaculum tali
Groove for flexor hallucis longus tendon
Peroneal trochlea

Lateral tubercle
Medial tubercle
Posterior process
Head

Talus

Transverse tarsal joint

Navicular bone
Tuberosity

Cuboid bone
Tuberosity
Groove for peroneus longus tendon

Tuberosity of 5th metatarsal bone

Base

Lateral
Intermediate
Medial

Cuneiform bones

Tarsometatarsal joint

Metatarsal bones

1 2 3 4 5

Body
Head
Base
Body
Head
Base
Head
Base
Tuberosity

Sesamoid bones
Medial
Lateral

Phalanges
Proximal
Middle
Distal

PLATE 492

Lateral view

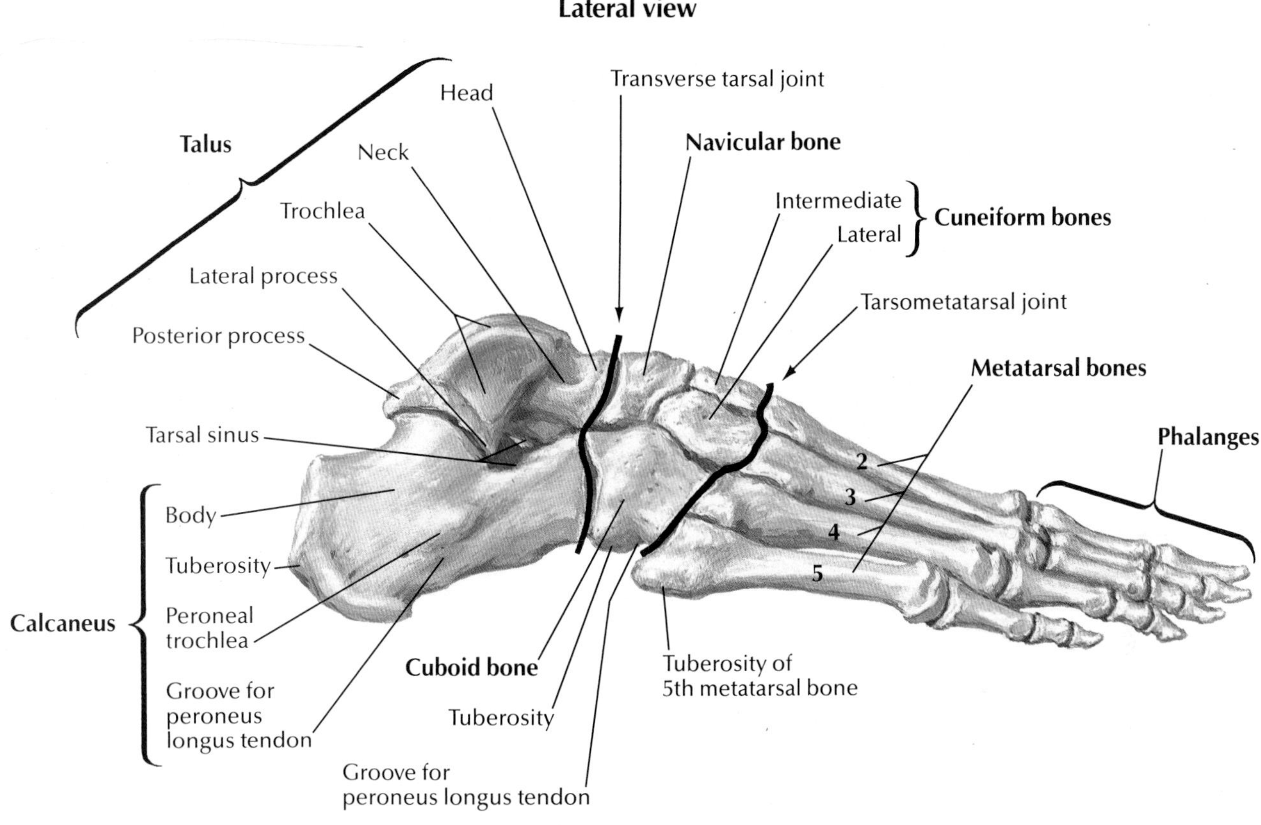

Talus
- Head
- Neck
- Trochlea
- Lateral process
- Posterior process

Transverse tarsal joint

Navicular bone

Intermediate } **Cuneiform bones**
Lateral

Tarsometatarsal joint

Metatarsal bones

Phalanges

Tarsal sinus

Calcaneus
- Body
- Tuberosity
- Peroneal trochlea
- Groove for peroneus longus tendon

Cuboid bone

Tuberosity

Groove for peroneus longus tendon

Tuberosity of 5th metatarsal bone

2
3
4
5

Medial view

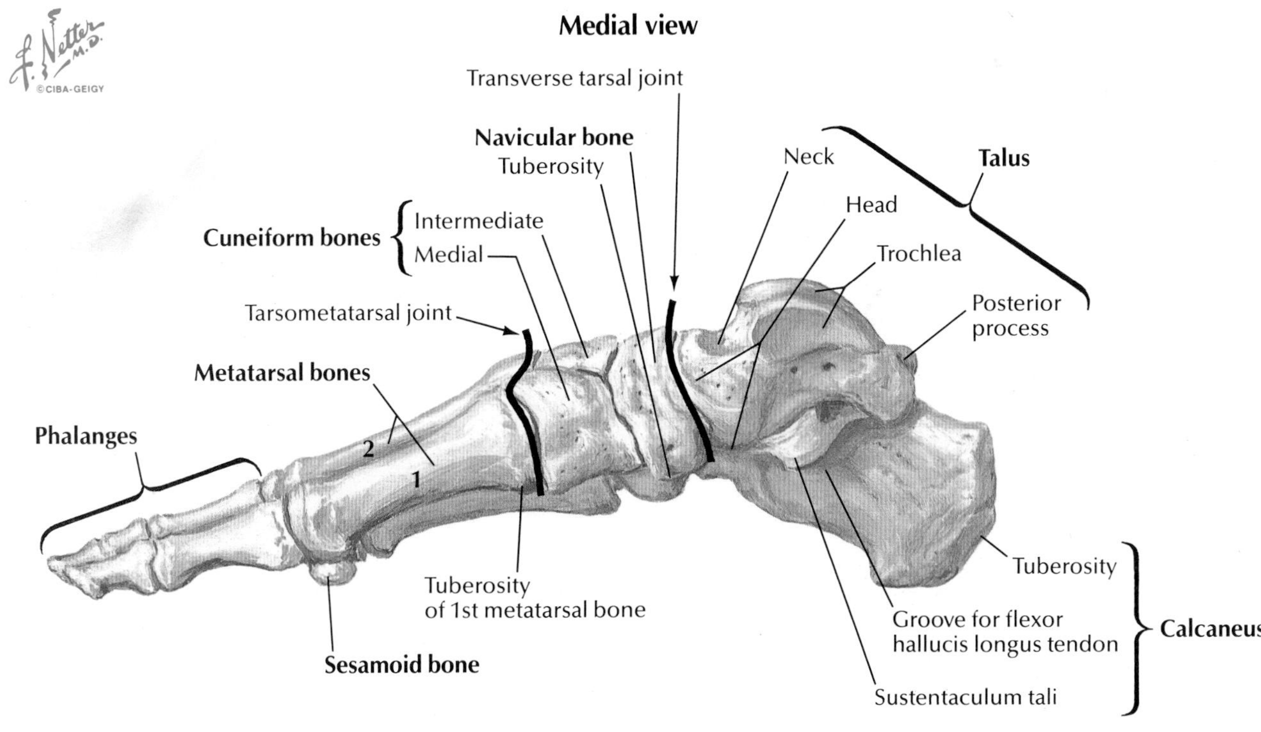

Transverse tarsal joint

Navicular bone
Tuberosity

Neck

Talus

Head

Trochlea

Posterior process

Cuneiform bones {
Intermediate
Medial

Tarsometatarsal joint

Metatarsal bones

Phalanges

2
1

Tuberosity of 1st metatarsal bone

Sesamoid bone

Tuberosity

Groove for flexor hallucis longus tendon

Sustentaculum tali

Calcaneus

Calcaneus

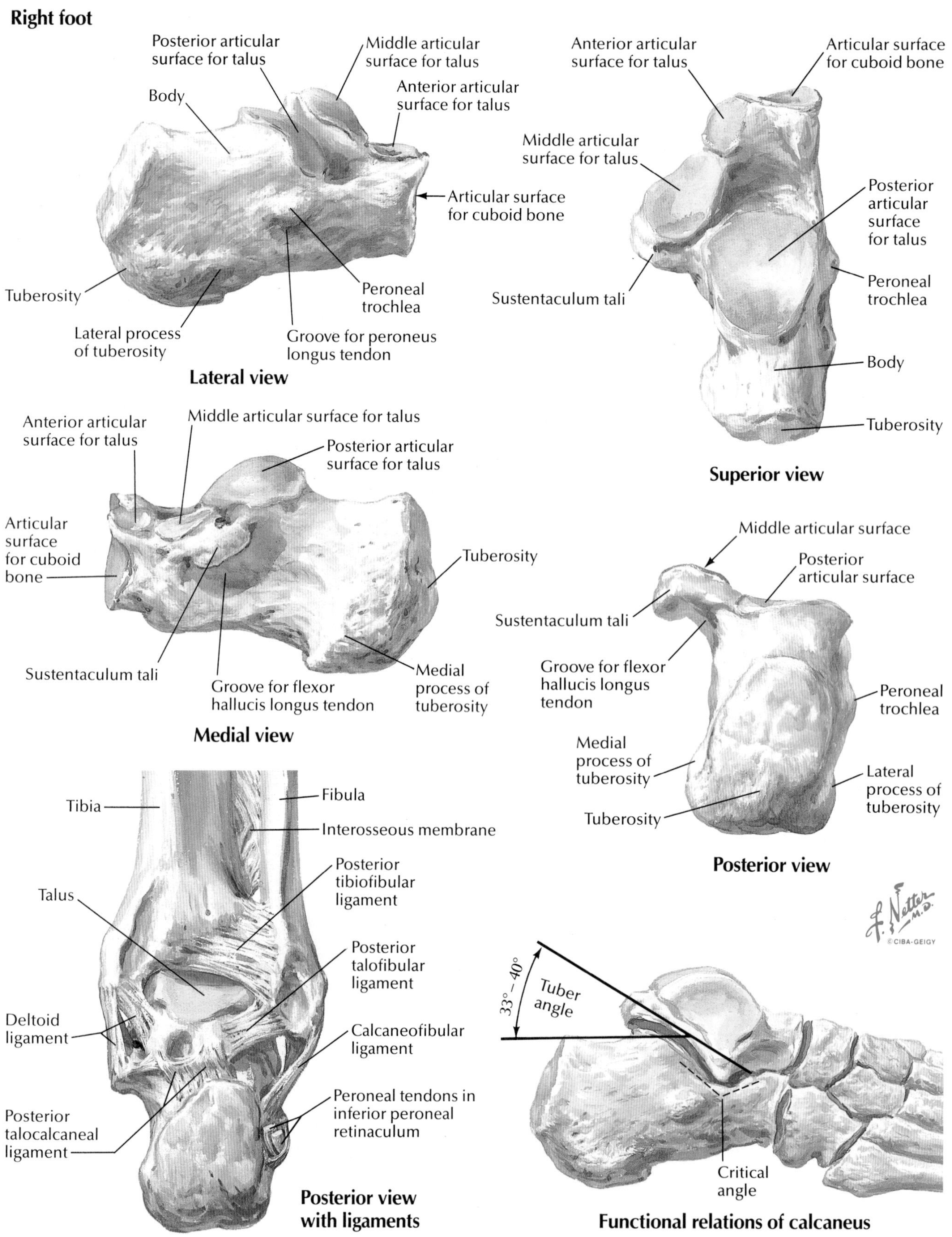

Posterior articular surface for talus

Middle articular surface for talus

Body

Anterior articular surface for talus

Articular surface for cuboid bone

Tuberosity

Peroneal trochlea

Lateral process of tuberosity

Groove for peroneus longus tendon

Lateral view

Anterior articular surface for talus

Articular surface for cuboid bone

Middle articular surface for talus

Posterior articular surface for talus

Sustentaculum tali

Peroneal trochlea

Body

Tuberosity

Superior view

Anterior articular surface for talus

Middle articular surface for talus

Posterior articular surface for talus

Articular surface for cuboid bone

Tuberosity

Sustentaculum tali

Groove for flexor hallucis longus tendon

Medial process of tuberosity

Medial view

Middle articular surface

Posterior articular surface

Sustentaculum tali

Groove for flexor hallucis longus tendon

Medial process of tuberosity

Tuberosity

Peroneal trochlea

Lateral process of tuberosity

Posterior view

Tibia

Fibula

Interosseous membrane

Posterior tibiofibular ligament

Talus

Posterior talofibular ligament

Deltoid ligament

Calcaneofibular ligament

Posterior talocalcaneal ligament

Peroneal tendons in inferior peroneal retinaculum

Posterior view with ligaments

33° – 40°

Tuber angle

Critical angle

Functional relations of calcaneus

PLATE 494

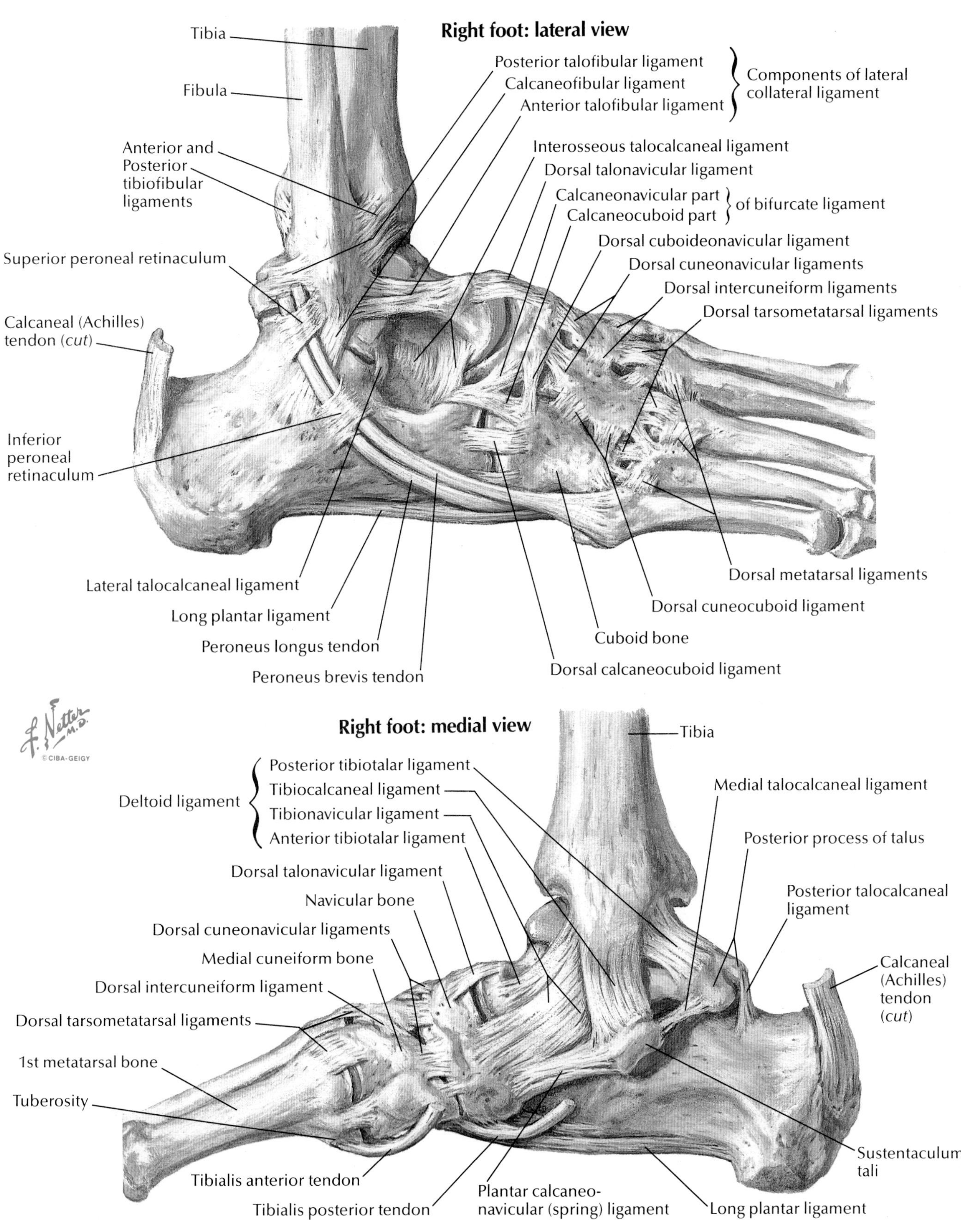

Right foot: lateral view

Tibia

Fibula

Posterior talofibular ligament
Calcaneofibular ligament
Anterior talofibular ligament

} Components of lateral collateral ligament

Interosseous talocalcaneal ligament

Dorsal talonavicular ligament

Anterior and Posterior tibiofibular ligaments

Calcaneonavicular part
Calcaneocuboid part

} of bifurcate ligament

Dorsal cuboideonavicular ligament

Superior peroneal retinaculum

Dorsal cuneonavicular ligaments

Dorsal intercuneiform ligaments

Dorsal tarsometatarsal ligaments

Calcaneal (Achilles) tendon (*cut*)

Inferior peroneal retinaculum

Lateral talocalcaneal ligament

Long plantar ligament

Peroneus longus tendon

Peroneus brevis tendon

Dorsal metatarsal ligaments

Dorsal cuneocuboid ligament

Cuboid bone

Dorsal calcaneocuboid ligament

Right foot: medial view

Tibia

Deltoid ligament {

Posterior tibiotalar ligament
Tibiocalcaneal ligament
Tibionavicular ligament
Anterior tibiotalar ligament

Medial talocalcaneal ligament

Posterior process of talus

Posterior talocalcaneal ligament

Dorsal talonavicular ligament

Navicular bone

Dorsal cuneonavicular ligaments

Medial cuneiform bone

Dorsal intercuneiform ligament

Dorsal tarsometatarsal ligaments

1st metatarsal bone

Tuberosity

Calcaneal (Achilles) tendon (*cut*)

Sustentaculum tali

Tibialis anterior tendon

Tibialis posterior tendon

Plantar calcaneo-navicular (spring) ligament

Long plantar ligament

Ligaments and Tendons of Foot: Plantar View

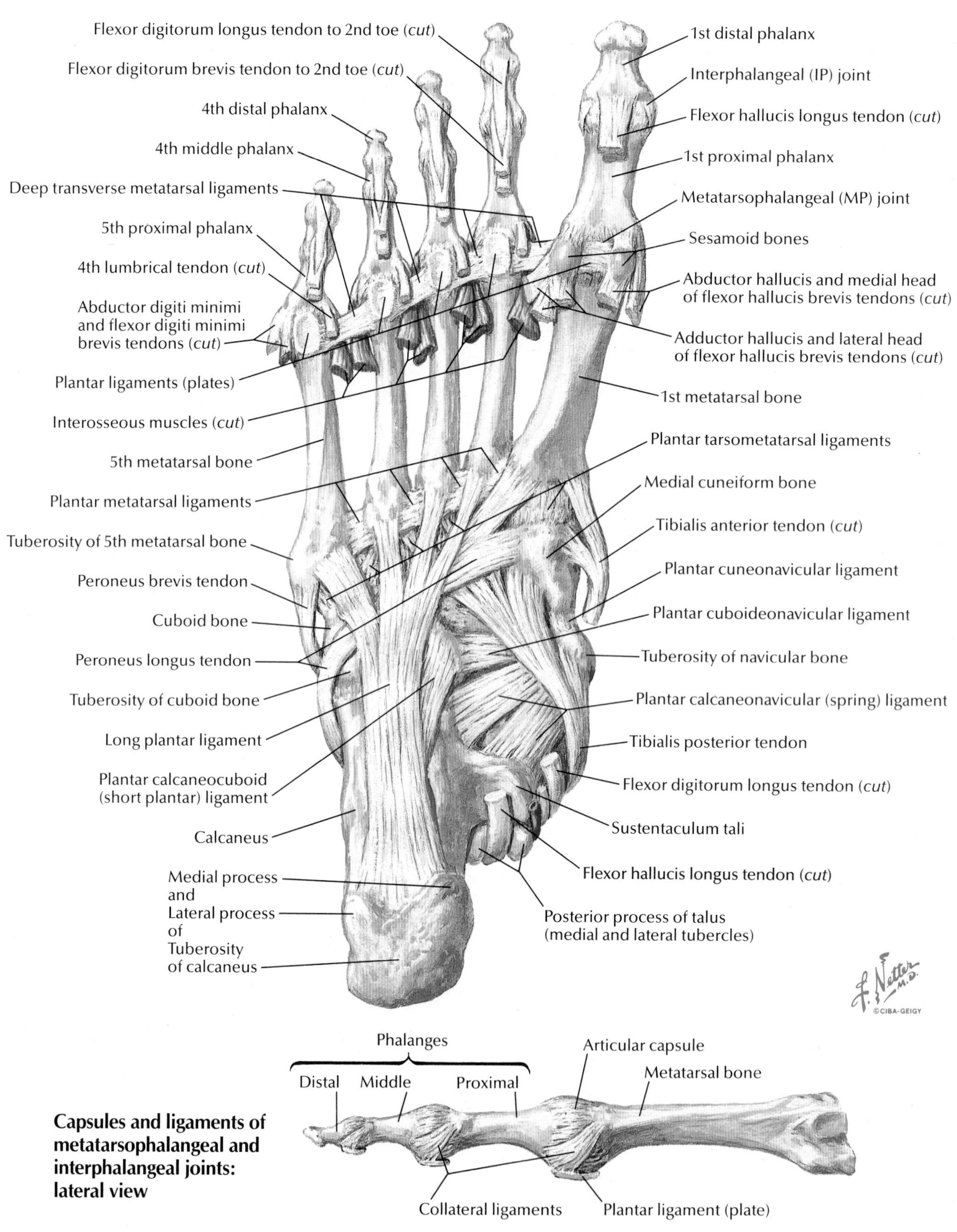

Flexor digitorum longus tendon to 2nd toe (cut)

Flexor digitorum brevis tendon to 2nd toe (cut)

4th distal phalanx

4th middle phalanx

Deep transverse metatarsal ligaments

5th proximal phalanx

4th lumbrical tendon (cut)

Abductor digiti minimi and flexor digiti minimi brevis tendons (cut)

Plantar ligaments (plates)

Interosseous muscles (cut)

5th metatarsal bone

Plantar metatarsal ligaments

Tuberosity of 5th metatarsal bone

Peroneus brevis tendon

Cuboid bone

Peroneus longus tendon

Tuberosity of cuboid bone

Long plantar ligament

Plantar calcaneocuboid (short plantar) ligament

Calcaneus

Medial process and Lateral process of Tuberosity of calcaneus

1st distal phalanx

Interphalangeal (IP) joint

Flexor hallucis longus tendon (cut)

1st proximal phalanx

Metatarsophalangeal (MP) joint

Sesamoid bones

Abductor hallucis and medial head of flexor hallucis brevis tendons (cut)

Adductor hallucis and lateral head of flexor hallucis brevis tendons (cut)

1st metatarsal bone

Plantar tarsometatarsal ligaments

Medial cuneiform bone

Tibialis anterior tendon (cut)

Plantar cuneonavicular ligament

Plantar cuboideonavicular ligament

Tuberosity of navicular bone

Plantar calcaneonavicular (spring) ligament

Tibialis posterior tendon

Flexor digitorum longus tendon (cut)

Sustentaculum tali

Flexor hallucis longus tendon (cut)

Posterior process of talus (medial and lateral tubercles)

Phalanges

Distal   Middle   Proximal

Articular capsule

Metatarsal bone

Capsules and ligaments of metatarsophalangeal and interphalangeal joints: lateral view

Collateral ligaments

Plantar ligament (plate)

PLATE 496

LOWER LIMB

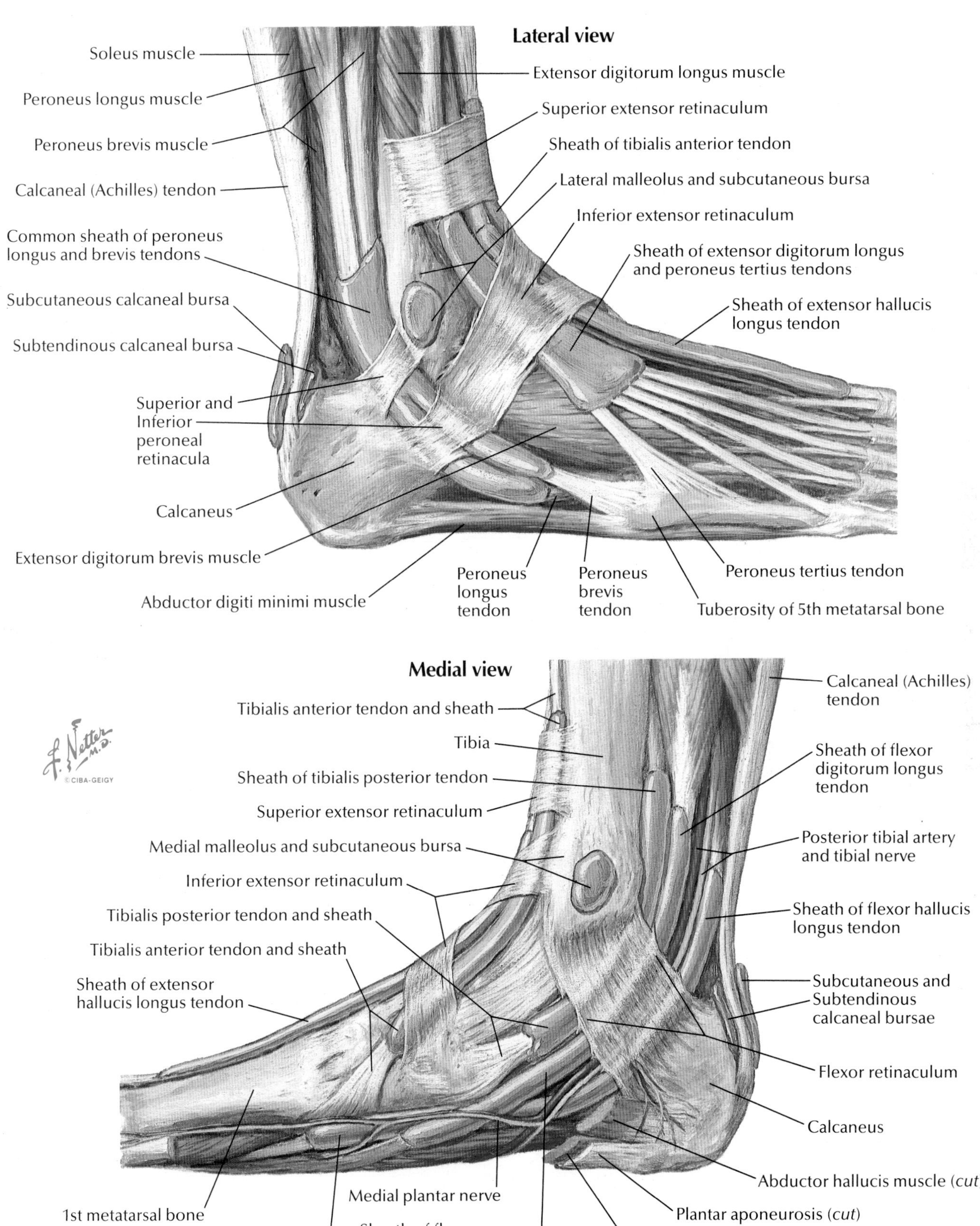

Lateral view

Soleus muscle

Peroneus longus muscle

Peroneus brevis muscle

Calcaneal (Achilles) tendon

Common sheath of peroneus longus and brevis tendons

Subcutaneous calcaneal bursa

Subtendinous calcaneal bursa

Superior and Inferior peroneal retinacula

Calcaneus

Extensor digitorum brevis muscle

Abductor digiti minimi muscle

Extensor digitorum longus muscle

Superior extensor retinaculum

Sheath of tibialis anterior tendon

Lateral malleolus and subcutaneous bursa

Inferior extensor retinaculum

Sheath of extensor digitorum longus and peroneus tertius tendons

Sheath of extensor hallucis longus tendon

Peroneus longus tendon

Peroneus brevis tendon

Peroneus tertius tendon

Tuberosity of 5th metatarsal bone

Medial view

Tibialis anterior tendon and sheath

Tibia

Sheath of tibialis posterior tendon

Superior extensor retinaculum

Medial malleolus and subcutaneous bursa

Inferior extensor retinaculum

Tibialis posterior tendon and sheath

Tibialis anterior tendon and sheath

Sheath of extensor hallucis longus tendon

1st metatarsal bone

Sheath of flexor hallucis longus tendon

Medial plantar nerve

Sheath of flexor digitorum longus tendon

Calcaneal (Achilles) tendon

Sheath of flexor digitorum longus tendon

Posterior tibial artery and tibial nerve

Sheath of flexor hallucis longus tendon

Subcutaneous and Subtendinous calcaneal bursae

Flexor retinaculum

Calcaneus

Abductor hallucis muscle (*cut*)

Plantar aponeurosis (*cut*)

Flexor digitorum brevis muscle (*cut*)

F. Netter M.D.

©CIBA-GEIGY

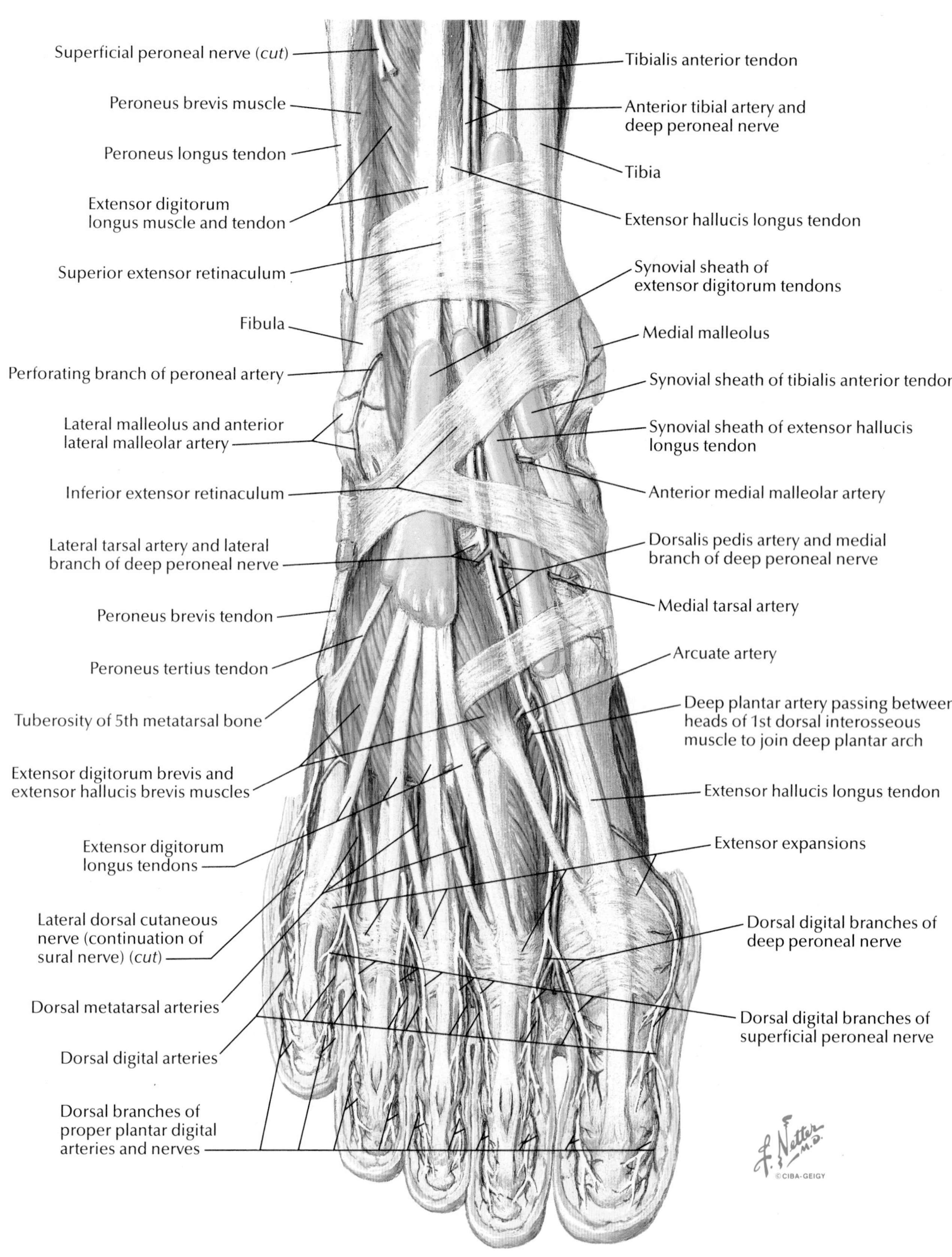

Superficial peroneal nerve (*cut*)

Peroneus brevis muscle

Peroneus longus tendon

Extensor digitorum longus muscle and tendon

Superior extensor retinaculum

Fibula

Perforating branch of peroneal artery

Lateral malleolus and anterior lateral malleolar artery

Inferior extensor retinaculum

Lateral tarsal artery and lateral branch of deep peroneal nerve

Peroneus brevis tendon

Peroneus tertius tendon

Tuberosity of 5th metatarsal bone

Extensor digitorum brevis and extensor hallucis brevis muscles

Extensor digitorum longus tendons

Lateral dorsal cutaneous nerve (continuation of sural nerve) (*cut*)

Dorsal metatarsal arteries

Dorsal digital arteries

Dorsal branches of proper plantar digital arteries and nerves

Tibialis anterior tendon

Anterior tibial artery and deep peroneal nerve

Tibia

Extensor hallucis longus tendon

Synovial sheath of extensor digitorum tendons

Medial malleolus

Synovial sheath of tibialis anterior tendon

Synovial sheath of extensor hallucis longus tendon

Anterior medial malleolar artery

Dorsalis pedis artery and medial branch of deep peroneal nerve

Medial tarsal artery

Arcuate artery

Deep plantar artery passing between heads of 1st dorsal interosseous muscle to join deep plantar arch

Extensor hallucis longus tendon

Extensor expansions

Dorsal digital branches of deep peroneal nerve

Dorsal digital branches of superficial peroneal nerve

PLATE 498

LOWER LIMB

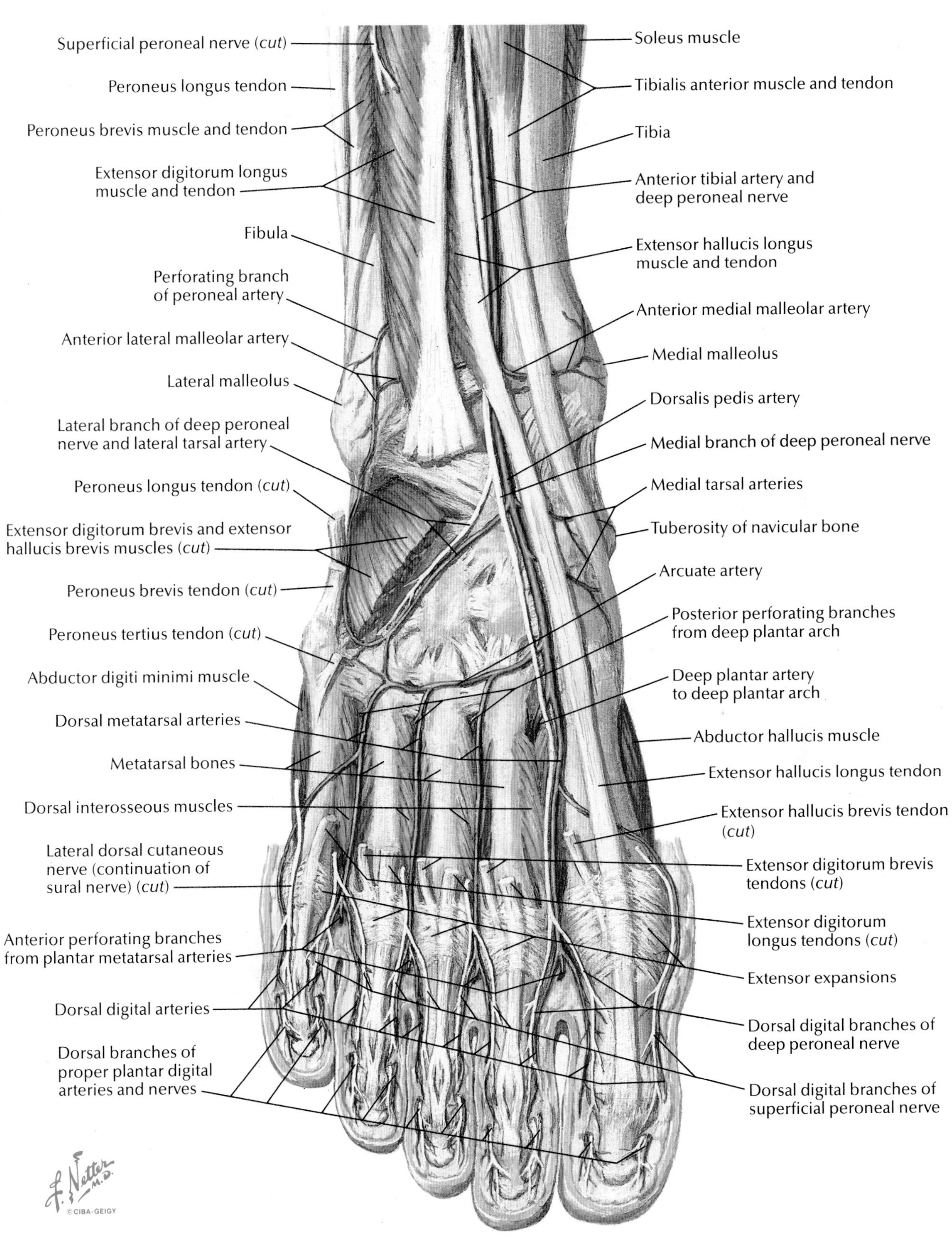

Superficial peroneal nerve (cut)

Peroneus longus tendon

Peroneus brevis muscle and tendon

Extensor digitorum longus muscle and tendon

Fibula

Perforating branch of peroneal artery

Anterior lateral malleolar artery

Lateral malleolus

Lateral branch of deep peroneal nerve and lateral tarsal artery

Peroneus longus tendon (cut)

Extensor digitorum brevis and extensor hallucis brevis muscles (cut)

Peroneus brevis tendon (cut)

Peroneus tertius tendon (cut)

Abductor digiti minimi muscle

Dorsal metatarsal arteries

Metatarsal bones

Dorsal interosseous muscles

Lateral dorsal cutaneous nerve (continuation of sural nerve) (cut)

Anterior perforating branches from plantar metatarsal arteries

Dorsal digital arteries

Dorsal branches of proper plantar digital arteries and nerves

Soleus muscle

Tibialis anterior muscle and tendon

Tibia

Anterior tibial artery and deep peroneal nerve

Extensor hallucis longus muscle and tendon

Anterior medial malleolar artery

Medial malleolus

Dorsalis pedis artery

Medial branch of deep peroneal nerve

Medial tarsal arteries

Tuberosity of navicular bone

Arcuate artery

Posterior perforating branches from deep plantar arch

Deep plantar artery to deep plantar arch

Abductor hallucis muscle

Extensor hallucis longus tendon

Extensor hallucis brevis tendon (cut)

Extensor digitorum brevis tendons (cut)

Extensor digitorum longus tendons (cut)

Extensor expansions

Dorsal digital branches of deep peroneal nerve

Dorsal digital branches of superficial peroneal nerve

Sole of Foot: Superficial Dissection

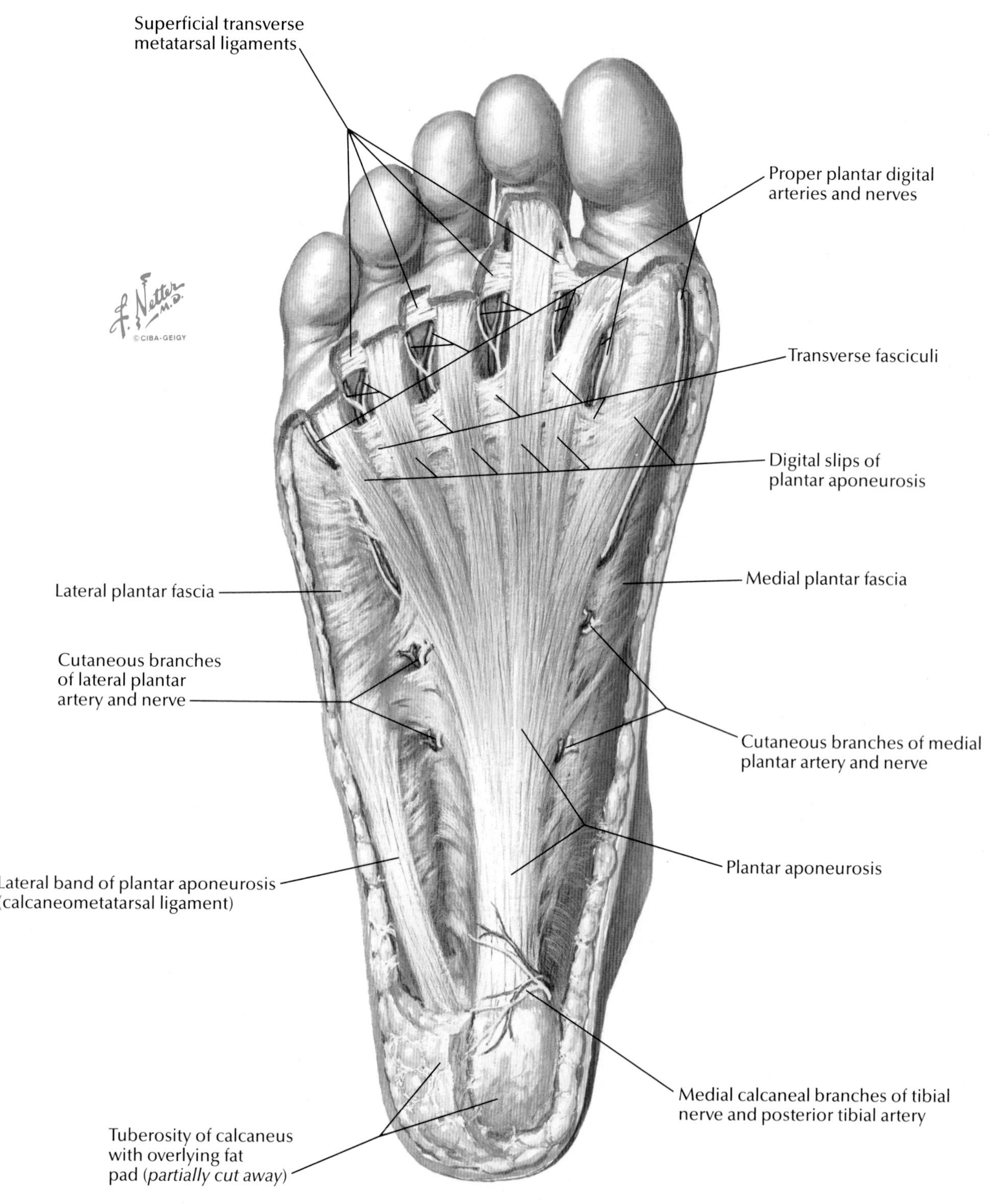

Superficial transverse metatarsal ligaments

Proper plantar digital arteries and nerves

Transverse fasciculi

Digital slips of plantar aponeurosis

Medial plantar fascia

Cutaneous branches of medial plantar artery and nerve

Plantar aponeurosis

Medial calcaneal branches of tibial nerve and posterior tibial artery

Lateral plantar fascia

Cutaneous branches of lateral plantar artery and nerve

Lateral band of plantar aponeurosis (calcaneometatarsal ligament)

Tuberosity of calcaneus with overlying fat pad (*partially cut away*)

PLATE 500

LOWER LIMB

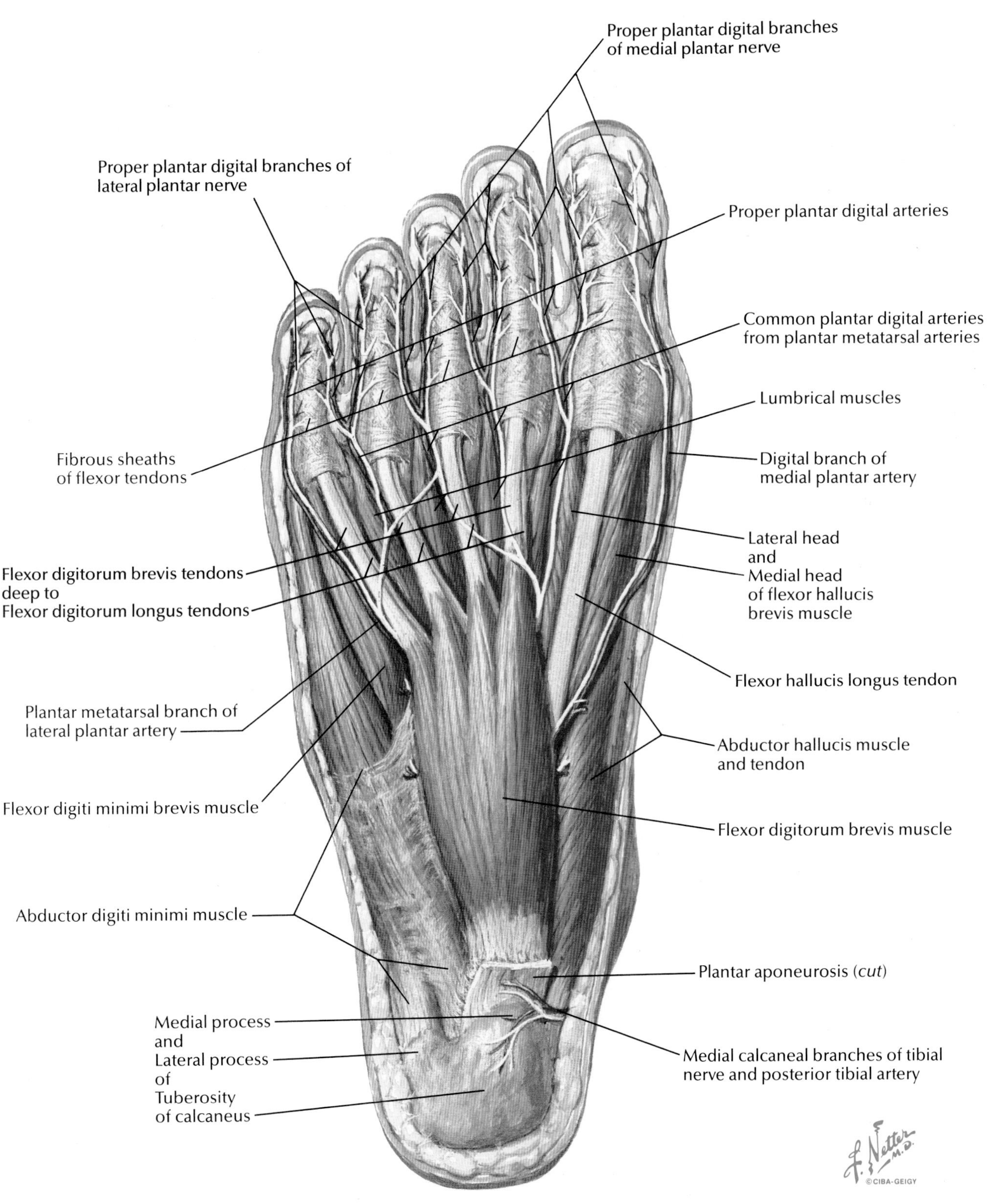

Proper plantar digital branches
of medial plantar nerve

Proper plantar digital branches of
lateral plantar nerve

Proper plantar digital arteries

Common plantar digital arteries
from plantar metatarsal arteries

Lumbrical muscles

Fibrous sheaths
of flexor tendons

Digital branch of
medial plantar artery

Lateral head
and
Medial head
of flexor hallucis
brevis muscle

Flexor digitorum brevis tendons
deep to
Flexor digitorum longus tendons

Flexor hallucis longus tendon

Plantar metatarsal branch of
lateral plantar artery

Abductor hallucis muscle
and tendon

Flexor digiti minimi brevis muscle

Flexor digitorum brevis muscle

Abductor digiti minimi muscle

Plantar aponeurosis (*cut*)

Medial process
and
Lateral process
of
Tuberosity
of calcaneus

Medial calcaneal branches of tibial
nerve and posterior tibial artery

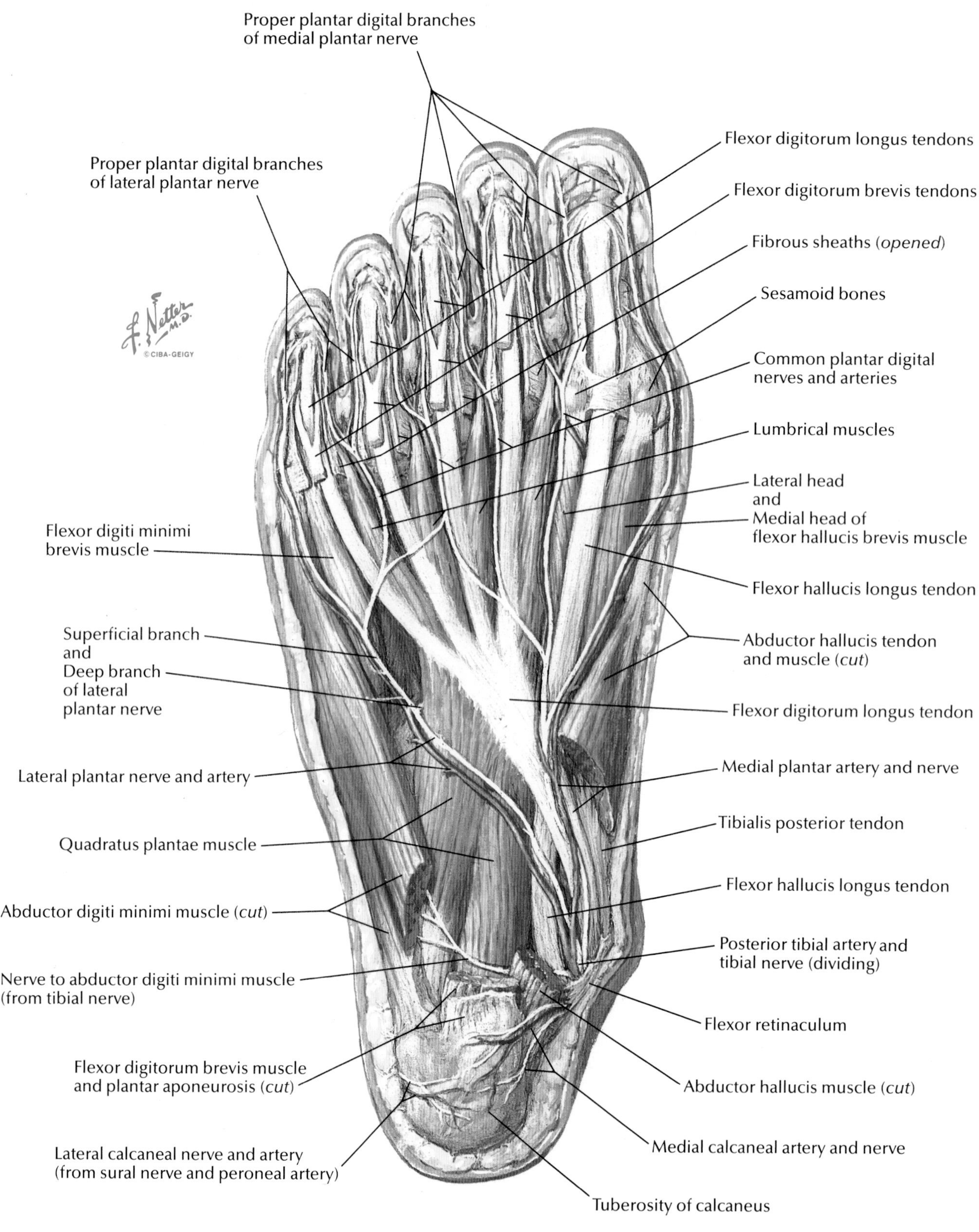

Proper plantar digital branches
of medial plantar nerve

Proper plantar digital branches
of lateral plantar nerve

Flexor digitorum longus tendons

Flexor digitorum brevis tendons

Fibrous sheaths (*opened*)

Sesamoid bones

Common plantar digital
nerves and arteries

Lumbrical muscles

Lateral head
and
Medial head of
flexor hallucis brevis muscle

Flexor digiti minimi
brevis muscle

Flexor hallucis longus tendon

Abductor hallucis tendon
and muscle (*cut*)

Superficial branch
and
Deep branch
of lateral
plantar nerve

Flexor digitorum longus tendon

Lateral plantar nerve and artery

Medial plantar artery and nerve

Tibialis posterior tendon

Quadratus plantae muscle

Flexor hallucis longus tendon

Abductor digiti minimi muscle (*cut*)

Posterior tibial artery and
tibial nerve (dividing)

Nerve to abductor digiti minimi muscle
(from tibial nerve)

Flexor retinaculum

Flexor digitorum brevis muscle
and plantar aponeurosis (*cut*)

Abductor hallucis muscle (*cut*)

Lateral calcaneal nerve and artery
(from sural nerve and peroneal artery)

Medial calcaneal artery and nerve

Tuberosity of calcaneus

PLATE 502

LOWER LIMB

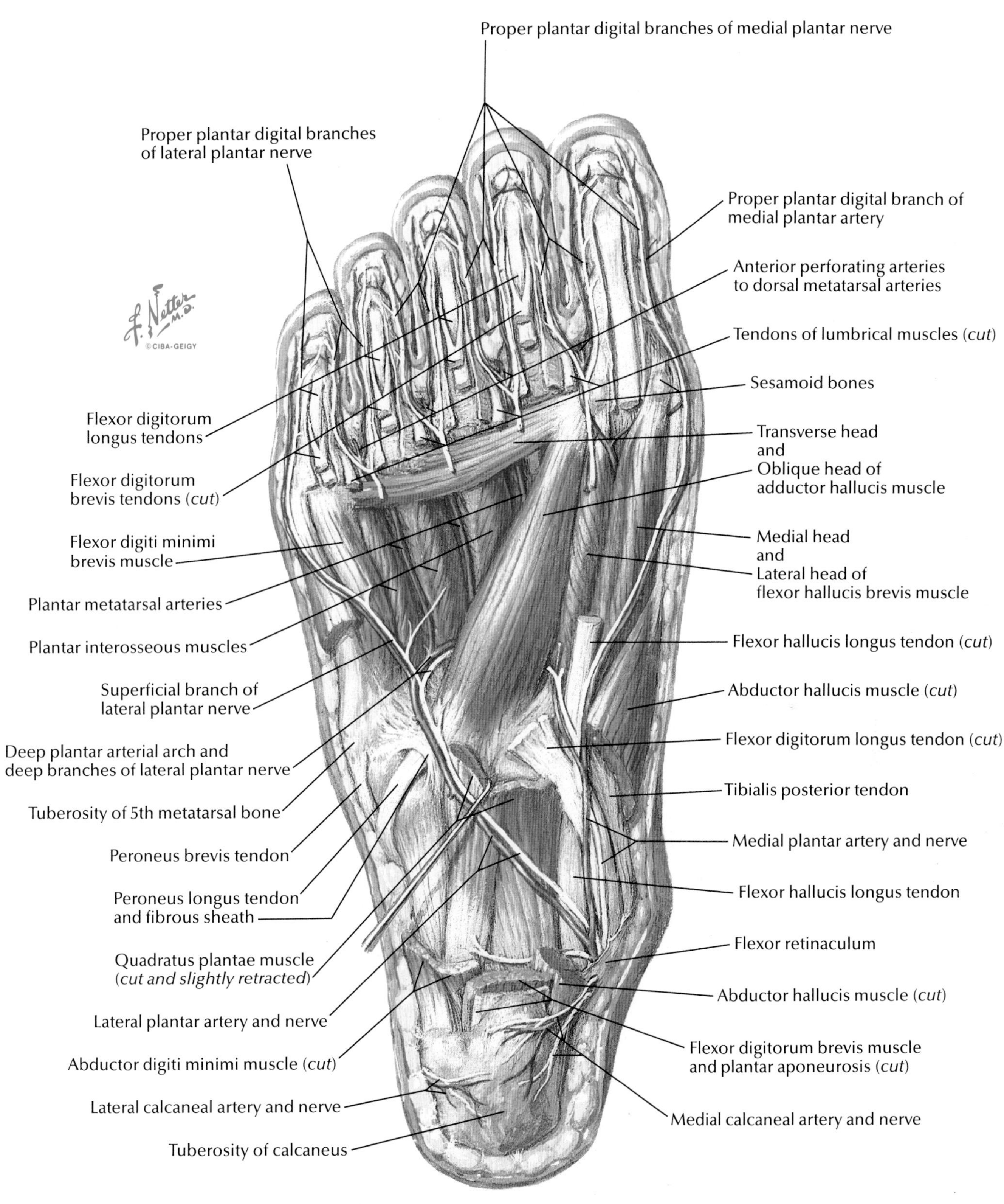

Proper plantar digital branches of medial plantar nerve

Proper plantar digital branches of lateral plantar nerve

Proper plantar digital branch of medial plantar artery

Anterior perforating arteries to dorsal metatarsal arteries

Tendons of lumbrical muscles (cut)

Sesamoid bones

Flexor digitorum longus tendons

Flexor digitorum brevis tendons (cut)

Transverse head and
Oblique head of adductor hallucis muscle

Flexor digiti minimi brevis muscle

Medial head and
Lateral head of flexor hallucis brevis muscle

Plantar metatarsal arteries

Flexor hallucis longus tendon (cut)

Plantar interosseous muscles

Abductor hallucis muscle (cut)

Superficial branch of lateral plantar nerve

Flexor digitorum longus tendon (cut)

Deep plantar arterial arch and deep branches of lateral plantar nerve

Tibialis posterior tendon

Tuberosity of 5th metatarsal bone

Medial plantar artery and nerve

Peroneus brevis tendon

Flexor hallucis longus tendon

Peroneus longus tendon and fibrous sheath

Flexor retinaculum

Quadratus plantae muscle (cut and slightly retracted)

Abductor hallucis muscle (cut)

Lateral plantar artery and nerve

Flexor digitorum brevis muscle and plantar aponeurosis (cut)

Abductor digiti minimi muscle (cut)

Lateral calcaneal artery and nerve

Medial calcaneal artery and nerve

Tuberosity of calcaneus

Interosseous Muscles and Deep Arteries of Foot

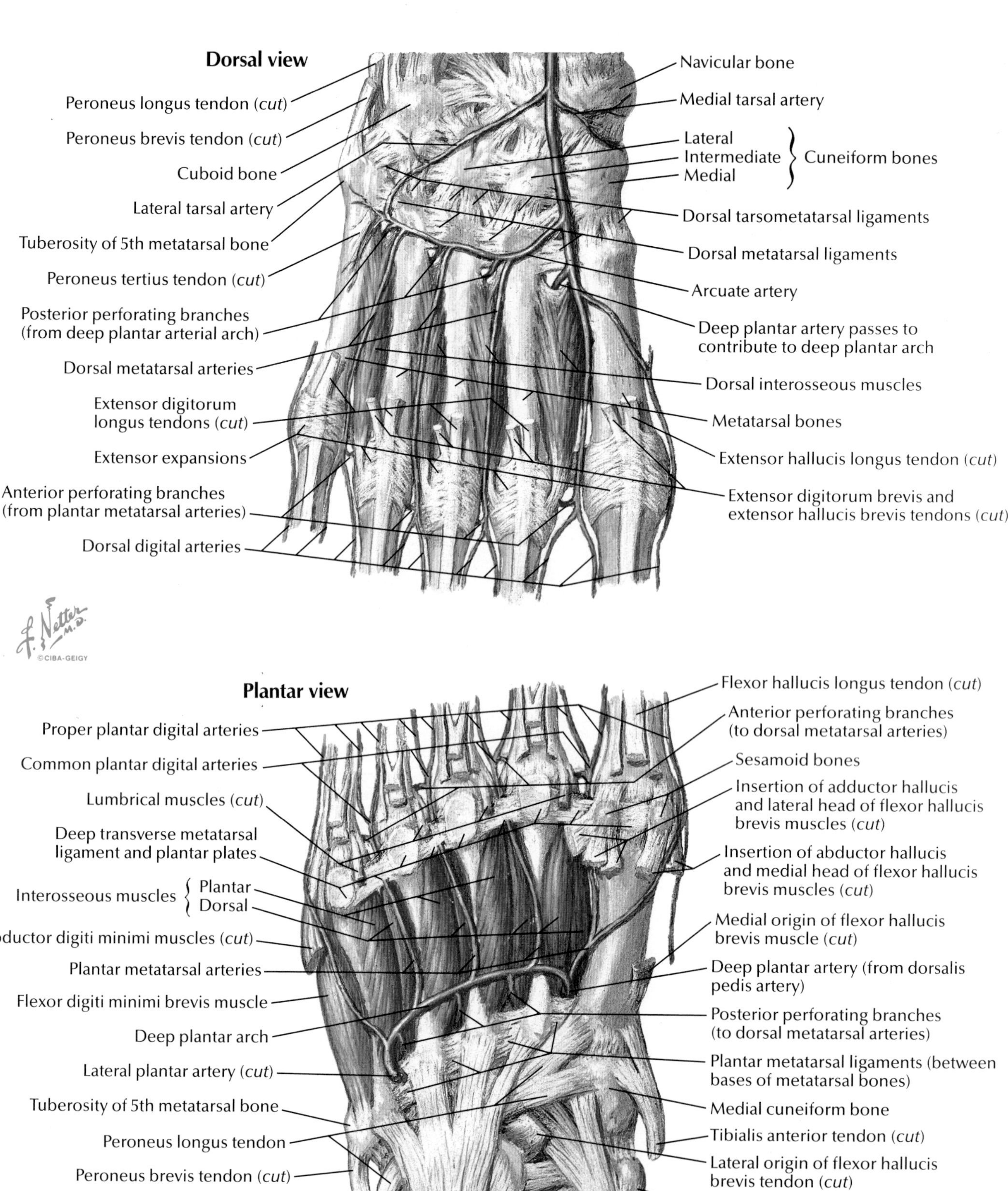

Dorsal view

Peroneus longus tendon (*cut*)

Peroneus brevis tendon (*cut*)

Cuboid bone

Lateral tarsal artery

Tuberosity of 5th metatarsal bone

Peroneus tertius tendon (*cut*)

Posterior perforating branches (from deep plantar arterial arch)

Dorsal metatarsal arteries

Extensor digitorum longus tendons (*cut*)

Extensor expansions

Anterior perforating branches (from plantar metatarsal arteries)

Dorsal digital arteries

Navicular bone

Medial tarsal artery

Lateral
Intermediate } Cuneiform bones
Medial

Dorsal tarsometatarsal ligaments

Dorsal metatarsal ligaments

Arcuate artery

Deep plantar artery passes to contribute to deep plantar arch

Dorsal interosseous muscles

Metatarsal bones

Extensor hallucis longus tendon (*cut*)

Extensor digitorum brevis and extensor hallucis brevis tendons (*cut*)

Plantar view

Proper plantar digital arteries

Common plantar digital arteries

Lumbrical muscles (*cut*)

Deep transverse metatarsal ligament and plantar plates

Interosseous muscles { Plantar
Dorsal

Abductor digiti minimi muscles (*cut*)

Plantar metatarsal arteries

Flexor digiti minimi brevis muscle

Deep plantar arch

Lateral plantar artery (*cut*)

Tuberosity of 5th metatarsal bone

Peroneus longus tendon

Peroneus brevis tendon (*cut*)

Tuberosity of cuboid bone

Long plantar ligament

Calcaneocuboid (short plantar) ligament

Flexor hallucis longus tendon (*cut*)

Anterior perforating branches (to dorsal metatarsal arteries)

Sesamoid bones

Insertion of adductor hallucis and lateral head of flexor hallucis brevis muscles (*cut*)

Insertion of abductor hallucis and medial head of flexor hallucis brevis muscles (*cut*)

Medial origin of flexor hallucis brevis muscle (*cut*)

Deep plantar artery (from dorsalis pedis artery)

Posterior perforating branches (to dorsal metatarsal arteries)

Plantar metatarsal ligaments (between bases of metatarsal bones)

Medial cuneiform bone

Tibialis anterior tendon (*cut*)

Lateral origin of flexor hallucis brevis tendon (*cut*)

Tuberosity of navicular bone

Tibialis posterior tendon (*cut*)

Plantar calcaneonavicular (spring) ligament

©CIBA-GEIGY

PLATE 504

LOWER LIMB

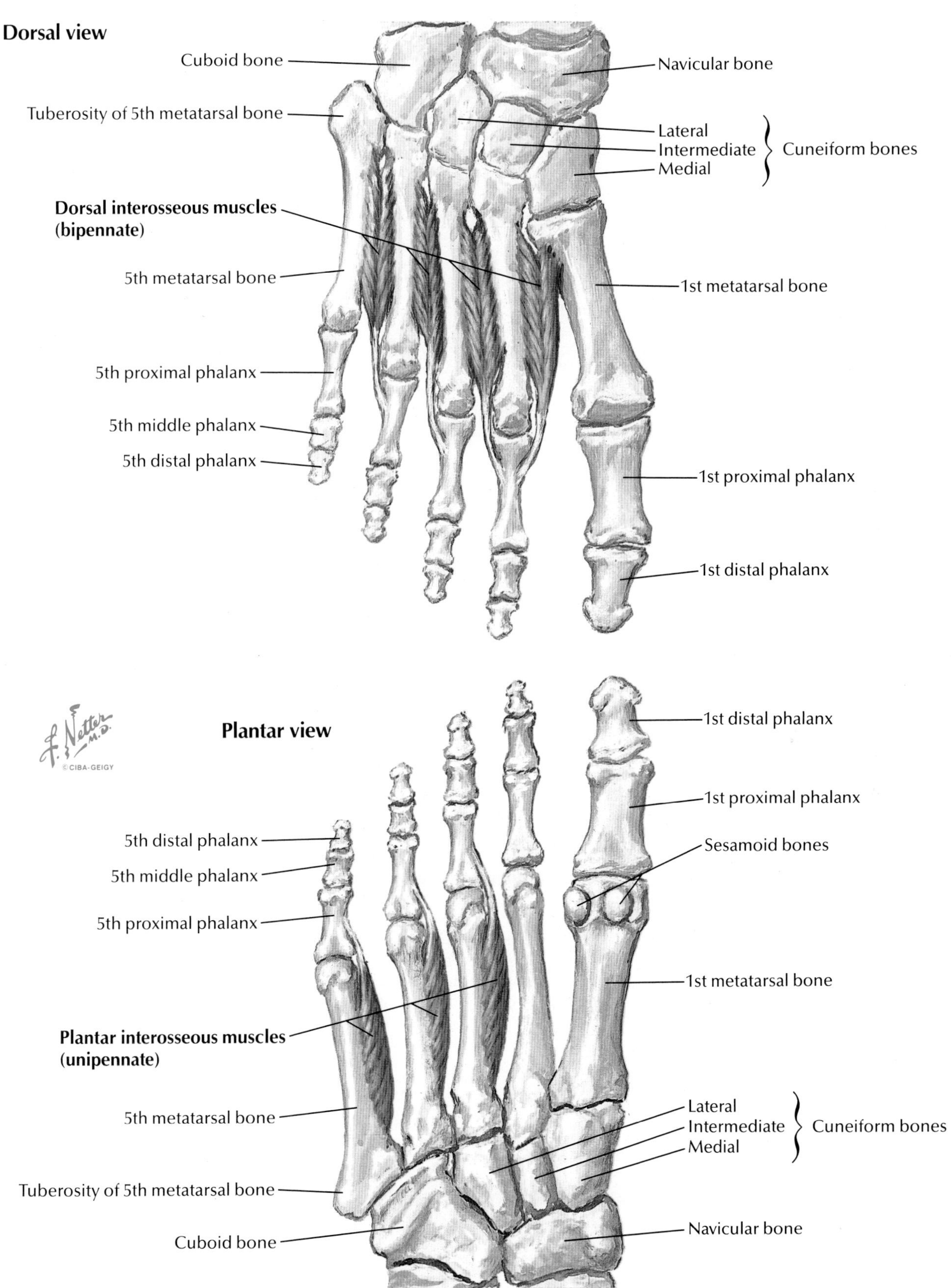

Dorsal view

Cuboid bone

Tuberosity of 5th metatarsal bone

Navicular bone

Lateral
Intermediate } Cuneiform bones
Medial

**Dorsal interosseous muscles
(bipennate)**

5th metatarsal bone

1st metatarsal bone

5th proximal phalanx

5th middle phalanx

5th distal phalanx

1st proximal phalanx

1st distal phalanx

Plantar view

1st distal phalanx

5th distal phalanx

1st proximal phalanx

5th middle phalanx

Sesamoid bones

5th proximal phalanx

**Plantar interosseous muscles
(unipennate)**

1st metatarsal bone

5th metatarsal bone

Lateral
Intermediate } Cuneiform bones
Medial

Tuberosity of 5th metatarsal bone

Cuboid bone

Navicular bone

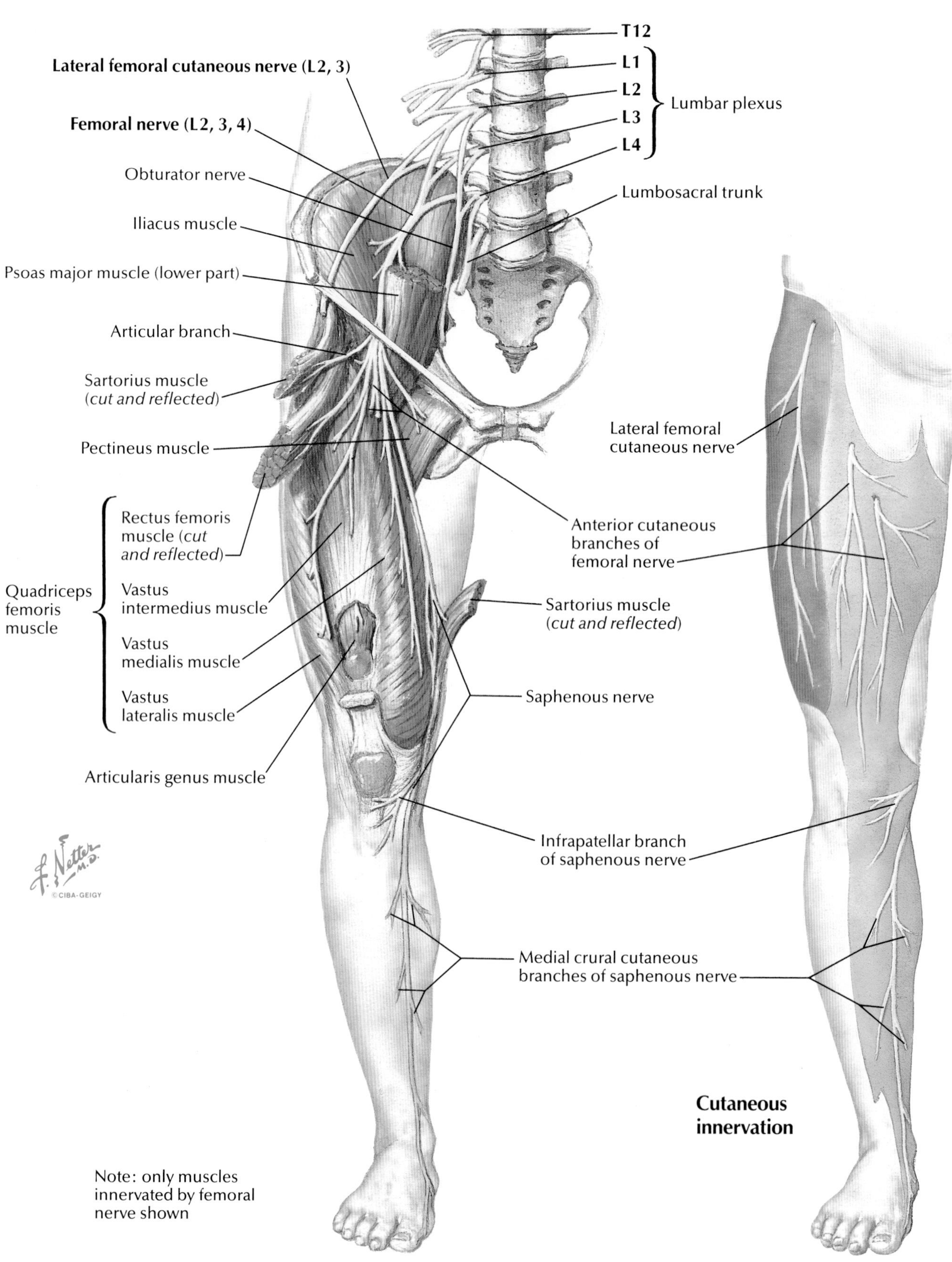

Lateral femoral cutaneous nerve (L2, 3)

Femoral nerve (L2, 3, 4)

Obturator nerve

Iliacus muscle

Psoas major muscle (lower part)

Articular branch

Sartorius muscle
(*cut and reflected*)

Pectineus muscle

Rectus femoris
muscle (*cut
and reflected*)

Quadriceps
femoris
muscle

Vastus
intermedius muscle

Vastus
medialis muscle

Vastus
lateralis muscle

Articularis genus muscle

Note: only muscles
innervated by femoral
nerve shown

T12

L1
L2
L3
L4

Lumbar plexus

Lumbosacral trunk

Lateral femoral
cutaneous nerve

Anterior cutaneous
branches of
femoral nerve

Sartorius muscle
(*cut and reflected*)

Saphenous nerve

Infrapatellar branch
of saphenous nerve

Medial crural cutaneous
branches of saphenous nerve

Cutaneous
innervation

PLATE 506

LOWER LIMB

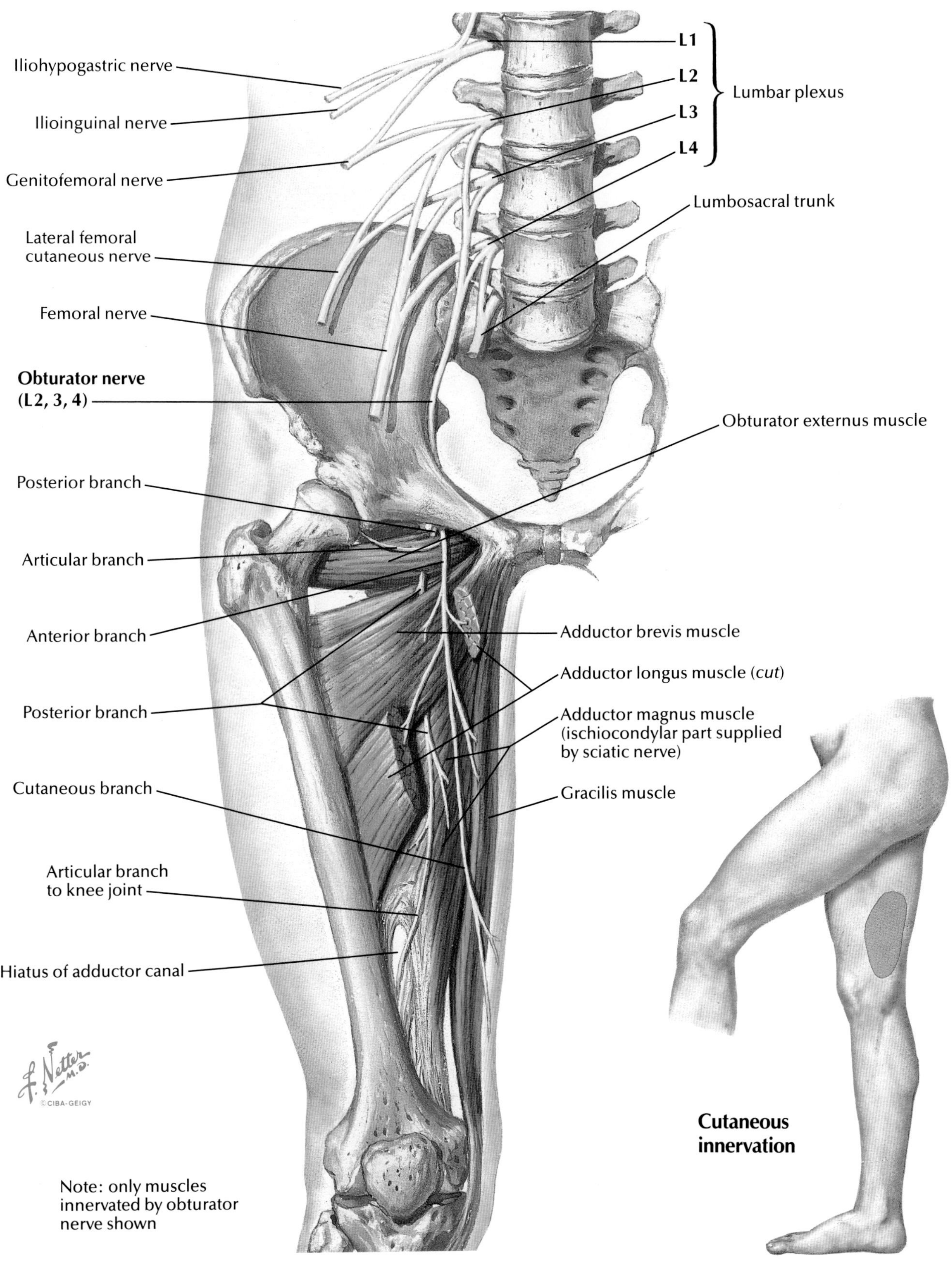

Iliohypogastric nerve

Ilioinguinal nerve

Genitofemoral nerve

Lateral femoral cutaneous nerve

Femoral nerve

Obturator nerve (L2, 3, 4)

Posterior branch

Articular branch

Anterior branch

Posterior branch

Cutaneous branch

Articular branch to knee joint

Hiatus of adductor canal

L1

L2

L3

L4

Lumbar plexus

Lumbosacral trunk

Obturator externus muscle

Adductor brevis muscle

Adductor longus muscle (*cut*)

Adductor magnus muscle (ischiocondylar part supplied by sciatic nerve)

Gracilis muscle

Cutaneous innervation

Note: only muscles innervated by obturator nerve shown

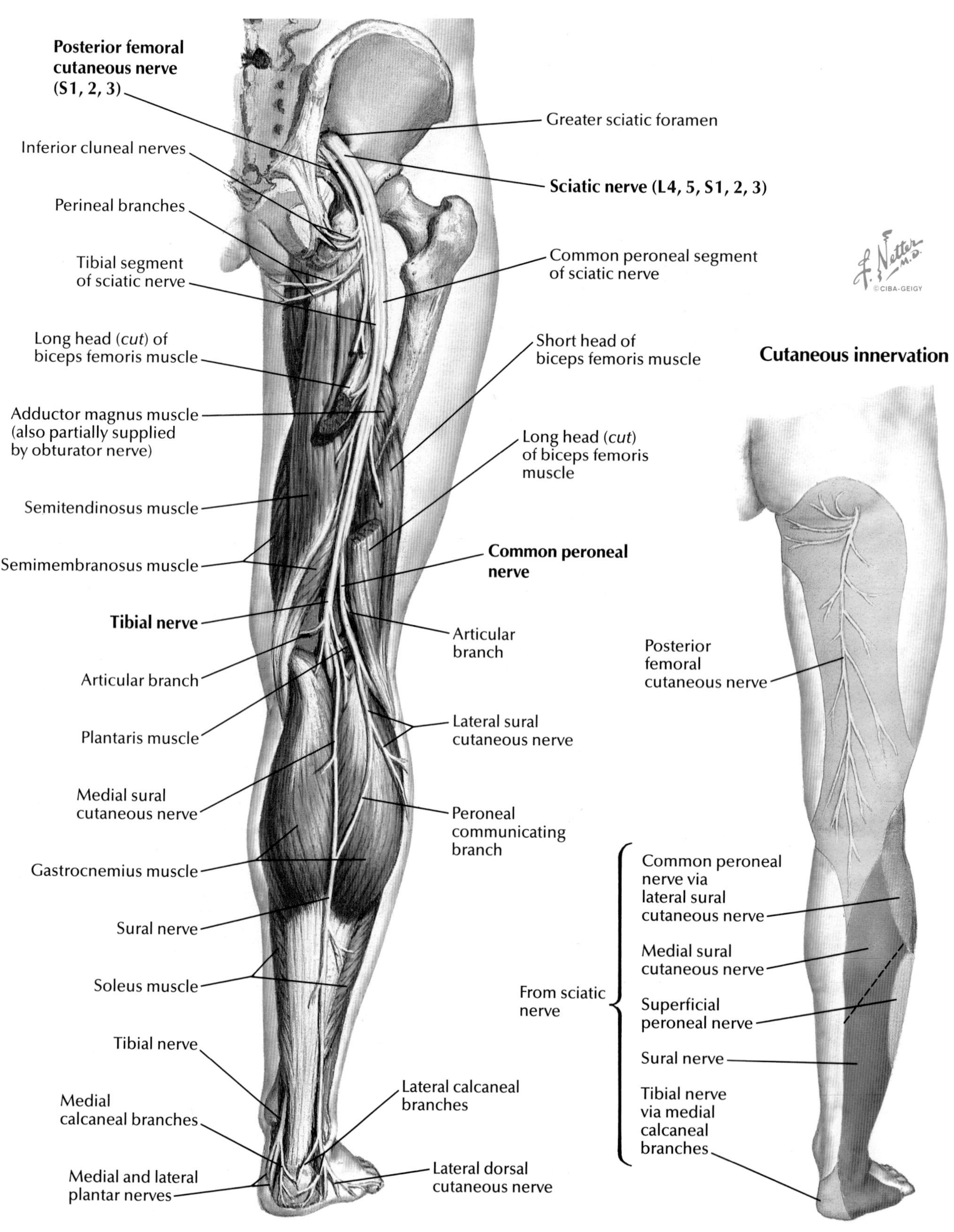

Posterior femoral
cutaneous nerve
(S1, 2, 3)

Inferior cluneal nerves

Perineal branches

Tibial segment
of sciatic nerve

Long head (cut) of
biceps femoris muscle

Adductor magnus muscle
(also partially supplied
by obturator nerve)

Semitendinosus muscle

Semimembranosus muscle

Tibial nerve

Articular branch

Plantaris muscle

Medial sural
cutaneous nerve

Gastrocnemius muscle

Sural nerve

Soleus muscle

Tibial nerve

Medial
calcaneal branches

Medial and lateral
plantar nerves

Greater sciatic foramen

Sciatic nerve (L4, 5, S1, 2, 3)

Common peroneal segment
of sciatic nerve

Short head of
biceps femoris muscle

Long head (cut)
of biceps femoris
muscle

Common peroneal
nerve

Articular
branch

Lateral sural
cutaneous nerve

Peroneal
communicating
branch

Lateral calcaneal
branches

Lateral dorsal
cutaneous nerve

Cutaneous innervation

Posterior
femoral
cutaneous nerve

Common peroneal
nerve via
lateral sural
cutaneous nerve

Medial sural
cutaneous nerve

From sciatic
nerve

Superficial
peroneal nerve

Sural nerve

Tibial nerve
via medial
calcaneal
branches

PLATE 508

LOWER LIMB

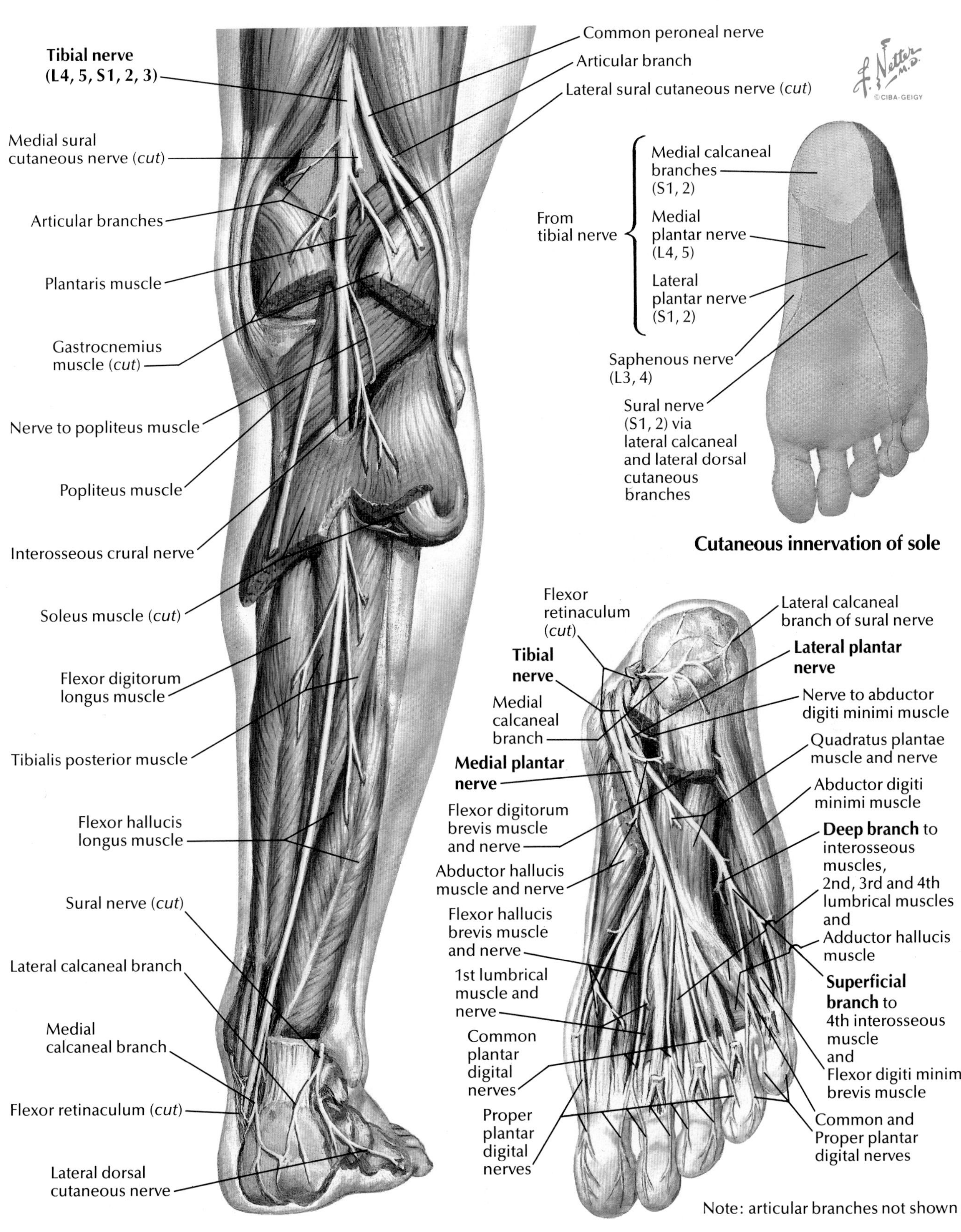

Tibial nerve (L4, 5, S1, 2, 3)

Medial sural cutaneous nerve (*cut*)

Articular branches

Plantaris muscle

Gastrocnemius muscle (*cut*)

Nerve to popliteus muscle

Popliteus muscle

Interosseous crural nerve

Soleus muscle (*cut*)

Flexor digitorum longus muscle

Tibialis posterior muscle

Flexor hallucis longus muscle

Sural nerve (*cut*)

Lateral calcaneal branch

Medial calcaneal branch

Flexor retinaculum (*cut*)

Lateral dorsal cutaneous nerve

Common peroneal nerve

Articular branch

Lateral sural cutaneous nerve (*cut*)

From tibial nerve
Medial calcaneal branches (S1, 2)
Medial plantar nerve (L4, 5)
Lateral plantar nerve (S1, 2)

Saphenous nerve (L3, 4)

Sural nerve (S1, 2) via lateral calcaneal and lateral dorsal cutaneous branches

Cutaneous innervation of sole

Flexor retinaculum (*cut*)

Tibial nerve

Medial calcaneal branch

Medial plantar nerve

Flexor digitorum brevis muscle and nerve

Abductor hallucis muscle and nerve

Flexor hallucis brevis muscle and nerve

1st lumbrical muscle and nerve

Common plantar digital nerves

Proper plantar digital nerves

Lateral calcaneal branch of sural nerve

Lateral plantar nerve

Nerve to abductor digiti minimi muscle

Quadratus plantae muscle and nerve

Abductor digiti minimi muscle

Deep branch to interosseous muscles, 2nd, 3rd and 4th lumbrical muscles and Adductor hallucis muscle

Superficial branch to 4th interosseous muscle and Flexor digiti minimi brevis muscle

Common and Proper plantar digital nerves

Note: articular branches not shown

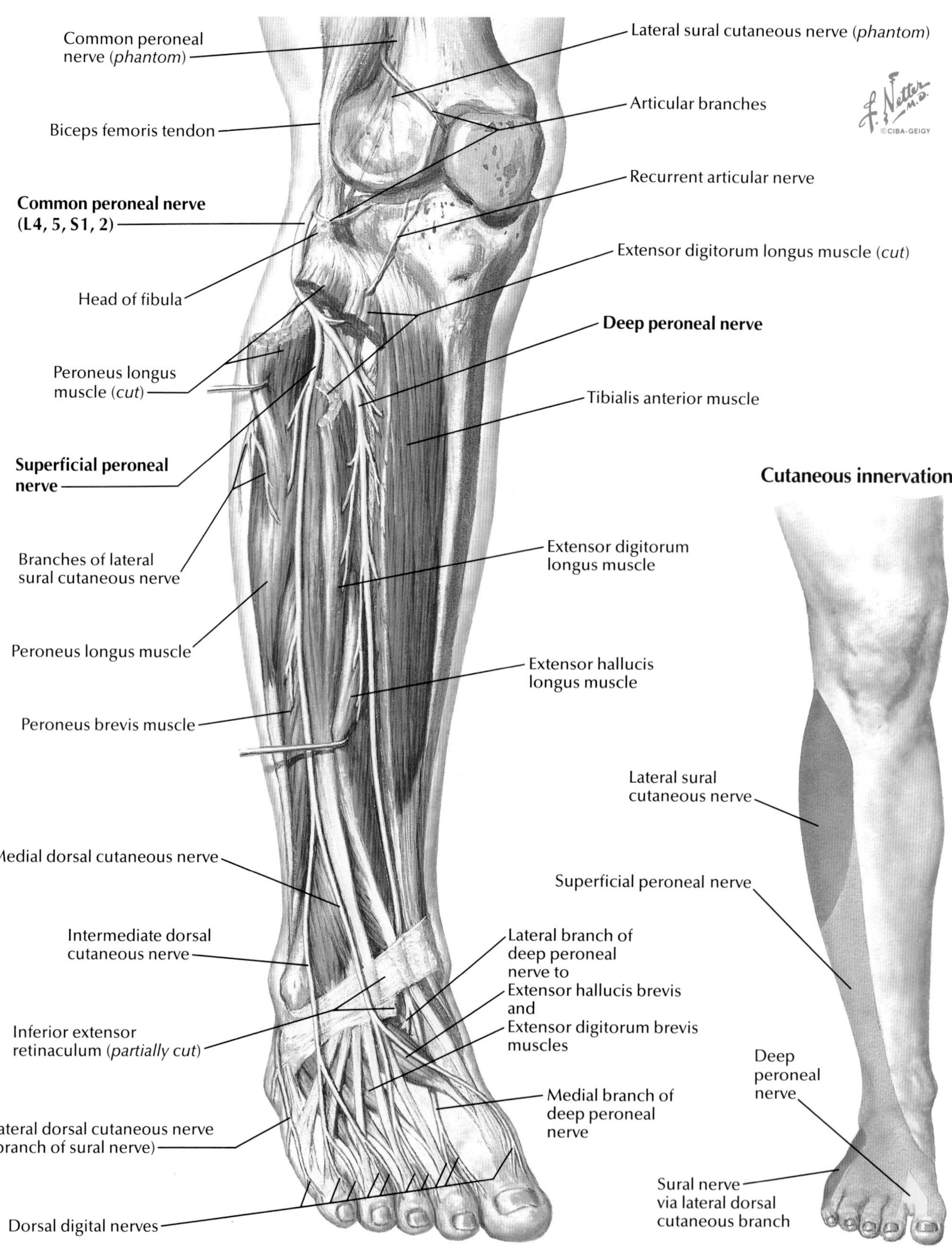

Common peroneal nerve (*phantom*)

Biceps femoris tendon

Common peroneal nerve (L4, 5, S1, 2)

Head of fibula

Peroneus longus muscle (*cut*)

Superficial peroneal nerve

Branches of lateral sural cutaneous nerve

Peroneus longus muscle

Peroneus brevis muscle

Medial dorsal cutaneous nerve

Intermediate dorsal cutaneous nerve

Inferior extensor retinaculum (*partially cut*)

Lateral dorsal cutaneous nerve (branch of sural nerve)

Dorsal digital nerves

Lateral sural cutaneous nerve (*phantom*)

Articular branches

Recurrent articular nerve

Extensor digitorum longus muscle (*cut*)

Deep peroneal nerve

Tibialis anterior muscle

Extensor digitorum longus muscle

Extensor hallucis longus muscle

Lateral branch of deep peroneal nerve to Extensor hallucis brevis and Extensor digitorum brevis muscles

Medial branch of deep peroneal nerve

Cutaneous innervation

Lateral sural cutaneous nerve

Superficial peroneal nerve

Deep peroneal nerve

Sural nerve via lateral dorsal cutaneous branch

PLATE 510

LOWER LIMB

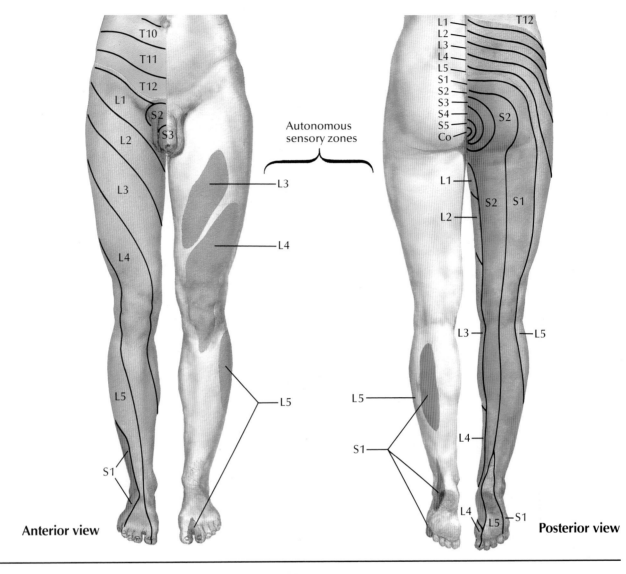

Autonomous
sensory zones

Anterior view

Posterior view

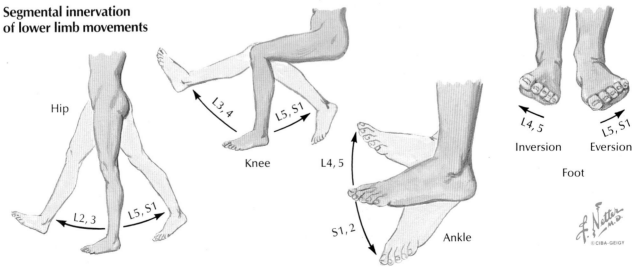

**Segmental innervation
of lower limb movements**

Hip

L2, 3   L5, S1

Knee

L3, 4   L5, S1

Ankle

L4, 5

S1, 2

Inversion   Eversion

L4, 5   L5, S1

Foot

Superficial Nerves and Veins of Lower Limb: Anterior View

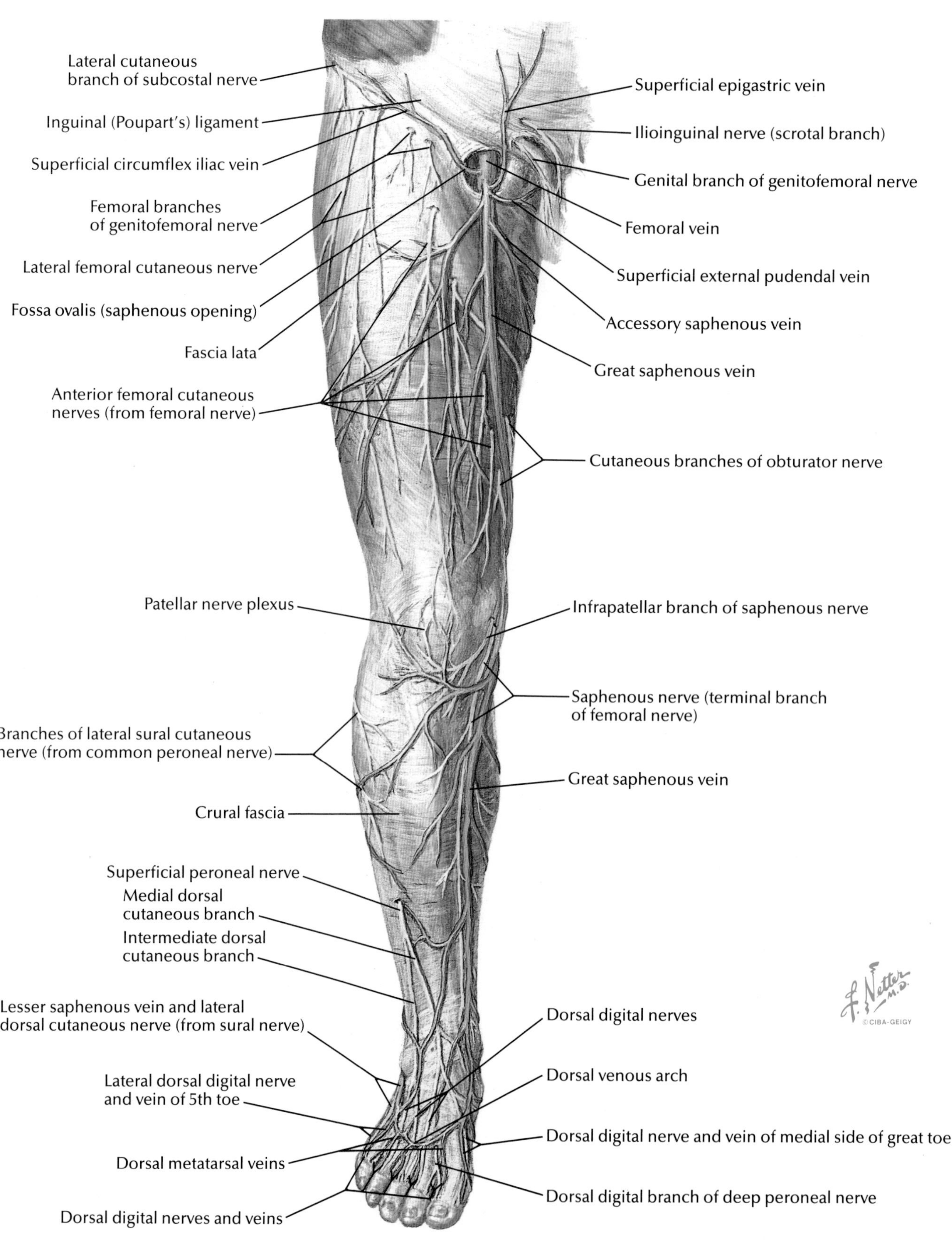

Lateral cutaneous branch of subcostal nerve

Inguinal (Poupart's) ligament

Superficial circumflex iliac vein

Femoral branches of genitofemoral nerve

Lateral femoral cutaneous nerve

Fossa ovalis (saphenous opening)

Fascia lata

Anterior femoral cutaneous nerves (from femoral nerve)

Patellar nerve plexus

Branches of lateral sural cutaneous nerve (from common peroneal nerve)

Crural fascia

Superficial peroneal nerve
Medial dorsal cutaneous branch
Intermediate dorsal cutaneous branch

Lesser saphenous vein and lateral dorsal cutaneous nerve (from sural nerve)

Lateral dorsal digital nerve and vein of 5th toe

Dorsal metatarsal veins

Dorsal digital nerves and veins

Superficial epigastric vein

Ilioinguinal nerve (scrotal branch)

Genital branch of genitofemoral nerve

Femoral vein

Superficial external pudendal vein

Accessory saphenous vein

Great saphenous vein

Cutaneous branches of obturator nerve

Infrapatellar branch of saphenous nerve

Saphenous nerve (terminal branch of femoral nerve)

Great saphenous vein

Dorsal digital nerves

Dorsal venous arch

Dorsal digital nerve and vein of medial side of great toe

Dorsal digital branch of deep peroneal nerve

PLATE 512

LOWER LIMB

Superficial Nerves and Veins of Lower Limb: Posterior View

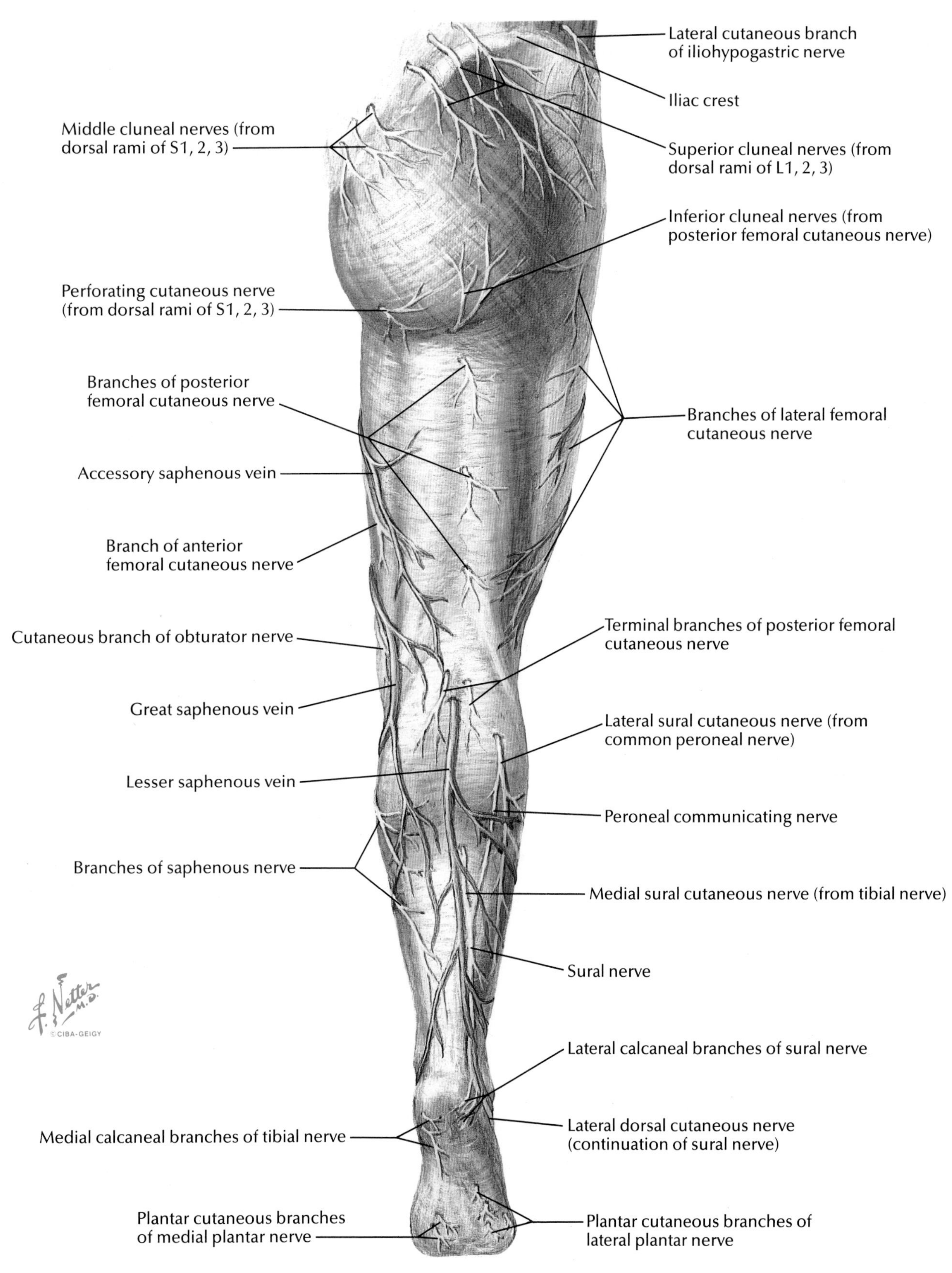

Lateral cutaneous branch of iliohypogastric nerve

Iliac crest

Middle cluneal nerves (from dorsal rami of S1, 2, 3)

Superior cluneal nerves (from dorsal rami of L1, 2, 3)

Inferior cluneal nerves (from posterior femoral cutaneous nerve)

Perforating cutaneous nerve (from dorsal rami of S1, 2, 3)

Branches of posterior femoral cutaneous nerve

Branches of lateral femoral cutaneous nerve

Accessory saphenous vein

Branch of anterior femoral cutaneous nerve

Cutaneous branch of obturator nerve

Terminal branches of posterior femoral cutaneous nerve

Great saphenous vein

Lateral sural cutaneous nerve (from common peroneal nerve)

Lesser saphenous vein

Peroneal communicating nerve

Branches of saphenous nerve

Medial sural cutaneous nerve (from tibial nerve)

Sural nerve

Lateral calcaneal branches of sural nerve

Medial calcaneal branches of tibial nerve

Lateral dorsal cutaneous nerve (continuation of sural nerve)

Plantar cutaneous branches of medial plantar nerve

Plantar cutaneous branches of lateral plantar nerve

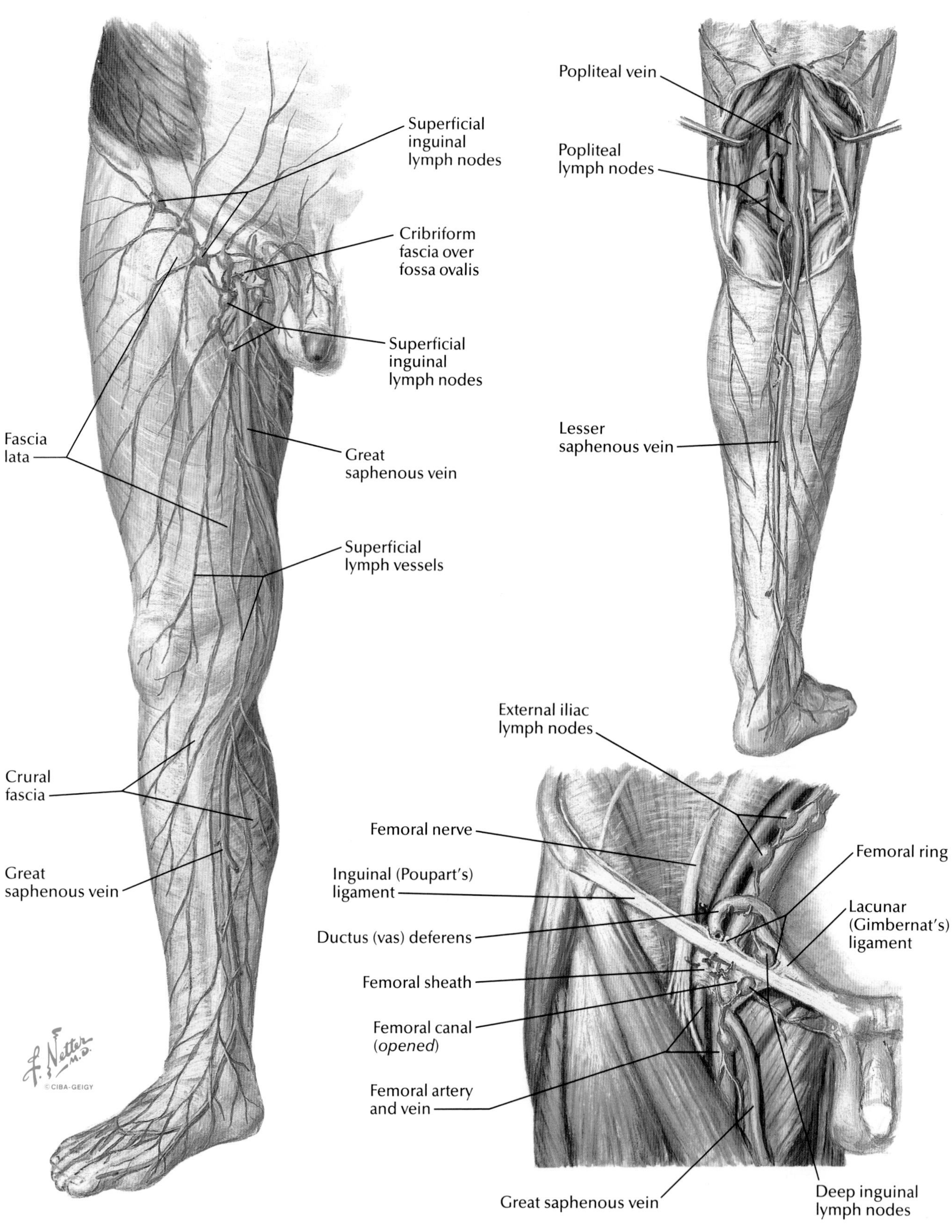

Superficial inguinal lymph nodes

Cribriform fascia over fossa ovalis

Superficial inguinal lymph nodes

Fascia lata

Great saphenous vein

Superficial lymph vessels

Crural fascia

Great saphenous vein

Popliteal vein

Popliteal lymph nodes

Lesser saphenous vein

External iliac lymph nodes

Femoral nerve

Inguinal (Poupart's) ligament

Ductus (vas) deferens

Femoral sheath

Femoral canal (*opened*)

Femoral artery and vein

Femoral ring

Lacunar (Gimbernat's) ligament

Great saphenous vein

Deep inguinal lymph nodes

PLATE 514

LOWER LIMB

REFERENCES

Plate 52

Braus H. Anatomie des Menschen. Berlin, Verlag von Julius Springer, 1924

Plate 85

Nishida S. The Structure of the Eye. New York, Elsevier North-Holland, 1982

Plate 150

Keegan JJ. J. Neurosurg 1947;4:115

Plate 158

Turnbull IM. Blood supply of the spinal cord. In Vinken PJ, Bruyn GW (eds). Handbook of Clinical Neurology, XII. Amsterdam, North-Holland, 1972, pp 478–491

Plates 188, 189

Jackson CL, Huber JF. Correlated applied anatomy of the bronchial tree and lungs with a system of nomenclature. Dis Chest 1943;9:319–326

Plate 191

Ikeda S, Ono Y, Miyazawa S, et al. Flexible bronchofiberscope. Otolaryngology (Tokyo) 1970;42:855–861

Plate 265

DiDio LJA. Anatomo-Fisiologia do Piloro ileo-ceco-colica no homem, Actas das Primeiras Jornadas Inter-universitarías Argentinas de Gastroenterologia, Rosario, 1954

———. Dados anatomicos sobre o "piloro" ileo-ceco-colico. (Com observacao direta in vivo de "papila" ileo-ceco-colica.) (English summary). Thesis, Fac Med, Univ de São Paulo, 1952

Plate 273

Healey JE Jr, Schroy. Anatomy of the biliary duct within the human liver; analysis of the prevailing pattern of branchings and the major variations of the biliary ducts. Arch Surg 1953;66:599

———, Sörensen. The intrahepatic distribution of the hepatic artery in man. J Int Coll Surg 1953;20:133

Plates 274, 275

Elias H. Liver morphology. Biol Rev 1955;30:263

———. Origin and early development of the liver in various vertebrates. Act Hepat 1955;3:1

———. Morphology of the liver. In "Liver Injury," Trans 11th Conference. New York, Macy Foundation, 1953

———. A re-examination of the structure of the mammalian liver; the hepatic lobule and its relation to the vascular and biliary system. Am J Anat 1949;85:379

———. A re-examination of the structure of the mammalian liver; parenchymal architecture. Am J Anat 1949;84:311

Plates 288, 289

Michels NA. Blood Supply and Anatomy of the Upper Abdominal Organs, With a Descriptive Atlas. Philadelphia, JB Lippincott, 1955

Plate 312

Thomas MD. In The Ciba Collection of Medical Illustrations, Vol 3, Part II. Summit NJ, CIBA, p 78

Plate 378

Flocks RH, Kerr HD, Elkins HB, et al. Treatment of carcinoma of the prostate by interstitial radiation with radio-active gold (Au198): A preliminary report. J Urol 1952;68(2):510–522

Plate 455

Keegan JJ, Garrett FD. The segmental distribution of the cutaneous nerves in the limbs of man. Anat Rec 1948;102:409–437

Plate 511

Keegan JJ. J Bone Joint Surg 1944;26:238

Last RJ. Innervation of the limbs. J Bone Joint Surg 1949;31(B):452

Index

References are to plate numbers; numbers in bold refer to primary sources. In most cases, structures are listed under singular nouns

A

Abdomen
arteries of 238, 247—see also arteries of individual organs
bones of 231
cross sections of 331, 332
lymph nodes of 249, 299–301, 325—see also lymph nodes of individual organs
muscles of 232–237, 246
nerves of 240, 241, 250—see also nerves of individual organs
veins of 239, 248—see also veins of individual organs
viscera of—see individual organs
Acetabulum 334, 457
Achilles—see Tendon, Achilles; calcaneal
Acinus 192
Acromion 22, 170, 174, 178, **396–402**, 404, 406, 407
Action of
extrinsic eye muscles 79
infrahyoid muscles 24
intrinsic laryngeal muscles 73
jaws 11
suprahyoid muscles 24
wrist 427
Adam's apple—see Prominence, laryngeal
Adamkiewicz—see Artery, of Adamkiewicz
Adenohypophysis 133, 140
Adenoid—see Tonsil, pharyngeal
Adhesion, interthalamic 100, 102, 105, 109, 139
Aditus of larynx 57, 60, 223
Adrenergic neurons 154
Agger nasi 32, 33
Air cell—see Cell (air)
Ala of
central cerebellar lobule 107
ilium 231, 334, 339, 457
sacrum 145
vomer 5
Albini—see Nodule, Albini's
Alveolus of
lung 192, 193
pancreas 279

Alveus of hippocampus 106
Ampulla
of ductus deferens 362
of duodenum 262, 276
hepatopancreatic 278
of inner ear 87
labyrinthine 90, 118
of lactiferous duct 167
of semicircular duct 90, 118
of uterine tube 350
of Vater—see Ampulla, of duodenum
of vestibule 91
Anastomosis
between
carotid and vertebral arteries 131
cervical and occipital arteries 28
circumflex femoral arteries 474
external and internal carotid arteries 80, 131
intercostal and lumbar arteries 218, 238
median and ulnar nerves 446, 448, 449
pancreatic arteries 284–286
pubic branches of obturator and inferior epigastric arteries 344
subclavian and carotid arteries 131
subclavian and vertebral arteries 131
at elbow 409
paravertebral 158
portacaval 297
prevertebral 158
scapular 402
Angiogram, coronary—see Arteriogram of coronary arteries
Angle
anterior chamber, of eye 82, 83, 86
iridocorneal—see Angle, anterior chamber, of eye
of Louis—see Joint, sternomanubrial
of mandible 9, 10, 60
of mastoid 6
of rib 170, 171
scapular 396, 397
of sternum 170
subpubic 336
Ankle
bones of 482, 483, 492–494
ligaments of 495
lymph nodes of 514
Annulus fibrosus of
heart 210, 213
intervertebral disc 144
Anoderm 369
Anomaly of
cervical ribs 173

Anomaly *cont.*
right inferior laryngeal nerve 74
right subclavian artery 74
Ansa
cervicalis 26, **27**, 29, 65, 68, 122, 123
hypoglossi—see Ansa cervicalis
subclavia 124, 198, 214, 215, 228
Anteflexion of uterus 352
Antihelix of external ear 88
Antitragus of external ear 88
Antrum
mastoid 89
pyloric 258
tympanic 89
Anus 341, 354, 358, 360, 371, 373, 393
Aorta
abdominal 165, 181, 217, 220, 246, **247**, 253, 256, 257, 261, 279, 282, 284, 290, 310, 313, 315, 316, 318, 324, 328, 329, 331–333, 343, 344, 348, 373, 375–378, 387
arch of 30, 68, 69, 74, 131, 184, 195, 196, 199–203, 208, 209, 213, 217, 219, **220**, 221, 225
ascending 131, 194, 203, 208, 211, 212
descending 131, 180, 194, 196, 219, 220, 225, 230
thoracic 156, 158, 179, 217, 219, 221, **225**
Aperture—see also Opening
lateral, of 4th ventricle 102, 103, 139
median, of 4th ventricle 102, 103, 109, 139
Apex of
bladder 342
fibula 482, 483
heart 201, 202
lung 184, 185, 187
sacrum 145
tongue 52
Aponeurosis
bicipital 406, 408, 420, 446, 453
external abdominal oblique 232–235, 240, 242, 244, 331, 332
gluteal 316, 464, 465, 472
internal abdominal oblique 234, 235, 240, 332
palatine 46, 59
palmar 416, 420, 421, 428, 432, 433, 435, 453
pharyngeal 59, 61, 223
plantar 497, 500–503
of scalp 17, 20, 21, 164—see also Galea aponeurotica
transversus abdominis 161, 162, 165, 235, 237, 238, 316, 328, 332

Artery, of penis *cont.*
deep 359, 361, 363, 380
dorsal 238, 359, 361, 376, 378, 380
perforating branches of
Circle of Willis 133
deep plantar arch 503
femoral 481
deep 471, 472, 481
internal thoracic 168, 176, 177, 179
plantar metatarsal 503
pericallosal 134, 135
posterior 135, 136
pericardiacophrenic 176, 180, 182, 195, 200, 201, 203, 218, 219, 230, 238
perineal 349, 361, 378–380
transverse 379, 380
of perineum 379, 380
peroneal 481, 485–487, 491, 498, 499
pharyngeal, ascending 29, 35, 63, 130, 131
phrenic, inferior **181**, 220, 225, 228, 247, 255, 257, 282–284, 286, 304–306, 308, 309, 318, 320, 329, 330, 385
plantar
deep 489, 498, 499, 504
lateral 487, 502–504
medial 487, 500–502
metatarsal 501, 503, 504
pontine 132–134, 136
popliteal 465, 472, 475, 481, 485–487
postcentral sulcal 135
posterior auricular 17, 29, 35, 63, 95, 130, 131, 164
precentral sulcal 134, 135
precuneal 135
pre-Rolandic 134, 135
princeps pollicis 439
prostatic 378
pterygoid 35
of pterygoid canal 35
pubic branches from
inferior epigastric 234, 236, 244, 247, 344, 345
obturator 243
pudendal
external
deep 238, 247, 376, 470, 481
superficial 232, 234, 238, 247, 376, 470, 481
internal 247, 287, 324, 361, 373, 374, 377–380, 469
pulmonary 187, 193, **194**, 195, 201, 202, 208, 209, 217–219
radial 408, 409, 419–**421**, 422, 423, 428, 433, 434, 438–440, 442, 443, 446
superficial palmar branch of 421, 422, 428, 433, 438, 439
radialis indicis 439
radicular 131, 179
anterior 157, 158
posterior 157, 158
rectal
inferior 287, 373, 377–380

Artery, rectal *cont.*
middle 247, 287, 309, 323, 324, 345, 373, 375, 377, 378
superior 247, 257, 287, 304, 309, 310, 323, 345, 373, 375, 385
rectosigmoid 287, 309, 373
recurrent
anterior
tibial 481, 489
ulnar 409, 421, 422
esophageal 181, 282, 283, 308
of Heubner 132–135
interosseous 409, 419
meningeal (lacrimal) 95
posterior
tibial 481, 487
ulnar 409, 418, 419, 422
radial 408, 409, 421, 422
renal 247, 304, 307, 309, 315, 317, **318**–320, 324, 327–329, 333, 375, 376, 385, 392
accessory 320
pelvic 319
of retina
central 80, 82, 86
macular 86
nasal 86
temporal 86
retinacular, of femur 474
retroduodenal—see Artery, pancreaticoduodenal, posterior superior
retroesophageal right subclavian 74
of round ligament of
femur 474
uterus 379
Rolandic 134, 135
sacral
lateral 157, 247, 373, 377, 378
middle 157, 247, 287, 345, 348, 373, 375, 377, 378
saphenous 470, 471, 481
scapular
circumflex 402, 404, 409
dorsal 402, 404
scrotal, posterior 378, 380
septal, nasal 35, 36
of shoulder 28
sigmoid 247, 257, 287, 309, 323, 332, 373
sinoatrial 204, 206, 213
sphenopalatine 35, 36, 63
spermatic, internal—see Artery, testicular
spinal
anterior 131, 132, 134, 136, 157, 158
posterior 132, 134, 136, 157, 158
splenic 225, 247, 257, 261, 279, 281, 282, **283**–286, 288–290, 292, 304–307, 313, 314, 331, 333
sternocleidomastoid 29
of stomach 282, 283
straight (arteria recta) 263, 286, 287, 312
striate, medial—see Artery, recurrent, of Heubner

Artery *cont.*
subclavian 25, 27, **28**, 63–65, 68–70, 74, 120, 124, 130, 131, 157, 168, 173, 175–177, 182, 186, 195, 200–202, 218–220, 225, 238, 402, 404
subcostal 238, 247
sublingual 53, 55
submental 35, 63
subscapular 238, 401, 402, 404, 409
sulcal
central 134, 135
of spinal cord 158
supraduodenal 282–286
suprahyoid 53, 63
supraorbital 17, 31, 35, 63, 76, 80, 131
suprarenal
inferior 247, 318, 319, 324, 329
middle 247, 318, 329
superior 181, 247, 318, 329
suprascapular 27, 28, 63, 68–70, 131, 401, 402, 404
supratrochlear 17, 31, 35, 63, 76, 80, 131
of tail of pancreas—see Artery, pancreatic, caudal
tarsal
lateral 489, 498, 499, 504
medial 489, 498, 499, 504
of teeth 35
temporal
branches of
maxillary 35, 63, 94
middle cerebral 134, 135
posterior cerebral 136
superficial 17, 29, 35, 55, 63–65, 80, 94, 95, 128, 130, 131
tentorial 95, 98
testicular 238, 243–245, 247, 257, 296, 304, 315, 318, 323, 324, 326, 332, 344, 365, **376**, 378, 384, 391
thalamogeniculate 136
thalamoperforating 136—see also Artery, thalamostriate
thalamostriate 133
of thigh 470–472, 481
thoracic
internal 28, 69, 130, 131, **168**, 174–**176**, 179, 180, 182, 186, 195, 200, 201, 218–220, 225, 230, 238
lateral 168, 174, 175, 177, 238, 402, 404, 409
superior 175, 177, 402, 404, 409
thoracoacromial 174, 175, 402–404, 409
thoracodorsal 238, 401, 402, 404, 409
thyrocervical—see Trunk (arterial), thyrocervical
thyroid
inferior 27, 28, 63, 68–70, 130, 131, 176, 214, 225, 402
superior 26, 27, 29, 63, 68–70, 130, 131
of thyroid gland 68, 70
tibial
anterior 481, 487, 489, 491, 498, 499
posterior 481, 485–487, 491, 497, 501–503

Bone *cont.*
talus 492–494
tarsal—see Bone, of foot
temporal 1–3, 5, 6, 8, 9
of thigh 475, 458
of thorax 170, 171
tibia—see Tibia
trapezium 426, 427, 430, 431, 434, 440
trapezoid 426, 427, 429, 430
triquetral 426–430
vertebra—see Vertebra
vomer—see Vomer
of wrist 426, 427, 430
zygomatic 1, 2, 5, 8, 76
Bowel—see Colon
Bowman—see Capsule, Bowman's
Boyden—see Sphincter, of common bile
duct
Brachium of
inferior colliculus 105, 108
superior colliculus 105, 108
Brain 96, 99, 109
Brainstem 108, 110, 111
Bregma 4
Brim, pelvic 145, 349—see also Linea,
terminalis of pelvis
Bronchiole 192, 193
Bronchus
anteromedial basal 191
cardiac (left lung) 191
eparterial 187, 190, 191, 194, 195, 220
extrapulmonary 190
intermediate 191, 195
intrapulmonary 190, 192
lingular 190, 191
lobar 191
lower lobe 187, 190, 191, 194
main **190**, 191, 194–196, 198, 218–222, 230
middle lobe 190, 191, 194
nomenclature of 191
2nd order 191—see also Bronchus, lobar
3rd order 191—see also Bronchus,
segmental
4th order 191
primary 190, 195, 196, 198—see also
Bronchus, main
segmental 192
subsegmental 192
superior division 190, 191
upper lobe 187, 190, 191, 194, 195
right—see also Bronchus, eparterial
Brunner—see Gland, duodenal
Buck—see Fascia, Buck's
Bulb
of corpus spongiosum 360
duodenal 259, 262
olfactory 101, 113
of penis 347, 360–363
urethral 347, 361, 362
vestibular 349, 355–357, 379
Bulla, ethmoidal 32, 33
Bundle
atrioventricular 213
Bachmann's 213

Bundle *cont.*
of His 213
interatrial conduction—see Bundle,
Bachmann's
of Kent (accessory atrioventricular) 213
oval 151
Burns—see Space, of Burns
Bursa
anserine 476, 477
of biceps femoris tendon 476, 477, 480
of fibular collateral ligament 476–478,
480
of gastrocnemius muscle 480
iliopectineal 458, 466
of iliotibial tract 476–478
olecranon 412
omental 256, 331, 333—see also Sac,
lesser peritoneal
radial 433–436
of semimembranosus muscle 476, 480
subcutaneous
calcaneal 497
infrapatellar 480
lateral malleolar 497
medial malleolar 497
prepatellar 480
subdeltoid 398, 406
subscapular 398
subtendinous
calcaneal 490, 497
infrapatellar 480
suprapatellar 477, 478, 480
ulnar 433–436, 439

C

Calcaneus 492–**494**, 496, 497
Calcar avis 105, 106
Calot—see Lymph node, of Calot;
Triangle, cystic
Calvaria 4, 96
Calyx of kidney 317
Camper—see Fascia, Camper's
Canal
adductor 470, 471, 475
Alcock's 287, 296, 368, 373, 374, 377,
379, 380, 386, 388
anal 341, 368, 369
carotid 5, 93
central, of spinal cord 102, 103, 109
cervical, of uterus 350
condylar 5, 7
dental root 51
facial 118
femoral 244, 514
gastric 259
of Hering 274, 275—see also Ductule,
bile
Hunter—see Canal, adductor
hyaloid, of eye 82
hypoglossal 3, 5, 7, 16, 122
incisive 3, 32–37
infraorbital 40

Canal *cont.*
inguinal 244
mandibular 54
nasofrontal 33
nasolacrimal 33
obturator 236, 334, 337, 339, 345, 346,
348, 377
optic 1, 3, 7, 78
pudendal 287, 296, 368, 373, 374, 377,
379, 380, 386, 388
pyloric 258
sacral 145
of Schlemm 82–84, 86
semicircular 90–92
spinal—see Canal, vertebral
vertebral 13, 143, 144
Canaliculus
bile 275
lacrimal 77
mastoid 5
tympanic 5
Cap of duodenum 259, 262
Capillary
intrapulmonary 193
subpleural 193
Capitate—see Bone, capitate
Capitulum of
humerus 396, 411
mandible—see Caput of mandible
Capsule—see also Ligament; Joint
atlantoaxial 14, 15
atlantooccipital 14, 15
of basal ganglia
external 104
internal 102, 104, 134
Bowman's 321
glomerular 321
of kidney 317, 321, 322, 328
lens 82, 83, 85
of liver 273
of suprarenal gland 329
temporomandibular 11
Tenon's 78, 82
of vertebral joint, lateral 14, 15
zygapophyseal 14, 15, 146
Caput of mandible 2, 10
Carpal—see Bone, carpal
Cartilage
alar 31, 33, 34
arytenoid 59, 71, 72
of auditory tube 46, 49, 59, 61, 93
corniculate 59, 71
costal 170, 171, 180, 184, 231, 241
cricoid 9, 23, 24, 57, 59, 62, 68, **71**, 72,
184, 190, 195, 221–223
laryngeal 71
nasal
lateral 31, 33, 34
septal 31, 34
thyroid 9, 23, 24, 26, 57, 59, 62, 68, **71**,
72, 184, 190, 195, 221–223
tracheal 190
Caruncle
hymenal 354

Fascia cont.
  of pelvic diaphragm
    deep—see Fascia, of pelvic
        diaphragm, superior
    inferior 349, 355, 356, 368, 370, 372,
        380
    superficial—see Fascia, of pelvic
        diaphragm, inferior
    superior 345, 346, 348, 349, 355, 368,
        370, 372
  of penis
    deep (Buck's) 232–234, 238, 239, 333,
        342, 358, **359**–361, 363, 365, 371,
        372, 376, 378, 380
    superficial (dartos) 232–234, 333, 342,
        358–360, 365
  perineal
    investing (Gallaudet's) 342, 347, 349,
        355, **356**, 357, **359**–361, 367, 372
    superficial (Colles') 333, 342, 347, 349,
        355–**357**, **358**–361, 367, 371, 372,
        379, 380, 386
  pharyngobasilar 32, 46, 53, 57–59, 61,
        62, 67
  plantar 500
  presacral 333, 345, 372
  pretracheal 23, 30, 57
  prevertebral 30, 54, 57, 59
  prostatic 342, 347, 362
  psoas 165, 328
  rectal 333, 345, 348, 355, 362, 367–370,
        372
  rectovesical 333, 340, 342, 362, 367,
        372
  renal 165, **328**, 329
  Scarpa's 232, 235, 333, 342, 355, 358,
        359
  of scrotum 232–234, 333, 342, **358**, 365,
        366, 371, 380
  Sibson's 218, 219
  spermatic
    external 232–234, 243, 245, 342,
        358–360, **365**, 366, 380
    internal 234, 244, 245, 365, 366
  sternocleidomastoid 21
  subcutaneous
    of abdomen 232, 235, 333, 342, 355,
        358, 359
      fatty—see Fascia, Camper's
      fibrous—see Fascia, Scarpa's
      membranous—see Fascia, Scarpa's
    of neck 30
  subserous 165, 234, 235, 244, 245, 387
  superficial
    of abdomen—see Fascia, subcu-
        taneous, of abdomen
    cervical (investing) 21, 23, 30, 57
  supradiaphragmatic 224
  temporalis 21, 41, 48
  of thigh—see Fascia lata
  thoracolumbar **160**–163, 165, 177, 178,
        237, 316, 332
  transversalis 165, 224, 234–**236**, 243–245,
        247, 257, 328, 331–333, 342–346, 355

Fascia cont.
  trapezius 21
  umbilical prevesical 234–236, 244, 245,
        333, 342, 345, 346
  of urogenital diaphragm
    deep—see Fascia, of urogenital
        diaphragm, superior
    inferior 333, 337, 349, 355, **356**, 357,
        359–**361**, 371, 379, 380, 386
    superficial—see Fascia, of urogenital
        diaphragm, inferior
    superior 246, 333, **337**, **339**, 349,
        355–357, 361, 362, 379
  uterine 345, 348, 349, 355
  vaginal 348, 349, 355, 367
  vesical 333, 342, 345, 347, 348, 355, 367,
        372
Fascicle—see Fiber
Fasciculus—see also Fiber
  cuneatus 108, 109, 151
  dorsal longitudinal 140
  dorsolateral 151
  gracilis 108, 109, 151
  interfascicular 151
  mamillothalamic 100
  medial longitudinal 107, 109, 151
  proprius 151
  septomarginal 151
  sulcomarginal 151
  transverse, of
    palmar aponeurosis 432
    plantar aponeurosis 500
Fat
  of breast 167
  in epidural space 156
  extraperitoneal 387
  in ischiorectal fossa 355, 358
  orbital 42, 78
  pararenal 165, 328
  perirenal 165, 328
  in prevesical space 234
  subcutaneous—see Fascia,
        subcutaneous
  of subhiatal ring 224
Fauces 58
Femur 231, **459**, 474, 475, 477, 480
Fenestra
  cochleae—see Window, round
  vestibuli—see Window, oval
Fiber—see also Fasciculus
  Bachmann's 213
  of ciliary zonule 82, 83, 85, 86
  of His 213
  of Kent 213
  intercrural inguinal 232, 242, 245
  of Luschka 340—see also Muscle,
        levator ani, prerectal fibers of
  of Mahaim 213
  to olfactory bulb 113
  Purkinje 213
  vaginorectal 345
  vesicocervical 345
  zonular 85, 86—see also Fiber, of ciliary
        zonule

Fibula 482, 483, 488, 490, 491, 494, 495,
        498, 499
Filum
  terminale
    dural 148, 149
    pial 148, 149, 156
Fimbria of
  hippocampus 100, 102, 104–106, 113
  uterine tube 350
Finger 437, 444
Fingernail 444
Fissure—see also Sulcus
  of cerebellum 107
  cerebral
    lateral—see Sulcus, cerebral, lateral
    longitudinal 101, 136, 138
    Sylvian—see Sulcus, Sylvian
  for ligamentum teres of liver 270
  for ligamentum venosum 270
  of lung 184–187
  orbital
    inferior 1, 2, 78
    superior 1, 7, 78
  petrosquamous 8
  petrotympanic 5
  pterygomaxillary 2
  ventral median, of spinal cord 151
Flexure
  colic
    hepatic 252, 254, 255, 258, 261, 267,
        271, 279, 328
    left 252–255, 258, 261, 267, 271, 279,
        329
    right 252, 254, 255, 258, 261, 267, 271,
        279, 328
    splenic 252–255, 258, 261, 267, 271,
        279, 329
  duodenal 262
  duodenojejunal 253, 261, 262, 279, 328,
        329
Flocculus of cerebellum 107, 108
Floor of mouth 47
Fluid, cerebrospinal 103
Fold—see also Ligament; Plica
  alar, of knee 477
  aryepiglottic 60, 61, 72, 75
  bloodless, of Treves 264
  cecal 264, 343, 344
  circular, of
    duodenum 262
    ileum 263
    jejunum 263
  duodenal 253, 261, 262, 278
  fimbriated, of tongue 45
  gastric 224, 259
  gastropancreatic 255
  glossoepiglottic 52, 75
  ileocecal 264
  infrapatellar 477
  inguinal 394
  interureteric 347
  of iris 83
  of Kerckring—see Fold, circular, of
        duodenum; ileum; jejunum

Glomerulus of
   kidney 321, 322
   olfactory nerves 113
Glottis 75
Goldmann gonioscopic mirror—see
      Mirror, Goldmann gonioscopic
Gonad 364, 394—see also Ovary; Testis
Graafian follicle—see Follicle, Graafian
Granulation, arachnoid 94–96, 103
Granulosa of ovarian follicle 353
Groove—see also Sulcus
   for anterior meningeal vessels 6
   of auditory tube 5
   chiasmatic 6
   for circumflex scapular vessels 397
   costal 171
   of digastric muscle 5
   of greater petrosal nerve 6, 92
   of inferior petrosal sinus 3, 6
   infraorbital 1
   intermuscular anal 368–370
   of internal carotid artery 6
   intertubercular, of humerus 396
   of lesser petrosal nerve 6
   mastoid 5
   for middle meningeal vessels 3, 4,
      6
   of middle temporal artery 2, 4
   mylohyoid 10
   nasopalatine 34
   obturator 457
   of occipital artery 5
   of occipital sinus 6
   for posterior meningeal vessels 6
   of radial nerve 397
   of sigmoid sinus 3, 6
   of subclavian artery 171
   of subclavian vein 171
   of superior petrosal sinus 3, 6
   of superior sagittal sinus 4, 6
   of transverse sinus 3, 6
   of ulnar nerve 397, 411
   urogenital 393
   of vertebral artery 12
Gubernaculum 364, 394
Gum 51
Gutter, paracolic 254, 264, 332, 343,
      344
Gyrus
   angular 99
   cingulate 100, 101
   dentate 100, 102, 105, 106, 113
   frontal 99, 100
   of insula 99
   lingual 100, 101
   occipitotemporal 100, 101
   orbital 101
   parahippocampal 100–102, 106, 113
   paraterminal 100
   postcentral 99
   precentral 99
   straight 101
   supramarginal 99
   temporal 99, 101

H

Habenula 104
Hair follicle 153, 154
Haller—see Artery, to falciform ligament
      (from superior epigastric)
Hamate—see Bone, hamate
Hamulus of
   cochlea 90
   hamate bone 416, 422, 426, 428, 430,
      431, 439
   pterygoid 2, **3**, 5, 8, 9, 33, 41, 44, 46, 49,
      58, 59, 62, 93
Hand
   arteries of 439, 442, 446
   bones of 430
   ligaments of 431
   lymph nodes of 456
   muscles (intrinsic) of 432–438, 443
   nerves of 439–443, 445, 446, 448, 449,
      451
   veins of 441, 453
Hartmann—see Infundibulum, of
      gallbladder
Haustra of large intestine 267
Head—see also individual regions
   of caudate nucleus 104–106, 136,
      138
   of femur 458, 459
   of fibula 462–464, 476, 477, 479, 480,
      482, **483**, 486–490, 510
   of humerus 396, 397
   of malleus 89, 118
   of mandible 2, 10
   of pancreas 279
   of radius 406, 411, 413
   of rib 170, 171
Heart 120, 153, 154, 200–202, 204, 205,
      209–211, **212–215**
Helicotrema of cochlea 87, 90, 91
Helix of external ear 88
Helvetius—see Collar of Helvetius
Hemisphere, cerebral 96, 99–101, 104
Henle—see Loop, Henle's
Hering—see Canal, of Hering; Ductule,
      bile
Hering-Breuer—see Reflex, Hering-Breuer
Hesselbach—see Triangle, inguinal
Heubner—see Artery, recurrent, of
      Heubner
Hiatus—see also Opening
   adductor 463, 471, 472, 481, 507
   anorectal 339
   of deep dorsal vein of penis 339
   esophageal 181
   of greater petrosal nerve 7
   of lesser petrosal nerve 7
   sacral 145
   saphenous—see Fossa, ovalis, of fascia
      lata
   semilunar, of ethmoid bone 32, 33, 43,
      44
   of urethra 339
Hilton—see Line, Hilton's white

Hilus of
   kidney 317
   lung 187
Hip
   arteries of 474
   bones of 457
   ligaments of 458, 459
   muscles of 464–466
   nerves of 473
Hippocampus 102, 104–106
His—see Bundle, of His
Homologues
   external genitalia 393
   internal genitalia 394
Hook—see Hamulus
Horn
   coccygeal 145
   of gray matter 151
   of hyoid bone
      greater 9, 62
      lesser 9
   of lateral ventricle
      anterior 102
      frontal 102
      inferior 102, 105, 106, 139
      occipital 102, 104–106, 136, 139
      posterior 102, 104–106, 136, 139
      temporal 102, 105, 106, 139
   sacral 145
   of thyroid cartilage 62, 71, 223
Houston—see Valve, rectal
Hunter—see Canal, adductor
Humerus 396, 397, 408, 410–412, 424,
      425
Hydatid of Morgagni 350—see also
      Appendix, vesicular
Hymen of vagina 349, 354
Hyoid—see Bone, hyoid
Hypopharynx 60—see also
      Laryngopharynx
Hypophysis 32, 98, 100, 101, 140
Hypothalamus 102, 129, 140, 310

I

Ileum 252, 254, 263–265, 267, 332, 343, 344
Ilium 231, 334–336, 339, 457—see also
      individual landmarks
Impressions on
   liver 270
   lung 187
Incisure—see also Notch
   angular, of stomach 258
   cardiac 258
Incus 87, 88, 91, 118
Infundibuliform—see Fascia, spermatic,
      internal
Infundibulum of
   ethmoid bone 32, 33
   gallbladder 276
   hypophysis 108, 133
Innervation, cutaneous 240, 241, 445—see
      also individual nerves

Inscriptions, tendinous, of rectus
abdominis muscle 233
Insertion of
arm muscles 396, 397
forearm muscles 424, 425
hip muscles 460, 461
leg muscles 484
scalene muscles 25, 171
shoulder muscles 395–397
thigh muscles 460, 461
Inspection of
larynx 75
mouth 45
Inspiration 75, 183
Insula 99, 104, 134
Intestine
large 252, 254, 267—see also Colon
small 120, 252, 263, 332, 333—see also
Duodenum; Ileum; Jejunum
Iris 76, 82, 84–86
Ischium 457—see also individual
landmarks
Island of
Langerhans 279
Reil 99—see also Insula
Isthmus of
cingulate gyrus 100, 101
prostate 362
thyroid gland 68

J

Jacobson—see Nerve, tympanic
Jaws 11—see also Mandible
Jejunum 252–254, 261–263, 332
Joint
acromioclavicular 400
atlantoaxial 14, 15
atlantooccipital 14–16
of back 146, 147
carpometacarpal 427, 429
costovertebral 172
elbow 411, 412, 446
glenohumeral 398, 401, 407
hip 458, 462, 463, 466, 474
intercarpal 427, 429
intermetacarpal 429
interphalangeal (finger) 431, 437, 444
interphalangeal (toe) 496
knee 476–480, 488, 514
lateral vertebral 13–15
medial vertebral 13
metacarpophalangeal 431, 496
midcarpal 427, 429
radiocarpal 426–429
radioulnar
distal 426–429
proximal 411–413
sacroiliac 336, 339
shoulder 398, 401, 407
sternoclavicular 171, 184, 395
sternocostal 171, 395
sternomanubrial 171

Joint *cont.*
tarsometatarsal 492, 493
temporomandibular 11, 35, 48, 49
of thorax 171, 172
transverse tarsal 492, 493
vertebral body 13
zygapophyseal 13–15, 146—see also
Facet of, vertebra for, vertebral
facet
Jugum of sphenoid bone 6
Junction
atlantooccipital 16
duodenojejunal 165—see also Flexure,
duodenojejunal
esophagogastric 224, 259
pharyngoesophageal 223
rectosigmoid 267, 367, 369, 370

K

Kent—see Bundle, of Kent
Kerckring—see Fold, circular, of
duodenum; ileum; jejunum
Kidney 165, 185, 217, 255–258, 261, 270, 271,
281, **315–317**, 323, 328, 329, 331, 364, 375
Klippel-Feil—see Syndrome, Klippel-Feil
Knee 476–480, 488
arteries of 481
lymph nodes of 514

L

Labbé—see Vein, of Labbé
Labium—see also Lip
majus 341, 346, 349, 354, 357, 393
minus 341, 346, 349, 354, 357, 393
Labrum
of acetabulum 334, 458, 474
glenoid, of scapula 398
Labyrinth
membranous 90–92
osseous 90–92
Lacertus fibrosus—see Aponeurosis,
bicipital
Lacuna
of Morgagni 363
of urethral gland 357
venous 94, 95
Laimer—see Area, of Laimer
Lake, lacrimal 76, 77
Lambda 4
Lamina
affixa 105
cribrosa, of sclera 82
medullary, of thalamus 105
osseous spiral, of cochlea 91
propria, of gingiva 51
quadrigeminal 100, 109
tectal 100, 109
terminalis 100, 101, 109, 140
of thyroid cartilage 61, 71
of vertebra 13, 143, 144, 146, 147

Langerhans—see Island, of Langerhans
Laryngopharynx 56, 57, 60
Laryngoscope 75
Larynx 75, 129, 154, 199
arteries of 70
cartilage of 71
muscles of 72, 73
nerves of 68, 70, 74
Layer—see also Lamina
nuclear, of medulla oblongata 107
odontoblast 51
of rectus sheath 235
Leg—see also Thigh
arteries of 485–489
bones of 482, 483
cross sections of 491
lymph nodes of 514
muscles of 485–490
nerves of 485–489, 508–510
veins of 485–489
Lens 76, 82–86
Ligament—see also Fold; Raphé
acetabular, transverse 334, 458
alar 15
of ankle 483, 495, 497
annular, of
digital tendon sheath 433, 435
elbow 412
trachea 190
anococcygeal 338, 355, 356, 371, 372
anterior, of head of fibula 483
apical, of dens 15, 16, 57, 59
arcuate
of diaphragm 181, 246
popliteal 478, 480
pubic 231, 337–342, 345, 346, 355,
361
of atlas 15, 16
bifurcate (ankle) 495
broad 323, 341, 343, 348–350, 394
calcaneocuboid 495, 504
dorsal 495
long 495, 496, 504
plantar 496
calcaneofibular 483, 494, 495
calcaneometatarsal 500
calcaneonavicular, plantar 495, 496,
504
capitotriquetral 428
cardinal 345, 348–351
carpal 420, 421, 428, 431–434, 439, 453
carpometacarpal 428, 429, 431
cervical
lateral 345—see also Ligament,
Mackenrodt's; cardinal
check, palpebral 78
collateral, of
ankle 495
elbow 412
fibula 463, 464, 476–480, 483, 486,
487, 489, 490
finger 431, 437
knee 463, 464, 476–480, 483, 486–490
radius 412, 428, 429

Nerve *cont.*
  mandibular 11, 18, 40, **41**, 56, 65, 81, 98, 112, 115, 116, 119, 125, 127–129
  marginal mandibular branch of facial 19, 26, 117
  masseteric 35, 41, 48, 49, 65, 116
  maxillary 18, 38–**40**, 41, 56, 65, 81, 98, 112, 115, 116, 125, 127–129
  to medial pterygoid muscle 41, 65, 116
  median 404–406, 408, 410, 420–423, 428, 432–434, 438, 439, 445–**448**, 453, 454
  meningeal branches of
    hypoglossal 122
    mandibular 41, 81
    maxillary 40, 81, 116
    ophthalmic 81, 116
    spinal 241
    vagus 120
  mental 18, 41, 65, 116
  motor
    branch of median, to thenar muscles 432, 438, 439, 446
    root of trigeminal 41, 125
  of mouth 56, 65
  musculocutaneous 404–406, 408, 410, 422, 445–**447**, 448
  mylohyoid 11, 35, 41, 47, 49, 54, 65, 116
  nasal branches of
    anterior ethmoidal 18, 31, 37, 38, 40, 116
    anterior superior alveolar 37
    greater palatine 37, 38, 125, 127
    infraorbital 37, 39, 40
    maxillary 116
    pterygopalatine ganglion 37–39, 125, 127
  of nasal cavity 37–39
  nasociliary 40, 78, 81, 115, 116, 125, 126
  nasopalatine 37–39, 116
  of neck 23, 26, 27, 65, 123, 124
  obturator 236, 250, 323, 375, 385, 467–469, 471, 475, 506, **507**, 512, 513
    accessory 250, 467, 468
    anterior branch of 471, 507
    posterior branch of 471, 507
  to obturator internus muscle 467, 469, 472, 473
  occipital
    greater 18, 123, 163, 164
    lesser 18, 27, 123, 163, 164
    third 18, 163, 164
  occipital branch of posterior auricular 117
  oculomotor 78, 79, 81, 98, 108, 110–112, **115**, 125, 152, 153
  olfactory 37, 38, 112, 113
  to omohyoid muscle 27—see also Ansa cervicalis
  ophthalmic 18, **40**, 41, 81, 98, 112, 115, 116, 125–129
  optic 42, 78, 79, 81, 82, 86, 98, 101, 112, **114**, 126, 136, 137
  of orbit 40, 81

Nerve *cont.*
  palatine
    descending 127
    greater 37–40, 46, 56, 65, 116, 125, 127
    lesser 37–40, 46, 56, 65, 116, 125, 127
  palmar branch of
    median 420, 421, 432, 433, 439, 445, 448, 453, 454
    ulnar 421, 432, 433, 439, 445, 449, 453, 454
  palpebral branch of lacrimal 18
  of pancreas 153, 313, 314
  parasympathetic 39, 115–117, 119, 120, 126–128, 152–154, 199, 215, 307, 310, 311, 313, 314, 327, 389–392
  parotid branch of auriculotemporal 116
  of parotid gland 153
  pectoral
    lateral 174, 403–405
    medial 174, 403–405
  pelvic splanchnic 152–154, 250, 304, 310, 326, 327, 385, 387, 389–392, 467, 469
  of pelvic viscera 385, 387, 390, 391
  of penis, dorsal 250, 359, 361, 380, 384–386, 391, 467, 473
  perforating cutaneous 386, 388, 467, 469, 473, 513
  pericardial branch of phrenic 182
  perineal branch of
    posterior femoral cutaneous 388, 473, 508
    pudendal 385, 386, 388, 467, 473
    4th sacral 467, 469
  of perineum 386, 388, 390, 391
  of peripheral blood vessels 153
  peroneal
    common 465, 467, 469, 472, 475–477, 485–490, 508–**510**
    deep 488, 489, 491, 498, 499, 510
    dorsal intermediate cutaneous 510, 512
    dorsal medial cutaneous 510, 512
    superficial 488–491, 498, 499, 508, 510, 512
  petrosal
    deep 38, 39, 117, 119, **125**, 127
    greater 38, 39, 56, 81, 89, 117–119, 125, 127, 129
    lesser 41, 81, 116, 117, 119, 128
  pharyngeal branch of
    glossopharyngeal 119
    pterygopalatine ganglion 38, 56, 116, 127
    vagus 119, 120, 124, 152, 228
  of pharynx 56, 65
  phrenic 25, 27, 28, 30, 63, 65, 68, 123, 124, 175–177, 180–182, 186, 195, 200, 201, 203, 214, 218–220, 230, 238, 304, 306, 313, 330, 404
  to piriformis muscle 467, 469
  plantar
    lateral 487, 500, 502, 503, 508, 509, 513
    medial 487, 497, 500–503, 508, 509, 513

Nerve *cont.*
  posterior
    division of
      mandibular 41
      obturator 471, 507
    femoral cutaneous 148, 467, 469, 472, 473, 475, 508, 513
    labial 388
    tibial 497, 502
  presacral—see Plexus (nerve), hypogastric, superior
  of prostate 153
  to psoas muscle 467, 468
  to pterygoid muscles 41, 65, 116
  of pterygoid canal (Vidian) 37–40, 116, 117, 119, 125, 127, 129
  pterygopalatine branch of maxillary 40
  pudendal 148, 250, 310, 326, 385–392, 467, 469, 472, 473
    perineal branch of 385, 386, 388, 467, 473
    posterior
      labial branch of 388, 467, 473
      scrotal branch of 385, 386, 467, 473
  of pupil
    dilator 115, 153
    sphincter 115, 153
  pyloric branch of hepatic plexus 120
  to quadratus femoris muscle 467, 469, 473
  quadratus plantae 509
  radial 401, 404, 405, 407, 410, 418, 419, 421–423, 432, 440–442, 445–448, **450, 451**, 454
  rectal
    inferior 310, 385, 386, 388, 389, 467, 473
    superior 310
  to rectus capitis muscles 27, 123
  of rectum 153
  recurrent
    branch of deep peroneal 489
    branch of mandibular—see Nerve, meningeal branches of mandibular
    esophageal branch of left inferior phrenic 308
    laryngeal 28, 30, 65, 68–70, 74, 120, 124, 152, 182, 195, 198, 200, 201, 214, 219, 220, 223, 228
    meningeal branch of spinal 311
  sacral splanchnic 152, 153, 309, 310, 326, 385, 387, 392, 469
  saphenous 470, 471, 475, 488, 489, 491, 506, 509, 512, 513
  to scalene muscles 27, 123, 405
  scapular, dorsal 404, 405, 450
  sciatic 148, 465, 467, 469, 472, 473, 475, **508**
  scrotal—see Nerve, ilioinguinal, anterior branch of; pudendal, posterior branch of
  of sebaceous gland 153
  sensory root of trigeminal 41, 125

Notch *cont.*
  of stomach
    angular 258
    cardiac 224, 258
  superior
    of thyroid cartilage 71
    vertebral 143, 144
  supraorbital 1, 2, 8
  suprasternal 184—see also Notch,
      jugular
  of thyroid cartilage 71
  trochlear, of ulna 411, 413
  of ulna
    radial 411, 413
    trochlear 411, 413
  ulnar, of radius 413
  vertebral
    inferior 143, 144
    superior 143, 144
Nucleus
  abducens 110, 111, 115
  accessory oculomotor 110, 111, 115, 126
  ambiguus 110, 111, 119–121
  anterior
    olfactory 113
    thalamic 105
  caudal—see Nucleus, inferior,
      salivatory; vestibular
  caudate 102, 104–106, 134, 138
  cochlear 110, 111, 118
  of cranial nerves **110, 111**, 115–122
  dentate, of cerebellum 107, 109
  dorsal
    cochlear 110, 111, 118
    vagal 110, 111, 120, 215, 310, 327
  dorsomedial, of hypothalamus 140
  Edinger-Westphal—see Nucleus,
      accessory oculomotor
  emboliform, of cerebellum 107
  facial 110, 111
  fastigial, of cerebellum 107
  geniculate, lateral 114
  globose, of cerebellum 107
  gracile 110
  hypoglossal 110, 111, 122
  hypothalamus, posterior 140
  inferior
    salivatory 110, 111, 119, 128
    vestibular 118
  intralaminar, of thalamus 105
  lateral
    geniculate 114
    olfactory tract 113
    thalamic 105
    vestibular 118
  lens 83, 85
  lentiform 102, 104, 134
  mamillary, of hypothalamus 140
  medial
    thalamic 105
    vestibular 118
  median, of thalamus 105
  mesencephalic, of trigeminal nerve 110,
      111, 116, 129

Nucleus *cont.*
  motor, of
    facial nerve 117
    trigeminal nerve 110, 111, 116, 129
  oculomotor 115
    accessory 110, 111, 115, 126
  olfactory 113
  paraventricular, of hypothalamus
      140
  pontine, of trigeminal 110, 111, 116
  posterior, of hypothalamus 140
  principal, of trigeminal 110, 111, 116
  pulposus 144
  red 101, 110, 111
  reticular 105
  rostral—see Nucleus, superior,
      salivatory; vestibular
  ruber—see Nucleus, red
  salivatory
    inferior 110, 111, 119, 128
    superior 39, 110, 111, 117, 127
  septal (pellucidum) 113
  of solitary tract 110, 111, 117, 119, 120,
      129, 215, 327
  spinal, of
    accessory nerve 110, 111
    trigeminal nerve 110, 111, 116, 119,
      120
  superior
    salivatory 39, 110, 111, 117, 127
    vestibular 118
  supraoptic, of hypothalamus 140
  thalamic 105
  trigeminal
    principal 110, 111, 116
    spinal 110, 111, 116, 119, 120
  trochlear 110, 111, 115
  tuberal, of hypothalamus 140
  vagus, dorsal 110, 111, 120, 215, 310,
      327
  ventral
    cochlear 110, 111, 118
    posteromedial, of thalamus 129
  ventromedial, of hypothalamus 140
  vestibular 110, 111, 118

O

Oddi—see Sphincter, of hepatopancreatic
    ampulla
Olecranon of ulna 407, 411, 413, 415, 418,
    419, 450
Omentum
  greater 252, 255, 256, 258, 271, 332, 333
  lesser 258, 271, 279, 305, 306, 331, 333
Opening—see also Hiatus
  of alveolar duct 192
  of auditory tube 32, 57, 58, 60, 61, 119
  of Bartholin's gland 354
  of bladder 346
  of bulbourethral duct 362, 363
  of coronary arteries 211, 212
  of coronary sinus 208

Opening *cont.*
  of ejaculatory duct 362, 363, 394
  of ethmoidal cells 32, 33, 44
  of greater vestibular gland 354
  ileocecal 267
  of internal acoustic meatus 92
  of maxillary sinus 32, 33, 42–44
  of nasolacrimal duct 32, 33, 43,
      77
  of paraurethral duct 354, 357
  of parotid duct 45
  of preputial gland 360
  of prostatic duct 362, 363
  of pylorus 262
  saphenous—see Fossa ovalis, of fascia
      lata
  of Skene's ducts 354, 357
  of sphenoidal sinus 32, 33, 43
  of stomach
    cardia 259
    pyloris 262
  of sublingual duct 45, 55
  of submandibular duct 45, 55
  of superior cerebral vein 95
  of Tyson's glands 360
  of ureter 347, 357, 362
  of urethra 341, 342, 354, 357, 360, 363,
      371, 393
  of urethral gland 357
  of uterine tube 350
  of uterus 350
  of vagina 341, 354
  of vermiform appendix 265
  of vestibular aqueduct 90
Ora serrata 82, 85, 86
Orbit 1, 2, 8, 42, 44, 76–81
  arteries of 80
  fascia of 78
  muscles of 79
  nerves of 40, 81
  veins of 80
Organ, spiral, of Corti 91
Orifice—see Opening
Origin of
  arm muscles 396, 397
  cremaster muscle 233, 242
  diaphragm 181
  forearm muscles 424, 425
  genioglossus muscle 47
  hip muscles 460, 461
  leg muscles 484
  scalene muscles 25
  serratus anterior muscle 171
  shoulder muscles 395–397
  subclavius muscle 171
  thigh muscles 460, 461
Oropharynx 30, 45, 56–58, 60, 61
Os—see Bone; Opening
Os odontoideum 16
Ossicles, auditory 88
Ostium—see Opening
Ovary 341, 343, 348–350, **353**, 375, 387,
    390, 394
Ovum 353

Symphysis, pubic **231**, 243, 245, 246,
 334–340, 342, 345, 346, 355, 358, 361,
 377
Synchondrosis 395
Syndrome
 Down's 16
 Klippel-Feil 16
 Morquio's 16
Systole 210

T

Tag, epithelial, of glans 393
Tail of
 caudate nucleus 102, 104, 106
 pancreas 279, 281, 315
Talus 492–494
Tarsus—see Bone, of foot
 of eyelid 76, 78, 79
Taste 52, 56, 117, 119, 129
Tectum—see Lamina, quadrigeminal;
 tectal
Teeth 44, 50, 51, 221
Tegmen tympani 87
Tela choroidea of 3rd ventricle 102, 105,
 138
Tendon—see also individual muscles
 Achilles 485–487, 490, 495, 497
 of ankle 495, 497–499
 annular, common 78, 79, 81, 115
 calcaneal 485–487, 490, 495, 497
 central, of
  diaphragm 180, 181, 246
   perineum 342, 346, 355, 356, 360–362,
    367, 371, 380
 common
  annular 78, 79, 81, 115
  extensor 415, 418, 419
  flexor 416, 417, 420
 conjoined 233, 234, 236, 243
 digastric intermediate 23, 24, 47, 53, 54
 extensor, common 415, 418, 419
 flexor, common 416, 417, 420
 patellar—see Ligament, patellar
 plantaris 465, 485, 486, 491
 quadriceps femoris 471, 475–477, 480,
  488–490
Tenia
 free 254, 264, 265, 267, 367, 370
 libera 254, 264, 265, 267, 367, 370
 mesocolic 264, 265, 267
 omental 264, 267
 of 4th ventricle 109
Tenon—see Capsule, Tenon's
Tentorium cerebelli 81, 97, 98, 100, 137, 138
Testis 333, 342, 364–366, 380, 391, 394
Thalamus 100, 102, 104, **105**, 106, 108, 109,
 137, 138, 140, 310
Thebesian valve—see Valve, Thebesian
Theca of ovarian follicle 353
Thigh
 arteries of 470–472, 481
 bones of 459–461

Thigh *cont.*
 cross section of 475
 lymph nodes of 514
 muscles of 462–466
 nerves of 470–472, 506–508
Thorax
 arteries of 176, 179, 225—see also
  arteries of individual organs
 bones of 170, 171
 cross section of 230
 joints of 171, 172
 lymph nodes of 169, 197, 227
 muscles of 174–178, 183
 nerves of 174, 178, 179, 198—see also
  nerves of individual organs
 veins of 176, 226—see also veins of
  individual organs
 viscera of—see individual organs
Tibia 478, 480, **482, 483**, 488, 489, 491,
 494, 495, 497–499
Tissue
 adipose 30, 232—see also Fascia,
  subcutaneous
 alar fibrofatty 31, 33
Tongue 32, 34, 42, **52–55**, 57, 58, 60, 67,
 119, 122, 129
Tonsil
 of cerebellum 107, 109, 137
 lingual 52, 57, 58, 75
 palatine 45, 46, 52, 54, 57, 58, 60
 pharyngeal 32, 57, 58, 60, 61
Topography of
 abdominal viscera 251
 autonomic nervous system 152
 esophagus 221
 kidney 316
 liver 269
 lung 184, 185
 perineum 358
 thyroid gland 68
Torus tubarius 32, 58, 60
Trabecula
 carneae 208
 fibrous, of adenohypophysis 140
 septomarginal 208, 211, 212
Trachea 9, 23, 24, 30, 57, 59, 62, 69–71, 75,
 120, 154, 184, 186, **190**, 191, 194–196,
 200, 218, 220–222, 225
Tract
 comma 151
 corticospinal 151
 dorsolateral 151
 gastrointestinal 154
 hypothalamohypophyseal 140
 iliotibial 462, **464**, 465, 472, 475–478,
  483, 485, 488–490
 internodal 213
 of Lissauer 151
 mamillothalamic 140
 olfactory 38, 100, 101, 108, 113
 optic 101, 102, 106, 108, 114, 132, 137
 pyramidal 151
 reticulospinal 151
 rubrospinal 151

Tract *cont.*
 of spinal cord 151
 spinal, of trigeminal nerve 110, 111, 116,
  119, 120
 spinocerebellar 151
 spinoolivary 151
 spinoreticular 151
 spinotectal 151
 spinothalamic 151
 supraopticohypophyseal 140
 tectospinal 126, 151
 tuberohypophyseal 140
 vestibulospinal 151
Tragus of external ear 88
Trapezium—see Bone, trapezium
Trapezoid—see Bone, trapezoid
Treves—see Fold, bloodless, of Treves
Triad, portal 273, 302
Triangle
 anal 358
 of auscultation 237, 399
 of Calot 284—see also Triangle, cystic
 cervical 21, 30, 160, 164, 174, 178
 cystic 284, 290
 deltopectoral 399
 Hesselbach's 236, 243
 inguinal 236, 243
 lumbar 160, 178, 237
 perineal 358
 Petit's 160, 178, 237
 suboccipital 164
 urogenital 358
Trigone—see also Triangle
 collateral 105
 fibrous, of heart 210
 habenular 105, 109
 hypoglossal 109
 lumbocostal 181
 olfactory 113
 of urinary bladder 342, 346, 347, 357,
  362, 363
 vagal 109
 vertebrocostal 181
Triquetrum—see Bone, triquetral
Trochanter
 of femur
  greater 231, 458, 459, 462, 463, 465,
   466, 472, 473
  lesser 231, 246, 458, 459, 466
Trochlea
 of humerus 396, 397, 411
 of orbit 79
 peroneal 492–494
 of talus 492, 493
Trolard—see Vein, of Trolard
Tropism—see Facet, tropism
Trunk (arterial)
 brachiocephalic 28, 68–70, 130, 131, 176,
  182, 195, 200–202, 220, 225
 celiac 152, 181, 217, 220, 225, 247, 253,
  257, 261, 279, **282–286**, 288–290,
  292, 307, 310, 314, 315, 318, 333, 385
 celiacomesenteric 288
 costocervical 27, 28, 63, 130, 131